THE AMERICAN PSYCHIATRIC PUBLISHING

Textbook of Psychoanalysis

THE AMERICAN PSYCHIATRIC PUBLISHING

Textbook of Psychoanalysis

EDITED BY

ETHEL S. PERSON, M.D.

Professor of Clinical Psychiatry
College of Physicians and Surgeons, Columbia University
Training and Supervising Analyst, Columbia University Center for
Psychoanalytic Training and Research, New York, New York

ARNOLD M. COOPER, M.D.

Stephen P. Tobin and Dr. Arnold M. Cooper Professor Emeritus
in Consultation-Liaison Psychiatry, Weill Cornell Medical College
Training and Supervising Analyst, Columbia University Center for
Psychoanalytic Training and Research, New York, New York

GLEN O. GABBARD, M.D.

Brown Foundation Chair of Psychoanalysis and Professor
Department of Psychiatry and Behavioral Sciences
Director of the Baylor Psychiatry Clinic, Baylor College of Medicine
Training and Supervising Analyst
Houston/Galveston Psychoanalytic Institute, Houston, Texas

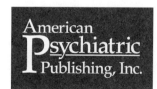

American Psychiatric Publishing, Inc.

Washington, DC
London, England

Manufactured in the United States of America on acid-free paper
09 08 07 06 05   5 4 3 2 1
First Edition

Typeset in Adobe's Janson Text and Frutiger

American Psychiatric Publishing, Inc.
1000 Wilson Boulevard
Arlington, VA 22209-3901
www.appi.org

Library of Congress Cataloging-in-Publication Data
The American Psychiatric Publishing textbook of psychoanalysis / edited by Ethel S. Person, Arnold M. Cooper, Glen O. Gabbard.—1st ed.
　　p. cm.
　Includes bibliographical references and index.
　ISBN 1-58562-152-8 (hardcover; alk. paper)
　1. Psychoanalysis. I. Title: Textbook of psychoanalysis. II. Title: Psychoanalysis. III. Person, Ethel Spector. IV. Cooper, Arnold M. V. Gabbard, Glen O.
　[DNLM: 1. Psychoanalysis. 2. Psychoanalytic Theory. 3. Psychoanalytic Therapy. WM 460 A5129 2005]
　RC504.A48 2005
　616.89'17—dc22
　　　　　　　　　　　　　　　　　　　　　　　　　　　　　　　2004021206

British Library Cataloguing in Publication Data
A CIP record is available from the British Library.

Contents

Contributors ix

Introduction xiii
    Ethel S. Person, M.D., Arnold M. Cooper, M.D., and Glen O. Gabbard, M.D.

P A R T   I

Core Concepts
Section Editor: Salman Akhtar, M.D.

1   Theories of Motivation in Psychoanalysis 3
    Fred Pine, Ph.D.

2   The Dynamic Unconscious: Psychic Determinism, Intrapsychic Conflict,
    Unconscious Fantasy, Dreams, and Symptom Formation. 21
    W. W. Meissner, S.J., M.D.

3   Early Relationships and Their Internalization. 39
    Salman Akhtar, M.D.

4   Object Relations Theories and Technique. 57
    Otto F. Kernberg, M.D.

5   Intersubjectivity 77
    Daniel Stern, M.D.

6   Gender and Sexuality 93
    Muriel Dimen, Ph.D., and Virginia Goldner, Ph.D.

P A R T   I I

Developmental Theory
Section Editor: Mary Target, Ph.D.

7   A Developmental Orientation for Contemporary Psychoanalysis. 117
    Robert N. Emde, M.D.

8   Psychoanalytic Developmental Theory 131
    Peter Fonagy, Ph.D., F.B.A.

9   Interface Between Psychoanalytic Developmental Theory and Other Disciplines 147
    Linda C. Mayes, M.D.

10 Attachment Theory and Research 159
Mary Target, Ph.D.

11 The Psychoanalytic Understanding of Mental Disorders:
The Developmental Perspective 173
Efrain Bleiberg, M.D.

P A R T   I I I

Treatment and Technique

Section Editor: Henry F. Smith, M.D.

12 What Is Psychoanalysis? What Is a Psychoanalyst? 189
Paul Williams, Ph.D.

13 Transference, Countertransference, and the Real Relationship 201
Adrienne Harris, Ph.D.

14 Theories of Therapeutic Action and Their Technical Consequences 217
Jay Greenberg, Ph.D

15 Process, Resistance, and Interpretation. 229
Eslee Samberg, M.D., and Eric R. Marcus, M.D.

16 Termination and Reanalysis. 241
Martin S. Bergmann, Ph.D.

17 Psychoanalysis and Psychopharmacology 255
Steven P. Roose, M.D., and Deborah L. Cabaniss, M.D.

18 Technique in Child Analysis 267
Judith A. Yanof, M.D.

19 Ethics in Psychoanalysis 281
Ernest Wallwork, Ph.D.

P A R T   I V

Research

Section Editor: Judith Kantrowitz, M.D.

20 Outcome Research 301
Robert S. Wallerstein, M.D.

21 Process Research 317
Wilma Bucci, Ph.D.

22 Developmental Research 335
Stanley I. Greenspan, M.D., and Stuart G. Shanker, D.Phil.

23 Conceptual Research 361
Anna Ursula Dreher, Dr.Phil.
Translation by Eva Ristl

P A R T   V

History of Psychoanalysis
Section Editor: Robert Michels, M.D.

24 Psychoanalysis: The Early Years 375
Daria Colombo, M.D., and Sander M. Abend

25 Psychoanalysis in North America From 1895 to the Present 387
Sanford Gifford, M.D.

26 Psychoanalysis in Great Britain and Continental Europe 407
David Tuckett, M.A., M.Sc., F.Inst.Psychoanal.

27 Psychoanalysis in the French Community 423
Dominique Scarfone, M.D.

28 Psychoanalysis in Latin America 435
Cláudio Laks Eizirik and Mónica Siedmann de Armesto

P A R T   V I

Psychoanalysis and Related Disciplines
Section Editor: Morris Eagle, M.D.

29 Freud and His Uses of Interdisciplinary Sources 453
John Kerr

30 Psychology 463
Joel Weinberger, Ph.D., and Kenneth N. Levy, Ph.D.

31 Anthropology 479
Robert A. Paul, Ph.D.

32 Literature 491
Emanuel Berman, Ph.D.

33 The Arts 501
Ellen Handler Spitz, Ph.D.

34 Philosophy 513
Jonathan Lear, Ph.D.

35 Politics and International Relations...525
Vamık D. Volkan, M.D.

36 Neuroscience...535
Mark Solms, Ph.D.

Glossary..547
Richard Zimmer, M.D., Editor
Peter M. Bookstein, M.D., Associate Editor; Edward Kenny, M.D., Associate Editor; and
Andreas K. Kraebber, M.D., Associate Editor

Name Index...563
Subject Index..571

Contributors

Sander M. Abend

Training and Supervising Analyst, New York Psychoanalytic Institute, New York, New York

Salman Akhtar, M.D.

Professor of Psychiatry, Jefferson Medical College; Training and Supervising Analyst, Psychoanalytic Center of Philadelphia, Philadelphia, Pennsylvania

Martin S. Bergmann, Ph.D.

Clinical Professor of Psychology, Postgraduate Programs in Psychoanalysis, New York University, New York, New York

Emanuel Berman, Ph.D.

Professor of Psychology, University of Haifa, Haifa, Israel; Visiting Professor, Postdoctoral Program, New York University, New York, New York; Training and Supervising Analyst, Israel Psychoanalytic Institute

Efrain Bleiberg, M.D.

Alicia Townsend Friedman Professor of Psychiatry and Developmental Psychopathology and Vice Chair and Director, Division of Child and Adolescent Psychiatry, The Menninger Department of Psychiatry, Baylor College of Medicine, Houston, Texas; Training and Supervising Analyst, Houston–Galveston Psychoanalytic Institute, Houston, Texas

Peter M. Bookstein, M.D.

Faculty, Columbia University Center for Psychoanalytic Training and Research; Assistant Clinical Professor of Psychiatry, Columbia University College of Physicians and Surgeons, New York City

Wilma Bucci, Ph.D.

Professor and Director of Research, Derner Institute of Advanced Psychological Studies, Adelphi University, Garden City, New York

Deborah L. Cabaniss, M.D.

Associate Clinical Professor of Psychiatry, College of Physicians and Surgeons, Columbia University; Training and Supervising Analyst, Center for Psychoanalytic Training and Research, Columbia University, New York, New York

Daria Colombo, M.D.

Assistant Professor, Department of Psychiatry, Weill Medical College of Cornell University, New York, New York

Arnold M. Cooper, M.D.

Stephen P. Tobin and Dr. Arnold M. Cooper Professor Emeritus in Consultation-Liaison Psychiatry, Weill Cornell Medical College; Training and Supervising Analyst, Columbia University Center for Psychoanalytic Training and Research, New York, New York

Muriel Dimen, Ph.D.

Adjunct Clinical Professor of Psychology, Postdoctoral Program in Psychotherapy and Psychoanalysis, New York University, New York, New York

Anna Ursula Dreher, Dr.Phil.

Psychoanalyst in Private Practice, Frankfurt am Main, Germany

Morris Eagle, M.D.

Professor of Psychology, Derner Institute of Advanced Psychological Studies, Adelphi University, Garden City, New York

Cláudio Laks Eizirik

Training and Supervising Analyst, Porto Alegre Psychoanalytic Society; Adjunct Professor, Department of Psychiatry and Legal Medicine, Federal University of Rio Grande do Sul, Porto Alegre, Brazil

Robert N. Emde, M.D.

Professor of Psychiatry, University of Colorado Health Sciences Center; Adjunct Professor, University of Denver, Denver, Colorado

Peter Fonagy, Ph.D., F.B.A.

Freud Memorial Professor of Psychoanalysis, University College London; Chief Executive, The Anna Freud Centre, London, England; Director, Child and Family Program, Baylor College of Medicine, Houston, Texas

Glen O. Gabbard, M.D.

Brown Foundation Chair of Psychoanalysis and Professor, Department of Psychiatry and Behavioral Sciences, and Director of the Baylor Psychiatry Clinic, Baylor College of Medicine; Training and Supervising Analyst, Houston/Galveston Psychoanalytic Institute, Houston, Texas

Sanford Gifford, M.D.

Associate Clinical Professor of Psychiatry, Harvard Medical School; Senior Physician, Brigham and Women's Hospital; Director of Archives, Hanns Sachs Library, Boston

Psychoanalytic Society and Institute, Boston, Massachusetts; Chairman, History and Archives Committee, American Psychoanalytic Association

Virginia Goldner, Ph.D.
Adjunct Clinical Associate Professor of Psychology, Postdoctoral Program in Psychotherapy and Psychoanalysis, New York University, New York, New York

Jay Greenberg, Ph.D.
Training and Supervising Analyst, William Alanson White Institute, New York, New York

Stanley I. Greenspan, M.D.
Clinical Professor of Psychiatry and Pediatrics, George Washington University Medical Center, Washington, D.C.

Adrienne Harris, Ph.D.
Faculty, Program in Psychoanalysis and Psychotherapy, New York University, New York, New York

Judith Kantrowitz, M.D.
Associate Clinical Professor of Psychology, Harvard Medical School; Training and Supervising Analyst, Boston Psychoanalytic Society and Institute, Boston, Massachusetts

Edward Kenny, M.D.
Candidate, Columbia University Center for Psychoanalytic Training and Research; Assistant Clinical Professor of Psychiatry, Columbia University College of Physicians and Surgeons, New York City

Otto F. Kernberg, M.D.
Director, Personality Disorders Institute, The New York–Presbyterian Hospital, Westchester Division, White Plains, New York; Professor of Psychiatry, Joan and Sanford I. Weill Medical College of Cornell University; Training and Supervising Analyst, Columbia University Center for Psychoanalytic Training and Research, New York, New York

John Kerr
Senior Consulting Editor, The Analytic Press; Research Associate, Institute for the History of Psychiatry, Weill Cornell Medical Center, New York, New York

Andreas K. Kraebber, M.D.
Faculty, Columbia University Center for Psychoanalytic Training and Research; Instructor in Psychiatry, Columbia University College of Physicians and Surgeons, New York City

Jonathan Lear, Ph.D.
John U. Nef Distinguished Service Professor, Committee on Social Thought and Department of Philosophy, The University of Chicago, Chicago, Illinois

Kenneth N. Levy, Ph.D.
Assistant Professor, Clinical and Developmental Psychology Doctoral Programs, Graduate School and University Center, Department of Psychology, Hunter College, City University of New York

Eric R. Marcus, M.D.
Clinical Professor of Psychiatry and Social Medicine, Columbia University College of Physicians and Surgeons; Training and Supervising Analyst, Columbia University Center for Psychoanalytic Training and Research, New York, New York

Linda C. Mayes, M.D.
Arnold Gesell Professor of Child Psychiatry, Pediatrics, and Psychology, Yale Child Study Center, New Haven, Connecticut

W.W. Meissner, S.J., M.D.
Training and Supervising Analyst Emeritus, Boston Psychoanalytic Institute; University Professor of Psychoanalysis, Boston College, Boston

Robert Michels, M.D.
Walsh McDermott University Professor of Medicine and Psychiatry, Cornell University; Training and Supervising Analyst, Columbia University Center for Psychoanalytic Training and Research, New York, New York

Robert A. Paul, Ph.D.
Charles Howard Candler Professor of Anthropology, Emory University; Training and Supervising Analyst Emory University Psychoanalytic Institute, Atlanta, Georgia

Ethel S. Person, M.D.
Professor of Clinical Psychiatry, College of Physicians and Surgeons, Columbia University; Training and Supervising Analyst, Columbia University Center for Psychoanalytic Training and Research, New York, New York

Fred Pine, Ph.D.
Emeritus Professor, Albert Einstein College of Medicine; Adjunct Professor, New York University Postdoctoral Program; Faculty, Columbia University Center for Psychoanalytic Training and Research, New York City

Steven P. Roose, M.D.
Professor of Clinical Psychiatry, College of Physicians and Surgeons, Columbia University; Chairperson, Research Committee, Center for Psychoanalytic Training and Research, Columbia University, New York, New York

Eslee Samberg, M.D.
Clinical Associate Professor of Psychiatry, Cornell University Medical College; Training and Supervising Analyst, The New York Psychoanalytic Institute, New York, New York

Dominique Scarfone, M.D.
Professor, Department of Psychology, University of Montreal; Training Analyst, Société et Institut psychanalytique de Montréal, Montreal, Quebec, Canada

Stuart G. Shanker, D.Phil.
Professor of Philosophy and Psychology and Distinguished Research Professor, York University, Toronto, Ontario, Canada

Mónica Siedmann de Armesto
Training and Supervising Analyst, Argentine Psychoanalytic Association, Buenos Aires, Argentina

Henry F. Smith, M.D.
Training and Supervising Analyst, Psychoanalytic Institute of New England, East (PINE), Needham, Massachusetts; Member, Boston Psychoanalytic Society and Institute, Boston, Massachusetts

Mark Solms, Ph.D.
Director, Arnold Pfeffer Center for Neuropsychoanalysis, New York; Director, Neuropsychoanalysis Centre, London; Chair of Neuropsychology, University of Cape Town, Cape Town, South Africa

Ellen Handler Spitz, Ph.D.
Honors College Professor of Visual Arts, University of Maryland, Baltimore, Maryland

Daniel Stern, M.D.
Professeur Honoraire, Université de Genève, Geneva, Switzerland; Adjunct Professor, Department of Psychiatry, Cornell Medical School; Faculty, Columbia University Center for Psychoanalytic Training and Research, New York, New York

Mary Target, Ph.D.
Reader in Psychoanalysis, University College London; Professional Director, The Anna Freud Centre, London, England

David Tuckett, M.A., M.Sc., F.Inst.Psychoanal.
Training and Supervising Analyst, British Psychoanalytical Society; Visiting Professor, Psychoanalysis Unit, University College, London, England

Vamık D. Volkan, M.D.
Professor Emeritus of Psychiatry, University of Virginia, Charlottesville, Virginia; Training and Supervising Analyst Emeritus, Washington Psychoanalytic Institute, Washington, D.C.; Senior Erik Erikson Scholar, Austen Riggs Center, Stockbridge, Massachusetts

Robert S. Wallerstein, M.D.
Emeritus Professor and Former Chair, Department of Psychiatry, University of California, San Francisco School of Medicine; Emeritus Training and Supervising Analyst, San Francisco Psychoanalytic Institute, San Francisco, California

Ernest Wallwork, Ph.D.
Professor of Ethics, Syracuse University, Syracuse, New York; Psychoanalyst, Private Practice, Washington, D.C., and Syracuse, New York

Joel Weinberger, Ph.D.
Professor, Derner Institute of Advanced Psychological Studies, Adelphi University, Garden City, New York

Paul Williams, Ph.D.
Visiting Professor of Psychoanalysis, Anglia Polytechnic University, Cambridge, England

Judith A. Yanof, M.D.
Training and Supervising Analyst and Child Supervisor, Boston Psychoanalytic Society and Institute; Instructor, Harvard Medical School, Boston, Massachusetts

Richard Zimmer, M.D.
Training and Supervising Analyst, Columbia University Center for Psychoanalytic Training and Research; Assistant Clinical Professor of Psychiatry, Weill Medical College of Cornell University, New York City

Introduction

ETHEL S. PERSON, M.D.

ARNOLD M. COOPER, M.D.

GLEN O. GABBARD, M.D.

FREUD DESCRIBED PSYCHOANALYSIS as a theory, a treatment, and a method of research. In Western culture, it has become much more than that. It is a way of looking at individual psychology and events in the world through a psychoanalytically oriented lens. Psychoanalysis has strong ties to psychiatry and psychotherapy, on the one hand, and to many other different disciplines, ranging from international relations to neuroscience, on the other. For these reasons, this textbook focuses on not only psychoanalytic theory and treatment but also developmental issues, psychoanalytic research, and the multiple ways psychoanalytic theory intersects with contiguous fields. It addresses differences in psychoanalysis in different parts of the world and is intended for a wide variety of professionals, not only psychoanalysts but also psychiatrists, psychotherapists, academics, people from other disciplines, and students.

The philosopher William James (1890/1952) maintained that the greatest discontinuity in nature was that between two minds. It is clear what he was talking about. Subjective experience tells us that we cannot enter another's mind. Yet the separateness of mind each of us experiences may not be so absolute as James suggests. The barrier between minds is perhaps both narrower and more porous than he describes. Although it is true that experiential reality, as a function of a separate brain, is indeed solitary, the "ownership" of the content of our minds is partly illusory. It is in looking at how the organization of mind is shaped that we begin to see evidence for the porosity of

the barriers separating minds from one another—whether through shared ideas or emotional, affective "contagion."

The major organization of mind occurs within the first 5 years of life. For Tolstoy, the distance "from the child of five to myself is but a step" (quoted in Troyat 1988, p. 15). In contrast, Tolstoy described the distance from the newborn baby to the child of 5 as appalling and the distance from the embryo to the infant as an abyss. Here Tolstoy presages Freud's great insights into early development. This is not to say that change ceases after early childhood. While there are profound conservative tendencies in the adult personality, there are also greater or lesser proclivities to change. Many observe that the personality undergoes continual changes (or at least refining), and Ralph Waldo Emerson contended that people may be more like their peers than like their progenitors. Although the rate of change in the adult is slower than in the child, and the basic structure of the mind is much more stable in the adult, change can and does occur. Were this not the case, psychoanalytic therapy could not be effective; all psychoanalytic theories recognize the potential for significant change, even relatively late in life.

Although the major emphasis in the psychoanalytic approach to the mind has been on the already-structured personality (particularly on intrapsychic conflict), there has always been a subtextual concern with the problem of understanding the development of the mind. Virtually all schools of psychoanalysis recognize the existence of unconscious and preconscious minds. But different theories emphasize different dynamics. Libido theory emphasizes the biologically preordained drives. Structural theory emphasizes relationships among id, ego, and superego. Object relations theory focuses more on an internalized relational world. There has been a strong trend in contemporary psychoanalysis toward emphasizing that all mental life is a result of social interactions. Technically, this is often referred to as a "two-person psychology," emphasizing that the events in analysis must be understood as involving interactions of the patient and analyst rather than as pure data coming from the patient. Postmodern schools such as those based on interpersonal, relational, intersubjective, and constructivist theories emphasize the two-person field, its emotional impact, and the co-construction of the transference-countertransference dimensions of the analytic dyad. But all psychoanalytic schools recognize the potential for significant change, even relatively later in life.

Prior to Freud, patients who appeared to suffer from physical disabilities but in whom no underlying physical cause could be found were diagnosed as malingerers or as having a weakened nervous system. Freud's great discovery was that some of these patients suffered from disorders of the mind, not of the brain or the nervous system.

If there is a founding case in psychoanalysis, it is generally considered to be Anna O.'s treatment by Breuer, during the course of which the "talking cure," an early precursor of psychoanalysis, developed almost by accident. Anna O. had initiated the process of a kind of free association, which she referred to as "chimney sweeping," in which her speaking of the origins of each of her symptoms and the affect that emerged at that time magically caused them to disappear. But her therapy was ultimately disrupted by events outside the consulting room, generally believed to be the objection of Breuer's wife to his immersion in the treatment. Whatever the actual facts, the case of Anna O. was pivotal in the course of early psychoanalytic theory.

In 1895, Breuer and Freud published what many regard as the first psychoanalytic text, *Studies on Hysteria*, in which they discussed the case of Anna O. and similar cases. Their central insight was that "hysterics suffer mainly from reminiscences" (Breuer and Freud 1893–1895/1955, p. 7). The importance of this text is that it established the etiology of hysteria as psychosocial rather than organic. In the concluding chapter of that initial volume, Freud defined some of his basic tenets of psychoanalysis: transference, resistance, interpretation, reconstruction of the past, and making of unconscious memories conscious in words.

Between 1895 and 1905, Freud's creativity simply exploded. Within those 10 years, he wrote the aforementioned *Studies on Hysteria* (Breuer and Freud 1893–1895/ 1955), *The Interpretation of Dreams* (Freud 1900/1953), *The Study of the Dora Case* (Freud 1905/1901), and *Three Essays on the Theory of Sexuality* (Freud 1905/1953). By 1912, Freud had formulated fairly explicit concepts about transference, linking the patient's reaction to the therapist to previous reactions that the patient had experienced to one or more significant figures from his childhood (Freud 1912).

While Freud first proposed instincts of self-preservation and species preservation as major motivators, he later proposed that infantile sexuality and aggression were the two primary instincts (Freud 1915a/1957). By 1915, he had outlined many of the major theoretical and therapeutic propositions that have survived in classical psychoanalysis, including "On Narcissism: An Introduction" (1914a/ 1957); "Remembering, Rethinking and Working Through" (1914b/1958); "Observations on Transference-Love" (1915[1914]/1957); "Instincts and Their Vicissitudes" (1915a/1957); "Repression" (1915a/1957) and "The Unconscious" (1915c/1957); and *Introductory Lectures on Psycho-analysis*, Parts I and II (1916/1957). For many years, it was specifically the acceptance or rejection of instinct theory that separated what was known as Freudian psychoanalysis from the so-called culturalist schools.

In 1926, with the publication of *Inhibitions, Symptoms and Anxiety*, Freud (1926/1959) introduced a major shift in the way he viewed the origins of anxiety. In contrast to his earlier hypothesis that anxiety was the product of dammed-up libidinal energy, he now saw anxiety as the ego's response to the perception of danger. Thus, anxiety served as a signal to mobilize the use of defensive mechanisms.

In 1929, Freud introduced the structural model of the mind, encompassing the id, ego, and superego, which advanced his theory from its original formulation based on the conscious and unconscious minds. The structural model also marked a transition from a primarily id psychology to the analysis of the ego. Ego psychology suggests that some behaviors originate in the ego's autonomous activities and the gratifications that accompany them.

With this new formulation, which emphasized the ways in which the individual coped with both the internal and the external environments, the concept of adaptation assumed greater importance. Although Freud's instinct or drive theory remained at the heart of his metapsychology, he also described the dynamic unconscious and the principles of psychic determinism and overdetermination.

Freud is both the founding father of psychoanalysis and the originator of an astonishing number of insights into psychic life. However, psychoanalytic theory and treatment have not remained static since his original formulations. Given Freud's astonishing creative outpouring, it is not too surprising that his entire work would present some contradictions and inconsistencies. Whereas libido theory remains central for some theorists, others emphasize different theories of motivation and structuralization. Although all schools of psychoanalysis trace their roots to Freud, there have been important differences. For example, if Freud's instinct model were to be strictly adhered to, personal attachment would be seen as motivated solely by the wish for instinctual gratification. What has been called classical or orthodox psychoanalysis still rests on drive theory, but such exclusive focus on drive theory has come to be challenged by an increasing emphasis on a two-person psychology.

As described in this volume, the growing knowledge of attachment theory; studies of developmental processes that emphasize the fine attunement of mother and child, leading to "mentalization"; and the emphasis on the sense of safety, on fantasy, and on the fact that fantasy generally involves interaction with another person and expected feelings between them—all these and more have led to profound new elaborations of Freud's original instinct theory.

The shift toward validating and sometimes prioritizing a two-person psychology was propelled through the work of Bowlby (1969) and others, who demonstrated that attachment is independent of sex and aggression and should be viewed as an independent drive. Bowlby's thinking found validation in Harlow's classic studies on monkeys, in which infant monkeys became attached to a terry cloth surrogate mother who provided "contact comfort" even when another surrogate mother was recruited to satisfy their needs for hunger and thirst (Harlow 1958, 1959). Bowlby's insight, along with Harlow's experiments, stoked the psychoanalytic emphasis on what came to be recognized as a primary attachment system. The importance of exploring interpersonal attachment and interaction has been further demonstrated by a cadre of psychoanalytic researchers and theorists, among them Greenberg and Mitchell (1983), Eagle (1984), Stern (1985), and Fonagy (2001).

Put simply, the observations of many different analysts coalesced to suggest that our interest in other people and our development of affectionate bonds are not simply derivatives of sexual libido, but constitute an independent developmental line grounded in inborn propensities. Experimental and clinical observations, taken together, constituted the basis for the rise of a two-person psychology. Fairbairn put the nature of this dramatic shift succinctly: "libido is primarily object-seeking rather than pleasure-seeking" (Fairbairn 1952).

Object relations theorists view the individual's internal world as the amalgam of attachment needs, self and object representations, and the affects associated with them. They explain behavior as, at least in large part, a consequence of the projection onto the external world of aspects of the internalized representational world. Whereas some object relational analysts have integrated their views with drive theory, others view object relations theories as an extension beyond drive theory or even as a replacement for it. The work of a generation of infant researchers has shown in fine detail precisely how mother and infant shape each other. Joseph Sandler emphasized that the needs for safety and satisfaction are powerful motivators of behavior that are not drive determined.

There may well be still another mode of interpersonal interaction: emotional contagion between two people. Lichtenstein (1977) alluded to this form when speaking of the emotional imprinting of a child by its mother (such emotional contagion is perhaps viewed as a precursor of identification).

Ego psychology suggests that some behaviors originate in the ego's autonomous activities and the gratifications that accompany them. As noted above, Sandler emphasized that the needs for safety and satisfaction are powerful motivators of behavior that are not drive determined. Sandler takes an even broader view of such motivating factors: "We find that we cannot be sure whether the term *motive* refers to drives, drive derivatives, affects, feelings, needs, wishes, aims, intentions, reasons, or causes....[The term *motive*] reflects a multidimensional concept" (Sandler 1989, p. 91).

Self psychologists view behavior as originating out of the very nature of the developing self to realize its own potential. Kohut (1977) identified this as an additional primary drive, not merely as an aspect of libido. Again, the "mirroring" of the mother is essential if this push to selfhood is to flourish.

In addition, affect theory has been distinguished as having a focus that is distinct from the original emphasis on instinctual drives. Affect can be viewed not only as an expression of an innate state but also as a signal in response to external events that can alert us to danger or to the promise of pleasurable gratification or a wish. Thus, it is not exclusively a product of our interior lives; rather, it is key in adaptation to the external world.

Needless to say, different theoretical insights and preferences have developed in different parts of the world. The evolution of psychoanalysis in North America has taken several different trajectories. While for some psychoanalysts, object relations theory has replaced Freud's ego psychology, other psychoanalysts maintain a commitment both to Freud's early theories and to more contemporary theories—a trend toward viewing drive theory in conjunction with object relations theory. However, some psychoanalysts still adhere almost entirely to drive theory, whereas others cleave almost exclusively to object relations theory. At this time, psychoanalysts throughout the world are not unified in a single view of mental life. "Theoretical pluralism" dominates the psychoanalytic scene. Whatever their biases (or preferences) as to theory, most analysts recognize that the many modifications and additions to Freud's canon have served to fill in some of the inevitable gaps in his rich formulations. Attention to preoedipal and object relational aspects of psychic life has revolutionized psychoanalytic thinking. These latter contributions also include advances in ego psychology, self psychology, interpersonal psychology, and internalization and a burgeoning interest in intersubjectivity. Group psychology has also received greater attention, in relation not only to groups but also to hierarchies.

Perhaps the most recent, and in some ways most radical, revisions in theory have taken place in the way we theorize sex and gender. These changes were propelled by the various sex and gender liberation movements of the second half of the twentieth century. Sex and gender studies have de facto introduced—or if not introduced, enlarged upon—psychoanalytic insights into the impact of culture and power hierarchies on the psyche. As a consequence, there is much more attention paid to the role of cultural directives and their intersection with preconscious fantasies (Person 2004).

All these various views have yet to be integrated into a single overarching analytic theory. Yet there is a greater willingness to consider more than one theoretical perspective. Moreover, although the core of psychoanalytic theory remains the clinical situation, psychoanalytic thought has been enriched through ideas and discoveries of infant research, anthropology, ethology, cognitive psychology, philosophy, narrative studies, and neuroscience. While these studies may or may not contribute to psychoanalytic theory per se, they do place limits on existing theories. For example, the psychoanalytic theory of development has to dovetail to some degree with consistent findings in infant studies. Reciprocally, psychoanalysis has had a profound effect on neighboring disciplines.

Since technique follows theory, the proliferation of theories necessarily dictates the demise of any one "standard" technique within the field. Particularly in the United States, theory is marked by the rise of an emphasis on intersubjectivity (i.e., a two-person psychology), by an interest in interdisciplinary psychoanalysis, and by the diminution of Freud's iconic status within psychoanalysis. Yet virtually all schools of psychoanalysis in the United States emphasize the importance of the transference-countertransference, their interactions, and their analysis.

This textbook, first conceived within American Psychiatric Publishing, Inc. (APPI), is designed to be a broad-based and comprehensive resource, valuable equally to the scientific specialist and to the curious student. We have tried to ensure that each chapter is written with a minimum of professional jargon, while including a reasonably comprehensive bibliography that allows readers to pursue their specific interest further if they so wish.

The reader will note that a psychiatric publisher decided to produce this volume at a time when some psychiatrists question the role of psychoanalysis as a preferential treatment within psychiatry. We strongly believe that psychoanalytic approaches continue to play a vital role in the treatment of specific psychiatric disorders. Rigid indications for psychoanalysis are eschewed by most clinicians, because assessing suitability for psychoanalytic treatment involves evaluating the patient's personality structure as well as making a descriptive diagnosis. A psychoanalytic assessment would include evaluation of such features as psychological mindedness, curiosity, motivation, significant suffering, capacity to regress in the service of the ego, ability to form a therapeutic alliance, and sufficient impulse control and frustration tolerance to persevere in a treatment that takes years.

The psychiatric diagnoses that are often suited for psychoanalytic treatment include neurotically organized personality disorders, such as obsessive-compulsive, masochistic (self-defeating), depressive, dependent, hysterical, and, in some cases, histrionic personality disorders (Gunderson and Gabbard 1999). In addition, for most patients with narcissistic personality disorder, psychoanalysis is the treatment of choice. Patients with borderline personality disorder can sometimes be analyzed with modifications in technique, and most can be treated with psychoanalytically informed psychotherapy. The same is true for some schizoid personality disorder patients and avoidant patients who do not respond to brief behavioral or other treatments. Although the classic neuroses have fallen out of the official diagnostic manual, many of the patients with such neuroses (now classified as generalized anxiety disorder) may benefit greatly from psychoanalysis. In addition, some patients with recurrent major depressive disorder or dysthymia respond well to psychoanalysis (often in conjunction with medication) as a way of understanding their underlying vulnerability to respond to certain stressors with depressive mood. Some sexual disorders and some psychosomatic conditions may also be treated effectively with psychoanalytic approaches.

Not all causes of human suffering are listed in standard diagnostic manuals. Many patients who come to analysis are plagued with work inhibitions, conflicts about love relationships, long-standing family problems, problems with authority, difficulties integrating themselves into group situations, and other difficulties in living that are not easily classifiable using diagnostic nomenclature. People with these concerns may be ideally suited for psychoanalytic treatment. Contraindications for psychoanalysis include obsessive-compulsive disorder and antisocial personality disorder. Many, if not most, psychoanalysts recognize that psychoanalysis can be carried out concurrently with other modalities, particularly in conjunction with psychopharmacological therapy. Although the caricature of psychoanalysis remains the doctor sitting behind the couch with a notebook in his hand (the standard cartoon setting), the reality is that psychoanalytic thinking infuses not just multiple forms of therapy, including group and family, but a broad research endeavor that has been immensely productive in increasing our knowledge of the significance of, for example, the nature of early attachment, the requirements for the capacity to develop mental life (i.e., the ability to imagine the mind of another), the complexity of gender, the significance of trauma, and the nature of early mother-infant attachment, as well as newer ideas concerning the conduct of psychoanalysis. An important addendum to note is that derivatives of psychoanalytic theory are threaded through popular culture in the United States, appearing in self-help books, fiction, theater, and daily conversation, in its most naive form in such widespread comments as "She's still hung up on her father."

While we have included different points of view in an effort to indicate the pluralism of psychoanalysis today both in the United States and abroad, this textbook necessarily has a North American bias. The fact is that different cultures have focused on different aspects of psychoanalytic theory and discovery. For example, the French are generally committed to the role of infantile sexuality and the automatic maternal seductiveness that is an essential part of infantile life. They have also been powerfully influenced by Lacan and his views on linguistic structure in forming the mind. The British, influenced by Melanie Klein, stress the significance of early infantile fantasy and the affects of paranoia and depression and the defense mechanisms of projective identification. They have given the closest attention to transference-countertransference interactions. As already suggested, the Americans, long devoted to an ego psychological and adaptational point of view, have more recently branched into multiple overlapping schools: self psychological, relational, interpersonal, and constructivist.

The focus in our six sections is as follows:

Part I: Core Concepts. This section is designed to introduce some basic concepts that are indispensable to approaching psychoanalytic theory. These concepts include motivational systems; the dynamic unconscious and intrapsychic conflict; symbol formation; fantasies and dreams; the importance of early relationships; internalization; object relations theory; intersubjectivity; and sex and gender.

Part II: Developmental Theory. This section addresses the developmental orientation in contemporary psychoanalysis; different kinds of developmental theory; the interface between developmental theory and other disciplines; attachment theory and related research; the development of the mind; and the psychoanalytic understanding of pathologies in development.

Part III: Treatment and Technique. This section defines what a psychoanalyst is and how a psychoanalyst is trained; transference, countertransference, and the real relationship; theories of treatment and the technical consequences of these different treatments; interpretation, resistance, and process; termination and reanalysis; psychoanalysis and psychopharmacology; child analysis; and psychoanalysis and ethics.

Part IV: Research. This section describes the burgeoning research in psychoanalysis, focusing on outcome research, process research, developmental research, and conceptual research.

Part V: History of Psychoanalysis. This section traces the history of psychoanalysis, beginning with the years of its inception and its development in North America, in Britain and Continental Europe, in France and the extended French community, and, finally, in Latin America. As with any other cultural and scientific endeavor, the sociology and politics of the profession have played their roles for better and worse. We have included in this text chapters that give some account of the history of psychoanalysis in each of the major geographical areas in order to help readers understand how individual personalities, world events, and cultural differences have led to varieties of discoveries and points of view.

Part VI: Psychoanalysis and Related Disciplines. This section opens with a chapter on how interdisciplinary sources were relevant to Freud's ideas from the beginning of his work. It then proceeds to discuss the interrelationships and reciprocal influences between psychoanalysis on the one hand and psychology, anthropology, philosophy, literature, the arts, politics and international relations, and neuroscience on the other.

Readers will undoubtedly find themselves wishing to know more about some areas and less about others. Some will wonder why we have emphasized certain aspects of the field while neglecting others. The field of psychoanalysis is vast and multifaceted, and any textbook is bound to fall short of being all things to all readers. We have sought to include thoughtful and extensive bibliographies in all sections so readers can be guided in pursuit of further knowledge on particular issues raised in the text. We hope we have accomplished our relatively modest goal of providing an up-to-date overview of the field concisely packaged in one volume.

References

Bowlby J: Attachment and Loss, Vol 1: Attachment. New York, Basic Books, 1969

Breuer J, Freud S: Studies on hysteria (1893–1895), in Standard Edition of the Complete Psychological Works of Sigmund Freud, Vol 2. Translated and edited by Strachey J. London, Hogarth Press, 1955, pp 1–319

Eagle M: Recent Developments in Psychoanalysis: A Critical Evaluation. New York, McGraw-Hill, 1984

Fairbairn WRD: Psychoanalytic Studies of the Personality. London, Tavistock, 1952

Fonagy P: Attachment Theory and Psychoanalysis. New York, Other Press, 2001

Freud S: The interpretation of dreams (1900), in Standard Edition of the Complete Psychological Works of Sigmund Freud, Vols 4 and 5. Translated and edited by Strachey J. London, Hogarth Press, 1953

Freud S: Three essays on the theory of sexuality, I: the sexual aberrations (1905), in Standard Edition of the Complete Psychological Works of Sigmund Freud, Vol 7. Translated and edited by Strachey J. London, Hogarth Press, 1953, pp 135–172

Freud S: The dynamics of transference (1912), in Standard Edition of the Complete Psychological Works of Sigmund Freud, Vol 12. Translated and edited by Strachey J. London, Hogarth Press, 1958, pp 99–108

Freud S: On narcissism: an introduction (1914a), in Standard Edition of the Complete Psychological Works of Sigmund Freud, Vol 14. Translated and edited by Strachey J. London, Hogarth Press, 1957, pp 67–102

Freud S: Remembering, repeating and working-through (further recommendations on the technique of psycho-analysis II) (1914b), in Standard Edition of the Complete Psychological Works of Sigmund Freud, Vol 12. Translated and edited by Strachey J. London, Hogarth Press, 1958, pp 145–156

Freud S: Instincts and their vicissitudes (1915a), in Standard Edition of the Complete Psychological Works of Sigmund Freud, Vol 14. Translated and edited by Strachey J. London, Hogarth Press, 1957, pp 117–140

Freud S: Repression (1915b), in Standard Edition of the Complete Psychological Works of Sigmund Freud, Vol 14. Translated and edited by Strachey J. London, Hogarth Press, 1957, pp 146–158

Freud S: The unconscious (1915c), in Standard Edition of the Complete Psychological Works of Sigmund Freud, Vol 14. Translated and edited by Strachey J. London, Hogarth Press, 1957, pp 166–204

Freud S: Observations on transference-love (1915[1914]), in Standard Edition of the Complete Psychological Works of Sigmund Freud, Vol 12. Translated and edited by Strachey J. London, Hogarth Press, 1957, pp 159–171

Freud S: Introductory lectures on psycho-analysis, Parts I and II (1916), in Standard Edition of the Complete Psychological Works of Sigmund Freud, Vol 15. Translated and edited by Strachey J. London, Hogarth Press, 1957, pp 9–239

Freud S: Inhibitions, symptoms and anxiety (1926), in Standard Edition of the Complete Psychological Works of Sigmund Freud, Vol 20. Translated and edited by Strachey J. London, Hogarth Press, 1959, pp 75–175

Greenberg JR, Mitchell SA: Object Relations in Psychoanalytic Theory. Cambridge, MA, Harvard University Press, 1983

Gunderson JG, Gabbard GO: Making the case for psychoanalytic therapies in the current psychiatric environment. J Am Psychoanal Assoc 47:679–704, 1999

Harlow HF: The nature of love. Am Psychol 13:653–685, 1958

Harlow HF: Affectional responses in the infant monkey. Science 130:422–432, 1959

James W: The stream of thought, in The Principles of Psychology (1890). Reprinted in James W: Great Books of the Western World, Vol 53. Chicago, IL, Encyclopedia Britannica, 1952

Kohut H: The Restoration of the Self. New York, International Universities Press, 1977

Lichtenstein H: The Dilemma of Human Identity. New York, Jason Aronson, 1977

Person E: Personal power and the cultural unconscious: implications for psychoanalytic theories of sex and gender. J Am Acad Psychoanal Dyn Psychiatry 32:59–75, 2004

Sandler J: Toward a reconsideration of the psychoanalytic theory of motivation, in Psychoanalysis: Toward a Second Century. Edited by Cooper AM, Kernberg OF, Person ES. New Haven, CT, Yale University Press, 1989

Stern DN: The Interpersonal World of the Infant: A View from Psychoanalysis and Developmental Psychology. New York, Basic Books, 1985

Troyat H: Tolstoy. Translated by Amphonx N. New York, Harmony Books, 1988

PART I

Core Concepts

SECTION EDITOR: SALMAN AKHTAR, M.D.

1

Theories of Motivation in Psychoanalysis

FRED PINE, Ph.D.

THEORIES OF MOTIVATION IN psychoanalysis have undergone a century of debate initiated by Freud's original conception—a conception that, under the title "instinctual drives," was itself a theory of motivation. The debated proposals have left a legacy of internal opposition and significant modification, all in a context of continuity. This continuity gives psychoanalysis its identity, the expansive modifications give it its breadth, and the ongoing opposition gives it its spur to continued theoretical growth. Nowhere is this trio—continuity, modification, and continued debate—more evident than in the psychoanalytic view of the driving forces of mental life.

The "driving forces of mental life"—a mental life that finds expression in thought, affect, and behavior—define the central subject matter of this chapter, motivation, as well as the subject matter of psychoanalysis itself, mental life and its derivatives. Biological processes, interpersonal processes, and cultural forces all influence the human being profoundly, but it is their representation and activity in individual mental life that lies at the heart of psychoanalytic theorizing, data gathering, and clinical process.

The steady modification of psychoanalytic ideas reflects psychoanalysis's status as an empirically and evidentially based enterprise, and it is that modified view that shall be detailed here. The focus will be on a contemporary psychoanalytic theory of motivation—one that draws on psychoanalytic history as needed to expand understanding and to highlight the evolution of the theory. Some discussion of individual human history will also be given because, whatever the nature of the initial built-in evolutionary and biological bases of human motivations—and these are indeed central—their final forms are the result of complex, personalized shaping processes that take time to occur; this time is provided in the unique histories of individual lives. Thus, the overall focus will be on how motivational status evolves over time—in human beings in general and in individual persons in particular. To define the territory (motivation) of this chapter simply: when behavior (including thought) seems to be sustained and organized around specific aims of the individual, we think of it as motivated. What are these sustaining and organizing motives as seen by psychoanalysis today?

Preliminary Considerations

In this section, I offer a historical view, giving a sense of what Freud came to by way of motivational theory, how he got there, and how his original conception is viewed today. But first I present a more contemporary view in order to address what was left undeveloped by Freud and remained to be accomplished. In subsequent sections, I detail how the gaps were filled in: where we have come to in motivational theory, and how we got to where we are.

The Present

To anticipate: I shall describe a set of proactive, reactive, and homeostatic motivations under four headings: motivations in the sphere of *human relations*, notably attachment and the repetition of internalized object relations; motivations in the sphere of *ego function*, notably the exercise of capacities, holding on to attained stability, and responding to affect signals of danger; motivation in the sphere of *self experience*, notably self-corrective "righting" responses (holding on to preferred subjective self-states); and motivations in the *drive* sphere, notably though not exclusively sexuality and aggression. For each, I shall note aspects of their biological and evolutionary roots, their individual and adventitious histories, and their clinical relevance. I end the presentation with a discussion of a superordinate issue in the motivational sphere (unconscious motivation) and two refinements of it (agency and developmental needs).

I begin with comments from two highly regarded theorists who wrote against the backdrop of Freud's "instinctual drive" theory with recognition of directions in which it was becoming modified.

In his 1971 paper "On Motivation and Instinct Theory," Hans Loewald, a man whose psychoanalytic theorizing was widely viewed as transformative, wrote:

> [In the development of psychoanalytic theory over the years], motivation had become instinctual, as had repression and defense, in contrast to the early notion of personal will. Psychic life is motivated by sometimes conflicting, sometimes confluent, sometimes fused, sometimes defused instinctual forces. There seems to be no room for *personal* motivation. Yet I have claimed that personal motivation is the fundamental assumption of psychoanalysis. We now seem to see that, on the contrary, psychoanalytic psychology postulates instinctual, unconscious, impersonal forces as the motives of our psychic life. Where is the person? Where is the ego or self that would be the source and mainstay of personal motivation? (Loewald 1971/1980, p. 110)

And in 1981, Joseph Sandler, another highly influential theorist, wrote:

> Because psychoanalytic theory and practice has placed so much emphasis on sexual and aggressive wishes, and because psychoanalysis has had to defend its findings in regard to the prevalence of such wishes, there has been a tendency to see *all* wishes as instinctual. With developments in ego psychology after the war, psychoanalytic theoreticians have gone through the most tremendous intellectual contortions to try to derive *all* wishes from sexual and aggressive impulses, and have attempted to maintain a position in which any unconscious wish is seen as being powered by instinctual energy or by a desexualized or neutralized form of that energy. (Sandler 1981, p. 187)

Loewald asks where the ego or self is in motivation. He makes clear within that same paper that he finds the source of personal motivation in individual history—in the infant's interactions with the more highly organized persons in his or her environment. This interaction puts its stamp on the growing person, changing the universal driving forces into organized and individually characteristic ones. Sandler, in other writings (not quoted here), leaving behind the "intellectual contortions" that he refers to, has also looked at the motivational power of relationships with others, on the one hand, and of affective states, prototypically feelings of safety (and of its absence), on the other. In subsequent sections of this chapter, we shall see how Loewald's call for a place for the ego and self in motivation theory, and Sandler's for a place for object relations and affects, have each achieved a place of importance today.

The Past

But first to origins and to Freud, where we shall end up pointed in the same directions: For reasons that may have been no more than matters of personal intellectual style, Freud tended to think in terms of motivational dualisms. Or perhaps we get this impression because, from early on, he firmly believed in the centrality of sexuality ("libido") as a core motivational force and later considered first one, and then another, and then yet another counterforce as operating alongside of it (see Freud 1915/1957). Be this as it may, Freud theorized at one early point about the presence of sexual (species-preserving) and ego (self-preserving) instincts; the links to evolutionary theory in the post-Darwinian climate of his intellectual development are clear. At a subsequent point (see Freud 1914a/1957), struck by a variety of phenomena that seemed to reflect self-preoccupation in contrast to genuine (even if conflicted) connection to others, he contrasted narcissistic (self-directed) and libidinal (other-directed) motives. And still later, witness to the horrors of World War I, and to the aftermath of the traumatic neuroses of war (such as "shell shock" and the repetitive dreams that follow it), he began the development of a theory of aggression alongside of sexuality. But, in doing this last, he took a long detour through philosophical speculations regarding a "repetition compulsion" (see Freud 1920/1955) that operates "beyond the pleasure principle," a speculation that, in altered form, has had profound implications within psychoanalytic theorizing regarding motivation. This requires a short explanation to prepare the ground for much of what follows herein.

Freud (1911/1958) thought the central principle guiding human function was the "pleasure principle"—that is, seeking pleasure and avoiding unpleasure. Repetition of trauma (as in posttraumatic dreams) seemed a contradiction to the pleasure principle—hence, repetition as a force "beyond the pleasure principle." But there was an additional dilemma that Freud never succeeded in resolving: the question of what produced pleasure. He early on thought in terms of tension reduction, but that idea never worked successfully enough—take for example the tension *buildup* sought in sexuality (though, granted, optimally followed by tension relief). Nonetheless, his observations on repetition of painful experiences led him into philosophical speculations (which shall not be rendered here) that ultimately brought him to the idea of a "death instinct," which was more or less equivalent to the aim of reducing all tension and returning to an inanimate state. For Freud, this death instinct, when turned outward on others, becomes the source of aggression and thus keeps him within the region that started his speculations: the horrors and destructiveness of World War I. Though a not insignificant number of psychoanalysts took the death instinct concept and used it centrally in their thinking about human psychic life, Freud himself did not do much more with it. In the United States, and for that matter everywhere in the world, psychoanalysts did pick up on the importance of aggression as a powerful motivational force alongside of sexuality as yet another dualism, though one not necessarily involving any role of a death instinct.

However, as will be seen, the question of tension buildup as opposed to tension reduction, the concept of repetition, and the role of aggression come to play significant roles in contemporary psychoanalytic motivational theory, but in conceptually diverse domains and without the philosophical superstructure that Freud brought to them. And, not so incidentally, these developments leave behind his concept of a death instinct—a concept that is totally at variance with evolutionary theory (*survival* of the fittest) and makes no sense as something that would suddenly appear in human evolution, as though we had stepped off the evolutionary ladder and gone our own way. Human destructiveness has to be accounted for in other ways.

Sex and aggression, two sets of (often interrelated) urges that any self-observant human being knows to be central for our species, remained the leitmotifs, the firsts among equals, of psychoanalytic motivational theory. But what of all those other pieces left suspended and relatively undeveloped in Freud's series of dualistic forays into motivation theory? They turned out to be both strikingly related to aspects of theory that have been developed since Freud's death and, hardly coincidentally, just the regions of motivation referred to in the opening quotations from Loewald and Sandler.

Recall that Freud had an early place for ego motives in one of his motivational dualisms (ego or self-preservative instincts vs. libidinal or species-preservative ones). But, with time, he came to think of the ego (that set of functions in human mental life related to defense, adaptation, and reality testing) primarily in terms of its role in defense against expression of the (sexual and aggressive) instinctual drives. His stated defining attribute of a psychoanalytic treatment (Freud 1914b/1957) was that it recognized the clinical phenomena of resistance and transference. But resistance was nothing other than the role of that same ego-as-defense as it appeared in the treatment process. Freud did not think in terms of the independent motivational status of certain aspects of ego functioning, which today we cannot ignore, though one very significant motive, maintenance of sameness, turns out to be implicit in the resistance concept itself, as shall be seen.

Freud, as any psychoanalytic clinician of necessity must, listened to patients talk a great deal about their relationships with the other persons in their lives—past and present, imagined and real, wished for and rejected—an aspect of human function that has come to be known as "object relations." But, while this is a constant focus of psychoanalytic clinical work, Freud did not self-consciously theorize about these relationships—an aspect of psychoanalytic theorizing that has come to be known, self-evidently enough, as "object relations theory." Perhaps he did not theorize because his main focus was the instinctual drives, or perhaps because object relations seemed infinitely variable and he sought more general, if not universal, concepts. Nevertheless, object relations theory today has important motivational considerations built into it, and among them there is a central place, in partially revised and partially continued form, for Freud's concept of the significance of repetition, the very concept that had a central place in one of his later dualisms (pleasure principle vs. repetition compulsion). In fact, in that definition of psychoanalysis just given, a treatment that recognizes the phenomena of resistance and transference, the reference to transference was an unrecognized move into object relations theory. It remained unrecognized because transference *could* be defined in terms of a sexual or aggressive drive psychology as the expression of those drives displaced to the person of the psychoanalyst. In this formulation, its other component, the repetition of old *relationships* through the relationship with the analyst, could be attended to less.

Freud (1914a/1957) also came close to a concept of the self and its motivational aspects with his narcissism (self-related) versus object libido (other-related) dualism. But "self" is a conceptually soft term, and Freud had scientific aspirations (and James Strachey, the English translator of the standard edition of Freud's works, largely replaced the word "self" with the word "ego," in line with that same aim). But with the writings of certain psychoanalytic infant observers—Rene Spitz (1959), Donald Winnicott (1960), and

Margaret Mahler (Mahler et al. 1975)—and, from a clinical vantage point, Heinz Kohut (1977), and subsequently others in additional ways, the word *self*, and in particular a self with motivational status, took on legitimacy, and in fact necessity, in psychoanalytic writings. Jacobson's (1964) use of the term *self-representation* rather than "self," thus underscoring its intrapsychic aspect, further added to its psychoanalytic "legitimacy." Today the concept "self," in various aspects, plays an important role in our understanding of the broad sweep of human motivation.

And so, abandoned or relatively undeveloped pieces of Freud's early motivational dualisms, as well as the ideas of contemporary critical theorists, have pointed us in the direction of motives in the spheres of object relations, ego functioning, and self experience, in addition to powerful sexual and aggressive urges or drives.

An Important Note

Before proceeding to an array of motives as currently understood, we need to reconsider Freud's continuing focus on sexuality as *a* (whether or not *the*) core human motivation. Was he wrongheaded? In fact, psychoanalysis has added to and altered but not replaced his formulation. How did Freud arrive at that formulation? First, by listening to his patients—that is, to people like any of us who know sexuality to be a powerful and often conflicted force in our lives. Probably also by attending to himself and discovering the same thing. Probably also he was influenced by his culture, that of late-19th-century Vienna in the Victorian age, in a place and at a time when sexuality was officially a silent subject but where the hypocrisy of affairs, mistresses, and prostitution were set against official morality and contributed to sexual conflict in individuals.

There were less personal aspects as well. Sexuality was a biological force, built-in and guaranteed by evolution, and hence marked Freud's attempt to formulate as scientific a basis as possible for his developing psychological views. And he made a major observation (Freud 1905/1953) that colored his thinking powerfully about "infantile sexuality": namely, the early, and thus potentially formative, role of sexual motivations (and the wishes and fantasies that spring from them) in psychic life. The observation was that of a close parallel between three areas: sexual foreplay, perversion, and the early bodily development and care of the young child. In each of the three, one could see the centrality of the mouth, the anal region, the genitals, the skin surface altogether, looking, being looked at, and experiencing or rendering moderate (and in some instances perhaps not so moderate) degrees of pain. This parallel with the phenomena of foreplay and of perversion led Freud to consider the child's early bodily experiences as protosexual—sexual here in a much expanded meaning of the term—and thus to grant these experiences a centrally formative role.

Freud evolved a theory of "instinctual drive"—of a fixed quantity of sexual energy that is centered in different bodily activities or regions (erotogenic zones) as the growing child moves through various "psychosexual phases." But with or without his instinct theory (the theory of the phases and a constant amount of libidinal energy), the role of the sensual experiences inherent in early bodily care calls out for recognition. The oral, anal, and genital zones are sensitive areas and profoundly important sites of both stimulation by and interaction with the primary caretaker. As such, they become formative sites of major interaction (relationship) tendencies. We know that human relationships become habitual, getting repeated, elicited, sought, and remaining with us—sometimes throughout a life. Hence, however we conceive of sexuality's development, the biologically grounded urges and sensual experiences of sexuality, broadly defined as in Freud's conception, and played out and personally shaped in the earliest infant-caregiver experiences, remain a major focus in human life.

However, giving continued recognition to motivations in the spheres of object relations, ego function, self, and aggression as well, one important point should be kept in mind about sexuality that may also have influenced Freud's giving it starring status in the motivational hierarchy (a point that he failed to note and state conceptually). Sexuality can be a final common pathway for the expression of almost anything in human mental life. It can repeat old object relations; it can hide (or meet) primal attachment needs under the veneer of sexual relations; it can temper negative affects such as anxiety, depression, or grief; it can elevate or lower self-esteem; it can be used to express aggression. Thus, while sex is always sexual, it need not be *only* sexual; it need not even be *mainly* sexual. An observer can be deceived into gliding over some of the hidden motivational and nonsexual functions for which sexuality serves as the final common expressive pathway.

Motivation in Psychoanalytic Theory: A Broad View

Heinz Hartmann (1939/1958) sought to expand Freud's psychoanalysis into "a general psychology." By this he meant one that focuses on aspects of ego functioning, including adaptation to the external surround, the built-in tools for such adaptation (thought, memory, perception, motility, and affect), and a "conflict-free" sphere of human mental life—all of this supplementing the psychoanalytic focus on instinctual drives and conflict. Today, offering a discussion of motivation within a general psychology of the mind, one can and indeed must also consider not only ego functioning and adaptation but also regions of emotionally intense, often conflicted, functioning that are beyond the instinctual driving forces—that is, the regions of object relations and self as well as the functioning of the ego itself.

Freud sought to develop a grand theory of the mind, within which certain motivations had premier status. Today it seems more cautious not to reach for such a grand theory. The motivations I describe here are part of a "practical" theory of mind in the sense that they grow within the observations of clinical practice. Perhaps one day a grand theory will subsume them all. Or perhaps they are simply additive aspects of the human repertoire.

One point should be made explicit, however: the motivations listed herein reflect and embody the developmental history of psychoanalytic theory itself. For decades, and certainly at least through the first two-thirds of the 20th century, psychoanalytic thinking in the United States was dominated by Freud's "structural theory": the conception that the mind can most usefully be looked at as divided into an id (the seat of the drives), an ego (the seat of the defenses), and a superego (the seat of conscience)—the whole often referred to, alternatively, as "ego psychology." The discussion below of motivations in relation to the drives, and, in some cases, in relation to the ego, reflects that theoretical paradigm. But, beginning in the last third of the 20th century, an "object relations" theoretic paradigm came into a prominence at least equal to that of ego psychology and the structural theory. This paradigm is built on the relations between people and the distinctive ways these relationships operate in human minds; it readily extends to concerns with the person (the "self") as a whole person, and not just as the site of the drive–defense–superego conflicts. Motivations relevant to those domains of psychic function are equally represented in what follows.

A few provisos: First, by no means would all psychoanalysts agree with all that I shall present, though the motivations I describe are central in the thinking of one or another significant set of analysts. Second, the motives I describe would not be given equal centrality by all psychoanalysts, and it is not my intent here to imply such equivalence; one or another will be more central in different persons or in the same person at different moments (Pine 1990). And third, the groupings through which I approach these motivations here are not sharply divided, but in fact overlap. At the least, the groupings serve expository purposes, though they also serve to make explicit the gaps in past theories and to show how the gaps have been filled.

Motivations in Object Relations

The term *object relations* has a history. Freud originally thought of the "object" as that thing through which the libidinal drive was gratified. Since the "thing" could be a person (say, the mother), a part of a person (say, the mother's breast or the infant's thumb), or an inanimate object (say, a teddy bear for an infant or black leather for a fetishist), the term "object" seemed appropriate. Later, when primary human relationships began to achieve their importance in psychoanalytic *theorizing* (they were always important in psychoanalytic *work*), the term "object relations" was nonetheless retained. But the term is not meant to objectify or dehumanize such relations. It is a remnant of history.

Internalized Object Relations

Evolution has brought our species to the point where we are not fully preadapted at birth. It requires months and years for neuromuscular and brain development to be more or less complete. During that long postbirth but preautonomous period, the human infant is heavily dependent on his or her caregivers for survival. This period of dependence guarantees the significance of those "objects," the primary caregivers, in the mental life of the child. Attempts to describe regularities in the way the infinitely variable array of individual relationships work in mental life are referred to as *object relations theories*. There are numerous such theories, but two core concepts with major motivational significance that run through them all will be extracted here: attachment and the repetition of internalized object relations. We shall start with the latter, not because it is more basic (it is not), but because 1) it achieved centrality in psychoanalytic thinking earlier and 2) it underlies one of the most common forms of interpretation of motivation offered to patients by their analysts during the course of clinical psychoanalysis.

To make it vivid and immediate, I present here some forms that such interpretations may take (all are drawn from actual clinical work). Note that these are all motivational statements in the sense given earlier: they attempt to explain what impels particular behaviors that are sustained and organized around the aims of the individual. In each of these, the analyst is speaking to a patient.

"You felt your parents were rejecting of you, but they were the only parents you had, and so you keep them with you by provoking rejection at the hands of each person in your life."

"The pain of their negligence was so great that you continually try to master it by inflicting it on others."

"Everyone becomes your father to you in your mind's eye, and then you relate to them as you did to him—challenging, defiant, and terrified underneath."

"Whenever anyone in your life treats you with kindness, you flee from it, expecting it to be followed by the same kinds of seductions that you felt to be your experience in your own family."

In each of these, we are saying that a person is behaving to repeat, to anticipate, to elicit, to demonstrate, to turn onto others, or to reverse some pattern of behavior (an object relationship) that was experienced, imagined, feared, or wished for within early relations with others. In these repetitions, the individual may play the role of himself or herself or the role of the other. This is the "stuff" of much human interaction. In fact, we can take as one measure of psychopathology the extent to which current relationships are rigidly and unrealistically experienced and dealt with as carbon copies of past relationships. To the degree that relationships are experienced in terms of current reality (no matter how difficult that reality may or may not be), we cannot think of them as psychopathological. But to the degree that they are rigidly distorted in terms of the past, the reverse holds true.

How do we conceive of such relationship patterns, and how do they originate? From the standpoint of internal object relations, each of us is seen as carrying around an internal drama, within which we enact one or more (or even all) of the roles, and within which also roles can be "assigned" to those around us in the way that we perceive them. Developmentally, these dramas are understood to have been created through the recording (as memories) of interactions between the person and his or her caregivers. But what is laid down as memory need not be, and almost certainly is usually not, veridical. It is the child's *experience* that is laid down as memory, and that experience is a product of the inner state in the child that meets the external inputs. Such states, which will be wishful, fearful, and expectant in many forms, color the way the parental inputs are received. For example, a child in physical pain, whose mother is sensitively ministering to the pain but cannot relieve it, may experience the mother at that moment as noncomforting, though the outside observer will see her as comforting.

How do we understand the motivational status of such happenings, the tendency to *repeat* these interactions in the forms in which they were experienced? Let us look at a concept that will be useful in developing an answer. Ernst Kris (1956) offered a distinction between shock trauma and strain trauma—and recall that it was shock trauma (the "shell shock" of soldiers in World War I) that led Freud

into his discussion of *repetition* in the first place. *Shock traumas* are big, all at once, overwhelming. A bomb blows up and kills people near us; we undergo major surgery; a beloved dies suddenly; the World Trade Center disaster occurs. In each of these situations, there is more stimulation than can be processed at that time and with the person's available resources (this being the psychoanalyst's working definition of trauma). We know that, following such events, there is a strong tendency to talk about them again and again, to dream about them, to fantasize about them—that is, to repeat them in one form or another. *Strain traumas*, the other form, contrast with shock trauma, but not in the tendency toward repetition (which is common to both). Strain traumas grow on us and get under our skin through the fact of their continual recurrence; they are not "all at once" shocks, but rather cumulatively, and at times retrospectively, destructive traumas (Khan 1963/1974). If a parent fails to notice us once, it passes; but if this not noticing is the habit of a lifetime, it grinds away at us; it achieves a traumatizing effect (an inability to be processed with available resources) over time. Or if we are constantly silenced at moments of joy, we can manage it once, or even twice, but again something crushing happens when this is the habit of a lifetime. As with shock trauma, we notice that *strain trauma produces tendencies toward repetition*. We understand this to be *repetition in efforts toward mastery* of the (strain) trauma—efforts to work them through. But clinically what we usually see are *failed* efforts at mastery—repetitions that are incited, reimagined, and going nowhere. Psychoanalysis is clinically based for its theorizing, and these tendencies toward repetition seem to be prominent in every psychoanalysis, often expressed in relation to the person of the analyst (transference).

This motivation is *proactive* in the immediate present. That is, internal discomforts, frustrations, fears, and longings in the sphere of relationships spontaneously impel new behaviors that repeat these internal experiences. Self-defeating? Yes. But nonetheless highly characteristic. Of course one can also view these repetitions as *reactive* to the whole history of childhood; but in the present the tendency to repeat impels behavior proactively.

In a contribution to motivational theory that has been highly influential, Kernberg (1982) has in fact derived Freud's libidinal and aggressive drives from such early internalized object relationships and the affects associated with them. He suggests that a first organization develops in terms of good and bad experiences, eventuating in love and hate, and that it is from these that libido and aggression derive: "Affects, in short, are the building blocks or constituents of drives" (p. 908).

An elegant example of the motivational power of such forms of painful object relationship appears in Edward

Albee's play *The Zoo Story* (1960). In it a man, a loner, is describing the struggle he goes through each day to avoid being bitten by a vicious dog in the hallway of his tenement building. The listener, increasingly horrified as he hears the story, finally shouts out the question why the man does not move elsewhere. And suddenly, the mood changes. The loner, the storyteller, looks to his questioner in condescension and surprise. He explains (in an "Isn't it obvious?" tone) that everyone has to have a relationship, and his is with the dog. And yes, we all do have to have relationships, but with the primary caregivers of our childhood, no matter how noxious, humiliating, or hurtful these relationships were. Such is the power and source of the repetition of internalized object relationships as a central human motivation.

Attachment

The story of the loner with his dog brings us naturally to the arena of attachment as a second primary motive in the object relations domain. The question of why abused children hold on to their parents, and why battered wives hold on to their mates, has long been of interest. And linked to that, the huge importance of separation and loss in human mental life cannot be denied. (I recall my own internal sense of dissatisfaction when, early in my psychoanalytic career, I tried to understand separation anxiety in terms of Freud's oral phase, in terms of the mother-as-provider who, like a conditioned stimulus, becomes a necessary object for the child. But it seemed forced; separation anxiety did not fit well into the procrustean bed of oral-drive theory.)

Into this arena, starting in the 1940s but especially with his later work on attachment and loss, came John Bowlby (1969), subsequently to be followed by a still growing flood of empirical researchers. Bowlby sought to explain separation anxiety, stranger anxiety, clinging to even abusive parents, fear of the dark, and more in terms of what he thought of as a primary, biologically built-in, attachment motive. Humans simply *are* attached to their primary caretakers, just as Lorenz's geese follow the first living, moving creature they see. But human infants demonstrate it through the various phenomena just listed, not through locomotor tracking, of which they are incapable at birth. Bowlby's proposal was that the evolutionary value of a primal attachment tendency is best understood in terms of "the environment of evolutionary adaptedness" (Bowlby 1969, pp 58–64)—the time when survival for early humans, living in the wild and under the threat of animal attack, would be enhanced by attachment to the group that lessened the danger of wandering off into darkness and being in danger from other animals. Stern's (1985) review of the infant literature, and his own work, make clear that object attachment, of remarkable subtlety and substantiality, is present so early as to render forced and artificial any attempt to explain this as being *derived* from drive gratification in some secondary way. Quite the reverse in fact: it is in the few quiet and satiated moments of the newborn's day that these signs of built-in attachment, of differential and preferential perceptual connection and attunement to the mother, are evident. Whatever the tie to mother from the fact of her feeding, and it is powerful, there seems to be a biological base to attachment to begin with.

The presence of a primal attachment need in human beings seems no longer to be contested. While Bowlby, a psychoanalyst himself, found his ideas excluded from the psychoanalytic canon for many years, the tide has turned, and his overall view is simply taken for granted now. And attachment, too, operates as a proactive motivation. The infant's distress cry that summons the mother, as well as the infant's (and child's and adult's) anxiety in the face of separation and loss, testifies to attachment-seeking. When the need is met, and even later in development when the attachment can be carried mentally (so-called object constancy [Fleming 1975; Pine 1985]), the attachment need is quiescent, not noticeable. But if it is unmet, or not securely achieved internally, then the attachment need becomes apparent.

Clinically, attachment needs work differently from internalized object relations. Every person is always carrying internalized object relations; how much these are repeatedly played out in destructive forms is, as I noted, one of the measures of psychopathology, but it is also one of the basic phenomena of every clinical psychoanalysis. Such internalized object relations are constituents of every personality and are always played out, the differences being only in how problematic they are. Attachment needs are different (as we shall see below; see also Akhtar 1999 for a discussion of needs versus wishes). To some extent, in the ordinary range of challenges of everyday living, attachment needs may be successfully resolved in some individuals (by present attachments and by internal object constancy, carrying our loved ones in mind in memory) and therefore may recede into the background. These needs may also be met by the very presence of the psychoanalyst in the patient's life and thus go almost unnoticed, part of what Freud (1912/1958) referred to as "the unobjectionable positive transference." The attachment needs, *when more or less satisfied*, become a secure base inside the person; this base can be seen as the stage on which the drama of the internalized object relations is played out. But, in those patients in whom the attachment needs have not been met and are not securely established by object constancy, *these needs* become the primary phenomena of an analysis (Pine

1976). They are then "noisy," not quiescent, and show themselves in separation anxiety and generalized neediness, or, contrariwise, in defense against these needs: isolation, emotional aloofness, hyper-independence or hyper-autonomy.

So, attachment as a primary, built-in motivation, and the internalization and repetition of object relations as an inevitable consequence of the long period of biological dependency on others, are two powerful motivations in the sphere of object relations that are recognized within psychoanalysis today.

Motivations in Ego Functioning

The term *ego* is a *concept* within psychoanalysis; it does not refer to the whole person. It is a summary term used to refer to those aspects of the person's functioning having to do with adaptation, reality testing, and defense. While the term *defense* referred originally to defense against the instinctual drives, it can readily be extended to refer to any regions of the person's functioning that produce conflict and/or painful negative affects that have to be coped with intrapsychically in some way ("defended against"). Thus, Anna Freud (1936/1966) referred to defense against affects, and Modell (1984) to defense against object relations.

Just as object relations are guaranteed significance in human life by our position in evolution—that is, not fully preadapted and hence dependent on others for many years—so too does ego function reflect our place in evolution. While humans are not fully preadapted, no creature survives in evolutionary terms without being at least partially preadapted. The built-in capacities for adaptation come to have motivational significance in at least two major ways (that will be discussed here as the exercise of capacities and the anxiety signal), and the adaptations that they bring about in turn bring into being a third motivational force (that will be discussed here as resistance to change).

Exercise of Capacities

As already noted, Hartmann (1952) brought analytic attention to what he referred to as the "ego apparatuses"—thought, perception, memory, motility, and affect—the built-in tools for adaptation. Hartmann of course did not discover these forms of function, but he discovered their relevance for psychoanalysis, for understanding more about how (in terms of the central theory at the time) the drives operated and were managed by the person. Although Hendrick (1942) wrote about "functionlust" long ago (i.e., urges for, and pleasure in, exercise of capacities), and Klein (1976) delineated the pleasures in the use of ego capacities, systematic attention to this phenomenon has

not been forthcoming (but see White 1963 for an exception). That attention shall be given here, theoretically in terms of the proactive motivational significance of the built-in tendency to exercise these capacities, and clinically in terms of the role of such exercise in forming a foundation for developments that have always been of central concern to psychoanalytic clinicians and theorists.

Contrary to Freud's focus on the centrality of tension reduction, we can no longer fail to recognize that the human infant is governed by tendencies toward stimulus-seeking as well as tension reduction (see Lichtenberg 1983; Stechler and Halton 1987; White 1963). Indeed a flood of experimental research has made clear that, virtually from the start of life, the infant's perceptual apparatus is attuned to the outside with consequences for memory, learning, and cognition more broadly. That is, what we conceive of as reality attunement and adaptation is built on prewired aspects of the infant organism. So, too, is defense (defined broadly as tension regulation). Lichtenberg (1983) summarized it thus: "What is suggested by the research [on the neonate] is that rather than a stimulus barrier and simple [tension] reduction mechanism, the infant is innately equipped to *regulate* stimuli and tension within optimal threshold limits" (p. 6). *Competence* (White 1963), starting as the capacity to make things happen (as simple as squeezing a rubber toy and making it squeak), is an outgrowth of such prewired tendencies and is a bedrock of self-esteem and of personal agency.

The relevant point for motivation theory, then, is that the exercise of capacities—and, through them, reality testing and adaptation—has a self-propelled quality. Although conflict, strivings for drive gratification, and ties to the object affect the development of reality testing, defense, and self-esteem profoundly, it all starts from a built-in base. Put otherwise, the built-in tendency for exploration, play, and consequent learning leads to a base for, say, reality testing (through perception and memory) and for self-esteem (through the ability to produce an effect, to make things happen); therefore, when these (e.g., reality testing, self-esteem) develop in affectively powerful, conflicted, and object relational settings, there is already a core present; they do not have to develop from scratch. We have learned that psychoanalytic listening will often reveal conflict- and affect-related components in the exercise of particular skills and talents, but this insight need not lead to a reductionist view. There is every reason to assume that the complex neurological apparatus given to us by evolution is preset to function in important ways in relation to the environment in which it evolved.

The functioning of these basic apparatuses becomes clinically relevant when they are *not* reliably in evidence. Like attachment tendencies, apparatus function is barely noticeable clinically and is taken for granted, when it has developed well. But when early affective flooding in the context of nongratification and disturbed relations to caregivers is too much present, or when illness and pain characterize an infant's experience, they may drown out the "leisure time" in which infants can explore and play (White 1963). In that setting, gaps in function that would otherwise have been served by such exploratory play and learning become evident clinically. And they do so because they form the basis not only for reality testing and self-esteem but for pathways to personal agency and to sublimation or alternative routes to adaptation and pleasure that serve the person well when they are present.

Anxiety (or Affect) Signal

The capacity to experience affect is one of the built-in ego apparatuses or tools of function. Of course, affect is also the final common pathway of what it is that the infant has to *cope with*. Ultimately, it is when stimuli from within or without produce negative affect that the infant needs or seeks help. Negative affect is the across-the-board end state of distress.

But it is also the *signal* of distress. The infant's built-in cry summons (signals) the mother. This may not initially be *intended* by the infant, but the signal value of the cry is soon learned and becomes intentional. The cry comes in the face of affective distress, either from hunger, cold, lack of physical support, or a rise in some built-in need to be held. Ultimately, for each one of us, that signal comes to work in interior ways—signaling *ourselves* regarding the need to protect ourselves (from internal phenomena that are experienced as dangers).

Freud (1926/1959) confronted this duality with regard to affect experience. Though at first he thought of anxiety as the result of undischarged libidinal tension, he later placed the experience of anxiety within the concept "ego"—as a tool of psychic function. In this second theory of anxiety Freud saw affect flooding as a first stage, a "traumatic anxiety" (i.e., more stimulation than the infant could cope with); but he suggested that under normal developmental conditions, anxiety becomes a "signal." Put simply, feelings (affects) are put in us by evolution to tell us how we feel, thus giving us information necessary for guiding our functioning. *Signal anxiety* alerts the infant to a situation of (real or psychically imagined) danger; and the infant, at first through calling the mother, and later through adaptive/defensive tools of his or her own, wards off the danger in some way (say, by a shift of attention or a flight into activity, and later by more sophisticated and subtle means). The failure to develop such a signal function of anxiety—that is, the tendency to remain at a point where the anxi-

ety rapidly rises to a traumatic level—is most difficult to deal with clinically and is a center of psychic pain for the affected individual.

In this model, anxiety (and negative affect altogether, including fear, shame, embarrassment, and guilt) becomes a tool of ego function—a signal to avoid, cope with, or ward off danger by some means. As such, the anxiety (or broader negative affect) signal is a powerful incitement, another proactive motivation within the sphere of ego function. Along with resistance to change, it is one of the central foci of psychoanalytic clinical work. Its motive force serves the person poorly or well, depending both on what it is that prompts the signal (i.e., how anxiety-prone the person is) and on what follows the anxiety signal (i.e., how well the coping mechanisms work). Much of psychoanalytic clinical work can be described as the effort to enable the patient to narrow the scope of experienced threat and to deal with the residue in more advanced, adaptive ways.

Resistance to Change

Freud (1914b/1957) labeled a recognition of resistance (along with transference) as the defining feature of a psychoanalytic treatment. Resistance turns out to be the tip of the iceberg of one of the most powerful motive forces in human functioning. It is a homeostatic motivational force.

The infant's early work of reality testing, adaptation, and defense against painful states is just that: *work*. Because the infant is responsive to stimuli from within and without, he or she experiences distress again and again as efforts are made to meet and regularize (make predictable) that world of stimulation. Once some order, some predictability, some way of anticipating and mastering stimulation are achieved, we can expect that that achievement will not readily be given up. This is what gives motive force to the homeostatic press for sameness; change risks danger in the form of psychic pain.

Over time, various theorists have remarked on this phenomenon. Freud (1923/1961) wrote: "What it is that the ego fears either from an external or from a libidinal danger cannot be specified; we know that it is in the nature of an overthrow or an extinction, but it is not determined by analysis" (p. 57). And Waelder (1936) described "the danger that the ego's whole organization may be destroyed or submerged" (p. 48). Cooper (1987) suggests that "the prospect of change is viewed as a danger by the neurotic ego not only because it threatens the awakening of forbidden impulses, but because any change of ego function or attitude threatens the sense of safety and coherence represented by the habitual and familiar" (p. 135). Recognition of the homeostatic motivational power of resistance to change has been around for decades.

It may be a characteristic of organized states (as of organizations altogether) that they tend toward a certain inertia (i.e., a steady state) unless actively forced to change. Once a particular and characteristic form of organization, a way of modulating stimuli, is achieved by the individual, the maintenance of that organization (within limits, and slowly changing) itself becomes an independent motivational force. The personal view of reality, and the mode of adaptation and defense, tend to be self-sustaining—to be maintained by the individual (sometimes, it seems, at all costs). It is perhaps most clear in the fragile individual's desperate clinging to his or her preferred internal order, no matter that that order has proven to be ineffective. But the general tendency is central to the clinically relevant understanding of motivation in the sphere of ego function as it develops during the person's life history.

So, the spontaneous exercise of capacities (with their profound developmental and indirect clinical significance) and the homeostatic press for sameness, as well as the fate of the anxiety signal (each with their profound clinical significance), are recognized as central motivational features in the sphere of ego function. That is, they sustain and organize behaviors around the aims of the individual.

Motivations in Self Experience

A number of prefatory comments are necessary with regard to the seemingly self-evident concept of *self*. In fact, the concept's very everydayness probably contributed to its having been largely ignored by theorists for many decades. As noted earlier, when the term appeared in Freud's writings, it was largely replaced (in the English translation) by the term *ego*, a term with a more technical ring to it (and not the same meaning). And yet the term "self" *is* part of everyday language; it must reflect something of psychological importance that we can aspire to capture in our theories.

A first formal recognition of the term was offered by Hartmann (1950), who defined self as a personal *concept* that, like any concept (a thought), is within the domain of the theoretical concept "ego." Thus, if a person says, "I wasn't myself when I did that," or "I can't believe I'm doing this," it implies that the person has a self concept that does not include whatever it is that is being referred to as different. "I'm a kind person," or "I'm not the sort of person who always plays it safe," or "I don't see myself as someone who ever gets really angry"—these are all concepts about a self as the person defines it (accurately, wishfully, with denial and blindness, or however).

Kohut (1977) pressed for a second arm in the definition of the term self—and it is that second arm that shall be my focus here (though not his theories in particular), as I believe its motivational relevance is both more subtle and more powerful. That second arm is the *experiential* aspect of self: self as a subjective experience. Even if the person can put that experience into words (thus, in a sense making it a concept), it is experience-near, reflecting lived feelings, and is very different from an idea about the self. The *idea* is the self seen from afar as it were; it is not the subjective experience. The *experiential* aspect of the self is also readily distinguishable from the *concept* "ego," an hypothesized set of functions having to do with defense, adaptation, and reality testing.

We take an experiential self for granted. And it, too, is a reflection of where human beings are in evolution. For we are self-conscious animals. Evolution has given us a brain that not only allows for self-awareness but renders it obligatory. We cannot escape an experiential self. Experiences tend to be carried inside and carried self-referentially. They nurture this sense of self, including how others treat us, whether they respond to us, and experiences stemming from our own achievements and failures to achieve. When the mother smiles joyfully at the young child, for example, her smile ordinarily produces a state of well-being, an inner state that can become more ongoing if the interpersonal experience is a regularly recurring one; if the mother looks on the child with hate or affectlessness, the process is similar, but in reverse.

A look at the current psychoanalytic literature suggests at least five variables that have received theoretic attention as clinically significant defining features of these subjective experiences of self. Although full discussion of these five will not be undertaken here, they shall at least be listed. Each is significant as a defining subjective quality of self experience, and each not infrequently is a center of disturbance that becomes central in a particular clinical psychoanalysis.

1. A sense of *boundaries between self and other*, from well differentiated through vague or obscure
2. *Self-esteem or self-worth*, from exaggeratedly high to comfortable to abysmally low
3. A sense of *wholeness and continuity*, with reference to a sense that one is one's own self through time and in different regions of function, and ranging at the other extreme to experiences of fragmentation or of an ad hoc self
4. *Genuineness*, the sense that what one is publicly and privately mesh with each other, as opposed to the sense of pretend, of a self in hiding, protected in its hiding perhaps because of a danger of humiliation, rejection, or nonresponse by the other
5. A sense of *agency*

Discussion of the last, a component of the experience of self, shall be deferred until later in relation to the superordinate concept of unconscious motivation and its refinements.

Clinically, one sees common and repeated thematic variations of self experience in each patient; each person "specializes," so to speak, in one or another (sometimes more than one) variation that is problematically central. The particular variation(s) expressed depends on the accidents of personal history. Clinically, again as with attachment needs and exercise of capacities, aspects of the subjective states of self that have developed well do not appear centrally in clinical work. They fade into a comfortable-enough background. It is the problematic subjective states that are clinically "noisy."

To illustrate some of these aspects of self experience with actual interpretive interventions drawn from clinical practice: "You got frightened when I used the word 'we' because it made you feel I was invading you, just as it used to feel with your mother" (boundaries). And, "Your parents' failure to respond to you was disorienting and made you lose touch with who you were, and so when I didn't greet you sufficiently when you walked in you can't feel that you and I are the same people who worked together in yesterday's session" (continuity). And, "You're showing me what your parents thought of themselves and of you by behaving in such a way as to advertise how worthless you are" (esteem). Each of these interventions has an educative aspect, an aspect that touches on the patient's subjective inner reality, and an aspect that addresses the patient's history and dynamics. Many of these subjective states of self are precipitates of early object relations as *experienced* by the person. They are *carried*, however, not simply as memories but as familiar, though painful, subjective states.

With these prefatory remarks as background, let us turn to one prominent and clinically relevant motivation in the sphere of subjective self experience.

The Righting Response and the Inner Subjective State of Self

Just as each person has certain primary problematic (to varying degrees problematic, of course), and therefore psychologically central, defining features of self experience, each person has a certain range of comfort with respect to those subjective states. When the subjective state varies outside that range, the person acts to reset the balance in what shall be referred to here as a "righting response." This response is the motivational feature by which behavior is sustained and organized around the aims of the individual—in this case to recalibrate the internal subjective experience of self.

Clearly, the righting response has similarities to at least two of the motive forces that were described within the domain of ego function: resistance to change and the anxiety signal. The resistance to change here, however, has reference to a consciously experienced, even if unformulated, subjective state; in the ego domain, the resistance to change had reference to automatic, nonconscious modes of defense and regulation of stimuli. And the subjective discomfort that I am describing here is indeed a subcategory of the anxiety signal described earlier; in each case it is an affect signal that triggers the response—here, to "correct" the subjective state; earlier, to set defenses in motion against threatening eruptions from within or experienced dangers from without.

The comfortable state of self is not necessarily one that would be viewed as "healthy" from the outside. Individual psychological histories produce different needs and different solutions. One person may live comfortably with a clear set of self–other boundaries; another is acutely and disturbingly alert to any sense of incursion on those boundaries; and yet another requires a certain vagueness in boundaries, feeling too alone or too threateningly autonomous if the experience is of a well-differentiated self. And similarly with any of the others. Some persons require a grandiose self feeling, while others create and seem to need situations that confirm their worthlessness. This is simply the way different lives are. How unstable these inner balances are, how insatiable the individual's need for a particular state, how active the search for (or the sensitivity to) inputs that confirm that state, and how much the person imagines and creates situations that disrupt the preferred state—these are all matters of individual difference. But, clinically, for some patients, the homeostatic motivation in this domain is a central guiding force in much of their lives.

Motivations in Drives

Freud's "libido theory," a theory of "instinctual drives" that was the starting point in his specifically psychoanalytic views of human biopsychological functioning, is perhaps (especially since it subsumes the Oedipus complex) the most widely known concept associated with him. Nonetheless, although sexuality retains a central place in the thinking and the clinical work of psychoanalysts (and indeed, with easy introspection, in the lives of each one of us), the libido theory itself is rarely referred to today. It was a theory based in a concept of a fixed amount of energy, expressed primarily in differing bodily zones and in progressive "psychosexual phases," with less energy available if any of it was stuck ("fixated") at an earlier phase; this libidinal energy was initially seen as virtually *the* original source of all other motivational forces in the person. We no longer have such a closed-system view of available energies nor such a unilinear view of motivation. But sex itself has not gone away, and will not. In the "important note" toward the beginning of this chapter, routes to the centrality of sexuality in human lives outside of the specifics of the libido theory were described.

More clearly even than any of the other motivations described thus far, sexuality reflects not just our particular place in evolution but evolution itself. We are part of evolution, and sexuality (plus natural selection) is evolution's vehicle. But the psychoanalytic conception of sexuality goes well beyond heterosexual genital intercourse in adults—the operative force in reproduction and hence in evolution—to include that set of phenomena (also discussed earlier in this chapter) that Freud (1905/1953) saw in the child, in sexual foreplay in adults, and in the perversions—all involving a multitude of acts in different bodily zones having an intense sensual component—and that led him to the theory of "infantile sexuality." Sexuality, thus broadly conceived, is a prototype of those forces that lead to behavior sustained and organized around the aims of the individual (i.e., motivations). It is also the prototype of the core defining features of motivations as proposed by David Rapaport (1960): they are cyclic, peremptory, and, of particular significance in human motivation (through the complexities of the human mind), *displaceable*. That is, they can be expressed in bodily, mental, and behavioral forms that are altered, disguised, and indirect. This latter feature is central to psychoanalytic findings with respect to both normal and pathological development of sexuality.

Now to some specific comments about both sexuality and aggression, the final dual-drive theory that Freud settled on and that psychoanalysts by and large work with (regarding motivations in the "drive" sphere).

Sexuality

Though the sexual drives can readily be seen as a prototype of those motives that sustain, direct, and organize behavior, the motivational picture in this domain is neither clear nor simple. Human beings are often notoriously single-minded in their pursuit of sexual gratification once arousal is initiated. That is sexuality's phenomenological "driving" feature. The sense of urgency and sensations of pleasure form its biological substrate. And this urgency can be felt with regard to oral, anal, and genital zones, as well as to the skin surface altogether. But this substrate is clearly just the start of the developed human motivational system around sexuality.

First, it is in the nature of human mind that all such sensations and urges receive mental representation; they are recorded in perception and memory and organized around specific experiences. Although they start as biological universals, they become individually specific. They become "wishes" in Freud's (1900/1953) sense: a wish is the connection of an urge to specific memories of prior situations of gratification. As these wishes in turn become subject to all other forces of mind, memories get distorted and altered by imagination and are therefore probably better described ultimately as fantasies. Thus, bodily urges get wrapped in a complex of wishful thoughts that set particular conditions for gratification. Sex is not like breathing, which must be met by oxygen intake if death is not to follow. Sexual needs can be repressed or be met vicariously; they are, in this sense, displaceable. And second, again as noted earlier, sex comes to serve diverse aims, well beyond the singularly sexual. Sex can repeat object relations and thus hold on to wished-for others; can serve attachment needs; can boost, lower, define, or weaken the sense of self (according to individual need or disturbance); and can be used to modulate a wide range of problematic affects, among them anxiety, depression, and longing.

In its least overdetermined form, sexual drive is relatively proactive (self-initiating), though it can of course be triggered by external stimuli. Its cyclic and peremptory quality stems from its bodily base, and the especially intense quality of its pleasure ensures its repetition (though, with development, conflict and defense alter this significantly). Behavior will often be organized in terms of sexual wish until satisfaction or some other route to quiescence is found, and this is its motivational feature. But that the omnipresence of sexual aims owes much to sex's capacity to carry latent aims within the spheres of object relations, ego functioning, and self experience is common knowledge within the interpretive work of psychoanalysis. In this sense, sex, as noted, is a major final common pathway for the expression of almost all motivations.

Aggression

Parallel considerations—a built-in biological base; the place of learning and an attachment to specific defining memories; and an expansion of functions to regions of object relatedness, ego mastery, and self experience—apply to aggressive drives as well as to sexuality. Aggressive urges, too, can sustain and direct (motivate) behavior around individual aims.

The proactive versus reactive status of aggression is not as clear as for sexuality. Aggression is certainly built-in and serves indispensable functions in species survival—in food gathering, mate selection, protection of the young, and territoriality. But it can be argued that those are all reactive or situational settings for aggression, still not quite proactive ones. Aggression in humans, like sexuality, can certainly be peremptory and is equally certainly displaceable—expressed in disguised ways or repressed altogether. But the cyclic feature characterizing sexuality is not as clearly seen in aggression. Parens (1979) argues that distinctions should be drawn among nonhostile aggression (say, exploratory behavior—which *is* proactive), nonhostile yet destructive aggressiveness (say, biting and chewing), and hostile destructiveness. (Stechler and Halton [1987] separate the first of these entirely from aggression.) But what *is* clear is that aggression, even if entirely reactive in humans (and the conceptual arguments regarding this are unresolved), is universal, because there is no way in human life for events that will trigger aggressive responses to be entirely avoided. Aggressive reactions come in response to physical restraint and to later interferences with directed activity (e.g., taking a toy away, preventing an activity). They also come in response to frustrations and nonsatisfactions of all kinds—of food, of maternal holding, of "narcissistic injuries" (hurts to the sense of self such as failures of recognition and approval). Such sources of aggression are omnipresent, and there is no way for development to proceed without a never-ending array of frustrations, deprivations, and environmental "failures" (from the point of view of the infant's and child's—or adult's—experience).

A significant question is how reactive aggression can become proactive, acquiring a more clearly sustained and "driving" quality. Stechler and Halton (1987) find an answer in the idea that when active exploratory behavior, which *is* proactive, is interfered with, it can lead to an aggressive reaction that is then carried, so to speak, by the proactivity of the active and exploratory tendencies themselves. From a quite different angle, Kernberg's work (1982 and passim), referred to earlier, which ties the development of aggression to internalized object relations that *do* get repeated, is another attempt at an answer to this question. McDevitt (1983) provided a closely related answer, one tied to actual developmental observation. And here we come to one of the mixed blessings of the human psyche—colloquially, the capacity to hold a grudge. McDevitt reported a pivotal set of infant observations and an important inference. He noted that early aggressive outbursts are reactive and short-lived; they end when the frustration is eliminated or the infant is distracted. But in the middle of the second year, this changes. Aggressive reactions are then sustained over time. McDevitt linked these observations to the development of object constancy. That is, now the toddler can hold on to the idea of the "other," in this instance the specific frustrating other, after the frustration ends. The aggressive response, operating now within a more advanced cognitive system capable of differentiated perception of the source of the injury, can be sustained over time. Beginning reactively, it can now be carried in mind and become self-initiating (proactive) in the angry response to the object.

Aggression, too, like sexuality, becomes subject to all the complexities of mind. It can be sustained, displaced, expressed symbolically, or defended against; and it can come to serve functions with respect to other motives as well. Aggression can become a form of sexual arousal and pleasure; it can play out internalized object relations; it can sustain or defend against attachment needs; and it can express or compensate for various needs and deficiencies in self state. (This tying of aggression to sexuality, to certain self states, to maintenance of sameness, and the like is a further route to the shift from reactive to proactive status.) Thus, both sexual and aggressive "drives," starting from a biological base, become part of individual human histories over their course of development.

A Superordinate Motivational Concept and Its Refinements

Unconscious Motivation

Freud saw himself in a line with Copernicus and Darwin as having shaken humankind's narcissistic view of our place in nature. Copernicus showed that we are not the center of the universe with the heavens rotating around us. Darwin showed that, even here on earth, we are not separate from all other living forms but on a continuum with them. And Freud believed that he had shown that humankind is not even in control in its own house: the mind. In this statement, he was referring to unconscious motivation.

The distinctive and overriding feature of psychoanalytic motivational theory is its postulate of unconscious motivation. While conscious motivation cannot and need not be ignored, it is the focus on unconscious motives, ordinarily organized in terms of repressed or disguised wishes, that is the centerpiece of psychoanalytic thinking. This concept was first brought to bear in relation to posthypnotic suggestion, and it rapidly came to shape the whole approach to free association, the singularly psychoanalytic "talking cure." This was not because talk alone would free the analysand from conflict, but rather free association itself was tied to the concept of unconscious motivation. "Free association" was not conceived of as "free." If the aims of ordinary human discourse were removed, the mind's flow of ideas would come to be governed by motivations of which the person was not aware. The listening analyst could then "hear" (infer) those motives and bring them to consciousness at the appropriate time.

While sexual desire as a motivational force is known to each of us, it is clearly not such desire that Freud refers to by the term *unconscious* motivation. Rather he refers both to the continued impact of such motives even when they are repressed and to a person's general (though not necessarily complete) unawareness of these motive forces in their multiple displaced, symbolic, and sublimated forms. Additionally, the person behaves in accord with such disguised and unrecognized motives in automatic, habitual ways, so that, in a somewhat different meaning of the term *unconscious*, the person is unaware of what drives him or her, even if awareness were possible if attention were to be drawn to the actual behavior. Many of these motives take shape so early in development as to be unrememberable; they are in fact often described as "unforgettable, though unrememberable." And they may have taken shape so early that they have never been processed in verbal terms, and again therefore are ordinarily not reachable in conscious memory.

As motivational theory moved on to the broad array I have described herein, one or the other or both of these concepts of unconscious motivation—a) repressed/disguised or b) acted on automatically/habitually with no attention paid—were generally found to apply. To name some of the concepts I have introduced: repetition of internalized object relationships, holding on to forms of adaptation that have been achieved to cope with psychic pain, righting responses to preserve familiar (comfortable or not) subjective states of self—all of these are ordinarily acted on without awareness, automatically. It becomes a hard-won accomplishment of clinical psychoanalysis for such awareness to be achieved.

In this sense, to the extent that the individual acts on powerful and centrally organizing motivations that serve unconscious aims, we sometimes say that the person is "lived by" his or her motives—that is, driven by them, "taking orders" from them, so to speak—and not living by choice, by "I want." It is in this sense that, as Freud said, the person is not master in his or her own house.

Two ideas that have subsequently found their way into the psychoanalytic literature—agency and developmental needs—can be conceptualized as correctives to the concept of the singular dominance of unconscious motivation.

Agency

Just as developments in motivation theory can be seen as having filled in the gaps in Freud's instinctual drive theory, so can the concept of agency be seen as filling in the gap left by the concept of unconscious motivation. For, in briefest form, the concept of agency can be thought of as the person's capacity to live by the terms "I want" or "I shall seek" or "I shall not"—that is, *awareness* of and behavioral implementation of personal aims. The person "lives" his or her aims rather than being "lived" by them.

The term *agency* began appearing in psychoanalytic writings with increasing frequency over the last half-century. Rapaport (1953/1987) in his concept of ego activity, Schafer (1976) in his "action language," Klein (1976) in his focus on the person in motivation, and Person (2002) in the centrality she gives to personal power and agency—each is thinking in ways related to this domain. The concept of agency gives recognition to an inner state describable as "being an active agent," a *source* of activity, rather than a passive actor driven by inner states. It thus refers to awareness, choice, and capacity to act. Winnicott (1960) described how early urges (the prototype being hunger) can be experienced as "impingements," not part of the "self," but how, in time and if development goes well, the child can develop recognition of these urges, a sense of ownership of them, familiarity with how they work, a trust that they will be satisfied (and therefore need not be disruptive), and a sense of choice about their gratification. In this sense they become parts of or even enrichments of the self rather than impingements. Much about the infant's need satisfaction is passive; the infant's needs are met from the outside. Agency refers to the growing capacity to be active in relation to need satisfaction and elsewhere.

But such issues of agency, of the representation of motives in full consciousness, can apply to any of the motivations described herein. The destructiveness of unconscious and automatically lived-out motivations lies, usually, in their unconscious and automatic qualities, not necessarily in the aims themselves. With awareness, with the capacity for judging appropriateness of expression and timing, some of these same motives may enrich the self, become part of us, and be expressive of our aims: they come to define our sense of "agency." As noted in the discussion of qualities of self experience (boundaries, esteem, genuineness, and wholeness and continuity), agency, too, can be considered a defining quality of subjective self feeling. Speaking in a spatial metaphor, agency can be seen as occupying a place "above" (more conscious than) unconscious motivation.

Developmental Needs

The distinctive and superordinate feature of psychoanalytic motivation theory has been not only the idea of unconscious motivation but the more specific idea that such motivation is organized around unconscious wishes for particular forms of gratification, unconscious guilt in relation to those wishes, and equally unconscious defenses against the wishes. But with the introduction of "deficit" views of human psychopathology, wishes have (for some theorists) lost their place as *the* organizing forces in the unconscious mind, and needs—specifically unmet needs—have taken a place alongside them. This view is associated with Kohut's (1977, 1984) writings more lately, and with Winnicott's (1960) writings before that. Lichtenberg (1989) has included ideas like these centrally in his theoretical writings, and Akhtar (1999) has thoroughly reviewed the whole area and the conceptual issues inherent in it.

Unmet needs have a variant status with regard to consciousness. The basic needs for feeding and care, for personal recognition, for a sense of safety (Sandler 1960), and for activity, exploration, and play (White 1963), *when unmet*, often become more "noisy." Ungratified *wishes* seem more repressible or displaceable than unmet *needs*. However, it is not always the case that unmet needs are thus noticeable to the patient; they too can be warded off and sometimes only reemerge during a psychoanalytic treatment when something about the work revives the sense of an unmet need (Pine 1994). But their status is different from wishes; they are *felt* as developmental necessities, and for the optimal development of the young child they probably are.

This has come to be seen as a central aspect of the clinical work with some or many patients, and the technical challenges it presents are indeed formidable (Pine 2003). Again speaking spatially, needs can be seen as occupying a space "underneath"—more basic than—unconscious motivation organized around wishes.

Conclusion

What I have presented here is largely a conceptual exposition of motivation theory as it has developed within psychoanalysis. While touches of the clinical work on which it is based have appeared, the degree to which this is a clinically based theory cannot be fully shown. To personalize this for just a moment, I remember well the various points at which, to my surprise, I found that I had to give due respect to major motive forces in my patients that "were not dreamed of in my philosophy" up to that point. This occurred with regard to motivations in the object relations sphere, the ego sphere, and the self sphere, more or less in that order, and most recently with regard to a particular patient and the centrality of attachment motives. In each case, the ground had been prepared by writings extant in the psychoanalytic literature, but conviction came only when I had to find my way with one or another patient.

Freud's original theory of instinctual drives can feel just right as a core motivational theory; we can resonate with it.

Not only are sex and aggression powerful and often conflicted forces in each of us, but they have a "driving," motivational quality. But this does not rule out the presence and significance of other motivational forces—some (such as attachment needs, the beginnings of the anxiety signal, and the exercise of capacities) inborn and some (such as repetition of internalized object relations, further developments in the anxiety signal, clinging to sameness in ego function, and maintenance of preferred subjective states of self) coming into being during the course of development—though even the former (inborn) are subsequently shaped by individual history. Any of them can operate unconsciously, "giving orders" to the person, or can be transformed into owned and directed motives, answerable to the person's "agency."

Nonetheless, whatever their developmental source and history, each of these motivational forces becomes represented in mind and can be expressed in automatic/habitual behavior and is thereafter subject to all of the vicissitudes of mental life. These forces are clung to, warded off, defended against, and acted out. In addition, they come to be endowed with additional psychological "meanings" within each person's system of dominant fantasies and wishes, and as such they get fully involved in intrapsychic conflict. As such, they become instigators of mental life—they impel mental activity and its affective and behavioral offshoots, whether homeostatic or reactive or proactive—and thus must be recognized in any full psychoanalytic theory of human motivation.

And so now, in ending, we are ready to return to the issue raised in the quoted material from Loewald (1971/1980) at the outset: "There seems to be no room for *personal* motivation [in psychoanalytic theory as it had developed before the era of his writing]....Where is the person? Where is the ego or self that would be the source and mainstay of personal motivation?" (p. 110). Our answer today must be: *the person is everywhere.*

Thus, sexual and aggressive tendencies become personalized. They reflect not just the expression of mechanical energic forces; they are embedded in individual wishes, fantasies, histories, and preferred forms of gratification, expression, or displacement. Where is the personal in psychoanalytic motivational theory? It is in individual history. Motives in the object relational sphere, like attachment and the repetition of internalized object relations, are inherently personal—built around the histories of personal relationships and their satisfactions and failings. And affectively driven motives, like those triggered by the anxiety signal or by attempts to maintain sameness (of defensive or adaptative style or of subjective state of self), all have an inherently subjective, and therefore personal, aspect.

Another significant source of the personal in motivation theory lies in the impact of cultural forces. Freud's original aim was to develop a scientific view of mind, and his theory of instinctual drives was embedded in evolutionary theory as its background and in personal biology as its site. Hartmann's (1939/1958) concept of the "average expectable environment" was one that permitted study of the person without attention to the environment, holding it constant (in theory) as "average." This was no doubt a useful device at one stage in the development of the theory. But of course people develop and function in a "specific personal environment," not an "average expectable" one, and family personalities and history, as well as broad cultural forces, make up that specific personal world.

In our era, for example, we have seen significant changes in personal motivation, in the degree of awareness of motives, and in motivation theory itself as a function of the large cultural forces captured by the terms "women's liberation" and "gay liberation." Interestingly, "consciousness raising," itself a spin-off from the psychoanalytic view of unconscious motivation, of being "lived" by unconscious forces or, in this instance, by unverbalized cultural forces, was one of the rallying cries of the women's movement. Chodorow (1978), Benjamin (1988), and Person (1995) have spoken to these effects.

And yet ultimately, in psychoanalysis from the very outset, motivations were always seen to be personal and idiosyncratic—for they were seen this way in the clinical situation, with individual persons, whether or not theory had yet succeeded in representing the personal adequately. Today, theory has caught up.

References

Akhtar S: The distinction between needs and wishes: implications for psychoanalytic theory and technique. J Am Psychoanal Assoc 47:113–151, 1999

Albee E: The Zoo Story. New York, Coward, 1960

Benjamin J: The Bonds of Love: Psychoanalysis, Feminism, and the Problem of Domination. New York, Pantheon, 1988

Bowlby J: Attachment and Loss, Vol 1: Attachment. New York, Basic Books, 1969

Chodorow NJ: The Reproduction of Mothering. Berkeley, University of California Press, 1978

Cooper A: Comments of Freud's "Analysis terminable and interminable," in On Freud's Analysis Terminable and Interminable. Edited by Sandler J. International Psychoanalytic Association Educational Monographs 1:127–148, 1987

Fleming J: Some observations on object constancy in the psychoanalysis of adults. J Am Psychoanal Assoc 23:743–759, 1975

Freud A: The ego and the mechanisms of defense (1936), in The Writings of Anna Freud, Vol 2. New York, International Universities Press, 1966

Freud S: The interpretation of dreams (1900), in Standard Edition of the Complete Psychological Works of Sigmund Freud, Vols 4 and 5. Translated and edited by Strachey J. London, Hogarth Press, 1953

Freud S: Three essays on the theory of sexuality, I: the sexual aberrations (1905), in Standard Edition of the Complete Psychological Works of Sigmund Freud, Vol 7. Translated and edited by Strachey J. London, Hogarth Press, 1953, pp 135–172

Freud S: Formulations on the two principles of mental functioning (1911), in Standard Edition of the Complete Psychological Works of Sigmund Freud, Vol 12. Translated and edited by Strachey J. London, Hogarth Press, 1958, pp 218–226

Freud S: The dynamics of transference (1912), in Standard Edition of the Complete Psychological Works of Sigmund Freud, Vol 12. Translated and edited by Strachey J. London, Hogarth Press, 1958, pp 99–108

Freud S: On narcissism: an introduction (1914a), in Standard Edition of the Complete Psychological Works of Sigmund Freud, Vol 14. Translated and edited by Strachey J. London, Hogarth Press, 1957, pp 67–102

Freud S: On the history of the psychoanalytic movement (1914b), in Standard Edition of the Complete Psychological Works of Sigmund Freud, Vol 14. Translated and edited by Strachey J. London, Hogarth Press, 1957, pp 7–66

Freud S: Instincts and their vicissitudes (1915), in Standard Edition of the Complete Psychological Works of Sigmund Freud, Vol 14. Translated and edited by Strachey J. London, Hogarth Press, 1957, pp 111–116

Freud S: Beyond the pleasure principle (1920), in Standard Edition of the Complete Psychological Works of Sigmund Freud, Vol 18. Translated and edited by Strachey J. London, Hogarth Press, 1955, pp 1–64

Freud S: The ego and the id (1923), in Standard Edition of the Complete Psychological Works of Sigmund Freud, Vol 19. Translated and edited by Strachey J. London, Hogarth Press, 1961, pp 12–66

Freud S: Inhibitions, symptoms and anxiety (1926), in Standard Edition of the Complete Psychological Works of Sigmund Freud, Vol 20. Translated and edited by Strachey J. London, Hogarth Press, 1959, pp 75–175

Hartmann H: Ego Psychology and the Problem of Adaptation (1939). Translated by Rapaport D. New York, International Universities Press, 1958

Hartmann H: Comments on the psychoanalytic theory of the ego. Psychoanal Study Child 5:74–96, 1950

Hartmann H: The mutual influences in the development of ego and id. Psychoanal Study Child 7:9–30, 1952

Hendrick I: Instinct and the ego during infancy. Psychoanal Q 11:33–58, 1942

Jacobson E: The Self and the Object World. New York, International Universities Press, 1964

Kernberg O: Self, ego, affects, and drives. J Am Psychoanal Assoc 30:893–918, 1982

Khan MMR: The concept of cumulative trauma (1963), in The Privacy of the Self. New York, International Universities Press, 1974, pp 42–58

Klein GS: Psychoanalytic Theory: An Exploration of Essentials. New York, International Universities Press, 1976

Kohut H: The Restoration of the Self. New York, International Universities Press, 1977

Kohut H: How Does Analysis Cure? Chicago, IL, University of Chicago Press, 1984

Kris E: The recovery of childhood memories in psychoanalysis. Psychoanal Study Child 11:54–88, 1956

Lichtenberg JD: Psychoanalysis and Infant Research. Hillsdale, NJ, Analytic Press, 1983

Lichtenberg JD: Psychoanalysis and Motivation. Hillsdale, NJ, Analytic Press, 1989

Loewald HW: On motivation and instinct theory (1971), in Papers on Psychoanalysis. New Haven, CT, Yale University Press, 1980, pp 102–137

Mahler MS, Pine F, Bergman A: The Psychological Birth of the Human Infant: Symbiosis and Individuation. New York, Basic Books, 1975

McDevitt JB: The emergence of hostile aggression and its defensive and adaptive modifications during the separation-individuation process. J Am Psychoanal Assoc 31:273–300, 1983

Modell AH: Psychoanalysis in a New Context. New York, International Universities Press, 1984

Parens H: The Development of Aggression in Early Childhood. Northvale, NJ, Jason Aronson Press, 1979

Person ES: Fantasy and cultural change, in By Force of Fantasy: How We Make Our Lives. New York, Basic Books/HarperCollins, 1995, pp 197–218

Person E: Agency: Authoring Our Own Life Stories, in Feeling Strong: The Achievement of Authentic Power. New York, William Morrow/HarperCollins, 2002, pp 183–211

Pine F: On therapeutic change: perspectives from a parent-child model. Psychoanalysis and Contemporary Science 5:537–569, 1976

Pine F: Developmental Theory and Clinical Process. New Haven, CT, Yale University Press, 1985

Pine F: Drive, Ego, Object, and Self: A Synthesis for Clinical Work. New York, Basic Books, 1990

Pine F: Conflict, defect, and deficit. Psychoanal Study Child 49:222–240, 1994

Pine F: Diversity and Direction in Psychoanalytic Technique. New York, Other Press, 2003

Rapaport D: Some metapsychological considerations concerning activity and passivity (1953), in Collected Papers of David Rapaport. Edited by Gill MM. New York, Basic Books, 1987, pp 530–568

Rapaport D: On the psychoanalytic theory of motivation, in Nebraska Symposium on Motivation. Edited by Jones MR. Lincoln, University of Nebraska Press, 1960, pp 173–247

Sandler J: The background of safety. Int J Psychoanal 41:352–356, 1960

Sandler J: Unconscious wishes and human relationships. Contemp Psychoanal 17:180–196, 1981

Schafer R: A New Language for Psychoanalysis. New Haven, CT, Yale University Press, 1976

Spitz RA: A Genetic Field Theory of Ego Formation. New York, International Universities Press, 1959

Stechler G, Halton A: The emergence of assertion and aggression during infancy. J Am Psychoanal Assoc 35:821–838, 1987

Stern DN: The Interpersonal World of the Infant: A View From Psychoanalysis and Developmental Psychology. New York, Basic Books, 1985

Waelder R: The principle of multiple function: observations on overdetermination. Psychoanal Q 5:45–62, 1936

White RW: Ego and Reality in Psychoanalytic Theory. Psychological Issues Monograph 11, Vol 3, No 3. New York, International Universities Press, 1963

Winnicott DW: Ego distortion in terms of true and false self, in The Maturational Processes and the Facilitating Environment. New York, International Universities Press, 1960, pp 140–152

2

The Dynamic Unconscious

Psychic Determinism, Intrapsychic Conflict,
Unconscious Fantasy, Dreams, and
Symptom Formation

W. W. MEISSNER, S.J., M.D.

SIGMUND FREUD MADE MANY significant and important contributions to the understanding of the functioning of the human mind, but among the most enduring and influential is the concept of the *dynamic unconscious*. We should be clear from the beginning that Freud's efforts to provide an explanatory framework or a theory of how the mind works as a way of understanding the organization and functioning of the unconscious—specifically his theory of instinctual drives as the organizing and driving forces of the mind—have no more than limited value and have in the ensuing years come under increasing scrutiny, criticism, and challenge—to the point of considerable doubt on the part of many and even outright rejection on the part of others. At the same time, Freud's model of the economics of mental functioning remains bedrock for many analysts. Despite controversies regarding the theoretical underpinnings of the unconscious, the substantial discovery of a level of unconscious functioning of the mind has remained as valid and unscathed as ever.

The enduring essence of Freud's concept of the unconscious is, first, that the human mind operates on more than one level and, second, that these levels are more or less, to one degree or other, accessible to conscious awareness and, inasmuch as some of them remain unconscious because of the repressive and defensive work of the rest of the mind, are simultaneously active and continually contributing to the ongoing flow of conscious mental activity and behavior. The evidence for levels of unconscious mental activity can be discerned only under specific conditions of observation; the levels are never directly experienced as such. To the extent that any mental event is experienced, it must be conscious, and therefore not unconscious. But unconscious mental processing is presumed to take place constantly, probably involves the major part of the activity of the mind at any point in time, and remains active and effective, operating in parallel with other parts of the mind that are occupied with conscious thoughts or experiences.

The revolutionary advances of modern neuroscience seem to be converging on this basically analytic understanding of the organization and functioning of the mind, particularly in terms of concepts of multiple and parallel processing as fundamental aspects of the patterns of brain information processing. For the most part, the neurobehavioral view of unconscious processes is merely descriptive—that is, focused on what is not conscious, largely omitting dynamic considerations and their related affective and motivational concerns. More recently, neuroscientific interest has begun to focus more directly on affective and motivational contributions to mental functioning, defining separate neural systems effecting motivational desire and craving, reward and punishment, and affective processing, and to acknowledge that these processes may take place on less-than-conscious levels.

An essential aspect of the analytic understanding of the mind is that all mental processes are motivated, and specifically that unconscious mental processes are motivated. Thus, the concept of motivation lies at the heart of the dynamic unconscious. In fashioning his theory, Freud ascribed the motivational aspect to the instinctual drives, which he regarded not only as sources of motivational attraction but as driving forces impelling the subject to action in the service of fulfilling the aim and attaining the goal satisfaction of any given desire. In the wake of doubts regarding the validity of the drive theory, it has become clear that drives are not necessary for understanding motivational dynamics. As Mitchell (1997), for one, observed:

> Freud's most important contribution was not the specific content he ascribed to the unconscious at any particular time (sexual, aggressive, oedipal, preoedipal), but the discovery of an enriched mode or method of explanation and meaning-making itself. Thus even though the relevance of many specific features of Freud's theory has faded, the principle of unconscious intentions linking present and past, rational and fantastic, and interaction and interiority has become a constitutive feature of contemporary Western culture. (p. 211)

We can draw a distinction between motivation as such and the agency that allows the subject to pursue and attain the desired object. The function of a motive is to draw that agent into action by providing an attraction to and the intention or purpose of reaching a goal, attaining an object, accomplishing an ambition, completing a task, and so on. The motive takes the form, then, of something one wishes for, desires, or seeks to accomplish, or of gaining some form of satisfaction. Its function is to elicit a response from the agent. The effectiveness of motives comes from a combination of internal need states, variously described, and external contexts and stimulus conditions answering in some fashion to the need. The juicy red apple serves as a source of motivation when it combines with an inner state of hunger or a wish for a gratifying taste. To the extent that these factors are conjoined, the agent is prompted to action—that is, I am moved to pick up the apple and eat it. Or on a more intellectual level, my desire to learn to read Middle English poetry motivates me to take a course in Middle English and to expend the effort to study and learn the material. Thus, motives do not cause anything, in the sense of efficient causality—that is, causality that involves action and the production of effects; rather they act to elicit causal action on the part of the agent. The agent in these examples is the human person.

Unconscious Aspects of the Mind

Unconscious Motivation

The dynamic unconscious has its own characteristic patterns of motivation. Freud originally described these as patterns of instinctual motivation and ascribed them to the corresponding drives. Without appealing to drives, however, we can still describe these motivational components as "instinctual" and as organized primarily in libidinal (or sexual), aggressive, and narcissistic modes. The term *instinctual* here is simply descriptive, connoting the basic and elemental quality of these motives in their undiluted and primitive form, without any connotation of the existence of instinctual drives as such. Libidinal motives connote attraction to or desire for any sexual or sensual object, one that offers the promise of sexual or sensual gratification. Aggressive motives in turn indicate the capacity of the organism to overcome obstacles, whether internal or external, whether conscious or unconscious, standing in the way of obtaining any given purpose or goal (Rizzuto et al. 2003). And narcissistic motives, in turn, have as their characteristic note the preservation, protection, or enhancement of the self. Freud (1905b/1953, 1915/1957) also described levels of organization of these motivational patterns in developmental terms corresponding to oral, anal, phallic, and genital states of developmental progression.

The complex patterns of psychosexual and psychosocial integration of these motivational themes were further developed by Erikson (1963), who postulated a parallel relationship between specific phases of ego or psychosocial development and specific phases of libidinal development. During libidinal development, particular erotogenic zones become the loci of stimulation for the development of particular modalities of ego functioning. Thus, the first modality of oral psychosexual development is related to the stimulus and motivational qualities of the oral zone: for example, the earliest stage is dominated by an oral-incorporative mode, involving the modality of "taking in." This modality extends to include the whole skin surface and the sense organs, which thus become receptive and increasingly hungry for proper stimulation. Other auxiliary modes are also operative, including a second oral-incorporative (biting) mode, an oral-retentive mode, an oral-eliminative mode, and finally, an oral-intrusive mode. These modes become variably important according to individual temperament but remain subordinated to the first incorporative mode unless the mutual regulation of the oral zone with the providing breast of the mother is disturbed, either by a loss of inner control in the infant or by a defect in reciprocal and responsive nurturing behavior on the part of the mother. Erikson put the emphasis in this stage of development on the modalities of "getting" and "getting what is given," thus laying the necessary ego groundwork for "getting to be a giver." But these same modalities correspond to and involve patterns of motivation to get, get what is given, and even to get to be a giver.

A second oral stage is marked by a biting modality because of the development of teeth. This phase is marked by the development of interpersonal patterns centering on the social modality of "taking" and "holding" on to things. Thus, incorporation by biting becomes a motivational theme that dominates the oral zone at this stage, and the child's libidinal needs and desires move on to a second organ mode, integrating a new social modality, "taking." The interplay of zones and modalities, needs and motives, that characterize this complex oral stage of development forms the basis for a basic sense of "trust," or, conversely, of a basic sense of "mistrust," that remains the basic element in the most fundamental nuclear conflict in the development of personality.

Similarly, with the advent of the anal-urethral-muscular stage, the "retentive" and "eliminative" modes and their correlative motives come into play. The extension and generalization of these modes over the whole of the developing muscular system enable the 18- to 24-month-old child to gain some form of self-control in the matter of conflicting impulses, such as "letting go" and "holding on." Where this control is disturbed by developmental defects in the anal-urethral sphere, a fixation on the modalities of retention or elimination can be established that can lead to a variety of disturbances in the zone itself (spastic), in the muscle system (flabbiness or rigidity), in obsessional fantasy (paranoid fears), and in social spheres (attempts at controlling the environment by compulsive routinization). Erikson extended this analysis to include the full scope of psychosexual and psychosocial development, of which the oral and anal phases are but the first in the series. However, in each case important motivational needs, themes, and patterns are involved and continue to play themselves out, particularly on the level of unconscious dynamic processing, in varying patterns of activation and integration throughout the life cycle.

These motivational patterns can be activated in any combination and integration depending on the circumstances and contexts of motivational activation. Libidinal and aggressive motives may come into play in the context of sexual attraction in which attempts on the part of the desiring subject are opposed or rejected by the desired object. The subject must find some way to overcome the obstacle to his or her desire in order to fulfill the libidinal aim. Thus, aggression can come into play in overcoming such an obstacle. Or narcissistic and aggressive motives may enter into conjunction in circumstances in which some threat is posed to the preservation or self-esteem of the self.

The threat of physical attack and possible injury or loss of life can arouse motives of self-preservation and call up corresponding motives of self-defense, activating aggressive motivation to overcome the obstacle to well-being of the self posed by the threatening object. Or, along similar lines, threats to self-esteem—as in failures to measure up to one's ego-ideal, or in becoming the object of criticism or being treated as the object of disdain or disrespect—are equivalently narcissistic assaults that can stimulate the self to respond defensively and aggressively (Kohut 1972; Rochlin 1973). It is also not uncommon in love relations that both libidinal and narcissistic needs are involved in the relation between lovers. If there is libidinal attraction and desire between lover and beloved, there is always a second current of narcissistic gratification and enhancement secondary to the acceptance by the beloved and mutual love—both loving and being loved. Consequently, the analytic view of instinctual motives sees them as constantly active and interactive, in largely unconscious and constantly shifting and varying patterns, in the process of influencing the course and variability of human behavior.

Regulatory Principles

Freud insisted that these motives could be unconscious as well as conscious, and in consequence all unconscious mentation was correspondingly motivated. Freud's training in neuroscience and his interest in science persuaded him to put his explanations of the unconscious in terms as close to currently accepted scientific standards as he could. It also persuaded him to formulate the basic principles by which the unconscious system operated in the form of regulatory principles. Among these principles, some have retained their validity and some have not. We can focus on a few that remain pertinent to understanding the operation of unconscious processes: psychic determinism (along with its related concepts of multiple determination and multiple function), the pleasure principle and the reality principle, repetition compulsion, and primary and secondary processes.

Psychic Determinism

The first such primary principle Freud appealed to was *psychic determinism*, by which he meant—following the model of physical science—that every action of the mind, even unconscious actions, is caused. Subsequent psychoanalytic thinking has been plagued by the further question,

Caused by what and how? This relates immediately to the questions of agency and motivation. To what extent should psychic determinism be interpreted in terms of causes in the mental apparatus, as opposed to reasons or meanings involved in motivation? For Freud, determination of mental life meant that there was nothing trivial, arbitrary, or haphazard about mental processes, but also that psychoanalysts could expect to be able to find sufficient motives for any given piece of behavior without exception. Even so, the tension persisted in Freud's thinking between the view of the man as an object moved by natural forces (causes as in other sciences) versus the view of man as motivated by meanings and reasons (Holt 1972). Even though his clinical experience drew him closer to the latter view, he could not altogether abandon the former.

Consequently, the problem persists whether and to what extent the determining factors involve causes or meanings or both. For some the distinction is radical—science deals with causes, humanities with reasons (Home 1966; Schafer 1976). Arlow (1959), for example, wrote, "Essentially psychic determinism implies the application to the phenomena of mental life of the same criteria for causality and relatedness that apply to the phenomena of nature in other sciences" (p. 205). On these terms, metapsychology would be regarded as a natural science, the realm of causes and not reasons; motives and meanings would have no place in such a theory. Thus, goal-directed actions can be distinguished from physically determined movements—actions were related to reasons, and movements to causes (Sherwood 1969). But the human organism experiences both actions and movements in various degrees of integration. Reasons have more to do with purposes, causes with mechanisms. Thus, reasons and causes both play a role in determining the outcome of a given piece of behavior.

But the principle of determination plays a somewhat different role in different causal settings. Psychic causality is not linear. Psychic determination in these terms would be difficult to reconcile with stricter notions of physical determination and cause-effect relations. The problem of determination in psychoanalysis becomes more complex because it does not deal simply with physical or behavioral events, but involves human actions and intentions involving meaning. Thus, psychic determinism within psychoanalysis has more to do with meanings and the relations of meanings than with causal connections. In Freud's early approach, determinism was absolute and particular; that is, every mental event, no matter how trivial, had to have meaning and be determined. Today, many analysts would not apply the principle in this rigid and mechanical sense, and many would raise serious doubts whether mental structure can be adequately viewed in the rigidly deterministic manner Freud originally suggested.

Determinism in psychoanalysis can be conceived more broadly and flexibly. In his original formulations, for example, Freud (1901/1960) tried to explain every instance of the psychopathology of everyday life, every forgetting or slip of the tongue, as related to a specific unconscious wish. Even in his analysis of jokes (Freud 1905a/1960), the same universal and specific determinism applied. Present-day analysts, however, would accept that one might not be able to explain each individual act in terms of its immediate determination. For example, in early development a general tendency might be established to lose things, which might have become part of the individual's character structure—as Anna Freud (1955/1968) suggested. The central issue would be the general trait, the tendency to lose things, rather than the determinants of every specific loss. Such a notion would imply a form of determinism at the level of character formation and development rather than the sort of rigid and absolute linear determinism of Freud's thinking. Moreover, it would take into account the history, developmental and otherwise, of the personality and the internal motivational conditions contributing to the behavior outcome, and not merely the immediate causal context.

Currently most analysts regard psychic determinism as meaning that all psychic actions are determined—that is to say, motivated. In other words, no psychic action, whether conscious or unconscious, occurs without reasons, with the reasons serving as statements of motivational purpose. Such conceptualization does not eliminate the occurrence of chance or ambiguous events. Keeping in mind that our focus here is on psychic actions, external chance events may be caused but not determined—the mudslide that destroys my house and threatens my life results from complex physical forces but it is not motivated. Similarly, as Werman (1977) pointed out, ambiguous events, because of the imprecision, uncertainty, or vagueness of their meaning or conversely the presence of more than one meaning, may provoke the subject to select or supply a clarifying personal meaning. He argues quite properly that the inability to accept chance and to tolerate ambiguity reflects a deficit in reality testing that underlies a lack of psychological mindedness. Thus, the primitive animistic mind might attribute the mudslide to the wrath of the gods. But such an attribution fails to take into account the distinction between cause and determinism, and this can lay the basis for wishful or magical thinking—the gambler, who believes he can overcome the odds of probability and chance stacked against him, provides a good example. Werman further cautions that if such magical thinking is too pervasive, it may serve as a powerful resistance in therapy.

Correspondingly, every psychic action has a causal source in some form of agency that performs the action in question. The question of agency remains somewhat un-settled in analytic thinking, but at least one solution is to locate agency in the self (i.e., in the self-as-agent), which is regarded as the source of all action of the organism, psychic and physical, conscious and unconscious, voluntary and involuntary (Meissner 1993, 2003). The self thus acts through the intermediary of its component functionally organized subsystems: psychically through id, ego, and superego, and their various combinations and integrations, and physically through the complex processes and mechanisms of the body and brain—all of which are components of the self (Meissner 2001).

Multiple Determination

Freud (1900/1953) himself introduced the notion of *multiple determination* (overdetermination), meaning that a particular psychic event could be explained in terms of more than one set of determining factors. In this sense, he envisioned a sort of "layering" of determinations in the patient's psychic life. The patient's behavior could be understood not only in terms of the determining events and motives in his or her present life but also, concurrently, in terms of the determining events and motives of the past. Thus, psychic formations, particularly those expressing unconscious determinants, could be the result of multiple motivational influences rather than only one. Further, such psychic events could also be related to a multiplicity of unconscious elements that could be organized in different meaningful contexts, each having its own coherent and specifiable meaning.

Such overdetermination is seen most clearly in the study of dreams (see section "Dream Formation" later in this chapter). The analysis of dream content suggests that each element of the dream, as well as the dream as a whole, is overdetermined. A number of different latent trains of thought may be combined into one manifest dream content that lends itself to a variety of interpretations. Such determining sequences of meaning need not be mutually independent, but may intersect at one or other point, as suggested by the patient's associations. The dream, or the symptom in the case of hysteria, reflects a compromise out of the interaction of such determining significances, which may in themselves be relatively diverse. In this sense, the classical paradigm for hysteria reflects the convergence of more than one opposing current of wishes, each arising from a different motivational system but finding fulfillment by convergence in a single symptomatic expression.

The principle of multiple determination lends itself readily to an understanding of determination in terms of meaning and motive, as delineated above, but less readily

to a sense of causal determination as it is understood in linear cause-effect models. If overdetermination is to be consistent with the determinist perspective in psychoanalysis, it must be formulated in terms of motives and meanings rather than causal sequences. The issues of psychic causality and multiple determinism can be integrated into a more complex perspective involving multiple and complex forms of causality and motivation that intersect in varying forms and proportions in the genesis of any psychic activity or behavior (Wallace 1985). The perspective of multicausality lends itself to an understanding of behavior as the resultant of multiple and variant influences, each of which exercises a determining effect, but no one of which can be regarded as the sole determinant.

Multiple Function

While the principle of multiple determination is concerned with causal origins or determining sequences of meaning, the principle of *multiple function* looks in the direction of results or purposes. Thus, any piece of psychic activity or action may have more than one purpose as part of its intention. Waelder (1936) originally formulated the principle to mean that no solution of a problem is possible that does not at the same time in some way or other represent an attempted solution of other problems. By implication, a psychic event or human action is not directed simply to one outcome or to the attaining of a single purpose or goal, but may, in fact, serve multiple purposes and be governed by varying and diverse intentions, both conscious and unconscious—a psychoanalytic version of parallel processing.

Pleasure and Reality Principles

Freud based his view of the *pleasure principle* directly on the constancy principle, according to which the unconscious system was governed by the tendency to respond to any excitatory stimulus by immediate discharge, thus lowering the level of tension to a presumably constant or homeostatic level of excitation. This state of lowered tension was interpreted as pleasure, and the state of heightened tension was interpreted as unpleasure or pain. Accordingly, in this view all psychic activity aims at avoiding unpleasure and achieving pleasure. We should note that this is no merely hedonistic doctrine, according to which human activity is viewed as intending or seeking affective pleasure. Rather, Freud's postulate is a statement about energic regulation, to the effect that psychic acts are determined by the balance of pleasure and unpleasure (levels of energic tension and discharge) involved in the immediate context of stimulation. The principle, however, is quite independent of conscious experiences of pleasure or pain. The pleasure principle is thus an expression of the rule-based order imposed on mental processes (Rapaport 1960). As Smith (1991) put it, "laws of nature are simply clear statements about how things work, how elements of a system interact, perhaps how they interact to go in a certain direction. The pleasure principle is just such a statement" (pp. 34–35).

We can suggest that a motivationally based version of the pleasure principle might represent the degree of functional satisfaction and efficacy derived from the effective operation of psychic functions and systems. This "pleasure" would be a function of the success of the transition from potential to active operation of any psychic system and the extent to which the operation of such a system— in isolation or in combination with other functional systems—works successfully to achieve purposeful and wished-for goals. The system would thus move from disequilibrium to homeostasis through directionality and intentionality, whether the goal-achievement carried a measure of affective satisfaction with it or not. As Smith (1991) points out, "The ultimate rule of behavior, the rule inclusive of all action, all universes of discourse, is the pleasure principle, which simply states that behavior in all structural conditions moves from high to low potential" (p. 3).

The companion to the pleasure principle is the *reality principle*, which is no more than an extension of the pleasure principle under modified structural conditions (Smith 1977). If the pleasure principle accompanies the accomplishment of effective system functioning, the reality principle interposes itself between the motive for functional satisfaction and its objective. In this classic sense, the reality principle dictated a modification, an inhibition of the inherent tendency for immediate and direct discharge, thus regulating that basic instinctual tendency according to the limitations and demands of reality. In this sense, the reality principle is less a separate principle and more the pleasure principle operating under structural conditions.

In Freud's schema, the reality principle in one sense operates in opposition to the pleasure principle, but in another sense it acts as the collaborator and the facilitator of the pleasure principle. The inherent dictates of the pleasure principle would require immediate discharge of instinctual tensions and thus the achievement of the aim of the motives seeking satisfaction. If the satisfaction cannot be gained by access to real objects, the mental apparatus can presumably fulfill its need in some form of hallucinatory substitution—as in dreams, for example. The principles serve as statements of how the system works—whether or not the operations of the system are associated with experiences of pleasure or unpleasure. The difficulty, of course, is that reality does not always correspond to the needs or wishes of the organism. While reality can offer its measure of gratification, it never measures up to the inherent instinctual demand for immediate satisfaction or for complete and unalloyed satisfaction of the wish. In order for the organism to deal with this state of affairs, a new principle must be appealed to, which both sets appropriate limits on the intensity and range of instinctual demands and correspondingly serves a more adaptive function in modifying instinctual demands so that they are more appropriately modulated and attuned to the real context of their fulfillment.

In Freud's view of the development of the mental apparatus, the pleasure principle reigns supreme at the very beginning of the infant's experience. Only gradually, as the capacities for encountering and interacting with reality emerge and develop, does the impact of reality force itself on the infant's search for gratification, and thus the reality principle increasingly asserts itself. The reality principle gradually imposes on the pleasure principle the necessity for delay, detour, inhibition, and compromise. Its functioning goes hand in hand with a developmental series of adaptations, which require the development and functioning of certain ego functions—attention, judgment, memory, the capacity for delay, and the increasing ability to substitute the alloplastic transformation of reality (to suit the organism's needs and wishes) for a tendency to immediate motor discharge. Nonetheless, the transition from the pleasure principle to the reality principle does not override the pleasure principle. The reality principle operates in contexts where satisfactions are sought and attained in relation to external objects and environments, while the pleasure principle continues to hold sway over the intrapsychic realm, the realm of fantasy, unconscious wishes, and dreams.

The reality principle consequently is effective in the operation of all psychic functions in coordination and conjunction with the pleasure principle. The operation of any psychic system is conditioned and mutually modified by the internal context of intra- and intersystemic operation within the mental apparatus; no system functions independently or in isolation from other simultaneously operating systems. The limiting conditions for the operation of individual functions and for more complex organizations of intrapsychic functions are set by the reality factors that determine the context of activity. One cannot chew nails. Consequently, the reality principle comes into play by setting the conditions for effective operation of psychic systems as they impinge on and intersect with external reality through both activating and inhibitory signals. The influence of reality factors on the operation of psychic systems is thus basically informational.

Repetition Compulsion

In dealing with neurotic symptoms, Freud encountered a repetitive quality, not merely descriptively, as in the recurrent behaviors of obsessional rituals, but also in the tendency to reproduce elements of past unresolved conflicts. The return of the repressed was familiar not only in dreams and symptoms but also in the acting out or reliving of the past in the transference. But other phenomena, such as the fate neuroses and the traumatic neuroses, seemed to emphasize the existence of a compulsion to repeat. In both cases, unpleasant experiences from the past were recreated and repeated, seemingly in the irresistible and compulsive form that is the hallmark of neurosis and unconscious determination. But it was difficult to see how such phenomena could fulfill the requirements of the pleasure principle or of the dynamics of wish fulfillment. Freud concluded that these phenomena had to have their source in some principle beyond the pleasure principle (Freud 1920/1955; Schur 1966). In trying to salvage the pleasure principle, he argued that what might produce unpleasure for one psychic agency may simultaneously be pleasurable for another. Thus, in the traumatic neuroses, the repetition of the traumatic experience in dreams or flashbacks may seem to violate the principle of unpleasure but may also serve for mastery of the trauma.

The explanation was less than completely satisfying, and the ambiguity in Freud's thinking has continued to plague psychoanalytic efforts to understand the repetition compulsion. One view of repetition sees it as the most demonic and resistive dimension of the instinctual forces, reflecting ultimately the impact of the death instinct. Other analytic thinkers distinguish between the repetitive tendency of instinctual forces and a restitutive tendency as a function of the ego. While the repetitive tendency can be said to go beyond the pleasure principle in its repetition of painful experiences, the restitutive tendency functions in parallel to reestablish the conditions prior to the trauma. It thus exploits the experience of repetition in the interests of ego adaptation and mastery.

In a motivational framework, repetition may have more to do with the stability of psychic functions and structural integrations. In this sense, the tendency to repetition has an adaptive aspect, playing an important role in development and in the unending process of assimilating and accommodating reality. In this sense, repetition is never identical but tends more to express variations on a theme. Repetition may play a role in the maintenance of personal schemata reflecting our personal experience and enabling us to preserve a cohesive self in the face of the flux of internal and external stimuli. Once a resolution has been established to deal with a given stimulus complex, the

structural integration tends to persist unless forced out of balance by subsequent stimulus inputs. The stability of such resolutions is particularly marked in traumatic contexts in which exceptional demands are placed on defensive psychic systems to manage excessive stimulus overload. Under similar or analogous stimulus conditions, similar response patterns are called into play. Thus, the repetition compulsion refers to structural conditions beyond the reach of a simple wish-fulfillment model and may operate in the interest of maintaining and reinforcing levels of self-organization and integration.

Primary and Secondary Process

Another distinction, fundamental to Freud's view of the functioning of the mental apparatus, that has remained one of the staples of the psychoanalytic view of the mind is that between *primary* and *secondary process*. In terms of the primary process, mental processes were viewed as flowing freely and spontaneously, without hindrance or impediment, from one thought content to another by means of mechanisms of condensation and displacement (discussed in relation to dreams in the section "Dream Formation" later in this chapter), thus achieving a more or less immediate satisfaction of unconscious wishes. Cognitive processes in primary process were seemingly disorganized, irrational, illogical, and even bizarre and contradictory. This pattern of more primitive mental activity was attributed to primitive hallucinations and to dream formation. In secondary process, however, mental activity was no longer free-flowing but was more controlled, integrated with other mental functions (as, e.g., with constraints imposed by the reality principle), thus allowing for delay and postponing of action and making room for experimental testing of real potentialities and consequences. Secondary process mentation was, then, more rational, realistic, organized, and logical. In these terms, then, the primary process system was concerned with the release of mental energy under direction of the pleasure principle, while secondary process concerned itself with the inhibition and control of mental energy and recognition and adaptation to reality under direction of the reality principle (McIntosh 1986).

But Freud carried the argument a step further. He made it clear that he felt he had discovered a basic characteristic of human mental functioning, both unconscious and conscious. His formulation of these systems still stands as an important fundamental insight into the organization of mental processes. He suggested that the organization of thought exhibited in dreams reflects the pattern of thought that took place in the unconscious levels of the mind, while the less primitive and more normal and logical organization of the secondary process was more characteristic of conscious and preconscious levels of mental functioning.

Current psychoanalytic thinking no longer regards the dichotomy between primary-unconscious processes and secondary-conscious processes as being as radical or thoroughgoing as Freud envisioned, but rather sees the manifestations of primary and secondary process reverberating in varying degrees through the entire realm of human psychic functioning as descriptive forms of cognitive organization and functioning (Noy 1969). In other words, the dichotomy of primary and secondary process is viewed as a continuum of differentiating degrees of primary and secondary process intermingling, extending from the absolute or pure pole of undiluted primary process activity to the opposite extreme of highly abstract, logical scientific thought. It should be noted parenthetically that undiluted primary process activity is a phenomenon that is rarely, if ever, identified and that may be conceptualized only in a pure form of primitive hallucinatory gratification, which in itself may be little more than a thought experiment and may never in fact occur except in primitive psychotic states. As our knowledge of scientific thinking (in the mind of the actual scientist) increases, we may even question whether secondary process thinking in its absolute form ever really exists either. In between lies the vast range of human activity and experience, which is expressive of both primary and secondary process modalities in varying degrees of balance and integration.

Intrapsychic Conflict

It became clear to Freud not only that these patterns of motivation could operate on different levels but that not infrequently they come into opposition to one another. In other words, at separate levels and in different forms of organization of the mind, different and at times opposing motives could be called into action. Mobilization of defense mechanisms countering undesirable motivational impulses of an instinctual variety, as in the classic theory of conflict and defense, is itself motivated, a point emphasized by Schafer (1968). Moreover, these motivational themes could remain active on an unconscious level so that an underlying motivational conflict could play a role in determining the course of conscious choice and behavior without any awareness on the part of the subject. Classic examples are the unconscious incestuous desire of the son for sexual intimacy with the mother in conflict with moral taboos opposing such behavior, or the ambivalent conflicts of both loving and hating the same object, with the

loving and hating, one or the other, often remaining active entirely on an unconscious level.

These aspects of unconscious dynamics were among the reasons for Freud's proposing the structural theory of id, ego, and superego. Intrapsychic conflicts could be analyzed as arising between these structural entities in the mind. Incestuous desire for the mother could be ascribed to the id, and the contravening prohibition against incest could be attributed to the superego—all operating on an unconscious level. Further, as Anna Freud (1965/1974) pointed out, introjections related to superego formation are based on relations with external authorities and give rise to a situation in which external forces opposing the child's sexual and aggressive motives are internalized and become intersystemic conflicts between ego and superego so that anxieties of object loss or separation give way to superego guilt. When such conflicts arise between one's own wishes and motives and the ideals and prohibitions of external authorities that are *not* fully internalized and remain attached to their respective object representations (usually but not exclusively parental representations), they constitute forms of object relations conflicts (Dorpat 1976).

These intersystemic conflicts between psychic structures could be complemented by intrasystemic conflicts within each of them—conflicts between loving and hating could be basically intrasystemic id conflicts; deciding to do or not do some task could be a form of ego conflict; and in the superego, conflicts between divergent values and their related motives could be largely intrasystemic (Rangell 1963). Or, from another perspective, conflicts could be described as "conflicts of defense" arising usually between structures and "conflicts of ambivalence" deriving from conflicting libidinal or aggressive aims or either-or dilemmas in intrasystemic terms (Kris 1984). Such conflicts, we should note, can arise in an endless variety of forms and patterns, conscious and unconscious, intrasystemic and intersystemic, and they are rarely if ever encountered in pure form. Some of the most effective work in analytic therapy centers on the recovery of such complex motivational schemes from the unconscious and on enabling the patient to recognize and acknowledge them and to begin to resolve them in one way or another. Obviously, the failure to resolve such hidden conflicts can create impediments and difficulties not only in interpersonal relations but in the effectiveness and satisfaction of living itself.

The persistence of such conflicts can also give rise to anxiety, particularly when one or another aspect of the conflict poses a threat intrapsychically. After much hesitation and indecision, Freud (1926/1959) finally distinguished two kinds of anxiety-provoking situations. In the first, which Freud took as its prototype the phenomenon of birth, anxiety occurs as a result of powerful threats to the basic needs of the organism against which the organism is powerless to defend against or handle. This type of situation arises because of the helpless state of the individual in the face of overwhelming threats to basic motivational needs for self-preservation and self-integrity. Such traumatic states are most likely to occur in infancy or childhood, when the ego is relatively immature and less capable of effective defense. They may also occur in adult life, however, particularly in states of psychotic turmoil or panic states, when the ego organization is overwhelmed by the threatening danger. In this sense, external trauma can serve as the basis for psychic impairment, whether in itself, if sufficiently intense, or in conjunction with unconscious conflict.

In the more common situation, which occurs typically after defensive organization of the psyche has matured, anxiety arises from anticipating danger rather than as its result. The anxiety may be evoked by circumstances similar to a previously experienced danger. The anxiety can serve a protective function by signaling the approach of danger. The signal of danger may arise because the individual has learned to recognize, at a preconscious or unconscious level, aspects of a situation that once proved to be or can be anticipated to be traumatic. Thus, the anxiety signals the ego to mobilize protective measures, which can then be directed toward averting the danger and preventing a traumatic situation from arising. The dangers may arise from both external and internal sources; for example, the threat to the ego from unconscious instinctual motives that endanger ego integrity, ego values, or defenses. The individual may use avoidance mechanisms to escape from a real or imagined danger from without, or the ego may bring to bear psychological defenses to guard against or reduce the level or intensity of instinctual motivation, as Anna Freud (1936/1966) pointed out.

Each stage of the child's development is accompanied by characteristic danger situations that are phase-specific or "appropriate" to the developmental issues of that particular phase. Thus, the earliest danger situation, which occurs when the child is most immature and psychologically and physiologically vulnerable and helpless, is the loss of the primary object—that is, the caretaking and nurturing person on whom the child is entirely dependent. Later, when the value of the object itself begins to be perceived, the fear of losing the object's love exceeds the fear of losing the object itself. The whole developmental effort of the child to separate physically and psychologically from dependence on the primary symbiotic objects, and the necessary developmental steps toward increasing individuation, are subject to the concomitant threats of loss of the object or loss of the object's love (Mahler et el. 1975).

In the phallic phase of development, however, the fear of bodily injury or castration assumes a prominent influ-

ence. This fear may be thought of as a variety of fear of loss; in this instance, though, the loss is that of a highly narcissistically invested part of the body. Further on, in the latency period, the characteristic fear is that parental representatives, in the internalized form of the superego, will be angry with, punish, or cease to love the child.

Consequently, in each of these phases, anxiety arises in the ego. Freud also noted that although each of these determinants of anxiety is phase-related and functions in reference to a particular developmental period, they can exist side by side in the contemporaneous self. Furthermore, the individual's anxiety reaction to a particular danger situation might occur after the emergence from the developmental phase with which that situation was associated. The persistence in later years of anxiety reactions that were appropriate to various pregenital or genital phases of development has important implications for the understanding of psychopathology. The persistence of such earlier forms of anxiety in later stages of development is a reflection of neurotic fixations at earlier stages of development, as well as a persistence of the characteristic conflicts of such earlier stages. Similar analyses can be made for the broad spectrum of defense-related affective states, including guilt, shame, anger, envy, and jealousy, all of which, like anxiety, can operate on an unconscious level.

Unconscious Fantasy

Among the by-products of the activity of the dynamic unconscious are unconscious fantasies. Fantasies are common experiences when they are conscious—everyone has moments of imagining a set of images or a daydream in which wishes of one kind or other are gratified. Fantasies of what I should have said in an argument, how I should have handled that discussion with my wife, what it would be like to have sex with some luscious beauty, and so forth. Walter Mitty was the hero of many such imagined adventures. Imagination can serve in many productive and creative ways as an aspect of scientific or artistic or literary creativity. Unconscious fantasies are analogous to such conscious processes, except that they are carried on at an unconscious level and reflect unconscious strata of motivation. Thus, the underlying patterns of motivation are basically instinctual, reflecting libidinal, aggressive, and narcissistic motifs. The classic patterns of unconscious fantasy reflect these basic motivational dynamics and related psychosexual developmental stages and can be shaped by patterns of experience and their internalized configurations (Arlow 1969).

As Klein (1976) commented, "The principle of the motivational activity of repressed schemata has been an enormously generative one in psychoanalytic thought and has led to a number of vital analytic propositions, e.g., the notion of an inner reality of unconscious fantasy in which introjected relationships hemmed in by contradictory affects and conflicts are nonetheless active in producing and responding to replicas of such relationships in inter-personal encounters" (p. 255). Common themes include birth and pregnancy fantasies, primal scene (fantasies of parental intercourse), beating, castration, bisexuality (play-ing the part of both sexes in the sexual act), family ro-mance (being the child of idealized parents)—all of which reflect in some way relatively infantile and instinctual mo-tives.

An important aspect of such fantasies pertains to the view the subject takes toward himself or herself. How one views oneself on an unconscious level goes a long way to-ward influencing how one sees the world around one and how one reacts with other persons in that world. To cite one example, one young man entertained the fantasy that he was a very special and entitled person for whom special opportunities and exceptions should be made available, and that in every undertaking others should bend every effort to accommodate and facilitate his purposes. When such compliance on the part of others did not occur, his response was full of rage and envious bitterness. He was well aware of his enraged and frustrated responses and the almost paranoid quality of his perception of and interac-tion with others, but the underlying suppositions that de-termined these responses remained hidden. Only gradu-ally and slowly in the course of analytic work was he able to gain access to these unconscious fantasies about him-self and to begin to deal with them. One variant of this theme was his conviction that he was destined to receive a Nobel Prize without having to expend the effort or prove himself by any concrete accomplishment or success. The pattern here was akin to that described by Freud (1916/1957) as the "exceptions" in which such powerful, narcis-sistically motivated fantasies play such a meaningful role in shaping the individual's character and patterns of inter-action and response to the outside world. They serve as a primary determining component of the individual's psy-chic reality, whether they are expressed in entirely uncon-scious terms or in some relatively conscious derivative form.

Such self-reflective fantasies find expression in self im-ages and self representations, reflecting the way in which the self-as-subject (Meissner 1999a, 1999b) knows the self-as-object (Meissner 1996)—such imaginings and rep-resentings being modes of such self-knowledge. In struc-tural terms, however, the self-as-object is in some part formed through the accretion of internalizations, prima-rily in the form of introjects, derived from relations with external objects. These introjective configurations are de-rived in the first instance from parental and caregiving objects and are shaped by instinctual motivations embedded in these relationships. In the case of the above "exception," the patient's self image was cast in terms of narcissistically determined themes deriving from his growing up as an only child who was the object of excessive maternal idealiza-tion and paternal expectations for outstanding perfor-mance.

Such unconscious fantasies are ubiquitous and pro-vide a constant underlying pattern of mental processing that pervasively influences the ongoing pattern of con-scious experience. Beating fantasies, deriving from and related to introjected self configurations having to do with a view of the self as passive and helpless victim, and re-flecting basically masochistic motives, can undergird sub-servient, self-sacrificing, and self-denying patterns of be-havior (Blum 1980; Freud 1919/1961, 1924/1961). The unconscious pattern and dynamic, however, remain hid-den, and the behavior is justified and rationalized on other grounds. For the most part, such unconscious fantasies are warded off by psychic defenses when they give rise to a threat to other unconscious motives or to other aspects of the psychic economy. Fantasies of sexual gratification may run counter to moral value-systems of the superego. In such cases, unconscious fantasies may be repressed, de-nied, or sublimated; may serve as the basis for projection; may contribute to patterns of splitting; and so on. These reflect areas of intrapsychic conflict between opposing mo-tivations—for example, between motives leading to grati-fication and motives to delay, substitute for, or reject grat-ification. Such conflictual patterns can also be resolved by compromise formation of one kind or another in which both sets of motives are satisfied in some relative fashion with-out the domination or elimination of either. Fantasies of sexual gratification, for example, can be resolved in some degree and motives forbidding such physical gratification can be accommodated, for example, by reading a sexy novel or watching a sexy movie.

Symbol Formation

A unique capacity of the human mind is its ability to form symbols to express meaning. *Symbols* are forms of indirect representation by which one mental representation takes the place of another, conveying its meaning by some acci-dental or conventional form. A symbol can thus substitute for some other idea from which it derives a secondary sig-nificance that it does not itself possess. While such repre-sentational substitutes have wide-ranging cultural uses, psychoanalysis focuses on the use of signs and symbols to express levels and varieties of meaning. Signs are usually regarded as conscious and as conveying the meaning of a particular concept by certain arbitrary and conventional connections. Language makes use of this relation, stipulating the connection between a signifier (a word) and the signified (mental content or concept) in more or less conventional terms. The use of any given word to express any given content—"water" to connote water—is both arbitrary and conventional.

Symbols operate somewhat differently in that the symbol can be a conscious and manifest representation that stands for an unconscious and latent thought content. Moreover, the symbolic relation is not arbitrary but rests on some form of similarity or analogy or common element shared between symbol and referent. Symbols are characteristically sensory and concrete in nature, as distinguished from the ideas they represent, which may be relatively abstract and complex. A symbol thus usually provides a more condensed expression of the idea represented. Thus, the image of a house can represent the body, money can symbolize feces, a pillar can refer to a phallus, or a bowl of flowers or a window can represent the female genitals. But also, as in the case of dream symbols, a given symbol can, by displacement or substitution, come to represent more than one thing—balloons can symbolize breasts, but because of their lightness and playful quality, they may also represent states of manic elation (Winnicott 1935/ 1992).

As forms of communication, symbols allow for the expression of unconscious content in a way that is sufficiently disguised by defensive processes to keep the latent meaning relatively hidden or disguised and thus consciously acceptable. Symbolic modes of unconscious thought consequently tend to be more primitive and represent forms of regression to earlier stages of mental development and to function in more regressed conditions. Symbols provide one vehicle for the "return of the repressed" and play a significant role in dreaming and dreamlike processes, but they can also find expression in a broad range of mental activity. The arts, whether the visual arts such as painting or in literary forms such as poetry, are a primary area for such expression. Something similar can be said of religious symbolism: the cross becomes a symbol of sacrifice and salvation, the menorah a symbol of the faith of Israel in a god of light and life. On these terms, symbol formation is motivated along the same lines as discussed in the previous section with regard to unconscious dynamics and thus represents a form of compromise formation mediating between unconscious motivations and conscious mental processing. Further, symbols tend to center on the same themes and motifs that are found in unconscious

fantasies: body parts and functions, birth and death, sexuality, family relations, and so on. To the extent that some symbols enjoy a degree of trans- or cross-cultural expression, they would seem to reflect the common themes of human life and experience found in all human cultures.

Dream Formation

Sleep and dream activity are some of the most intensely studied aspects of psychological functioning in recent neurobehavioral research. The discovery of rapid eye movement (REM) cycles and the definition of the various stages of the sleep cycle have stimulated a flurry of research into the neurobiology of dreaming. This activity has opened up a whole new realm of fresh questions, allowing us to draw much closer to a more comprehensive understanding of the links between patterns of dream activity and underlying neurophysiological and psychodynamic variables and to understanding the nature of the dream process and the dream experience itself.

In this context, we can appreciate the uniqueness and originality of Freud's analysis of the dream experience. Only when Freud's attention had been refocused to the significance of inner fantasy experiences, by reason of his abandonment of the seduction hypothesis and in the context of his developing the technique of free association (see below), did the significance and value of the study of dreams impress itself on him. Freud realized that in the process of free association, his patients would frequently report their dreams along with associative material connected with them. He discovered little by little that dreams had a definite meaning, although that meaning was often quite hidden and disguised. Moreover, when he encouraged his patients to associate freely to the dream fragments, he found that what they frequently reported was more closely connected with repressed material than with events of their waking experience. Somehow the dream content seemed to be closer to unconscious memories and fantasies of the repressed, and associations to dream content seemed to facilitate disclosure of this latent material. He came to view the dream experience as a relatively conscious expression of unconscious fantasies or wishes not readily accessible to ordinary consciousness. Thus, dream activity was considered by Freud to be one of the normal manifestations of unconscious processes, although it is also clear that similar mechanisms are at work in conscious fantasies and daydreams (see section "Unconscious Fantasy" earlier in this chapter).

The manifest content, experienced in dreaming in the form of dream images and thoughts, represented for Freud unconscious wishes or thoughts, disguised through a process of symbolization and other distorting mechanisms, which constituted the dream work. The mechanisms of the dream work, specifically processes of displacement, condensation, symbolism, and repression, were regarded not only as characteristic of the formation of dreams but as basic to the operation of the unconscious in all its manifestations. Thus, dreams contained content, the so-called latent content, that had been repressed or excluded from consciousness by defensive activities of the ego, and, as consciously recalled by the dreamer, was simply the end result of unconscious mental activity taking place during sleep. In the analytic process, dream interpretation moved by way of associative exploration from the manifest content of the dream to the latent dream content that lay behind the manifest dream and that provided its core unconscious meaning. From a more contemporary viewpoint, it is known that cognitive activity during sleep has a great deal of variety. Some cognitive activity follows the description that Freud provided of dream activity, but much of it is considerably more realistic and more consistently organized along logical lines. The dreaming activity that Freud analyzed and described is probably more or less associated with the stage 1 REM periods of the sleep-dream cycle (Hartmann 1967, 1982; Reiser 1994).

Freud thought that dreaming activity could be initiated by a variety of stimuli. Contemporary understanding of the dream process, however, suggests that dreaming activity takes place more or less in conjunction with cyclic patterns of central nervous system activation that characterize certain phases of the sleep cycle. What Freud thought to be initiating stimuli may in fact not be initiating at all, but may be merely incorporated into the dream content, determining to that extent the material in the dream thoughts. A variety of sensory impressions, such as pain, hunger, thirst, or urinary urgency, may play a role in determining dream content. Thus, instead of disturbing one's sleep and leaving a warm bed, a sleeper who is in a cold room and who urgently needs to urinate may dream of awaking, voiding, and returning to bed. The pattern of dream thoughts could also be shaped by residues of thoughts, ideas, and feelings left over from experiences of the preceding day. These residues remain active in the preconscious and, like sensory stimuli, can be incorporated by the sleeper into thought content of the manifest dream. Such day residues could be amalgamated with unconscious infantile and instinctual motives, thus effectively disguising the infantile motive and allowing it to find expression in the dream material. Day residues may in themselves be quite superficial or trivial, but they acquire added meaning and significance as dream instigators through unconscious connections with deeply repressed instinctual motives and wishes.

In Freud's schema, the ultimate motivating factors stimulating dream activity and dream formation were the wishes stemming from infantile levels of psychic development. These motives took their content specifically from oedipal and preoedipal levels of psychic integration. Thus, nocturnal sensations and day residues, however intense, had to be associated with and connected with one or more repressed wishes from the unconscious to give rise to the dream content. This point of view needs some revision because it now seems that in some phases of nighttime cognitive activity, the mind is able to process residues of daytime experience without much indication of connection with unconscious repressed content. In addition, the point of view advanced by Fairbairn (1952)—that figures appearing in the dream represent parts of the dreamer's own personality—suggests that some dreams, at least those he described as "state of affairs" dreams, reflect the actual endopsychic situation and its related conflicts. Along similar lines, Kohut (1977) described "self-state dreams" in which the manifest content and related associations reveal a healthy part of the psyche reacting with anxiety to disturbances in the self. One characteristic of these dreams is that associations do not lead to deeper levels of meaning but tend to focus on the anxiety itself, so that links to underlying or repressed levels of motivation remain indirect and often implicit. However, in those phases of cognitive activity during sleep that bear the stamp of dreaming activity as Freud described and defined it, this essential link to the repressed probably still retains its validity.

Mechanisms of Representation in the Dream Work

The unconscious processes that Freud discovered in the study of dreams were regarded as characteristic of primary process mentation reflecting the organization of mental processes in the dynamic unconscious. The theory of the nature of dream work, developed in *The Interpretation of Dreams* (1900/1953), became the fundamental description of the operation of unconscious processes. Freud applied the important distinction between primary and secondary process in his analysis of the dream process. The secondary process produced perfectly rational dream thoughts comparable to those experienced in normal waking thinking, while the primary process produced a quite different organization of dream thoughts, which seemed at first bewildering and irrational but became understandable in the light of the disguising mechanisms of the dream work.

The basic problem of dream formation is to determine how it is that latent dream content finds representation in the manifest content. As Freud saw it, the state of sleep brought with it relaxation of repression, and concomitantly, latent unconscious motives were permitted wider amplitude of influence. Because motoric pathways were blocked in the sleep state, these repressed wishes and motives had to find other means of representation, by way of mechanisms of thought and fantasy. These mechanisms included symbolism, displacement, condensation, projection, and secondary revision.

Symbolism

Symbolism in dream work is the same as described above in regard to symbol formation and was described and defined more or less by study of the dream work. In his examination of dream content, Freud discovered that the ideas or objects represented in this way were highly charged with inappropriate feelings and burdened with conflict. It was the forbidden meanings of these symbols, derived from instinctual levels of motivation, that remained unconscious. Many questions still persist about the origins of symbolic processes, the stage of development in which they become organized, the extent to which they require altered states of consciousness such as the sleep state for their implementation, and the degree to which symbolic expression is related to underlying conflicts.

Displacement

The mechanism of displacement refers to the transfer of motivational interest from an original object to a substitute object or objects or to a symbolic representation of the object. Because the substitute object is in itself relatively neutral—that is, less motivationally and affectively invested—it allows for a lessened degree of containment by repression. Thus, whereas symbolism can be taken to refer to the substitution of one object for another, displacement facilitates distortion of unconscious wishes through transfer of affective and motivational investment from one object to another. Despite this substitution, the aim of the unconscious motivation remains unchanged. For example, in a dream, the mother may be represented visually by an unknown female figure (at least one who has less emotional significance for the dreamer), but the naked content of the dream nonetheless continues to derive from the dreamer's unconscious instinctual impulses toward the mother. Displacement probably accounts for the greater part of the distortion of dream content in the dream work.

Condensation

In condensation, several unconscious wishes, impulses, or attitudes can be combined into a single image in the manifest dream content. In a child's nightmare, for example,

an attacking monster may represent not only the dreamer's father but also some aspects of the mother and even, at the same time, some of the child's own primitive hostile impulses. The converse of condensation can also occur in the dream work, namely, the diffusion of a single latent wish or impulse through multiple representations in the manifest dream content. The combination of mechanisms of condensation and diffusion provides the dreamer with a highly flexible and economic device for facilitating, compressing, and diffusing or expanding the manifest dream content, thus further disguising it.

Projection

The process of projection allows dreamers to rid themselves of their own unacceptable wishes or motives and experience them in the dream as coming from other persons or independent sources. Not surprisingly, the figures to whom these unacceptable motives are ascribed in the dream often turn out to be those toward whom the subject's own unconscious impulses are directed. For example, someone with a strong repressed wish to be unfaithful to his wife may dream that his wife has been unfaithful to him; or a patient may dream that she has been sexually approached by her analyst, although she is reluctant to acknowledge her own repressed wishes toward the analyst. Similarly, the child who dreams of a destructive monster may be unable to acknowledge his or her own destructive impulses and the fear of the father's power to hurt the child. The figure of the monster consequently would be a result of both projection and displacement.

Secondary Revision

The mechanisms of symbolism, displacement, condensation, and projection all reflect operation of the primary process. But in the organization of the manifest dream content, primary process forms of organization are supplemented by an additional process that organizes the absurd, illogical, and bizarre aspects of the dream thoughts into a more logical and coherent form. The distorting effects of symbolism, displacement, and condensation thus acquire, through a process of secondary revision, a degree of coherence and pseudorationality that is necessary for acceptance on the part of the subject's more mature and reasonable ego. Secondary revision thus uses intellectual processes that more closely resemble organized secondary thought processes governing rational states of consciousness. It is through secondary revision, then, that the logical mental operations characteristic of the secondary process are introduced into and modify dream work. The dream as recounted in analysis is thus in some part the result of secondary revision.

Affects in the Dream

In addition to the manifestations just described, dreams also express various affective states or emotions. Repressed emotions, associated with the latent content, may not appear in the manifest dream content at all, or may be experienced in considerably altered form. Thus, for example, repressed hostility or hatred toward another individual may be modified into a feeling of annoyance or mild irritation in the manifest dream expression, or it may even be converted into its absence or even into its opposite. The latent affect may possibly be directly transformed into an opposite in the manifest content, as when a repressed longing is represented by a manifest repugnance or vice versa. Thus, the vicissitudes of affect and the transformation by which latent affects are disguised introduce another dimension of distortion into the content of the manifest dream, in addition to and in parallel with processes of indirect representation that characterize the vicissitudes of dream content.

These mechanisms, however, have only limited capacity to disguise and channel unconscious instinctual motives. When anxiety in the dream content became so severe that it resulted in nightmares or night terrors or even a partial awakening, this suggested to Freud some failure in the primitive defensive operations of the ego. An element of the latent dream content had succeeded, despite the dream work and the repressing functions of the ego, in finding its way into the manifest dream content in a form that was too direct, too little disguised, and too readily recognized for the self to tolerate. The self-as-ego reacted to this breakthrough of repressed impulses with anxiety. Thus, even in *The Interpretation of Dreams*, Freud foreshadowed later developments in his thinking about anxiety—namely, that anxiety seems to serve a warning function alerting the ego to the breakthrough of instinctual and repressed motives and impulses.

The punishment dream is related to the anxiety dream. In the punishment dream, the ego, in its role as self-related function, anticipates condemnation on the part of the superego (conscience) if part of the latent content, derived from repressed impulses, should find its direct expression in the manifest dream content. Specifically, in reaction to the anticipation of the dire consequences of the loss of ego control in sleep and the threat of instinctual breakthrough, there develops a compromise between the repressed wish and the repressing agency, specifically involving superego functions. Thus, the demands of the superego for punishment are satisfied in the dream content by giving expression to punishment fantasies.

Symptom Formation

Freud drew an analogy between the formation of dreams and the formation of neurotic symptoms. Symptoms are usually regarded as more ego-dystonic (more disruptive and contrary to ego functioning) and transient than character traits, which are usually more ego-syntonic and enduring qualities of personality functioning. In many instances, however, the distinction between symptoms and traits is not all that clear—compulsive behavior or inhibitions, for example, can be either. As in the mechanisms of dreaming, Freud viewed symptoms as arising from the influence of unconscious motives and conflicts, usually infantile in origin and more often than not specifically related to oedipal conflicts. When such motives are activated, defensive measures arise to either repress the associated fantasies or impulses or otherwise defend against their coming to consciousness. Such stable defensive patterns can play a role in character formation or may find degrees of partial or compromise gratification through forms of sublimation. When such adaptive resolutions fail or when the balance between repressing and repressed components falters, the threat of emergence of unconscious wishes or desires into consciousness brings with it a related experience of anxiety, guilt, shame, or other symptomatic affect corresponding to the nature or quality of the motivational stimulus.

When the intensity of the motivational impulse overrides defensive measures, symptoms can result. Consequently, psychoneurotic symptoms are equivalently compromise formations that allow partial and substitute gratification of unconscious motives and fantasy wishes on one hand and a degree of control and regulation by defensive and adaptive capacities of the self on the other. Such symptomatic compromises are far from desirable, since they give rise to significant degrees of neurotic suffering and impairment. The compromise formation itself may be further motivated by a need to avoid even more threatening alternatives, often enough some form of unconscious guilt or shame. The anxiety and impairment involved in the symptom are tolerated in the interest of avoiding even more painful or self-diminishing motives.

In this sense, neurotic symptoms, such as phobias, reflect a partial defect in the psychic apparatus. Specifically, in phobias defensive functions of the ego have not succeeded in adequately coping with the unconscious motivational threat. Consequently, mental conflict persists, and the danger actually arising from within is now externalized and treated as if originating in the external world, at least in part. Thus, neurosis represents a failure in the defensive function of the ego, resulting in distortion of the ego's relationship to reality. In psychotic states the failure of defensive function is more complete, and the potential threat to the fragile ego and its permeable defenses is all the more overwhelming and annihilating. Thus, greater portions of external reality are perceived as overwhelming and threatening, and greater distortions of the ego become necessary to accommodate distortions in the patient's view of the outside world.

Free Association

One of the cornerstones of the psychoanalytic technique is free association. The patient is encouraged to use this method to whatever extent is possible throughout the treatment. The primary function of free association, besides the obvious one of providing content for the analysis, is to help to induce the necessary regression and passive dependence connected with establishing and working through the transference neurosis. Freud developed the method of free association gradually and as a result of experimenting with a variety of other methods. In the *Interpretation of Dreams* (1900/1953), he described the method in the following terms:

> This [technique] involves some psychological preparation of the patient. We must aim at bringing about two changes in him: an increase in the attention he pays to his own psychical perceptions and the elimination of the criticism by which he normally sifts the thoughts that occur to him. In order that he may be able to concentrate his attention on his self-observation[,] it is an advantage for him to lie in a restful attitude and to shut his eyes. It is necessary to insist explicitly on his renouncing all criticism of the thoughts that he perceives. We therefore tell him that the success of the psychoanalysis depends on his noticing and reporting whatever comes into his head and not being misled, for instance, into suppressing an idea because it strikes him as unimportant or irrelevant or because it seems to him meaningless. He must adopt a completely impartial attitude to what occurs to him, since it is precisely his critical attitude which is responsible for his being unable, in the ordinary course of things, to achieve the desired unravelling of his dream or obsessional idea or whatever it may be. (p. 101)

Our interest in free association here is not so much as a technique of analysis, but as a medium for expression of the dynamic unconscious. One of the purposes of the associative approach is to facilitate access to unconscious and repressed mental content. While the technique has undergone a variety of modifications over the years, the method remains one of the principal means of access to unconscious material in the analytic process. We have also come to regard the process of free association less as something taking place in isolation in the patient, and more as a com-

plex process reflecting the quality of the relationship between analyst and patient. The patient's free associating is a function of the more basic relationship (Kris 1982). In the classic method devised by Freud, this process focused on dream symbols, but not exclusively. Any symbolic content that offers promise of revealing unconscious content might reveal its mysteries in the course of free associating. Then again it might not. As Freud noted, symbols in dreams often do not give rise to associations, but when such symbols have a commonly accepted reference, the analyst's judicious questioning of such possible implications can stimulate further associations or open areas of further inquiry that address unconscious connections and conflicts.

In the classic view, the usefulness of free associating depended on the understanding of symbol formation. Under conditions of regressive inducement in analysis, relaxation of defensive barriers to the expression of unconscious motives was expected to ease the access of such repressed material to conscious awareness. In the uncensored and minimally defended process of free associating, such content was thought to find its way to consciousness more readily and thus to open the way to further exploration and understanding. Under the guiding supposition of psychic determinism—namely, that all mental content was motivated—and the regulative effects of the pleasure and reality principles, the manifest material of the patient's associations was conceived as reflecting to one or another degree the underlying current of unconscious latent content. The model of the mind operating in this conception of free associative processes was analogous to that of the dreaming process. The model served as an idealized purecase scenario, from which the actual course of analytic work deviated more or less—often more than less. Some of the most important aspects of analytic work are concerned with understanding not only the process of free associating but also the causes and reasons for the impediments, failures, and distortions affecting the process both intrapsychically and in the context of the analytic relation.

Conclusion

While the interest of analysts tends to center on the role of the dynamic unconscious in the clinical context—each of the aspects of the unconscious discussed in this chapter plays a unique role in the analytic process—the basic principles governing the operation of the dynamic unconscious are by no means restricted to that setting and context. The dynamic unconscious, as conceived by Freud and envisioned in more explicitly motivational terms by contemporary analysts, is ubiquitous, constantly operating below and beyond the reach of conscious awareness, and continually exercising its influence in motivating behaviors, choices, preferences, attitudes, patterns of feeling and belief, and values. All human actions, certainly beyond the level of pure physiology and reflex, are motivated both consciously and unconsciously. We can conclude, therefore, that all our choices and decisions (as well as behaviors, attitudes, beliefs, feelings, and thoughts)—the choices that constitute the fabric of our lives, such as the choices we make in selecting a marriage partner or a job or career—are in some degree, whether directly or indirectly, influenced by unconscious dynamic motives.

References

Arlow JA: Psychoanalysis as scientific method, in Psychoanalysis, Scientific Method, and Philosophy. Edited by Hook S. New York, New York University Press, 1959, pp 201–211

Arlow JA: Unconscious fantasy and disturbances of mental experience. Psychoanal Q 38:1–27, 1969

Blum HP: Paranoia and beating fantasy: an inquiry into the psychoanalytic theory of paranoia. J Am Psychoanal Assoc 28:331–361, 1980

Dorpat TL: Structural conflicts and object relations conflict. J Am Psychoanal Assoc 24:855–874, 1976

Erikson EH: Childhood and Society, 2nd Edition. New York, WW Norton, 1963

Fairbairn WRD: Psychoanalytic Studies of the Personality. London, Tavistock, 1952

Freud A: The ego and the mechanisms of defense (1936), in The Writings of Anna Freud, Vol 2. New York, International Universities Press, 1966

Freud A: About losing and being lost (1955), in The Writings of Anna Freud, Vol 4. New York, International Universities Press, 1968, pp 302–316

Freud A: Normality and pathology in childhood (1965), in The Writings of Anna Freud, Vol 6. New York, International Universities Press, 1974, pp 25–63

Freud S: The interpretation of dreams (1900), in Standard Edition of the Complete Psychological Works of Sigmund Freud, Vols 4 and 5. Translated and edited by Strachey J. London, Hogarth Press, 1953

Freud S: The psychopathology of everyday life (1901), in Standard Edition of the Complete Psychological Works of Sigmund Freud, Vol 6. Translated and edited by Strachey J. London, Hogarth Press, 1960

Freud S: Jokes and their relation to the unconscious (1905a), in Standard Edition of the Complete Psychological Works of Sigmund Freud, Vol 8. Translated and edited by Strachey J. London, Hogarth Press, 1960, pp 1–247

Freud S: Three essays on the theory of sexuality, I: the sexual aberrations (1905b), in Standard Edition of the Complete Psychological Works of Sigmund Freud, Vol 7. Translated and edited by Strachey J. London, Hogarth Press, 1953, pp 135–172

Freud S: Instincts and their vicissitudes (1915), in Standard Edition of the Complete Psychological Works of Sigmund Freud, Vol 14. Translated and edited by Strachey J. London, Hogarth Press, 1957, pp 109–140

Freud S: Some character types met with in psychoanalytic work, I: the exceptions (1916), in Standard Edition of the Complete Psychological Works of Sigmund Freud, Vol 14. Translated and edited by Strachey J. London, Hogarth Press, 1957, pp 309–315

Freud S: 'A child is being beaten' (1919), in Standard Edition of the Complete Psychological Works of Sigmund Freud, Vol 17. Translated and edited by Strachey J. London, Hogarth Press, 1961, pp 175–204

Freud S: Beyond the pleasure principle (1920), in Standard Edition of the Complete Psychological Works of Sigmund Freud, Vol 18. Translated and edited by Strachey J. London, Hogarth Press, 1955, pp 1–64

Freud S: The economic problem of masochism (1924), in Standard Edition of the Complete Psychological Works of Sigmund Freud, Vol 19. Translated and edited by Strachey J. London, Hogarth Press, 1961, pp 155–170

Freud S: Inhibitions, symptoms and anxiety (1926), in Standard Edition of the Complete Psychological Works of Sigmund Freud, Vol 20. Translated and edited by Strachey J. London, Hogarth Press, 1959, pp 75–175

Hartmann E: The Biology of Dreaming. Springfield, IL, Charles C Thomas, 1967

Hartmann E: From the biology of dreaming to the biology of the mind. Psychoanal Study Child 37:303–335, 1982

Holt RR: Freud's mechanistic and humanistic image of man. Psychoanalysis and Contemporary Science 1:3–24, 1972

Home HJ: The concept of mind. Int J Psychoanal 47:42–49, 1966

Klein GS: Psychoanalytic Theory: An Exploration of Essentials. New York, International Universities Press, 1976

Kohut H: Thoughts on narcissism and narcissistic rage. Psychoanal Study Child 27:360–400, 1972

Kohut H: Restoration of the Self. New York, International Universities Press, 1977

Kris A: Free Association: Method and Process. New Haven, CT, Yale University Press, 1982

Kris A: The conflicts of ambivalence. Psychoanal Study Child 39:213–234, 1984

Mahler MS, Pine F, Bergman A: The Psychological Birth of the Human Infant: Symbiosis and Individuation. New York, Basic Books, 1975

McIntosh D: The economy of desire: psychic energy as a purely psychological concept. Psychoanalysis and Contemporary Thought 9:1–31, 1986

Meissner WW: The self-as-agent in psychoanalysis. Psychoanalysis and Contemporary Thought 16:459–495, 1993

Meissner WW: The self-as-object in psychoanalysis. Psychoanalysis and Contemporary Thought 19:425–459, 1996

Meissner WW: The self-as-subject in psychoanalysis, I: the nature of subjectivity. Psychoanalysis and Contemporary Thought 22:155–201, 1999a

Meissner WW: The self-as-subject in psychoanalysis, II: the subject in analysis. Psychoanalysis and Contemporary Thought 22:383–428, 1999b

Meissner WW: The self-as-person in psychoanalysis. Psychoanalysis and Contemporary Thought 23:479–523, 2001

Meissner WW: The Ethical Dimension of Psychoanalysis: A Dialogue. Albany, State University of New York Press, 2003

Mitchell S: Influence and Autonomy in Psychoanalysis. Hillsdale, NJ, Analytic Press, 1997

Noy P: A revision of the psychoanalytic theory of the primary process. Int J Psychoanal 50:155–178, 1969

Rangell L: Structural problems in intrapsychic conflict. Psychoanal Study Child 18:103–138, 1963

Rapaport D: On the psychoanalytic theory of motivation, in The Collected Papers of David Rapaport. Edited by Gill MM. New York, Basic Books, 1960, pp 530–568

Reiser MF: Memory in Mind and Brain: What Dream Imagery Reveals. New Haven, CT, Yale University Press, 1994

Rizzuto A-M, Meissner WW, Buie DH: The Dynamics of Human Aggression: Theoretical Foundations, Clinical Applications. New York, Brunner-Routledge, 2003

Rochlin G: Man's Aggression: The Defense of the Self. Boston, MA, Gambit, 1973

Schafer R: Mechanisms of defense. Int J Psychoanal 49:47–62, 1968

Schafer R: A New Language for Psychoanalysis. New Haven, CT, Yale University Press, 1976

Schur M: The Id and the Regulatory Principles of Mental Functioning. New York, International Universities Press, 1966

Sherwood M: The Logic of Explanation in Psychoanalysis. New York, Academic Press, 1969

Smith J: The pleasure principle. Int J Psychoanal 58:1–10, 1977

Smith J: Arguing with Lacan: Ego Psychology and Language. New Haven, CT, Yale University Press, 1991

Waelder R: The principle of multiple function: observations on over-determination. Psychoanal Q 5:45–62, 1936

Wallace ER: Historiography and Causation in Psychoanalysis: An Essay on Psychoanalytic and Historical Epistemology. Hillsdale, NJ, Analytic Press, 1985

Werman DS: Normal and pathological nostalgia. J Am Psychoanal Assoc 25:387–398, 1977

Winnicott DW: The manic defense (1935), in Through Paediatrics to Psycho-Analysis: Collected Papers. New York, Brunner/Mazel, 1992, pp 29–144

3

Early Relationships and Their Internalization

SALMAN AKHTAR, M.D.

SINCE ITS INCEPTION 100 years ago, psychoanalytic developmental theory has steadily moved from the economics of drive-defense energy to the internalized ecology of mutual relations between child and caregivers. Preoccupation with erogenous zones and psychosexual phases has given way to interest in growth needs, attachment styles, and object relations. Many reasons account for this shift. First, the burgeoning child-observational studies over the past 50 years demonstrated the profound importance of early child-parent interactions for the later growth of the personality. Second, the "widening scope of psychoanalysis" led to encounters with individuals whose deeply troubled lives were undeniable results of highly frustrating and traumatizing early interpersonal relationships. Third, the increasing recognition of the importance of noninterpretive elements in clinical work led to a search for what had gone wrong in those relational configurations earlier on. Finally, the modern conceptualization of drives (a central motivating agent in psychoanalytic theory) as collated derivatives of affects, and therefore object relations, also resulted in greater attention paid to the early relationships of the growing child developmental theory. These diverse influences resulted in the early interpersonal surround becoming the focus of psychoanalytic developmental theory, although attention toward the child's nonhuman environment remained inoptimal.

In this chapter, I delineate the impact of a child's relationships with his or her mother and father (and with the two as the parental couple) on his or her personality development and mental functioning. I also offer brief comments on the developmentally facilitating role of siblings, grandparents, and even nonfamilial persons such as maids, housekeepers, friends, clergy, and schoolteachers. The role of animals, inanimate objects, and religious deities in the child's mental growth is elucidated. I conclude the chapter with some synthesizing remarks. However, to avoid oversimplification as well as undue reductionism, some caveats need to be offered at the very outset.

Some Caveats

The formative influence of early relationships on mental functioning and behavior is indeed profound. However, cause and effect, impact and outcome, and preformation and epigenesis are neither sharply demarcated nor linearly correlated in this realm. Retrospective inferences regarding a particular behavioral trait, having emanated from this or that childhood experience, are especially prone to errors of heuristic enthusiasm. Prospective observations are sparse, especially when it comes to long-term follow-up studies that could shed light on how relational experiences shape internal affects and fantasies and how these, in turn, regulate overt behavior. Given such limitations of data, generalizations about the lifelong psychic impact of early relationships should be regarded as just that, namely, generalizations. A lot remains unknown, and what *is* known seems subject to many intervening variables.

Constitutional Factors

Child-observational studies of the past 50 years (A. Freud 1963, 1965/1974; Kagan and Moss 1962; Mahler et al. 1975; Spitz, in Emde 1984; Stern 1977, 1985; Thomas and Chess 1977; Thomas et al. 1963) have established that an infant is not a psychic tabula rasa. The infant brings affective-motor sensitivities of his or her own to bear on the interactions he or she evokes and receives from early caregivers. As a result, a psychic amalgam of the child's inherent potentials and conscious or unconscious maternal evocations of them (Jacobson 1964; Lichtenstein 1963; Mahler et al. 1975) constitutes the "basic core" (Weil 1970) of the human infant.

Endowment and experience enter into complex interactions from the very start of life. For instance, a constitutionally retiring baby evokes different responses from the mother than does a more active infant. Similarly, a child gifted with talent or beauty often receives more indulgence from parents than a child who lacks such attributes. And genotypal propensities themselves lead children to seek experiences most suited to their needs. Moreover, the assimilation of environmental input alters the inner world of the child, and this, in turn, elicits somewhat changed reactions from the external reality. While psychoanalytic developmental theory emphasizes the centrality of early experience for the emergence of mental structures and function, it cannot overlook the fact that such early experience is, at least in part, dependent on, and at times prominently shaped by, the child's inherent affective-cognitive assets and liabilities. Freud's early warning that "we must give up the unfruitful contrast between external and internal factors, between experience and constitution" (1912/1958, p. 238) must be heeded.

Element of Subjectivity

Faced with the patient's transferences, the psychoanalyst constantly struggles with disentangling what might be his or her (intended or unwitting) contribution to the experience and what is emanating from the internal world of the patient. Of course, making such distinctions might not always be possible or even necessary; Sandler's (1976) concept of "role responsiveness" and Renik's (1993) emphasis on the inevitability of countertransference enactments speak to this point.

While clearer in his thinking vis-à-vis matters of transference, the analyst is prone to gullibility when it comes to the patient's reports of childhood experiences with his or her parents. Ill-conceived notions of "schizophrenogenic mothers" and autism-causing "Frigidaire environment" are results of confusing the patient's subjective reports with objective facts about unseen others from decades ago. The following example highlights this point. A colicky child, finding no relief through mother's ministrations, might subjectively construe her to be "bad," at least at that moment; this might happen despite the mother's trying everything in her control to soothe the baby, and feeling terrible about his or her distress. Here the objective facts and subjective experience appear to diverge considerably. Take another example. A mother who is uncomfortable with physical closeness seems more rejecting to her daughter than to her son, since girls tend to stay physically closer to the "symbiotic orbit" (Mahler et al. 1975) and need greater "emotional refueling" than boys, who, in general, thrive on separateness and motor freedom. One and the same mother is thus intrapsychically felt and constructed in a different manner by her two children. The point to remember here is that relationships are subjective by nature.

Unreliability of Recall

In a related vein, it must be acknowledged that psychoanalytic reconstructions are at best tentative. Transference patterns, especially in the setting of severe psychopathology, and reports of childhood interactions with parents often turn out to be defensively altered and narcissistically tailored memories. A middle-aged man undergoing analysis, for instance, offered the memory of a tennis match in which his father badly defeated him after losing a game to him, as a proof of his father's vindictiveness. Further analytic work, spread over months, however, revealed that the patient had actually let his father win because the father had recently had a heart attack. Still later in the course of this patient's treatment, it became evident that the two games (in which the father lost and won, respectively) had been played on different days and had little to do with each other. It was this patient's need to see his father as dangerously retaliatory (in order to keep his own powerful competitive impulses in check) that had led to the conflation of the two memories. A "historical truth" had defensively been changed into a false "narrative truth" (Spence 1982).

Multiplicity of Roles and Developmental Overlays

In the course of development, the child's relationship with his or her caregivers undergoes constant evolution, change, and revision. There are shifts in instinctual demands and developmental needs over time. Intense closeness with mother, for instance, is needed during the "symbiotic phase," and ample distance from her is sought during the "practicing phase" of toddlerhood (Mahler et al. 1975). The same mother who is experienced as "good enough" (Winnicott 1960b) during the preoedipal phase might seem seductive and dangerous during the oedipal phase. In other words, there is hardly a static "relationship with mother" or "relationship with father." A more meaningful way of searching for answers is to ask the question "Relationship with mother at what phase of life and in the context of which instinctual wishes and ego needs?" Another important point to remember is that object relations from different developmental periods get layered in the mind, with various scenarios of satisfactions and dissatisfactions either becoming condensed or being used as defenses against one another. The situation is complicated by the fact that a "good enough mother" might come across as being not "good enough" toward a sibling or as being a terrible wife to one's father. The synthesis of these diverse roles can pose a burden for the growing child's ego, especially if the contradictions are too stark.

Cultural Factors

Consideration of early relationships must also take their cultural context into account. To be sure, dyadic preoedipal and triadic oedipal issues seem to be universal configurations. However, their dramatis personae, their affective intensities, their durations, and the extent to which regressive movements between various developmental phases are permissible vary from culture to culture and even in subcultures within a given nation. No hard and fast rules exist, and declared claims or privately held beliefs to the contrary belie intellectual colonialism. In the context of psychoanalysis, this has, at times, resulted in regarding the male, the white, and the Western psyche as paradigms and the female, the dark-skinned, and the Eastern as esoteric variants. Notions of "prolonged breast feeding," and "insufficient individuation" in the East, for instance, characterize such an attitude. The implication here is that the Western notions of the optimal length of breastfeeding and the desirable extent of individuation are both well established and correct. That this is far from being true becomes apparent in clinical analytic encounters with immigrant patients from diverse cultures, if the analyst, in his or her listening, can retain dispassionate empathy and capacity for surprise.

■ ■ ■

It is with these five caveats—namely, the nature-nurture interaction, subjective nature of relationships, pitfalls of memory and reconstruction, overlays of multiple and evolving roles, and cultural context of relationships—in mind that the following descriptions of early relationships should be approached.

Relationship With Mother

The relationship of a human infant to his or her mother is so profoundly integral to the former's psychic survival and functioning that it led Winnicott (1971) to declare that "there is no such thing as an infant." Or, to put it more explicitly, there is no such thing as an infant alone; a human infant exists as a member of the infant-mother dyad. This relationship lays the foundation of the child's self experience, capacity for "basic trust" (Erikson 1950), identity, and ability to maintain "optimal distance" (Akhtar 1992; Mahler et al. 1975) between the self and its objects throughout the life span. So complex and rich is this relationship that it defies simplification, and yet that is precisely what needs to be done for didactic purposes. At no point in this process, though, should it be overlooked that what is being described is just one aspect of an elaborate tapestry, one note in a symphony. With this proviso, the child's relationship with his or her mother can be divided into four categories.

Mother's Body

A child's relationship to his or her mother's body is psychologically significant in a number of ways.

1. The intrauterine experience of the child, though according to Freud (1918/1961) largely a matter of "retrospective phantasizing" (p. 103), seems to leave dim residues that are unrememberable but might play a silent, baseline role in one's preference for closed versus open spaces (Balint 1959) and one's sleeping postures and overall proprioceptive sensitivities (Piontelli 1987, 1988).
2. Breastfed infants can distinguish the smell of their mother's milk by the first month of life and use this olfactory bridge for attachment and bonding.
3. Exposure to mother's skin (the breast at first and later her face, hands, and so on) lays down the groundwork for lifelong skin-color preferences and "skin-color anxiety" (McDonald 1970) that is their converse.
4. The growing child uses mother's body for self-soothing and seeking of safety, especially when faced with situations of real or imagined danger. Physically hurt, the child darts back to mother to be held and kissed. Saying goodbye to the waking world of external objects, the

sleepy child longs for mother's caress. As he or she grows more, the child learns to soothe himself or herself via objects (e.g., a teddy bear) and activities (e.g., thumb sucking) that become proxy mothers.

5. Mother's eyes, and especially the way a child feels being looked at by them, play an extremely important role in the earliest estimations of one's self-worth (Wright 1991). Sparkling and kind glances from the mother inform the child of his loved status. Dull, pasty, and indifferent maternal glances make one dread that one is uninteresting, even invisible. Contemptuous glares by the mother can pierce a child's soul and sow the seeds of self-hatred and retaliatory rage.

6. The cadence of mother's voice, especially as it is experienced during the infantile period when one is being introduced to spoken words (and also in mother's singing lullabies to the baby), lays the sonic foundations for experiencing and expressing empathy and for the capacity to hum and sing to soothe oneself.

7. The mother's body has slightly different functions for her children of two sexes. The boy needs a greater distance from mother's body, and their anatomical difference helps in this aspect of the necessary "disidentification" (Greenson 1968) on the boy's part. The girl possesses a body similar to mother's, and the latter's intuitive knowledge of her body enhances their mutual empathy and the potential for emulation.

8. Fantasies about the insides of mother's body and about mother's genitals constitute a powerful dimension of the growing child's "theories" about childbirth, the sexual act, and anatomical differences between the sexes, all of which have enormous psychical consequences (Freud 1908/1959, 1925/1961; Klein 1937/1975, 1940/1975), including, later, for adult attitudes of comfort or discomfort vis-à-vis female sexuality.

Mother's Presence

Closely related to the issue of the mother's body is that of her presence and availability. Both physical and mental availability are important here. Some aspects of the former have already been covered. Other aspects include mother's physical presence, which offers a potential safeguard against "stranger anxiety" (Spitz 1963/1983)—since the child looks at the mother for approval to go or not go to an unfamiliar person. This forms a rudimentary step in the direction of separation, with mother's availability being a paradoxical requirement for the development of autonomy. Furman's (1982) celebrated phrase that "mothers have to be there to be left" speaks to this very point.

However, the importance of mother's availability goes beyond its physical dimensions. The child also needs mother

to be available in four "mental" ways. The first applies to her being available to her infant as a "subjective object" (Winnicott 1962), one that is experienced as an environmental provision and ego coverage rather than as a separately existing object of desire. Such an object meets physiological needs, is reliable, takes into account the infant's proprioceptive sensitivity, and is scarcely noticed by the infant. When such "holding goes well, there is built up in the infant a continuity of being which is the basis of ego strength" (Winnicott 1960b, p. 52).

The second aspect of mother's mental availability refers to her offering "mental space" to the growing child. The infant, preverbal and inchoate in subjectivity, especially needs this. However, the more "grown up" child also needs mother's blank reverie to "contain" (Bion 1967) his or her unbearable affects, incomprehensible mental links, and unverbalizable fantasies, if only to return them after a palatable translation. This not only deepens the child's self knowledge but also enhances his or her capacity to elaborate and process his or her own spontaneous thoughts by internalizing mother's capacity to do so. A mother who is unable to listen to her child with interest (i.e., fails to lend him or her "mental space") not only deprives the child of learning more about his or her own self but also weakens the child's capacity to "mentalize" (Fonagy and Target 1997) his or her inner experiences.

The third aspect of maternal availability is evident in the "survival of the object" (Winnicott 1971). The mother tolerates and absorbs the child's aggression and yet remains unaltered in her benevolent attitude toward the child. Her maternal devotion "survives" the assaults and helps the child mend the split between his or her loving and hostile views of her (Klein 1940/1975).

Finally, the mother takes an active interest in buffering, regulating, and organizing the extent of inner and outer stimuli for the infant. This external function is gradually internalized by the child, who then develops a "protective shield" (Freud 1895/1955) that determines the threshold of stimulation optimal for him or her. The child can be vigorous without being exhausted and sedate without experiencing deadness.

Mother's Mental Contents

The contents of mother's mind are of profound importance in determing the nature of child-mother relationship. On the basis of her mental contents, the mother might allow or disallow her child access to her body. Also, based on her mental contents, the mother might make herself more or less mentally available to her child.

More specifically, the content of mother's mind affects the formation of the "basic core" (Weil 1970) of the child's psyche. Of all the potentialities offered by the inherent temperament of her infant, the mother selectively evokes some, which then become the bedrock of her specific child's identity (Lichtenstein 1963). The impact of maternal mental content, however, extends beyond infancy. It affects her estimation of the child's abilities and intentions as well as her willingness and ability to be meaningfully engaged with her child. Her attitude and fantasies about her body especially affect her relationship with her daughter. A mother who is self-deprecating and masochistic in this regard can considerably damage her daughter's sense of femininity and bodily pride.

Mother's Relationships

Children are also affected by the manner in which their mother relates to others in the environment. Her attitude about her other children teaches the child the capacity to share and sensitizes him or her to the issues of fairness and unfairness. Her relationship with their father, while painful in so far as it leads to feelings of exclusion, imparts to her children a sense of generational boundaries and the need to respect parental privacy. Her relationship to her own mother allows her to let go of her adolescent children as she turns back to their grandmother to "fill" the near-somatic lacuna created by their departure (Furman 1982).

At a more subtle level, mother's fantasy life and the ongoing dialogue she has with her internal objects affect the child in complex and often "unknown" ways. This was evident in the case of a middle-aged male analysand who was very attached to a gramophone left behind by his mother. She had died when he was only 7 years old, and he ascribed his attachment to the machine to the fact that it had once belonged to her. Later in the course of his treatment, however, he began to be curious about its importance to *her* and what role that unspoken importance might have played in his own positive feelings for the grammophone.

■ ■ ■

In summary, it is safe to say that a child's relationship with his or her mother is deep, complex, varied, and subject to evolution and change over time. If matters go well, this relationship leads to the foundations of a coherent self, a healthy sense of optimism and confidence, a capacity to tolerate frustrations without losing love for those causing them ("object constancy"), core gender identity, and capacities for reparation, sharing, and accepting generational differences. Relationship with mother is fundamentally transformative, and identification with her gives rise to transformational capacities toward one's self and toward others.

Relationship With Father

Despite Freud's painstaking delineation of the father's ontogenetic role in establishing the incest barrier (1909a/1955, 1924/1961), his speculations regarding the phylogenetic origins of the father-son struggle (1913/1958), his emphasis that a boy's preoedipal development includes "identification of an affectionate sort with his father" (1925/1961, p. 250), and his explicit declaration that he "can not think of any need in childhood as strong as the need for a father's protection" (1930/1957, p. 72), psychoanalytic developmental theory did not pay adequate attention to the father's role in child development till the 1950s. Perhaps, this inattention was a counterpart to the great interest, developing at that time, in the mother's role in the child's emotional life. Perhaps, the silence also reflected the profession's mourning of its own father.

Nearly two decades after Freud's (1930/1957) last comments about the father's importance, Loewald (1951) noted that the father's role is not restricted to the vicissitudes of the oedipal phase, but includes his acting as a protector against the threat of reingulfment by the mother of a child of either sex. Mahler and Gosliner (1955) further elucidated the father's role in the development of the child's ego as well as the superego precursors. Mahler (1967) noted that the child reacted to the father as to a "breath of fresh air," one who was different from the mother and was more playful. He pulls the child out of the "symbiotic orbit" (Mahler et al. 1975) he or she inhabits with the mother. In essence, the father functions as a bridge between the internal world and the external reality for the child (Abelin 1971). He thus becomes an object of fascination, and the accompanying shift in the child's attention toward the outer rind of his psychosocial life is highly salutary. Through involvement with father, the child develops greater exploratory skills and social responsiveness.

In a series of contributions spanning two decades, Blos (1962, 1965, 1967, 1974, 1985) demonstrated that the early preoedipal son-father relationship critically affects the boy's self image and worldview for a lifetime. The little boy seeks father's approval and praise, thus establishing a deep and lasting bond between them. Father's approval instills in the son "a modicum of self-possession and self-assertion—distilled, as it was, out of mutual sameness or shared maleness—which renders the wider world not only manageable and conquerable but infinitely alluring" (Blos 1985, p. 11). At the end of adolescence, father's affirmation of his son's manhood allows the latter to assume adult prerogatives. Blos noted that the last psychic structure to crystallize is the ego ideal, and this happens as a result of renouncing negative oedipal strivings at the end of adolescence. A young man must replace his tender and submissive ties to his protective father by his own sense of ideals and moral injunctions. Still, as a young adult he returns, one last time, to seek "father's blessing" (Blos 1985, p. 30) before entering into matrimony.

Ross (1979) comprehensively reviewed the literature on the father's developmental contributions, adding significant insights of his own. He posited the concept of the "Laius complex" (1982) (i.e., father's hostile competitiveness with his son), traced the vicissitudes of men's need for father figures over the life span (1994), and noted that escape from a forbidding paternal transference on a spouse is often the unconscious motive for male infidelity in long marriages (1996).

In light of this literature, the father's multifaceted role in child development can be seen as consisting of the following four tasks:

1. Being a protective, loving, and collaborative partner to the mother, the father facilitates and enhances her ability to devote herself to the child.
2. Offering himself as a relatively neutral, ego-oriented, new object during the rapprochement subphase of separation-individuation, the father provides the child with stability, a haven from conflict, and (in the case of a boy) an important measure of "dis-identification" (Greenson 1968) from the mother.
3. Appearing on the evolving psychic horizon of the child as the romantic partner of the mother, the father helps consolidate the child's capacity to experience, bear, and benefit from the triangular familial relationship and the conflicts attendant on it.
4. Presenting himself as an admirable model for identification to his son and by reflecting the budding femininity of his daughter with restrained reciprocity, the father enriches his children's gender identities and gives direction to their later sexual object choices.

The question of how early in the child's development the father acquires an independent psychic importance still lacks a satisfactory answer. At first, psychoanalytic developmental theory regarded father as important mainly during the phallic-oedipal phase of development. He was the giver of law, the founder of incest barrier, and the inspiring agent of ego ideal. With the advent of child-observational studies, psychoanalytic developmental theory began to acknowledge the importance of the "preoedipal father." He helped the child separate from the mother and became a bridge to the external world. More recently, it has been observed that patterns of infant-father interaction are different from those of the infant-mother interaction from as early as the first month of life (Yogman 1982). The father

is an alternate attachment figure for the infant (Lamb 1997; Muir 1989). Infants are capable of forming multiple attachments and can have an insecure attachment to the mother but a secure one to another nurturing figure, including the father (Fox 1991).

The difference in child-mother and child-father interaction is also evident in Herzog's (1984) elucidation of the "homeostatic" and "disruptive" attunements of parents to their growing child. Through video-monitored child-observational studies, Herzog demonstrated that mothers usually join in with a toddler in his or her ongoing play (e.g., building a tower with wooden blocks), thus giving the child a "continuity of being" (Winnicott 1960a), validity, and harmony with the environment ("homeostatic attunement"). Fathers, on the contrary, characteristically disrupt the playing toddler's equilibrium by cajoling him or her into joining them in a new activity ("disruptive attunement"). Homeostatic attunement has affirming qualities necessary for sustenance and consolidation of self experience. Disruptive attunement has enhancing qualities necessary for broadening and deepening of self experience. The influence of the two types of attunements is additive and contributes to the fluid solidity of healthy self experience.

Herzog further observed that fathers distract the child away from the game he or she is playing only when the mother is with the child. In her absence, and especially with younger children, fathers too start playing the child's own game (i.e., resort to homeostatic attunement). This suggests that homeostatic attunement is an experiential prerequisite for disruptive attunement. Such conceptualization finds a parallel in the clinical situation wherein the analyst's holding and affirmative (i.e., homeostatic) functions have to be securely in place for his interpretive (i.e., disruptive) efforts to be fruitful. The patient's inner sense of the analytic relationship must be stable (or should be stabilized) for him or her to utilize the destabilizing impact of interpretation, which, by definition, brings something new to the patient's attention.

Interestingly, the difference in the ways growing children relate to their two parents includes their use of their parents' respective bodies. Pruett (1988, 2000) notes that the child draws nurturance, safety, and soothing from the mother's body. In contrast, the child uses the father's body for playing and aggressively testing the extent (and safety) of his or her own physical strength and prowess. When scared or injured, the child seeks haven at the mother's bosom. When enthusiastic and curious, he or she enlists father's body for horseplay.

All this is clearer in the case of boys than girls. Indeed, the psychoanalytic literature on the child-father relationship has been tilted toward boys. Notable exceptions in this regard are the contributions of Lax (1977), Tessman (1982), Bernstein (1983), Benjamin (1988), Ross (1990), Chodorow (1994), and Garfield (2004). Together these authors underscore that a child's relationship with father is not hard-wired and develops in accordance with psychological and cultural factors specific for the growing girl and boy. These authors delineate the dialectics of distance and intimacy in the developmental dialogue between fathers and daughters. They note the longing in a girl for a close and collaborative relationship with her father that exists parallel to her oedipal desire for him.

Bernstein (1983), in a seminal contribution to the topic of female superego, noted the problems faced by a growing girl—and, later, woman—when the father is available as an object of desire and idealization but not as a model of efficacy and object for identification. In Tessman's (1982) phraseology, the girl's "erotic excitement" is validated while her "endeavor excitement" is not. Explicating this matter further, Garfield (2004) notes that

> [t]he father's unique contribution here is to accept his daughter's femininity, sexuality, and her interest and competence in work. If he denigrates her endeavor excitement, and or demands compliance as a part of her femininity, she will experience great conflict about work. If he can only value her achievements, her identity as a loving girl and woman will be compromised. (p. 41)

A girl who lacks a father supportive of both her efficacy and her erotic strivings feels hurt; the resulting anger can give rise to defensive idealization on the one hand and helplessness and masochistic submission on the other. Benjamin (1988) has poignantly described such an impact of a missing father on female development, and Chodorow (1994) has elucidated the cultural factors operating in this realm.

Relationship With the Parental Couple

The aggregate of a child's independent relationships with mother and father is not synonymous with his or her relationship with the parental couple. Indeed, the dawning awareness of the parents' being a couple is a hallmark of a child's entry into the oedipal phase. This awareness lays the groundwork for all sorts of affective experience, fantasy, and structure formation. Prominent among these are painful feelings of exclusion, defiant aspirations of breaking through the fence separating the child from the couple, curiosities and fantasies about parental sexuality ("primal scene"), and, finally, grudging (though highly beneficial)

acceptance of generational boundaries and the incest barrier. Acceptance of parents as a couple leads to the child's "entrance into a temporal order" (Chasseguet-Smirgel 1985, p. 28), generational filiation (i.e., becoming a son or daughter, not merely a boy or girl), and, through that, a sense of historical continuity.

During the latency phase (from ages 6–7 to 13–14 years), the growing child leans on each individual parent for a different kind of support while also drawing a silent ego nourishment from their stability as a couple. Their disagreements about intellectual and social matters (e.g., the meaning of a movie or a novel, the reasons for a school or neighborhood ordinance), if voiced without derogation of each other, enrich the child's mind by offering him multiple perspectives on external reality. Moreover, the fact that their couplehood "survives" such arguments strengthens the child's conviction that all assertiveness is not dangerous and that one can live with, and indeed love, individuals with whom complete agreement is not possible.

During adolescence, the upsurge of libidinal drive and the resultant search for sexual objects create the necessity to defensively distance oneself from the parental couple. At the same time, the opportunity to witness affectionate, and even some limited sensual, exchanges between parents diminishes the feared dangerousness and dirtiness of sexual impulses. The adolescent boy especially benefits from the exposure to the mother's pleasant acceptance of father's flirtatiousness, since it helps him to mend the Madonna-whore split of the maternal imago developed during early childhood (Freud 1912/1958).

Such salutary vicissitudes of the child's relationship with the parental couple must not overshadow the fact that too little distinction between parental figures in the child's mind, especially if the home environment is one of strife and if the parents totally exclude the child from their mental lives, can give rise to a menacing "parental couple" introject in the latter's psyche. This, in turn, can breed lifelong fear of authority figures and a tendency to experience them as conspiring against oneself.

Relationship With Siblings

A child's relationship with his or her siblings includes a wide range of experiences. Not having any siblings prevents the child from sharing the material and emotional provisions offered by parents but also leaves him lonely and excessively dependent on parental whims. Having siblings has its own pros and cons. On the positive side, it offers the child an opportunity to share secrets, cooperate in ego-building endeavors, elaborate day dreams, and socialize beyond the parental orbit (Provence and Solnit 1983). On the negative side, the relationship provides a fertile soil for envy, jealousy, resentment, and hatred. History, legend, mythology, and literature from all parts of the world are replete with striking tales of love and hate in this relational matrix. More often, ambivalence prevails and the relationship continues to evolve throughout childhood, adolescence, and even during adult life. Its nature and intensity are governed by a number of factors.

Before addressing them, however, I should note that while the importance of sibling rivalry and its consequences in mental life were discovered early on in psychoanalysis (Freud 1900/1953, 1910/1955, 1917/1961), the theoretical and clinical tendency, till about two decades ago, was to view sibling attachments largely as displacements from parental objects. A number of investigators (Ainslie 1997; Neubauer 1983) have raised doubts about such an assumption and noted that sibling relationships "tend to be more vital to development than is often suggested" (Parens 1988, p. 32). These bonds can influence evolving character traits and exert lifelong impact on object choices. Indeed, analysts have reported patients whose selection of lovers was "profoundly influenced by persistent unconscious attachment to older siblings" (Abend 1984, p. 425). Sharpe and Rosenblatt (1994) have argued that

> in families with multiple siblings, oedipal-like triangles develop among siblings and between siblings and parents that exhibit many of the characteristics of the oedipal "parental" triangle. Such relationships are not solely displacements of parental oedipal constellations, but may exist parallel to and relatively independent of the oedipal parental triangle. Moreover, they often exert a definitive influence on the individual's later identifications, choice of adult love object, and the patterns of object-relating. (p. 492)

A number of factors, however, affect the nature and outcome of the sibling relationship; these factors have been discussed in detail elsewhere (Akhtar and Kramer 1999). Here it might suffice to note the following:

1. Absence of parents often intensifies the sibling relationship.
2. Loving relationship between parents solidifies sibling relationship.
3. Parental favoritism can poison the sibling relationship.
4. The presence of adopted siblings poses special challenges for both the adopted siblings and their "biological" counterparts.
5. The relationship between twins is more complex and highly vulnerable to the parental attitudes toward them (Ainslie 1997; Volkan and Ast 1997).
6. Having opposite-sex siblings can deprive a child of some play activities but can also be utilized as a second theater to work through oedipal fantasies by displacement.
7. The "developmental distance" (Solnit 1983, p. 283) between siblings is often more important than the count of calendar months (however, an age difference of less than 2 years can complicate the older child's separation individuation [Mahler et al. 1975] and an age difference of more than 5 years can cause marked resentment or estrangement).
8. The presence of a positively (e.g., via extraordinary beauty or talent) or negatively (e.g., via congenital defect or serious illness) "special" sibling can lead to the other sibling's needs being overlooked; this, in turn, results in the healthy child's becoming resentful, unduly self-sufficient, and rejecting of his strivings for attachment.

Subject to a number of variables, the sibling relationship nonetheless offers the growing child an arena for practicing ego skills, a chamber of shared secrets, a conduit for role modeling, and a haven from the complexities of the ongoing dialogue with parental objects.

Relationship With Grandparents

Psychoanalytic exploration of adult development, set in motion by Erikson's (1950) delineation of lifelong psychosocial tasks, has recently paid attention to grandparenthood. However, this literature has largely focused on the grandparent's psychic use of the grandchild and makes only passing comments about the importance of this relationship for the latter. Cath (1989) noted that the grandchild might benefit by his or her relationship with grandparents since "both may be struggling with autonomy from the middle or 'sandwich' generation, both searching for newer identities, greater independence, and new anchorages" (p. 104). And Colarusso (1997) observed that relationship with a grandparent might satisfy the toddler's developmental need for fusion with an idealized object before venturing into the world beyond the symbiotic membrane.

Long before these contemporary observations, Abraham (1913/1955), in an early and largely unread paper, highlighted the useful role of grandparents for the child. He observed that interaction with grandparents in general, and seeing the parents interact with grandparents in particular, demonstrate to the growing child that "even the father on whom, by reason of his unconscious fixation, he feels wholly dependent is not omnipotent, but is himself in turn subject to a higher power" (p. 47). That the word "father" here can (and should) be seen as standing for "parent" goes without saying. It is the spirit of the sentence that counts. It declares that the growing child is helped in "depersonification" (Jacobson 1964) of superego introjects and development of abstract morality by his or her relationship with the grandparents.

All in all, therefore, it seems that a child's relationship with grandparents benefits him or her by 1) strengthening the child's burgeoning ego capacities for separation from parents, 2) offering the child blissful merger states while his or her parents are gently nudging him or her to "grow up," and 3) refining his or her superego functions. Replication of such experiences can be witnessed in clinical situations as well, especially in treatments with older analysts. An important thing to learn here is that triangulated transferences not only represent oedipal scenarios and sibling triangles but also pitting of parents against grandparents, with the analyst being cast in one or the other role.

Relationship With Animals

The "average expectable environment" (Hartmann 1939/ 1958) necessary for harmonious psychological growth is populated not only by reliable parents, siblings, and grandparents but also by nonhuman objects that remain consistent. Emotions and fantasies not verbalized with human figures in the environment are often mastered through enactments with animals (Searles 1960). In societies where the human-animal separation is less pronounced than in the urbanized West, the growth-facilitating role of animals is greater.

Such essential kinship between the child and animal received considerable attention from Freud. He observed that as man evolved he

> acquired a dominating position over his fellow-creatures in the animal kingdom. Not content with this supremacy, however, he began to place a gulf between his nature and theirs. He denied the possession of reason to them, and to himself he attributed an immortal soul, and made claims to a divine descent which permitted him to break the bond of community between him and the animal kingdom. (1913/1958, p. 140)

Freud went on to say that this "piece of arrogance" does not exist in children. They are not surprised by fairy tales in which animals talk or think like human beings. Indeed, they "have no scruples in allowing to rank animals as their full equals. Uninhibited as they are in the avowal of their bodily needs, they no doubt feel themselves more akin to animals than to their elders, who may well be a puzzle to them" (Freud 1913/1958, p. 127). Animals may also represent power and courage for the child. That they bite,

bark, sting, claw, and devour makes animals ready recipients for conflict-ridden aggressive drives (Akhtar and Brown 2005; Fenichel 1945; Schowalter 1983). Because their sexual organs and reproductive lives are often visible to children (Jelliffe and Brink 1917), animals may readily become the objects of projected libidinal derivatives. Because many animals are warm, soft, and available on an as-needed basis, they come to be substitutes for emotionally absent parents.

Children's use of animals as part of normal development is most evident in their attachment to transitional objects (Winnicott 1953) in the shape of stuffed animals, their love of actual pets (Sherick 1981), their playful mimicry of animals, their concoction of imaginary animals, and, above all, their fondness for storybooks and movies with animals as protagonists (see Burland 2005; Krueger and Krueger 2005). Together, these diverse child-animal "interactions" offer the child symbolic reservoirs for projection, agreeable objects for trial action, containers for fantasy, and targets for instinctual release. The role of animals in a child's mental development, though not fully appreciated, is profound. Not surprisingly, three of Freud's "famous" cases—namely, those of Little Hans (1909a/ 1955), Rat Man (1909b/1955), and Wolf Man (1918/ 1961)—involved human fantasies and preoccupation with animals.

Relationship With the Inanimate Surround

The inanimate world also plays a crucial role in the development and sustenance of the human personality. From the very beginning of life physical objects have an impact on the human mind, which, in turn, utilizes them to express, consolidate, and enhance itself. Such an "ecological dimension of the self" (Akhtar 2001) first makes its appearance in the infant's acquiring the distinction between animate and inanimate objects. The distinction evolves along many axes, ranging from the simple perceptual one to the most complex one of conceptual interpretation (Lichtenberg 1983; Stern 1977). The timing of such development, however, remains unclear. Spitz (1963/1983) observed that it was around the sixth month of life that "the child will no longer accept the inanimate object in place of the living partner, however briefly. Endowing the inanimate with the privileged gestalt (of human face) and with movement is no avail" (p. 149). Spitz added that around 8 months of age, when "stranger anxiety" appears, many children show "anxiety reactions in response to toys and other inanimate objects" (p. 150) as well. He held that the "second organizer of the psyche" is the capacity to distinguish not only the primary love object (mother) from strangers but also the animate from the inanimate.

With increasing capacity for making such distinctions, the capacity for "object permanence" (Piaget 1936/1952) evolves. Such stability of representation, initially restricted to what is at hand, gradually spreads to cover a larger terrain. Frosch's (1964) concept of "reality constancy" is important in this context. This capacity enables the individual to "tolerate alterations and changes in environment without psychic disruptions and adaptational dysfunctions" (p. 350). It forms the background of perceptual experience of physical reality throughout life. Pacella's (1980) concept of "waking screen" is an elaboration of this very notion. The "waking screen" plays "an active role in scanning, integrating, rejecting, or modifying all the new percepts of object representations throughout life" (p. 130).

The "waking screen" at the deepest level, the capacity for "reality constancy" at the intermediate level, and the need for an "average expectable environment" (Hartmann 1939/1958) at the surface form the basis for the self's relationship with its physical surround. When these three are intact, the use of inanimate objects is largely for drive, fantasy, or ego-related instrumental purposes. When they are disturbed, the use of inanimate objects is largely for psychic structuralzation and stability of the self.

The use of physical objects in the process of psychic growth is most strikingly evident in the concept of the "transitional object" (Winnicott 1953). Significantly, Winnicott (1953) emphasized that such an object "comes from without from our point of view, but not from the point of view of the baby. Neither does it come from the within; it is not an hallucination" (p. 233). This vitally important object, which is affectionately cuddled and excitedly mutilated but must never change, is neither repressed not mourned over the course of later life. It simply loses meaning, since this "intermediate area of experience" (p. 30), which is neither real nor unreal and which lies between the internal world and external reality, gradually spreads over the cultural field at large. Capacity to play and to enjoy poetry, movies, fiction, and music thus develops.

Inanimate objects are used in other ways as well during the process of separation-individuation. Winnicott (1960/1965) and Fischer (1991) have referred to the older child's use of a string and the fantasy of a transatlantic cable, respectively, to overcome separation anxiety. Much earlier than them, Freud (1920/1955) had described the "fort-da" game, employing a wooden reel and string, played by his 18-month-old grandson to master separation related concerns.

Physical objects also help the growing child master oedipal anxieties. The little girl puts on mother's necklace and coquettishly uses her lipstick to woo daddy, and the little boy wears father's large shoes in symbolic competitiveness with him. Such stolen pleasure of using adult physical objects, however, diminishes with the resolution of Oedipus complex. The subsequent involvement with external reality is striking. Board games, toys, amusement parks, and video arcades help the latency-age child rework both separation-individuation related and oedipal concerns in an aim-inhibited and ego-dominated way (Balint 1959; Erikson 1950; Glenn 1991; Waelder 1936; Winnicott 1971). Such excursions into the physical surround (and their electronic, "virtual" counterparts) encourage the child to leave a zone of safety, court danger, and then return to a secure "home base." They permit the player the vicarious enjoyment of merger and separation, rivalry and competitiveness, and a counterphobic management of castration anxiety.

The forging of identity during adolescence also enlists physical objects for its purposes. For disengaging from parental mores, cutout jeans, nose and tongue rings, and T-shirts with outrageous declarations are used. For consolidating new ego ideals, posters of athletes and musicians and ever-growing CD collections are used. Together, the two types of "neo-generational objects" (Akhtar 2003) help in disengagement from earlier parental dictates internalized in the form of a strict superego and enhance the parallel reliance on the value of one's peers and, ultimately, of oneself.

All in all, it seems that from infancy to adolescence, the physical environment offers the growing child instruments and vessels for expressing and containing his or her inner goings-on. The dependence on such provision is taken for granted. However, when this background screen gets lacerated, the experiential rupture is profoundly painful. Analysts who deal with immigrant patients are all too familiar with their nostalgic search for retrospectively idealized versions of the formative ecology of their childhood (Akhtar 1999).

Other Important Relationships

This survey of the growing child's formative relationships has left four areas unaddressed. First, the discussion of familial ties here has not included stepparents and stepsiblings. The fact is that in today's world, where divorce and reconstructed families are commonplace, relationships with steprelatives has acquired marked significance. Psychoanalytic observations of such scenarios (Brenner 2001; Cath and Shopper 2001) are just beginning to accrue and deserve serious attention.

Second, the growing child's relationship with his or her extended family (including uncles, aunts, cousins) can offer compensations and corrections for conflicts and deficits in his or her experience with the nuclear family. This might be of greater significance in certain cultural groups. In India and Japan, for instance, the developing self stays forever in emotionally close and interdependent relationships with the extended family (Akhtar 1999; Roland 1988; Yamamoto and Wagatsuma 1980). The intertwined developmental tracks of separation and individuation remain farther apart from each other than they are in the West. In other words, the Eastern self can achieve high degrees of individuation without comparable achievement of separateness: "Infantile objects are relinquished very gradually, and this process does not take place to the degree necessary in cultures where the child is being prepared to live an adult life that is independent of the extended family" (Bonovitz 1998, p. 178).

Third, the growing child is also influenced by individuals who are related to him or her neither by blood nor by second marriages of his or her parents. Babysitters, nannies, and housekeepers can, at times, play a profoundly important developmentally facilitating role in the child's life. The founder of psychoanalysis, Freud himself, was very attached to a childhood nursemaid and would occasionally dream of her even as an adult. Such attachment is especially intense if the child is neglected by parents and seeks solace elsewhere. It is not infrequent, in clinical practice, to see adults whose main childhood source of emotional nourishment was a maid or a housekeeper. Similar sustenance can at times be provided by a neighboring family, school teachers, and even childhood friends. Clergy can also play a significant role. The role of such "non-related" individuals is often strikingly evident in the lives of orphans and children displaced as a result of political turmoil and war.

Finally, there is the issue of the child's relationship with God. Putting aside the debate regarding the validity of God's existence, the fact remains that most children have a lively spiritual life (Coles 1990) and evolve an unconscious, and frequently conscious, intrapsychic "God representation" (Rizzuto 2001) over the course of their development. This representation and the hopes, wishes, and fears attached to it are deeply connected with the child's "real" object relations, narcissistic balance, metabolism of aggression, and defensive structure. Under libidinally fortunate circumstances, the God representation provides a sense of union and belonging (like a mother) and reinforces the dictates of superego and aspirations of ego ideal (like a father). In the setting of a severely frustrating childhood, however, it is difficult to develop and sustain such a soothing internal object. The God representation then becomes hyperinvested with threatening powers. Belief in God can thus be emotionally sustaining or narcissistically injurious depending on the intrapsychic libido-aggression economy. In fact, both the child's (and subsequent adult's) belief in God and disbelief in God have normal and pathological variants.

> Belief in God seems healthy and normal if it emanates from identification with loving parents who were God-believing and if such belief provides personal soothing and intrapsychic coherence. Belief in God seems pathological if harshness assigned to him is used by a punitive superego to torment the ego or if the specificity and intensity of a particular religion leads to prejudice and loathing of those belonging to a different faith. Disbelief in God seems healthy if it emanates from identification with loving, atheistic parents and is accompanied by the capacity for faith in the secular institutions of nation, love, work, parenting, and so on. Disbelief in God seems pathological if it represents cynicism, inner faithlessness, and psychic unbelonging on a wider basis. (Parens and Akhtar 2001, p. 15)

From Interaction to Internalization

The foregoing passages describe a multitude of relationships that a child develops as he or she travels along his or her formative years. While the intrapsychic impact of these has been noted, the descriptive slant so far has been toward interactions in reality. Now the other pole of this spectrum—namely, the internalization of these interpersonal relationships and its role in the formation of the intrapsychic world—will be highlighted. In order to do so, the forms, processes, and metabolism of such internalization need to be taken into account.

Formal Aspects of Internalization

As far as the form is concerned, originally it was thought that the attitudes and dictates of important others in the environment become part of the growing child's psyche. This gives content to the individual's conscience ("superego") and a characteristic style ("ego") to his or her way of managing the demands of internal and external reality. Freud's celebrated phrase that the "ego is a precipitate of abandoned object cathexes" (1923, p. 29) refers to this last-mentioned point. As psychoanalytic theory evolved, however, it became clear that it is not only the dictates of early objects that are internalized but also the objects themselves. The purpose of this process was to bring the dialogue with the object under one's omnipotence. The notion of "internal objects" (Klein 1940/1975) was thus born.

In a further development of theory, it was noted that all internalizations are essentially dyadic in nature. In other words, each unit of internalization consists of an object and a portion of ego, with the two being engaged in an affectively significant interaction. Fairbairn (1940/1952) was the first to propose this idea in the context of his conceptualizations of schizoid phenomena. He posited that when an internalized object is repressed, the portion of ego that is in dialogue with that object also gets repressed. With Hartmann's (1950/1964) distinction of the "self" and the "ego," the wording of this conceptualization moved from ego-object constellation to self-object constellation. Finally, the notions of self representation and object representation (emphasizing that these were intrapsychic constructs and not externally observable entities) were introduced by Jacobson (1964). As a result, the unit of internalization came to be viewed as comprising a self representation engaged in an affective dialogue with an object representation. More recently, the emphasis has begun to shift from the two structural components to the affective or cognitive relational exchange between them.

Processes of Internalization

In order to meaningfully internalize object relationships, the early ego must accomplish two essential tasks (Kernberg 1967, 1975, 1987). The first is the differentiation of self images from object images. The accomplishment of this task depends on the maturation of primary autonomous functions, as well as on the gratification and/or frustration of early instinctual needs, since "libidinal gratification draws attention cathexes to the interaction between self and objects and fosters the differentiation in that area, and because frustration brings to awareness the painful absence of the fulfilling objects and thus contributes to differentiate self from non-self" (Kernberg 1975, p. 26).

The second task for the developing ego is to integrate the self and object images built under the libidinal drives with self and object images built under the influence of aggressive drives. In the beginning, the self and object images formed under the loving influences exist separately from those built under depriving influences. The experience of the self is simplistic and often contradictory, being overly dependent on the affects related to gratification or the lack of it from an external object. However, with growing memory skills, increasing synthetic ability of the ego, manageable amounts of constitutional aggression, and a predominance of "good" introjects, the two contradictory self images are mended. Partial introjections and identifications along libidinal and aggressive lines coalesce. The resulting ambivalent but deeper and realistic view of the self forms the rudimentary substratum of one's identity.

The concomitant deepening of the awareness of others as distinct and unique individuals facilitates more varied interactions with them than were hitherto possible. Meanwhile, the discovery of anatomical differences between the sexes lays the foundation of gender identity, and the vicissitudes of the oedipal phase give that identity a more refined object-related direction. Through these developments and interactions in later childhood, the earlier concrete identifications with parents are replaced by more selective identifications with parental roles, ideals, and prohibitions. In other words, identifications are now not with an object per se but with a particular relation to an object within which the child internally preserves the respective roles of both the self and the object while developing the capacity to reenact either of these roles later on. Identity, thus enriched, is finally consolidated in adolescence, when further individuation takes place through "disidentification" with primary objects, role clarification, and psychosexual self-definition. In this process, individual identifications become "depersonified" (Jacobson 1964)—that is, they lose their concrete similarities with their original sources. This selective repudiation and mutual assimilation of earlier identifications leads to a new psychic configuration, the ego identity.

Metabolism of Internalization

Though all object relations theorists agree that the intrapsychic world is constructed from the internalization of self-object relations, there is disagreement over the extent to which actual experiences of childhood are transformed by internal affects, drives, and unconscious fantasy. At one conceptual pole of the controversy is Klein (1937/1975, 1940/1975), who emphasizes the drive-impelled, "phantasy" nature of the internalized world of object relations. At the other pole are interpersonal analysts like Sullivan (1953), who view the internalized object relations as an unmodified reflection of actual childhood relationships. Occupying an intermediate place in this spectrum of theorizing are Jacobson (1964) and Kernberg (1975, 1987), who propose that while actual relationships of the child do give rise to them, internal object relations in an adult personality are not an exact replica of the former. Internalizations are affected by the state of the ego apparatuses and the economy (e.g., intensity, neutralization) of drives. Indeed, the drives themselves might be superordinate motivational systems derived from the coalescence of peak affective exchanges between self and object during the earliest periods of development (Kernberg 1987). Psychic structures therefore only partially reflect the external reality contributing to them. A strict superego, for instance, is as readily traceable to harsh parents as it is to the child's hostility toward them that leads their injunctions to appear excessively rigid and frightening in the first place.

Two other matters—possibly overlapping but having different domains and purposes—need to be taken into account: the concepts of "fitting together" (Hartmann 1939/1958) and "unconscious fantasy" (Arlow 1969). The synthetic function of the ego always seeks to construct as harmonious a gestalt as possible from the various introjections and identifications. Ill-fitting parts, if not huge and powerful, are repressed and a relatively smooth, conscious, central core of psychic reality is established. Rationalization is employed to give this conscious topography a nod from logic and reason. After all, the individual has got to ensure not only a sense of safety (Sandler 1960a, 1960b) but also a sense of sanity for himself or herself. One way or the other, things have to "fit together."

Next is the role of fantasy. While in Kleinian theory the term "phantasy" is used for a metaphorical description of instinctual activity (Hayman 1989), the customary ego psychology use of "fantasy" is different. It refers to the imaginative elaboration of existential statements ("I am...") or discursive stories ("I do..." or "He/She does...") that respectively express narcissistic and object-related agendas. Such audiovisual scenarios are evolved in order to fill gaps in actual knowledge of causes of events as well as to defend against anxiety, discharge instinctual tensions, and practice growth strivings. They incorporate actual tidbits of childhood experience as well as concessions to the pleadings of instinctual desire. Moral dictates can also be incorporated into the fantasy, and so can aspects of current realities. However, these are often diluted and circumvented in order to fulfill self- and object-related needs and wishes. The resultant compromise formations appear as palatable versions of organizing fantasies (e.g., daydreams, life goals) in the consciousness. The unrealistic, archaic, and morally repugnant aspects undergo repression. They often continue to exert dynamic influence on affect and behavior in the form of an organizing unconscious fantasy (Arlow 1969). The impact of such subterranean convictions and longings on subsequent choices of vocation and life partners is often striking.

Conclusion

In this chapter, I have provided a wide-ranging survey of the growing child's relationship with a multitude of objects in his or her animate and inanimate surround. In delineating these relationships and their impact on the child, I have paid equal attention to the actual external events during the formative years and their intrapsychic storage ("internalization") and elaborations. The relationship with the mother and father has been noted to be at the developmental center

of the child's life, with mother providing union, safety, validity, esteem and trust, and father offering separateness, exploratory vigor, moral restraint, and future orientation. Of course, the psychic contributions of the two parents overlap and the sharpness of above-mentioned distinctions is largely for didactic purposes. In addition, the parental couple, as an entity in its own right, offers the child a measure of tolerance of exclusion while laying the groundwork of incest barrier and respect for generational differences.

The growing child is also affected by his or her relationships with siblings, grandparents, and extended family members. These relationships offer their own psychological benefits, including the potential for ameliorating the deficiencies and disturbances in the child-parent relationship. Steprelatives, non–family members, and even the animals and ecological surround of the child help him or her grow, express, mentalize, and metabolize his or her intrapsychic goings-on. The child's inner dialogue with representation of divine figures also provides an avenue for working out conflicts and sustaining hope in face of difficult developmental tasks.

All these internal objects together give form, style, strength, and content to the child's psychic reality. While certainly undergoing revision and updating as the development continues, these very internal objects (and the relational dialogue between them and the child) are replicated in choices of friends and lovers, in work and sublimations, and in clinical transferences. However, such re-creations are not linearly traceable to childhood, since adult charcterological process are infinitely more subtle, have accommodated much "change of function," and are vulnerable to defensive compromises of memory when it comes to their alleged origins.

In the end, therefore, we are left with an existential paradox. On the one hand, the early relationships of a child have indelible impact on him or her. They give his or her character its specific texture and its unique coloration. They seem to dictate his or her destiny. On the other hand, if early relationships have been largely favorable, they also give rise to the potential for autonomy, individuation, spontaneity, new learning, and change. In other words, belonging produces freedom. A solid psychic anchor frees one to float on the waves of life's ocean. A loved and loving child grows up to meet the world with that hallmark of mental health: disciplined fearlessness.

References

Abelin EL: The role of the father in the separation-individuation process, in Separation-Individuation: Essays in Honor of Margaret Mahler. Edited by McDevitt JB, Settlage CF. New York, International Universities Press, 1971, pp 229–253

Abend S: Sibling love and object choice. Psychoanal Q 38:425–430, 1984

Abraham K: Some remarks on the role of grandparents in the psychology of the neuroses (1913), in Clinical Papers and Essays on Psychoanalysis. New York, Brunner/Mazel, 1955, pp 44–47

Ainslie R: The Psychology of Twinship. Northvale, NJ, Jason Aronson, 1997

Akhtar S: Tethers, orbits, and invisible fences: clinical, developmental, socio-cultural and technical aspects of optimal distance, in When the Body Speaks: Psychological Meanings in Kinetic Clues. Edited by Kramer S, Akhtar S. Northvale, NJ, Jason Aronson, 1992, pp 21–57

Akhtar S: Immigration and Identity: Turmoil, Treatment, and Transformation. Northvale, NJ, Jason Aronson, 1999

Akhtar S: Things are us: a friendly rejoinder to Marianne Spitzform's paper "The ecological self: metaphor and developmental experience." Journal of Applied Psychoanalytic Studies 3:205–210, 2001

Akhtar S: Things: developmental, psychopathological, and technical aspects of inanimate objects. Canadian Journal of Psychoanalysis 11:1–44, 2003

Akhtar S, Brown J: Animals in psychiatric symptomatology, in The Mental Zoo: Animals in the Human Mind and Its Pathology. Madison, CT, International Universities Press, 2005, pp 3–38

Akhtar S, Kramer S: Brothers and Sisters: Developmental, Dynamic, and Technical Aspects of the Sibling Relationship. Northvale, NJ, Jason Aronson, 1999

Arlow J: Unconscious fantasy and disturbances of conscious experience. Psychoanal Q 38:1–27, 1969

Balint M: Thrills and Regressions. London, Hogarth Press, 1959

Benjamin J: The Bonds of Love: Psychoanalysis, Feminism, and the Problem of Domination. New York, Pantheon, 1988

Bernstein D: The female superego: a different perspective. Int J Psychoanal 64:187–200, 1983

Bion WR: Second Thoughts. New York, Jason Aronson, 1967

Blos P: On Adolescence. New York, Free Press, 1962

Blos P: The initial stage of male adolescence. Psychoanal Study Child 20:145–164, 1965

Blos P: The second individuation process of adolescence. Psychoanal Study Child 22:162–186, 1967

Blos P: The genealogy of the ego ideal. Psychoanal Study Child 29:43–88, 1974

Blos P: Son and Father: Before and Beyond the Oedipus Complex. New York, Free Press, 1985

Bonovitz J: Reflections of the self in the cultural looking glass, in The Colors of Childhood: Separation-Individuation Across Cultural, Racial, and Ethnic Differences. Edited by Akhtar S, Kramer S. Northvale, NJ, Jason Aronson, 1998, pp 169–188

Brenner I: The contemporary stepfather's search for legitimacy, in Stepparenting: Creating and Recreating Families in America Today. Edited by Cath SM, Shopper M. Hillsdale, NJ, Analytic Press, 2001, pp 69–80

Burland A: A cinematic zoo, in The Cultural Zoo: Animals in the Human Mind and Its Sublimations. Edited by Akhtar S, Volkan VD. Madison, CT, International Universities Press (in press)

Cath SH: Readiness for grandfatherhood and the shifting tide, in Fathers and Their Families. Edited by Casth S, Gruwitt A, Gunsberg L. Hillsdale, NJ, Analytic Press, 1989, pp 99–120

Cath SH, Shopper M: Stepparenting: Creating and Recreating Families in America Today. Hillsdale, NJ, Analytic Press, 2001

Chasseguet-Smirgel J: The Ego Ideal: A Psychoanalytic Essay on the Malady of the Ideal. New York, WW Norton, 1985

Chodorow NJ: Femininities, Masculinities, Sexualities. Lexington, The University Press of Kentucky, 1994

Colarusso CA: Separation-individuation processes in middle adulthood, in The Seasons of Life: Separation-Individuation Perspectives. Edited by Akhtar S, Kramer S, Northvale, NJ, Jason Aronson, 1997, pp 73–94

Coles R: The Spiritual Life of Children. Boston, MA, Houghton Mifflin, 1990

Emde R (ed): Rene A. Spitz, Dialogues From Infancy: Selected Papers. New York, International Universities Press, 1984

Erikson EH: Childhood and Society. New York, WW Norton, 1950

Fairbairn WRD: Schizoid factors in the personality, in An Object-Relations Theory of the Personality. New York, Basic Books, 1954, pp 3–27

Fenichel O: The Psychoanalytic Theory of Neurosis. New York, WW Norton, 1945

Fischer N: The psychoanalytic experience and psychic change. Paper presented at the 27th Congress of International Psychoanalytical Association, Buenos Aires, Argentina, August 1991

Fonagy P, Target M: Attachment and reflective function: their role in self-organization. Dev Psychopathol 9:679–700, 1997

Fox ND, Kimmerly NC, Schafer WD: Attachment to mother/attachment to father: a meta-analysis. Child Development 67:541–555, 1991

Freud A: The concept of developmental lines. Psychoanal Study Child 18:245–265, 1963

Freud A: Normality and pathology in childhood (1965), in The Writings of Anna Freud, Vol 6. New York, International Universities Press, 1974, pp 25–63

Freud S: Project for a scientific psychology (1895), in Standard Edition of the Complete Psychological Works of Sigmund Freud, Vol 1. Translated and edited by Strachey J. London, Hogarth Press, 1955, pp 283–398

Freud S: The interpretation of dreams (1900), in Standard Edition of the Complete Psychological Works of Sigmund Freud, Vols 4 and 5. Translated and edited by Strachey J. London, Hogarth Press, 1953

Freud S: On the sexual theories of children (1908), in Standard Edition of the Complete Psychological Works of Sigmund Freud, Vol 9. Translated and edited by Strachey J. London, Hogarth Press, 1959, pp 205–226

Freud S: Analysis of a phobia in a five-year-old boy (1909a), in Standard Edition of the Complete Psychological Works of Sigmund Freud, Vol 10. Translated and edited by Strachey J. London, Hogarth Press, 1955, pp 1–149

Freud S: Notes upon a case of obsessional neurosis (1909b), in Standard Edition of the Complete Psychological Works of Sigmund Freud, Vol 10. Translated and edited by Strachey J. London, Hogarth Press, 1955, pp 151–318

Freud S: A special type of object choice made by men (1910), in Standard Edition of the Complete Psychological Works of Sigmund Freud, Vol 11. Translated and edited by Strachey J. London, Hogarth Press, 1955, pp 163–175

Freud S: Types of onset of neurosis (1912), in Standard Edition of the Complete Psychological Works of Sigmund Freud, Vol 12. Translated and edited by Strachey J. London, Hogarth Press, 1958, pp 231–238

Freud S: Totem and taboo (1913), in Standard Edition of the Complete Psychological Works of Sigmund Freud, Vol 13. Translated and edited by Strachey J. London, Hogarth Press, 1958, pp 1–161

Freud S: A childhood memory from Dichtung und Wahrheit (1917), in Standard Edition of the Complete Psychological Works of Sigmund Freud, Vol 17. Translated and edited by Strachey J. London, Hogarth Press, 1961, pp 145–156

Freud S: From the history of an infantile neurosis (1918), in Standard Edition of the Complete Psychological Works of Sigmund Freud, Vol 17. Translated and edited by Strachey J. London, Hogarth Press, 1961, pp 1–122

Freud S: The psychogenesis of a case of homosexuality in a woman (1920), in Standard Edition of the Complete Psychological Works of Sigmund Freud, Vol 18. Translated and edited by Strachey J. London, Hogarth Press, 1955, pp 145–174

Freud S: The ego and the id (1923), in Standard Edition of the Complete Psychological Works of Sigmund Freud, Vol 19. Translated and edited by Strachey J. London, Hogarth Press, 1961, pp 1–66

Freud S: The dissolution of the Oedipus complex (1924), in Standard Edition of the Complete Psychological Works of Sigmund Freud, Vol 19. Translated and edited by Strachey J. London, Hogarth Press, 1961, pp 173–182

Freud S: Some psychical consequences of the anatomical distinction between the sexes (1925), in Standard Edition of the Complete Psychological Works of Sigmund Freud, Vol 19. Translated and edited by Strachey J. London, Hogarth Press, 1961, pp 241–258

Freud S: Civilization and its discontents (1930), in Standard Edition of the Complete Psychological Works of Sigmund Freud, Vol 21. Translated and edited by Strachey J. London, Hogarth Press, 1957, pp 57–145

Frosch J: A note on reality constancy, in Psychoanalysis: A General Psychology—Essays in Honor of Heinz Hartmann. Edited by Loewenstein RM, Newman LM, Schur M, et al. New York, International Universities Press, 1964, pp 349–376

Furman E: Mothers have to be there to be left. Psychoanal Study Child 37:15–41, 1982

Garfield R: Making a case for father hunger in girls, in Real and Imaginary Fathers: Development, Transference, and Healing. Edited by Akhtar S, Parens H. Northvale, NJ, Jason Aronson, 2004, pp 34–44

Glenn J: Transformations in normal and pathological latency, in Beyond the Symbiotic Orbit: Advances in Separation-Individuation Theory—Essays in Honor of Selma Kramer. Edited by Akhtar S, Parens H. Hillsdale, NJ, Analytic Press, 1991, pp 171–188

Greenson RR: Disidentifying from the mother. Int J Psychoanal 49:370–374, 1968

Hartmann H: Ego Psychology and the Problem of Adaptation (1939). Translated by Rapaport D. New York, International Universities Press, 1958

Hartmann H: Comments on the psychoanalytic theory of the ego (1950), in Essays on Ego Psychology. New York, International Universities Press, 1964, pp 113–141

Hayman A: What do we mean by "phantasy?" Int J Psychoanal 70:105–114, 1989

Herzog J: Fathers and young children: fathering daughters and fathering sons, in Foundations of Infant Psychiatry, Vol 2. Edited by Call JD, Galenson E, Tyson R. New York, Basic Books, 1984, pp 335–343

Jacobson E: The Self and the Object World. New York, International Universities Press, 1964

Jelliffe SE, Brink AB: The role of animals in the unconscious with some remarks on theriomorphic symbolism as seen in Ovid. Psychoanal Rev 4:253–271, 1917

Kagan J, Moss HA: Birth to Maturity. New York, Wiley, 1962

Kernberg OF: Borderline personality organization. J Am Psychoanal Assoc 15:641–685, 1967

Kernberg OF: Borderline Conditions and Pathological Narcissism. New York, Jason Aronson, 1975

Kernberg OF: Ego psychology: object relations theory of transference. Psychoanal Q 56:197–213, 1987

Klein M: Love, guilt, and reparation (1937), in Love, Guilt, and Reparation and Other Works. New York, Free Press, 1975, pp 306–343

Klein M: Mourning and its relation to manic-depressive states (1940), in Love, Guilt, and Reparation and Other Works. New York, Free Press, 1975, pp 344–369

Krueger D, Krueger L: Animals in children's stories, in The Cultural Zoo: Animals in the Human Mind and Its Sublimations. Edited by Akhtar S, Volkan VD. Madison, CT, International Universities Press (in press)

Lamb MD: The development of father-infant relationships, in The Role of the Father in Child Development. Edited by Lamb MD. New York, Wiley, 1997, pp 459–488

Lax R: The role of internalization in the development of certain aspects of female masochism. Int J Psychoanal 58:289–300, 1977

Lichtenberg JD: Psychoanalysis and Infant Research. Hillsdale, NJ, Analytic Press, 1983

Lichtenstein H: The dilemma of human identity: notes on self-transformation, self-objectivation, and metamorphosis. J Am Psychoanal Assoc 11:173–223, 1963

Loewald HW: Ego and reality. Int J Psychoanal 32:10–21, 1951

Mahler MS: On human symbiosis and the vicissitudes of individuation. J Am Psychoanal Assoc 15:740–763, 1967

Mahler MS, Furer M: On Human Symbiosis and the Vicissitudes of Individuation. New York, International Universities Press, 1968

Mahler MS, Gosliner BJ: On symbiotic child psychosis: genetic, dynamic, and restitutive aspects. Psychoanal Study Child 10:195–212, 1955

Mahler MS, Bergmann A, Pine F: The Psychological Birth of the Human Infant: Symbiosis and Individuation. New York, Basic Books, 1975

McDonald M: Not by the Color of their Skin. New York, International Universities Press, 1970

Muir R: Fatherhood from the perspective of object relations theory and relational systems theory, in Fathers and Their Families. Edited by Cath SH, Gurwitt A, Gunsberg L. Hillsdale, NJ, Analytic Press, 1989, pp 47–61

Neubauer PB: The importance of the sibling experience. Psychoanal Study Child 38:325–336, 1983

Pacella B: The primal matrix configuration, in Rapprochement: The Critical Subphase of Separation-Individuation. Edited by Lax RF, Bach S, Burland JA. New York, Jason Aronson, 1980, pp 117–131

Parens H: Siblings in early childhood: some direct observational findings. Psychoanalytic Inquiry 8:31–50, 1988

Parens H, Akhtar S: Is God a subject for psychoanalysis? in Does God Help? Developmental and Clinical Aspects of Religious Belief. Northvale, NJ, Jason Aronson, 2001, pp 1–17

Piaget J: Origins of Intelligence in Children (1936). New York, International Universities Press, 1952

Piontelli A: Infant observation from before birth. Int J Psychoanal 68:453–463, 1987

Piontelli A: Prenatal life reflected in the analysis of a psychotic girl at age two. International Review of Psychoanalysis 15:73–81, 1988

Provence S, Solnit AJ: Development-promoting aspects of the sibling experience. Psychoanal Study Child 38:337–351, 1983

Pruett K: The Nurturing Father. New York, Warner Books, 1988

Pruett K: Fatherhood. New York, Free Press, 2000

Renik O: Analytic interaction: conceptualizing technique in light of the analyst's irreducible subjectivity. Psychoanal Q 62:553–571, 1993

Rizzuto A-M: Does God help? What God? Helping whom? The convolutions of divine help, in Does God Help? Developmental and Clinical Aspects of Religious Belief. Edited by Akhtar S, Parens H. Northvale, NJ, Jason Aronson, 2001, pp 19–52

Roland A: In Search of Self in India and Japan: Toward a Cross Cultural Psychology. Princeton, NJ, Princeton University Press, 1988

Ross JM: Fathering: a review of some psychoanalytic contributions on paternity. Int J Psychoanal 60:317–327, 1979

Ross JM: Oedipus revisited: Laius and the Laius complex. Psychoanal Study Child 37:169–192, 1982

Ross JM: The eye of the beholder: on the developmental dialogue between fathers and daughters, in New Dimensions in Adult Development. Edited by Nemiroff RA, Colarusso CA. New York, Basic Books, 1990, pp 47–72

Ross JM: What Men Want. Cambridge, MA, Harvard University Press, 1994

Ross JM: Male infidelity in long marriages: second adolescences and fourth individuations, in Intimacy and Infidelity: Separation-Individuation Perspectives. Edited by Akhtar S, Kramer S. Northvale, NJ, Jason Aronson, 1996, pp 107–130

Sandler J: Countertransference and role-responsiveness. Int Rev Psychoanal 3:43–47, 1960a

Sandler J: The background of safety. Int J Psychoanal 41:352–363, 1960b

Sandler J: Countertransference and role-responsiveness. Int Rev Psychoanal 3:43–47, 1976

Schowalter J: The use and abuse of pets. J Am Acad Child Psychiatry 22:68–72, 1983

Searles HF: The Non-Human Environment in Normal Development and Schizophrenia. New York, International Universities Press, 1960

Sharpe SA, Rosenblatt AD: Oedipal sibling triangles. J Am Psychoanal Assoc 42:491–523, 1994

Sherick I: The significance of pets for children. Psychoanal Study Child 36:193–215, 1981

Solnit AJ: The sibling experience. Psychoanal Study Child 38:281–284, 1983

Spence DP: Narrative Truth and Historical Truth. New York, WW Norton, 1982

Spitz R: Life and the dialogue (1963), in Rene A. Spitz, Dialogues From Infancy: Selected Papers. Edited by Emde R. New York, International Universities Press, 1983, pp 147–160

Stern DN: The First Relationship: Infant and Mother. Cambridge, MA, Harvard University Press, 1977

Stern DN: The Interpersonal World of the Infant: A View From Psychoanalysis and Developmental Psychology. New York, Basic Books, 1985

Sullivan HS: The Interpersonal Theory of Psychiatry. Edited by Perry HS, Gawel ML. New York, WW Norton, 1953

Tessman LH: A note on the father's contribution to the daughters way of loving and working, in Father and Child. Edited by Cath S, Gurwitt A, Ross JM. Boston, MA, Little Brown, 1982, pp 13–37

Thomas A, Chess S: Temperament and Development. New York, Brunner/Mazel, 1977

Thomas A, Chess S, Birch H, et al: Behavioral Individuality in Early Childhood. New York, New York University Press, 1963

Volkan VD, Ast G: Siblings in the Unconscious and Psychopathology. Madison, CT, International Universities Press, 1997

Waelder R: The psychoanalytic theory of play. Psychiatr Q 2:208–212, 1936

Weil AM: The basic core. Psychoanal Study Child 25:442–460, 1970

Winnicott DW: Transitional objects and transitional phenomena: a study of the first not-me possession. Int J Psychoanal 34: 89–97, 1953

Winnicott DW: Ego distortion in the terms of true and false self (1960a), in The Maturational Processes and the Facilitating Environment. New York, International Universities Press, 1965, pp 140–152

Winnicott DW: The theory of parent-infant relationship. Int J Psychoanal 41:585–595, 1960b

Winnicott DW: String: a technique of communication (1960c), in The Maturational Processes and the Facilitating Environment. New York, International Universities Press, 1965, pp 153–157

Winnicott DW: Ego integration in child development (1962), in The Maturational Processes and the Facilitating Environment. New York, International Universities Press, 1965

Winnicott DW: Playing and Reality. New York, Basic Books, 1971

Wright K: Vision and Separation: Between Mother and Baby. Northvale, NJ, Jason Aronson, 1991

Yamamoto J, Wagatsuma H: The Japanese and the Japanese American. Journal of Operational Psychiatry 11:120–135, 1980

Yogman MW: Observations on the father-infant relationship, in Father and Child: Developmental and Clinical Perspectives. Edited by Cath SM, Gurwitt A, Gunsberg L. Boston, MA, Little, Brown, 1982, pp 101–122

4

Object Relations Theories and Technique

OTTO F. KERNBERG, M.D.

Object Relations Theories

Basic Concepts

The basic assumption of contemporary object relations theories is that all internalizations of relationships with significant others, from the beginning of life on, have different characteristics under the conditions of peak affect interactions and low affect interactions. Under conditions of low affect activation, reality-oriented, perception-controlled cognitive learning takes place, influenced by temperamental dispositions (i.e., the affective, cognitive, and motor reactivity of the infant), leading to differentiated, gradually evolving definitions of self and others. These definitions start out from the perception of bodily functions, the position of the self in space and time, and the permanent characteristics of others. As these perceptions are integrated and become more complex, interactions with others are cognitively registered and evaluated, and working models of them are established. Inborn capacities to differentiate self from nonself, and the capacity for cross-modal transfer of sensorial experience, play an important part in the construction of the model of self and the surrounding world.

In contrast, under conditions of peak affect activation—be they of an extremely positive, pleasurable or an extremely negative, painful mode—specific internalizations take place framed by the dyadic nature of the interaction between the baby and the caretaking person, leading to the setting up of specific affective memory structures with powerful motivational implications. These structures are constituted, essentially, by a representation of self interacting with a representation of significant other under the dominance of a peak affect state. The importance of these affective memory structures lies in their constituting the basis of the primary psychic motivational system, in the direction of efforts to approach, maintain, or increase the conditions that generate peak positive affect states, and to decrease, avoid, and escape from conditions of peak negative affect states.

Positive affect states involve the sensuous gratification of the satisfied baby at the breast, erotic stimulation of the skin, and the disposition to euphoric "in tune" interactions with mother; peak negative affective states involve situations of intense physical pain or hunger, or painful stimuli that trigger intense reactions of rage, fear, or disgust, that may motivate general irritability and hypersensitivity to frustration and pain. Object relations theory assumes that these positive and negative affective memories are built up separately in the early internalization of these experiences and, later, are actively split or dissociated from each other in an effort to maintain an ideal domain of experience of the relation between self and others and to escape from the frightening experiences of negative affect states. Negative affect states tend to be projected, to evolve into the fear of "bad" external objects, while positive affect states evolve into the memory of a relationship with "ideal" objects. This development evolves into two major, mutually split domains of early psychic experience, an idealized and a persecutory or paranoid one—idealized in the sense of a segment of purely positive representations of self and other, and persecutory in the sense of a segment of purely negative representations of other and threatened representation of self. This early split experience protects the idealized experiences from "contamination" with bad ones, until a higher degree of tolerance of pain and more realistic assessment of external reality under painful conditions evolve.

This early stage of development of psychic representations of self and other, with primary motivational implications (i.e., move toward pleasure and away from pain), eventually evolves toward the integration of these two peak affect determined segments, an integration facilitated by the development of cognitive capacities and ongoing learning regarding realistic aspects of self and others interacting under circumstances of low affect activation. The normal predominance of the idealized experiences leads to a tolerance of integrating the paranoid ones, while neutralizing them in the process. In simple terms, the child recognizes that it has both "good' and "bad" aspects, and so do mother and the significant others of the immediate family circle, while the good aspects predominate sufficiently to tolerate an integrated view of self and others.

This state of development, referred to by Kleinian authors (Klein 1940/1948; Segal 1964/1988) as the shift from the paranoid-schizoid to the depressive position, and by ego psychological authors as the shift into object constancy, presumably takes place somewhere between the end of the first year of life and the end of the third year of life. Here Margaret Mahler's (Mahler and Furer 1972a, 1972b) research on separation-individuation is relevant, pointing to the gradual nature of this integration over the first 3 years of life. At the same time, however, in the light of contemporary infant research, Margaret Mahler's notion of an initial autistic phase of development followed by a symbiotic phase of development seems contradicted by the nature of the evidence. Rather than an emphasis on the symbiotic stage of development, what seems relevant are "symbiotic" moments of fantasized fusion between self representation and object representation under peak affect conditions, momentary fusions that are counteracted by the inborn capacity to differentiate self from nonself, and the real and fantasized intervention of "third excluded others," particularly the representation of father disrupting the states of momentary symbiotic unity between infant and mother. Here mother's capacity to represent a "third excluded other" becomes important: French authors have stressed the importance of the image of the father in the mother's mind.

Peter Fonagy's (Fonagy and Target 2003) referral to the findings regarding mother's capacity to "mark" the infant's affect that she congruently reflects to the infant points to a related process: mother's contingent (accurate) mirroring of the infant's affect, which, as a marked (differentiated) signaling that she does not share it and yet empathizes with it, contributes to the infant's assimilating his or her own affect while marking the boundary between self and other. Under normal conditions, then, an integrated sense of self ("good and bad"), and the surrounding integrated representations of significant others ("good and bad") that are also differentiated in terms of their gender characteristics as well as their status/role characteristics, jointly determine normal identity.

The concept of ego identity originally formulated by Erikson (1950/1959, 1956/1959) included in its definition the integration of the concept of the self. An object relations approach expands this definition with the corresponding integration of the concepts of significant others. In contrast, when this developmental stage of normal identity integration is not reached, the earlier developmental stage of dissociation or splitting between an idealized and a persecutory segment of experience persists. Under these conditions, multiple, nonintegrated representations of self split into an idealized and a persecutory segment, and multiple representations of significant others split along similar lines, jointly constituting the syndrome of identity diffusion. One might argue that, to the extent that Erikson considered confirmation of the self by the representations of significant others as an aspect of normal identity, he already stressed the relevance of that relationship between the self concept and the concept of significant others. However, he did not as yet conceive of the intimate connection between the integration or lack of it on the part of the concepts of self and the parallel achievement or failure in the corresponding concepts of others. It was the work of Jacobson (1964) and the work of Ronald Fairbairn (1954) in Great Britain, who pointed to the dyadic nature of the development of early internalizations, that created the basis for the contemporary psychoanalytic object relations theory.

This formulation of the internalization of dyadic units under the impact of peak affect states has significant implications for the psychoanalytic theory of drives, for the understanding of the etiology of identity diffusion, and for the psychoanalytic psychotherapy of severe personality disorders or borderline personality organization. Regarding the psychoanalytic theory of drives, this formulation supports the proposal I have formulated in recent years (Kernberg 1984, 1992) that affects are the primary motivational system and that Freud's dual-drive theory of libido and aggression corresponds, respectively, to the hierarchically supraordinate integration of positive and negative affect states. The integration of affects determines the functions of the drives, and the drives, in turn, are manifest in each concrete instance in the activation of an affect state that links a certain representation of self with a certain representation of object. These include the wishful and frightening erotic fantasies of highly desired and potentially forbidden relationships between self and others, as well as highly threatening and potentially disorganizing fantasies of aggressive relationships.

Alternative Object Relations Theories

Psychoanalytic object relations theories include so broad a spectrum of approaches that it might be said that psychoanalysis itself, by its very nature, is an object relations theory: all psychoanalytic theorizing deals, after all, with the impact of early object relations on the genesis of unconscious conflict, the development of psychic structure, and the reactualization or enactments of past pathogenic internalized object relations in transference developments in the current psychoanalytic situation. The narrowest definition would restrict object relations theory to the so-called British School, particularly as exemplified in the work of Melanie Klein (1940/1948, 1946, 1957), Ronald Fairbairn (1954), and Donald Winnicott (1958, 1965, 1971).

A third definition of what constitutes object relations theory—my own—would include the British School and the contributions from ego psychology by Erik Erikson (1950/1959, 1956/1959), Edith Jacobson (1964, 1971), Margaret Mahler (Mahler and Furer 1968; Mahler et al. 1975), Hans Loewald (1980), Otto Kernberg (1976, 1980, 1984), and Joseph Sandler (1987), as well as the interpersonal approach of Harry Stack Sullivan (1953, 1962) and Greenberg and Mitchell (1983; Mitchell 1988). Psychoanalytic object relations theories could then be defined as those that place the internalization, structuralization, and clinical reactivation (in the transference and countertransference) of the earliest dyadic object relations at the center of their motivational (genetic and developmental), structural, and clinical formulations. Internalization of object relations refers to the concept that in all interactions of the infant and child with the significant parental figures, what the infant internalizes is not an image or representation of the other ("the object"), but *the relationship between the self and the other* in the form of a self image or self representation interacting with an object image or object representation. This internal structure replicates in the intrapsychic world both real and fantasized relationships with significant others. This third definition constitutes the frame for what follows.

The various object relations theorists differ on several major issues. The most important is the extent to which the theory is perceived as harmonious with or in opposition to Freud's traditional drive theory (Freud 1920/1955, 1923/1961, 1933/1964)—that is, whether object relations are seen as supplementing or supplanting drives as the motivational system for human behavior. From this perspective, Klein, as well as Mahler and Jacobson, occupies one pole, combining Freud's dual-drive theory with an object relations approach. For Fairbairn and Sullivan, on the other hand, object relations replace Freud's drives as the major motivational system. Contemporary interpersonal psychoanalysis as represented by Greenberg and Mitchell (1983; Mitchell 1988), based on an integration of principally Fairbairnian (Fairbairn 1954) and Sullivanian (Sullivan 1953, 1962) concepts, asserts the essential incompatibility of drive-based and object relations–based models of psychic motivational systems. Winnicott (1958, 1965, 1971), Loewald (1980), and Sandler (1987) maintain an intermediate posture (for different reasons); they perceive the affective frame of the infant-mother relationship as a crucial determinant in shaping the development of drives: Although I adhere to Freud's dual-drive theory, I consider drives to be supraordinate motivational systems, with affects their constituent components (Kernberg 1976, 1984).

A related controversy has to do with the origin and role of aggression as a motivator of behavior. Those theoreticians who reject the idea of inborn drives (Sullivan) or who equate libido with the search for object relations (Fairbairn) conceptualize aggression as secondary to the frustration of libidinal needs, particularly traumatic experiences in the early mother-infant dyad. (It should be noted, however, that although Fairbairn in theory rejected the idea of an inborn aggressive drive, in clinical practice he paid considerable attention to the structuralization of aggressively invested internalized object relations and their interpretation in the transference.) Theoreticians who adhere to Freud's dual-drive theory, in contrast, believe that aggression is inborn and plays an important part in shaping early interactions; this group includes Klein in particular and to some extent Winnicott and the ego psychology–object relations theoreticians.

Another controversy concerns the extent to which actual experiences with significant others in infancy and early childhood are seen as transformed by the combination of unconscious fantasy and the building of psychic structure that reflects intrapsychic conflicts. For the British School—in spite of the heavy emphasis of Winnicott and Fairbairn on the reality aspects of the early interactions between infant and mother—the effects of unconscious fantasy on the development of psychic structures and the defensive reshaping of structuralized internalized object relationships result in a significant gap between actual early experience and unconsciously reactivated object relations in the transference; the Kleinians insist on the fantastic nature of the internalized world of object relations. For interpersonal psychoanalysts, particularly Sullivan (1953, 1962), Fromm-Reichmann (1950), and Guntrip (1961, 1968), early internalized object relations are maintained with relatively little structural change, so that these theorists tend to interpret transference developments as fairly close reflections of actual traumatic object relations of the past. Along with Jacobson, Mahler, and Sandler, I occupy an intermediate realm in this respect, with a particular emphasis on the characterological transformations and fixations of internalized object relations.

The various theorists also differ in the extent to which they interpret transference enactments in terms of the activation of the patient's intrapsychic conflicts or as shaped in part by countertransference and the analyst's personality. The interpersonal or relational school views the patient-analyst dyad as a new, potentially growth-promoting experience that makes an important contribution to the resolution of the patient's unconscious conflicts.

Klein and her followers, as well as Jacobson, Mahler, and myself, are close to the classical position in emphasizing the intrapsychic conflicts aspects of the transference and making limited use of countertransference elements. (I focus more sharply than the others, however, on countertransference, especially in my treatment of severe character pathology.) Interpersonal psychoanalysis, as represented by Guntrip (1961, 1968) (who was influenced by Fairbairn and Winnicott) and Greenberg and Mitchell (1983; Mitchell 1988), places heavy emphasis on the mutual influence of transference and countertransference and the reality aspects of the therapeutic interactions derived from the analyst's personality.

Certain characteristics distinguish object relations theory in general from other approaches. My ego psychological–object relations theory differs from traditional ego psychology in emphasizing the indissoluble integration of drives with object relations. For Jacobson, Mahler, and myself, affects are not simply discharge manifestations of drives but sustained tension states that represent the drive derivative embedded in the relationship between self and object representation. In contrast, traditional ego psychology assumes a much looser relationship between drive derivatives and their investments in objects.

Ego psychology–object relations theory also focuses strongly on the early, preoedipal stages of development, while traditional ego psychology stresses oedipal conflicts. And while traditional ego psychology stresses the interplay of impulse and defense in terms of impersonal defense mechanisms directed against diffuse drive derivatives, ego psychology–object relations theory describes the impulse-defense equilibrium in terms of impulsively and defensively activated object relations in the transference

(and countertransference) (Kernberg 1987a, 1988). In addition, ego psychology–object relations theory focuses on the structural characteristics of the early ego-id matrix before the consolidation of the tripartite structure, particularly in exploring severe psychopathologies; in contrast, traditional ego psychology tends to explore all psychopathology within the frame of the tripartite structure.

Interpersonal object relations theory has significant similarities to Kohut's (1971, 1977) self psychology. In fact, Fairbairn, Winnicott, Kohut, and Sullivan all stress the reality aspects of good versus bad mothering and the influence of satisfactory early relationships of the infant and the mother in setting up the structure of the normal self. However, a basic difference between all object relations theories—including interpersonal psychoanalysis—and Kohut's self psychology is that Kohut's developmental model centers on the gradual consolidation of an archaic grandiose self in relation to idealized "self-objects," while all "bad" relationships are not conceptualized as internalized object relations; in Kohut's view, aggression is a disintegration product and not part of structured internalized object relations. In contrast to self psychology, object relations theories, even those that deny aggression as a drive (Fairbairn and Sullivan), stress the importance of the internalization of "bad" object relations—that is, aggressively invested, dissociated representations of self and objects. These differing formulations have significant impact on technique, particularly on the conceptualization and management of negative transferences.

Finally, object relations theory may be contrasted to French approaches, both Lacanian (Roudinesco 1990) and mainstream psychoanalysis (Oliner 1988). The latter has maintained close links with traditional psychoanalysis, including the British object relations theories. Insofar as Lacan (1966) conceptualized the unconscious as a natural language and focused on the cognitive aspects of unconscious development, he underemphasized affect—a dominant element of object relations theories. At the same time, however, in postulating a very early oedipal structuralization of all infant-mother interactions, Lacan emphasized archaic oedipal developments; this implicitly links his formulations with those of Klein. French mainstream psychoanalysis also focuses on archaic aspects of oedipal developments but places much more emphasis on Freud's dual-drive theory and on the affective nature of the early ego-id (Chasseguet-Smirgel 1986). But in that neither mainstream nor Lacanian psychoanalysis spells out specific structural consequences of dyadic internalized object relations, neither would fit the definition of object relations theory proposed in this chapter.

Object relations theories have several additional characteristics in common. They all focus on the influence of the vicissitudes of early developmental stages in the formation of the psychic apparatus. They are all interested in normal and pathological development of the self and in identity formation, and they all accept an internalized world of object relations as part of their conceptualization of the psychic apparatus. To the extent that object relations theories deal with the relationship of past and present intrapsychic and interpersonal object relations, they also provide links to family structure and group psychology. Their interest in the affective aspects of the relationship between self and object, between self representations and object representations, leads object relations theories to a particular concern with the origin and vicissitudes of early affect. This, in turn, provides a linkage between object relations theory, empirical research on affect development, and neurophysiology.

All object relations theories focus heavily on the enactment of internalized object relations in the transference and on the analysis of countertransference in the development of interpretive strategies. They are particularly concerned with patients with severe psychopathologies, including psychotic patients who are still approachable with psychoanalytic techniques and those with borderline conditions, severe narcissistic character pathology, and the perversions. Object relations theories explore primitive defensive operations and object relations both in cases of severe psychopathology and at points of severe regression with all patients.

Melanie Klein

Melanie Klein's (1940/1948, 1946) object relations theory fully incorporates Freud's dual-drive theory, emphasizing, in particular, the importance of inborn aggression as a reflection of the death instinct. Both the death instinct and the life instinct operate from birth onward and influence the development of earliest object relations; these will determine the structure of early ego and early superego formation. Both instincts find mental expression in the form of unconscious fantasy, the content of which represents the self and objects under the influence of primitive emotions reflecting the drives. Envy, greed, and, to some extent, jealousy later on are specific emotions derived from oral aggression.

The life instinct is expressed from birth onward in pleasurable contacts with gratifying objects, primarily the "good breast." Those objects are invested with libido and are introjected as internal objects infused with emotions representing libido. The projection of the good inner object onto new objects is the basis of trust, the wish to explore reality, and learning and knowledge. Gratitude is the predominant emotion linked with the expression of libido.

The death instinct, expressed in primitive emotions, particularly envy, is projected outward in the form of fears of persecution and annihilation. All early experiences of tension and displeasure are expelled in an effort to preserve purified pleasure within the ego; these experiences are projected into what become persecutory objects. From the beginning of life, an ego is in operation, developing defenses against anxiety, processes of introjection and projection, and carrying out integration and synthesis. Anxiety constitutes the ego's response to the expression of the death instinct; it is reinforced by the separation caused by birth and by frustration of oral needs.

Anxiety becomes fear of persecutory objects and, later, through the introjection of aggression in the form of internalized bad objects, fear of being persecuted from within and outside. Inner persecutors constitute the origin of primitive superego anxiety. The projection of inner tension states and of painful external stimuli constitutes the origin of paranoid fears, but the projection of pleasurable states, reflecting basically the life instinct, gives rise to basic trust. External stimuli invested with libido or aggression become primitive objects.

Objects are at first split-off or part objects and only later become total or whole objects. The tendency to perceive objects as either ideal (all good) or persecutory (all bad) is the consequence of the defense of splitting. The predominance of part-object relationships in earliest life is a consequence of the maximal operation of splitting mechanisms. Only later, when splitting mechanisms decrease, is a synthesis of good and bad aspects of objects possible; ambivalence toward whole objects can now be tolerated and acknowledged.

Klein described two basic constellations of defenses and object relations that constitute, beginning in the first year of life, recurring polarities of human experience, at all stages of psychosexual development. She called these the *paranoid-schizoid position* and the *depressive position*. The paranoid-schizoid position is the earliest developmental stage; it culminates within the first half of the first year of life and is characterized by the predominance of splitting and other related mechanisms, by part-object relations, and by paranoid fears about the preservation or survival of the ego, stemming from oral-sadistic and anal-sadistic impulses. Excessive persecutory fears can result in pathological strengthening and fixation at this first position, which underlies the development of schizophrenia and paranoid psychosis. The principal defenses of the paranoid-schizoid position are splitting, idealization, denial of internal and external reality, stifling and artificiality of emotions, and projective identification. Projective identification, originally described by Klein, is of fundamental importance in this group of primitive defenses.

The depressive position dominates during the second half of the first year of life. Splitting processes begin to diminish, as the infant becomes more aware that the good and bad external objects are really one and that mother as a whole object has both good and bad parts. The infant's recognition of its own aggression toward the good object, which had been perceived as bad, reduces projection. In contrast to the persecutory fears of external attack characteristic of the paranoid-schizoid position, the predominant fear in the depressive position is of harming the good internal and external objects. This basic fear constitutes depressive anxiety or guilt, the primary emotion of the depressive position. The preservation of good objects now becomes more important than the preservation of the ego. Internal bad objects that are no longer projected constitute the primary superego, which attacks the ego with guilt feelings. Within the superego, bad internal objects may contaminate good internal objects that, because of their demanding or standard-setting nature, have also been internalized into the superego, bringing about cruel demands for perfection.

Under normal conditions, the following mechanisms permit the working through of the depressive position: reparation (the origin, in Klein's thinking, of sublimation); increased reality testing; ambivalence: the capacity to become aware of and to tolerate love and hate toward the same object, with love predominating over hate in emotional reactions to whole objects; and gratitude, which is reinforced by guilt. Normal mourning, for Klein, always implies guilt, reactivating the guilt of the depressive position and the introjection not only of the lost external object but also of the internal good object that was felt to be threatened, and the gratification at being alive, including the activation of manic triumph and secondary guilt over it.

Pathological developments of the depressive position are represented by the *manic defenses*, which include reactivation of idealization as a way of preserving the good internal and external objects in the face of ambivalence toward them, a sense of triumph over the lost object, and contempt. Another major development of the depressive position is *pathological mourning*, characterized by the loss of the good external and internal objects caused by the fantasized destructive effects of the hatred directed toward them, failure of the efforts of compensation by means of idealization, and a circular reaction of guilt, self-reproach, and despair. Depressive psychosis constitutes the final outcome of pathological mourning, while hypomanic syndromes reflect the pathological predominance of the constellation of manic defenses. Such manic syndromes include, in addition to the manic defenses mentioned, identification with the superego, compulsive introjection, manic triumph, and extreme manic idealization.

In Kleinian theory, both the ego and the early superego are constituted of internalized object relations. All conflict-laden situations and developmental stages reactivate paranoid-schizoid and depressive object relations and defenses; the systematic analysis of these mechanisms in the transference is a central aspect of Kleinian technique (Segal 1967).

Klein (1945/1948) also proposed that the oedipal complex is activated toward the end of the first year of life. She believed that these early oedipal developments were secondary to the displacement from mother to father of the infant's paranoid-schizoid and depressive positions. The transfer of oral dependency from mother to father dominates the early positive oedipal complex in girls and the early negative oedipal complex in boys; the transfer of aggressive fears and fantasies from mother to father produces fantasies of dangerous sexual organs and destructive parental sexual relations. The projection of oral and anal sadistic fantasies onto the genitals of both sexes colors early castration anxiety in both sexes. Oral envy of mother is the origin of penis envy in girls and oedipal jealousy and rivalry in both sexes. The transfer of good object relations to the oedipal object and to the fantasized sexual relations of the parents determines the capacity for normal oedipal identifications and development and the capacity for good sexual relations. The aggressive infiltration of the fantastic views of the primal scene and of the relations with both parents results in severe oedipal inhibitions and conflicts.

Kleinian technique, in addition to focusing on the analysis of primitive object relations and defenses, strongly insists on the primacy of the analysis of the transference from very early in the treatment and on the analysis in depth of transference developments to their dominant and often primitive levels of anxiety. The early Kleinian tendency to interpret most transference reactions as reflecting developments in the first year of life, however, has gradually shifted; contemporary Kleinian technique emphasizes the analysis of unconscious meaning in the "here and now" and takes a more gradual and cautious approach to genetic reconstructions. Segal (1981), Rosenfeld (1987), and Spillius and Feldman (1989) represent the mainstream Kleinian approach. Bion (1967, 1970) and Meltzer (1973; Meltzer et al. 1975) have developed what may be characterized as more radical transformations of classical psychoanalysis in the light of Kleinian developments.

Ronald Fairbairn

Ronald Fairbairn's (1954) object relations theory is closely related to Klein's. He proposed that an ego is present from birth, that libido is a function of the ego, and that there is no death instinct, aggression being a reaction to frustration or deprivation. For Fairbairn, the ego (and therefore libido) is fundamentally object seeking, and libido is essentially reality oriented in promoting attachment of the infant to the earliest objects—first, mother's breast, and later, mother as a total person. The earliest and original form of anxiety, Fairbairn suggested, is separation anxiety, activated when frustrations—largely temporary separations from mother—occur. These frustrations bring about the internalization of the object and also ambivalence toward it.

Fairbairn proposed that both the exciting and the frustrating aspects of the internalized object are split off from the main core of the object and repressed by the ego. There thus come to be two repressed internal objects, the exciting (or libidinal) and the rejecting (or antilibidinal). Both carry with them into repression parts of the ego by which they are cathected, leaving the central ego unrepressed but acting as the agent of repression. In consequence, the original ego is split into three egos: a central (conscious) ego attached to an ideal object (ego ideal), a repressed libidinal ego attached to the exciting (or libidinal) object, and a repressed antilibidinal ego attached to the rejecting (or antilibidinal) object.

This concept differs from Freud's tripartite structure in that there is no id and all three components are fundamentally ego structures. Fairbairn considered this splitting of the ego to be in the service of defense: the splitting of a fundamental core object that was libidinally invested and yet frustrating at the same time—a basic "schizoid" operation—leads to the repression of the frustrating aspect of the object as a bad internal object (the antilibidinal object) and of the exciting aspect as an unavailable, libidinal object.

In psychoanalytic treatment, the patient's initial relationship to the analyst as an ideal object reflects the activation of the central conscious ego as a defense against the repressed libidinal and antilibidinal internalized object relationships; these, however, gradually emerge in the transference as well. Fairbairn suggested that the exaggerated development of such an impoverished central ego as a product of excessive schizoid operations is characteristic of both the schizoid and the hysterical personalities.

Fairbairn believed that the infant's original fear was that its love for mother would empty her out and destroy her, which made the infant feel futile and depleted. Fairbairn considered this fantasy an essential emotional experience of schizoid personalities, which imparted an aggressive quality to their dependent needs. Only later on, Fairbairn suggested, was the frustration from mother experienced as a consequence of the individual's own aggressive impulses, now projected onto mother as a bad object and leading to the internalization of a bad internal object. Fairbairn saw these split-off internalized object relations not simply as fantasies but as endopsychic structures, the basic structures of the psychic apparatus.

For Fairbairn, the various erotogenic zones represented not the origin of libidinal stimuli but the channels available for expression of libidinal needs directed to objects; he defined anal and phallic conflicts not in terms of libidinal stages but as particular "techniques" activated in a sequence of interactions and conflicts with parental objects.

Fairbairn saw the development of masochistic tendencies in the treatment as a basic manifestation in the transference of previously split-off bad internalized object relations; he considered the interpretation of such masochistic needs to be a key phase in the resolution of pathological schizoid states. He described the "masochistic defense" as a consequence of unconscious efforts to preserve the relationship with frustrating yet needed objects: the "absolution of blame" of the object on the part of the self transformed the unconditional badness of the object into a conditional one, and the experience of unconscious guilt expressed this effort to maintain a relationship with the frustrating object. He proposed that the psychoanalytic resolution of unconscious guilt feelings might bring about an intensification of the patient's resistances and of negative therapeutic reactions because the patient then would be faced with the need to come to terms with the libidinal attachment to bad, ambivalently loved objects, a crucial aspect of internalized object relations.

Fairbairn maintained a rather classical psychoanalytic technique throughout most of his professional life, adopting only minor modifications, late in his career, of the psychoanalytic setting to enable the patient to see the analyst if he or she so desired. His principal followers include Sutherland (1989) and Guntrip (1961, 1968). The latter introduced significant changes in Fairbairn's approach, with an even more radical rejection of drive theory than Fairbairn's original formulations.

Donald Winnicott

Donald Winnicott's (1958, 1965, 1971) object relations theory is less systematized than those of Klein and Fairbairn. His writings have an evocative quality that has had a profound influence on psychoanalytic theory and practice. But, although he maintained his allegiance to many of Freud's and Klein's formulations, there are potential contradictions between his ideas and some of theirs. While his approach is eminently compatible with Fairbairn's, he did not fully work out these relationships; Guntrip attempted to achieve such an integration of Fairbairn's and Winnicott's thinking.

Winnicott's emphasis is on the concept and origin of the self, the development of the infant's subjective sense of reality in the context of its relationship to mother. Winnicott suggested that the infant's primary experience is an oscillation between integrated and unintegrated affective states and that the protective environment provided by the empathic presence of the "good enough mother" permits the infant to experience a nontraumatic gratification of its needs. The repeated availability of mother's gratifying presence in response to the activation of its internal needs gradually shapes a normal self experience. Mother's capacity for appropriate physical handling of the infant's instinctive needs and her emotional "holding" of its affective needs—a capacity derived from her "primary maternal preoccupation" during the latter stage of pregnancy and the first few months of the infant's life—fosters the infant's omnipotent fantasy that it is able to create the reality required for satisfaction. The infant's subjectively experienced initiative "impinges" on the "environment-mother," bringing about her empathic response and gratification of its needs. The sense of omnipotence—the infant "created" the needed object at the point of need—strengthens the early self experience and creates the basis for the later development of transitional objects and transitional experiences.

When mother is not empathic to the infant's needs, fails to react to them, or reacts in a faulty way, the infant's experience is that of an external "impingement," which is traumatic. A basic defensive operation then occurs in the form of splitting between the infant's nascent, "true self"—which now withdraws into an internal world of fantasy—and an adaptive "false self." The true self relates to an internal world of gratifying and frustrating object representations, roughly corresponding to Klein's internal world of object relations; the false self deals with adaptation to external reality. Under excessively traumatic circumstances, with chronic failure in the mothering function, an exaggerated false self may lead to a chronic sense of inauthenticity and even to severe psychopathology, including antisocial behavior. Cognitive functions may be recruited to rationalize the operation of the false self and to promote a defensive, intellectualized version of self and others that does not correspond to the authentic object-related needs of the true self.

Under optimal mothering conditions, the infant is able to adapt to a shared reality with mother. The infant at first assumes this reality to be omnipotently created; gradually, when its tolerance for unavoidable environmental frustration and failure increases, it creates what Winnicott called a "transitional object," a concrete object that is the infant's "first possession"—that is, is recognized as not part of the self and yet as not part of external reality either. The transitional object fulfills the functions of a fantasized relationship that is unchallenged by mother and infant alike; it constitutes the origin of future "illusion," creating an intermediate "space" between internal reality and external reality that will evolve first into the illusional space of play and eventually into the creative areas of art, culture, and religion. The transitional object is "created" by the infant with mother's silent agreement during the second half of the first year of life. It gradually "dissolves" without a sense of loss or mourning during the second or third year of life. Winnicott posed a connection between the normal development of transitional objects and subsequent psychopathology of fetishism and fetishistic object relations.

The infant's relation with the transitional object replicates the relation with mother in reality and in its internal world. In expressing both libidinal and aggressive needs toward that transitional object and in that object's "survival," the infant is reassured that its aggression has not destroyed the object. Winnicott saw the origin of aggression in the child's initial "ruthlessness" in treating the object, roughly corresponding to the time of Klein's paranoid-schizoid position. He modified Klein's transition from the paranoid-schizoid into the depressive position in his concept of the development of the "capacity for concern"—namely, the infant's gradual recognition that its ruthlessness corresponds to aggression directed to a bad object that is also a good object. Mother, at that stage, exercises her "holding function" in the sense of her symbolic "survival" following the onslaught of her infant's aggression. Winnicott described the infant's capacity to both "use" an object ruthlessly and relate to it in dependent, lovingly gratifying ways; he described the "capacity to be alone" as derived from the infant's capacity to be alone in the presence of mother, assured of her potential availability, a capacity corresponding to Klein's concept of the consolidation of a good internal object and the related capacity for trust.

Winnicott considered patients who had achieved consolidation of a true self and the capacity for concern—the equivalent of Klein's consolidation of the depressive position—suitable for psychoanalysis. He considered those in whom a false self dominates and the normal trusting relationship to external objects has not become consolidated—particularly those with severely schizoid pathology and antisocial behavior—as requiring modifications in analytic technique. For these severely ill patients, Winnicott proposed that the analytic setting itself, in its stability, reliability, and soothing quality, represents the "holding environment" that was prematurely disrupted. He contended that the psychoanalyst must provide, by his or her own stability, reliability, and availability, the "environment mother" that the patient lacked in the past. Optimally, this will permit the patient's benign regression to an early state of nonintegration, which replicates the early state of the infant-mother relationship, when there was as yet no clear boundary between mother and infant. The analyst's tolerance for interpretation of the patient's need to regress, to be understood in regression, and, symbolically speaking, to be "held" by the analyst may permit the reactivation of early traumatic circumstances, the undoing of the defensive withdrawal of the true self, and the beginning of the consolidation of object relations involving the true self and the early gratifying and frustrating maternal object.

Winnicott significantly influenced mainstream French psychoanalytic thinking, as well as ego psychology–object relations theories such as Modell's (1976), and interpersonal psychoanalysis as represented by the work of Greenberg and Mitchell (1983). There are important potential correspondences between Winnicott's approach and Kohut's (1971, 1977) self psychology, such as their stress on the therapeutic importance of a good analytic relationship, but also very significant differences: Winnicott's conceptualization of a complex internal world includes aggressively determined internalized object relations.

Harry Stack Sullivan

Harry Stack Sullivan (1953, 1962) was the chief proponent of interpersonal psychoanalysis. The cornerstone of his approach was the belief that all psychological phenomena are interpersonal in origin and that psychic life starts out as the internalization of relations with significant others. Sullivan classified the essential human needs as "needs for satisfaction," corresponding to instinctively anchored biological needs, and "needs for security," implying the need for gratifying experiences with others that would consolidate a sense of an effective and safe self and a basic sense of goodness. Gratification of the needs for satisfaction would increase security, bring about a sense of euphoria, and facilitate emotional growth. But undue frustrations of the needs for satisfaction would affect the need for security as well. Undue frustration of the emotional need to relate to significant others—even given gratification of basic needs for satisfaction—determines the experience of anxiety and, if exaggerated, its extension to a sense of personal "badness." Excessive anxiety is the fundamental cause of emotional illness, and the frustration of essential security needs is its origin.

For Sullivan, the development of a healthy sense of self depended on the "reflected appraisal by others"; acceptance by others creates a sense of good self and promotes the integration of the self in satisfying security needs. Sullivan described stages in the capacity for appraisal of the interactions with others. The original or "prototaxic" experiences are characteristic of the first months of life, before the development of the capacity for differentiating self from others. "Parataxic" experience corresponds to the development of distortions in early experiences with oth-

ers that are reflected in the transference developments in psychotherapeutic treatment. The mature capacity for realistic assessment of one's relations with others is expressed in the "syntaxic" mode of experience.

These are alternative ways of formulating Freud's primary and secondary processes, just as Sullivan's classification of the needs for satisfaction and security replaced Freud's drive theory. Sullivan also proposed early defensive operations of "selective inattention"—roughly corresponding to Freud's preconscious—and "dissociation" as a more radical elimination of self-awareness—equivalent to Freud's mechanism of repression. Sullivan described three levels of development derived from normal and conflictual early object relations. Gratifying internalized object relations lead to a sense of "euphoria" and inner goodness, which facilitates emotional growth and the deepening of an external and internalized world of object relations. They are the source of the "good me." Unsatisfactory relations with others, characterized by anxiety and frustrations of the need for security, lead to setting up a sense of a "bad me." The psychopathology of a dissociated "bad me" may lead, by projection, to paranoid development. In intimate relations to the "good me" and the "bad me," the individual develops "personifications" of significant others, particularly "good mother" and "bad mother"; here Sullivan described the intrapsychic structures common to all object relations theories. Extremely frustrating experiences leading to commensurate anxiety and profound personal disorganization are expressed in a sense of "not me," a primitive distortion and destruction of intrapsychic experience characteristic of psychosis. Sullivan described extreme conditions under which, by a process of "malevolent transformation," all object relations would be interpreted as essentially bad and dangerous, characteristic of paranoid psychoses.

Sullivan's treatment approach focused on the need to reactivate the patient's dissociated "bad me" and "not me" experiences in the transference by providing an empathic, stable, sensitive interpersonal environment in which the patient would be able to tolerate activation of dissociated parataxic relationships. For practical purposes, Sullivan focused on the understanding, ventilation, and interpretive resolution of negative transferences, on the assumption that this would permit the patient to unblock his or her capacity for gratifying object relations and enable the development of positive growth experiences in the psychotherapeutic relationship, the resumption of a basic sense of goodness, a consolidation of the self, and emotional growth.

Sullivan profoundly influenced Frieda Fromm-Reichmann (1950), Otto Will (1959), and Harold Searles (1965), who further developed his approach to the psychoanalytic treatment of psychotic, particularly schizophrenic, patients. In developing a general theory of the treatment of patients with psychotic and borderline illness, Searles has integrated Kleinian concepts, particularly those of Rosenfeld and Bion (both of whom had worked with psychotic patients within a Kleinian frame of reference), with his Sullivanian background. Sullivanian thinking, together with Fairbairn's approach, has profoundly influenced contemporary interpersonal or relational psychoanalysis as represented by the work of Greenberg and Mitchell (1983).

Edith Jacobson

Starting out with an ego psychological approach strongly influenced by Hartmann (1964), Edith Jacobson (1971) focused on affect development. She proposed that affects were not simply discharge processes but the representations of drives intimately integrated with self and object representations from the earliest stages of development. Her conceptualization of affective processes explained how affects carry out fundamental intrapsychic regulatory functions by means of this investment of self and object representations; it also clarified the relationships between setting up affectively invested self and object representations, on the one hand, and the vicissitudes of ego and superego development, particularly their constituent constellations of self and object representations, on the other.

In her treatment of patients with affective disorders and adolescents with severe identity problems and narcissistic conflicts, Jacobson integrated her findings with Mahler's (Mahler and Furer 1968) regarding autistic and symbiotic psychosis in childhood and separation-individuation. Mahler, in turn, had interpreted her own findings in the light of Jacobson's (1964) earlier formulations.

Jacobson (1964) proposed that intrapsychic life starts out as a psychophysiological self within which ego and id are not differentiated. She suggested that the first intrapsychic structure is a fused or undifferentiated self-object representation that evolves gradually under the impact of the relationship of mother and infant. This fused self-object representation (corresponding to Mahler's symbiotic stage of development) ends with the gradual differentiation of the self representation from the object representation, contributing to the capacity for differentiating the self from the external world.

Jacobson saw the defensive refusal of self representation and object representation under severely traumatic circumstances as the origin of subsequent psychotic identifications characteristic of symbiotic psychosis of childhood and of affective psychosis and schizophrenia in adulthood. She also described the defensive dissociation of fused or undifferentiated self-object representations

invested with aggressive drive derivatives as the counterpart to the libidinally invested ones, so that, particularly under pathological circumstances, fused self-object representations of an "all good" and an "all bad" nature coexist while being mutually dissociated.

Gradually, during the stage of separation-individuation that dominates the second part of the first and the second years of life, differentiation of self and object representations in both the "good" and the "bad" segments of experience is achieved. This is followed, first, by the integration of the "good" and "bad" self representations and object representations and, later, by the development of ideal-self representations and ideal-object representations, which crystallize in order to restore a sense of an ideal relationship with mother. It is the toned-down, ambivalent relation to mother in reality that evokes the psychological need to recreate an ideal relationship in fantasy.

Efforts to deny and devalue the bad aspects of self and of mother may lead to the exaggerated fixation of dissociated "bad" self and object representations that dominates the psychopathology of borderline conditions. Under optimal circumstances, in contrast, good and bad self representations are integrated into a consolidated concept of self, and good and bad representations of mother, father, and siblings evolve into integrated constellations of real and idealized objects and object relations, which become part of ego structures.

Jacobson suggested that the superego also evolves out of successive layers of internalized object relations. The first layer is represented by "bad" object representations with a prohibitive, punishing quality. This is followed by a second layer of ideal-self and ideal-object representations that will enact idealized superego demands. Again, under normal circumstances, the gradual integration of these bad and ideal layers of superego precursors leads to their toning down and to the consequent internalization and integration of a third layer of the more realistic superego introjects of the oedipal period. The gradual individualization, depersonification, and abstraction of these three layers lead to the healthy integrated superego of latency, puberty, and adolescence, when a partial reorganization brings about the transformation into the adult superego. Jacobson applied this model to the treatment of neurotic, borderline, and psychotically depressed patients.

It is tempting to trace parallels in the theories of Jacobson, Mahler, Klein, and Fairbairn. All of them focused on the vicissitudes of the internalization and gradual integration of self and object representations, on splitting or primitive dissociation and integration, and on the gradual building up of the overall psychic structures under the influence of the integration of early object relations.

Margaret Mahler

As a result of her observations of children with autistic and symbiotic psychoses and of the mother-child relationships in the first few years of life, Margaret Mahler (Mahler and Furer 1968; Mahler et al. 1975) developed a theory of the psychostructural preconditions of autistic psychosis, symbiotic psychosis, normal and pathological separation-individuation, and, as the culmination of early development, object constancy and a consolidated tripartite structure.

Mahler hypothesized an earliest stage of development, the autistic phase, during the first month of life, predating the establishment of the symbiotic phase (which develops between the second and the sixth month of life). In the last part of her life, however, as a result of the findings of neonatal observations, she revised this idea and concluded that a normal autistic phase probably did not exist and that cases of autistic psychosis with strong psychological determinants were pathological developments.

The symbiotic phase of development is characterized by cueing and matching between infant and mother, in which the infant experiences blissful states of merger with mother. The infant anticipates and initiates pleasurable responses in interacting with mother and develops a sense of confidence and basic trust in mother, expressed in smiling and direct eye contact; this leads to the capacity to be alone as well as with mother.

In the second half of the first year of life, the stage of separation-individuation sets in, to be completed toward the end of the third year. The first subphase of separation-individuation, between about 6 and 10 months, is *differentiation* or *hatching*, characterized by an increase in the infant's scanning of the environment and checking back to mother for "visual refueling." The infant now is capable of easily being comforted by mother substitutes, but he or she also develops stranger anxiety, "custom inspection" in intensive visual interaction with mother's and others' faces, and a gradual differentiation between what is animate and inanimate, good and bad.

The *differentiation* subphase is followed by "practicing," from roughly 11 to 16 months, characterized by the mastery of upright locomotion, pleasure in exploring and in asserting "free will," and the tendency to take mother for granted except when prolonged separation leads to "low keyedness." Now the toddler develops a "love affair with the world," with a sense of omnipotence and an active, even aggressive autonomy, darting and running away from mother but also wishing to share with her, to control by means of "shadowing."

Practicing leads into the subphase of *rapprochement*, between 18 months and the third year, when the toddler makes intense efforts to control mother while clinging to her anxiously. This subphase culminates in what Mahler called the "rapprochement crisis," characterized by an intensification of darting away alternating with temper tantrums. There is aggressive control of mother, insistence on autonomy in responses to her, and manifestations of sharp splitting characterized by idealizing clinging to mother and aggressive separation from her. The pathology of the rapprochement crisis is marked by excessive separation anxiety, passivity or demandingness, depressive mood, pathological coercion and possessiveness of mother, pathological envy, and temper tantrums. It is related to severely disappointing, unavailable, or overintrusive mothers; to painful and sudden dissolutions of the child's fantasized omnipotence; and to traumatic circumstances causing excessive narcissistic frustration.

Over the fourth and fifth years of life, in the process Mahler called "toward object constancy," the child develops an integrated sense of self, a differentiated relation with other adults and peers, awareness in depth of mother, and tolerance for ambivalence. During this phase, oedipal conflicts become clearly dominant.

Mahler's understanding of the underlying nature of internalized object relations, drawing on Jacobson's developmental model, implied dealing with mutually dissociated or split-off idealized and persecutory relationships within which self and object representations were fused, typically activated in the transference of psychotic patients. The psychoanalytic exploration of borderline conditions, in contrast—reflecting particularly the pathology of internalized object relations during the subphase of rapprochement—implied the analysis of mutually dissociated or split-off idealized and persecutory relationships within which the patient had achieved a clear capacity to differentiate between self and object representations in both segments. Harold Searles's (1965) description of the stages in the psychoanalytic treatment of psychotic patients—1) the early, out-of-contrast phase, 2) intense symbiotic involvement, 3) separation, and 4) integration—also reflects Mahler's concept of symbiotic psychosis and separation-individuation development. I have drawn on both Mahler's observations regarding pathological rapprochement crises and Jacobson's developmental schemata to provide a theoretical background for an approach to the psychoanalytic psychotherapy of borderline conditions.

Otto Kernberg

Like Jacobson and Mahler, I adhere to Freud's dual-drive theory and consider drives indissolubly linked to object relations. I believe that libidinal and aggressive drive derivatives are invested in object relations from very early in life—namely, in temporary symbiotic states under the influence of peak affect activation. I propose that the ideational and affective representations of drives are originally undifferentiated from one another and that (following Jacobson in this regard) affect states representing the most primitive manifestations of drives are essential links of self and object representations from the very beginning.

I propose that affects are the primary motivational system and that, internalized or fixated as the very frame of internalized "good" and "bad" object relations, they are gradually integrated into libidinal and aggressive drives to form hierarchically supraordinate motivational systems. In other words, primitive affects are the "building blocks" of the drives (Kernberg 1990). I see unconscious intrapsychic conflicts as always between, on the one hand, certain units of self and object representations under the impact of a particular drive derivative (clinically, a certain affect disposition reflecting the instinctual side of the conflict) and, on the other hand, contradictory or opposing units of self and object representations and their respective affect dispositions reflecting the defensive structure. Unconscious intrapsychic conflicts are never simply between impulse and defense; rather, both impulse and defense find expression through certain internalized object relations.

At levels of severe psychopathology—in patients with borderline personality organization—splitting mechanisms stabilize such dynamic structures within an ego-id matrix and permit the contradictory aspects of these conflicts (predominantly condensed oedipal-preoedipal conflicts infiltrated with primitive aggression) to remain at least partially conscious, in the form of primitive transferences. In contrast, patients with neurotic personality organization present impulse-defense configurations that contain specific unconscious wishes reflecting sexual and aggressive drive derivatives embedded in unconscious fantasies relating to well-differentiated oedipal objects. Repressed unconscious wishes, however, always come in the form of corresponding units composed of self representation and object representation and an affect linking them (Kernberg 1987a, 1988).

Patients with neurotic personality organization present with well-integrated superego, ego, and id structures. In the psychoanalytic situation, the analysis of resistances brings about the activation in the transference, first, of relatively global characteristics of these structures and, later, of the internalized object relations of which they are composed. The analysis of drive derivatives occurs in the context of the analysis of the relation of the patient's infantile self to significant parental objects as projected onto the analyst.

The borderline personality organization shows a predominance of preoedipal conflicts, and psychic representations of preoedipal conflicts condensed with representations of the oedipal phase. Conflicts are not predominantly repressed and therefore unconsciously dynamic: rather, they are expressed in mutually dissociated ego states reflecting the defense of primitive dissociation or splitting. The activation of primitive object relations that predate the consolidation of ego, superego, and id is manifest in the transference as apparently chaotic affect states, which have to be analyzed in sequential steps as follows:

1. Clarification of a dominant primitive object relation in the transference, with its corresponding self and object representations and the dominant affect linking them

2. Analysis of the alternative projection of self and object representations onto the therapist while the patient identifies with a reciprocal self or object representation of this object relationship, leading to the gradual development of awareness of this identification with self and object in that relationship

3. The interpretive integration of mutually split-off, idealized, and persecutory part-object relations with the characteristics mentioned

Analysis may gradually bring about transformation of part-object relations into total object relations and of primitive transferences (largely reflecting Mahler's stages of development predating object constancy) into the advanced transferences of the oedipal phase. The analyst's exploration of his countertransference, including concordant and complementary identifications (Racker 1957), facilitates transference analysis, and the analysis of primitive defensive operations, particularly splitting and projective identification, in the transference also contributes to strengthening the patient's ego.

I have also described 1) the pathological condensation of idealized internalized object relations in the pathological grandiose self of narcissistic personalities, and 2) the gradual resolution of the pathological grandiose self in the transference as its component part-object relationships are clarified and the corresponding dominant primitive defensive operations are interpreted (Kernberg 1984).

To the extent that I have drawn on findings regarding primitive defenses and object relations stemming from the Kleinian school, Fairbairn's ideas about the essential dyadic structures involving self representation–object representation–affect, and Jacobson's and Mahler's theoretical frames, my approach may be considered an effort to integrate several object relations theories within an ego psychology–object relations theory model.

Technique

General Principles

An object relations focus is not geared exclusively to the understanding and treatment of patients with severe regression in the transference; it has applications for the standard psychoanalytic technique, as many have long been integrated into that technique.

Within an object relations framework, unconscious intrapsychic conflicts always involve self and object representations, or rather, conflicts between certain units of self and object representations under the impact of determined drive derivative (clinically, a certain affect disposition) and other contradictory or opposing units of self and object representations and their respective affect dispositions, reflecting the defensive structure. As I noted earlier, unconscious intrapsychic conflicts are never simple conflicts between impulse and defense; rather, the drive derivative finds expression through a certain primitive object relation (a certain unit of self and object representations), and the defense, too, is reflected by a certain internalized object relation. The conflict is between these intrapsychic structures. Thus, all character defenses really reflect the activation of a defensive constellation of self and object representations directed against an opposite and dreaded, repressed self and object constellation. For example, in obsessive, characterological submissiveness, a chronically submissive self image in relating to a powerful and protective parental image may defend the patient against the repressed, violently rebellious self relating to a sadistic and castrating parental image. Thus, clinically, both character defense and repressed impulse involve mutually opposed internal object relations.

While, therefore, the consolidation of the overall intrapsychic structures (ego, superego, and id) results in an integration of internalized object relations that obscures the constituent units within these overall structures, in the course of psychoanalysis one observes the gradual redissolution of pathogenic superego and ego structures and, in this context, the activation and clarification of the constituent internalized object relations in the transference. In this regard, the classical formulation of the transference as reflecting an impulse and an identification may easily be translated into the transference as always reflecting an object relation under the impact of a certain drive derivative.

In other words, the unconscious intrapsychic conflicts reflected in neurotic symptoms and pathological character traits are always dynamically structured; they reflect a relatively permanent intrapsychic organization consisting of opposite, contradictory, or conflictual internalized object relations. At severe levels of psychopathology for which psychoanalysis is usually contraindicated (certain types of severe character pathology, borderline conditions), dissociative mechanisms stabilize such dynamic structures within an ego-id matrix and permit the contradictory aspects of these conflicts to remain—at least partially—in consciousness.

On the other hand, with patients presenting less severe character pathology and psychoneurosis, the dynamically structured intrapsychic conflicts are truly unconscious and are predominantly intersystemic conflicts involving ego, superego, and id and their advanced, high-level or "neurotic" defense mechanisms. Here, in the course of the psychoanalytic process, the development of a regressive transference neurosis will gradually activate in the transference the constituent units of internalized object relations that form part of ego and superego structures, and of the repressed units of internalized object relations that have become part of the id. At first, rather global expressions of ego and superego functions, such as generalized guilt feelings about unacceptable impulses, or broadly rationalized ego-syntonic character traits, make their appearance. Eventually, however, the transference is expressed more and more directly by means of a certain object relation that is used defensively against an opposing one reflecting the repressed drive derivatives. In the case of both defense- and impulse-determined object relations, the patient may reenact the self representation of that unit while projecting the object representation onto the analyst, or, at other times, project his or her self-representation onto the analyst while identifying with the object representation of the unit.

Because in the ordinary psychoanalytic case these transitory identifications emerge in the context of a well-integrated tripartite structure and a consolidated ego identity, with integration of both the patient's self concept and his or her concepts of significant others—including the psychoanalyst, the patient can maintain a certain distance from, or perspective on, this momentary activation of a certain distortion of self and object representations without losing, at least potentially, the capacity for reality testing in the transference. This permits the analyst to deal with the regressive transference neurosis from a position of technical neutrality, by interpretive means; it also permits the patient to deal with interpretations introspectively, searching for further self-understanding in the light of the analyst's interpretive comments. In spite of temporary weakening of reality testing during affect storms and transference acting out, this quality of the psychoanalytic process is one of its outstanding, specific features.

The analyst, while empathizing by means of a transitory or trial identification with the patient's experience of himself and his object representations, also explores empathically the object relation that is currently predominant in the interactional or nonverbal aspects of the transference and, in this context, the nature of self or object representations that the patient is projecting onto him or her. The analyst's subjective experience, at that point, may include a transitory identification either with the patient's self experience—as is the case in concordant identification—or with the patient's currently dissociated or projected self or object representations—as is the case in complementary identification (in which the analyst, rather than identifying with the patient's self or ego, identifies with his object representation or the superego in global terms [Racker 1957]).

Throughout this process, the analyst first transforms his or her empathic understanding into intuitive formulations; he later ventures into a more restrictive formulation that incorporates a general understanding in the light of all available information. The empathy with and intuitive understanding of the patient's affect states during this process, as well as the integrative formulation of the affect states, clarifies the nature of the drive derivative activated and defended against in the object relation predominating in the transference.

It needs to be stressed that what I have just outlined is a focus, from an object relations standpoint, on the theory of psychoanalytic technique that permits us to maintain this same theory for varying technical approaches. This theory of technique takes into consideration the structural characteristics, defensive operations, object relations, and transference developments of patients who are fixated at or have regressed to a structural organization that antedates the integration of intrapsychic structures, as well as of patients whose tripartite structure has been consolidated (i.e., the standard psychoanalytic case that we have examined in detail). I am suggesting that this focus on the theory of psychoanalytic technique for the entire spectrum of patients for which a psychoanalytic approach may be considered the treatment of choice facilitates the application of a nonmodified psychoanalytic technique to some patients with severe psychopathology, clarifies certain modifications of the standard psychoanalytic technique in cases for which psychoanalysis is contraindicated for individual reasons, and, most importantly, implies a reconfirmation of standard psychoanalytic technique for the well-organized patient with solid integration of the tripartite structure.

Oedipal and Preoedipal Conflicts and Their Condensation

The earlier the development, fixation, or regression of psychopathology, the more seriously it affects not only the development of ego and superego structures (which is reflected in the treatment in a premature activation of the constituent internalized object relations that ordinarily are integrated within more global ego and superego functions in early stages of psychoanalysis), but also the capacity for entering a normal oedipal situation. Under these conditions, preoedipal conflicts, particularly a predominance of conflicts around preoedipal aggression, infiltrate all object relations. In addition to reinforcing and fixating primitive defensive operations centering around splitting, excessive aggression also contaminates the later object relations characteristic of the oedipal complex.

This contamination by excessive aggression creates characteristic distortions in the oedipal constellation, reflected in the following frequent findings: Excessive splitting of the preoedipal maternal image may be complicated later on by defensive devaluation, fear, and hatred of the oedipal mother and an unstable idealization of the oedipal father that easily breaks down and is replaced by further splitting of father's image. This reinforces oedipal rivalry in men and penis envy in women, excessive fear and guilt over sexuality in both sexes, and the search for desexualized and idealized relationships that influence the development of very early forms of homosexuality in both sexes. A predominance of sadistic and masochistic components in genital strivings is another consequence of this situation. Under these circumstances, the differentiation of parental images along sexual lines, typical for triangular oedipal relationships, may be complicated by splitting mechanisms, which make one sex good and the other bad, or by pathological fusion of the respectively idealized or threatening aspects of both sexes, so that unrealistic combined father/mother images develop (the "phallic mother" is only one example of these developments).

Oedipal conflicts condensed with pathological preoedipal object relations contribute to creating fantastic transference developments. The predominance of partial, nonintegrated self and object representations when early ego defenses predominate also contributes to creating fantastic transference developments. Therefore, the earlier the points of fixation or regression of the psychopathology, the greater is the gap between actual childhood experience, the structuring of these intrapsychic elaborations, and the nature of transference developments.

Although in all patients the predominant transference paradigm may be conceived as a "personal myth" that condenses conflicts from various stages of development, when there is a predominance of total object relations and intersystemic conflicts in the transference, the genetic link between the transference and the antecedent childhood experiences is more direct and more readily available and lends itself to earlier reconstructions than in cases of severe psychopathology or when severe regression occurs in the transference. In these latter cases, the road from present transference developments to the genetic or intrapsychic history of organization of the material is more indirect, and paradoxically, early childhood experiences can be reconstructed only in advanced stages of the treatment—hence, the danger of equating primitive transference with "early" object relations in a mechanical, direct way, and the misleading temptation to "reconstruct" the earliest intrapsychic development on the basis of primitive transference manifestations.

It is important to differentiate patients who have not reached object constancy, in whom the syndrome of identity diffusion and the chronic predominance of primitive defense mechanisms indicate the presence of borderline personality organization, from patients with stable ego identity and, therefore, the preconditions of object constancy, total object relations, and the capacity for maintaining reality testing in the transference even under conditions of severe regression. In the latter, when primitive transferences are activated in advanced stages of the treatment, the analyst can maintain an interpretive stance and technical neutrality, while utilizing the understanding that object relations theory provides as one important viewpoint for the resolution through interpretation of primitive transferences.

Transference Regression and Reconstruction of the Past

In many neurotic patients and in patients with nonborderline character pathology, regressions to primitive transference do occur in the analysis. Because of the intense affective development, the temporary weakening of reality testing, the projective tendencies, and the chaotic interactions that develop at such points, the analyst is sometimes tempted to move away from a technically neutral and strictly interpretive attitude. Such moves away from an analytic attitude are often rationalized with the assumption that the patient has reached a stage of "ego deficit" or "fragility of the self" or "maturational arrest." In fact, what occurs at such points of regression is that the patient has regressed from some stage of his infantile (yet integrated) self relating to an infantile (yet integrated) parental object to a stage that predates object constancy. Now, both the self and object representations activated in the transference are partial and reflect dissociated or split-off aspects of a warded-off, integrated object relations that the patient experiences as intolerable because of the intense ambivalence or contradiction between love and hatred involved.

By the same token, the analysis of intrapsychic conflict in terms of defense and impulse is no longer facilitated by the organizing features of intersystemic conflict,

but, rather, contradictory ego states—or ego-id states—constitute the polarities of the conflict. Both sides include primitive impulse derivatives imbedded in a primitive unit of internalized object relation. Under these circumstances, defense and content can rapidly be interchanged in shifting equilibria of such activated part-object relations, and contradictory impulses are conscious and mutually dissociated or split off rather than unconscious (i.e., repressed). Here the nature of consciousness and unconsciousness no longer coincides with what is on the surface and what is deep, what is defense and what is content.

At such stages, the analysis of the nature of the immediate predominant object relations in the transference, and of the predominant defensive operations connected with its dissociation from other, contradictory, object relations, helps the analyst to clarify the predominant meaning of the transference, the defensive aspects of the object relations it activates, its motivation in protecting the patient against a contradictory or opposite object relation, and the implicit conflict between primitive ego structures. If, at this point, the analyst first interprets the part-object relation activated and its affect state, and later its defensive function against other, contradictory, parallel or previously conscious affect states linked to other part-object relations, dramatic change and new understanding may be gained while the patient's reality testing returns to normal. This interpretative approach, however, requires that the analyst first ascertain whether the patient is still able to maintain some degree of self-observation and reality testing in the transference. Otherwise, it is crucially important to start out by clarifying the reality aspects of the psychoanalytic situation and then to focus on the patient's "interpretation" of the analyst's interpretative comments, before interpreting the defensive function of one object relation in the transference against the impulsive or instinctual function of the opposite one.

The more the transference developments present the characteristics of activation of part-object relations, predominance of primitive defensive operations, and condensation of preoedipal and oedipal conflicts, the more it is indicated to interpret the transference in an "as if" (i.e., nongenetic) mode. For example, I interpreted a patient's chronic frustrations with me at a certain advanced stage of her treatment as a search for a warm and giving, endlessly patient and understanding father with strong maternal features, "as if" she were reliving a time in which she would have wished to have a father with breasts and a penis from which milk would flow endlessly. This interpretation stemmed from many dreams, masturbatory fantasies, and complex interactions in the transference, and I did not "place it historically" because of the reasons mentioned before. Such an "as if" qualification to genetic reconstructions permits a more natural sorting out of the initially condensed, mixed, compressed material stemming from various stages of development, and a gradual crystallization, on the basis of this same repetitive primitive transference pattern, of a sequence of early and later stages of development as issues within the same transference constellation.

The basic contribution of object relations theory to the analysis of the transference is an expansion of the frame of reference within which transference manifestations are explored, so that the increasing complexities of transference regression at severe levels of psychopathology may be understood and interpreted. In practice, the transference of patients with classical psychoneurosis and character pathology with neurotic personality organization may still be understood as the unconscious repetition in the here-and-now of pathogenic relations from the past—more concretely, the enactment of an aspect of the patient's unconscious infantile self in relating to (also unconscious) infantile representations of his parental objects.

The fact that in neurotic psychopathology, regression is to a relatively integrated, though repressed, unconscious infantile self, connected to relatively integrated, though unconscious, representations of the parental objects, makes such transferences fairly easy to understand and interpret: it is the unconscious relation to the parents of the past, including realistic and fantasied aspects of such relationships and the defenses against both of them, that is activated in the transference. That unconscious aspect of the infantile self carries with it a concrete wish reflecting a drive derivative directed to such parental objects and a fantasied fear about the dangers involved in the expression of this wish. But ego psychology–object relations theory stresses the fact that even in these relatively simple transference enactments, such activation always implies the activation of basic dyadic units of a self representation and an object representation, linked by a certain affect, which reflect either the defensive or the impulsive aspects of the conflict. More precisely, any concrete unconscious fantasy that reflects an impulse-defense organization is typically activated first in the form of the object relation representing the defensive side of the conflict and only later in the form of one reflecting the impulsive side of the conflict.

For example, a patient with masochistic personality structure, an architect in her late thirties, misinterpreted my comments as devastating criticism at precisely those moments when she felt our working relationship was good. She then became enraged with me and challenging and defiant, accusing me of trying to control her as had her mother. I understood her behavior to mean that our realistic working together had activated in her unconscious fantasy that I, as her father, was sexually seducing her (derived, in turn, from her projection onto me of underlying positive oedipal wishes). She defended herself masochistically by experiencing me as her nagging mother and herself as an impotent child.

My interpretation focused on her view of me as her critical mother after she felt I had helped her and she had expressed her appreciation; this gradually permitted the emergence of more direct positive feelings with a mixture of erotic excitement and fear over my becoming a seductive father. Now I interpreted her fear of my becoming the seductive father as an expression of her projection onto me of sexual impulses toward me that she did not dare experience directly. This was followed, in turn, by more direct expression of positive oedipal fantasies toward me.

What does an object relations approach add to these relatively simple formulations regarding the transference? First, it highlights that a consistent set of units—a self representation interacting with an object representation under the dominance of a certain affect—frames the experience of concrete unconscious fantasies, wishes, and fears. Second, each defense-impulse organization is reflected in two mutually opposed units, so that both defense and impulse are reflected in a fantasied relation between self and object. Third, even at the high or neurotic level of pathology, a process may be observed that becomes prevalent with more severe psychopathology: the rapid reversal or alternation between a) the activation of the patient's self representation while the object representations are projected onto the analyst, and b) other moments in which the patient enacts an identification with that object representation while projecting the self representation onto the analyst. When the masochistic patient referred to before was experiencing me as aggressively scolding, which resulted in her feeling hurt and mistreated, she then lashed out at me in angry, sarcastic, ironic ways that clearly reflected her description of her mother's behavior, while I experienced myself as temporarily identified with her infantile self, paralyzed by this onslaught, which made it very difficult for me to interpret the situation at hand to the patient. In other words, at points of temporary regression there is both an intensification and a primitivization of the affect reflecting the corresponding drive derivative, and a proneness to rapid reversals of identifications with self or object that may be understood and interpreted more easily within the organizing frame of internalized object relations.

Here I am examining afresh the very nature of identifications in the transference. I am reiterating that, at bottom, all identifications are not with an object but with a relation to an object within which the patient identifies with both self and object and their roles in this relationship, with the possibility of reenacting either of the two roles in it.

For practical purposes, then, instead of interpreting the vicissitudes of a "pure" impulse-defense configuration, we interpret the transference in terms of the activation of an internalized object relation that determines alternating activations of the same conflict in what, at the surface, may seem contradictory experiences and behavior. This approach enriches the interpretation with clarifying nuances and details. Thus, I was able to point out to my masochistic patient that, in treating me as aggressively as she felt treated by her mother, she was identifying with mother and simultaneously implicitly submitting to mother's image inside of her and becoming like mother as an expression of unconscious guilt over the feared sexualized relation with me as father. Thus, the time-honored clinical observation that one affect may be employed as a defense against another (repressed or dissociated) affect should be reformulated as the defensive use of one internalized object relation and its corresponding affect against another internalized object relation and its affect.

The general principles of transference interpretation in the treatment of borderline personality organization include, in short, the following tasks (Kernberg 1984): 1) to diagnose the dominant object relation within the overall chaotic transference situation; 2) to clarify which is the self representation and which is the object representation(s) and what is the dominant affect linking them; and 3) to interpretively connect this primitive dominant object relation with its split-off opposite one.

An object relations frame of reference permits the analyst to organize what looks like complete chaos and gradually to clarify the various condensed part-object relations in the transference. Such clarification will bring about the integration of self and object representations, which in turn will lead to the more advanced neurotic type of transference described earlier.

Countertransference

Racker's (1957) description of concordant and complementary identifications in the countertransference is a most helpful contribution to the technical application of object relations theory. Racker distinguished between *concordant identification*, in which the analyst identifies with what is activated in the patient, and *complementary identification*, in which the analyst identifies with the agency that is in conflict with the agency the patient is identifying with. This latter is usually one the patient cannot tolerate and hence projects. In object relations terms, we might say that, in concordant identification, the analyst identifies with the same representation activated in the patient,

self with self, object with object. Concordant identification in the countertransference is of central importance as the source of ordinary empathy under conditions in which the patient is in a self-reflective mood, but also under conditions in which the analyst may be tempted to share, by proxy, a patient's acting out.

In complementary identification, in object relations terms, the patient and the analyst enact, in their temporary identifications, the self representation and the object representation, respectively, of a certain internalized object relation. Under conditions of sexualized transferences, for example, the analyst may respond seductively to the patient's fear of and temptation toward an oedipal acting out. More frequently, under the predominance of particularly negative transference, the analyst becomes the patient's aggressive and threatening object, while the patient becomes his frightened self; or, a reversal takes place in which the analyst may experience himself paralyzed by the patient's aggression, reacting with fear and impotent hatred; here, the patient identifies himself with his threatening object, while the analyst identifies himself with the patient's threatened self representation.

In general, under complementary countertransference, the analyst is identified with an internal imago that the patient, at that point, cannot tolerate and has to dissociate and project. In fact, the mechanism of projective identification is a central defensive operation of the patient that tends to evoke complementary countertransference reactions in the analyst: the analyst now feels empathic with what the patient cannot tolerate in himself, and, by the same process, the analyst may acquire significant information regarding the total object relationship that has been activated in the transference. Here lies a potentially most rewarding use of the countertransference on the part of the psychoanalyst. The danger, of course, is the temptation to act out this complementary identification in contrast to using it as material to be integrated into the interpretive process (Kernberg 1987b).

If the analyst tolerates his countertransference, he can use it to clarify the dominant object relations in the transference, provided, of course, that professional boundaries are maintained. If, under conditions of extreme transference regression, countertransference reactions are so intense that they become, at least partly, observable to the patient, the analyst should acknowledge honestly what the patient has observed. It is important that the analyst refrain from providing explanations beyond acknowledging what the patient has observed, and follow up this acknowledgement with an interpretation of the total object relation now activated in the therapeutic interaction.

Conclusion

Psychoanalytic object relations theory has significantly expanded and enriched psychoanalytic technique and its application to derived psychoanalytic approaches to a broad spectrum of severe psychopathology. It has provided new ways to conceptualize and carry out transference interpretations. Within psychoanalytic theory at large, it has linked the mechanisms and structures of the tripartite psychoanalytical model with the structures and mechanisms of early developmental stages of psychic life.

References

Bion WR: Second Thoughts: Selected Papers on Psychoanalysis. New York, Basic Books, 1967

Bion WR: Attention and Interpretation. London, Heinemann, 1970

Chasseguet-Smirgel J: Sexuality and Mind: The Role of the Father and the Mother in the Psyche. New York, New York University Press, 1986

Erikson EH: The problem of ego identity (1956), in Identity and the Life Cycle: Selected Papers. New York, International Universities Press, 1959, pp 101–164

Erikson EH: Growth and crises of the healthy personality (1950), in Identity and the Life Cycle: Selected Papers. New York, International Universities Press, 1959, pp 50–100

Fairbairn R: An Object-Relations Theory of the Personality. New York, Basic Books, 1954

Fonagy P, Target M: Psychoanalytic Theories: Perspectives From Developmental Psychopathology. London, Whurr Publishers, 2003, pp 270–282

Freud S: Beyond the pleasure principle (1920), in Standard Edition of the Complete Psychological Works of Sigmund Freud, Vol 18. Translated and edited by Strachey J. London, Hogarth Press, 1955, pp 1–64

Freud S: The ego and the id (1923), in Standard Edition of the Complete Psychological Works of Sigmund Freud, Vol 19. Translated and edited by Strachey J. London, Hogarth Press, 1961, pp 12–66

Freud S: New introductory lectures on psycho-analysis (1933 [1932]) (Lectures XXIX–XXXV), in Standard Edition of the Complete Psychological Works of Sigmund Freud, Vol 22. Translated and edited by Strachey J. London, Hogarth Press, 1964, pp 1–182

Fromm-Reichmann F: Principles of Intensive Psychotherapy. Chicago, IL, University of Chicago Press, 1950

Greenberg JR, Mitchell SA: Object Relations in Psychoanalytic Theory. Cambridge, MA, Harvard University Press, 1983

Guntrip H: Personality Structure and Human Interaction. London, Hogarth Press, 1961

Guntrip H: Schizoid Phenomena, Object Relations, and the Self. New York, International Universities Press, 1968

Hartmann H: Essays on Ego Psychology. New York, International Universities Press, 1964

Jacobson E: The Self and the Object World. New York, International Universities Press, 1964

Jacobson E: Depression. New York, International Universities Press, 1971

Kernberg OF: Object Relations Theory and Clinical Psychoanalysis. New York, Jason Aronson, 1976

Kernberg OF: Internal World and External Reality: Object Relations Theory Applied. New York, Jason Aronson, 1980

Kernberg OF: Severe Personality Disorders: Psychotherapeutic Strategies. New Haven, CT, Yale University Press, 1984

Kernberg OF: An ego-psychology object relations theory approach to the transference. Psychoanalytic Q 56:197–221, 1987a

Kernberg OF: Projection and projective identification: developmental and clinical aspects. J Am Psychoanal Assoc 35: 795–819, 1987b

Kernberg OF: Object relations theory in clinical practice. Psychoanal Q 57:481–504, 1988

Kernberg OF: New perspectives in psychoanalytic affect theory, in Emotion: Theory, Research and Experience. Edited by Plutchik R, Kellerman H. New York, Academic Press, 1990, pp 115–130

Kernberg OF: Aggression in Personality Disorders and Perversions. New Haven, CT Yale University Press, 1992

Klein M: Notes on some schizoid mechanisms. Int J Psychoanal 27:99–110, 1946

Klein M: Mourning and its relation to manic-depressive states (1940), in Contributions to Psychoanalysis, 1921–1945. London, Hogarth Press, 1948, pp 311–338

Klein M: The Oedipus complex in the light of early anxieties (1945), in Contributions to Psychoanalysis, 1921–1945. London, Hogarth Press, 1948, pp 379–390

Klein M: Envy and Gratitude. New York, Basic Books, 1957

Kohut H: The Analysis of the Self: A Systematic Approach to the Psychoanalytic Treatment of Narcissistic Personality Disorder. New York, International Universities Press, 1971

Kohut H: The Restoration of the Self. New York, International Universities Press, 1977

Lacan J: Ecrits 1. Paris, Editions du Seuil, 1966

Loewald H: Papers on Psychoanalysis. New Haven, CT, Yale University Press, 1980

Mahler M, Furer M: On Human Symbiosis and the Vicissitudes of Individuation. New York, International Universities Press, 1968

Mahler M, Furer M: On the first three subphases of the separation-individuation process. Int J Psychoanalysis 53:333–338, 1972a

Mahler M, Furer M: Rapprochement subphases of separation-individuation process, in Psychoanal Q 41:487–506, 1972b

Mahler M, Pine F, Bergman A: The Psychological Birth of the Human Infant: Symbiosis and Individuation. New York, Basic Books, 1975

Meltzer D: Sexual States of Mind. Perthshire, Scotland, Clunie Press, 1973

Meltzer D, Brenner J, Hoyter S, et al: Explorations in Autism. Aberdeen, Scotland, Aberdeen University Press, 1975

Mitchell SA: Relational Concepts in Psychoanalysis: An Integration. Cambridge, MA, Harvard University Press, 1988

Modell A: "The holding environment" and the therapeutic action of psychoanalysis. J Am Psychoanal Assoc 24:285–307, 1976

Oliner MM: Cultivating Freud's Garden in France. Northvale, NJ, Jason Aronson, 1988

Racker H: The meaning and uses of countertransference. Psychoanal Q 26:303–357, 1957

Rosenfeld H: Impasse and Interpretation: Therapeutic and Anti-Therapeutic Factors in the Psychoanalytic Treatment of Psychotic, Borderline and Neurotic Patients. London, Tavistock/Routledge/Institute of Psycho-Analysis, 1987

Roudinesco E: Jacques Lacan and Co: A History of Psychoanalysis in France, 1925–1985. Chicago, IL, University of Chicago Press, 1990

Sandler J: From Safety to Superego: Selected Papers of Joseph Sandler. New York, Guilford, 1987

Searles H: Collected Papers on Schizophrenia and Related Subjects. New York, International Universities Press, 1965

Segal H: Melanie Klein's techniques, in Psychoanalytic Technique: A Handbook for Practicing Psychoanalysts. Edited by Wolman BB. New York, Basic Books, 1967, pp 168–190

Segal H: The Work of Hanna Segal. New York, Jason Aronson, 1981

Segal H: Introduction to the Work of Melanie Klein (1964). London, Karnac Books/Institute of Psycho-Analysis, 1988

Spillius EB, Feldman M (eds): Psychic Equilibrium and Psychic Change: Selected Papers of Betty Joseph. London, Tavistock/Routledge, 1989

Sullivan HS: The Interpersonal Theory of Psychiatry. Edited by Perry HS, Gawel ML. New York, WW Norton, 1953

Sullivan HS: Schizophrenia as a Human Process. New York, WW Norton, 1962

Sutherland JD: Fairbairn's Journey into the Interior. London, Free Association Books, 1989

Will OA: Human relatedness and the schizophrenic reaction. Psychiatry 22:205–223, 1959

Winnicott DW: Collected Papers: Through Paediatrics to Psychoanalysis. New York, Basic Books, 1958

Winnicott DW: The maturational processes and the facilitating environment, in Studies in the Theory of Emotional Development. New York, International Universities Press, 1965

Winnicott DW: Playing and Reality. New York, Basic Books, 1971

5

Intersubjectivity

DANIEL STERN, M.D.

BROADLY SPEAKING, *intersubjectivity* concerns the ability to share in another's lived experience. More specifically, Dunn provides a convenient summary definition of intersubjectivity in psychoanalysis as "the dynamic interplay between the analyst's and the patient's subjective experience in the clinical situation" (Dunn 1995, p. 723). The issue of intersubjectivity entered the psychoanalytic discourse through the doors of transference (Freud 1905 [1901]/1953, 1912a/1958) and countertransference (Freud 1912b/1958), with a large influence from Ferenczi (Aron and Harris 1993). But alongside these specific contributions, intersubjectivity has permeated psychoanalysis since its beginning as a hidden basic assumption. After all, persons would never even bother to talk to others about their personal subjective experiences if they did not assume that the others could share or see the mental landscape they were describing. In this sense, intersubjectivity has been almost like the oxygen we breath but never see or think of.

In the last decades, however, intersubjectivity not only has been made visible but is assuming a foreground position in the theories and practice of psychoanalysis. It has emerged as one of the major underpinnings of several new schools in psychoanalysis: the broad category of intersubjectivist schools (Aron 1991; Atwood and Stolorow 1984; Beebe and Lachman 2002; Benjamin 1988, 1995; Ehrenberg 1982, 1992; Greenberg 1988; Hoffman 1991; Jacobs 1991; Knoblauch 2000; Modell 1993; Ogden 1994; Renik 1993; Spezzano 1995; Stolorow et al. 1987, 1992, 1994), the interactional school (Boesky 1990; Chused 1991; Chused

and Raphling 1992), the relational schools (Bollas 1987; Greenberg and Mitchell 1983; Mitchell 1988, 1993, 1997, 2000), and schools based on aspects of self psychology (Goldberg 1988, 1994; Kohut 1959, 1977; Wolf 1988). All have highlighted some of the basic intersubjectivist assumptions that set these approaches apart from classical Freudian psychoanalysis, at least theoretically (see Aron 1991; Dunn 1995; Mitchell 2000 for critical reviews).

Classical Versus Intersubjective Views of Psychoanalysis

The differences between the intersubjective and the classical conceptions of the nature and process of psychoanalysis can be summarized along three major lines.

First, the classical approach assumes that the analyst can be objective (with effort and care)—that he or she can observe from a "third person perspective" and, from this objective vantage point, discover the psychic reality that resides in the patient's mind, consciously or unconsciously. Not only does the patient's psychic reality lie as an object to be discovered as in any natural science, but it exists (in the main) independently of the observer (the analyst) and of the therapeutic relationship. The patient's subjective reality is determined intrapsychically by the interaction of psychobiological tendencies (e.g., drives, original phantasies, psychosexual stages) with earlier experience—earlier than walking into the analyst's office that day.

In contradistinction, the intersubjective approach posits that neither the analyst nor the patient can ever take a "third person perspective" because the material that emerges in a session is inevitably co-created by the mingling of both the patient's and the analyst's subjectivities. In the extreme, there is no objective reality that stands outside the intersubjective matrix of a session. In this view, the patient's subjective reality as it emerges in a session is not independent of the intersubjective matrix with the analyst. The patient's psychic reality is not discovered or brought forward in time; rather, it is determined by interactive and relational phenomena prevailing at the moment. The intrapsychic origins assumed by the classical position have been replaced by social origins. From this perspective, transference and countertransference get subsumed under the larger category of intersubjectivity (Ogden 1992a, 1992b, 1994). It is in the light of this interplay of the patient's and analyst's subjectivities that Green (1975) describes the "analytic object."

Several authors with a classical approach take into account the inevitably intersubjective nature of the happenings during a session but find that doing so does not totally undermine the classical position (Brenner 1968; Whitebook 1993, 1995). Others suggest that the theoretical distinctions between schools become less apparent in actual practice (Dunn 1995).

Second, underlying these two positions is a divergence in what is conceived of as the main tendency of the psyche. In the classical view, it is to discharge energy and achieve pleasure. With this as a central goal, the immediate context becomes relatively nonspecific. This view leads toward a one-person psychology, in which the subjectivity of the analyst can be relegated to a secondary position. In the intersubjective view, the main tendency of mind is to establish object relationships. To do this, the subjectivity of the object, as well as that of the subject, becomes crucial, and a two-person psychology emerges.

Third, the thinking behind the classical approach is causal and positivistic in that one searches for presumably findable causal links already existing in someone's mind. This is the classical model for proceeding in any natural science. Even in the more hermeneutic tradition, one searches for the pieces of subjectivity that make the most coherent narrative. In the intersubjective approach, the classical model of science has been partially replaced by a more nonlinear mode of conceptualizing that is inspired by dynamic systems theory (Prigogine 1997; Prigogine and Stengers 1984), complexity theory (Waldrop 1992), or chaos theory (Gleick 1987). This switch in models is necessary if the primary data in a session arise by virtue of the unpredictable interplay of two subjectivities. Clinical data become an emergent property that did not exist before, in that form, in either's mind until they interacted and that pops up in a nonlinear, noncausal, relatively unpredictable manner.

In many of the fields that explore the mind, there has been a pendulum swing from the individual to the social, and the linear to the nonlinear. This change in perspective has necessitated different scientific models that address the nonlinear rather than the causal and that can deal with the spontaneous emergence of happenings from an interactive matrix. For instance, in developmental thinking, alone, the role of the social environment has become more emphasized in the emergence of language (Vygotsky 1934/1962), meaning (Bruner et al. 1966), morality (Rochat 1999), consciousness (Stern 2003), identity (Feldman and Kalman 1996), and the self—all of which are now seen largely in the light of their social co-creation. Trends in psychoanalysis are part of this same movement. In psychoanalysis this shift has taken the form of moving from the intrapsychic to the relational and intersubjective.

Psychoanalysis was never blind to this perspective. The classical conceptualizations of transference, countertransference, projective identification, identification, internalization, object relations, empathy, and superego formation all touch the essence of the intersubjective perspective. However, the classical theory did not alter to more fully take into account what it already knew about intersubjectivity. The reasons that intersubjectivity as a central phenomenon, in itself, remained hidden for so long will become apparent.

With this in mind, I examine in this chapter some of the fundamental notions and findings behind the intersubjective perspective and some of the clinical implications. I also describe some of the recent findings and observations that provide the bases for thinking along intersubjectivist lines. But first let us return to definitions.

Definitions

Intersubjectivity is the capacity to share, know, understand, empathize with, feel, participate in, resonate with, and enter into the lived subjective experience of another. It is a form of nonmagical mindreading via interpreting overt behaviors such as posture, tone of voice, speech rhythm, and facial expression, as well as verbal content. Such a capacity is, of course, a crucial aspect of the work of psychoanalysis, which assumes that the analyst can come to share, know, and feel what is in the mind of a patient, in the sense of what the patient is experiencing. And the analysand expects (hopes and fears) that the analyst can and will do this.

We first turn to a more complete definition of inter-subjectivity, in which we can distinguish its various forms and other related terms, especially as they are used in psychoanalysis.

How is intersubjectivity different from empathy or sympathy? For all practical purposes, psychoanalysis has used the term *empathy* in the place of intersubjectivity. (Actually, the original meaning of *sympathy* comes closer to the current sense of intersubjectivity.) The problem with comparing empathy and intersubjectivity is that empathy, as used in the context of psychoanalysis, has come to have so many meanings (Lichtenberg et al. 1984). Reed (1984) noted that the concept of empathy in psychoanalysis not only has multiple meanings but also has several antithetical usages. The active use (grasping meanings, understanding, interpreting) and the passive use (resonating, loosing the self in the other, illumination) are two examples. There is a tension in usages of the term between those in which empathy appears to be basically rational and those in which it is ultimately mysterious, having a completely intuitive basis. In a similar vein, there is a tension between empathy as a process belonging essentially to art (where it had its origin in aesthetics) and one belonging to science (a dichotomy long evident in psychoanalysis). In the totality of its usages, there is also confusion as to whether empathy refers more, or even exclusively, to emotional experience or feelings than to explicit, verbal, propositional content. Furthermore, empathy has been antithetically viewed as penetration (phallic and masculine) or as creation (nurturing and feminine). There is also the confusion about the nature and scope of empathy. Is it a tool, instrument, clinical mechanism, a way of listening, a condition of humanness, or a basic principle of therapeutic technique? Where are its limits? Or, in a similar vein, is empathy periodic, only being activated from time to time, or a continuous process? Is it empathy only when it evokes a response or action toward the person empathized with? Or can it be silent and motionless? This summary does not exhaust all the meanings and uses of the concept of empathy, but it gives an idea of the complexity and weight of the intellectual and historical baggage that the concept carries in psychoanalysis.

In short, *empathy* has become the term in psychoanalysis that has been used to encompass the many facets of the concept of intersubjectivity. For this reason I will not try to explore where the definitions of empathy and intersubjectivity overlap or diverge. It would be useless. Instead, I plan to take the term and concept of *intersubjectivity* and establish it as the fundamental human process that empathy borrows from in creating its multiple meanings.

This isolating of intersubjectivity (both the term and the concept) from empathy is justified on several grounds. First, as discussed in the next section, we are beginning to have a solid, unified, scientific, and developmental basis for understanding intersubjectivity. Other disciplines (philosophy, development psychology, consciousness studies, academic psychology, neuroscience) are all actively studying intersubjectivity, and the term *intersubjectivity* has become the coinage of the larger realm. If psychoanalysis would use it too, we could better note where psychoanalysis, because of its particular nature, may need other terms to distinguish concepts clearly from the base concept of intersubjectivity. It would also clarify and systematize the multiple meanings sought after in psychoanalysis.

Is consciousness required for intersubjectivity? In philosophy, intersubjectivity refers only to mental material that is conscious (this can include material that was preconscious or unconscious just before). This restriction is necessary because intersubjectivity addresses the subjectivity of the other, and subjectivity concerns only what is now being experienced on the mental stage of consciousness. Indeed, as noted at the opening of this chapter, Dunn (1995) defines intersubjectivity in the psychoanalytic situation as the interplay of two subjectivities. For other psychoanalysts, on the contrary, intersubjectivity also includes mental material that is unconscious or simply out of awareness. The knowable mental stage of the other has been extended, and one can know what is happening in the wings as well as on the stage of consciousness. To push it even further, Heller and colleagues (2001) suggest that a therapist can know another's mind implicitly and nonconsciously through their nonverbal behaviors—that is, without consciously knowing that he or she knows. It is clear that intersubjectivity requires an awareness of subjective states but not necessarily a reflective consciousness of these states.

Is intersubjectivity symmetric in the analytic setting (symmetry or asymmetry; one-way or two-way intersubjectivity)? If the analyst understands or feels what is going on in the mind of the patient but the patient does not know that (or if the patient understands or feels the analyst's experience but the analyst does not know that), we have a situation of one-way, asymmetric intersubjectivity. Neither knows that the other knows. This is the situation that prevails in psychoanalysis much of the time. In two-way intersubjectivity, both analyst and patient are viewing a similar mental landscape together and they know it and mutually validate each other's knowledge. It permits them to sense or to say, "I know that you know that I know," or, "I feel that you feel that I feel." This also happens during sessions but is a rarer, more circumscribed event. The two-way experience often results during interpretive activities, especially immediately after an interpretation has been made and the impact is being absorbed by the patient.

Many psychoanalysts (Stolerow et al. 1992) focus mainly on the one-way intersubjectivity of the analyst's knowing the patient's subjective experience; this focus is congruent with an emphasis on the transference. Others (e.g., Benjamin 1995; Jacobs 1991) focus more on the one-way intersubjectivity going in the other direction; here the emphasis is more on the countertransference. Still others (Boston Process of Change Study Group 2003a, 2003b; Stern et al. 2002) talk in terms of a roughly symmetrical field, or at least one whose direction fluctuates frequently.

Is intersubjectivity about understanding or about feeling? Some analysts focus on the understanding of what is going on in another's mind—understanding in the sense of knowing, describing, and even explaining. Others (e.g., Kohut 1977) focus on the empathic immersion, the participation in the other's experience. Intersubjectivity includes both. This distinction can also be seen through the lens of verbal versus nonverbal sources of intersubjectivity. While talking has a very special place in psychoanalysis, it is always accompanied by gestures, changes in body tonus, shifts in posture, and changes in tone of voice and other paralinguistic features such as spacing of silences and rhythm. These nonverbal features are the other source for intersubjectivity, along with the content of speech. Without the nonverbal it would be hard to achieve the empathic, participatory, and resonating aspects of intersubjectivity. One would only be left with a kind of pared down, neutral "understanding" of the other's subjective experience. One reason this distinction is drawn is that in many cases the analyst is consciously aware of the content of speech while processing the nonverbal aspects out of awareness. With an intersubjectivist perspective, a more conscious processing by the analyst of the nonverbal is necessary. A second reason for distinguishing between verbal and nonverbal sources is that the purely verbal source for intersubjectivity operates in a different time frame and by way of a different process than the nonverbal sources (Stern 2003).

Can intersubjectivity be imaginary? In projective identification the patient, for example, imagines that he or she feels or knows what is in the therapist's mind, but in fact these mental contents belong to the patient and were projected onto the other's mind. If that were all, it would be a false or imagined intersubjectivity. However, the projection is not made of whole cloth; it is usually built around a piece of truth about the analyst, however small. In addition, it is frequently noted that a countertransference may begin to emerge in the analyst that complements the transference of the patient. Even if the truth is small, we end up with a complex mixture of "true" and imagined intersubjectivity.

Intersubjectivity comprises a large set of phenomena. It seems unnecessary at this point to restrict its usage with too tight a definition, especially in clinical matters. Nonetheless, the distinctions noted above should be kept in mind in order to think and communicate more clearly.

The Nature and Development of Intersubjectivity

Intersubjectivity has a developmental course that raises many fundamental questions for psychoanalysis. The first is, When does intersubjectivity begin? It cannot begin until there is sufficient self-other differentiation so that one can reasonably speak of some kind of awareness of entering another's mind or sharing between two minds. Among psychoanalytic thinkers there is a divergence about when this becomes possible. Mahler stated the traditional position that during an initial phase of "normal autism" (which englobes primary narcissism), there is no self-other differentiation (Mahler et al. 1975). Thus, intersubjectivity even of a most primitive kind could not exist. Fusion is not intersubjectivity; the existence of two separate minds must be sensed. Others argue that self-other differentiation begins at birth, thus opening the door for a primative form of intersubjectivity, a "core intersubjectivity" which is present in all the later forms (Stern 1985; Trevarthen 1993; Trevarthen and Hubley 1978). What might a core intersubjectivity be like?

Recent neurobiological findings suggest a neural foundation for a core intersubjectivity, a "primary intersubjectivity" (Trevarthen and Hubley 1978)—a core on which key clinical phenomena such as empathy, identification, and internalization ultimately rest. A crucial recent finding, the discovery of "mirror neurons," provides possible neurobiological mechanisms for understanding the capacity for core intersubjectivity (e.g., Gallese 2001; Rizzolatti et al. 2001).

Mirror neurons sit adjacent to motor neurons and fire in an observer who is doing nothing but watching another person behave (e.g., reaching for a glass). The pattern of firing in the observer mimics the exact pattern that would occur in the observer if she were reaching for the glass herself. In brief, the visual information received when we are watching another person act gets mapped onto the equivalent motor representation in our own brain by the activity of these mirror neurons. It permits us to directly participate in another's actions, without having to imitate them. We experience the other *as if* we were executing the same action or feeling the same emotion. This "participation" in another's mental life creates a sense of sharing with and understanding the other, and in particular their intentions and feelings.

Clearly, the mirror neuron system may take us far into understanding (at the neural level) intersubjectivity and the other phenomena that rest on it. At this point, the evidence for such a resonance system is good for hand, mouth, face, and foot actions. It also functions for paralinguistic vocal behaviors, facial expressions, and touch. We know what it feels like to be another who has made a certain sound, moves their face into a certain expression, or has been touched by someone else. This mode of participating in another's experience is clearly built into the system and must be present in babies from the beginning.

Experiments on very early imitation by neonates suggest that this is true. Early imitation has been another major route to proposing early forms of intersubjectivity (Kugiumutzakis 1999; Maratos 1973; Meltzoff 1995; Meltzoff and Moore 1977, 1999). Meltzoff and colleagues began by focusing on neonates imitating actions seen on an experimenter's face (e.g., sticking the tongue out). This is not a reflex. How could one explain such behaviors when the infants did not know they had a face or tongue; when they only saw a visual image of the experimenter's act, yet responded with a motor act guided by their own proprioceptive (not visual) feedback; and when there had been no previous learning trials to establish such an (invisible) imitation? The answer lies in an early form of intersubjectivity based on mirror neurons and a cross-modal transfer of form and timing.

The central idea is that we are born with a capacity to participate in the experience of others. This base is a given, a mental primative, and the developmental starting point of a core intersubjectivity

An experiment with a preverbal infant bears on this idea. The infant watched an experimenter act as if he wished to pull the bulb off one end of a dumbbell-like object, but he failed. Later, when the infant was given the object, he immediately tried to pull the bulb off. He succeeded and seemed pleased. When, however, the "experimenter" was a robot that performed the same failed actions as the real experimenter, the infant, when given the chance, did not try to pull the knob off. The infant seemed to assume that only people, not robots, have intentions that are worth inferring and imitating. Robots are not like me (Meltzoff 1995). Meltzoff and colleagues concluded that infants take in something of the other in the act of imitation, which solidifies the sense that the other is "like me" and "I am like them." They further speculated that for an infant to learn about (make internal representations of) inanimate objects, he must manipulate or mouth them, but to learn about (and represent) people he must imitate them. The infant's mind uses different channels for people.

The infant, even as a neonate, has the minimal basic capacities for a limited core intersubjectivity. As develop-

ment proceeds, then, and the infant acquires new capacities, she can (intersubjectively) experience another executing those same capacities. For instance, infants very early acquire the ability to infer intentions in others. This is in fact what they go after in parsing people's behavior. For instance, preverbal infants grasp the intention of someone acting, even when they have never seen the intention fully enacted (i.e., never reaching its intended goal). In such a situation, grasping the intention requires an inference about what is in someone else's mind. In one experiment, the preverbal infant watched an experimenter pick up an object and "try" to put it into a container. But, the experimenter dropped the object en route, so it never got to the intended goal. Later, when the infant was brought back to the scene and given the same material, he picked up the object and directly put it into the container. In other words, he enacted the action that he assumed was intended, not the one he had seen. The infant chose to privilege the unseen, assumed intention over the seen, actual action (Meltzoff 1995; Meltzoff and Moore 1999). Others (e.g., Gergely and Csibra 1997) have demonstrated the same inferring of intentions, a form of "mind reading" or intersubjectivity. This finding is particularly interesting in that it accords with the psychoanalytic notion that the wish/motive is the basic unit of psychodynamic life, not only for the one who is wishing but also for the one who is interpreting the other's wishes/motives.

In brief, the developmental evidence suggests that beginning at birth the infant enters into an intersubjective matrix. That this occurs is assured because basic forms of intersubjectivity are manifest right away. As new capacities are developed and new experiences become available, they are swept into the intersubjective matrix, which has its own ontogenesis. At first actions, then intentions and affects, then sharing attention, and then, as the infant reaches the second year and is capable of new experiences such as language, the "moral" emotions of shame, guilt, and embarrassment get drawn into the intersubjective matrix as something the child can now experience within himself or herself and in others.

During middle childhood, another cognitive leap occurs, making dyadic (two-way) intersubjectivity clearer and explicit. This leap, referred to as acquiring a "theory of mind," entails developing a representation of other minds as separate from one's own and as entertaining different contents from one's own mind (Baron-Cohen 1995; Fodor 1992; Leslie 1987). This developmental leap allows an explicit, recursive participation in the intersubjective process. Now, one can say not only that "I know that you know" but also "I know that you know that I know."

The breadth and complexity of the possible contents of the intersubjective matrix expand developmentally. At each phase of the life course, the intersubjective matrix grows deeper and richer. We develop our mind and sustain its integrity in a matrix of other people's wishes, feelings, intentions, actions, thoughts, and beliefs.

Autism provides another line of vision on intersubjectivity. What strikes one most about autistic individuals is that they are not immersed in an intersubjective matrix. There appears to be a failure of "mindreading" (Grandin 1995; Hobson 1993). Even more, one gets the impression that there is no interest in reading another's behavior or mind, as if it has no special attractions or possibilities, any more than an inanimate object does. Others, such as Francis Tustin (1990), claim that this "disinterest" to things human is defensive, to protect these children with their painfully low thresholds for human stimulation. Even if this explanation is correct, in whole for some cases and in part for others, the result is the same. The human world is not treated as special and "like them." There is a massive failure of intersubjectivity. Autistic persons appear to be "mind blind." It is this that makes them often appear odd or from another world. The existence of autism is not in itself evidence for the intersubjective matrix. However, the picture of people living without being immersed in an intersubjective matrix gives a perspective on the matrix we normally live in and take for granted.

Another view on intersubjectivity comes from phenomenological philosophy. Historically, we, in the modern, scientifically oriented West, have isolated the mind from the body and from other minds. Our experience of other minds has to be constructed privately, slowly, and perhaps quite idiosyncratically within our own mind. Until recently this view has been dominant and largely unchallenged except by philosophers. In Greek antiquity, minds were thought to be far more permeable to other minds. We are now experiencing a revolution—not back to the views of antiquity, but closer to them. This revolution has been inspired largely by the work of philosophers of phenomenology, especially Edmund Husserl (1960, 1962, 1964, 1980, 1989). The phenomenological approach has been revitalized by contemporary philosophers and incorporated by some scientists into current alternative views of human nature that are rapidly gaining strength (e.g., Clark 1997, 1999; Damasio 1994, 1999; Freeman 1999; Gallagher 1997; Marbach 1999; Sheets-Johnstone 1999; Thompson 2001; Varela et al. 1993; Zahavi 2001). This new view assumes that the mind is always embodied in and made possible by the sensorimotor activity of the person and that it is interwoven with and co-created by its interactions with other minds. The mind takes on and maintains its form and nature from this open traffic. It emerges and exists only from the ongoing interaction of intrinsic self-organizing brain processes with the environment of other minds, including the culture. Without these constant interactions, there would be no recognizable mind.

One of the consequences of this phenomenological view of "embodied cognition" is that the mind is, by nature, "intersubjectively open" because it is partially constituted through its interaction with other minds (Husserl 1960; Thompson 2001; Zahavi 2001). Such openness is possible only because human beings possess a mental primative described as "the passive (not voluntarily initiated), pre-reflected experience of the other as an embodied being like oneself" (Thompson 2001, p. 12).

Recent neurobiological findings support this philosophical position. The intersubjective openness seen so early in development in the form of primary intersubjectivity (synchrony, imitation, attunement, etc.) also supports this philosophical view. It is in this sense that Bråten (1999) speaks of the infant being made by nature to encounter "virtual others," a sort of empty original phantasy, ready to be filled. We are preprepared to enter into the intersubjective matrix, which is a condition of humanness.

Intersubjectivity as a Basic and Independent Tendency of Mind

A consequence of the basic subjectivist view concerns the fundamental tendencies of mind: the drives and motivational systems. As stated earlier (see section "Classical Versus Intersubjective Views of Psychoanalysis" in this chapter), in the classical view discharge of psychic energy, with its accompanying gratification, is the fundamental tendency of mind from which all other motivations flow. On the contrary, if intersubjectivity is given a primary place, an object-related need to share experiences must be identified. The history of modern psychoanalysis is full of efforts to establish object-related drives as having a primary status, not dependent on or variations of the sexual drive, and not describable in terms of physiological satisfaction. The British object relations school (e.g., the Kleinian school [Heimann 1950]) made a major step in that direction. The advent of attachment theory (Bowlby 1969) pushed these notions further. Now, with the growing importance of intersubjectivity, an object-related need for intersubjectivity is required. Such a need goes well beyond a need for physical proximity or contact, psychological security, or sexual contact. It involves a need for psychological intimacy—for the sharing of worlds of subjective experience. This need is so pervasive and important it may be best considered a basic, independent tendency of mind (Stern 2003).

The notion of a primary need for intersubjectivity, in the psychobiological sense of a drive or instinct, requires justification in terms of its necessary role in the survival of the species. Species survival was a not insignificant theoretical underpinning of the importance Freud gave to the sexual drive and the importance Bowlby gave to the attachment motivation.

A drive or basic motivational system must meet certain criteria. It should be a universal tendency to behave in a way characteristic of a species. This tendency should strongly favor species survival. It should be universal and innate, though it can receive important environmental shaping. It must have a peremptory quality, a push in the form of wish, so its value to the organism can take precedence. And it must be able to enlist, assemble, and organize behaviors and mental events rapidly as needed.

Does a tendency toward intersubjectivity meet these criteria? Several authors have argued that the answer is yes (Stern 2003; Trevarthen 1998). In brief, intersubjectivity makes three main contributions to assuring survival: promoting group formation, enhancing group functioning, and ensuring group cohesion. The same impulse that contributes to species survival can also serve to make psychotherapy move forward.

Humans are a relatively defenseless species. We survive because of our brains and coordinated group activity. Human survival depends on group formation (dyads, families, tribes, societies) and almost constant group cohesion. Many different capacities and motivations act together to form and maintain groups: attachment ties, sexual attraction, dominance hierachies, love, and sociability. Intersubjectivity can be added to the list.

Broadly speaking, the intersubjective motivational system concerns regulating psychological belongingness versus psychological aloneness. At the extremes, there is, at one pole, cosmic loneliness and, at the other pole, mental transparency, fusion, and disappearance of the self. The intersubjective motivational system regulates the zone of intersubjective comfort somewhere between the two poles. The exact point of comfort depends on one's role in the group, whom one is with, and the personal history of the relationship leading up to that moment. The point on the continuum must be negotiated continually with second-to-second fine tuning. Too much is at stake for it not to be.

What is at stake is psychological intimacy and belongingness, which play a powerful role in group formation and maintenance. Psychological belongingness is different from physical, sexual, attachment, or dependency ties. It is a separate order of relatedness—a form of group belonging that either is unique to humans or has taken an enormous quantitative and qualitative leap in our species. One might argue that the leap is language. But without intersubjectivity, language could not develop.

The intersubjective motivational system can be considered separate from and complementary to the sexual and attachment drives—and equally fundamental. Clinically, we see sexual or attachment behaviors in the service of intersubjective belonging (and vice versa). (For a more detailed discussion of such issues of motivational systems, see Dornes 2002 and Lichtenberg 1989.) In attachment theory, there are two contradictory motives and poles: proximity/security and distance/exploration-curiosity. The attachment system mediates between these two poles. The basic survival advantage is in physically staying close together for protection against environmental dangers—be they those posed by tigers, automobiles, electric plugs, or other people—and yet being able to explore in order to learn about the world. Attachment is designed for physical closeness and group bonding rather than for psychological intimacy. Many people who are "strongly" attached do not share psychological closeness or intimacy (but, in fact, the opposite). Another system is needed for that. Dissociating the two motivational systems is important both theoretically and clinically. The same applies to the sexual impulse relative to intersubjectivity. These three motivations—sex, attachment, intersubjectivity—can become mixed or serve one another in multiple combinations while remaining independent.

Humans need to act together to survive. The ability to read others' intentions and feelings allows for an extremely flexible coordination of group action. The ability to communicate quickly and subtly within the group, through the use of intention movements, signals, and language, expands the group's efficiency and speed of action—in other words, its adaptability.

In addition to language, humans have the most highly developed and richest repertoire of facial and vocal (paralinguistic) expressions. These too assume an intersubjective capacity within the group that goes beyond simple sign decoding or instrumental communication.

Humans spend an enormous amount of time becoming proficient in intersubjectivity and practicing it developmentally. We are the most imitative species. Nadel (1986) reported that reciprocal imitation constitutes the main form of play between children up to 3 or so years of age. And it continues beyond that age, just less so. After 3 years, teasing, kidding, tricking, and so forth become major activities (Dunn 1999; Reddy 1991). These too have an intersubjective basis. You can only tease or trick someone if you know in advance what they are going to experience. We are the most playful species and spend years refining these skills.

Cohesion within human groups is greatly enhanced by moral suasion. I argue, as many have, that intersubjectivity is the basic condition for morality. The "moral emotions" (shame, guilt, embarrassment) arise from being able to see yourself in the eyes of another—that is, as you sense the other sees you. Freud, in his account of the origin of morality via the superego—the internalized regard of the parent—makes the same assumption.

Intersubjectivity plays an essential role in the appearance of reflective consciousness. The idea of reflective consciousness having its origin in social interaction is not new. Some form of an "other" is the essential feature. The "other" can be external or internal, but the primary experience must be shared from a second point of view (Stern 2003). The advent of reflective consciousness, together with the development of language, is considered key to the evolutionary success of the human species. Both reflective consciousness and language enhance adaptability by giving birth to new options that can transcend fixed action patterns, habit, and some past experience.

In brief, intersubjectivity contributes advantages for group survival. It promotes group formation and coherence and permits more efficient, rapid, flexible, and coordinated group functioning. It also provides the basis for morality's role in maintaining group cohesion and language's role in facilitating group communication.

A motivational system must contain subjectively a felt motive or motives that organize and direct behaviors to a valued goal. While searching for and moving toward the goal, there is a subjective experience of peremptoriness, felt as desire or need. When the goal is achieved, there is the subjective feeling of gratification or relative well-being. Can we speak of an intersubjective motive with the subjective quality of peremptoriness?

There are two such motives. The first felt need for intersubjective orientation is a need to read the intentions and feelings of another in order to sound that person out—a process carried out in the service of figuring out "where we two are at," "what is going on," "where things stand," and "where they are likely to go." This sounding of the immediate dyadic situation and its possibilities occurs upon meeting and then is continually updated, often second by second or minute by minute as needed. It is a form of orientation. If we cannot orient ourselves in time and space, there is confusion and anxiety, and searching behaviors are put in motion. The same is true for intersubjective orientation in psychic space. We need to know where we stand in the intersubjective field with an individual, family, or group. "Intersubjective orientation" is also a vital ongoing event in psychotherapy. It is sought after, and a high affective value is attached to it. The intersubjective field is constantly probed to discover or create "where you are." The need to be intersubjectively oriented is felt as a peremptory force that mobilizes action, thought, and feeling.

Intersubjective orientation is a basic need in the context of direct social contact. When we are not thus oriented, anxiety arises and coping or defense mechanisms are mobilized. This anxiety could be called "intersubjective anxiety." Psychoanalysis has richly explored what are best called the basic fears or anxieties. Being alone or being isolated is on the list, but it is usually not specified whether the aloneness or isolation means physically or mentally. The intersubjective position suggests that two different fears are involved and that the anxiety/fear of psychic loneliness is a separate entry, one that belongs to our intersubjective condition.

A second felt need for intersubjective orientation is to define, maintain, or reestablish self identity and self cohesion—to make contact with our self. We need the eyes of others to form and hold ourselves together. Here, too, the need for the other's regard can be peremptory. Male prisoners with very long or life sentences present an interesting example. By talking they will not get early parole, nor will they be absolved. Yet, they often want to talk to someone. Such prisoners keep coming to talk, to share their inner world. Why? One receives the clinical impression that many of these individuals need intersubjective encounters to remain in contact with themselves. Under the isolating conditions of prison, they need the intersubjective regard of the other to find their identity once again and maintain it (C. Simonet and P. Jaffe, personal communication, 2001).

Without some continual input from an intersubjective matrix, human identity will dissolve or veer off in odd ways. It does not matter whether this contact is in the form of dyadic mind sharing, engaging in group rituals, or having internal dialogues with internalized others or parallel selves.

In this regard, it is interesting to consider that the majority of children ages 6 to 12 in the several cultures studied have "imaginary companions" (Pearson et al. 2001). The figure is higher for girls, but very likely there is underreporting for boys. Why do so many children this age have imaginary companions? Most often there is some form of dialogue with these companions. Children apparently create these companions to complement or stabilize, to validate, or to orient the their identity by way of an "inter-intra" subjective relationship.

Falling in love provides another situation for exploring the power of the intersubjective push. Falling in love has wide cultural and historical variability but is sufficiently pervasive and has enough common features to warrant examination. First, it is a mental state that could be called a special state of mental organization because it pulls together so many diverse behaviors, feelings, and thoughts into an integrated assembly that is readily recognized. Some of the elements of falling in love that are driven by an intersubjectve motive are as follows.

Lovers can look into each other's eyes, without speaking, for minutes on end, a sort of plunging through the "window of the soul" to find the interior of the other. On the contrary, nonlovers in this culture cannot tolerate the mounting intensity of silent mutual gaze for more than 7 seconds or so without turning away or fighting. There is also exquisite attention among lovers to the other's intentions and feelings, allowing them not only to read the other's intentions and feelings correctly but also to anticipate them. There is a playfulness that involves much facial, gestural, and postural imitation. There is the creating of a private world, a sort of privileged intersubjective space to which they alone have the keys. The keys are special words with specific meanings, secret abbreviations, sacred rituals and spaces, and so on—all the things that create a psychological niche in which intersubjectivity can flourish.

Ethel Person (1988) has pointed out that in the process of falling in love, the lover creates a two-person world, in which the couple forms, and also re-creates himself. The lover is thrown into a turbulent process of self-change (whether permanent or not is another question). The situation is almost the opposite of the life prisoner's, in which nothing can change and the prisoner can just stay the same, albeit with effort. The lover too needs the eyes of the other to verify and validate his metamorphosis, to keep him in contact with himself, with his shifting identity. The regard of the other also helps maintain self cohesion in the face of the desire for communion and fusion.

A basic motivational system should be innate and universal and diverse in its modes of expression. The evidence for the neurobiological and developmental foundations of intersubjectivity presented above goes a certain distance in addressing the issue of innateness—at least the capacity for intersubjectivity.

Concerning the primary motivational status of intersubjectivity, some might argue that intersubjectivity is a human condition, not a motivational system in itself, because it is nonspecific and is brought into play in the service of almost all motivational systems. A counterargument is that while intersubjectivity can come into play in the service of other motivational systems, it is strongly activated in highly specific and important interhuman situations in which it becomes the goal state unto itself:

- When the threat of intersubjective disorientation with accompanying intersubjective anxiety arises
- When the desire for psychic intimacy is great (as in falling in love)
- When rapidly coordinated group functioning is needed and the coordination must be spontaneously, rapidly, and flexibly altered from moment to moment (e.g., hunting a dangerous wild animal)

- When self-identity is threatened and dipping into the intersubjective matrix is needed to prevent self dissolution or fragmentation

In these situations, intersubjective contact is the goal state. For our purposes, the intersubjective motive is also at play in directing the second-by-second regulation of the therapeutic process in which the sharing of mental landscapes is desired and must be sought.

Intersubjectivity Seen Clinically

Many of the therapeutic implications of the intersubjectivist approach can be found in the references to this approach in the introductory section of this chapter. Here, I present an extended view of the intersubjectivist assumptions that comes from the work of the Boston Change Process Study Group (BostonCPSG) (2002, 2003; Stern et al. 1998; Tronick et al. 1998). (The current BostonCPSG members are N. Bruschweiler-Stern, K. Lyons-Ruth, A. Morgan, J. Nahum, L.S. Sander, and D.N. Stern.)

The basic premise of the intersubjectivist approach is that the central psychoanalytic subject matter consists of the material that emerges during a session from the co-creative interplay of two subjectivities. If one accepts this premise, several consequences follow. First, greater attention must be given to the "here and now"—namely, the present moment in which the material emerges. This focus requires a more phenomenological approach that addresses experience as it unfolds during a session, because the material in a session as actually experienced by patient and analyst is happening in the present moment. The analyst adopts the viewpoint of being in the middle of an ongoing session; what will happen next, in the seconds that follow, is not yet known. This is a different perspective than the more common one of retrospectively viewing the session either alone or as part of several sessions taken together.

Elsewhere (Stern 2003) I have adopted this phenomenological perspective in viewing therapy and in considering the subjective experience of the present moment as therapy unfolds. One of the implications of this shift in perspective is that the present starts to play a more central role relative to the past. Memories are seen as experiences that are happening now. They are chosen and reassembled under the present remembering context of the momentary intersubjective field co-created by patient and analyst. In this sense, the experienced present determines the functional past (not the historical past) as much as the past determines the experience of the present. As Edelman (1990) has described, one assembles pieces of the past to "remember the present."

Another implication is that the *process* of a session moves more into the foreground, relative to the content. This emphasis involves a greater attention to the microevents that are the raw data of a session (a phrase, a speaking turn, a silence, a shift in posture, etc.). Such events are the small moves (relational moves and present moments) that constitute the stuff of the therapeutic interaction. They are also the only moments that are directly lived before being abstracted into narrative meanings. These moves—each lasting only several seconds as a rule—regulate the intersubjective field. What happens from move to move is largely unpredictable as to the exact form and timing of its appearance. The psychodynamic content of the session is largely permitted to emerge or prevented from emerging by the nature of the immediately prevailing intersubjective field. The likelihood of the emergence of the material, the timing of its emergence, the form of its expression, and even the content itself are importantly dependent on the immediate status of the intersubjective field.

With these assumptions in mind, it is clear that the process, compared with the verbal content, of the analytic session takes on greater importance. Attention to the micro-level process must occur in parallel with attending to the meaningful content of the verbal flow. In brief, it is necessary to take a more phenomenological perspective of the analytic process in which the ending of the session is not yet known.

Three main intersubjective motives push the clinical process:

1. *Sounding out the other to see where one is in the intersubjective field.* This motive, a form of intersubjective orienting, involves the moment-by-moment testing, mostly out of consciousness, of where the relationship between patient and therapist is and where it is going. Orienting oneself in this way is a precondition of working together.
2. *Sharing (or avoiding sharing) experience in order to be known (or not known).* Each time the intersubjective field is enlarged, the relationship is implicitly altered. The patient then is experiencing a new way of being-with the therapist and hopefully others. The change is implicit; it need not be made explicit and talked about; it becomes part of the patient's implicit relational knowing. Another consequence is that whenever the intersubjective field is enlarged, new paths for explicit exploration open up. More of the patient's world becomes consciously, verbally understandable.
3. *Defining and redefining one's self by using the reflection of the self from the analyst's "eyes."* One's own identity gets reformed or consolidated in this process.

These goals are realized at the local level by the sequences of relational moves and present moments that make up the session.

An example serves best to illustrate a dialogue of relational moves and present moments that lead to continual adjustment of the intersubjective field. This description comes from the clinical experience of a member of the BostonCPSG (cited in Boston Change Process Study Group 2002, 2003; Stern 2003). The example is quite banal in the sense of being largely devoid of psychodynamically meaningful content of the usual kind. The emphasis, rather, is on describing the process of creating and adjusting the intersubjective field. It is the kind of adjustment that analysts make with their patients all the time but that usually passes unremarked (but not unregistered). From the intersubjective perspective, attending to adjustments in the intersubjective field moves into the foreground. The session is driven forward, in large part, by the need to establish intersubjective contact. This is why the general intersubjective motive is considered as particularly relevant to the clinical situation.

Dialogue of Relational Moves: Clinical Example

Relational Move 1 (Opening of the Session)

PATIENT: *"I don't feel entirely here today."*

The intersubjective intention is to announce the immediate state of her position in the relationship. It establishes a certain distance and reluctance to do much intersubjective work, at least for the moment. She is saying that she is not yet available for or desirous of such joint work.

Relational Move 2

ANALYST: *"Ah."*

Said with a pitch rise at the end. This serves as a recognition of the patient's declaration. It is not clear whether it is a full acceptance of the intersubjective state the patient has put forward, a mild questioning of it, or both. In either case, it represents a small step toward working together—small but significant compared with a silence or even a "Hmm" (with a terminal pitch fall). The "Ah" is more open/questioning than a "Hmm" and implies a future event.

Relational Move 3

BOTH PATIENT AND ANALYST: *A silence of six seconds ensues.*

The patient is signaling her hesitancy to jump right in to change the immediate intersubjective status quo. In letting the silence evolve, the analyst puts forward an implicit intention not to change things for the moment, or an implicit invitation and perhaps mild pressure on the patient to break the silence, or both. In either event, patient and therapist are together co-creating a sort of mutual acceptance of the immediate status quo—namely, to do or say nothing. Whether it is a solid or unstable acceptance remains to be seen.

Relational Move 4

PATIENT: *"Yeah."*

The patient reinstates the original intersubjective position. She is not yet ready to move forward or closer. Yet, she indicates that she wishes to maintain contact by saying something. She has not approached, but she has also not withdrawn.

Relational Move 5

BOTH PATIENT AND ANALYST: *Again a silence intervenes.*

The patient still does not take up the implicit invitation to continue from the last move. But since contact has been maintained with the "Yeah," the silence can proceed without any important loss of intersubjective ground. The analyst is holding to his ground, but since his exact position has been left unclear, the relationship can tolerate it. They are loosely being-together in this somewhat unstable state.

Relational Move 6

ANALYST: *"Where are you today?"*

The analyst now makes a clear move toward the patient in the form of an invitation to open wider the intersubjective field.

Relational Move 7

PATIENT: *"I don't know, just not quite here."*

The patient takes a step forward and a half-step back. The forward step is probably the larger because she does share something—namely, the not knowing where she is today. (Which proves not to be true. She does know but is not ready to talk about it. The intersubjective conditions are not yet right.) Her "just not quite here" serves to restate her first relational move (no. 1). Also there is the continued partial refusal by the patient of the analyst's invitation to enlarge the intersubjective field.

Relational Move 8

BOTH PATIENT AND ANALYST: *A longish silence.*

The analyst indicates by silence that he does not intend a re-invitation, at least not now. Nor will he push her harder. He will wait for the patient's initiative and to see what will come up. This silence, too, is a sort of invitation and pressure, weak or strong, depending on the handling of silences that is their habitual pattern of working together. The patient keeps distance but also contact so that a sense of her deciding hangs in the air. It is clear their intersubjective position vis-à-vis each other is unstable. But they have signaled that they can tolerate this limited, temporary way of being-together for the moment. The sharing of this joint toleration, in itself, brings a slight shift in the intersubjective field. It is implicitly known by both of them that something must happen soon.

Relational Move 9

PATIENT: *"Something happened last session that bothered me …[pause], but I'm not sure I want to talk about it."*

The patient takes a big step forward toward the analyst in the sense of sharing experience and expanding the intersubjective field. She also takes a hesitant step backward. The preexisting tension is broken and a new tension is created. An opening has been made that promises to further expand the intersubjective field. This qualifies as a small "now moment" (Boston Change Process Study Group 2002; Stern et al. 1998) because it concentrates attention on new implication of the present moment and its resolution.

Relational Move 10

ANALYST: *"I see…so is the other place where you are now our last session?"*

The analyst validates what the patient said as now intersubjectively shared—namely, that she is not fully there, being still occupied by something [unsettling] that happened last session. He has moved closer to her but without pressing her.

Relational Move 11

PATIENT: *"Yeah…I didn't like it when you said…"*

The patient explains what she did not like about last session. A larger field of intersubjectivity now starts to be claimed and shared.

We can stop the account here to avoid discussing the content belonging to the verbal outflow and stay with the process of regulating the micro-intersubjective environment. So little seems to have happened, so far, yet patient and analyst are positioning themselves intersubjectively so that something can emerge at the content level. Even more important from our point of view, they are establishing a body of implicit knowing about how they work together. They are establishing complicated implicit patterns, unique to them, of how to regulate their intersubjective field. This regulation amounts to experiencing and learning ways-of-being-with another—ways that may not have been in their repertoire before. These ways include the accumulation of a history of being able to resolve such moments and the confidence that goes with having such a history; the experience of tolerating silences together and learning what durations of silence signify what; and the experience of learning to tolerate unstable dyadic states without rushing to premature closure or flight. Any one of these is a potential theme for creating a narrative and working at the level of verbalization and meaning in the usual psychodynamic sense. However, these themes come from the process of regulating the intersubjective field.

There is a second clinical implication of the above intersubjectivist assumptions—one that might best be labeled "sloppiness and co-creation" in the analytic process. The moving along in a session, while it is happening, is largely a spontaneous, unpredictable process at the local level of moment to moment. The analyst cannot know exactly what the patient is going to say next, let alone what she is going to do next, until she says it or does it. And the same applies to the patient. Even when the analyst knows in advance that the patient will soon have to talk about *x*, he cannot know when *x* will come up, nor the exact form that it will take. Often the theme at hand is well known, but one still doesn't know what will happen next.

For this reason, psychotherapy (as experienced from within) is a "sloppy" process. Sloppiness results from the interaction of two minds working in a "hit–miss–repair–elaborate" fashion to co-create and share similar worlds. Because the process is largely spontaneous and unpredictable from move to move, there are a lot of mismatches, derailments, misunderstandings, and indeterminacy. These "mistakes" require a process of repair. Observations of parents and infants reveal that there are "missteps" every minute in the best of interactions. The majority of them are quickly repaired by one or both partners. For certain stretches of interaction, rupture and repair constitute the main activity of mother and baby (Stern 1977; Tronick 1986). Missteps are most valuable because the manner of negotiating repairs and correcting slippages is one of the more important ways-of-being-with another that become implicitly known. They amount to coping or defense mechanisms. The rupture-repair sequence thus is an important learning experience for the infant in negotiating the imperfect human world.

The BostonCPSG found a parallel sloppiness in observing the therapeutic process at the local level from moment to moment (Boston Change Process Study Group 2003). There are several sources of sloppiness:

- The difficulty in knowing your own intentions, in transmitting them, and in another's reading them correctly (a kind of intrinsic "intentional fuzziness")
- Defensive distortions
- Unpredictability
- Redundancy (a large amount), most often with evolving variations
- The improvisational nature of the moving-along process (albeit within larger theoretical guidelines)

"Sloppiness" plays a crucial role. It can be viewed not as error or noise in the system, but rather as an inherent feature of intersubjective interactions. The sloppiness of the process throws new, unexpected, often messy elements into the dialogue. But these can be, and are, used to create new possibilities. Sloppiness is not to be avoided or regretted; rather it is necessary for understanding the almost unlimited co-creativity of the moving-along process.

Sloppiness would be of little value if it did not occur in a context of co-creativity. Both the sloppiness and its repair or unexpected usage are the product of two minds working together to maximize coherence. Note that I use the word "co-create" rather than "co-construct." The latter carries the suggestion that a prior plan is being put in place, with already formed pieces being assembled according to a known model.

The intersubjective process leads to the idea that whatever happens in a session is co-created, or co-adjusted. Several aspects make that clear. First, each move or moment creates the context for the one that follows. So, if the patient (or analyst) enacts a relational move, the subsequent relational move by the partner has already been constrained and partially prepared for. Note that if the patient says something and the analyst is silent while the patient is talking and in the moment right after, that silence, too, is a relational move, as it creates a micro-intersubjective context for what will happen next. This mutual context-creating goes on and on, one relational move after the next, such that the direction of where patient and analyst go together is very largely dyadically determined. It is not the result of following a structure already existing intrapsychically. Second, each relational move or present moment is designed to express an intention relative to the inferred intentions and desires of the other. The two end up seeking, chasing, missing, finding, and shaping each other's intentionality. In this sense also, the moving-along process of a session is co-created—which is significantly true even of free association paths.

To carry this line of thinking further, sloppiness can be seen, in a two-person psychology, as being analogous to eruptions of unconscious material in a one-person psychology (e.g., free association, slips of the tongue, dreams). Both sloppiness and eruptions of unconscious material, along with other unplanned-for emergent events, create the surprise discoveries that push the dyad to its uniqueness. Potentially, they are among its most creative elements.

It is important to emphasize that sloppiness is potentially creative only when it occurs within a well-established framework. Without that, it is only disorder. Accordingly, the analyst can work within the basic techniques and theoretical guidelines of psychoanalysis. Furthermore, within the idiosyncratic style that each analyst uses when applying the method, there is a wide degree of freedom for the co-creation of sloppiness, tailor-made to the dyad.

The BostonCPSG has commented that the processes of intersubjective sloppiness and co-creativity also contribute to the emergence of special moments between the analyst and patient, called "now moments" (Boston Change Process Study Group 2002; Stern 2003; Stern et al. 1998; Tronick et al. 1998). At such moments, the existing understanding between the two participants about the nature of their relationship or the status of their intersubjective sharing is thrown into question or opened out into question. These moments, which are affectively charged and full of potential consequences for the therapeutic relationship, require some resolution. An example (quoted from Stern 2003) serves best:

> Suppose that a patient has been in analytic therapy on the couch for a few years and has expressed concern from time to time that she does not know what the analyst is doing back there, sleeping, knitting, making faces. Then, one morning, without warning, the patient enters, lies down, and says, "I want to sit up and see your face." And with no further ado, she sits up and turns around. The analyst and patient find themselves starring at each other in startled silence. That is a "now moment." (The fact that it can also be called "acting in" is not the point.) The patient did not know she was going to do it, right before, certainly not that day, that moment. It was a spontaneous eruption. Nor did the analyst anticipate it, just then, in that way. Yet, they now find themselves in a novel, charged, interpersonal, and intersubjective situation.

The current state of the implicitly known relationship is sharply thrown into question and placed at stake. The shift is brought about by the unpredictable arising of an emergent property—one that was being prepared for, unseen, in the moving-along process. It threatens to throw the entire intersubjective field into a new state, for better or worse.

The resolution of a now moment comes in the form of a "moment of meeting"—a moment in which the two parties achieve an intersubjective meeting. When this happens, the two become aware of what each other is experiencing in that moment. They share a sufficiently similar mental landscape so that a sense of what Sander (1995a, 1995b, 2002) refers to as "specific fittedness" is achieved. Moments of meeting usually follow immediately after "now moments" that set them up. The moment of meeting then resolves the perturbation created in the now moment. A continuation of the example of the analysand who suddenly sat up to look at her therapist serves well here. (This is a clinical anecdote from a case conducted by Lynn Hofer, a psychoanalyst in New York.)

> Right after the patient, a woman, sat up, the patient and analyst found themselves looking at each other intently. A silence prevailed. The analyst, without knowing exactly what she was going to do, softened her face slowly and let the suggestion of a smile form around her mouth. She then leaned her head forward slightly, raised her eyebrows a little, and said, "Hello."

The patient continued to look at the analyst. They remained locked in a mutual gaze for a moment. After a moment, the patient lay down again and continued her work on the couch, but more profoundly and in a new key opening up new material. The change in their analytic work together was dramatic.

The "hello" (with facial expression and head movement) was a "moment of meeting" when the therapist made an authentic personal response beautifully adjusted to the situation immediately at hand (the now moment). It altered the therapy markedly. It was a nodal point at which a quantum change in the intersubjective field was achieved. In dynamic systems theory, the moment represents an irreversible shift into a new state. After a successful moment of meeting, the therapy resumes its process of moving along, but it does so in a newly expanded intersubjective field that opens up different possibilities.

The "hello" is a specific fitted match; it is shaped to the immediate local context. This is why most standard technical maneuvers do not work well in these situations. Imagine that instead of saying "Hello" to her patient, the therapist had said, "Yes?" or "What are you thinking now?" or "What do you see?" or "Do you see what you expected?" or "Hmmm?" or let the silence continue. All of these are technically acceptable (not necessarily optimal) within a psychoanalytic framework and may lead to interesting places, but they are inadequate to the specific situation.

What is most interesting about the intersubjective event of the "now moment–moment of meeting linkage" is that it does not need to be verbalized or analyzed in the usual sense to have its therapeutic effect. The intersubjective field gets implicitly changed, and this alters the therapeutic relationship, transference, and countertransference. Analytic work begins again from a new starting place. In the case example, the patient knew differently that the analyst was "open" to her and "on her side." It did not have to be said.

Moments of meeting provide some of the most nodal experiences for change in a psychotherapy. They are very often the moments most remembered, years later, as changing the course of therapy, and they get elevated as a sort of peak amid the other surrounding moves and present moments. There is a spectrum of such moments, from momentous to trivial. They are the points of nonlinear change in the patient's implicit knowledge, just as an interpretation can create a change in the patient's explicit knowledge. The two are complementary and very often act together, with the moment of meeting confirming the interpretation.

Now moments and moments of meeting are products, par excellence, of the intersubjective dialogue. They are the fruit of the sloppy, nonlinear process of two people working within an intersubjective matrix. It is in this way that the intersubjective perspective widens, complements, and, on some points, challenges the classical approach, both clinically and theoretically.

Conclusion

As psychoanalysis moves further from a one-person psychology toward a two-person psychology, intersubjectivity has emerged as a major concept for understanding this shift. New schools of psychoanalysis (e.g., the "intersubjective" and the "relational" approaches) have appeared. They are based on the notion that a main subject matter of psychoanalysis is the interplay of two subjectivities and the unpredictable material that is co-created by this encounter. This new emphasis transcends the traditional concepts of transference and countertransference, which now become special cases of the more pervasive matrix of intersubjectivity. The intrapsychic gives some ground to the interpsychic. The assumptions of the linearity and causality of mental activity are now complemented by notions of dynamical systems. And there is a greater emphasis on process relative to content and on the smaller-scale, local level relative to overarching narratives. In general, intersubjectivity presents new challenges to psychoanalytic theory and practice and opens up new opportunities.

References

Aron L: The patient's experience of the analysis's subjectivity. Psychoanal Q 49:678–692, 1991

Aron L, Harris A (eds): The Legacy of Sandor Ferenczi. Hillsdale, NJ, Analytic Press, 1993

Atwood G, Stolorow R: Structures of Subjectivity: Explorations in Psychoanalytic Phenomenology. Hillsdale, NJ, Analytic Press, 1984

Baron-Cohen S: Mindblindness: An Essay on Autism and Theory of Mind. Cambridge, MA, MIT Press, 1995

Beebe B, Lachman F: Infant Research and Adult Treatment: Co-Constructing Interactions. Hillsdale, NJ, Analytic Press, 2002

Benjamin J: The Bonds of Love: Psychoanalysis, Feminism, and the Problem of Domination. New York, Pantheon, 1988

Benjamin J: Like Subjects, Love Objects. New Haven, CT, Yale University Press, 1995

Boesky D: The psychoanalytic process and its components. Psychoanal Q 49:527–531, 1990

Bollas C: The Shadow of the Object: Psychoanalysis of the Unknown Thought. New York, Columbia University Press, 1987

Boston Change Process Study Group: Explicating the implicit: the local level and the microprocess of change in the analytic situation. Int J Psychoanal 83:1051–1062, 2002

Bowlby J: Attachment and Loss, Vol 1: Attachment. New York, Basic Books, 1969

Boston Change Process Study Group: Something more than the "something more than interpretation" is needed: a comment on the paper by the Process of Change Study Group. Int J Psychoanal 84:109–118, 2003

Bråten S: Infant learning by altero-centric participation: the reverse of egocentric observation in autism, in Intersubjective Communication and Emotion in Early Ontogeny. Edited by Bråten S. Cambridge, England, Cambridge University Press, 1999

Brenner C: Psychoanalysis as science. J Am Psychoanal Assoc 16:675–696, 1968

Bruner J, Olver RR, Greenfield PM: Studies in Cognitive Growth. New York, Wiley, 1966

Chused JF: The evocative power of enactment. J Am Psychoanal Assoc 39:615–640, 1991

Chused JF, Raphling DL: The analyst's mistakes. J Am Psychoanal Assoc 40:89–116, 1992

Clark A: Being There: Putting Brain, Body, and World Together Again. Cambridge, MA, MIT Press, 1997

Clark A: An embodied cognitive science? Trends Cogn Sci 3:345–351, 1999

Damasio A: Decartes' Error: Emotion, Reason, and the Human Brain. New York, Putnam, 1994

Damasio A: The Feeling of What Happens: Body and Emotion in the Making of Consciousness. San Diego, CA, Harcourt, 1999

Dornes M: Psychanalyse et Psychologie du Premier Age. Paris, Presses Universitaires de France, 2002

Dunn J: Intersubjectivity in Psychoanalysis: Critical Review. Int J Psychoanal 76:723–738, 1995

Dunn J: Making dense of the social world: mind reading, emotion, and relationships, in Developing Theories of Intention. Edited by Zelazo PD, Astington JW, Olson DR (eds). Mahwah, NJ, Lawrence Erlbaum, 1999

Edelman GM: The Remembered Present: a Biological Theory of Consciousness. New York, Basic Books, 1990

Ehrenberg DB: Psychoanalytic engagement: the transaction as primary data. Contemp Psychoanal 10:535–555, 1982

Ehrenberg DB: The Intimate Edge: Extending the Reach of Psychoanalytic Interaction. New York, WW Norton, 1992

Feldman CF, Kalmar D: Autobiography and fiction as modes of thought, in Modes of Thought: Explorations in Culture and Cognition. Edited by Olson D, Torrence N. Cambridge, England, Cambridge University Press, 1996

Fodor J: A theory of the child's theory of mind. Cognition 44:283–296, 1992

Freeman WJ: How Brains Make Up Their Minds. London, Weidenfeld & Nicholson, 1999

Freud S: Fragment of an analysis of a case of hysteria (1905 [1901]), in Standard Edition of the Complete Psychological Works of Sigmund Freud, Vol 7. Translated and edited by Strachey J. London, Hogarth Press, 1953, pp 1–122

Freud S: The dynamics of transference (1912a), in Standard Edition of the Complete Psychological Works of Sigmund Freud, Vol 12. Translated and edited by Strachey J. London, Hogarth Press, 1958, pp 99–108

Freud S: Recommendations to physicians practising psycho-analysis (1912b), in Standard Edition of the Complete Psychological Works of Sigmund Freud, Vol 12. Translated and edited by Strachey J. London, Hogarth Press, 1958, pp 109–120

Gallagher S: Mutual enlightment: recent phenomenology and cognitive science. Journal of Consciousness Studies 4:195–214, 1997

Gallese V: The "Shared Manifold" Hypothesis: From Mirror Neurons to Empathy. Journal of Consciousness Studies 8:33–50, 2001

Gergely G, Csibra G: Teleological reasoning in infancy: the infant's naive theory of rational action. A reply to Premack and Premack. Cognition 63:227–233, 1997

Gleick J: Chaos: Making a New Science. New York, Viking, 1987

Goldberg A: A Fresh Look at Psychoanalysis. Hillsdale, NJ, Analytic Press, 1988

Goldberg A: Farewell to the objective analyst. Int J Psychoanal 75:21–30, 1994

Grandin T: Thinking in Pictures. New York, Doubleday, 1995

Green A: The analyst, symbolization and absence in the analytic setting. Int J Psychoanal 56:1–22, 1975

Greenberg J: Oedipus and Beyond. Cambridge, MA, Harvard University Press, 1988

Greenberg J, Mitchell SA: Object Relations in Psychoanalytic Theory. Cambridge, MA, Harvard University Press, 1983

Heimann P: On countertransference. Int J Psychoanal 31:81–84, 1950

Heller M, Haynal-Reymond V, Haynal A, et al: Can faces reveal suicide attempt risk? in The Flesh of the Soul: the Body We Work With. Edited by M. Heller. Bern, Switzerland, Peter Lang, 2001, pp 231–256

Hobson P: Autism and the Development of Mind. Hove/Hillside, NJ, Lawrence Erlbaum, 1993

Hoffman I: Discussion: toward a social-constructivist view of the psychoanalytic situation. Psychoanalytic Dialogues 1:74–105, 1991

Husserl E: Cartesian Meditations. Translated by Cairns D. The Hague, Martinus Nijohff, 1960

Husserl E: Ideas Pertaining to a Pure Phenomenology and to a Phenomenological Philosophy, First Book: General Introduction to Pure Phenomenology. Translated by Gibson B. New York, Collier, 1962

Husserl E: The Phenomenology of Internal Time-Consciousness. Translated by Churchill JS. Bloomington, Indiana University Press, 1964

Husserl E: Ideas Pertaining to a Pure Phenomenology and to a Phenomenological Philosophy, Third Book: Phenomenology and the Foundation of the Sciences. Translated by Klein TE, Pohl WE. The Hague, Martinus Nijhoff, 1980

Husserl E: Ideas Pertaining to a Pure Phenomenology and to a Phenomenological Philosophy, Second Book. Translated by Rojcewicz R, Schuwer A. Dordrecht, The Netherlands, Kluwer Academic Publishers, 1989

Jacobs TS: The use of self: countertransference and communication in the analytic setting. Madison, CT, International Universities Press, 1991

Knoblauch SH: The Musical Edge of Therapeutic Dialogue. Hillsdale, NJ, Analytic Press, 2000

Kohut H: Introspection, empathy and psychoanalysis: an examination of the relationship between mode of observation and theory. J Am Psychoanal Assoc 14:243–272, 1959

Kohut H: The Restoration of the Self. New York, International Universities Press, 1977

Kugiumutzakis G: Genesis and development of early human mimesis to facial and vocal models, in Imitation in Infancy. Edited by Nadel J, Butterworth G. Cambridge, England, Cambridge University Press, 1999, pp 36–59

Leslie AM: Pretence and representation: the origins of "theory of mind." Psychol Rev 94:412–426, 1987

Lichtenberg JD: Psychoanalysis and Motivation. Hillsdale, NJ, Analytic Press, 1989

Lichtenberg J, Bornstein M, Silver D (eds): Empathy I. Hillsdale, NJ, Analytic Press, 1984

Mahler MS, Pine F, Bergman A: The Psychological Birth of the Human Infant: Symbiosis and Individuation. New York, Basic Books, 1975

Maratos O: The origin and development of imitation in the first six months of life. Unpublished doctoral dissertation, University of Geneva, 1973

Marbach E: Building materials for the explanatory bridge. Journal of Consciousness Studies 6:252–257, 1999

Meltzoff AN: Understanding the intentions of others: re-enactment of intended acts by 18-month-old children. Dev Psychol 31:838–850, 1995

Meltzoff AN, Moore MK: Imitation of facial and manual gestures by human neonates. Science 198:75–78, 1977

Meltzoff AN, Moore MK: Persons and representations: why infant imitation is important for theories of human development, in Imitation in Infancy. Edited by Nadel J, Butterworth G. Cambridge, England, Cambridge University Press, 1999, pp 9–35

Mitchell S: Relational Concepts in Psychoanalysis: An Integration. Cambridge, MA, Harvard University Press, 1988

Mitchell S: Hope and Dread in Psychoanalysis. New York, Basic Books, 1993

Mitchell S: Influence and Autonomy in Psychoanalysis. Hillsdale, NJ, Analytic Press, 1997

Mitchell S: Relationality: From Attachment to Intersubjectivity. New York, Analytic Press, 2000

Modell A: The Private Self. Cambridge, MA, Harvard University Press, 1993

Nadel J: Imitation et Communication Entre Jeune Enfants. Paris, Presses Universitaires de France, 1986

Ogden T: The dialectically constituted/decentered subject of psychoanalysis, I: the Freudian subject. Int J Psychoanal 73: 517–526, 1992a

Ogden T: The dialectically constituted/decentered subject of psychoanalysis, II: the contributions of Klein and Winnicott. Int J Psychoanal 75:613–626, 1992b

Ogden T: Subjects of Analysis. Northvale, NJ, Jason Aronson, 1994

Pearson D, Rouse H, Doswell S, et al: Prevalence of imaginary companions in a normal child population. Child Care Health Dev 27:13–22, 2001

Person ES: Dreams of Love and Fateful Encounters: The Force of Romantic Passions. New York, WW Norton, 1988

Prigogine I: The End of Certainty. New York, Free Press, 1997

Prigogine I, Stengers I: Order Out of Chaos: Man's New Dialogue With Nature. New York, Bantum Books, 1984

Reddy: Playing with other's expectations: teasing and mucking about in the first year, in Natural Theories of Mind: Evolution, Development, and Simulation of Everyday Mindreading. Edited by Whiten A. Oxford, England, Blackwell, 1991, pp 143–158

Reed GS: The antithetical meaning of the term "empathy" in psychoanalytic discourse, in Empathy I. Edited by Lichtenberg JD, Bornstein M, Silver D. Hillsdale, NJ, Analytic Press, 1984, pp 7–24

Renik O: Analytic interaction: conceptualizing technique in light of the analyst's irreducible subjectivity. Psychoanal Q 62:533–571, 1993

Rizzolatti G, Fogassi L, Gallese V: Neurophysiological mechanisms underlying the understanding and imitation of action. Nat Rev Neurosci 2:661–670, 2001

Rochat P (ed): Early Social Cognition. Mahwah, NJ, Lawrence Erlbaum, 1999

Sander L: Thinking about developmental process: wholeness, specificity, and the organization of conscious experiencing. Invited address, annual meeting of the Division of Psychoanalysis. American Psychological Association, Santa Monica, CA, 1995a

Sander L: Identity and the experience of specificity in a process of recognition. Psychoanalytic Dialogues 5:579–593, 1995b

Sander LW: Thinking differently: principles of process in living systems and the specificity of being known. Psychoanalytic Dialogues 12:11–42, 2002

Sheets-Johnstone M: The Primacy of Movement. Philadelphia, PA, John Benjamins Publishing Company, 1999

Spezzano C: Classical vs contemporary theory: differences that matter clinically. Contemp Psychoanal 31:20–46, 1995

Stern DN: The First Relationship: Infant and Mother. Cambridge, MA, Harvard University Press, 1977

Stern DN: The Interpersonal World of the Infant: A View From Psychoanalysis and Developmental Psychology. New York, Basic Books, 1985

Stern DN: The Present Moment in Psychotherapy and Everyday Life. New York, WW Norton, 2003

Stern DN, Sander LW, Nahum JP, et al: Non-interpretive mechanisms in psychoanalytic therapy: there "is something more" than interpretation. The Boston Change Process Study Group. Int J Psychoanal 79:903–921, 1998

Stolorow R, Brandchaft B, Atwood G: Psychoanalytic Treatment: An Intersubjective Approach. Hillsdale, NJ, Analytic Press, 1987

Stolorow R, Brandchaft B, Atwood G: Contexts of Being: The Intersubjectivist Foundation of Psychological Life. Hillsdale, NJ, Analytic Press, 1992

Stolorow RD, Atwood GE, Bandschaft B (eds): The Intersubjective Perspective. Northvale, NJ, Jason Aronson, 1994

Thompson E: Empathy and consciousness. Journal of Consciousness Studies 8:1–32, 2001

Trevarthen C: The self born in intersubjectivity: an infant communicating, in The Perceived Self. Edited by Neisser U. New York, Cambridge University Press, 1993, pp 121–173

Trevarthen C: The nature of motives for human consciousness. Special issue: the place of psychology in contemporary sciences, part 2. Edited by Velli T. Psychology: The Journal of the Hellenic Psychological Society 4:187–221, 1998

Trevarthen C, Hubley P: Secondary intersubjectivity: confidence, confiders, and acts of meaning in the first year, in Action, Gesture, and Symbol. Edited by Lock A. New York, Academic Press, 1978

Tronick EZ: Interactive mismatch and repair challenges to the coping infant. Zero to Three 6:1–6, 1986

Tronick EZ, Bruschweiler-Stern N, Harrison AM, et al: Dyadically expanded states of consciousness and the process of theraputic change. Infant Ment Health J 19:290–299, 1998

Tustin F: The Protective Shell in Children and Adults. London, Karnac Books, 1990

Varela FJ, Thompson E, Rosch E: The Embodied Mind: Cognitive Science and Human Experience. Cambridge, MA, MIT Press, 1993

Vygotsky LS: Thought and Language (1934). Translated by Hanfmann E, Vakar G. Cambridge, MA, MIT Press, 1962

Waldrop MM: Complexity: The Emerging Science at the Edge of Order and Chaos. New York, Simon & Schuster, 1992

Whitebook J: A scrape of indepencence: on the ego's autonomy in Freud. Psychoanalysis and Contemporary Thought 16: 359–382, 1993

Whitebook J: Perversion and Utopia: A Study in Psychoanalysis and Critical Theory. Cambridge, MA, MIT Press, 1995

Wolf ES: Treating the Self Elements of Clinical Self-Psychology. New York, Guilford, 1988

Zahavi D: Beyond empathy: phenomenological approaches to intersubjectivity. Journal of Consciousness Studies 8:151–167, 2001

6

Gender and Sexuality

MURIEL DIMEN, PH.D.

VIRGINIA GOLDNER, PH.D.

UNLIKE ANY OTHER GREAT theory of mind, Freud's invention of psychoanalysis placed the category of sexuality and the question of gender at theoretical ground zero. As a result, despite its oft-documented limitations, psychoanalysis remains a point of origin—and of return—for generations of investigators concerned with the relations between psyche and culture.

Not surprisingly, given its shared preoccupations, feminism has been part of the psychoanalytic backstory from the beginning, serving as its sometimes muffled, sometimes obstreperous interlocutor. Almost 100 years later, while the content of the controversies has shifted from questioning the nature of women to questioning the very category of gender itself, the tensions still swirl, and the stakes, remarkably, seem as high as ever.

Thus, it is important to make clear from the outset that psychoanalytic theories about sexuality and gender never lie flat on the page. However neutral and descriptive they may appear to the uninitiated reader, they are century-old rejoinders, still freighted with the painful affects of unresolved conflict. Perhaps because the history of these debates, both doctrinal and political, has been written so often and so well, it is easier to see how theories are never innocent or detached, how concepts do not mirror reality so much as construct it. As Einstein put it, "The theory determines what we can observe."

Ever since the twentieth-century revolution in the sciences met up with the postmodern turn in cultural stud-ies, uncertainty has been on the rise and authority in decline. Yet textbooks continue to speak in an omniscient voice, one that emanates from "everywhere and [thus] nowhere" (Bourdieu and Eagleton 1992, p. 115). The invisible narrator, unbiased and all-knowing, tells a version of the story in question that now becomes *the* story, the canonical statement against which all others are downgraded to competing or "alternative" status.

Since there is no "above and outside" from which to make our claims, no one sees reality through a lens free from the imprint of one's own subjectivity and milieu—ourselves included. Under these conditions, the credibility of authorial expertise requires transparency, not omniscience. Thus, in introducing the ideas that make up this chapter, we will try to specify our personal coordinates rather than seek to transcend them.

Having written and practiced at the intersection of clinical psychoanalysis, feminism, and their multiple, cross-disciplinary interlocutors for the past 30 years, we are committed to a perspective that honors the founding position of Freud by seeking to dislodge his radically disruptive vision and method from the normative, misogynistic framework in which it was embedded. Such a project necessitates building bridges to other kinds of scholarship, where questions of gender and sexuality have also been critically engaged. Our chapter tells the story of this collective effort, which unfolded over the course of the last century and shows no signs of slowing down in this, the new millennium.

Gender: Conflated, Critiqued, Deconstructed, Reassembled

The terms *gender* and *sexuality* have had distinct conceptual and lexical histories in psychoanalytic theory and in the culture at large. Sexuality was not articulated as a unique aspect of individual psychology until late in the nineteenth century (Katz 1996), while the concept of gender (though not yet the term itself) emerged as a site of critical awareness much later, with the publication of Simone de Beauvoir's *The Second Sex* in 1949 (Young-Bruehl 1996). It was not until John Money's empirical work on hermaphroditic children in the 1950s (Money et al. 1955) that gender and sexuality were formally conceived as separate and distinct categories of analysis and experience.

The term *gender* comes even later to psychoanalysis. While it was obviously central in and to Freud's thinking, it is not to be found in the *Standard Edition* or in *The Language of Psychoanalysis* (Laplanche and Pontalis 1973), a canonical reference work of psychoanalytic concepts. Indeed, gender did not emerge as a psychoanalytic category in its own right until Robert Stoller (1968), elaborating and extending Money's research into the clinical domain, conceptualized it as a central dimension of self-organization, a move that launched the contemporary field of empirically grounded, psychoanalytic gender studies.

Psychoanalytic Feminism

With the advent of psychoanalytic feminism, Dinnerstein (1976), Chodorow (1999a), and Benjamin (1988) complicated psychoanalytic gender theory by conceptualizing gender as an analytic and social category, not merely a psychological one. With this move, the psychoanalytic study of gender became increasingly multidisciplinary, as cultural, philosophical, literary/linguistic and sociopolitical theories intersected with those being developed in clinical psychoanalysis (see Stimpson and Person 1980 for an early, still classic interdisciplinary collection). It has become a major challenge and source of enrichment to hold the tension between "theoretical gender," as it has been constructed in the academy, and the "psychological gender" of lived experience that is theorized in the clinic (Chodorow 1999b).

Feminist theories conceptualize gender as a culturally instituted, normative ideal (Butler 1990) that sexes the body and genders the mind in compliance with the hegemonic principle of gender polarity. Throughout history and across cultures, gender categories (male/female, masculine/feminine) have been almost universally construed as mutually exclusive oppositions, with each side defined by what the other was not. Butler demonstrated that gen-

der actually *creates* subjectivity itself, since "persons only become intelligible through becoming gendered," and, thus, that "gender and sexual identities that fail to conform to norms of cultural intelligibility appear only as developmental failures or logical impossibilities" (Butler 1990, p. 16). One of the core projects and accomplishments of psychoanalytic feminism has been to articulate the pathogenic implications of this regulatory regime.

Chodorow's (1999a) early work brought these questions into focus by situating gender in the object-relational matrix of mothering rather than in the phallic discourse of the sexual instincts. Beginning with the obvious, but untheorized, fact that women are children's primary caregivers ("every infant's first love, first witness and first boss" [Dinnerstein 1976, p. 28]), Chodorow considered the implications of the fact that (only) "women mother" (the first two words of her text). She showed how this culturally mandated kinship arrangement produced and reproduced genders hobbled by pathology, such that masculinity was defined by the "not me" experience of difference (from mother and mother's femininity), whereas femininity could never escape its origins in the "part of me" sameness with the mother.

Benjamin (1988), in her initial contributions, took up the question of gender domination. She argued that psychoanalysis took "women's subordination to men for granted, [making it] invisible" (p. 6), and went on to show how psychoanalytic theory could be used to make a special kind of sense out of this ubiquitous phenomenon. Arguing that the polarity masculinity/femininity was established and reproduced in each individual mind by the pathogenic action of splitting, Benjamin also demonstrated how the gender binary serves as template for other binaries, especially master and slave, subject and object. Goldner (1991) subsequently argued that the either/or structure of the gender paradigm was, in effect, a universal pathogenic situation that induces a traumatically compliant false-self system, which results in a multitude of symptoms and innumerable forms of suffering, unrecognized as such.

The Postmodern Turn

By the last decade of the twentieth century, the postmodern turn in gender studies had locked in on feminist theory's defining move: the monolithic, transhistorical category of gender itself. Work in cultural studies and queer theory established that gender was not a ubiquitous principle of polarity, unmoored from the conditions of its making, but was actually constituted and stabilized by other binary oppositions, especially those of race (black/white) and sexuality (gay/straight) (e.g., Domenici and Lesser 1995; Layton 1998; Leary 1997).

The historian Sander Gilman (1995) has shown how the symbolic slippage among the categories of race, gender, and sexuality operated in Freud's theory of mind. Freud's idealization of heterosexual masculinity echoed the cultural fantasy of masculine perfection embodied by the so-called Aryan male. By contrast, Freud equated femininity with castration, an inferior and humiliated genre of masculinity. Gilman proposed that Freud used this thesis to project the personal debasement he experienced as a Jewish male onto the categories of femininity and homosexuality, since, in the anti-Semitic European context of that time, it was actually the circumcised (= emasculated = homosexual) Jewish male who was defined as the debased, castrated figure. (The slang term for clitoral masturbation, for example, was "playing with the Jew.")

As postmodern academic theorists set about deconstructing the notion of gender as a pre-given, timeless cultural imperative, postmodern psychoanalytic clinicians began to shift the question from "Gender, what is it?" to "Gender, *is* it?" Instead of an essence or "thing in itself," Dimen (1991) argued that gender was "less a determinative category, than a force field [of dualisms]...consisting not of essences, but of shifting relations among multiple contrasts." (p. 43). Following Lacan, Harris (1991) called gender a "necessary fiction," Benjamin (1998), following Marx, called it a "real appearance," and Goldner (1991) characterized it as a paradoxical, "false truth." Each of these metaphors condenses the art of the double-take, making the point that while gender is not an identity or essence at the core of a person, it is still a *core experience* that comes to *constitute* identity. The challenge is neither to essentialize gender nor to dematerialize it.

This tension is especially important to maintain when theorizing the paradox of transsex and transgender identities, which simultaneously critiques and reinscribes traditional gender polarities. It is even more critical to hold the complexity of such contradictions in the treatment situation. (See, for example, the rich exchange between Stein [1995a, 1995b] and Chodorow [1995]; see also the monograph issue of the *Journal of Gay and Lesbian Psychotherapy* [Drescher 2004] devoted to questions of gender nonconformity and gender dysphoria.)

More recently, the theoretical focus of psychoanalytic gender studies has shifted from deconstructing gender to "re-assembling" it (Harris 2000) in ways that do not re-essentialize it (see also Kulish 2000). In some of these approaches, gender is being reformulated as an intersubjectively constituted "compromise formation" (Goldner 2003; Harris 2000); in others, the emphasis is on psychic representations of gendered embodiment (Bassin 1996; Elise 1997). But all contemporary perspectives emphasize that gender is a multilayered, dynamically inflected "per-

sonal idiom" (Bollas 1989), and theoreticians of varying persuasions have come together around the idea that psychological gender is assembled from the gender tropes that family, culture, and historical period make available (Chodorow 1997; Harris 2000; Layton 1998; Person 1999). In this theoretical turn, gender has become a "symbolic resource" (Gagnon 1991) that not only acts "on" us but also is available "to" us—which perturbs our question yet again, from "How does gender work" to "How is gender work*ed*?"

Freud's Legacy

In his introduction to the final revision of Freud's revolutionary opus, *Three Essays on the Theory of Sexuality* (Freud 1905/1953), literary critic Steven Marcus (1975) pared the essential insight about Freud's thinking down to one pithy statement: "[I]t's impossible to make a statement about Freud being right or wrong, since he is always both" (p. xli).

Many commentators have shown how the radical Freud set sail at the outset of *Three Essays* but then retired below deck to the footnotes, where he produced a shadow canon that undermined the heteronormative positions that Freud, the bourgeois physician, was producing above the line (see, e.g., Bersani 1986; Dimen 2003; May 1986). While the bourgeois Doctor concluded that heterosexual reproductive coitus was the inevitable telos of sex and the ultimate statement of maturity, his alter ego countered that there was nothing inevitable about the developmental outcome of sexual object choice. When Freud-the-Doctor opined that gender splitting (masculinity = activity, femininity = passivity) was necessary for procreative purposes (resulting from active, genital masculine heterosexuality, and passive, genital feminine heterosexuality), his alter maintained that "every individual...displays a combination of activity and passivity whether or not this tallies with their biological [sex]," and that there is nothing to inherently distinguish "procreative" from other kinds of sex (Freud 1905/1953, p. 220).

The two alters continually interrupted and undercut each other in a dialogue that Freud himself thought was unfinished and unsatisfactory. "[I] am under no illusion as to the deficiencies...of this little work," he wrote. "It is my earnest wish that [it] may age rapidly—that what was once new in it may become generally accepted, and that what is imperfect in it may be replaced by something better" (Freud 1905/1953, p. 130).

Many generations of analysts and scholars have taken up his invitation, and many of those have critiqued his casual misogyny, ambivalent homophobia, and traditional family values. But long before feminists, gay and lesbian scholars, and queer theorists staked out positions relative to Freud's particular vision, clinical psychoanalysts had set about revising his notions of sex and gender. Among Freud's contemporaries, Karen Horney (1924/1967, 1926/1967), supported by Ernest Jones (1935/1961), courageously challenged Freud's views of femininity as a kind of "defeated masculinity," while Melanie Klein (1928), along with Horney, moderated Freud's emphasis on penis envy by describing male envy of female reproductive organs, which she described as sites "of receptivity and bounty" (p. 190). (Fliegel [1986] and Chodorow [1989] provide detailed discussions of the intense debates around the psychology of femininity during the 1920s and 1930s.)

After a long fallow period, Chasseguet-Smirgel (1970), echoing and extending themes Horney had developed 40 years before, argued that Freud's view of femininity as a collection of "lacks" could be understood as a defensive reversal of the child's profound sense of helplessness in the face of the preoedipal mother's overwhelming power. Thus, she argued, the power of the father/penis/phallus derives not from any inherent superiority but from the child's need to "beat back the mother."

Nominal Gender, Subjective Gender, Ideological Gender

"*The* Anatomical Difference"

While Freud did, of course, write continuously about masculinity and femininity, he was not systematic or self-conscious about theorizing gender as a category or construct, tending to "oscillate...between the construction and deconstruction of gender categories" (Benjamin 1998, p. 38). But he was ultimately constrained by his early theorizing, in which he concretized masculinity and femininity as expressions of an individual's "mental sexual character," an unwieldy phrase that encodes the problems of conflation that have dogged the thesis ever since.

The first of his many missteps was the seemingly innocuous premise that gender was a "psychical consequence of the anatomical distinction between the sexes" (Freud 1925/1961). This ostensibly neutral but ultimately ideological statement served to ground his equation of masculinity with activity, femininity with passivity. While these social stereotypes worked at the level of common sense, he always knew they were problematic, both philosophically and psychologically.

Freud's gender theories leaned on what anthropologists call "folk science," the unexamined cultural assumptions that underlie common knowledge (Dimen 2003, p. 64). "*The* anatomical difference," for example, a phrase drenched

in a sense of the obvious, has lost its status as self-evident. Generations of scholars working in anthropology (Herdt 1992), history (Laqueur 1990), biology (Fausto-Sterling 1986), social psychology (Kessler and McKenna 1978) and postmodern theory (Butler 1990) have shown how the term fixates on the genitals, exaggerating and mythologizing the relatively small physical differences between the sexes, while effacing their obvious commonality and likeness (Rubin 1975).

This fetishization of the genitals undergirds the practice of "sex assignment" in most (but not all) cultures: the foundational act of categorization through which we are named and name ourselves "boy" or "girl," "man" or "woman." It has been a staple of feminist theory to demonstrate how this seemingly neutral cultural ritual is actually a form of social regulation that crams the sexes into two mutually exclusive categories. "Male and female it creates them," wrote Gayle Rubin (1975) in an instantly classic paper, "and it creates them heterosexual." (Empirical support for this thesis has been established by Kessler [1990], who showed how decision-making processes concerning surgical options for intersex children were uncritically directed toward ensuring their physical conformity with a binary, heterosexual system of gender relations.)

The Penis and Phallocentrism

Freud further fetishized the genitals (or more precisely the penis, the only genital that mattered [to him]) by defining sexual difference and psychical gender solely in terms of the have/have not status of the penis and the "castration complex" its presence or absence engendered. He ultimately made "penis envy" (female) and "castration anxiety" (male) biologically irreducible bedrock.

In this phallocentric narrative, the chance discovery in every childhood of genital difference(s) was made the founding moment of gender identity, because it installed the Great Divide between the sexes, grounding gender in the trauma of lack or fear of lack. ("Little girls recognize [genital difference] immediately, and are overcome by envy" [Freud 1905/1953, p. 122]; "No male human being is spared the fright of castration at the sight of the female genital" [Freud 1927/1957, p. 153].)

The rich variations in the way gender is experienced and performed *within* each sex, as well as the commonalities that cross the boundary between them, were entirely effaced by Freud's universalized, genitalized, phallicized theory of sexual difference. In this implausibly misogynistic account of gender development, masculinity and femininity are reduced to a reciprocal set of strategies that defend against narcissistic injury (femininity) and narcissistic threat (masculinity).

Fifty years later, Chasseguet-Smirgel (1976) coined the term "phallic monism" to pinpoint how Freud's thesis posited and valorized a primitive unisex/gender system in which there is only masculinity. Femininity does not "exist" on its own terms but comes into being only as the negative of masculinity and thus as "the sex that is not one" (Irigaray 1985). In psychodynamic terms, feminists have shown how Freud constituted femininity as the container for masculinity's detritus, as in the axiom, "Femininity *is* whatever masculinity repudiates." (Young-Bruehl [1990] discusses the inconsistencies in Freud's gender monism by tracking his contradictory positions that libido is masculine but humans are inherently bisexual.)

Nominal, Subjective, and Ideological Gender

Freud's gender theories are riddled with compounding and confounding assumptions. First, by deriving the gender binary (male/female) from the anatomical binary (man/woman), Freud naturalized the psychological process of gender splitting by mapping it onto the social process of sex assignment, an outcome he mistakes for a pregiven fact of nature. Second, by defining the gender binary male/female in terms of the psychically fraught antinomy active/passive, Freud conflated the distinctions between *nominal* gender, the category through which we are named and name ourselves male or female; *subjective* gender, the psychical meaning and experiential feeling of "being" male or female; and *ideological* gender, the evaluative, psychosymbolic categories of masculinity and femininity, which, as feminists and cultural theorists have shown, attribute all that is culturally valued to "masculinity" and project all that is hated and feared onto "femininity."

Freud himself was never satisfied with this formulation. While he was unable to recognize how his underlying misogyny was the psychodynamic engine driving the thesis off the tracks, he did conclude at the end of his life that "we have made use of…an obviously inadequate empirical and conventional equation, calling everything that is strong and active male, everything that is weak and passive female" (Freud 1940/1964, p. 188).

The Oedipus Complex

Ideological Gender and the Oedipus Complex

The oedipal narrative that dominates classical psychoanalytic theory tracks the boy's (and girl's) emergence into heterosexual masculinity (femininity) from his (and her) early embeddedness in what Freud, and later, with more theoretical fervor, Lacan, deemed a presymbolic, precultural maternal universe. The trip from preoedipal symbiosis and oedipal romance to the patriarchal order of reality/civilization is framed as cautionary tale. It illustrates how repression serves the needs of culture by installing the incest taboo in each mind and family. This prohibition prevents romantic/sexual love from flowering at the wrong time (between a child and his or her parents), the wrong place (inside instead of outside the family), and toward the wrong type of person (of the same sex instead of the opposite sex).

The Oedipus complex, Gayle Rubin (1975) argued, is the psychodynamic narrative that accords personal meaning and social legitimation for the cultural imperative that links the binary system of gender to the obligatory status of heterosexuality and to the implicit ("less articulate," in Rubin's [1975] words) prohibition of homosexuality. The tortuous oedipal journey Freud laid out for preoedipal boys and girls, whose nominal gender (male/female) had not yet taken on the ideological and psychologically charged meanings of masculinity and femininity, was designed in accordance with this invisible cultural a priori: gender must be an exclusionary (either/or) category that "brings about" procreative heterosexuality, as in "opposites attract."

But in Freud's phallic universe, the construction of a psychodynamic rationale for the erotic charge of gender opposites was neither simple nor obvious. He could not conjure a means whereby each gender could, for example, have "its own special libido," with one "pursuing the aims of a masculine sexual life, the other a feminine [one]…. There is only one libido," he wrote, "and following the conventional equation of activity and masculinity, it is masculine…. The juxtaposition, 'feminine libido' is without any justification" (Freud 1933, p. 131).

His theoretical challenge was thus far more complicated: to construct a developmental story that would culminate in the genders (male/female) lining up with the positions (active/passive) so as to endow the conventional imagery of heterosexual intercourse (the woman "receiving" the penis into the vagina so as to become pregnant) with an erotic, psychosexual inevitability. As a result, the long march to heterosexuality for girls would require an elaborate series of switchbacks, so that the active sexuality Freud observed in girls as well as boys would be turned back on itself, leaving femininity an empty shell.

Freud's oedipal drama is launched by the child's discovery of sexual difference, which, as we have seen, is the moment of realization that the girl is "castrated." The alignment of femininity with passivity begins here, with the girl's horror at her genital mutilation. This equation results in penis envy and hatred toward her mother for being deficient, which leads her to repudiate/repress her active (phallic, masculine, homoerotic) romantic tie to mother and her turn to the father. Tellingly, this "turn to the father" is already marked by the daughter's desexualization, since it is fueled not by desire but only by the goal of possessing father's penis for herself, in order to undo the narcissistic humiliation of her "castration." When the girl finds out she cannot have it, she defaults to passive feminine heterosexuality in order to have a (boy) baby as a substitute penis.

By contrast, the boy's oedipal odyssey tracks the underground path of his desire, whose repression is linked to his genital narcissism. Incited by his fear and disgust at the female genitals, the boy abandons his wish to overthrow or displace his father, repressing his romantic love for his mother until puberty. Having renounced his oedipal rivalry by identifying with his father's (hetero) masculinity, the boy now waits "his turn" to possess a woman like his mother, a woman of his own. (See Lewes's [1988] description of 12 possible oedipal constellations for the boy, only one of which conforms to this universalized, normative developmental narrative.)

Feminist Critiques of the Oedipal Paradigm

The Oedipus complex was a magnet for debate from the moment of its inception and continues to be a nodal point of contention among contemporary psychoanalytic traditions. Even Freud acknowledged that the circuitous route to what he called femininity was likely to fail, leaving the girl with a "masculinity complex." The term referred to the daughter's refusal to give up her active, preoedipal bond to the mother, and to the ongoing penis envy (understood in psychological as well as anatomical terms) that was its result.

In another unfortunate but all too common outcome, Freud described how girls would experience a "break on [their] sexuality" (Freud 1908/1959, p. 192) at puberty, prompting a retreat into sexual inhibition and revulsion. Since women possessed "a weaker sexual instinct" (Freud 9, 192) to begin with, it was no wonder that the ordeals of femininity left so many of them in a hysterical state, in which symptoms took the place of their sexuality.

Horney's (1924/1967, 1925/1967) critique of Freud's convoluted oedipal thesis revealed that the masculinity Freud idealized was not so much a state of excellence as it was the grandiose fantasy of a vulnerable male child ("What I have is great; what you have is nothing"). "Freud's devaluation of the female genital." she concluded, "differs in no case by a hair's breadth from the typical ideas that the little boy has of the little girl" (Horney 1926/1967, p. 58). She challenged the view that there was only one worthy

genital. Ernest Jones agreed: "I do not see a woman…as a permanently disappointed creature struggling to console herself with secondary substitutes alien to her nature" (Jones 1935/1961, p. 495).

Femininity and Masculinity

Primary Femininity

Both Horney and Jones refused Freud's phallic monism, arguing for the girl's "innate" femininity, which they believed was an expression of her innate, pleasure-oriented heterosexuality, brought into awareness by early vaginal sensations (an awareness Freud and his loyalists disputed). As their perspective evolved at the time and over the next half century, it became elaborated into a countervision of "primary femininity," which has documented and theorized the obvious fact that girls, as well as boys, have a primary awareness of and positive cathexis toward their genitals that precedes their awareness of sexual (genital) difference.

In contrast to the original Freudian conception of femininity as grounded in castration and progressing toward passive, vaginal heterosexuality, the postclassical primary femininity tradition has engaged the project of developing theoretical categories that establish "linkages between body sensation, body ego, and gender identity" (Lasky 2000, p. 1385). This strategy traces the experiential and psychosymbolic contours of a specifically female developmental line, grounded in the anatomical female body, with its particular pleasures and dangers.

The approach re-theorizes feminine psychosexual development, shifting from focusing in a phallic way on the girl's genital "lack" to elucidating her fear of losing or damaging what she already possesses and initially cherishes—her unique body and genitals. For example, in a classic paper, Mayer (1985) described both the little girl's initial narcissistic fantasy that "everybody must be just like me" (having an opening and an "inside space") and her later "castration anxiety," which Mayer creatively redefined as the fear of being "closed up" as boys are—physically and mentally.

The feminist impulse at work here also involves a particular critique of terms like "castration anxiety" and "penis envy," which are derived from imagery of the male body. It is argued that these phallocentric categories can obscure, if not erase, the particularity of female embodiment, rendering it theoretically and psychically unrepresentable (Bassin 1982; Goldberger 1999; Kulish 2000). This critique has led to the development of new terms and refinements of old ones, such as Kestenberg's (1982) "inner genital," Bernstein's (1990) replacement of "castration anxiety" with "genital anxiety," and Elise's (1997) substitution of primary "femaleness" for "primary femininity."

The French psychoanalytic tradition of *"écriture feminine"* ("writing femininity") proffers a literary strategy for representing the unrepresentable condition of embodied femininity. In this approach, language is used evocatively ("semiotically") rather than symbolically (Kristeva 1990). For example, Irigaray (1985) describes the labia as "two lips which embrace continually" (p. 345).

A central critique of this theoretical perspective has been its tendency toward essentialism: the presumption that a particular sexed anatomy "results" in, or produces, a particular gendered psyche. Many contributors to this approach have themselves addressed this issue, some enhancing the critique itself, which has resulted in more complex formulations of the relations between embodiment and gender (e.g., Balsam 2001; Elise 1997; Kulish 2000; Lasky 2000).

Phallic Masculinity/Personal Maleness

Freud's idealization of phallic masculinity not only erased and debased femininity as a category and as a lived, embodied self experience. It also delayed the theorization of masculinity in all its specificity and multiplicity. As Corbett (personal communication, 2004) has observed, men, like women, can be clinical subjects in psychoanalysis, but, unlike femininity, masculinity has rarely been taken up as a theoretical problem beyond Freud's original classical paradigm.

Phallic masculinity has been, in essence, "beyond analysis." Rather than a phenomenon to be explained, it has been an ideal to be achieved. Indeed, any maleness that does not "measure up" jumps the gender binary, becoming a degraded varietal of femaleness ("effeminacy"). (Chodorow [1998] and Corbett [2001a] have elaborated the mechanisms for this process, describing how the defensive construction of masculinity as "not femininity/not mother," "not small/not boy," and "never loser/only winner" can default into aggressive homophobia.)

Chodorow (1999a) and Benjamin (1988), building on the work of Stoller (1968), began the project of problematizing masculinity as a cultural category, identity position, and psychic phenomenon. Chodorow showed how, under the routine social conditions of father absence or distance, boys seek to identify with the category of (hyper) masculinity as a means to make a symbolic ("positional") identification with a father who is not personally available. This transference to, and identification with, the phallic imagery of masculinity eventuates in a familiar hypermasculine stance, a version of manhood that Ross (1986) eloquently critiques as "a screen, a sheath, an artificially aggressivized brittle, cardboard creation…[pointing toward] the unavailability early on of the father as a libidinal object and figure for internalization and identification" (p. 54) (See also articles by Kaftal [1991] on the pathogenic consequences of father-absence/hunger, and Pollack [1995] on the traumatic consequences of the cultural pressures requiring boys to separate too soon and too absolutely from the mother.)

The premature abandonment of boys by their mothers and fathers, and by a culture that valorizes the phallic illusions of machismo, produces men who tend to be lacking in empathy, are unskilled in relationality, and are unable to relate to others outside a dynamic of domination. These psychological wounds and deficits have serious social ramifications. It is a statistical fact that men and boys, not women and girls, engage in the vast majority of individual, domestic, and collective acts of violence. These behaviors are rooted in the affects of shame, humiliation, and narcissistic threat. Chodorow (1998) argued that humiliation from men (the man-boy dichotomy) and fears of feminization (the male-female dichotomy) are central ingredients fueling the rage driving male social violence (see Goldner 1998 for a discussion of the gender dynamics of domestic violence).

A Fork in the Road

Until the advent of the constructionist, postmodern turn, the primary demarcation distinguishing psychoanalytic gender theories lay between those that "analyzed the gender divide in terms of the structural relationship to the phallus…[and those that privileged] the object relation to the mother" (Benjamin 1998, p. 43). By making the castration complex and its heterosexual resolution foundational for gender development, oedipally centered, primarily Lacanian-inspired theories privilege the (law of the) father (phallus), who embodies and represents culture (symbolization) and hierarchy (see Mitchell and Rose 1982) over the "mother world" (Freud 1931/1961, p. 51) of nature and merger.

By contrast, object relations theories privilege the early, active primacy of the mother in shaping the child's subjectivity, grounding gender in processes of attachment and identification with her, and implicating gender in mechanisms of separation-individuation from her. Oedipal relations are still considered crucial to the psychic construction of masculinity and femininity, but they are now regarded as "superimposed" (Person and Ovesey 1983) on the earlier processes of gender formation that Freud did not recognize.

Whereas Freud rooted gender in the discovery of sexual (genital) difference, which he believed occurred at around age 4, researchers have since established that genital awareness, labeling, and symbolization begin much earlier, during the second year of life. Moreover, Person and Ovesey (1983) argued that gender self-designation *precedes* the child's discovery of the sexual distinction, and thus, reversing Freud, they further argued that genital experience does not *create* gender, but rather the child's rudimentary sense of gender shapes the experience of genital awareness and the personal meaning of sexual difference. However, De Marneffe's (1997) recent research investigating the cognitive sequencing of gender and genital labeling in very young children (15–36 months) suggests that the coordination of conceptions of genital difference with those of gender difference follows no universal fixed sequence (see also Senet 2004).

Attachment-Individuation Theories of Gender

Core Gender

Speculating that all infants initially identify with their mother's (female) gendered body and psyche, Stoller (1968) theorized an initial phase of "proto-femininity" for both boys and girls. With this move he was reversing Freud yet again, by substituting a version of primary femininity for the phallic monism of primary masculinity, thus making masculinity, not femininity, the second, more precarious sex.

In the classical account, it is the girl whose gender development is doubly challenged, since she has to switch her love object from mother to father in order to abandon active masculinity in favor of passive femininity. In Stoller's (1976) account, it is the boy whose gender is doubly challenged, since he must abandon his "primordial" identification with his mother's femininity in order to become "male" like his father. Neither schema is theoretically adequate or plausible, since each proposes an essentialist theory of one gender and a constructionist theory of the other. In the classical trope, "man is born, woman is made"; in the revisionist account, "woman is born, man is made" (Person 1999).

Person and Ovesey (1983), in their historically influential critique, maintained that neither gender was "original," "natural," "innate," or "primordial" and that masculinity and femininity should therefore be theorized as "parallel constructs." They also disputed Stoller's (1968) notion that boys would need to "dis-identify" (Greenson 1968) from the mother in order to establish their masculinity. In line with Money (1973), they maintained that core gender (one's self-designation as male or female) is cognitively and experientially constructed in conformity with sex assignment and rearing, while the later development of gender role identity (the self-evaluation of one's maleness or femaleness: "I am masculine," "I am feminine") is a "psychological achievement...fraught with conflict" (Person and Ovesey 1983, p. 226). Since the catastrophic failure of Money's most famous case of sex-reassignment became public (Colapinto 2000), there has been both a reevaluation of the role of prenatal hormones in establishing core gender and a reconsideration of the relational psychodynamics shaping gender role identity (Fast 1999a, 1999b; Harris 1999).

Gender as Symbolic Resource and Relational Strategy

In Person and Ovesey's (1983) schema, gender role identity is not the product of a simple process of identifying with the nominal gender of the "same-sexed" parent, but is a work-in-progress, evolving in and through the rough and tumble processes of separation-individuation. From their perspective, gender does not simply unfold along its own developmental pathway, since it gets implicated in and is inflected by those early conflicts and losses.

It is important to note that gender is being theorized as more than "psychological achievement" (a constructionist but still static concept). Without any fanfare, and perhaps without theoretical self-consciousness, Person and Ovesey (1983) introduced a critical aspect of gender's protean dimensionality into the discourse of psychoanalytic gender studies. To use Gagnon's (1991) term, they showed how gender was a "symbolic resource" that could be deployed by the subject as a means to express and/or magically resolve psychic conflict and trauma. This conceptualization of gender as a vehicle, rather than an entity, and thus a means rather than an end in itself, was an unheralded, critical moment in the early development of object relations gender theory, one that shifted the discourse away from gender essentialism and reification (see also Coates 1997).

Person and Ovesey (1983) elaborated their perspective by discussing how both boys and girls can manifest "excessive femininity" as a psychic strategy to master separation anxiety. Being feminine "like" mother becomes a symbolically embodied means of both "being" and "having" her (within). (See Coates 1990 for an exegesis of the melancholic, relational dynamics of extreme boyhood femininity, and Corbett 1996 for a critical perspective that theorizes effeminacy in relation to the normative regime of phallic masculinity.)

Chodorow (1999a) and Benjamin (1988) elaborated this strategy by describing and theorizing how the child's experiences of, desires for, and likeness and difference with his or her parents get mapped onto the gender binary. Goldner (1991) explicated how these moves, which take many forms, could be understood as relational strategies for establishing, maintaining or denying crucial attachments. For example, whereas Coates's (1991) work on melancholic boyhood femininity highlights a "sameness" strategy, Chodorow's (1999a) description of how boys deploy the category of masculinity to separate from and repudiate the mother shows the use of a "difference" strategy: "I am *not* like my mother, I am *not* female."

Benjamin's (1988, 1995, 1998) relational theory of gender has brought this approach to profound fruition by showing how gender is not simply an individual strategy (deployed by mother, father, or child) to facilitate wishes for separation or merger, but is also a critical aspect of the intersubjective processes of recognition and negation circulating among them. In her thesis, the defensive use of the gender binary, concretely applied, does not exhaust its psychic possibilities. Her counterintuitive concept of "identification with difference," for example, conveys how the preoedipal girl seeks to identify with her father "homoerotically," as another "like subject" who embodies and represents self-originating desire, agency, and the "exciting outside." Benjamin's crucial contribution is the intersubjective dimension, which highlights the significance of the father's recognition of, and identification with, the child as a subject like himself. Because daughters often represent their fathers' disclaimed feminine identifications, fathers are less likely to recognize likeness in daughters than in their sons. In Benjamin's view, the father's negation/refusal of the girl's identificatory love, her "homoerotic love for like(ness)," is a key factor in the development of penis envy.

It is only a short step from thinking of gender as a dyadic process to thinking about it as part of the intersubjective matrix that comes into play in the crosscurrents of family relations. As Harris (2000) put it, there is a "unique dialectic [tying the] parent's experience of body, gender identity, and desire with the child's rudimentary sense of self-body-gender-desire....[This bidirectional tension] creates the relational matrix into which the child's gender comes into being and into use" (p. 243).

For better and worse, the child's multilayered experience and presentation of gender are tied to sustaining his or her primary object relations. In polarized families, in which gender becomes a heightened symbol of unrest and disquiet, the child's gender development can become implicated in double-binding injunctions that result in splitting and false-self operations (Goldner 1991). But at the same time, the child's gender can also "be a vehicle for a particular skilled task that a child needs to resolve...the securing of stable interactions, and the internal stability in another person. In the goal of keeping an internal object world alive (and originally an external scene alive and vital), gender can [also] be the brilliant solution" (Harris 2000, p. 244).

Toward a Decentered Gender Paradigm

Gender "Over-inclusiveness"

Fast's (1984) child observation studies led her to describe a period of "gender over-inclusiveness" following the phase of separation-individuation, when children inventively deploy gender identifications as a means of symbolizing previously unformulated aspects of their developing sense of self. During this time, they imaginatively identify with the traits and capacities of both (parents') genders and resist the cultural requirements of gender and sexual dichotomization.

With the advent of the oedipal period, when the either/or terms of the gender binary can no longer be evaded, as Fast describes it, children cope with the loss of "having it all" by defensive repudiation or envy of what the other sex "has." From her postclassical perspective, she regards the renunciation of psychic bisexuality (gender multiplicity) as a necessary loss of omnipotence that will be eventually ameliorated by the fantasy, and ultimately the reality, of heterosexual love.

An alternative perspective, put forth in closely related arguments by Aron (1995), Bassin (1996), and Benjamin (1995), contends that the multiplicity of gender identifications established in the preoedipal period can be a continuing source of psychic enrichment in adult life, just as it was for the developing child (see also Breen 1993 for a discussion of gender as "out of focus"). Looking beyond oedipal complementarity to a postoedipal position, these authors argue for the symbolic "recuperation of early bisexuality, gender overinclusiveness,...[gender discordant] body-ego representations and cross gender identifications" (Bassin 1999, p. 13; see also Elise 1997; Stimmel 1996).

The psychic and theoretical issue is not, therefore, gender per se, but how rigidly and concretely it is being used in an individual mind or family context, and what psychic and intersubjective work it is being deployed to do. The question is whether the subject experiences herself or himself as personally investing gender with meaning, or whether gender is a "meaning happening to her (him)" (see Aron 1995; Sweetnam 1996).

Gender as Personal Idiom

These arguments reflect a contemporary strategy/position in psychoanalytic gender studies that seeks ways to subvert the gender order rather than to transcend or defy it. (See the debate among Bassin [2000], Elise [2000], Layton [2000a, 2000b], and Stimmel [2000] about whether this approach actually "reinstates" rather than undermines gender polarities.)

Psychoanalytic feminism began by documenting the pathogenic processes and effects of psychological conformity to the culturally ubiquitous gender binary. Postmodern gender theories see through such compliance, showing how resistance to the either/or of gender is already present, under the radar, in psychic and cultural life (see also Dimen 2003). Thus, it is not enough to delineate how the dictates of gender are traumatically "absorbed" through various mechanisms of compliance. We must also be able to articulate how the subject engages these categories, indeed talks back. Gender, in other words, not only acts on (against) us but also is a cultural trope available *to* us, one that can actually be deployed by the subject in the service of its *own* aims, including the subversion of gender imperatives themselves.

The protean complexity of gender that has been unpacked in these pages gives the lie to the commonsense view of gender as an unremarkable aspect of character that "speaks for itself." Rather, gender is better understood as a social category and psychic identity position that is both a site of injury and a creative, potentially defiant idiom of the self. Thus, gender can be thought of as a compromise formation held in the tension between the pressures of conformity and compliance, on one hand, and the individual's continuous project of self-creation and self-protection.

Gender may be culturally mandated, but it is individually crafted. No individual's gender literally reproduces gender categories, since each is a personal interpretation *of* a gender category. To quote Clifford Geertz (1986), "it is the copying that originates" (p. 380).

Every individual creates a uniquely personal, dynamically driven, multilayered, relationally savvy version of gender, assembled from the gender tropes that each culture and each historical period make available. Put another way, gender is a uniquely personal, conscious and unconscious interpretation of a cultural archetype, an embodied expression of the statement "*This* is what *I* mean by femininity (masculinity)."

From Dualism to Multiplicity

Once we have established that gender is both fluid and embodied, inventive and defensive and crucially relational in its

design, it becomes obvious that the ideal of a unified gender identity makes sense only as a "resistance in terms of treatment, and an impoverishment in terms of character" (May 1986, p. 88). As Person (1999) has written, "[A]gainst what appears to be a 'dichotomously, categorical expression of gender,' there exists in each person a complicated, multi-layered interplay of fantasies and identifications, some 'feminine,' some 'masculine.'...In essence, conscious unity and unconscious diversity co-exist" (p. 314). If there is a goal toward which to aspire, why should it be the "hegemony of one, consciously coherent, sex-appropriate view of oneself" (May 1986, p. 183), as opposed to the capacity to "tolerate the ambiguity and instability of these profoundly personal and ideologically charged categories of experience" (Harris 1991)? Should gender be considered (only) an "achievement" or (also) a loss?

Sex Revived

As we shift gears from gender to sexuality, it is important to note how the historical narratives of gender and sexuality contrast. Although psychoanalysis started with sex, it is only through the critique of gender, effected, as has just been recounted, from both within and without the field, that sexuality becomes (re)problematized. It goes without saying that gender and sexuality are inextricable, extricated here only for the purposes of exposition. Their experiential "interimplication," to use Butler's (1990) felicitous coinage, has been and will continue to be evident throughout this chapter. The unpacking and theoretical reassembling of gender requires and allows us now to deconstruct sexuality: to peer into its construction and meanings, its reverberations and silences. What we will say is that although the term *sexuality* is no less complex than that of gender, the debates about it are much less thickly layered, its intellectual history is patchier. Before us lies the opportunity to enrich that history.

Inventing sex, psychoanalysis soon came to take for granted those early definitions that, even in 1905, Freud, as we have seen, in fact hoped would be revised. But many things conspire to petrify living ideas (see Dimen 1999), so that by 1995, nearly a century later, André Green (1996) would write: "Has sexuality anything to do with psychoanalysis?" Yet, although there was a desexualization, there was also, even as Green was firing his initial salvo, a flurry of psychoanalytic writing on sex from ego psychological, contemporary classical, French neoclassical, and queer, feminist, and postmodernist perspectives (e.g., Bach 1995; Kernberg 1995; Lesser and Domenici 1995; McDougall 1995). The anxiety that conventionally clouds thinking about sexuality, in psychoanalysis as elsewhere, may have started to lift as psychoanalysis has welcomed the insights of social, feminist, queer, and postmodernist critiques.

Sex, if it is a fact, is also an idea. Like most ideas, it has weight—a body, you might say—of its own. Ideas are commonly thought to be accurate recastings of the facts they represent, molds giving the true outlines of the reality they encase. We tend to assume a one-to-one relation between an idea and the thing that the idea is about. Through ideas we can see, as through transparent glass, the "real" truth. Or so goes the model of thought with which the West has been operating for 200 years or so (Flax 1990; Harvey 1989).

As we have been arguing, however, it makes sense, in the twenty-first century, to take into account an alternative way of thinking that has cohered of late: the postmodernist paradigm that, if the attacks now leveled at it by the academia that once adored it are any indication, has now joined the philosophical canon. What we, along with Freud and his critics, are unused to entertaining is that ideas have substance; they color and shape. When we write, talk, or think about "sex," we are engaging a reality even before we begin to study it. It is not so much that ideas distort a previously existing, true, and knowable reality. It is more that ideas possess a reality of their own. They constitute a sort of parallel universe that must be parsed so as to set in sharp relief the world it is meant to illuminate.

Libido, Drive, Instinct

Libido in One-Person and Two-Person Psychologies

Ideas about sexuality are nested in other sets of ideas. Indeed, the psychoanalytic, feminist, and cultural debates not only on gender but on self, body, language, and transference and countertransference reveal psychosexuality, and its problems, as controversial in unforeseen ways. Let us consider, to begin with, how libido, Freud's (1905/1953) cardinal concept of sexual desire, alters when viewed from the perspective of the first of these changes, the coalescence of a two-person psychology. According to Person's (1986) admirable summary, libido is, classically, not only an appetite demanding satisfaction. It also has psychological power. Libido is a force that registers sexual instincts in the mind and thereby partners the emotion of sexual longing. Alternatively conceived, libido is an energy that accumulates to produce "unpleasure." It mounts, surges, and seeks release. Existing outside awareness, libido nevertheless serves to excite consciousness, there to be trans-

formed into something the psyche wishes to get rid of. For pleasure, in Freud's view, consists in the reduction of unpleasure, that is, of tension.

Just about 50 years after Freud's *Three Essays on the Theory of Sexuality*, psychosexual theory took an unexpected turn. Classical, "one-person" psychology construes libido as a force that, drawing on the body but registered in the mind, drives individual developmental processes and behavior. In contrast, according to postclassical, "two-person," or relational, psychology, libido obtains between individuals. Libido, argues Fairbairn (1954), is not an impersonal force; rather, it is personal, seeking not discharge but objects.

If we think of the need for objects at the root of psyche, or self, then we need to reinterpret pleasure. "There is no such thing as an infant," proclaims Winnicott (1953, p. 39), only the mother-infant unit: no baby develops outside object relation. In this view, mind is inherently interpersonal, or, at least, the manifest divide between intrapsychic and interpersonal is no longer self-evident. Mind, in this perspective, develops not within an individual skin but between persons; psychic process and structure emerge out of early object relations. Likewise, pleasure inheres in attachment, issuing not from tension discharge but from the object relationships themselves. To put it more schematically, libido, circulating between as well as within persons, is a two-person phenomenon. (It seems important to point out, at this juncture, the historical "convergence of psychoanalysis and feminism" [Benjamin 1984]: recognizing the ineluctable twoness of psychic structure entails recognizing the presence and subjectivity of the mother in early object relations [Benjamin 1988; Chodorow 1999a; Dinnerstein 1976], a move that, from a feminist and antimisogynist perspective, requires psychoanalytic recognition of *women's* presence and subjectivity.)

Drive, Aim, Object

The argument that sexuality is interpersonal and intersubjective as well as intrapsychic applies also to psychosexual development. In the classical view, sexuality arrives in pieces rather than all at once, and comprises three innate but initially disparate elements: drive, aim, and object. *Drive*, according to Laplanche and Pontalis (1973, p. 214), refers to a dynamic process in which a pressure directs an organism toward an *aim*. Deriving from a corporeal "source," the drive aims to purge the tension this stimulus creates, while the *object* serves as the means by which this aim may be achieved.

By thus formulating the relations among drive, aim, and object, Freud challenged the prevailing consensus. Generally, the object—the loved one—was thought to be the stimulus that, at puberty, awakened the drive and directed it toward its aim of heterosexual and reproductive intercourse. Freud argued instead that the sexual instinct, albeit innate, lacks an inborn aim and object. Rather, aim and object are acquired, and pleasure can take many forms. Aims are therefore multiple and fragmented, and objects are "variable, contingent and only chosen in…definitive form in consequence of the vicissitudes of the subject's history" (Laplanche and Pontalis 1973, p. 215); we might note parenthetically how important, even in this classical formulation, is personal "history" to psychosexuality.

Component Instincts

Psychosexual development is "biphasic": if the first phase, infantile sexuality, is "polymorphously perverse," the second, puberty, concludes psychosexual development by using genital heterosexuality to "solder" together drive, aim, and object. These "transformations of puberty" also unite what have hitherto been the severally emerging component or partial instincts that sequence sexual development. Each of these has two parts: a bodily source and an aim. Even though, in Freud's ultimate view, the entire body is an erogenous zone, the mucus membranes, like the mouth or anus, vagina or urethra, are fundamental: "we must regard each individual as possessing an oral erotism [or instinct], an anal erotism, a urethral erotism, etc." (Freud 1905/1953, p. 205). These partial instincts are partnered by aims—for example, the scopophilic instinct, the instinct to master, and so on (Laplanche and Pontalis 1973, p. 74).

Serving, in Freud's view, as elements of foreplay, the component instincts remain disconnected from one another until brought under the sway of genital erotism. After this point, when the genitals gain functional and experiential dominance due to the emergence of the reproductive aim, all preparatory pleasure that results from the satisfaction of other erotic zones translates into genital excitement. In sum, then, "a new sexual aim appears, and all the component instincts combine to attain it, while the erotogenic zones become subordinated to the primacy of the genital zone" (Freud 1905/1953, p. 212).

Yet even erogenous zones and component instincts may participate in a two-person psychology. Corporeal erotogeneity, Fairbairn (1954) argued, flames as much from relatedness as from body chemistry (or epigenesis). Likewise, psychosexual stages are not just corporeal but also interpersonal moments. Sullivan's (1953) example is the most familiar and famous: the mouth is an erogenous zone not because its mucosity innately situates excitement, but because nursing makes it a primal site of attachment. Oral erotism, experienced within and by the individual organism, has two-person roots and resonances: it is exciting to get together with mother and get fed. Likewise, the anus is arousable because it situates toilet-training power struggles. Out of this phase of parent-child relatedness, which makes matters of control and will primary, anality acquires its close link to the component instincts of sadism and masochism.

Sex and the Single Narrative: Development and Identity

The Feminist Critique

Objects, it may be argued, are present, albeit back-burnered, in classic psychosexual theory. For the moment of genital union is also the moment of oedipal resolution, when, to use Kernberg's (1995) formulation, body-surface erotism and total object relation come together. Even if the oedipal narrative were an inevitable unfolding of biological destiny, it would still account for psychosexual development in terms of critical object relations (Fairbairn 1954). In Freud's view, sexual interests evolve from birth until they become the target of inhibitions during the fifth year and then reemerge in puberty, this time not polymorphous but ready to enter reproductive service. This process is described by the oedipal narrative, which, as we have seen, can no longer be uncritically accepted as a veridical account or accurate prediction of psyche, culture, or history.

These critiques, stemming from within classic psychoanalytic theory, object relational theory, and the feminist attention to gender, complicate the single narrative that constitutes the classical story of sexuality. Even within that narrative, it will be noted, there are already two routes to adult sexuality: one for males, the other for females. Conventionally, only the female story was thought complicated. Recall here the double repressive shift in *both* instinct *and* object that, taking corporeal form, was classically deemed necessary to femininity: The girl must switch her object from mother to father, and must also switch from "partial instinct" (the pleasure of clitoral masturbation) to genital erotism, in which the clitoris becomes "as kindling to the [putative] vaginal fire."

As it turns out, however, no one story of male psychosexual development exists either. It is not only that, among men as well as women, sexuality takes at least two forms, heterosexual or homosexual. Differences abide even within these categories. Consider the two binaries already critiqued earlier, the customary association of masculinity with activity and femininity with passivity, a caricature of gender that classically slides into a caricature of sexual identity: femininity=passivity=(male) homosexuality. Yet, among homosexual men, as Corbett (1993) demonstrates, masculine gender identity may remain intact whether the sexual aim is active—the wish to care for another man, the wish to fill up the other's erotogenic zones—or passive—the wish to be cared for by or have one's erotogenic zones filled up by the other. Reminding us, furthermore, that it is from fantasy rather than behavior that we are to deduce sexual orientation (A. Freud 1952), Corbett (1993) proposes that masculinities may be "differently structured" (p. 347): a man may alternate between passive and active aims—he may, in sex, be inserter or insertee—but nevertheless experience himself as male. Certainly the same sort of variation must apply to heterosexual masculinity.

Heterosexuality and Homosexuality

As has been shown with regard to gender, the very terms we use to describe sexuality are the terms that create it. Far from being transparent (Schafer 2003, p. 23), these terms are always culturally constructed as well as personally significant. Let us examine heterosexuality and homosexuality. Traditionally in psychoanalysis, *homosexuality* has usually been regarded not as a sexuality in its own right but as a neurotic distortion of a fundamental, normal, and natural heterosexuality. But *heterosexuality* itself is, as Dimen (2003, p. 179) says of gender, "a dense weave of significance"; in particular, as soon as it is invoked, so is procreativity, even though not all heterosexual people procreate or (wish to) become parents.

In revealing classical psychosexual theory's masculinism, the feminist critique also unveils its heterosexism and sexual prescriptivity. Sexuality, as described in the writings of Freud (1905/1953, 1924/1961, 1925/1961, 1931/1961, 1933/1964), presumes, as was noted earlier, a heterosexual outcome. Notably, Freud begins *Three Essays* with a chapter on "sexual aberrations." Here and elsewhere he argues that sexual desires for acts exceeding and transgressing reproductive heterosexual intercourse are ubiquitous, if also generally unconscious; as demonstrated by Freud in the second chapter of *Three Essays*, on "infantile sexuality," we are all more polymorphously perverse than otherwise. Each of us has homosexual as well as heterosexual wishes; indeed, we are bisexual from the start. But our sexual multiplicity must, in the end, become uniform. In *Three Essays'* final narrowing (Person 1986), sanity, society, and species survival all in the end depend on puberty's transformation of diffuse, diverse sexual aims into the reproductive discharge of semen into the vagina.

Sexuality, Illness, and Normality

Psychoanalysis, changing in response to contemporary social critiques (Roughton 2002), has begun to attend to a foundational contradiction. Freud notoriously waffled on sexual normality: sometimes you have to be heterosexual to be mentally healthy, and sometimes you can be homosexual. One lesbian patient, he confided in a footnote, was "in no way neurotic" (Freud 1920/1955, p. 158). As Freud (1935/1951) famously wrote in the letter to the American mother about her gay son, homosexuals are no more or less ill than anyone else; indeed, they have contributed greatly to civilization. Recent contributions pick up the thread; as Schafer (2003) says, "Many heterosexual analytic patients show the same or similar conflicts [found in homosexual or perverse patients], even the same intensity of conflict and defense, and the same or similar disturbing developmental circumstances" (p. 30) (see also Isay 1986). In 1973, psychoanalysis finally exhumed its buried-alive intellectual and civil open-mindedness when the American Psychiatric Association removed homosexuality from the *Diagnostic and Statistical Manual of Mental Disorders*.

Even though much prejudice quietly persists, this shift in psychosexual thinking mandates the recognition that there cannot be one single route to adult sexuality. In Coates's (1997) view, the concept of developmental lines, confining rather than expanding understanding, should be jettisoned (see also Corbett 2001b; Schuker 1996). Rather, if each person has unconsciously made both heterosexual and homosexual object choices, and if some go one way and others go another, then psychosexual development, and definitions of sexual health, must be many and various. "Normal" sexuality must always be written in quotation marks, because object choice can only be a compromise formation: "Any heterosexuality [like any homosexuality] is a developmental *outcome* [that] results from fantasy, conflict, defenses, regression, making and breaking relationships internally and externally, and trying to constitute a stable self and maintain self-esteem" (Chodorow 1994, p. 62). There is no other *psychoanalytic* way to view the matter: despite his allegiance to Darwin (Schafer 1977), Freud was writing a *psychology*, not a biology, of sex.

New Narratives of Sexuality

Sexual Idiom

As clinical practice attests, patients have sexual problems (Green 1996), but the paths to and outcomes of sexual development are multiple, not unitary (Breen 1993, p. 38). Desire itself is, to put it in different language, idiomatic. What Bollas (1989) writes of the personal idiom altogether must hold true for sexual desire in particular: "a set of unique person possibilities specific to this individual and subject in its articulation to the nature of lived experience in the actual world" (p. 9). These possibilities may include heterosexual object choice as a solution to the conflicts of the oedipal and preoedipal passages. But they may also include sadomasochism and other practices formerly dubbed "perversions" as adaptive solutions to disorders of self (Weille 2001), for which McDougall (1995) coined the term "neosexualities."

At times fixed and at times fluid, sexual idiom is a narrative subject to both coherence and discontinuity. Take sexual identity. Conventionally, this named sense of one's sexual preference, linked to the notion of object choice, is presumed to be homogeneous and stable. Postconventionally, this category loosens and multiplies. For example, a person anatomically female may identify as a woman and desire a woman, or may identify as a man and desire a woman (Harris 1991), and these identifications might vary in the course of a lifetime. Identities, as Layton (1998) says, may be "multiple, contradictory, fluid, constructed in relation to other identities, and constantly changing" (p. 3). But identities may also constitute fixed points, for while conscious object choice may shift, sexual fantasies are notably limited and fixed, thus serving as "mainstays of identity" (Person 1986). Moreover, although sexual identity lacks an essence, still it is socially informed and thereby constitutes a basis for connecting with those similarly identified and disconnecting from those differently identified (Layton 1998, p. 4). The multiple elements of which sexual identity is made render outcomes only possible, not determined.

Revising the Classical Narrative

The oedipal narrative, as classically told, is useful but is, after all, a story—and only one, at that—of how a person becomes heterosexual, not only of how a person becomes sexually and psychically mature. According to recent postmodernist thinking, especially Butler (1990), sex and gender contain rather more polyphony. This view, construing sexual desire and gender identity as socially, historically, and culturally variable constructs (Foucault 1976/1980), regards heterosexuality and the gender binary as opposite sides of a coin. Arguing that no object is ever truly given up, and regarding gender as an achievement rather than a given (positions taken alternately by Freud), Butler (2002) has put forth the provocative thesis that gender and heterosexuality constitute each other.

This new narrative reveals the multiplicity of desire hiding in the classical oedipal account (e.g., "what happens to the girls' [homosexual] desire for her mother?" as Rubin [1975] asked long ago). Meant to be left behind, homosexuality is in the new account retained as *gender*.

On the journey to heterosexual normality as it is culturally and hence unconsciously inscribed, desire and identification come to exclude each other: the child may not both identify with and desire the same parent. The girl's identification with mother, for example, requires a repudiation of desire for mother: if she is to be feminine, she will have to desire a man—her father—not a woman. If wanting a girl—being homosexual—puts being a girl into question, then the foreclosure of homosexual desire for girls is foundational to gender. *Mutatis mutandis*, the same holds for boys, whose gender identity is unfortunately but conventionally founded, we have seen, if not on disidentification then at least on repudiation: "If a man becomes heterosexual through the repudiation of the feminine, then where does that repudiation live except in an identification which his heterosexual career seeks to deny; indeed, the desire for the feminine is marked by that repudiation: he wants the woman he would never be; indeed, he wouldn't be caught dead being her: thus, he wants her" (Butler 2002, p. 7).

Challenging standard developmentalism, this postmodern narrative returns us to classical skepticism about sexual desire's genesis: "The synthesis is thus not so satisfactory as the analysis; in other words, from a knowledge of the premises we could not have foretold the nature of the result" (Freud 1920/1955, p. 167). Consider, for instance, the development of lesbian sexual identity, for which Schuker (1996) suggests we "identify [many] influential nodal points" (p. 496). Although her list builds linearly from the biological ground up, we might imagine instead a set of mutually determining possibilities laid out as on a map. These would include early object relations; gender identity's construction and negotiation; sexual trauma; temperament; desire as attachment and defense; feelings about and representations of procreativity, power, and gender; cultural imagery of sex and gender as transmitted through familial dynamics and fantasy; and identifications with parents, their sexuality, and their gender. *Ceteris paribus*, a similar map of sexual development could be drawn for men, and for hetero- and other-sexual people, for perversion as well as procreativity, and so on.

Multiplicities of Desire

Where the classical linear oedipal story makes homosexuality a brief stop on the way to (masculine) heterosexuality, the new narrative imagines homosexuality and heterosexuality as coevals and probes their common evolution. Two perspectives on this coexistence have cohered. In Butler's view, the excluded desire, whether homosexual or heterosexual, does not disappear; the object is instead registered as unconscious melancholy. (Interestingly, Meltzer [1973/1979, p. 32], following Melanie Klein, notes that good and bad objects are only "slowly and incompletely" integrated into the parental imagos of the superego.) If you cannot grieve what you have disavowed—"I never loved her/him, I never lost her/him"—melancholy ensues. Heterosexuality and homosexuality, femininity and masculinity, and therefore men and women in their gender identifications—all are "haunted by the specter of a certain... unthinkability:...the disavowal of loss by which sexual formation, including gay sexual formation, proceeds" (Butler 2002, p. 9).

Note, then, the contrast with the classical binary paradigms (oedipal vs. preoedipal, mother vs. father, identification vs. desire, "being" vs. "loving"): psychoanalytic theories influenced by the postmodern, constructionist turn conceptualize the relations between object love and identification as mutually determinative rather than linear, as multifaceted rather than binary, and thus as not merely oppositional but also congruent, interpenetrating, oscillating, and so forth. As we have seen, others (Aron 1995; Bassin 1996; Benjamin 1995) construe a postoedipal solution to this problem: the recovery of the gender multiplicity foregone in the oedipal passage. Bassin (1996) imagines that, one's core gender identity having found psychic coherence, one might then be able to play, to riff on alternate gender identifications much as a jazz musician riffs on fundamental themes. This inventiveness and playfulness rests on a postoedipal psychic configuration of paradox (Benjamin 1995), wherein opposites are not mutually exclusive, and polarities, like masculinity and femininity, or homosexual and heterosexual desire, may coexist without requiring resolution.

Sexual Subjectivity

Sexual Self States

The psychoanalytic ground beneath our feet, the standpoint from which "sexual subjectivity" (a concept that we introduce here) may be viewed, shifts. Classically, sex, like any phenomenon (indeed like any patient), was an object to be studied and known by a scientist's putatively disinterested mind. Claims to untrammeled objectivity hold no more. Implicated as we are in the subject matter we study, influenced by the people we treat, our definitions, explications, and interpretations of sexuality are informed by our sexual experiences, whether cognitive, affective, personal, familial, or cultural. Our task therefore shifts: if we want to know something of sexuality as an object of study, we need to know something of sexual subjectivity—unconscious and conscious registry of desire, identity, object choice, and practices—our own included.

The theorization of sexual self states may be the next task on our clinical and theoretical horizon. If the oedipal narrative historically organizes and creates sex and gender, new narratives generate the question of sexual self states: what, where, how is sex? Sexuality itself is no longer taken for granted as a self-evident drive, affect, or set of behaviors. Sexual desire is no longer a unisex model of tension, discharge, relief, of a straight shoot from polymorphous perversity to adult procreativity. Not only must femininity as well as masculinity, homosexuality as well as heterosexuality as well as bisexuality, be taken into account when it comes to desire. There may be as many sorts of desire as there are individuals who desire (Chodorow 1994); indeed, desire itself changes throughout life, to extend a point insisted on by the classical narrative.

Of what might sexual subjectivity consist? Certainly, like sexual identity, it must be built of multiple elements and function as a compromise formation. Chodorow (2003, pp. 12–17) has proposed that individual sexuality comprises several linked, interacting components that are universally occurring but idiosyncratically combined: erotization, sexual practices, an internal world, affective tonality, sexual object choice, sexual (and, we should add, gender) identity, culture, and fantasy, the last of which integrates in highly personal fashion all the preceding elements, marking them with aggression as well as lust.

Desire

To this list, or perhaps alongside it, should be added the general category of desire, which, not used so much as such by Freud, has entered the Anglophone psychoanalytic lexicon through the influence of Lacanian psychoanalysis. "Desire" is one of those terms at the foundation of a discipline that eludes definition. It designates a state of longing that receives, at least in Western culture, a primarily sexual expression entailing longing, arousal, and near satisfaction. The qualification is important. From Freud to Lacan, postcoital *tristesse* is something of a shibboleth: *"En attendant toujours quelque chose qui ne venait point"* ("Always waiting for something which never came") (Freud 1941/1964, p. 300, quoted by Green 1996, p. 872).

Concurring, Lacan sees satisfaction as a necessarily alluring impossibility critical to the crystallization of subjectivity, sanity, and culture. Lacanian theory has made this sad incompleteness revolve around what can only be written as "m/Other." Desire, symbolized by the Phallus (which is not intended to be the same as the biological penis; but see Flax 1990 [p. 104] and Grosz 1992 [p. 322] on the social and political context for this claim), is defined as the wish to be the object of the Other's desire. However, since, in point of fact, the first Other is a mother (who may, we would argue *contra* Lacan, be male or female), one's longing seeks an impossible state of grace and power accorded not even to father—it's *your* mother, not his own, who desires him. Her longing to be the object of his desire is, however, a displacement from her own primordial longing to be the object of her m/Other's desire. And the same poignant impossibility holds for him: his object of desire, his own m/Other, longs to be the object of her husand's—and m/Other's—desire. The object of desire is in this construal an eternal mirage: if each of us desires to be the object of the other's desire, desire's satisfaction always remains just out of reach. Recognition of this endless deferral constitutes entry into the Symbolic, the order of existence which one enters upon being able to recognize that no one, not even those endowed with a biological penis, possesses the Phallus: we all long for that which cannot exist. The Phallus also signifies the recognition that subjectivity is not self-identical: founded in a split—the illusion of a unitary self endowed only by the m/Other's recognition—subjectivity is always divided, a postulate at the basis of deconstructionist theories of gender multiplicity. "Only the concept of a subjectivity at odds with itself gives back to women the right to an impasse at the point of sexual identity, with no nostalgia whatsoever for its possible or future integration into a norm" (Rose 1986, p. 15; see also Dyess and Dean 2000).

Body and Bodymind

It is worth noting that Lacanian theory (re)introduces to psychosexual theory the object purged by one-person psychology. But that object is no longer only the object that at puberty stimulates desire. It is an object that desires, it is a subject; the m/Other desires someone other than you. Sexual subjectivity is therefore forever complicated by intersubjectivity, as may be seen in the postclassical body. In the classical view, the body was an object-body made of zones, organized by goals, traversed by a force, and knowable by science. It imprinted psyche, and psyche in turn mapped it. Postclassically, however, the body emerges in intersubjective (which is also cultural) space and, rather than being divided into parts, multiplies. The shift from then to now is from the body as object to embodiment—that is, the body as subjectively experienced. Embodiment may be conceptualized as "bodymind" (Wrye 1998), a both/and that we can employ in working through the Cartesian dualism between subjective mind and objective body. An interleaving of psyche and soma, private epochs, interpersonal history, and public convention, bodymind situates extreme individuality.

Opening that "frontier between the mental and the physical" where Freud (1905/1953, p. 168) situates the instincts, bodymind, as Dimen (2000) has shown, denotes not two polar functions but a third area: the body as subject to and subject of perception in conversation with the world, as Merleau-Ponty (1962) saw it. The body is neither subject nor object but both: my body, you might put it, is at once "an object for others and a subject for myself" (Merleau-Ponty 1962, p. 167). The body always involves other minds, existing simultaneously for self and for other. The body can be both subject and object, rather than one or the other, because (at least) two people are involved in it, each from a necessarily different relation to it. No one can know my own body from the inside as I do, nor can I perceive it as you can from the perspective of your own embodiment, which exists outside of mine. The body is therefore a site that expresses or communicates meaning and an emergent construction in intersubjective, interpersonal, and social life. Finally, key to the body's two-person construction is the preoedipal mother, active in what (in a one-person model) Anzieu (1989) calls the "skin-ego" but which (in a two-person model) we might dub the "touch-ego" (Dimen 2000, p. 30).

Transference and Countertransference

The multiplicity of bodies brings us to the matter of sexuality in the consulting room and the problems of sexual transference and countertransference. The recent discussion of these matters in the literature is not surprising, given the postclassical shift from an authoritarian to a more democratic psychoanalysis. As the once ominiscient, masculinized scientist knew his feminized subject, so the once all-knowing doctor knew his patient. But from Anna O. and Breuer onward, psychoanalysis might be thought of as the first of the scholarly disciplines to produce a new form of knowledge: the object of study, talking back to the doctor, becomes also the subject of study, rendering the doctor-observer a participant as well, whose subjectivity in terms becomes an object of study. Anna O. taught Breuer the talking cure. And Ferenczi (1933/1988) suggested the value of not running from the erotic countertransference, as Breuer is rumored to have done. Rather, he advised, and some have begun to follow, although not without debate, that we examine the analyst's sexual feelings, assessing them in particular and general (Davies 1994, 1998; Gabbard 1989; Maroda 1994). There is no longer one center of desire in the consulting room.

In one of those loop-de-loops that constitute intellectual history, we are returning to our classical starting point. Polymorphousness of theory—multiple narratives of desire, the two-person construal of the individual body, the equal importance of transference and countertransference, and so on—leads back to the polymorphousness of desire and its original situation: the preoedipal period. Classically, sexuality was theorized as general: despite Freud's masculinization of libido and his oedipal protagonist, he intended a theory of sex beyond gender. Then, with the feminist critique, the category of sexuality was reinvestigated through the question of gender (Benjamin 1998).

Enigmas of Sexuality

Recent work (e.g., Dimen 1999; Laplanche 1976; Stein 1998; Stoller 1979) has, however, led to a rethinking of sexual experience itself, not only its wordlessness, excessiveness, complicity with aggression, and mystery, but its gendering. In keeping with the classical sense of the unconscious as locus of strangeness and incomprehensibility, this revision takes sexuality as a site of difficulty, trauma, and enigma. At the same time, sexuality is no longer a one-person affair. Rather, it is at once intrapsychic, interpersonal, intersubjective, and social. In postmodern perspective, we can have it both ways. With the "seduction theory" (perhaps better termed the "molestation theory") having been corrected by impeccable evidence of sexual abuse and its sequelae, sexuality's place in phantasy can be recaptured as well. Plural and diverse in its manifestations, sources, delights, and troubles, sexuality can also be construed as existing simultaneously in material and psychic realities, having a place in both lived experience and unconscious fantasy.

Freud, we have seen, finds the source of sexual difficulty in the developmental necessity to weld drive, aim, and object into one—a precarious enterprise often likely to fail given the chthonic diffuseness of sexual experience and diversity of aims. Contemporary French psychoanalytic theory delves more deeply into sexual subjectivity. McDougall (1995) locates sexuality's traumatic quality in the necessity of loss: for her, the achievement of sexual and other identity and maturity means relinquishing the claim to gender "overinclusiveness." In Laplanche's (1976) view, sexual desire's origins render it an "alien internal entity." For him, as for Kristeva (1983), psychosexual development is strongly marked by the mother, for it is now seen to proceed in relation to her sexuality, which by definition consists in her unconscious. Given the concreteness of social change—now that men as well as women, gay as well as straight, are taking up the maternal role—such conceptions of psychic development will require some alteration.

If sex thus becomes an "enigmatic message," sexuality as an unconscious transmission to the infant from the maternal or, as we might now emend it, the parental unconscious, then sexuality is always already an inarticulable mystery, a site of excess caused in no small part by the in-tersubjectivity of sex. Agreeing with but going beyond Laplanche, Stein (1998) limns sexuality's excess, its sacred transcendence and loss of self that contrast with and even contradict the integrated state of mind, the profane connectedness, required for ordinary life. Making a further distinction, Benjamin (1998) finds excess to result from "failures in affective containment [that] may produce sexual tension rather than reflect some interpersonal transmission of unconscious sexual content" (p. 7). Davies (2001), unearthing yet another intersubjective effect of the unmetabolizable spillover of parent-child intimacy, suggests that the unavoidable absence of parents' empathy with their children's sexual feeling inevitably imbues sexuality with a sense of trauma. (Of course, such an absence depends on cultural context: in societies where parents and children share a sleeping space, children's presence during parental sex may afford mutual sexual empathy. The primal scene's significance is, in other words, culturally relative, not necessarily traumatic or even, as Aron [1995] proposes, generative).

In/Conclusion: Perversion and Normality

Let us conclude an admittedly incomplete entry on a rapidly evolving topic with an overview of a highly contestable category of sexuality, as a way of illustrating some continuing central dilemmas. Conventionally, sexual perversion is briefly defined as any deviation from coitus with a person of the opposite sex aimed at achieving orgasm through genital penetration (Laplanche and Pontalis 1973, p. 306). But under the bright lights of feminist inquiry, a two-person psychology, and (post)modern skepticism, the very concept of "perversion," and its presumed integrity, become suspect, inviting lively debate.

Perversion carries three meanings: that of illness, that of moral sanction, and that of human sexuality itself. Psychoanalysis is, Freud once said, at once a body of knowledge, a theory of human nature, and a method of cure. If, as a method of cure, it diagnoses illness and prescribes treatment, psychosexual theory is critical to the medical function of psychoanalysis. Indeed, the importance of sexual etiology lies precisely in psychoanalysis' disciplinary role in what Foucault (1976/1980) called a "technology of health and pathology." If sexual illness causes psychic illness, a standard of sexual health must exist: as we have seen, as soon as heterosexuality and procreation are invoked as the twinned telos of sexual development in a theory that otherwise pronounces on mental health—for example, the achievement of selfhood—they become the criteria for adult normality. By this standard, any deviation from the reproductive heterosexual path indicates the germ of psychic illness.

That calling a perversion an illness has functions over and above medical care is suggested by how well psychoanalysts have ignored disclaimers over the course of the last century. Freud (1905/1953) wrote that perverse practices permit "normal" heterosexual functioning; "neuroses are, so to say, the negative of perversion" (p. 165). Ninety years later, Kernberg (1995) prescribed that a healthy sexual relationship encompass occasional moments when one uses the other "as a pure sexual object" (p. 58). Yet the term "perversion" seems so important that even now it is in the course of being redefined. No longer, Dimen (2001) contends, does it refer to sexuality. Rather it designates the mutilated capacities to love (Bach 1995; Stoller 1975) and to survive loss and narcissistic injury (Chasseguet-Smirgel 1985); the creation of deadness in the psychoanalytic situation (Ogden 1996); or the anal mashing of all distinctions, of the sexes and the generations, as part of an effort to destroy civilization (Chasseguet-Smirgel 1985).

The cultural values and social sanctions contained in this effort to rehabilitate a category doomed from its inception are inevitable in a topic as hot as sexuality. It is no longer possible, since the Foucauldian critique, to view psychoanalysis as existing outside its cultural and political milieu (see also Person, in press). As such it possesses both facilitating and socially controlling functions, emancipatory and dominating clinical and theoretical practices. Psychoanalysis is implicated in a system of disciplinary power that facilitates healing by naming the illness, or helping the patient to name it. The power to name is, however, also the power to blame—the pervert as outlaw—and to shame—the pervert as, well, pervert.

Consider Laplanche and Pontalis's (1976) caution: "It is difficult to comprehend the idea of perversion otherwise than by reference to a norm" (p. 306). In other words, perversion and that inadequately specific term *normality* construct each other. But "normality" is not merely a scientific term: the very idea of a "norm" is always already filled with and prompted by cultural significance and custom. In the discourse of psychosexuality, perversion and heteronormality constitute each other's limits. Perversion marks the boundary across which you become an outlaw. Normality marks off the territory that, if stayed inside of, keeps you safe from shame, disgust, and anxiety.

The same may be said of sexuality *tout court*. All sexuality may, in fact, be considered a deviation, a swerving from a path that no longer may be traversed. If we are correct in thinking that sexuality, like the psyche itself, is simultaneously subjective and intersubjective, intrapsychic and interpersonal, then desire itself is inevitably

marked by the losses of the earliest object-relational experience—indeed, by the loss of that state of mind itself. Here we must agree with Lacan's view of desire as distinguished from need. Need, like hunger, must have one thing and one thing only: food. Desire thrives on substitutes. It may be satisfied or deferred—turned into pleasure or babies or buildings or bombs. It may accept a blow job or coitus or a beating, a fantasy or a body, a belt or a breast or a picture, a male or a female or a transvestite.

The reconstruction of psychosexual theory challenges other psychoanalytic fundamentals, notably the question of mental health, of sanity, and hence of treatment and cure. What, after all, is sexual pathology? If all sexualities may claim wholesomeness, if all have a valid psychic place, then all are subject to the same psychic vicissitudes. Put yet another way, sexuality has nothing inherently to do with mental health or mental illness. You may be ill if you are heterosexual, or transvestite, and healthy if you are homosexual or bisexual, or whatever.

The difficulty and variousness of perversion, as of sexuality itself, should make us hesitate before we proclaim or adhere to a single explanation for sexuality or a single developmental account. For much of the last century, the pull has been toward the normalizing and one-dimensionalizing pole of psychoanalytic theory: a single narrative of reproductive heterosexual desire as the gold standard by which mental health is measured. Yet even as conformism dominated psychoanalytic thought and clinical practice, an opposing pole existed and is, as we have seen, now receiving its due. Psychosexual theory is a work in process, and its results are not yet in. But we invite you to stay tuned.

References

Anzieu D: The Skin Ego. Translated by Turner C. New Haven, CT, Yale University Press, 1989

Aron L: The internalized primal scene. Psychoanalytic Dialogues 5:195–236, 1995

Bach S: The Language of Perversion and the Language of Love. Northvale, NJ, Jason Aronson, 1995

Balsam R: Integrating male and female elements in a woman's gender identity. J Am Psychoanal Assoc 49:1335–1360, 2001

Bassin D: Women's images of inner space: data towards expanded interpretive categories. Int Rev Psychoanal 9:191–203, 1982

Bassin D: Beyond the he and the she: toward the reconciliation of the masculine and feminine in the postoedipal female mind. J Am Psychoanal Assoc 44 (suppl):157–190, 1996

Bassin D: Working through our predecessors and our own readings, in Female Sexuality. Edited by Bassin D. Northvale, NJ, Jason Aronson, 1999, pp 5–21

Bassin D: On the problems(s) with keeping difference(s) where they belong. Studies in Gender and Sexuality 1:185–197, 2000

Benjamin J: The convergence of psychoanalysis and feminism: gender identity and autonomy, in Women Therapists Working With Women. Edited by Brody CM. New York, Springer, 1984, pp 37–45

Benjamin J: The Bonds of Love: Psychoanalysis, Feminism, and the Problem of Domination. New York, Pantheon, 1988

Benjamin J: Like Subjects, Love Objects. New Haven, CT, Yale University Press, 1995

Benjamin J: Shadow of the Other: Intersubjectivity and Gender in Psychoanalysis. New York, Routledge, 1998

Bernstein D: Female gender anxieties, conflicts, and typical mastery modes. Int J Psychoanal 71:151–165, 1990

Bollas C: Forces of Destiny. London, Free Association Books, 1989

Bourdieu P, Eagleton T: Doxa and common life. New Left Rev 191:111–121, 1992

Breen D: General introduction, in The Gender Conundrum. Edited by Breen D. London, Routledge, 1993, pp 1–39

Butler J: Gender Trouble. New York, Routledge, 1990

Butler J: Melancholy gender-refused identification, in Gender in Psychoanalytic Space. Edited by Dimen M, Goldner V. New York, The Other Press, 2002, pp 3–21

Chasseguet-Smirgel J: Freud and female sexuality: the consideration of some blind spots in the exploration of the "dark continent." Int J Psychoanal 57:275–286, 1976

Chasseguet-Smirgel J: Creativity and Perversion. New York, WW Norton, 1985

Chodorow NJ: Seventies questions for thirties women: gender and generation in a study of early women psychoanalysts, in Feminism and Psychoanalytic Theory. New Haven, CT, Yale University Press, 1989, pp 199–218

Chodorow NJ: Femininities, Masculinities, Sexualities. Lexington, University Press of Kentucky, 1994

Chodorow NJ: Multiplicities and uncertainties of gender: commentary on Ruth Stein's "Analysis of a Case of Transsexualism." Psychoanalytic Dialogues 5:291–299, 1995

Chodorow NJ: The enemy outside: thoughts on the psychodynamics of extreme violence with special attention to men and masculinity. Journal for the Psychoanalysis of Culture and Society 3:25–38, 1998

Chodorow NJ: The Reproduction of Mothering, 2nd Edition. Berkeley, University of California Press, 1999a

Chodorow NJ: The Power of Feelings: Personal Meaning in Psychoanalysis, Gender, and Culture. New Haven, CT, Yale University Press, 1999b

Chodorow NJ: Les homosexualités comme formation compromise. Revue Française de Psychanalyse 67:4–64, 2003

Coates S: Ontogenesis of boyhood gender identity disorder. J Am Psychoanal Assoc 18:414–438, 1990

Coates S: Is it time to jettison the concept of developmental lines? Commentary on de Marneffe's paper. Gender and Psychoanalysis 1:35–55, 1997

Colapinto J: As Nature Made Him. New York, HarperCollins, 2000

Corbett K: The mystery of homosexuality. Psychoanalytic Psychology 10:345–358, 1993

Corbett K: Homosexual boyhood: notes on girlyboys. Gender and Psychoanalysis 1:429–463, 1996

Corbett K: Faggot = loser. Studies in Gender and Sexuality 2:3–28, 2001a

Corbett K: More life: centrality and marginality in human development. Psychoanalytic Dialogues 11:313–335, 2001b

Davies JM: Love in the afternoon: a relational reconsideration of desire and dread in the countertransference. Psychoanalytic Dialogues 4:153–170, 1994

Davies JM: Between the disclosure and foreclosure of erotic transference–countertransference: can psychoanalysis find a place for adult sexuality? Psychoanalytic Dialogues 8:747–766, 1998

Davies JM: Erotic overstimulation and the co-construction of sexual meanings in transference and countertransference experience. Psychoanal Q 70:757–788, 2001

De Beauvoir S: The Second Sex (1949). Translated by Parshley HM. New York, Vintage Books, 1974

De Marneffe D: Bodies and words: a study of young children's genital and gender knowledge. Gender and Psychoanalysis 2:3–35, 1997

Dimen M: Deconstructing difference: gender, splitting, and transitional space. Psychoanalytic Dialogues 1:337–354, 1991

Dimen M: Between lust and libido: sex, psychoanalysis, and the moment before. Psychoanalytic Dialogues 9:415–440, 1999

Dimen M: The body as Rorschach. Studies in Gender and Sexuality 1:9–39, 2000

Dimen M: Sexuality, Intimacy, Power. Hillsdale, NJ, Analytic Press, 2003

Dinnerstein D: The Mermaid and the Minotaur. New York, Harper & Row, 1976

Domenici T, Lesser R (eds): Disorienting Sexuality: Psychoanalytic Reappraisals of Sexual Identities. New York, Routledge, 1995

Drescher J: Transgender subjectivities: a clinician's guide. Journal of Gay and Lesbian Psychotherapy 8:1–152, 2004

Dyess C, Dean T: Gender: the impossibility of meaning. Psychoanalytic Dialogues 10:735–757, 2000

Elise D: Primary femininity, bisexuality, and the female ego ideal: a re-examination of female developmental theory. Psychoanal Q 66:470–489, 1997

Elise D: Bye-bye to bisexuality: response to Lynne B. Layton. Studies in Gender and Sexuality 1:61–69, 2000

Fairbairn WRD: Observations on the nature of hysterical states. Br J Med Psychol 27:105–125, 1954

Fast I: Gender Identity: A Differentiation Model. Hillsdale, NJ, Analytic Press, 1984

Fast I: Aspects of core gender identity. Psychoanalytic Dialogues 9:633–663, 1999a

Fast I: Reply to commentary. Psychoanalytic Dialogues 9:675–683, 1999b

Fausto-Sterling A: Myths of Gender: Biological Theories of Women and Men. New York, Basic Books, 1986

Ferenczi S: The confusion of tongues between adults and children (1933). Contemp Psychoanal 24:196–206, 1988

Flax J: Thinking Fragments: Psychoanalysis, Feminism, and Postmodernism in the Contemporary West. Berkeley, University of California Press, 1990

Fliegel ZO: Women's development in analytic theory, in Psychoanalysis and Women: Contemporary Reappraisals. Edited by Alpert JL. Hillsdale, NJ, Analytic Press, 1986, pp 3–31

Foucault M: The History of Sexuality, Vol. 1 (1976). Translated by Hurley R. New York, Vintage, 1980

Freud A: Studies in passivity (1952), in Indications for Child Analysis and Other Papers. New York, International Universities Press, 1969

Freud S: Three essays on the theory of sexuality, I: the sexual aberrations (1905), in Standard Edition of the Complete Psychological Works of Sigmund Freud, Vol 7. Translated and edited by Strachey J. London, Hogarth Press, 1953, pp 135–172

Freud S: Civilized sexual morality and modern nervous illness (1908), in The Standard Edition of the Complete Psychological Works of Sigmund Freud, Vol 9. Translated and edited by Strachey J. London, Hogarth Press, 1959, pp 177–204

Freud S: The psychogenesis of a case of homosexuality in a woman (1920), in Standard Edition of the Complete Psychological Works of Sigmund Freud, Vol 18. Translated and edited by Strachey J. London, Hogarth Press, 1955, pp 145–174

Freud S: The dissolution of the Oedipus complex (1924), in Standard Edition of the Complete Psychological Works of Sigmund Freud, Vol 19. Translated and edited by Strachey J. London, Hogarth Press, 1961, pp 173–182

Freud S: Some psychical consequences of the anatomical distinction between the sexes (1925), in Standard Edition of the Complete Psychological Works of Sigmund Freud, Vol 19. Translated and edited by Strachey J. London, Hogarth Press, 1961, pp 241–258

Freud S: Fetishism (1927), in The Standard Edition of the Complete Psychological Works of Sigmund Freud, Vol 21. Translated and edited by Strachey J. London, Hogarth Press, 1957, pp 52–157

Freud S: Female sexuality (1931), in The Standard Edition of the Complete Psychological Works of Sigmund Freud, Vol 21. Translated and edited by Strachey J. London, Hogarth Press, 1961, pp 221–245

Freud S: On femininity (1933), in New Introductory Lectures, in The Standard Edition of the Complete Psychological Works of Sigmund Freud, Vol 22. Translated and edited by Strachey J. London, Hogarth Press, 1964, pp 112–134

Freud S: An outline of psycho-analysis (1940), in The Standard Edition of the Complete Psychological Works of Sigmund Freud, Vol 23. Translated and edited by Strachey J. London, Hogarth Press, 1964, pp 144–207

Freud S: Findings, ideas, problems (1941), in The Standard Edition of the Complete Psychological Works of Sigmund Freud, Vol 23. Translated and edited by Strachey J. London, Hogarth Press, 1964, pp 299–300

Freud S: Letter to an American mother (1935). Am J Psychiatry 107:787, 1951

Gabbard G (ed): Sexual Exploitation in Professional Relationships. Washington, DC, American Psychiatric Press, 1989

Gagnon J: Commentary on Goldner's "Toward a Critical Relational Theory of Gender." Psychoanalytic Dialogues 1:273–276, 1991

Geertz C: Making experiences, authoring selves, in The Anthropology of Experience. Edited by Turner V, Bruner E. Champaign, University of Illinois Press, 1986, pp 373–381

Gilman S: Freud, Race, and Gender. Princeton, NJ, Princeton University Press, 1995

Goldberger M: Obsolete terminology constricts thinking imaginative thinking. Psychoanal Q 68:462–466, 1999

Goldner V: Toward a critical relational theory of gender. Psychoanalytic Dialogues 1:249–272, 1991

Goldner V: The treatment of violence and victimization in intimate relationships. Family Process 37:263–286, 1998

Goldner V: Ironic gender/authentic sex. Studies in Gender and Sexuality 4:113–139, 2003

Green A: Has sexuality anything to do with psychoanalysis? Int J Psychoanal 76:871–883, 1996

Greenson R: Dis-identifying from mother: its special importance for the boy. Int J Psychoanal 45:220–226, 1968

Grosz E: Phallus: feminist implications, in Feminism and Psychoanalysis: A Critical Dictionary. Edited by Wright E. Oxford, England, Blackwell, 1992, pp 320–323

Harris A: Gender as contradiction. Psychoanalytic Dialogues 1: 197–220, 1991

Harris A: Making genders: commentary on paper by Irene Fast. Psychoanalytic Dialogues 9:663–675, 1999

Harris A: Gender as a soft assembly. Studies in Gender and Sexuality 1:223–251, 2000

Harvey D: The Condition of Postmodernity. Oxford, England, Oxford University Press, 1989

Herdt G, Stoller R: Intimate Communications: Erotics and the Study of Culture. New York, Columbia University Press, 1992

Horney K: On the genesis of the castration complex in women (1924), in Feminine Psychology. Edited by Kelman H. New York, WW Norton, 1967, pp 37–53

Horney K: The flight from womanhood (1926), in Feminine Psychology. Edited by Kelman H. New York, WW Norton, 1967, pp 54–70

Irigaray L: This Sex Which Is Not One. Translated by Porter C, Burke C. Ithaca, NY, Cornell University Press, 1985

Isay RA: Being Homosexual: Gay Men and Their Development. New York, Farrar, Straus, Giroux, 1989

Jones E: Early development of female sexuality (1935), in Papers on Psychoanalysis, 5th Edition. London, Maresfield Reprints, 1961, pp 485–495

Kaftal E: On intimacy between men. Psychoanalytic Dialogues 1:305–328, 1991

Katz JN: The Invention of Homosexuality. New York, Dutton, 1996

Kernberg O: Love Relations: Pathology and Normality. New Haven, CT, Yale University Press, 1995

Kessler S: The medical construction of gender. Signs 16:3–26, 1990

Kessler S, McKenna W: Gender: An Ethnomethodological Approach. Chicago, IL, University of Chicago Press, 1978

Kestenberg J: The inner genital phase, in Early Female Development: Current Psychoanalytic Views. Edited by Mendell D. Jamaica, NY, Spectrum Publications, 1982, pp 71–126

Klein M: Early stages of the Oedipus complex. Int J Psychoanal 9:167–180, 1928

Kristeva J: Tales of Love. Translated by Roudiez M. New York, Columbia University Press, 1983

Kristeva J: Women's time, in Essential Papers on the Psychology of Women. Edited by Zanardi C. New York, New York University Press, 1990, pp 374–400

Kulish N: Primary femininity: clinical advances and theoretical ambiguities. J Am Psychoanal Assoc 48:1355–1379, 2000

Laplanche J: Life and Death in Psychoanalysis. Translated by Mehlman J. Baltimore, MD, Johns Hopkins University Press, 1976

Laplanche J, Pontalis J-B: The Language of Psycho-Analysis. Translated by Nicholson-Smith D. New York, Norton, 1973

Laqueur T: Making Sex. Cambridge, MA, Harvard University Press, 1990

Lasky R: Body ego and feminine gender identity. J Am Psychoanal Assoc 48:1381–1412, 2000

Layton LB: Who's that Girl? Who's that Boy? Northvale, NJ, Jason Aronson, 1998

Layton LB: The psychopolitics of bisexuality. Studies in Gender and Sexuality 1:41–61, 2000a

Layton LB: Reply to Bassin, Stimmel, and Elise. Studies in Gender and Sexuality 1:85–97, 2000b

Leary K: Race in psychoanalytic space. Gender and Psychoanalysis 2:157–172, 1997

Lesser R, Domenici T (eds): Disorienting Sexuality. New York, Routledge, 1995

Lewes K: The Psychoanalytic Theory of Male Homosexuality. New York, Simon & Schuster, 1988

Marcus S (ed): Introduction, in Three Essays on the Theory of Sexuality by S. Freud. Translated and revised by Strachey J. New York, Basic Books, 1975

Maroda K: The Power of Countertransference. Northvale, NJ, Jason Aronson, 1994

May R: Concerning a psychoanalytic view of maleness. Psychoanal Rev 73:175–193, 1986

Mayer EL: Everybody must be just like me: observations on female castration anxiety. Int J Psychoanal 66:331–347, 1985

McDougall J: The Many Faces of Eros. New York, WW Norton, 1995

Meltzer D: Sexual States of Mind (1973). Perthshire, Scotland, Clunie Press, 1979

Merleau-Ponty M: The Phenomenology of Perception. Translated by Smith C. New York, Routledge, 1962

Mitchell J, Rose J (eds): Feminine Sexuality: Jacques Lacan and l'École Freudienne. Translated by Rose J. New York, Pantheon, 1982

Money J: Gender role, gender identity, core gender identity: Usage and definition of terms. J Am Acad Psychoanal 1:397–402, 1973

Money J, Hampson JG, Hampson JI: An examination of basic sexual concepts. Bulletin of the Johns Hopkins University Hospital 97:301–319, 1955

Ogden T: The perverse subject of analysis. J Am Psychoanal Assoc 44:1121–1146, 1996

Person E: A psychoanalytic approach, in Theories of Sexuality. Edited by Geer J, O'Donohue W. New York, Plenum, 1986, pp 385–410

Person E: The Sexual Century. New Haven, CT, Yale University Press, 1999

Person E: Something borrowed: how mutual influences among gays, lesbians, bisexuals, and straights changed women's lives and psychoanalytic theory. Annual of Psychoanalysis (in press)

Person E, Ovesey L: Psychoanalytic theories of gender identity. J Am Acad Psychoanal 11:203–226, 1983

Pollack SS: Deconstructing dis-identification: rethinking psychoanalytic concepts of male development. Psychoanalysis and Psychotherapy 12:30–45, 1995

Rose J: Sexuality in the Field of Vision. London, Verso, 1986

Ross JM: Beyond the phallic illusion: notes on man's heterosexuality, in The Psychology of Men. Edited by Fogel G, Lane F, Liebert R. New York, Basic Books, 1986, pp 49–70

Roughton R: The two analyses of a gay man: the interplay of social change and psychoanalytic understanding. Annual of Psychoanalysis 30:83–99, 2002

Rubin G: The traffic in women: notes on the political economy of sex, in Toward an Anthropology of Women. Edited by Reiter RR. New York, Monthly Review Press, 1975, pp 157–210

Schafer R: Problems in Freud's psychology of women, in Female Psychology: Contemporary Psychoanalytic Views. Edited by Blum H. New York, International Universities Press, 1977, pp 331–360

Schafer R: On male nonnormative sexuality and perversion in psychoanalytic discourse. Annual of Psychoanalysis 30:23–35, 2003

Schuker E: Toward further analytic understanding of lesbian patients. J Am Psychoanal Assoc 44 (suppl):485–508, 1996

Senet N: A study of preschool children's linking of genitals and gender. Psychoanal Q 73:291–335, 2004

Stein R: The poignant, the excessive and the enigmatic in sexuality. Int J Psychoanal 79:253–268, 1998

Stein R: Analysis of a case of transsexualism. Psychoanalytic Dialogues 5:257–289, 1995a

Stein R: Reply to Chodorow. Psychoanalytic Dialogues 5:301–310, 1995b

Stimmel B: From "nothing" to "something" to "everything": bisexuality and metaphors of the mind. J Am Psychoanal Assoc 44(suppl):191–214, 1996

Stimmel B: The baby with the bathwater. Studies in Gender and Sexuality 1:79–85, 2000

Stimpson C, Person E (eds): Women: Sex and Sexuality. Chicago, IL, University of Chicago Press, 1980

Stoller RJ: The sense of femaleness. Psychoanal Q 37:42–55, 1968

Stoller RJ: Primary femininity. J Am Psychoanal Assoc 24 (suppl): 59–78, 1976

Stoller RJ: Sexual Excitement. New York, Pantheon, 1979

Sullivan HS: The Interpersonal Theory of Psychiatry. Edited by Perry HS, Gawel ML. New York, WW Norton, 1953

Sweetnam A: The changing contexts of gender: between fixed and fluid experience. Psychoanalytic Dialogues 6:437–459, 1996

Weille KH: The psychodynamics of consensual sadomasochistic and dominant-submissive sexual games. Studies in Gender and Sexuality 2:131–160, 2001

Winnicott DW: Transitional objects and transitional phenomena. Int J Psychoanal 34:89–97, 1953

Wrye H: The embodiment of desire: relinking the bodymind within the analytic dyad, in Relational Perspectives on the Body. Edited by Aron L, Anderson FS. Hillsdale, NJ, Analytic Press, 1998, pp 97–116

Young-Bruehl E: Freud on Women: A Reader. New York, WW Norton, 1990

Young-Bruehl E: Gender and psychoanalysis: an introductory essay. Gender and Psychoanalysis 1:7–19, 1996

PART II

Developmental Theory

SECTION EDITOR: MARY TARGET, PH.D.

7

A Developmental Orientation for Contemporary Psychoanalysis

ROBERT N. EMDE, M.D.

A DEVELOPMENTAL ORIENTATION frames an approach to psychoanalytic treatment. A central feature of this approach is an appreciation for development as an ongoing, active, lifelong process that not only has a past but exists in a present and has a future. From the patient's viewpoint, a developmental orientation for psychoanalysis represents new beginnings (Balint 1952; Loewald 1960). One aim of this approach is to release developmental processes of adaptation so that there is less encumbrance by shadowed repetitions of conflict from one's past. In reexperiencing aspects of conflicted relationships from the past in the midst of a special new relationship—one steeped in an atmosphere of trust, security, and empathy—new connections are made by the patient, and new adaptive possibilities for living emerge and can be tried out.

The developmental orientation, with its forward-looking emphasis, supplements the other viewpoints of psychoanalysis. It makes use of many insights from the genetic viewpoint (concerned with psychoanalytic reconstructions of the past) and enlarges the adaptive viewpoint of psychoanalysis while working within a dynamic framework of unconscious defense and resistance. A further feature of this orientation is that it makes use of current knowledge

of the human developmental process, not only from the accumulated clinical experience of psychoanalytic practice but also from a range of other disciplines in the developmental sciences.

In this chapter, I highlight the additive features of the developmental orientation of psychoanalysis. The other working viewpoints are discussed in Sections I ("Core Concepts") and III ("Treatment and Technique") of this textbook.

Use of the Past in the Developmental Present

Psychoanalysis, in its approach to psychopathology, addresses suffering and maladaptive behavior, as do other treatments. But, in addition, psychoanalysis deals with unconscious conflict and fantasy as they become understood in an intimate, relatively long-lasting form of relationship treatment. As such it has a developmental orientation, not only in terms of the influence of the past but also in terms of understanding current influences and wider alternatives so as to avoid maladaptive repetitions in the future. As noted, the past is made use of through reexperiencing many of its conflicted aspects in the therapeutic encounter (i.e., in experiences of transference) so as to engage new possibilities and "new beginnings." In other words, what is useful about one's past is being able to understand it in terms of one's developmental present.

A goal of the patient in psychoanalytic treatment is to be able to make use of the past by arriving at a wider understanding of his or her biography (Erikson 1950), including ambivalent relationships with parents and others and of recurrent conflicts (including many aspects that were not conscious), and to be able to distinguish what was true and vital *then* from what is vital *now*. The patient comes to have more of a capacity for introspection and empathy (Kohut 1959) and for emotional appreciation for others, as well as for one's self in the past, what is currently referred to as *reflective functioning* (Fonagy et al. 2002). Some have described an aspect of this process in vivid literary terms as one in which the problematic ghosts of one's represented past can be converted, with psychoanalytic treatment, to useful ancestors for the present (Fraiberg et al. 1975; Loewald 1960).

And key to the developmental orientation is the appreciation of different developmental capabilities, limitations, opportunities, and challenges at different points in the life span. What can be accomplished now as a 20-year-old, for example, in the way of potency, sexual intimacy, and responsibility with a desired other is different from what one may have wished for and could not accomplish as a 5-year-old. The conflicted relationships and dreams one has as a 50-year-old with career and family are different from those of a 20-year-old. The particulars of adult development from a psychoanalytic perspective have occupied the attention of a number of authors (see Benedek 1970; Colarusso and Nemiroff 1981; Dewald 1980; Neugarten 1979; Pollock 1980; Vaillant 1977). Adult development includes responses to life events such as marriage, parenthood, loss of loved ones, retirement, and biological decline; it also includes initiatives in response to perceived possibilities of achieving better levels of adaptation (Settlage et al. 1988).

Psychoanalysis, from a developmental orientation, can be regarded as existential; it operates with an awareness of one's present position in the life cycle, affirming existence along with its limitations as well as its potentials. Although we are limited in terms of our capacities and what we can do in our circumstances, we are free within a range of possibilities and we are responsible for what we do. Psychoanalytic treatment can also be regarded as "tragic" (Kohut 1977; Schafer 1959), in that it takes into account the human predicament in terms of one's mortality, vulnerabil-

ity, and ambivalent relationships, conflicts, and unrealized dreams. It also takes into account disappointments that result when one reflects on the wished-for changes and betterments that have not occurred in a lifetime. The well-adapted person—whether assisted by psychoanalysis or not—accommodates to one's existential predicament and continues to participate in development. It is a characteristic of adaptive development that the individual assimilates new experiences and relationships, even in the midst of unfulfilled wishes and even in the midst of diminished capacities.

Adaptation, Forward-Looking Processes, and Early Relationships

Processes of adaptation are a central aspect of the developmental orientation for psychoanalysis. Perspectives about adaptation and mental organization in context have gained increasing prominence within psychoanalysis over the past 65 years, beginning with the work of Heinz Hartmann (1939/1958) and building on accumulated clinical experience as well as accumulated knowledge from other disciplines in the developmental sciences (Emde 1999; Mayes 1994; Rado 1953). The developmental orientation draws attention to the forward-looking aspects of adaptation that characterize an individual throughout life as well as the formative origins of such adaptive processes that take place in the context of early relationships. The forward-looking aspects of adaptation are apparent as we consider the anticipatory signaling functions of affects and the early formation of the cognitive representational world of self and others, a world that consists of expectations, planful schemas, and possibilities. These will be considered next.

Psychoanalysis gives prominence to experiences in infancy and early childhood that occur in the context of parental and caregiving relationships (see Chapter 3, "Early Relationships and Their Internalization"). Early relationship experiences are different from later ones because they are formative. Experiences in first relationships set patterns and prototypes for how to behave with a caring other and for what to anticipate in the way of satisfactions and frustrations in particular circumstances (Sameroff and Emde 1989; Stern 1985). Such experiences become internalized by the individual, continue as strong influences in development throughout childhood, and are activated in similar relationship contexts throughout life. A number of psychoanalytic observers have emphasized that affective representations of self in relation to others arise in early caregiving relationship experiences and set expectations, both adaptive and maladaptive, that continue afterward

(Bion 1962; Erikson 1959; Fairbairn 1963; Guntrip 1971; Klein 1967; Spitz 1959; Winnicott 1965). Otto Kernberg (1976, 1990; see also Chapter 4, "Object Relations Theory and Technique") has theorized that basic units of integrated motives arise in infancy that involve affect, self, and object—a notion that can also be thought of as emotion schemas of self in relation to others. Peak affective states of experienced pleasure or unpleasure with the caregiver, when internalized, motivate corresponding wishes either to repeat or to avoid similar affective experiences.

The psychoanalytic notion of *wish* is itself a forward-looking concept because it deals with an imagined state in the future. Sandler and Sandler (1978) have translated the psychoanalytic notion of "drive" or "need" into the terms of a represented wish, one that includes the desired or expected response of the significant other (i.e., the response of the "object"). In other words, the very notion of "wish" implies a set of expectations—with goals and actions of others in relation to self in an imagined scenario. Thus, experience is organized in a way that integrates the dynamic past and the future (i.e., according to expectations). Current theorizing in the cognitive sciences, as well as in some areas of psychoanalysis concerned with process research (see Chapter 21, "Process Research"), is making use of similar models that deal with sequences of expectation and dynamic themes of self in relation to others. (Noteworthy are the "core conflictual relationship themes" conceptualized by Luborsky [1977], the "role relationship models" conceptualized by Horowitz [1991], and the emotion schemas of self in relation to others of Bucci [1997].)

Perhaps the most poignant area linking forward-looking processes and models of early development is that of attachment theory and research (see Chapter 10, "Attachment Theory and Research"). Beginning in infancy, monitoring the accessibility of the attachment figure occurs according to what John Bowlby (1969, 1988a) conceptualized as "working models of attachment." Such models are expectation sets that result from early relationship experiences with primary caregivers; they include representations of self in relation to others that are linked by affects and that may be self-enhancing (as in secure attachment) or self-maintaining/defensive (as in insecure attachment). Moreover, working models of attachment relationships, with their concomitant expectations, persist over the course of development and are apt to be influential in adult love relationships (Shaver and Hazan 1985) as well as in parenting relationships (Fonagy et al. 1991; Grossmann 1987; Main 1985; Ricks 1985).

Similar models involving expectations have also been articulated by other psychoanalytic observers of early development. Daniel Stern (1985) has vividly described the intimate development of self in relation to others in infancy in which representations of interactions with primary caregivers become generalized and guide expectations and subsequent behavior. Ideas about reflective functioning or "mentalizing," as articulated by Peter Fonagy and Mary Target (1998), are recent psychoanalytic concepts linking self in relation to others that involve affect and by their nature are likely to influence adaptive expectations of others. *Reflective functioning* refers to the ability to appreciate mental states (i.e., feelings, beliefs, and intentions) in others as well as in one's self. This ability is envisioned as a skill that is learned early in development, with origins presumably linked to back-and-forth meaningful exchanges of affect with the parent (see detailed discussion in Fonagy et al. 2002). Assessing reflective functioning, working models of attachment (especially in the Adult Attachment Interview), and relationship configurations of conflict is currently an area of vigorous psychoanalytic process research (see Chapter 21).

Background of the Developmental Orientation

A developmental orientation and approach was articulated by a task force of clinicians chaired by Calvin Settlage and Selma Kramer and summarized by Goodman (1977) and also by Emde (1980), Shane (1977), and Settlage (1980). The task force brought the experience of child analysis and adult analysis to bear on contemporary knowledge of developmental processes, and it articulated much of the framework noted in the previous section. As Morton Shane put it, "[T]he use of the developmental approach implies that the analytic patient, regardless of age, is considered to be still in the process of ongoing development as opposed to merely being in possession of a past that influences his present conscious and unconscious life" (Shane 1977, pp. 95–96). Subsequent contributions describing the usefulness of a developmental orientation for psychoanalytic work were made by Abrams (1990), Tyson and Tyson (1990), and Wallerstein (1990).

In one sense, psychoanalysis, from its beginnings, has been developmentally oriented. It has given early development a central place in its clinical theory, it has described meaningful developmental sequences, and it has connected later repetitions of conflicts to earlier ones that were not understood or mastered. In another sense, however, the developmental orientation as reviewed in this chapter reflects dramatic changes in psychoanalytic thinking. Much of Freud's thinking had its origins in the zeitgeist of nineteenth-century biology, which was deterministic and at times reductionistic. Although its early theory often reflected these origins, psychoanalysis, in its theory and practice, increasingly moved beyond its deterministic origins as it dealt with expanding structures of meaning, with uncertainty, and with changing adaptive contexts. In so doing, it has become more consistent with contemporary developmental psychobiology.

Let us trace how this has occurred. Freud's concept of motivation was centered on his unpleasure-pleasure principle: unpleasure resulted from an increase in drive tension and pleasure from its decrease. This principle has often been referred to as the principle of *entropy* (Rapaport 1959), since motivation was seen in terms of a discharge of energy or a running down to a lower level of organization. Freud's psychobiological model was based on a physics that specified entropy as the second law of thermodynamics. But today's biology has brought us to a changed viewpoint. Organized complexity is now a central concept, and, correspondingly, contemporary developmental biology is considered a biology of increasingly organized complexity. In other words, *negentropy*, or increasing organization, characterizes developmental systems. Although it is rare for negentropy to be discussed directly, a number of models for psychoanalytic theorizing have changed in accordance with this viewpoint, particularly when a developmental orientation is adopted (see, e.g., Bowlby 1969, 1988b; Emde 1980; Lichtenberg 1989; Peterfreund 1971).

Freud, although he kept to his entropic model, gave us a background that we can see today in historical retrospect as in some ways developmentally oriented. An early version of increasingly organized complexity in development can be seen in his description of successive psychosexual stages and their transformations in puberty (Freud 1905/1953), as well as in his concerns with increasing structures of meaning (for a review, see Emde 1992). Subsequent psychoanalytic authors also provided a background for the developmental orientation before its articulation in the 1970s. Hartmann's (1939/1958) theory about increasing differentiation and structuralization of the ego can be seen as a theory of increasing organization and complexity in development. Similarly, Spitz (1959), following Hartmann, made use of concepts of successive differentiation in development and theorized about the sequential appearance of organizers of the ego in new fields of integration. Erikson (1950) formulated, along quite similar lines, his ideas of epigenesis throughout the life span, with changing and more complex levels of organization between self and society at each level.

The history of psychoanalytic thinking about affect provides an important background for the developmental orientation in that, before its articulation in 1972, clinicians increasingly saw affects not merely as maladaptive, disorganized, and discharge phenomena but instead as adaptive, organized, and anticipatory. Beginning with what might be called Freud's clinically based later views, affects began to be seen as composite states that include direct feelings of pleasure and unpleasure that are evaluative and include cognitions, and that function in an adaptive way both unconsciously and consciously (see Freud 1923/1961; 1926/1959; 1930/1957; 1933[1932]/1964; see also Brenner 1974; Engel 1962; Jacobson 1953; Schur 1969). An important feature of this line of thinking is instantiated by Freud's formulation that affects are signals, seated in the ego. The signal formulation describes how affects have a regulatory and anticipatory role, one that functions automatically to mobilize a mental defense or an adaptive action. Signal anxiety in a small dose prevents one from becoming overwhelmed by states of helplessness that may arise because of linkages to earlier developmental conflicts and experiences. Others have since described a developmental sequence involving signal depression or "helplessness" in which small doses of these affects function to regulate self-esteem and to avoid overt depression (Anthony 1975; Bibring 1953; Brenner 1975; Engel 1962; Kaufman 1977). Similarly, Sandler (1960) proposed that a feeling of safety has a regulatory anticipatory role as a signal affect, and others (Engel 1962; Jacobson 1953) proposed that positive affects may have signal functions.

The view that affects have a continuous regulatory role in our lives and are not usually disruptive has gained increasing psychoanalytic acceptance since Freud's day. There are, of course, extreme states, but in everyday life affects regulate interest, engagement, boredom, frustration, and related states of involvement with the world on a pleasure-unpleasure continuum. This idea was contained in Jacobson's (1953, 1957) idea of moods as a "barometer of ego functioning" and was subsequently made more explicit by others (Blau 1955; Castelnuovo-Tedesco 1974; Novey 1961; Rangell 1967). Along this line, affects came to be seen as vital for human social relatedness and central to object relations (Landauer 1938; Novey 1961; Rangell 1967; Schafer 1964; Spitz 1959). Correspondingly, affects were described as important social communicators in early development (Basch 1976; Rapaport 1953; Schur 1969) and as essential communications in the psychoanalytic process (Greenacre 1971; Spitz 1956).

There are many additional streams of influence that contribute to today's developmental orientation and approach. Within psychoanalysis, the clinical experience of analysts working with children has made a strong contribution. Noteworthy are that of Anna Freud (1965/1974), pointing to developmental lines going forward, as well as to the analyst's active role in participating in the child's development, and that of Margaret Mahler and her colleagues, pointing to processes of separation-individuation that recur throughout life (Mahler et al. 1975). Other analysts working with adults made contributions conceptualizing the psychoanalytic process itself as a developmental one, presenting opportunities for an opening of experience to new relationships (Balint 1952; Gitelson 1962; Loewald 1960) and corrective adaptive experiences (Alexander and French 1946). Perhaps more than anyone else, Hans Loewald (1960, 1971) provided a background for today's developmental orientation. Loewald, in theorizing about what he referred to as "therapeutic action," brought developmental concepts of higher levels of integration into the process of psychoanalytic therapy itself, regarding it as a special developmental experience. In his words, "Analysis is thus understood as an intervention designed to set ego-development in motion…not simply by the technical skill of the analyst, but by the fact that the analyst makes himself available for the development of a new 'object-relationship'" (Loewald 1960, p. 17).

Therapeutic action deals with understanding the influences that move psychoanalytic therapy forward. Clearly, specific factors related to individual goals, adaptive strengths, and circumstances, as well as the particulars of individuality and disorder, are most important. What Loewald addressed, however, are more general factors, highlighting that psychoanalytic treatment itself is an interactive, developmental process. Such a view is consistent with the recognition that psychoanalysis, as a relationship form of treatment, has moved in many ways from a one-person to a two-person psychology (Thomä and Kächele 1987). The analytic process is more than the reconstruction and analysis of a patient's past; it involves an ongoing interaction between patient and analyst within a special relationship, one in which internalized relationship patterns are repeated in the context of the analytic relationship that develops over time. This view has also intensified an interest in the processes of early development when relationships are formed.

Early Development and Developmental Motives

Earlier, we discussed psychoanalytic interest in early relationship experiences. The developmental orientation emphasizes that an interest in these experiences is not the result of any close similarity with later experiences or concerns with regression, but rather the result of an interest in formative and fundamental processes that are forward-looking. Thus, early relationship experiences lead to affective representations of self in relation to others, and these in turn set expectations about security as well as about con-

flicts. Early experiences set adaptive pathways. A related reason for interest is that early development may bring into focus general vital processes that appear early and continue throughout life, and thus may be relevant for therapeutic action. Both Loewald (1960) and Gitelson (1962) noted the possibility that strong developmental forces could be activated in treatment, similar to those observed in the infantile dyadic condition.

More recently, I summarized an extensive body of multidisciplinary infancy research and was led to a formulation strongly supportive of this possibility (Emde 1988a, 1988b, 1990). The overall formulation is as follows. Evidence suggests that certain early-appearing motivational features of developmental process are biologically prepared (i.e., inborn) and persist throughout life. Developing in the necessary adaptive context of the infant-caregiver relationship, these motivational features can be regarded as basic motives of development. As such, they can be mobilized through empathy so as to enhance therapeutic action with adults as well as children. Examples of these features, which can be referred to as "basic motives," are presented below.

The first basic motive of development consists of *activity*. Activity is presumed by all developmental theories. More specifically, immediately after birth, preprogrammed sensorimotor systems become activated in the expectable evolutionary environment of caregiving, and, as Marshall Haith's (1980) work with the visual motor system shows us, developmental agendas are apparent in visual activity that leads to increasing organization and knowledge of the world. Since this form of basic motivation does not depend on learning or reinforcement, we can think of it as an inborn propensity to exercise early sensorimotor systems. Moreover, hereditary influences in this propensity are species-wide; there is little room for individual differences. Propensities for such activity are what have been called "strong developmental functions" (cf. McCall 1979). The other basic motives illustrate the same principle.

A second basic motive concerns *self-regulation*. Modern biology has taught us that self-regulation of physiology is basic to all living systems. It is built into cardiorespiratory and metabolic systems and sustains life. But beyond this, there is self-regulation for behavioral systems—in the short-term sense, for arousal, attentiveness, and sleep-wake cycles, and in the long-term sense, for growth and vital developmental functions. The developing individual maintains an integrity during major hazards and environmental perturbations. Development is goal oriented, and there are multiple ways of reaching species-important developmental goals, a feature that von Bertalanffy (1968) referred to as "equifinality." This idea is illustrated by children who are congenitally blind (Fraiberg 1977), congenitally deaf (Freedman 1972), or born without limbs (Decarie 1969), all of whom go through infancy with different sensorimotor experiences but nonetheless typically develop object permanence, representational intelligence, and self-awareness in early childhood. Related to this idea are self-righting tendencies. For important functions, there is a strong tendency to get back on the developmental pathway after deficit or challenge (Sameroff and Chandler 1976; Waddington 1962). Well-documented observations of developmental resilience (e.g., severe infant retardation due to deprivation which is later corrected by environmental change) illustrate this kind of self-regulation (for examples, see Clarke and Clarke 1976).

A third basic motive of development concerns *social fittedness*. Developmental research has indicated the extent to which the human infant comes into the world preadapted with organized capacities for initiating, maintaining, and terminating interactions with other humans. At birth these capacities include a propensity for participating in eye-to-eye contact; a state responsivity for being activated and soothed by human holding, touching, and rocking; and a propensity for showing prolonged alert attentiveness to the stimulus features contained in the human voice and face (for reviews, see Campos et al. 1983; Emde and Robinson 1979; Papousek and Papousek 1982; Stern 1985). The integrative capacities of the young infant (for processing sequential information, for cross-modal perception, for an early form of social imitation and for orienting—to mention only some of these) also indicate preadaptations for the dynamic circumstances of human interaction (Meltzoff 1985; Papousek and Papousek 1981; Stern 1985). Bowlby (1969) indicated that the propensity for attachment is a biologically based motivational system, in many ways as important as feeding and sexuality. The term *social fittedness* is used here to emphasize the dyadic nature of this regulatory motivational process. Social fittedness is remarkable also from the parent side. A variety of parenting behaviors with young infants are done automatically, appear to be species-wide, are not conscious, and do not seem the product of individual experience. They have therefore been referred to as "intuitive parenting behaviors" (Papousek and Papousek 1979). Examples include parental behaviors supporting visual contact, such as positioning the infant so that eye-to-eye distance maximizes the newborn's ability to see the face, exaggerated greeting responses, parental imitation of the newborn's facial and vocal expressions, and "baby talk" (see also Snow 1972). Finally, research on behavioral synchrony also illustrates social fittedness in the biological predisposition of parent and infant to mesh their behaviors in timed mutual interchanges observed during social interaction (Als et al. 1979; Brazelton et al. 1979; Condon and Sander 1974; Haith 1977; Meltzoff 1985; Sander 1975).

A fourth basic motive concerns *affective monitoring*, a propensity to monitor experience according to what is pleasurable and unpleasurable. In other words, there is a preadapted organized basis in the central nervous system for guiding the direction of experience in early infancy. From the parent's point of view, infant affective expressions are predominant in guiding caregiving. Mother, for example, hears a cry and acts to relieve the cause of distress; she sees a smile and hears cooing and cannot resist maintaining a playful interaction. Research documents, from the infant's point of view, an increasing use of affective monitoring for guiding one's own behavior whether a mother intevenes or not (for reviews of the infant's developing emotions, see Campos et al. 1983; Emde 1988b, 1999).

A fifth basic motive of development builds on the first motive of activity to specify what can be designated as *cognitive assimilation*. Cognitive assimilation, which Piaget considered to be the "basic fact of life," refers to the biological propensity to process new information and to structuralize such information according to what is familiar. In other words, it refers to a fundamental forward-looking propensity to seek out the novel in order to make it familiar. Other researchers have considered cognitive assimilation to be the early and continuing tendency to reduce cognitive discrepancy (Kagan et al. 1978; McCall 1972), whereby the individual is motivated to act so as to resolve a perceived difference from what is expected. In either consideration there is a movement to expand knowledge with an increasingly organized view of the world.

(As with all other psychological domains, cognitive assimilation operates according to principles of regulation. Affects are central mediators in this regulatory activity. If the environmental event is mildly or moderately discrepant from what is known, it is experienced as interesting; if the event is extremely discrepant, it is experienced as frightening. Something familiar, appearing in an unexpected context (providing it is not too abrupt), is experienced as surprising and may even become joyful. Restriction of or restraint on one's plans to resolve a discrepancy can lead to frustration and anger. Finally, pleasure and mastery, in their various forms, can occur when a plan is carried out and a discrepancy is resolved [Morgan and Harmon 1984].)

Overall, these developmental motives, so salient in infancy, are presumed to operate as general background influences in analytic work, as silent aspects of the developmental process. They can be considered fundamental modes of development, part aspects of developmental regulation in general and in their operation interwoven and inseparable. It is further presumed that these motivational influences can be mobilized over time through the empathic and interpretive availability of the analyst. It is to the processes of empathy and interpretation that we turn next, as well as to the shared aspects of therapeutic action.

Therapeutic Availability

Psychoanalysis is a form of treatment that relies on availability of the analyst over time. In this section (modified from Emde 1990), I discuss the contributions of the developmental orientation to thinking about this availability in terms of the processes of therapeutic action involving affect regulation, empathy, interpretation, and shared meaning. In doing this, a caveat seems in order. At times the developmental orientation makes use of analogs between the processes of forming early relationships and the processes of beginning a new special relationship in analytic work. Although early relationship experiences may contribute to adaptive and maladaptive prototypes that recur throughout life and may need to be understood in their dynamic particulars, no straightforward equating of early experiences to the analytic experience is intended, nor are allusions to early experience intended to imply regression. Rather, these analogs, because they reflect aspects of development, are meant to inform thinking about the general processes of empathy, interpretation, and what is shared in the developing analytic relationship.

Analysts agree that the availability of the professional helper is what sets the stage for therapeutic action. Availability is what fosters trust, confidence, and a consistency of expectations; it is therefore a presupposition for the therapeutic alliance. Developmental analogs in infancy and in caregiving have been described, both in terms of the patient's experience—as "basic trust" (Erikson 1950), and "confidence" (Benedek 1970)—and in terms of the analyst's experience—as a "diatrophic attitude" (Gitelson 1962; Spitz 1956). It is noteworthy that availability, both in the early caregiving situation and in the analytic/therapeutic situation, becomes manifest through regulation. Regulation ensures balance, the avoidance of extremes, and the maintenance of individual integrity during the flow of life. From a developmental view, regulation functions to ensure optimal exploration against a background of safety. This view is consistent with that advanced by psychoanalytic and developmental theorists (Sameroff 1983; Sameroff and Emde 1989; Sander 1985; Sandler 1960; Sandler and Sandler 1978). The view is also consistent with the advice of textbook writers concerning analytic technique: the analyst needs to maintain a balance between affective experiencing and interpretive activity (see Fenichel 1941; Thomä and Kächele 1987). Correspondingly, in the following subsections, I discuss the developmental aspects of two main avenues of therapeutic availability: affect regulation and interpretation.

Affect Regulation and Empathy

The developmental orientation indicates that the analyst participates in a special developmental experience in the therapeutic action of analysis. How? It has been said that no therapy works unless you become part of the problem, and that psychoanalysis does not work unless you become most of the problem. In addition to the obvious reference to the centrality of intense transference experiences, the saying has reference—on the analyst's side—to such aspects as "role responsiveness," as discussed by Sandler (1976), and immersions in projective identifications and productive countertransferences, as discussed by Ogden (1979) and Fleming and Benedek (1966). Still, all of these developments occur in a contained—or regulated—sense. A special context allows for this kind of experience. The context is one in which there is a shared zone of understanding for both patient and analyst. In addition to a shared sense of openness about what can be expressed, there is a shared sense of safety and restraint about what will not happen.

In the therapeutic process, the analyst attends to current affective states and inferred signal affects. Additionally, the analyst uses his or her own signal affect processes in response to the patient and allows a resonance with what the patient is attempting to communicate. This reminds us of two other developmental analogs of affect regulation. The most obvious one, *affective mirroring*, is a confirmatory experience both in therapeutic action and in early caregiving that has been so well articulated by Kohut (1971, 1977). Another is what might be referred to as the *provision of affective "scaffolding"* by the therapist. As Kohut (1977) and Stolorow and colleagues (1987) pointed out, mother's soothing and comforting of negative affects provides a basis for the child's tolerance and for "dosing" of affects (cf. the "holding environment" of Winnicott [1960]). The patient, like the young child, learns from the therapeutic experience about how to "dose" particular affects in certain circumstances. One might carry this a step further and say, following the developmentalist Vygotsky (1978; see also Wertsch 1985), that this illustrates a process whereby one learns from another by means of "scaffolding" and pulling forward in development—in this case by the therapist (in analogy to mother) demonstrating and making possible the use of affects as internal signals.

Clinicians have come to recognize that empathy occupies an important role in psychoanalytic work alongside that of interpretation (see Beres and Arlow 1974; Freedman 1972; Kohut 1959; Schafer 1959; Shapiro 1981; Stolorow et. al. 1987). Partly because of such recognition, Kohut's formulation of what can be regarded as a "corrective empathic experience"—namely, that empathic failures of primary caregivers during earliest childhood are causes of psychopathology that require later corrective empathic experiences during analysis—has received considerable clinical attention (see Chapter 4).

What might be referred to as an empathic attitude of the analyst contains a number of dispositions. These include maintaining an ongoing attitude of encouraging exploration in the midst of negative affects and what is painful, as well as encouraging the discovery of the unexpected and the capacity for surprise (Reik 1936; Schafer 1959). There is an atmosphere of interest in errors and misperceptions. Major errors are, of course, introduced by transference distortions. But transference has its positive affirmative aspects in addition to its self-defeating aspects (Kohut 1977; Loewald 1980). Rothenberg (1987) has pointed to the positive value of creativity in the therapeutic process in which it is seen as a higher-order aspect of adult functioning. According to this view, the analyst envisions alternatives and can make use of metaphor, paradox, and, occasionally, humor, often with a sense of irony.

Most would agree that a goal of intensive psychotherapy and analysis is to obtain freedom from repeating the painful self-defeating patterns of the past. But there is also another important goal. This involves an affirmation of connections between past and current experience. While we seek to establish a sense of discontinuity (putting the past in its place), we also seek to establish a sense of continuity (gaining a sense of ownership and connectedness with one's past, including both its positive aspects and the struggles that one has overcome). We might refer to this feature of the therapeutic process as *affirmative empathy*. With successful treatment, the patient gains an affirmative sense of life continuity—both in terms of self and other representations. As stated by Beres and Arlow (1974), a goal of psychoanalytic work is to enable the patient to develop an empathy for his self of the past, to see himself on a continuum from his early life to his current life, along with an acceptance of formerly repudiated aspects of himself. As Erikson (1950) put it, the goal is one of helping the patient to make his own biography. This has to do with affirming individuality and basic values rooted in biology, family, and culture. Kohut (1971) placed an affirmative empathic attitude at the center of the therapeutic process in his self psychology.

Interpretation and Shared Aspects of Therapeutic Action

Therapeutic action also relies on the analyst's availability over time in terms of increasing understanding and interpretive activity. Indeed, interpretation of defense and of internal conflict in the context of transference is regarded as a sine qua non for analytic work. This chapter has given less attention to interpretation, since, in contrast to empathy, it has occupied center stage in analytic considerations (see Thomä and Kächele 1987; see also Chapter 15, "Process, Resistance, and Interpretation"). The developmental orientation endorses the analytic tradition that interpretations need to be appropriate to the level and context of the development of the individual to whom they are applied. Accordingly, empathy, although based on the analyst's emotional sensitivity and responsiveness, involves more than emotion. Empathy involves, as Kohut (1959) put it, "vicarious introspection." It depends on cognition, on perspective taking, and on knowledge about the other person and the situation. The knowledge required for empathy in therapeutic work can be thought of as a set of schemas or as a "working model" of the patient (including past, current, and transference aspects) that undergoes continual updating over the course of treatment (Basch 1983; Greenson 1960).

A theme of this chapter is that the developmental orientation is forward-looking as it points to making use of the past in the reflected-upon experience of the present within the analytic process. From this perspective, the analyst's availability includes an appreciation not only of complex affects but of complex intentions and of a wider cognitive range that contributes to the patient's feeling of "being understood." And such availability does more: it anticipates movement and encourages exploration. Rene Spitz used to say that a good psychoanalytic interpretation guides the patient to his or her next step. It helps the patient make new connections among affects, memories, and actions; it helps the patient move to new possibilities.

Some aspects of interpretation can be thought of as similar to a forward-looking process of what a parent or teacher does in child development. We are reminded again of what has been referred to as "scaffolding" (Vygotsky 1978); this amounts to an interpretive "pull" toward a higher level of understanding with both differentiation and integration (Loewald 1960). In Loewald's view, this reflects a positive aspect of the "neutrality" of the analyst that includes

> the capacity for mature object-relations, as manifested in the parent by his or her ability to follow and, at the same time, be ahead of the child's development....In analysis, a mature object relationship is maintained with a given patient if the analyst relates to the patient in tune with the shifting levels of development manifested by the patient at different times, but always from the viewpoint of potential growth, that is, from the viewpoint of the future. (Loewald 1960, p. 20)

The middle phase of analysis is when there is a deepening of transference experiences and their resistances, as well as some interpretive understanding of these experiences. In the course of concentrated work, there is an expanding sense of meaning. The analyst is available to the patient for a continuing experience in which there is an increasing respect for individuality, defensive struggling, and the quest for truth. Both participants engage in a contrasting of "now" versus "then" experiences in the light of varying transference manifestations. Exploration is valued in the face of conflict.

The sense of mutuality has now progressed within the patient-analyst relationship experience to the point that there is more of a sense of "we" that is affective as well as cognitive. Moments of intense feelings of togetherness and of shared meaning are extremely important for psychoanalytic work. Such moments often precede and surround productive work within interpretive activity, and they contribute to the regulation of previously warded-off affects. It is also the case that such moments occur at different levels of organization (and co-organization). In addition to the analyst's emotional availability providing a "background of safety" for overall analytic work (Sandler 1960), the analyst serves as a "beacon of orientation" (Mahler et. al. 1975), providing reassurance for new directions and more specific work. More reflective exploration can go on in the midst of uncertainty and painful emotions.

Moreover, from the vantage point of the basic motivational features of development reviewed earlier (see section "Early Development and Developmental Motives" earlier in this chapter), something further can be suggested in this process. Normative, biologically prepared developmental processes may become actualized that are fostered by the interactive, emotional availability of the analyst. This may lead to a resurgence of activity and cognitive exploration in which affects are more regulated, and to reflections about self and others in which new possibilities for adaptation are envisioned, discussed, and tried.

Two examples can illustrate the points about the analyst's availability and mutuality discussed above. The first example concerns a man in his 30s who had experienced a prolonged period of parental unavailability in early childhood. During the analysis, he repeatedly found himself yearning for a responsive presence—at times with memories of mother's unavailability and at times with memories of father's unavailability. After 3 years of analysis, he talked in one session about his experience during a recent vacation. He had felt lonely and anguished and found himself having imaginary dialogues with the analyst, and these gave him comfort. Patient and analyst then began to reflect on the progress that had occurred in the analysis; poi-

gnantly, the word "we" was used by each to describe shared understandings of both struggles and gains.

A second example is one that comes from the research study of a recorded analysis using the case of Mrs. C (Mayes and Spence 1994; Spence et al. 1994). This study illustrates a point made earlier that internalized relationship patterns are repeated in the context of the analytic relationship that develops over time. The researchers found that the analyst's interventions were correlated with a pattern of pronoun usage occurring in the patient's speech, a correlation that increased over the course of the analysis and was especially prominent in the final phases of treatment. From a detailed study of these patterns, the researchers concluded that the patterns indicated an increasing sensitivity of the analyst to a repeated special mode of interactive experience. They also speculated that this interactive experience may have reactivated a special form of developmental experience, one that was positive and shared, whose prototype was the contingent responsiveness experienced in the mother-infant relationship.

A sense of "we" that develops in analysis, in analogy to the early caregiving experience, organizes (by interpretation) what was previously less organized, as we discussed in the previous section. And in this the analyst, as Loewald (1960) stated, "functions as a representative of a higher stage of organization and mediates this to the patient" (p. 24). There is a gradient of knowledge and expertise in the analytic relationship just as there is in early caregiving relationships. Thus, cycles of increased organization and shared meaning occur with interpretive activity. But it should be emphasized that analytic work is not easy. Progress is not linear. Disorganization and reorganization are recurring processes within the analytic experience.

A few words about the termination process. In terminating, there is a necessary reworking not only of conflicts about leaving but also of what has been experienced throughout treatment. The patient needs to put in place the shared meaning of what has occurred. Correspondingly, the analyst needs to acknowledge the validity of the patient's increasing autonomy. We are reminded again of a basic feature of the development process: in early caregiving, secure attachment generates exploration (Bowlby 1969); in like manner, the capacity for intimacy and the capacity for autonomy develop alongside each other—they do not compete. The patient mentioned in the example above began increasingly to talk about his increased energy and interests outside of analysis that included new satisfying experiences in family relationships and at his job. He had come a long way in his analytic work and in his life. He was ready to move on.

Moving Beyond

The past is not forgotten. It was an early discovery of psychoanalysis that the conflicted past is remembered not only consciously but also nonconsciously by way of patterns of behavior and symptoms. The developmental orientation emphasizes that "the use of the past" can occur as a product of analytic work. As one understands more about past conflicts and struggles, and as one gains empathy for one's self in the past as contrasted with the present, one can appreciate the value of others and self in an ongoing representational world. One can then make a useful biography (as Erikson put it) and have useful ancestors instead of ghosts (as Fraiberg and colleagues put it). It is not enough, however, to reflect on and understand one's conflicted and painful past; nor is it enough to make a biography with a background of ancestors. New possibilities for living in the present must be envisioned and tried out.

Perhaps in the early days of psychoanalysis, when behavior was seen through a deterministic lens, the past was viewed more simply. Now we are in a different world, with science recognizing uncertainty and with influences on behavior seen as probabilistic. The developmental sciences have shown us that genetic influences are strong, but such influences typically depend on environmental interactions across the course of development and operate according to what developmental biologists refer to as "probabilistic epigenesis" (Gottlieb 1992). Thus, seeking alternatives and new possibilities seems more important in today's world.

As I have reviewed, the developmental orientation adds a forward-looking perspective for understanding the psychoanalytic treatment process. The psychoanalytic patient comes to treatment not only to regulate affect with more anticipatory signaling adaptive functions in the midst of conflict, and to be aware of new adaptive possibilities to old repetitive conflicts, but also to try out new alternative modes of being and interacting. In the later phases of analytic work, much of this trying out occurs within the newly experienced relationship with the analyst, and much of it, increasingly, also occurs in relationships outside the analytic treatment situation. In other words, in the course of the analytic developmental experience, the patient begins to put into action and practice the new possibilities that are realized and to find suitable replacements in life for old, repeated maladaptive patterns.

As mentioned earlier, the developmental orientation makes use of knowledge gained from other disciplines in the developmental sciences. Developmental psychology has recently become aware that future-oriented mental systems, such as anticipatory processes, expectations, and plans, although understudied, are essential for life and develop-ment; hence, they are now the subject of active investigation (Haith et al. 1994). Similarly, the developmental orientation of psychoanalysis indicates that forward-looking processes are essential for successful treatment. Hence, one hopes they will be the subject of increasing attention. More than envisioning alternatives to old maladaptive patterns, however, analytic patients need to practice new possibilities.

Contributions from other disciplines are also instructive and point to the importance of practicing. Both learning theory (Wachtel 1977) and the newer discipline of connectionism (Huether et al. 1999) emphasize the finding that extinction is an active process involving the acquisition of new responses, skills, or connections; it is not a passive one of decay. Thus, old painful memories, difficulties, expectations, and connections are not simply forgotten in successful clinical work; they are replaced. An implication for psychoanalysis is that new satisfying experiences need to be put into play in order to inhibit old maladaptive behavior patterns. It is not enough to understand or make connections with reasons for symptoms or reasons for self-defeating behavioral patterns. The developmental orientation indicates that new beginnings require not only cognitive explorations but also the practicing of new alternatives.

Much of this line of thought is new territory for psychoanalysis and will be seen as controversial and even unsettling by some who are less used to this approach. What the developmental orientation indicates is that psychoanalysis needs more useful theory and research related to practicing in the midst of new beginnings. It indicates that we need more knowledge about how to facilitate practicing experiences within analytic settings without being intrusive or directive and as patients become more autonomous and prepare to move beyond. Freud was concerned at the end of his life with issues of what could be accomplished, using the phrase "analysis terminable and interminable" (Freud 1937/1964). The developmental orientation rephrases issues for the ending of analysis as "development terminable and interminable."

References

Abrams S: The psychoanalytic process: the developmental and the integrative. Psychoanalytic Q 59:650–677, 1990

Alexander F, French TM: The Principle of Flexibility in Psychoanalytic Therapy: Principles and Application. New York, Ronald Press, 1946

Als H, Tronick E, Brazelton TB: Analysis of face-to-face interaction in infant-adult dads, in The Study of Social Interaction. Edited by Lamb M, Suomi S, Stephenson GR. Madison, WI, University of Wisconsin Press, 1979, pp 33–76

Anthony EJ: Childhood depression, in Depression and Human Existence. Edited by Anthony EJ, Benedek T. Boston, MA, Little, Brown, 1975, pp 231–277

Balint M: New beginning and the paranoid and the depressive syndromes. Int J Psychoanal 33:214–224, 1952

Basch MF: The concept of affect: a reexamination. J Am Psychoanal Assoc 24:759–777, 1976

Basch MF: Empathic understanding: a review of the concept and some theoretical considerations. J Am Psychoanal Assoc 31:101–126, 1983

Benedek T: Parenthood during the life cycle, in Parenthood: Its Psychology and Psychopathology. Edited by Anthony EJ, Benedek T. Boston, MA, Little, Brown, 1970, pp 185–206

Beres D, Arlow JA: Fantasy and identification in empathy. Psychoanal Q 43:26–50, 1974

Bibring E: The mechanism of depression, in Affective Disorders. Edited by Greenacre P. New York, International Universities Press, 1953, pp 13–48

Bion WR: Learning From Experience. New York, Basic Books, 1962

Blau A: A unitary hypothesis of emotion, I: anxiety, emotions of displeasure, and affective disorders. Psychoanal Q 24:75–103, 1955

Bowlby J: Attachment and Loss, Vol 1: Attachment. New York, Basic Books, 1969

Bowlby J: A Secure Base: Parent-Child Attachment and Healthy Human Development. New York, Basic Books, 1988a

Bowlby J: Developmental psychiatry comes of age. Am J Psychiatry 145:1–10, 1988b

Brazelton TB, Als H, Tronick E, et al: Specific neonatal measures: the Brazelton neonatal behavioral assessment scale, in Handbook of Infant Development. Edited by Osofsky J. New York, Wiley, 1979, pp 185–215

Brenner C: On the nature and development of affects: a unified theory. Psychoanal Q 43:532–556, 1974

Brenner C: Affects and psychic conflict. Psychoanal Q 44, 5–28, 1975

Bucci W: Psychoanalysis and Cognitive Science: A Multiple Code Theory. New York, Guilford, 1997

Campos JJ, Barrett KC, Lamb ME, et al: Socioemotional development, in Handbook of Child Psychology, Vol 2. Edited by Mussen PH (Haith MM, Campos J, vol eds). New York, Wiley, 1983, pp 783–915

Castelnuovo-Tedesco P: Toward a theory of affects. J Am Psychoanal Assoc 22:612–625, 1974

Clarke AM, Clarke ADB: Early Experience: Myth and Evidence. London, Open Books, 1976

Colarusso CA, Nemiroff RA: Adult Development: A New Dimension in Psychodynamic Theory and Practice. New York, Plenum, 1981

Condon WS, Sander LW: Neonate movement is synchronized with adult speech: interactional participation and language acquisition. Science 183:99–101, 1974

Decarie TG: A study of the mental and emotional development of the thalidomide child, in Determinants of Infant Behavior, Vol 4. Edited by Foss B. London, Methuen, 1969, pp 167–187

Dewald PA: Adult phases of the life cycle, in The Course of Life: Psychoanalytic Contributions Toward Understanding Personality Development, Vol 3: Adulthood. Edited by Greenspan SI, Pollock GH. Bethesda, MD, National Institute of Mental Health, 1980, pp 35–53

Emde RN: A developmental orientation in psychoanalysis: ways of thinking about new knowledge and further research. Psychoanalysis and Contemporary Thought 3:213–235, 1980

Emde RN: Development terminable and interminable, I: innate and motivational factors from infancy. Int J Psychoanal 69:23–42, 1988a

Emde RN: Development terminable and interminable, II: recent psychoanalytic theory and therapeutic considerations. Int J Psychoanal 69:283–296, 1988b

Emde RN: Mobilizing fundamental modes of development: an essay on empathic availability and therapeutic action. J Am Psychoanal Assoc 38:881–913, 1990

Emde RN: Individual meaning and increasing complexity: contributions of Sigmund Freud and Rene Spitz to developmental psychology. Dev Psychol 28:347–359, 1992

Emde RN: Moving ahead: integrating influences of affective processes for development and for psychoanalysis. Int J Psychoanal 80:317–339, 1999

Emde RN, Robinson J: The first two months: recent research in developmental psychobiology and the changing view of the newborn, in Basic Handbook of Child Psychiatry, Vol 1. Edited by Call J, Noshpitz J, Cohen R, et al. New York, Basic Books, 1979, pp 72–105

Engel G: Anxiety and depression-with-drawal: the primary affects of unpleasure. Int J Psychoanal 43:89–97, 1962

Erikson E: Childhood and Society. New York, WW Norton, 1950

Erikson E: Identity and the Life Cycle: Selected Papers. New York, International Universities Press, 1959

Fairbairn WRD: Synopsis of an object relations theory of the personality. Int J Psychoanal 44:224–225, 1963

Fenichel O: Problems of Psychoanalytic Technique. New York, The Psychoanalytic Quarterly, 1941

Fleming J, Benedek T: Psychoanalytic Supervision. New York, Grune & Stratton, 1966

Fonagy P, Target M: Mentalization and the Changing Aims of Child Psychoanalysis. Psychoanalytic Dialogues 8:87–114, 1998

Fonagy P, Steele M, Steele H: Maternal representations of attachment during pregnancy predict the organization of infant-mother attachment at one year of age. Child Development 62:880–893, 1991

Fonagy P, Gergely G, Jurist E, et al: Affect Regulation, Mentalization, and the Development of the Self. New York, Other Press, 2002

Fraiberg S, Adelson E, Shapiro V: Ghosts in the nursery: a psychoanalytic approach to the problems of impaired infant-mother relationships. J Am Acad Child Psychiatry 14:387–421, 1975

Fraiberg S: Insights From the Blind. New York, Basic Books, 1977

Freedman D: On hearing, oral language, and psychic structure, in Psychoanalysis and Contemporary Science, Vol 1. Edited by Holt R, Peterfreund E. New York, Macmillan, 1972, pp 57–69

Freud A: Normality and pathology in childhood (1965), in The Writings of Anna Freud, Vol 6. New York, International Universities Press, 1974, pp 25–63

Freud S: Three essays on the theory of sexuality, I: the sexual aberrations (1905), in Standard Edition of the Complete Psychological Works of Sigmund Freud, Vol 7. Translated and edited by Strachey J. London, Hogarth Press, 1953, pp 135–172

Freud S: The ego and the id (1923), in Standard Edition of the Complete Psychological Works of Sigmund Freud, Vol 19. Translated and edited by Strachey J. London, Hogarth Press, 1961, pp 12–66

Freud S: Inhibitions, symptoms and anxiety (1926), in Standard Edition of the Complete Psychological Works of Sigmund Freud, Vol 20. Translated and edited by Strachey J. London, Hogarth Press, 1959, pp 75–175

Freud S: Civilization and its discontents (1930), in Standard Edition of the Complete Psychological Works of Sigmund Freud, Vol 21. Translated and edited by Strachey J. London, Hogarth Press, 1957, pp 57–145

Freud S: New introductory lectures on psycho-analysis (1933[1932]) (Lectures XXIX–XXXV), in Standard Edition of the Complete Psychological Works of Sigmund Freud, Vol 22. Translated and edited by Strachey J. London, Hogarth Press, 1964, pp 1–182

Freud S: Analysis terminable and interminable (1937), in Standard Edition of the Complete Psychological Works of Sigmund Freud, Vol 23. Translated and edited by Strachey J. London, Hogarth Press, 1964, pp 209–253

Gitelson M: The curative factors in psychoanalysis: the first phase of psychoanalysis. Int J Psychoanal 43:194–204, 1962

Goodman S: Child analysis, in Psychoanalytic Education and Research. Edited by Goodman S. New York, International Universities Press, 1977, pp 1–407

Gottlieb G: Individual Development and Evolution. New York, Oxford University Press, 1992

Greenacre P: Emotional Growth. New York, International Universities Press, 1971

Greenson RR: Empathy and its vicissitudes. Int J Psychoanal 41:418–424, 1960

Grossmann K: Maternal attachment representations as related to child-mother attachment patterns and maternal sensitivity and acceptance of her infant, in Relations Between Relationship Within Families. Edited by Hinde RA, Stevenson-Hinde J. Oxford, England, Oxford University Press, 1987, pp 241–260

Guntrip H: Psychoanalytic Theory, Therapy, and the Self. New York, WW Norton, 1971

Haith MM: Eye contact and face scanning in early infancy. Science 198:853–855, 1977

Haith MM: Rules That Babies Look By. Hillsdale, NJ, Lawrence Erlbaum, 1980

Haith MM, Benson JB, Roberts RJ, et al: The Development of Future-Oriented Processes. Chicago, IL, University of Chicago Press, 1994

Hartmann H: Psychoanalysis and the Problem of Adaptation (1939). New York, International Universities Press, 1958

Horowitz MJ: Emotionality and schematic control processes, in Person Schemas and Maladaptive Interpersonal Patterns. Edited by Horowitz MJ. Chicago, IL, University of Chicago Press, 1991, pp 413–423

Huether G, Doering S, Ulrich R, et al: The stress-reaction process and the adaptive modification and reorganization of neuronal networks. Psychiatry Res 87:83–95, 1999

Jacobson E: The affects and their pleasure-unpleasure qualities in relation to the psychic discharge processes, in Drives, Affects, Behavior. Edited by Lowenstein R. New York, International Universities Press, 1953, pp 38–66

Jacobson E: Normal and pathological moods: their nature and functions. Psychoanal Study Child 12:73–126, 1957

Kagan J, Kearsley R, Zelaso P: Infancy: its place in human development. Cambridge, MA, Harvard University Press, 1978

Kaufman IC: Developmental considerations of anxiety and depression: psychobiological studies in monkeys. Psychoanalysis and Contemporary Science 4:317–363, 1977

Kernberg OF: Object Relations Theory and Clinical Psychoanalysis. New York, Jason Aronson, 1976

Kernberg, OF: New perspectives in psychoanalytic theory, in Emotion: Theory, Research, and Experience. Edited by Pluchik R, Kellerman H. New York, Academic Press, 1990, pp 115–131

Klein GS: Peremptory ideation: structure and force in motivated ideas, in Motives and Thought: Psychoanalytic Essays in Honor of David Rapaport. Edited by Holt RR. New York, International Universities Press, 1967, pp 80–182

Kohut H: Introspection, empathy, and psychoanalysis: an examination of the relationship between mode of observation and theory. J Am Psychoanal Assoc 7:459–483, 1959

Kohut H: The Analysis of the Self: A Systematic Approach to the Psychoanalytic Treatment of Narcissistic Personality Disorders. New York, International Universities Press, 1971

Kohut H: The Restoration of the Self. New York, International Universities Press, 1977

Landauer K: Affects, passions, and temperament. Int J Psychoanal 19:388–415, 1938

Lichtenberg JD: Psychoanalysis and Motivation. Hillsdale, NJ, Analytic Press, 1989

Loewald HW: On the therapeutic action of psychoanalysis. Int J Psychoanal 41:16–33, 1960

Loewald HW: On motivation and instinct theory. Psychoanal Study Child 26:91–128, 1971

Loewald HW: Reflections on the psychoanalytic process and its therapeutic potential, in Papers on Psychoanalysis. New Haven, CT, Yale University Press, 1980, pp 372–383

Luborsky L: Measuring a pervasive psychic structure in psychotherapy: the core conflictual relationship theme, in Communicative Structures and Psychic Structures. Edited by Freedman N, Grand S. New York, Plenum, 1977, pp 367–395

Mahler MS, Pine F, Bergman A: The Psychological Birth of the Human Infant: Symbiosis and Individuation. New York, Basic Books, 1975

Mayes L: Understanding adaptive processes in a developmental context. Psychoanal Study Child 49:12–35, 1994

Mayes LC, Spence DP: Understanding therapeutic action in the analytic situation: a second look at the developmental metaphor. J Am Psychoanal Assoc 42:789–817, 1994

McCall RB: Smiling and vocalization in infants as indices of perceptual-cognitive processes. Merrill-Palmer Q 18:341–348, 1972

McCall RB: The development of intellectual functioning in infancy and the prediction of later IQ, in Handbook of Infant Development. Edited by Osofsky J. New York, Wiley, 1979, pp 707–741

Meltzoff AN: The roots of social and cognitive development: models of man's original nature, in Social Perception in Infants. Edited by Field TM, Fox NA. Norwood, NJ, Ablex, 1985, pp 1–30

Morgan GA, Harmon RJ: Developmental transformations and mastery motivation: measurement and validation, in Continuities and Discontinuities in Development. Edited by Emde RN, Harmon RJ. New York, Plenum, 1984, pp 263–291

Neugarten B: Time, age, and the life cycle. Am J Psychiatry 136:887–894, 1979

Novey S: Further considerations on affect theory in psychoanalysis. Int J Psychoanal 42:21–31, 1961

Ogden TH: On projective identification. Int J Psychoanal 60:357–373, 1979

Papousek H, Papousek M: Early ontogeny of human social interaction: its biological roots and social dimensions, in Human Ethology: Claims and Limits of a New Discipline. Edited by Foppa K, Lepenies W, Ploog D. New York, Cambridge University Press, 1979, pp 456–489

Papousek H, Papousek M: Integration into the social world, in Psychobiology of the Human Newborn. Edited by Stratton PM. New York, Wiley, 1982, pp 367–390

Peterfreund E: Information, Systems, and Psychoanalysis: An Evolutionary Biological Approach to Psychoanalytic Theory. Psychological Issues Monograph No 25/26. New York, International Universities Press, 1971

Pollock GH: Aging and aged: development on pathology, in The Course of Life: Psychoanalytic Contributions Toward Understanding Personality Development, Vol 3: Adulthood. Edited by Greenspan SI, Pollock GH. Bethesda, MD, National Institute of Mental Health, 1980, pp 549–585

Rado S: Recent advances in psychoanalytic therapy, in Psychoanalysis of Behavior: Collected Papers, Vol 1. New York, Grune & Stratton, 1953, pp 251–267

Rangell L: Psychoanalysis, affects, and the human core: on the relationship of psychoanalysis to the behavioral sciences. Psychoanal Q 36:172–202, 1967

Rapaport D: On the psychoanalytic theory of affect. Int J Psychoanal 34:177–198, 1953

Rapaport D: The Structure of Psychoanalytic Theory: A Systematizing Attempt. Psychological Issues Monograph No 6. New York, International Universities Press, 1959

Reik T: Surprise and the Psychoanalyst. London, Kegan Paul, 1936

Ricks MH: The social transition of parental behavior: attachment across generations, in Growing Points in Attachment Theory and Research: Monographs of the Society for Research in Child Development, Vol 50. Edited by Bretherton I, Waters E. Ann Arbor, MI, Society for Research in Child Development, 1985, pp 211–227

Rothenberg A: The Creative Process of Psychotherapy. New York, WW Norton, 1987

Sameroff AJ: Developmental systems: contexts and evolution, in Handbook of Child Psychology, Vol 1. Edited by Mussen PH. New York, Wiley, 1983, pp 237–294

Sameroff AJ, Chandler MJ: Reproductive risk and the continuum of caretaking casualty, in Review of Child Development Research. Edited by Horowitz FD, Hertherington M, Scarr-Salapatek S, et al. Chicago, IL, University of Chicago Press, 1976, pp 187–244

Sameroff A, Emde EN: Relationship Disturbances in Early Childhood. New York, Basic Books, 1989

Sander L: Infant and caretaking environment: investigation and conceptualization of adaptive behavior in a series of increasing complexity, in Explorations in Child Psychiatry. Edited by Anthony EJ. New York, Plenum, 1975, pp 129–166

Sander LW: Toward a logic of organization in psychobiological development, in Biologic Response Styles: Clinical Implications. Edited by Klar K, Siever LJ. Washington, DC, Amererican Psychiatric Press, 1985, pp 20–36

Sandler J: The background of safety. Int Rev Psychoanal 41:352–365, 1960

Sandler J: Countertransference and role-responsiveness. Int J Psychoanal 3:43–47, 1976

Sandler J, Sandler A-M: On the development of object relationships and affects. Int J Psychoanal 59:285–296, 1978

Schafer R: Generative empathy in the treatment situation. Psychoanal Q 28:342–373, 1959

Schafer R: The clinical analysis of affects. J Am Psychoanal Assoc 12:275–299, 1964

Schur M: Affects and cognition. Int J Psychoanal 50:647–653, 1969

Settlage CF: Psychoanalytic developmental thinking in current and historical perspective. Psychoanalysis and Contemporary Thought 3:139–170, 1980

Settlage CF, Curtis J, Lozoff M, et al: Conceptualizing adult development. J Am Psychoanal Assoc 36:347–369, 1988

Shane M: A rationale for teaching analytic technique based on a developmental orientation and approach. Int J Psychoanal 58:95–108, 1977

Shapiro T: Empathy: a critical reevaluation. Psychoanalytic Inquiry 1:423–448, 1981

Shaver P, Hazan C: Compatibility and Incompatibility in Relationships. New York, Springer-Verlag, 1985

Spence DP, Mayes LC, Dahl H: Monitoring the analytic surface. J Am Psychoanal Assoc 42:43–64, 1994

Snow CE: Mother's speech to children learning language. Child Development 43:549–565, 1972

Spitz RA: Transference: the analytical setting. Int J Psychoanal 37:380–385, 1956

Spitz RA: A Genetic Field Theory of Ego Formation. New York, International Universities Press, 1959

Stern D: The Interpersonal World of the Infant: A View From Psychoanalysis and Developmental Psychology. New York, Basic Books, 1985

Stolorow RD, Brandchaft B, Atwood GE: Psychoanalytic Treatment: An Intersubjective Approach. Hillsdale, NJ Analytic Press, 1987

Thomä H, Kächele H: Psychoanalytic Practice. New York, Springer, 1987

Tyson P, Tyson R: Psychoanalytic Theories of Development: An Integration. New Haven, CT, Yale University Press, 1990

Vaillant GE: Adaptation to Life. Boston, MA, Little, Brown, 1977

von Bertalanffy L: General System Theory Foundations, Development, Applications. New York, Braziller, 1968

Vygotsky LS: Mind in Society: The Development of Higher Psychological Processes. Cambridge, MA, Harvard University Press, 1978

Wachtel PL: Psychoanalysis and Behavior Therapy: Toward an Integration. New York, Basic Books, 1977

Waddington CH: New Patterns in Genetics and Development XXI of the Columbia Biological Series. New York, Columbia University Press, 1962

Wallerstein RS: Foreword, in Psychoanalytic theories of development: An Integration. Edited by Tyson P, Tyson R. New Haven, CT, Yale University Press, 1990, pp ix–xiv

Wertsch JV: Vygotsky and the Social Formation of Mind. Cambridge, MA, Harvard University Press, 1985

Winnicott DW: The theory of the parent-infant relationship. Int J Psychoanal 41:585–595, 1960

Winnicott DW: Ego Distortion in Terms of True and False Self in the Maturational Processes and the Facilitating Environment. New York, International Universities Press, 1965

8

Psychoanalytic Developmental Theory

PETER FONAGY, Ph.D., F.B.A.

PSYCHOANALYSIS IS ALL ABOUT children. When Freud conceived of his "neurotica," he already had a model in mind fundamentally inspired by embryology. When the contemporary analyst addresses unreasonable relational expectations and disturbing preconscious fantasies with her patient, the assumption that she is focusing on childlike modes of thought runs right through the interaction. The key idea, unchanged since Freud's day, is the notion that pathology is rooted in and in critical respects made up of recapitulated ontogeny. Disorders of the mind are best understood as maladaptive residues of childhood experience—developmentally primitive modes of mental functioning. The developmental point of view is acknowledged by all genuinely psychoanalytic theories to some degree.

Notwithstanding the importance of the developmental perspective for all these theories, the application of knowledge from child development to theorization is centrally flawed by at least two related difficulties. The first concerns unjustified confidence in tracing the psychopathology of particular forms to specific phases (an example is the link sometimes made between borderline personality disorder and the rapprochement subphase of separation and individuation). The second relates to the overemphasis on early experience, which is frequently found to be at odds with developmental data. Westen (Westen et al. 1990a, 1990b) is particularly clear in his evidence that patholog-

ical processes of self representation and object relationships actually characterize developmental phases far later than those that have traditionally concerned psychoanalytic theoreticians. The emphasis on deficits in preverbal periods is a particular problem for psychoanalytic theory because it places so many of the hypotheses beyond any realistic possibility of empirical testing.

Recent longitudinal, epidemiological birth cohort studies (Hofstra et al. 2002; Kim-Cohen et al. 2003) have provided dramatic confirmation that psychoanalysts were on the right track when they emphasised the developmental perspective in their understanding of the clinical problems they faced with their adult patients. These studies show that in the vast majority of cases, adult psychopathology is antedated by diagnosable childhood disturbance. Across adult disorders, 75% of the affected individuals had a diagnosable childhood problem (Kim-Cohen et al. 2003). It is impossible to conceive of adult problems without considering the development of vulnerabilities, biological and psychosocial, that antedate the disturbance. In fact, there seems to be no realistic way of thinking of psychopathology other than developmentally (Munir and Beardslee 1999). However, this only makes the task of examining the status of psychoanalytic theorizing from a developmental perspective all the more urgent. In this chapter, I explore the developmental aspects of the major theoretical traditions within psychoanalysis.

Overview of Psychoanalytic Theories

Psychoanalytic theory is not a static body of knowledge; it is in a state of constant evolution. In the first half of the twentieth century, Sigmund Freud and his close followers worked to identify the roles of instinct in development and psychopathology (drive theory). Later, the focus evolved and shifted to the development and functions of the ego, more formally ego psychology, to a current interest in the early mother-infant dyad and its long-term effect on interpersonal relationships and their internal representation, embodied in object relations theories. Concurrently, a psychology of the self evolved as part of most psychoanalytic theories. With its integration into mainstream theories, there is a better conceptual basis for a comprehensive and phenomenological clinical theory. There has been a movement away from metapsychological constructs couched in a natural science framework, to a clinical theory closer to personal experience—one whose core focus is the representational world and interpersonal relationships. Contemporary theories attempt to trace the sometimes highly elusive link between formative emotional relationships and the complex interactions they involve, and the formation of mental structures.

Two factors, both intrinsically tied to development, have made this theoretical move possible: observation-based psychoanalytic developmental theories (A. Freud 1965/1974; Mahler et al. 1975; Spillius 1994) and the growth of object relations theory. The latter, when viewed within a developmental framework (see Pine 1985), explores the evolution of a differentiated, integrated representational world that emerges within the context of a mother-infant matrix, or what Winnicott (1960) termed "the holding environment." At its broadest, object relations theory concerns the development of schemas from a diffuse set of sensorimotor experiences in the infant, into a differentiated, consistent, and relatively realistic representation of the self and object in interaction. This evolution is toward increasingly symbolic levels of representation, but with the general assumption that earlier levels of representations of interactions are retained in the mind and continue to exert powerful influences.

Psychoanalytic models have evolved through diverse attempts to explain why and how individuals in psychoanalytic treatment deviated from the normal path of development and came to experience major intrapsychic and interpersonal difficulties. Each model reviewed in this chapter focuses on particular developmental phases and outlines a model of normal personality development derived from the analyst's clinical experience.

Freud and the "Classical" Psychoanalytic Tradition

Initially Freud saw pathology as the expression of developmental trauma (Breuer and Freud 1893–1895/1955) and elaborated this concept into a maturation-driven developmental model of psychological disturbance (Freud 1900/1953). Freud's (1905/1953) developmental principle was to try to explain all pathological behavior in terms of the failure of the child's mental apparatus to deal adequately with the pressures inherent in a maturationally predetermined sequence of drive states. Freud was the first to give meaning to mental disorder by linking it to childhood experiences (Breuer and Freud 1893–1895/1955) and to the vicissitudes of the developmental process (Freud 1900/1953). One of Freud's greatest contributions was undoubtedly the shift in his thinking toward recognition of infantile sexuality (Green 1985). Freud's discoveries radically altered our perception of the child from one of idealized innocence to that of a person (Freud 1933[1932]/1964) struggling to achieve control over his or her biological needs and to make them acceptable to society through the microcosm of the family (Freud 1930/1957). Freud's second major shift in thinking once again gave a prominent place to the influence of the social environment in shaping development (Freud 1920/1955, 1923/1961, 1926/1959). This revision recast the theory in more cognitive terms (Schafer 1983), restoring adaptation to the external world as an essential part of the psychoanalytic account.

There are many limitations to Freud's developmental model. It can be argued that the most important post-Freudian contributions have been in the domains that Freud neglected, in particular the cultural and social context of development; the significance of early childhood experiences; the significance of the real behavior of the real parents; the role of dependency, attachment, and safety in development alongside the role of instinctual drives; the synthesizing function of the self; and the importance of the nonconflictual aspects of development. However, the picture concerning empirical evidence for aspects of development within Freud's model is not as bleak as many critics think (e.g., Crews 1996). For example, Westen (1998) demonstrated that there exists substantial empirical support for Freud's core construct: that human consciousness cannot account for its maladaptive actions. Work on procedural, or implicit, memory demonstrates that we act in certain ways because of experience, despite our inability to recall those particular experiences (Schachter 1992; Squire and Kandel 1999). Importantly, the implicit memory systems develop before the explicit, declarative system, leaving open the possibility of influences of early experience without conscious knowledge of the nature of these experiences. Of course, neuroscience does not substantiate the full spectrum of Freud's developmental claims. For example, infantile amnesia, a key developmental concept in Freud's formulation of the Oedipus complex, is more parsimoniously explained by the delayed myelination of the hippocampus, which only becomes fully functional between the third and fourth years of life, than by Freud's concept of primal repression. There is evidence that infantile amnesia exists in other mammals, including rats and monkeys (Rudy and Morledge 1994).

The ego psychological approach represents an essential repositioning of psychoanalytic developmental ideas. Early ego psychologists balanced Freud's developmental emphasis on sexual and aggressive instincts by focusing on the evolution of the adaptive capacities (Hartmann 1939/1958), which the child brings to bear on her struggle with her biological needs. Hartmann's model (Hartmann et al. 1949) attempted to take a wider view of the developmental process, to link drives and ego functions, and show how very negative interpersonal experiences could jeopardize the evolution of the psychic structures essential to adaptation. He also showed that the reactivation of developmentally earlier ego functions (ego regression) was the most important component of all psychopathology. Fixation in development is as much, then, a property of the ego as it is of the id, and individual differences in cognitive function that pervade personality may be understood as the consequence of developmental arrests in specific phases of ego development (Arlow 1985; Brenner 1982). Hartmann (1955/1964, p. 221) was also among the first to indicate the complexity of the developmental process, stating that the reasons for the persistence of particular behavior are likely to differ from the reasons for its original appearance ("genetic fallacy"). Among the great contributions of ego psychologists are the identification of the ubiquity of intrapsychic conflict throughout development (Brenner 1982), and the recognition that genetic endowment, as well as interpersonal experiences, may be critical in determining the child's developmental path. The latter idea has echoes in the epidemiological concept of resilience (Luthar et al. 2000).

Pushing the "Classical" Developmental Envelope

A number of other "classical" psychoanalytic authors advanced the developmental perspective. An influential exponent of structural developmental theory, Erik Erikson (1950) was primarily concerned with the interaction of social norms and biological drives in generating self and identity. He was remarkable among psychoanalysts because of his attention to cultural and family factors and because he conceived of development as covering the entire life cycle. Erikson (1959) extended Freud's problematic erotogenic zone concept to a more subtle idea of "organ modes." The concept of mode of functioning enabled Erikson to stay within the drive model but introduce a whole series of constructs including identity and basic trust. Westen (1998) considered investigations of Eriksonian concepts of identity (Marcia 1994), intimacy (Orlofsky 1993), and generativity (Bradley 1997) to have been some of the most methodologically sound studies inspired by psychoanalytic theories of development. Spitz (1959) proposed that major shifts in psychological organization, marked by the emergence of new behaviors and new forms of affective expression, occur when functions such as smiling are brought into new relation with one another and are linked into a coherent unit. The way in which these organizers of development herald dramatic changes in interpersonal interactions was elaborated in a highly influential series of papers by Robert Emde (1980a, 1980b, 1980c). Spitz (1945, 1965) was one of the first to ascribe primary importance to the mother-infant interaction as a force that could quicken the development of the child's innate abilities, and to describe the self-regulatory processes, such as affect regulation, that could increase the child's resilience (Spitz 1957).

Edith Jacobson (1964), one of the great innovators of North American psychoanalytic developmental theory, assumed that, because early drive states shifted continuously between the object and the self, a state of primitive fusion existed between self and object representations. Jacobson suggested that introjections and identificatory processes replaced the state of primitive fusion and that, through these, traits and actions of objects became internalized parts of self images. Jacobson applied her developmental perspective to a wide variety of disorders, in particular to depression, which she associated with the gap between self representation and ego ideal.

Hans Loewald was probably the most influential reformist of the North American psychoanalytic tradition. Loewald (1971a/1980, 1973) proposed a developmental model that has at its center a motive force toward "integrative experience"; organizing activity defines the "basic way of functioning of the psyche." His fundamental assumption was that all mental activity is relational (both interactional and intersubjective; see Loewald 1971a/1980, 1971b/1980). Internalization (learning) is the basic psychological process that propels development (Loewald 1973). As Friedman (1996) noted, Loewald saw structures as processes. Loewald deemphasized metapsychology and proposed a subtle revision of the classical model to place internalization, understanding, and interpretation at its center, in place of drives and defenses against them (Cooper 1988).

Direct observers of children and psychoanalysts of children (e.g., Fraiberg 1969, 1980; A. Freud 1965/1974) have taught us that neither child nor adult symptomatology is fixed, but rather both constitute a dynamic state superimposed on, and intertwined with, an underlying developmental process. Anna Freud's study of disturbed and healthy children under great social stress led her to formulate a relatively comprehensive developmental theory, in which the child's emotional maturity could be mapped independently of diagnosable pathology. Particularly in her early work in the war nurseries (A. Freud 1973), she identified many of the characteristics that later research linked to "resilience" (Luthar et al. 2000). For example, her observations spoke eloquently of the social support that children could give one another in concentration camps, support that could ensure their physical and psychological survival. More recent research on youngsters experiencing severe trauma has confirmed her assumption of the protective power of sound social support (e.g., Laor et al. 1996). Anna Freud's work stayed so close to the external reality of the child that it lent itself to a number of important applications (Goldstein et al. 1973, 1979).

Anna Freud was also a pioneer in identifying the importance of an equilibrium between developmental processes (A. Freud 1965/1974). The first psychoanalyst to adopt a coherent developmental perspective on psychopathology (A. Freud 1965/1974), she provided a comprehensive developmental theory, using the metaphor of developmental lines to stress the continuity and cumulative character of child development (A. Freud 1962, 1963). For example, aspects of the child's relationship to the mother could be described as a line that moved from dependency to emotional self-reliance to adult object relationships. There are two major reasons to value the notion of developmental lines. First, the concept provides an evaluation of the stage of the child's emotional maturation alongside psychiatric symptoms. Second, unevenness of development may be regarded as a risk factor for psychiatric disturbance, and thus developmental lines have etiological significance. A child's problem may be understood in terms of an arrest or regression along a particular line of development (A. Freud 1965/1974).

Anna Freud should perhaps be described as a modern structural theorist. Her model is fundamentally developmental. The individual is seen as capable of moving back along developmental lines if necessary to deal with some current, potentially overwhelming challenge, at which point they can move forward again. Here there is no equa-

tion of behavior and pathology; a given behavior may not be a true symptom, but rather a temporary "blip." The notions of mobility of function and the meaning of behavior are key assumptions of broader developmental approaches to psychopathology (Cicchetti and Cohen 1995; Garmezy and Masten 1994).

Anna Freud's insistence on the literal use of her father's structural model of drives limits the usefulness of her model. She regarded the balance between id, ego, and superego, drive fixation, and so forth as the most scientific aspects of her father's contribution and was reluctant to abandon them. But her revision of the structural model is hidden behind her modesty about the significance of her innovations. Masten and Curtis (2000) have drawn attention to two historically rich traditions of study: the development of competence and psychopathology, both of which are present in the history of psychiatry and psychoanalysis but are not commonly integrated. Development of competence has remained the domain of developmental psychology, while disturbance and dysfunction have been explored in the realm of child and adult psychiatry. Perhaps Anna Freud's corpus is a notable exception to this tendency to separate competence from pathology (Masten and Coatsworth 1995).

Margaret Mahler, a pioneer of developmental observation in the United States, drew attention to the paradox of self development: that a separate identity involves giving up a highly gratifying closeness with the caregiver. Mahler's model assumes that the child develops from "normal autism" through a "symbiotic period" to the four subphases of the separation-individuation process (Mahler and Furer 1968). Each step is strongly influenced by the nature of the mother-infant interaction, in particular by such factors as early symbiotic gratification and the emotional availability of the mother. The separation-individuation process is thought to begin at 4–5 months, in the subphase of differentiation identified as hatching (differentiation of the body image) (Mahler et al. 1975), when the infant's pleasure in sensory perception can begin if his or her symbiotic gratification has been satisfactory. In the "rapprochement" subphase, from 15–18 to 24 months, the infant begins to have greater awareness of separateness and experiences separation anxiety, and consequently has an increased need to be with the mother. Mahler's observations of this "ambitendency" of children in their second year of life threw light on chronic problems of consolidating individuality. Mahler (1974) described her work as enabling clinicians treating adults to make more accurate reconstructions of the preverbal period, thereby making patients more accessible to analytic interventions. The pathogenic potential of withdrawal of the mother, when confronted with the child's wish for separateness, was further elaborated by Masterson (1972) and Rinsley (1977) and helps to account for the transgenerational aspects of psychological disturbance.

Evidence from infant research casts considerable doubt on Mahler's formulations about early development, particularly her notions of normal autism and selfobject merger (e.g., Gergely 2000). Mahler's original contributions to the understanding of borderline personality disorder have been the most lasting. Her view of these patients as fixated in a rapprochement—wishing to cling but fearing the loss of their fragile sense of self, wishing to be separate but also fearing to move away from the parental figure—has been crucial to both clinical intervention and theoretical understanding. Mahler's developmental framework, however, may well be appropriate to the truly psychological world of the infant. Fonagy and colleagues (1993) argue that whereas the infant is well aware of himself and the object in the physical domain, the same cannot be said of the infant's mental or psychological self, which represents mental states of belief and desire. Whereas the child may be fully aware of the cohesion and boundedness of the physical mother, he might well assume that psychological states extend beyond the physical boundaries.

In the United Kingdom, Joseph Sandler's development of Anna Freud's and Edith Jacobson's work represents the best integration of the developmental perspective with psychoanalytic theory. His comprehensive psychoanalytic model has enabled developmental researchers (Emde 1983, 1988a, 1988b; Stern 1985) to integrate their findings into a psychoanalytic formulation that which clinicians have been able to use. At the core of Sandler's formulation lies the representational structure that contains both reality and distortion and is the driving force of psychic life. Sandler differentiated the deeply unconscious hypothetical structures assumed by classical psychoanalysis to develop early in life and that have no chance of directly emerging into consciousness (the past unconscious) from the present unconscious, which also worked as Freud described (irrational, only partly observing the reality principle, but principally concerned with current rather than past experience) (Sandler and Sandler 1984). Sandler (1976) described how patients tend to create relationships to actualize unconscious fantasies by casting themselves and their therapists in specific relationship patterns; by extension, he offered an entirely new theory of internal object representations (Sandler and Sandler 1978). Sandler was one of the most creative figures in enabling psychoanalysis to be a psychology of feelings, internal representations, and adaptations closely tied to the clinical origins of psychoanalysis. Although his theories are still extensively used, those who use his ideas often are unaware of doing so. He advanced thinking by clarifying a range of psychoanalytic concepts but was unable to excite his colleagues with the novelty of his contributions.

Object Relations the British Way

The focus of object relations theories on early development and infantile fantasy represented a shift in worldview for psychoanalysis from one that was tragic to a somewhat more romantic one (see, e.g., Akhtar 1992). The classical view, rooted in a Kantian philosophical tradition, holds that striving toward autonomy and the reign of reason is the essence of being human. By contrast, the romantic view, to be found in Rousseau and Goethe, values authenticity and spontaneity above reason and logic. In the classical view, man is seen as inherently limited but able to, in part, overcome his tragic flaws, to become "fairly decent" (Akhtar 1992, p. 320). The romantic approach perhaps originates with the work of Ferenczi and is well represented in the work of Balint, Winnicott, and Guntrip in the United Kingdom and Modell and Adler in the United States. The romantic psychoanalytic view is undoubtedly more optimistic, seeing man as full of potential and the infant as ready to actualize his destiny (Akhtar 1989). In the classic psychoanalytic view, conflict is embedded in normal development. There is no escape from human weakness, aggression, and destructiveness, and life is a constant struggle against the reactivation of infantile conflicts.

Melanie Klein's (1935/1975, 1930, 1959/1975) work combines the structural model with an interpersonal, object relations model of development. Her papers on the depressive position (Klein 1935/1975, Klein 1940/1984), her paper on the paranoid-schizoid position (Klein 1946), and her book "Envy and Gratitude" (Klein 1957/1975) established her as the leader of an original psychoanalytic tradition. In the Kleinian model the human psyche has two basic positions: the paranoid-schizoid and the depressive (Klein 1935/1975, 1946, 1952/1975; Klein et al. 1946). In the *paranoid-schizoid position*, the psyche relates to part rather than whole objects. Relationships with important objects such as the caregiver are split into relations to a persecutory and to an idealized object; the ego (the self) is similarly split. In the *depressive position*, the relationship is with integrated parents, both loved and hated, and the ego is more integrated. The discovery of this ambivalence, and of the absence and potential loss of the attacked object, opens the child to the experience of guilt about his or her hostility to a loved object. Bion (1957) was the first to point out that the depressive position is never permanently achieved. In fact, the very term "position" suggests a permanence that this state of mind rarely has. It is now accepted that the mind cycles between the two positions, as the achievement of the depressive position creates anxiety that can only be handled in the paranoid-schizoid state (by more primitive defenses such as splitting).

Spillius (1993) suggested that the depressive position might be initiated by the child's perception of the parent as thinking and feeling (having a "theory of their mind" or "mentalizing"; see Fonagy et al. 1991; Morton and Frith 1995). Mentalizing is closely related to Bion's (1962a, 1962b) notion of "K," as getting to know oneself or the other person, and the evasion of the process, which he calls "minus K." Bion (1959) pointed to the need for projective identification in infancy, a time when the baby is unable to absorb all his or her intense experiences. By projecting the unprocessed elements into another human mind (a container) that can accept and transform them into meanings, the baby's mind can cope. Capable mothers experience and transform these feelings (Bion's "beta elements") into a tolerable form, combining mirroring of intolerable affect with emotional signals, indicating that the affect is under control (Bion's "alpha function").

Kleinian developmental concepts have become popular because they provide powerful descriptions of the clinical interaction between both child and adult patient and analyst. For example, projective identification depicts the close control that primitive mental function can exert over the analyst's mind. Post-Kleinian psychoanalysts (Bion 1962a; Rosenfeld 1971) were particularly helpful in underscoring the impact of emotional conflict on the development of cognitive capacities. But there is no evidence to support Klein's implicit claim that the infant relates to the object as a psychological entity. Melanie Klein constantly attributed awareness of minds to the baby, which we now know the child is most unlikely to have until at least the second year (Baron-Cohen et al. 2000). The question arises as to why Klein dates pathology to such early stages (Bibring 1947). The answer might be that the mental states of infancy are extremely hard to observe: the postulation of crucial pathogenic processes in infancy is extremely unlikely to be disproven. Psychoanalytic infant observation (Bick 1964) also permits widely differing interpretations. However, evidence is accumulating that most of the important mental disorders of adulthood are indeed foreshadowed in infancy (e.g., Marenco and Weinberger 2000). Furthermore, early brain development is increasingly seen as pivotal in the evolution of psychological disturbance (Schore 2003).

The early relationship with the caregiver emerged as a critical aspect of personality development from studies of severe character disorders by the object-relations school of psychoanalysts in Britain. Fairbairn's focus on the individual's need for the other (Fairbairn 1952) helped shift

psychoanalytic attention from structure to content and profoundly influenced both British and North American psychoanalytic thinking. As a result, the self as a central part of the psychoanalytic model emerged in the work of Balint (1937/1965, 1968) and Winnicott (1971). Winnicott (1962, 1965a) saw the child as evolving from a unity of infant and mother, which has three functions that facilitate healthy development: "holding," facilitating integration; "handling," leading to "personalization" or individuation; and object-relating. The concept of the caretaker or false self, a defensive structure created to master trauma in a context of total dependency, has become an essential developmental construct. Winnicott's (1965b) notions of primary maternal preoccupation, transitional phenomena, the holding environment, and the mirroring function of the caregiver provided a clear research focus for developmentalists interested in individual differences in the development of self structure. Winnicott (1965c, 1965d), in distinguishing between deprivation and privation, added to our understanding of environmental influence. Privation can only be experienced while the infant does not have an awareness of maternal care, in the phase of absolute dependence. Deprivation is experienced when the baby is in a state of relative independence, once he or she is sufficiently aware of both his or her own needs and the object that he or she can perceive a need as unmet or the other's care being lost (Winnicott 1952/1975).

In line with Winnicott's assumptions about development is a large body of evidence that infants from the earliest orient actively toward people in general and toward facial displays capable of mirroring their internal states in particular. Thus, they show neonatal imitation of facial gestures (Meltzoff and Moore 1997). A great deal in this literature is consistent with Winnicott's claim that "there is no such thing as a baby," only a dual unit of infant and mother in which, for example, the mother and the infant mutually create the infant's moods (Tronick 2001). The infant is thought to monitor and process the mother's affect to generate his or her own affective state, which in turn, through a more complex representational structure, triggers mood states in the mother. Research does not, however, support Winnicott's exclusive concern with the infant-mother relationship and the privileging of the mother-child relationship in etiological models (see, e.g., McCauley et al. 2000 for a discussion of research on childhood depression). Winnicott's assumption that the relationship between infant and mother provided the basis for all serious mental disorder runs counter to accumulating evidence for the importance of genetic factors (Rutter et al. 1999a, 1999b). Evidence suggests that Winnicott overstated the case for environmental influences on normal and pathological development. While psychoanalysts prior to Winnicott and the British Independents had been inclined to environmentalism and preferred nurture to nature explanations of pathology, the Freudian heritage was one of great respect for constitutional factors and the role of genetics, for example, in symptom choice and vulnerability to environmental stress. While never totally rejecting the role of constitutional factors, in psychosis for example, Winnicott's theory emphasized the exclusive role of the early environment to a degree that has turned out to be clearly incompatible with the behaviorial genetics data.

Object Relations in North America

There have been many attempts by North American theorists to incorporate object relations ideas into models that retain facets of structural theories. Two attempts stand out as having had lasting impact on developmental approaches. Self psychology, the work of Kohut (1971, 1977, 1984, Kohut and Wolf 1978), was based primarily on his experience of treating narcissistic individuals. His central developmental idea was the need for an understanding caregiver to counteract the infant's sense of helplessness in the face of the infant's biological striving for mastery. The mother who treats the child as though the child has a self initiates the process of self formation. The function of the selfobject is to integrate the child's affects through helping the child differentiate, tolerate, and think about affects (Stolorow 1997; Stolorow and Atwood 1991). To begin with, empathic responses from the mirroring selfobject (assumed to be the mother) allow the unfolding of exhibitionism and grandiosity.

Kohut emphasized the need for such understanding objects throughout life, and these notions are consistent with accumulating evidence for the powerful protective influence of social support across a wide range of epidemiological studies (Brown and Harris 1978; Brown et al. 1986). Frustration by caregivers, when phase-appropriate and not too intense, permits a gradual modulation of infantile omnipotence through "a transmuting internalization" of this mirroring function. Transmuting internalization of the selfobject leads gradually to consolidation of the nuclear self (Kohut and Wolf 1978, pp. 83 and 416). Drive theory becomes secondary to self theory, in that the failure to attain an integrated self structure both leaves room for, and in itself generates, aggression and isolated sexual fixation. However, the self remains problematic as a construct; in Kohut's model, it is both the person (the patient) and the agent that are assumed to control the person (Stolorow et al. 1987).

There is evidence that mothers speaking to their infants as if the baby had a self enhances the likelihood of secure attachment (Oppenheim and Koren-Karie 2002), even when mother-infant interaction is observed at 6 months and attachment at 12 months (Meins et al. 2001). A large body of evidence also supports the central role of self-esteem in the generation of psychological disturbance. For example, it is clear that life events that trigger feelings of humiliation and entrapment are particularly powerful in triggering episodes of depression (Brown et al. 1995). Tyson and Tyson (1990) take issue with Kohut's emphasis on pathogenic parents, neglecting the infant's constitution and capacity to modify his or her own environment. Kohut also leans heavily on Winnicott and British object relations theorists, although his indebtedness is rarely acknowledged. In an apparently helpful clarification, Wolf (1988) pointed out that selfobject needs are concrete only in infancy. In later development they can be increasingly abstract, with symbols or ideas serving selfobject functions. Anything that makes a person feel good may be considered to have a selfobject function, and the only way we know if an activity or person has a selfobject function is through observing its effects on well-being. Used this broadly, the concept has no explanatory power. Nevertheless, Kohut's descriptions of the narcissistic personality have been powerful and influential examples of the use of developmental theory in psychoanalytic understanding.

Otto Kernberg, who trained as a Kleinian analyst, has mainly worked in the environment of ego psychology and yet has achieved a remarkable level of integration between these two, quite possibly epistemologically inconsistent (Greenberg and Mitchell 1983), developmental frameworks (see Kernberg 1975, 1980a, 1980b, 1984, 1992). Kernberg does not fully adopt the Kleinian model of development, although he makes good use of Kleinian concepts (such as the model of early object relations and superego formation, aggression, envy, splitting, and projective identification) in understanding severe psychopathology. Ultimately, his model is a creative combination of the ideas of the modernizers of structural theory (Jacobson, Sandler, Loewald, Mahler) and the Klein-Bion model. This may account for Kernberg's being the most cited psychoanalyst alive and one of the most influential in the history of the field. The major psychic structures (id, ego, and superego) are integrations of internalizations (principally introjections) of object representations in self-object relationships under various emotional states. Thus, a superego may be harsh because of a prevailing affect of anger and criticism. Kernberg outlines a developmental sequence borrowed from Jacobson and Mahler but with a far less specific timetable. In essence, in early stages good and bad object images are split by the ego to protect images from the destructive power of bad ones. In the third year of life, the polarized good and bad representations are thought to become gradually more integrated so that total self and object representations are formed.

The elegance of Kernberg's theory lies in bringing together the metapsychological or structural (experience-distant) and phenomenological (what Kernberg called experience-near) levels of description. Kernberg goes beyond traditional ego psychology in that the explanation in terms of "ego weakness" is no longer circular. Ego weakness is coterminous with an active defensive process that leads to the split-ego organizations that cannot withstand close contact with bad object representations. In line with Kernberg's speculations, affect theorists suggest that a constitutional affect bias normally becomes consolidated through repetitions of discrete emotions and comes to be organized into rigid patterns. Psychopathology such as depression arises in association with a sadness bias that may arise as a consequence of constitutional characteristics (e.g., stress reactivity and hypothalamic-pituitary-adrenal axis arousal) and socialization experience (Zahn-Waxler et al. 2000).

Beyond Object Relations

In the 1980s and perhaps the early 1990s, there was once again theoretical hegemony in psychoanalysis. Most psychoanalysts felt comfortable with a broad object relations model of development more or less influenced by structural, Kleinian, or self psychology ideas. Consensus of this kind had probably not occurred since Freud's death. Alas, such agreement could not last, and the hegemony of object relations has begun to give way to new approaches. This shift is probably less due to any specific new problems uncovered in relation to the object relations approach and more due to what seems to be a reaction against "old" ideas driven by disappointment with the psychoanalytic approach in general in the United States and also in Western Europe.

With the gradual demise of ego psychology in the United States and the opening of psychoanalysis to psychologists and other nonmedically qualified professionals, a fresh intellectual approach to theory and technique gained ground in theoretical and technical discussions, rooted in the work of Harry Stack Sullivan (1953) and Clara Thompson (1964). The *interpersonalist approach*, represented by prolific contemporary writers such as Ogden (1994), McLaughlin (1991), Hoffman (1994), Renik (1993), Benjamin (1998), and Bromberg (1998), has revolutionized the role of the analyst in the therapeutic situation. Like all new

psychoanalytic approaches, this one too has powerful historical roots. It is a direct descendent of Harry Stack Sullivan's interpersonal psychiatry school (Sullivan 1953), linked with British object relations approaches by an influential volume coauthored by the most powerful advocate of this new approach (Greenberg and Mitchell 1983). The relational model has the interpersonal model, particularly the assumption of the interpersonal nature of subjectivity, as its starting point (Mitchell 1988). An individual human mind is a contradiction in terms, as subjectivity is invariably rooted in intersubjectivity (Mitchell 2000).

Whereas classical analytic theory stands or falls on its biological foundations (Sulloway 1979), the heritage of interpersonal relational theories is qualitatively different, more at home with postmodern deconstructive ideas than with brain-behavior integration. For example, the power of sexuality is derived not from organ pleasure but from its meaning in a relational matrix (Mitchell 1988). A similar relational argument was advanced by Mitchell for aggression (Mitchell 1993). The etiological emphasis is on the reality of early childhood experience that teaches the child about "the specific ways in which each of his object relationships will inevitably become painful, disappointing, suffocating, over-sexualised and so on" (Ogden 1989, pp. 181–182). Here and elsewhere, the emphasis is on observable behavior and a reluctance to privilege fantasy over actuality. Reality is not *behind* the appearance; it is *in* the appearance (Levenson 1981). Distortions are produced by interpersonal anxiety in the real world. Fantasy is accepted as formative in the sense that it makes reality relevant (Mitchell 2000).

Lewis (1998) reviewed empirical research in three areas relevant to this approach: studies of families and marriages, the role of adult relationships in undoing the adult consequences of destructive childhood experiences, and the relationship of marital variables and the onset and course of depressive disorder. Research results in all these areas are consistent with the relational assumption that current interpersonal relationships can determine the emergence and course of psychological disturbance. Even more impressive are outcome studies of brief psychotherapy, in which only trials with interpersonal psychotherapy are found to be consistently effective across a range of disorders (Roth and Fonagy 2004).

A second popular developmental model to emerge into the vacuum left by a more or less widespread disappointment with classical approaches has been *attachment theory*. Bowlby's (1969, 1973, 1980) work on separation and loss also focused psychoanalytic developmentalists' attention on the importance of the reality of security (safety, sensitivity, and predictability) of the earliest relationships. Attachment theory is almost unique among psychoanalytic theories in bridging the gap between general psychology and clinical psychodynamic theory. Attachment is a behavioral system that organizes behaviors that normally ensure a caregiving response from the adult. This is key to understanding the heated nature of the controversy between theorists of psychoanalysis and attachment theorists. A behavioral system involves inherent motivation; it is not reducible to another drive. While Bowlby takes forward three of the five metapsychological viewpoints (Rapaport and Gill 1959)—the genetic or developmental; the structural, elaborated substantially in the context of modern cognitive psychology; and the adaptive points of view—two aspects, economic and dynamic considerations, were explicitly discarded. To most psychoanalysts these latter features of psychoanalytic models were far more critical to the definition of the discipline than the first three. Bowlby's contribution was "denounced" as nonanalytic by the most influential psychoanalysts of the period (A. Freud 1960/1969; Hanley 1978). Yet his cognitive systems model of the internalization of interpersonal relationships (internal working models) is consistent with object relations theory (Fairbairn 1954; Kernberg 1975), and these psychodynamic ideas have been introduced beyond psychoanalysis. According to Bowlby, the child develops expectations regarding a caregiver's behavior and his or her own behavior. Bowlby's developmental model highlights the transgenerational nature of internal working models: our view of ourselves depends on the working model of relationships that characterized our caregivers. Empirical research on this intergenerational model is encouraging: an accumulating body of data confirms that there is intergenerational transmission of attachment security and insecurity (Main et al. 1985; see review by van IJzendoorn 1995) and that parental mental representations shaping this process may be assessed before the birth of the first child (Fonagy et al. 1991; Steele et al. 1996). A rapprochement between attachment theory and psychoanalysis has become possible because of the widening of the empirical base of attachment research to include key clinical problems that necessitated a more dynamic approach and because of dissatisfaction within psychoanalysis with the economic point of view (Fonagy 2001).

A number of theories have drawn deeply from the developmental research tradition, combining attachment theory ideas with psychoanalytic conceptions within general systems theory frames of reference (see, e.g., Tyson and Tyson 1990). For example, Daniel Stern's (1985) book *The Interpersonal World of the Infant* represented a milestone in psychoanalytic theorization concerning development. His work is distinguished by being normative rather than pathomorphic, and prospective rather than retrospective. His focus is the reorganization of subjective perspectives on self and other as this occurs with the emergence of new maturational capacities. Stern's four phases of the development of the sense of self (the emerging self, core self, subjective self, and narrative self) map neatly onto Damasio's (1999) neuropsychological descriptions: the "proto-self" (first-order neural maps), core consciousness (second-order neural maps), and extended consciousness (involving third-order neural maps), which links to Stern's subjective self. Stern (1993) describes the subjective integration of all aspects of lived experience as "emergent moments" that derive from a range of schematic representations (event representations, semantic representations, perceptual schemas, sensorimotor representations) in conjunction with a representation of "feeling shapes" (patterns of arousal across time) and "proto-narrative envelopes" that give a proto-plot to an event with an agent, an action, instrumentality, and context (see Bruner 1990). These schematic representations are conceptualized in combination as the "schema-of-a-way-of-being-with." It is distortions in this basic schema that lead to vulnerabilities to psychopathology. Stern (1993) offers a compelling example of a way-of-being-with a depressed mother and describes the baby trying repeatedly to recapture and reanimate her. He describes how depressed mothers, monitoring their own failure to stimulate, may make huge efforts to enliven their infant in an unspontaneous way, to which infants respond with what is probably an equally false response of enlivened interaction. He is perhaps closest to Sandler in his psychoanalytic model of the mind, but his formulation of object relations also has much in common with those of Bowlby, Kohut, and Kernberg. Stern's development of the "way-of-being-with" notion takes us closer to providing a neuropsychologically valid way of depicting a psychoanalytic model of the development of interpersonal experience (Read et al. 1997). Many of Stern's suggestions have proved to be highly applicable clinically in explanations of therapeutic change (Stern 1998; Stern et al. 1998).

A further psychodynamic model, closely linked to attachment theory, focuses on the developmental emergence of the agentive self, particularly as revealed by the vicissitudes of the unfolding of the capacity to mentalize (i.e., to conceive of mental states as explanations of behavior in oneself and in others) (Fonagy and Target 1997; Fonagy et al. 2002). This approach is rooted in attachment theory but claims a further evolutionary rationale for the human attachment system that goes beyond Bowlby's phylogenetic and ontogenetic claims for proximity to the protective caregiver (Bowlby 1969), in that it considers the major selective advantage conferred by attachment to humans to be the opportunity thereby afforded to develop social intelligence and a capacity for meaning-making (Fonagy

2003). The secure base provides experiences of being mirrored that promote the understanding of emotions, the singular organization of the self structure and effective attentional control systems, and facilitates the development of mentalization (see also Carpendale and Lewis, in press). Trauma (particularly attachment trauma), when combined with the sequelae of a deeply insecure early environment with enfeebled affect representation and poor affect control systems as well as a disorganized self structure, inhibits playfulness and interferes directly with affect regulation and attentional control systems. It also can bring about a total failure of mentalization as a defensive adaptive maneuver on the part of the child, who protects himself or herself from frankly malevolent and dangerous states of mind of the abuser by affectively decoupling this capacity to conceive of mental states, at least in attachment contexts (Fonagy 1991). The most serious impact of trauma occurs with the defensive identification of the victim with the abuser. The victim offers the dissociated, alien part of himself or herself as a space to be colonized by the traumatic experience. Externalization of this inevitably persecutory part of the self becomes an imperative of psychological survival and explains many of the puzzling behaviors of borderline personality organisation, including persistent projective identification and self-harm and persistent suicide attempts.

Conclusion

Early psychoanalytic theories have not been supplanted by later formulations, and most psychoanalytic writers assume that a number of explanatory frameworks are necessary to give a comprehensive account of the relationship of development and psychopathology (see Sandler 1983). So-called neurotic psychopathology is presumed to originate in later childhood at a time when there is self-other differentiation and when the various agencies of the mind (id, ego, superego) have been firmly established. The structural frame of reference (Arlow and Brenner 1964; Sandler et al. 1982) is most commonly used in developmental accounts of these disorders. Personality or character disorders (e.g., borderline personality disorder, narcissistic personality disorder, schizoid personality disorder), as well as most nonneurotic psychiatric disorders, are most commonly looked at in frameworks developed subsequent to structural theory. Here, a variety of theoretical frameworks are available, including the structural; most of these point to developmental pathology arising at a point in time when psychic structures are still in formation (see, e.g., Kohut 1971; Modell 1985).

But do theories matter at all? Do they really influence clinical work with patients? This is a difficult question to answer. Evidently, analysts from very different persuasions, with very different views of pathogenesis, are convinced of the correctness of their formulations and are guided in their treatments by convictions. Since we do not yet know what is truly mutative about psychotherapy, it might well be that for many patients the analyst's theory of their etiology is not so crucial. The complex relationship between clinical work and theoretical development, alongside a brief review of the evidence concerning the outcome of psychoanalysis, will be considered in Chapter 14 ("Theories of Therapeutic Action and Their Technical Consequences").

References

Akhtar S: Kohut and Kernberg: a critical comparison, in Self Psychology: Comparisons and Contrasts. Edited by Detrick DW, Detrick SP. Hillsdale, NJ, Analytic Press, 1989, pp 329–362

Akhtar S: Broken Structures: Severe Personality Disorders and Their Treatment. Northvale, NJ, Jason Aronson, 1992

Arlow JA: The structural hypothesis, in Models of the Mind: Their Relationships to Clinical Work. Edited by Rothstein A. New York, International Universities Press, 1985, pp 21–34

Arlow JA, Brenner C: Psychoanalytic Concepts and the Structural Theory. New York, International Universities Press, 1964

Balint M: Early developmental states of the ego, primary object of love, in Primary Love and Psychoanalytic Technique (1937). London, Tavistock, 1965, pp 90–108

Balint M: The Basic Fault. London, Tavistock, 1968

Baron-Cohen S, Tager-Flusberg H, Cohen DJ (eds): Understanding Other Minds: Perspectives From Developmental Cognitive Neuroscience. Oxford, England, Oxford University Press, 2000

Benjamin J: The Shadow of the Other: Intersubjectivity and Gender in Psychoanalysis. New York, Routledge, 1998

Bibring E: The so-called English School of Psychoanalysis. Psychoanal Q 16:69–93, 1947

Bick E: Notes on infant observation in psychoanalytic training. Int J Psychoanal 45:558–566, 1964

Bion WR: Differentiation of the psychotic from the non-psychotic personalities. Int J Psychoanal 38:266–275, 1957

Bion WR: Attacks on linking. Int J Psychoanal 40:308–315, 1959

Bion WR: Learning From Experience. New York, Basic Books, 1962a

Bion WR: A theory of thinking. Int J Psychoanal 43:306–310, 1962b

Bowlby J: Attachment and Loss, Vol 1: Attachment. New York, Basic Books, 1969

Bowlby J: Attachment and Loss, Vol 2: Separation: Anxiety and Anger. New York, Basic Books, 1973

Bowlby J: Attachment and Loss, Vol 3: Loss: Sadness and Depression. New York, Basic Books, 1980

Bradley C: Generativity-stagnation: development of a status model. Developmental Review 17:262–290, 1997

Brenner C: The Mind in Conflict. New York, International Universities Press, 1982

Breuer J, Freud S: Studies on hysteria (1893–1895), in Standard Edition of the Complete Psychological Works of Sigmund Freud, Vol 2. Translated and edited by Strachey J. London, Hogarth Press, 1955, pp 1–319

Bromberg PM: Standing in the Spaces. Hillsdale, NJ, Analytic Press, 1998

Brown GW, Harris TO: Social Origins of Depression: A Study of Psychiatric Disorders in Women. London, Tavistock, 1978

Brown GW, Harris TO, Bifuloc A: Long-term effects of early loss of parent, in Depression in Young People: Developmental and Clinical Perspectives. Edited by Rutter M, Izard CE, Read PB, New York, Guilford, 1986, pp 251–296

Brown GW, Harris TO, Hepworth C: Loss, humiliation and entrapment among women developing depression: a patient and non-patient comparison. Psychol Med 25:7–21, 1995

Bruner JS: Acts of Meaning. Cambridge, MA, Harvard University Press, 1990

Carpendale JIM, Lewis C: Constructing an understanding of mind: the development of children's social understanding within social interaction. Behav Brain Sci (in press)

Cicchetti D, Cohen DJ: Perspectives on developmental psychopathology, in Developmental Psychopathology, Vol 1: Theory and Methods. Edited by Cicchetti D, Cohen DJ. New York, Wiley, 1995, pp 3–23

Cooper AM: Our changing views of the therapeutic action of psychoanalysis: comparing Strachey and Loewald. Psychoanal Q 57:15–27, 1988

Crews F: The verdict on Freud. Psychol Sci 7:63–67, 1996

Damasio A: The Feeling of What Happens: Body and Emotion in the Making of Consciousness. New York, Harcourt Brace, 1999

Emde RN: Emotional availability: a reciprocal reward system for infants and parents with implications for prevention of psychosocial disorders, in Parent-Infant Relationships. Edited by Taylor PM, Orlando F. New York, Grune & Stratton, 1980a, pp 87–115

Emde RN: Toward a psychoanalytic theory of affect, Part 1: the organizational model and its propositions, in The Course of Life: Psychoanalytic Contributions Toward Understanding Personality Development, Vol 1: Infancy. Edited by Greenspan SI, Pollock GH. Bethesda, MD, National Institute of Mental Health, 1980b, pp 63–83

Emde RN: Toward a psychoanalytic theory of affect, Part 2: emerging models of emotional development in infancy, in The Course of Life: Psychoanalytic Contributions Toward Understanding Personality Development, Vol 1: Infancy. Edited by Greenspan SI, Pollock GH. Bethesda, MD, National Institute of Mental Health, 1980c, pp 85–112

Emde RN: Pre-representational self and its affective core. Psychoanal Study Child 38:165–192, 1983

Emde RN: Development terminable and interminable, I: innate and motivational factors from infancy. Int J Psychoanal 69:23–42, 1988a

Emde RN: Development terminable and interminable, II: recent psychoanalytic theory and therapeutic considerations. Int J Psychoanal 69:283–286, 1988b

Erikson EH: Childhood and Society. New York, WW Norton, 1950

Erikson EH: Identity and the Life Cycle: Selected Papers. New York, International Universities Press, 1959

Fairbairn WRD: Psychoanalytic Studies of the Personality. London, Tavistock, 1952

Fairbairn WRD: An Object-Relations Theory of the Personality. New York, Basic Books, 1954

Fonagy P: Thinking about thinking: some clinical and theoretical considerations in the treatment of a borderline patient. Int J Psychoanal 72:1–18, 1991

Fonagy P: Attachment Theory and Psychoanalysis. New York, Other Press, 2001

Fonagy P: The development of psychopathology from infancy to adulthood: the mysterious unfolding of disturbance in time. Infant Ment Health J 24:212–239, 2003

Fonagy P, Target M: Attachment and reflective function: their role in self-organization. Dev Psychopathol 9:679–700, 1997

Fonagy P, Steele H, Moran G, et al: The capacity for understanding mental states: the reflective self in parent and child and its significance for security of attachment. Infant Ment Health J 13:200–217, 1991

Fonagy P, Moran GS, Target M: Aggression and the psychological self. Int J Psychoanal 74:471–485, 1993

Fonagy P, Gergely G, Jurist E, et al: Affect Regulation, Mentalization, and the Development of the Self. New York, Other Press, 2002

Fraiberg S: Libidinal object constancy and mental representation. Psychoanal Study Child 24:9–47, 1969

Fraiberg S: Clinical Studies in Infant Mental Health. New York, Basic Books, 1980

Freud A: The Writings of Anna Freud, Vol 3: Infants Without Families: Reports on the Hampstead Nurseries (1939–1945). New York, International Universities Press, 1973

Freud A: Discussion of Dr. Bowlby's paper (Grief and mourning in infancy and early childhood) (1960), in the Writings of Anna Freud, Vol 1. New York, International Universities Press, 1969, pp 167–186

Freud A: Assessment of childhood disturbances. Psychoanal Study Child 17:149–158, 1962

Freud A: The concept of developmental lines. Psychoanal Study Child 18:245–265, 1963

Freud A: Normality and pathology in childhood (1965), in The Writings of Anna Freud, Vol 6. New York, International Universities Press, 1974, pp 25–63

Freud S: The interpretation of dreams (1900), in Standard Edition of the Complete Psychological Works of Sigmund Freud, Vols 4 and 5. Translated and edited by Strachey J. London, Hogarth Press, 1953

Freud S: Three essays on the theory of sexuality, I: the sexual aberrations (1905), in Standard Edition of the Complete Psychological Works of Sigmund Freud, Vol 7. Translated and edited by Strachey J. London, Hogarth Press, 1953, pp 135–172

Freud S: Beyond the pleasure principle (1920), in Standard Edition of the Complete Psychological Works of Sigmund Freud, Vol 18. Translated and edited by Strachey J. London, Hogarth Press, 1955, pp 1–64

Freud S: The ego and the id (1923), in Standard Edition of the Complete Psychological Works of Sigmund Freud, Vol 19. Translated and edited by Strachey J. London, Hogarth Press, 1961, pp 12–66

Freud S: Inhibitions, symptoms and anxiety (1926), in Standard Edition of the Complete Psychological Works of Sigmund Freud, Vol 20. Translated and edited by Strachey J. London, Hogarth Press, 1959, pp 75–175

Freud S: Civilization and its discontents (1930), in Standard Edition of the Complete Psychological Works of Sigmund Freud, Vol 21. Translated and edited by Strachey J. London, Hogarth Press, 1957, pp 57–145

Freud S: New introductory lectures on psycho-analysis (1933[1932]) (Lectures XXIX–XXXV), in Standard Edition of the Complete Psychological Works of Sigmund Freud, Vol 22. Translated and edited by Strachey J. London, Hogarth Press, 1964, pp 1–182

Friedman L: The Loewald phenomenon. J Am Psychoanal Assoc 44:671–672, 1996

Garmezy N, Masten A: Chronic adversities, in Child and Adolescent Psychiatry: Modern Approaches, 3rd Edition. Edited by Rutter M, Taylor E, Hersov L. Oxford, England, Blackwell Scientific Publications, 1994, pp 191–208

Gergely G: Reapproaching Mahler: new perspectives on normal autism, normal symbiosis, splitting and libidinal object constancy from cognitive developmental theory. J Am Psychoanal Assoc 48:1197–1228, 2000

Goldstein J, Freud A, Solnit AJ: Beyond the Best Interests of the Child. New York, Free Press, 1973

Goldstein J, Freud A, Solnit AJ: Before the Best Interests of the Child. New York, Free Press, 1979

Green R: Atypical psychosexual development, in Child and Adolescent Psychiatry: Modern Approaches, 2nd Edition. Edited by Rutter M, Hersov L. Oxford, England, Blackwell Scientific Publications, 1985, pp 638–649

Greenberg JR, Mitchell SA: Object Relations in Psychoanalytic Theory. Cambridge, MA, Harvard University Press, 1983

Hanley C: A critical consideration of Bowlby's ethological theory of anxiety. Psychoanal Q 47:364–380, 1978

Hartmann H: Ego Psychology and the Problem of Adaptation (1939). Translated by Rapaport D. New York, International Universities Press, 1958

Hartmann H: Notes on the theory of sublimation (1955), in Essays on Ego Psychology. New York, International Universities Press, 1964, pp 215–240

Hartmann H, Kris H, Loewenstein R: Notes on the theory of aggression. Psychoanal Study Child 3–4:9–36, 1949

Hoffman IZ: Dialectic thinking and therapeutic action in the psychoanalytic process. Psychoanal Q 63:187–218, 1994

Hofstra MB, van der Ende J, Verhulst FC: Child and adolescent problems predict DSM-IV disorders in adulthood: a 14-year follow-up of a Dutch epidemiological sample. J Am Acad Child Adolesc Psychiatry 41:182–189, 2002

Jacobson E: The Self and the Object World. New York, International Universities Press, 1964

Kernberg OF: Borderline Conditions and Pathological Narcissism. New York, Jason Aronson, 1975

Kernberg OF: Internal World and External Reality: Object Relations Theory Applied. New York, Jason Aronson, 1980a

Kernberg OF: Some implications of object relations theory for psychoanalytic technique, in Psychoanalytic Explorations of Technique: Discourse on the Theory of Therapy. Edited by Blum H. New York, International Universities Press, 1980b, pp 207–239

Kernberg OF: Severe Personality Disorders: Psychotherapeutic Strategies. New Haven, CT, Yale University Press, 1984

Kernberg OF: Aggression in Personality Disorders and Perversions. New Haven, CT, Yale University Press, 1992

Kim-Cohen J, Caspi A, Moffitt TE, et al: Prior juvenile diagnoses in adults with mental disorder: developmental follow-back of a prospective longitudinal cohort. Arch Gen Psychiatry 60:709–717, 2003

Klein M: A contribution to the psychogenesis of manic-depressive states (1935), in Love, Guilt, and Reparation: The Writings of Melanie Klein, Vol 1. London, Hogarth Press, 1975, pp 236–289

Klein M: The psychotherapy of the psychoses. Br J Med Psychol 10:242–244, 1930

Klein M: Mourning and its relation to manic-depressive states (1940), in Love, Guilt, and Reparation: The Writings of Melanie Klein, Vol 1. New York, Macmillan, 1984, pp 344–369

Klein M: Notes on some schizoid mechanisms, in Developments in Psychoanalysis. Edited by Klein M, Heimann P, Isaacs S, et al. London, Hogarth Press, 1946, pp 292–320

Klein M: The mutual influences in the development of ego and id (1952), in Envy and Gratitude and Other Works, 1946–1963. New York, Delacorte Press, 1975, pp 57–60

Klein M: Envy and gratitude (1957), in The Writings of Melanie Klein, Vol 3. Edited by Money-Kyrle R. London, Hogarth Press, 1975, pp 176–235

Klein M: Our adult world and its roots in infancy (1959), in The Writings of Melanie Klein. Edited by Money-Kyrle R. London, Hogarth Press, 1975, pp 247–263

Klein M, Heimann P, Issacs S, et al (eds): Developments in Psychoanalysis. London, Hogarth Press, 1946

Kohut H: The Analysis of the Self: A Systematic Approach to the Psychoanalytic Treatment of Narcissistic Personality Disorders. New York, International Universities Press, 1971

Kohut H: The Restoration of the Self. New York, International Universities Press, 1977

Kohut H: How Does Analysis Cure? Chicago, IL, University of Chicago Press, 1984

Kohut H, Wolf ES: The disorders of the self and their treatment: an outline. Int J Psychoanal 59:413–426, 1978

Laor N, Wolmer L, Mayes LC, et al: Israeli preschoolers under Scud missile attacks: a developmental perspective on risk modifying factors. Arch Gen Psychiatry 53:416–423, 1996

Levenson E: Facts or fantasies: on the nature of psychoanalytic data. Contemporary Psychoanalysis 17:486–500, 1981

Lewis JM: For better or worse: interpersonal relationships and individual outcome. Am J Psychiatry 155:582–589, 1998

Loewald HW: On motivation and instinct theory (1971a), in Papers on Psychoanalysis. New Haven, CT, Yale University Press, 1980, pp 102–137

Loewald HW: The transference neurosis: comments on the concept and the phenomenon (1971b), in Papers on Psychoanalysis. New Haven, CT, Yale University Press, 1980, pp 302–314

Loewald HW: On internalization, in Papers on Psychoanalysis. New Haven, CT, Yale University Press, 1973, pp 69–86

Luthar SS, Cicchetti D, Becker B: The construct of resilience: a critical evaluation and guidelines for future work. Child Development 71:543–562, 2000

Mahler MS: Symbiosis and individuation: the psychological birth of the human infant, in The Selected Papers of Margaret S. Mahler. New York, Jason Aronson, 1974, pp 149–165

Mahler MS, Furer M: On Human Symbiosis and the Vicissitudes of Individuation, Vol 1: Infantile Psychosis. New York, International Universities Press, 1968

Mahler MS, Pine F, Bergman A: The Psychological Birth of the Human Infant: Symbiosis and Individuation. New York, Basic Books, 1975

Main M, Kaplan N, Cassidy J: Security in infancy, childhood and adulthood: a move to the level of representation. Monogr Soc Res Child Dev 50:66–104, 1985

Marcia JE: The empirical study of ego identity, in Identity and Development: An Interdisciplinary Approach. Edited by Bosma HA, Graafsma TLG, Grotevant HD, et al. Thousand Oaks, CA, Sage, 1994, pp 67–80

Marenco S, Weinberger DR: The neurodevelopmental hypothesis of schizophrenia: following a trail of evidence from cradle to grave. Dev Psychopathol 12:501–527, 2000

Masten AS, Coatsworth JD: Competence, resilience and psychopathology, in Developmental Psychopathology, Vol 2: Risk, Disorder, and Adaptation. Edited by Cicchetti D, Cohen DJ. New York, Wiley, 1995, pp 715–752

Masten AS, Curtis WJ: Integrating competence and psychopathology: pathways towards a comprehensive science of adaptation and development. Dev Psychopathol 12:529–550, 2000

Masterson JF: Treatment of the Borderline Adolescent: A Developmental Approach. New York, Wiley Interscience, 1972

McCauley E, Pavidis K, Kendall K: Developmental precursors of depression: the child and the social environment, in The Depressed Child and Adolescent: Developmental and Clinical Perspectives. Edited by Goodyer I. New York, Cambridge University Press, 2000, pp 46–78

McLaughlin J: Clinical and theoretical aspects of enactment. J Am Psychoanal Assoc 39:595–614, 1991

Meins E, Ferryhough C, Fradley E, et al: Rethinking maternal sensitivity: mothers' comments on infants mental processes predict security of attachment at 12 months. J Child Psychol Psychiatry 42:637–648, 2001

Meltzoff AN, Moore MK: Explaining facial imitation: theoretical model. Early Development and Parenting 6:179–192, 1997

Mitchell SA: Relational Concepts in Psychoanalysis: An Integration. Cambridge, MA, Harvard University Press, 1988

Mitchell SA: Aggression and the endangered self. Psychoanal Q 62:351–382, 1993

Mitchell SA: Relationality: From Attachment to Intersubjectivity. Hillsdale, NJ, Analytic Press, 2000

Modell AH: Object relations theory, in Models of the Mind: Their Relationships to Clinical Work. Edited by Rothstein A. New York, International Universities Press, 1985, pp 85–100

Morton J, Frith U: Causal modeling: a structural approach to developmental psychology, in Developmental Psychopathology, Vol 1: Theory and Methods. Edited by Cicchetti D, Cohen DJ. New York, Wiley, 1995, pp 357–390

Munir KM, Beardslee WR: Developmental psychiatry: is there any other kind? Harv Rev Psychiatry 6:250–262, 1999

Ogden T: The Primitive Edge of Experience. New York, Jason Aronson, 1989

Ogden T: The analytic third: working with intersubjective clinical facts. Int J Psychoanal 75:3–19, 1994

Oppenheim D, Koren-Karie N: Mothers' insightfulness regarding their children's internal worlds: the capacity underlying secure child-mother relationships. Infant Ment Health J 23:593–605, 2002

Orlofsky J: Intimacy status: theory and research, in Ego Identity: A Handbook for Psychosocial Research. Edited by Marcia JE, Waterman AS, Matteson DR, et al. New York, Springer-Verlag, 1993, pp 111–133

Pine F: Developmental Theory and Clinical Process. New Haven, CT, Yale University Press, 1985

Rapaport D, Gill MM: The points of view and assumptions of metapsychology. Int J Psychoanal 40:153–162, 1959

Read SJ, Vanman EJ, Miller LC: Conectionism, parallel constraint satisfaction processes, and Gestalt principles: (re)introducing cognitive dynamics to social psychology. Pers Soc Psychol Rev 1:26–53, 1997

Renik O: Analytic interaction: conceptualizing technique in the light of the analyst's irreducible subjectivity. Psychoanal Q 62:553–571, 1993

Rinsley DB: An object relations view of borderline personality, in Borderline Personality Disorders: The Concept, the Syndrome, the Patient. Edited by Hartocollis P. New York, International Universities Press, 1977, pp 47–70

Rosenfeld H: Contribution to the psychopathology of psychotic states: the importance of projective identification in the ego structure and object relations of the psychotic patient, in Melanie Klein Today. Edited by Spillius EB. London, Routledge, 1988, 1971, pp 117–137

Roth A, Fonagy P: What Works for Whom? A Critical Review of Psychotherapy Research, 2nd Edition. New York, Guilford, 1994

Rudy JW, Morledge P: The ontogeny of contextual fear conditioning: implications for consolidation, infantile amnesia, and hippocampal system function. Behav Neurosci 108:227–234, 1994

Rutter M, Silberg J, O'Connor T, et al: Genetics and child psychiatry, I: advances in quantitative and molecular genetics. J Child Psychol Psychiatry 40:3–18, 1999a

Rutter M, Silberg J, O'Connor T, et al: Genetics and child psychiatry, II: empirical research findings. J Child Psychol Psychiatry 40:19–55, 1999b

Sandler J: Countertransference and role-responsiveness. Int Rev Psychoanal 3:43–47, 1976

Sandler J: Reflections on some relations between psychoanalytic concepts and psychoanalytic practice. Int J Psychoanal 64:35–45, 1983

Sandler J, Sandler A-M: On the development of object relationships and affects. Int J Psychoanal 59:285–296, 1978

Sandler J, Sandler A-M: The past unconscious, the present unconscious, and interpretation of the transference. Psychoanalytic Inquiry 4:367–399, 1984

Sandler J, Dare C, Holder A: Frames of reference in psychoanalytic psychology, XII: the characteristics of the structural frame of reference. Br J Med Psychol 55:203–207, 1982

Schachter DL: Priming and multiple memory systems: perceptual mechanisms of implicit memory. J Cogn Neurosci 4:244–256, 1992

Schafer R: The Analytic Attitude. New York, Basic Books, 1983

Schore A: Affect Regulation and the Repair of the Self. New York, WW Norton, 2003

Spillius EB: Developments in Kleinian thought: overview and personal view. Br Psychoanalysis Society Bulletin 29:1–19, 1993

Spillius EB: Developments in Kleinian thought: overview and personal view. Psychoanalytic Inquiry 14:324–364, 1994

Spitz RA: Hospitalism: an inquiry into the genesis of psychiatric conditions in early childhood. Psychoanal Study Child 1:53–73, 1945

Spitz RA: No and Yes: On the Genesis of Human Communication. New York, International Universities Press, 1957

Spitz RA: A Genetic Field Theory of Ego Formation: Its Implications for Pathology. New York, International Universities Press, 1959

Spitz RA: The First Year of Life: A Psychoanalytic Study of Normal and Deviant Development of Object Relations. New York, International Universities Press, 1965

Squire LS, Kandel ER: Memory: From Molecules to Memory. New York, Freeman Press, 1999

Steele H, Steele M, Fonagy P: Associations among attachment classifications of mothers, fathers, and their infants: evidence for a relationship-specific perspective. Child Development 67:541–555, 1996

Stern D: The Interpersonal World of the Infant: A View From Psychoanalysis and Developmental Psychology. New York, Basic Books, 1985

Stern D: Acting versus remembering in transference love and infantile love, in On Freud's "Observations on Transference-Love." Edited by Person ES, Hagelin A, Fonagy P. New Haven, CT, Yale University Press, 1993, pp 172–185

Stern D: The process of therapeutic change involving implicit knowledge: some implications of developmental observations for adult psychotherapy. Infant Ment Health J 19:300–308, 1998

Stern D, Sander L, Nahum J, et al: Non-interpretive mechanisms in psychoanalytic therapy: the "something more" than interpretation. Int J Psychoanal 79:903–921, 1998

Stolorow R: Review of "a dynamic systems approach to the development of cognition and action." Int J Psychoanal 78:620–623, 1997

Stolorow R, Atwood G: The mind and the body. Psychoanalytic Dialogues 1:190–202, 1991

Stolorow R, Brandschaft B, Atwood G: Psychoanalytic Treatment: An Intersubjective Approach. Hillsdale, NJ, Analytic Press, 1987

Sullivan HS: The Interpersonal Theory of Psychiatry. Edited by Perry HS, Gawel ML. New York, WW Norton, 1953

Sulloway FJ: Freud: Biologist of the Mind. New York, Basic Books, 1979

Thompson C: Transference and character analysis, in Interpersonal Psychoanalysis. Edited by Green M. New York, Basic Books, 1964, pp 22–31

Tronick EZ: Emotional connection and dyadic consciousness in infant-mother and patient-therapist interactions: commentary on paper by Frank M. Lachman. Psychoanalytic Dialogues 11:187–195, 2001

Tyson P, Tyson RL: Psychoanalytic Theories of Development: An Integration. New Haven, CT Yale University Press, 1990

van IJzendoorn MH: Adult attachment representations, parental responsiveness, and infant attachment: a meta-analysis on the predictive validity of the Adult Attachment Interview. Psychol Bull 117:387–403, 1995

Westen D: The scientific legacy of Sigmund Freud: toward a psychodynamically informed psychological science. Psychol Bull 124:333–371, 1998

Westen D, Ludolph P, Block MJ, et al: Developmental history and object relations in psychiatrically disturbed adolescent girls. Am J Psychiatry 147:1061–1068, 1990a

Westen D, Lohr N, Silk K, et al: Object relations and social cognition in borderlines, major depressives, and normals: a TAT analysis. Psychological Assessment 2:355–364, 1990b

Winnicott DW: Psychoses and child care (1952), in Through Paediatrics to Psychoanalysis. New York, Basic Books, 1975, pp 229–242

Winnicott DW: The theory of the parent-infant relationship, in The Maturational Process and the Facilitating Environment. New York, International Universities Press, 1960, pp 37–55

Winnicott DW: The theory of the parent-infant relationship: further remarks. Int J Psychoanal 43:238–245, 1962

Winnicott DW: Ego distortion in terms of true and false self, in The Maturational Processes and the Facilitating Environment. London, Hogarth Press, 1965a, pp 140–152

Winnicott DW: The Maturational Process and the Facilitating Environment. London, Hogarth Press, 1965b

Winnicott DW: Morals and education, in The Maturational Processes and the Facilitating Environment. New York, International Universities Press, 1965c, pp 93–105

Winnicott DW: Psychotherapy of character disorders, in The Maturational Processes and the Facilitating Environment. Edited by Winnicott DW. London, Hogarth Press, 1965d, 203–216

Winnicott DW: Playing and Reality. London, Tavistock, 1971

Wolf E: Treating the Self. New York, Guilford, 1988

Zahn-Waxler C, Klimes-Dougan B, Slattery MJ: Internalizing problems of childhood and adolescence: prospects, pitfalls, and progress in understanding the development of anxiety and depression. Dev Psychopathol 12:443–466, 2000

9

Interface Between Psychoanalytic Developmental Theory and Other Disciplines

LINDA C. MAYES, M.D.

THERE ARE MANY ROUTES to making a bridge between clinical psychoanalysis and empirical research. The examples most easily recognized as "psychoanalytic research" are those focusing on therapeutic efficacy and outcome and those emphasizing understanding details of the therapeutic process and, thus, ways to measure that process in an analytic therapy (Bellak 1961; Joseph 1975; Lustman 1963; Margolis 1989; Messer 1989). Each of these routes is an appropriate example of the all-too-difficult task of creating a freely traveled bridge between empirical methods and psychoanalysis as a therapeutic endeavor. Indeed, studies of this genre have taken the brunt of the critique of psychoanalysis as a science (or nonscience) and as a collected body of work, and the discipline has been called on to justify the efficacy of psychoanalysis, particularly with adults (Edelson 1989; Fonagy et al. 2002b; Galatzer-Levy et al. 2000; Wallerstein 1988, 1993, 2000, 2003).

Psychoanalysts are increasingly asked to justify their work with empirically validated theoretical propositions and positive, measurable therapeutic outcomes. There is also considerable discussion regarding the interface of so-called evidence-based treatments and psychodynamic approaches (Auchincloss 2002; Clements 2002; Corvin and Fitzgerald 2000; Fonagy 2002, 2003b; Gray 2002). Focusing on an empirical, evidence-based justification of

psychoanalytic treatments is important in particular for refining understanding of the therapeutic goals of psychoanalysis and the mechanisms of action of psychoanalytic interventions. These efforts have led down very productive paths, resulting in better understanding of issues, such as the impact of therapist-patient match (Kantrowitz 1995, 2002; Kantrowitz et al. 1990), better adaptations of specific psychodynamic treatment approaches to patients' diagnostic profiles and needs (Blatt and Auerbach 2003; Blatt et al. 2000; Fonagy et al. 2002b; Mortimore 2003), and increasingly sophisticated methods for studying psychoanalytic process (Jones 1995; Jones and Windholz 1990; Jones et al. 1993).

At the same time, however, progress in bolstering the empirical portfolio for the efficacy and effectiveness of psychoanalytic treatments has been inevitably slow. The reasons for this lack of progress are that there are many brands of psychoanalytic therapy (even within similar parameters of frequency or amount of treatment), few patients, long treatments, many possible domains of outcome, and various competing treatments that, at least in the short run, may produce similar levels of symptom relief and manifest psychological adaptation in either children or adults. Additional challenges include the difficulties of finding outcomes, suited to the goals of psychoanalysis, that are amenable to reliable measurement. That is, many of the currently accepted empirical methods for studying long-term psychological functioning and adaptation are simply not well suited to the complexity of psychoanalytic process and therapeutic goals.

In response to these well-documented challenges, a number of scientists and scholars have turned to what is often called *applied psychoanalytic research*—that is, studies that draw on analytic theory, and even methods or principles of psychodynamic treatment, but that are not primarily studies of psychoanalytic treatment or analytic case material. Studies in this genre seek to find parallels and proofs in contemporary neuroscience, cognitive and developmental psychology, and other scientific fields for the basic propositions of psychoanalytic theory (i.e., validation by association), or they draw on analytic theory for their basic research hypotheses. Finding theoretical harmony in other fields is a fruitful way to bring psychoanalysis to other disciplines and encourage collaborations, and it is intellectual bridging that is essential not only to the growth of psychoanalysis but to growth and intellectual ferment in any field. Indeed, a number of recent discussions regarding the corpus of research in psychoanalysis have pointed to studies in this broad applied genre as exemplars of both a tradition of scientific inquiry in psychoanalysis and a growing new spirit of psychodynamic inquiry (Sonnenberg 1993; Wallerstein 2003).

In this chapter, I discuss the challenges for developing new models of applied psychoanalytic research. An important question is why, within psychoanalysis, there is not a received, accepted, and passed-on culture of developmental empirical research, or at least a psychoanalytic version of developmental studies that facilitates active cross-disciplinary collaboration with other developmental scientists. One very important barrier arises because there are different, though not incompatible, epistemologies and, hence, different ways of asking questions and different methods of study. Making this epistemological barrier explicit is one step toward re-introducing a spirit of empirical inquiry into psychoanalysis and for bringing psychoanalytic perspectives and psychoanalysts into active discourse and collaboration with contemporary developmental, social, and brain sciences. Another barrier relates to perceptions within the established field of psychoanalysis about the professional risks of entering a culture of inquiry and assuming an investigative mind-set. I suggest that there are a number of ways that psychoanalysts may become full partners in investigative endeavors while at the same time maintaining the clinical depth and richness of their day-to-day work with patients.

To illustrate each of these points I present examples from relevant areas of developmental science, or from the work of active psychoanalytic investigators and of applied psychoanalytic bridging between the developmental sciences and psychoanalysis. The examples in the chapter are presented not as paradigmatic of the applied psychoanalytic research genre, for there is really no one model for this kind of applied bridging, but rather as models of how psychoanalysts can be active participants in basic research of great relevance to both developmental science and psychoanalysis.

Two Epistemologies: Psychoanalysis and Developmental Science

What areas of developmental and behavioral neuroscience research might be fertile ground for a psychoanalytically oriented investigation? Examples of such areas are developmental themes such as the transmission of patterns of parenting across generations; the impact of acute and chronic trauma in childhood; the relations among emotional experiences, learning, and memory; and early social development. Indeed, some of the most active areas of research in child psychiatry and developmental psychology are concerned with understanding the building-up of a representational world in early development, with how children enter into the fullness of social relationships, and with what the threats are to that social trajectory (Hesse and Cicchetti 1982). Although they are the province of active developmental research, these themes have long been of interest in psychoanalysis. The child psychoanalyst sees children's growth in terms of the building-up of complex internal mental structures and fantasies that integrate desire and action. Historically, child analysts have been interested in the ways in which a child takes in the social world and transmutes relationships into psychic structures and into a mental life.

At the same time, developmental investigators are defining the various modules that children develop, integrate, and revise as they grow into the social world (Fonagy et al. 2002a; Hesse and Cicchetti 1982). Decades of work on patterns of attachment have laid out the scaffolding for the central role from childhood to adulthood of early relationship templates (Belsky 2002; Fonagy 2003a; Fonagy and Target 2003). Similarly, many have productively defined the social cognitive precursors that a child needs in order to be able fully to comprehend and compute the complex transactions of social discourse: What was he really thinking? Did she not know what has happened? Does my mother's smile mean she really loves me? Without these most basic algorithms for the to-and-fro of mental life, children are as lost as if they were in a foreign country ignorant of the native language. And most recently, elegant interdisciplinary work is beginning to outline how highly socially specialized our brains have become; our species has evolved special brain regions dedicated to the recognition of faceness (George et al. 1999; McCarthy et al. 1997; Rossion et al. 2001), the differentiation of emotion, and the sorting and preservation of our most important, intimate relationships from relationships with casual acquaintances or even strangers. The process of becoming fully and socially human is written into human biology at the most fundamental levels. All of these areas, and more, are putting meat on the bones of that essential mystery: what does it mean to become a successfully adapted, loving, and working member of the human community?—a mystery that is at the core of psychoanalytic theory and clinical focus.

However, despite the depth and human complexity of these questions, few contemporary approaches in developmental psychology to children's social or emotional development have placed a primary emphasis on the emergence of a child's inner experiences, internal world, or the process of symbolization. For example, discussions of the capacity for imagination primarily emphasize the emerging metacognitive capacity to distinguish real from pretend as the essence of an ability for symbolization (Rosen et al. 1997; Taylor and Carlson 1997; Wellman et al. 2001). Similarly, only a few developmental studies have addressed how children's capacities for symbolization emerge in the context of their ongoing relationships with parents and other adults or in the context of psychosocial adversity (Cicchetti and Beeghly 1987). On the other hand, despite the close relation of these kinds of questions to the most central concerns of psychoanalysis, only a small number of psychoanalysts have joined in the discourse (Fonagy and Target 2003); attachment perspectives have been especially fruitful areas for bridging discourse between developmentalists and psychoanalysts (Aber et al. 1999; Fonagy 1999, 2001; Slade 2001; Steele et al. 1999).

That said, however, why is there not a more fruitful dialogue among developmental psychologists, neuroscientists, and analysts who are interested in these most basic aspects of early development? Are there general and specific barriers to analysts becoming more involved and contributing to these areas of developmental research? Obviously there are many possible responses to these questions—some are systemic to each field, some to the culture of research in general, and some to the individual practitioners. No single reply will either solve the dilemma or fully point to the salient issues and a solution. But one set of answers involves shifting epistemologies, or ways of knowing, in both psychoanalysis and developmental sciences that make it more difficult for developmentalists and analysts to find a compatible intellectual meeting ground in addressing issues of the nature of observation and knowl-edge, types of questions, conditions for proof, and sufficient evidence (Fajardo 1998; L.C. Mayes, W. Kessen: "Transparency in Science and Psychoanalysis: The Problem of the Unobservable," unpublished manuscript, 1999).

Parenthetically, these shifting epistemologies or methods for knowing are not only the agents of a widening chasm between psychoanalysis and an empirical tradition but also the product of how psychoanalysis developed in part outside the formal academy and, hence, outside the stimulation and critique of close contact with other disciplines (Mayes and Cohen 1996). In other words, psychoanalysis carries the legacy of always being on the outside looking in—a perception Freud found considerable credence for in, for instance, professorial status being withheld, but also one he imbued with vital urgency in warning his contemporaries to be wary of all critics of psychoanalysis. This organized set of beliefs about standing outside the official academy offers complex challenges for the field. On the one hand, freedom from the strictures of formal disciplines often encourages creativity. On the other, being in constant contact with divergent points of view encourages clarification, borrowing, constructive evaluation, and sharing of knowledge and methods.

Although both adult and child psychoanalysis emerged with little to no contact with formal academic psychology, both psychoanalysis and psychology in their beginnings were firmly grounded in a solid faith in methods based on the objectivity of observation of natural phenomena, a belief characteristic of the nineteenth-century scientific community. Learning to look was the standard of science at that time. Freud believed that "ideas are not the foundation of science, upon which everything rests: that foundation is observation alone" (Freud 1914b/1957, p. 77). He chastised Jung and Adler for "deciding to turn entirely away from observation" and contended that "enthusiasm for the cause even permitted a disregard of scientific logic" (Freud 1914a/1957, p. 62). And by the end of his career, he was perplexed, if not bitter, in his complaint that "I have always felt it a gross injustice that people have refused to treat psychoanalysis like any other natural science…[it is a] science based on observation" (Freud 1925[1924]/1959, p. 58).

Particularly in the social sciences, faith in the authority of observation and the basic empirical method extended well into the mid-twentieth century. Although in other sciences, newer epistemologies, including nonlinear dynamics, changed the primacy of observation as the source of data (Haken 1977, 1988; Prigogine and Stengers 1984), the social sciences stayed grounded in linear, observation-based methods (Mayes 2001). For academic psychology, this emphasis on observation of manifest behavior was integral to the mapping of stages of children's development, as in the work of Piaget, Gesell, and others of the early infant developmentalists (Mayes 1999). The linear, epigenetic theories of development, with past events having predictable, observable manifestations in the present, were readily compatible with psychoanalytic notions of reconstruction and understanding the dynamic etiologies of symptom configurations. Linking manifest behavior with latent meaning was also a compatible exercise for psychology and psychoanalysis, since both had a strong faith in the correspondence between internal experience and what could be observed. And in the early and middle years of psychoanalysis, empirical traditions in psychoanalysis were exemplified by Erikson, Lois Murphy, Bowlby, Ainsworth, Mahler, and Spitz. Investigators such as these blended their analytic and natural science traditions to study the most complex of psychological processes in the consulting room and in playgrounds, group homes, family homes, and villages. They studied play, defense and coping, separation, attachment, and internalization. Like their counterparts in academic psychology at the time, they observed small numbers of children up close in great detail and were comfortable with interpreting internal experiences from observable, measurable behavior. To wit, Erikson's interpretations of the internal fantasy life associated with children's prototypic play (Erikson 1995) or Bowlby's interest in how children's behavioral responses to separations was a window on the complexity and stability of their internal object world (Bowlby 1989). Also, among ego psychologists focused primarily on adults, there was a vital empirical tradition within psychoanalysis, as represented by the work of Gill (Gill and Hoffman 1982), Rappaport, George Klein, and others.

However, developmental psychology and psychoanalysis began to diverge as psychoanalysis shifted to a more individualistic perspective centered on a single patient and analyst and a less absolute, one-to-one correspondence between manifest, observable behavior and latent meaning or internal experience. With accumulated clinical experience with both children and adults, analysts became more cautious about reading internal experience from observable behavior. Any given behavior or symptom could be understood to have multiple meanings and multiple dynamic determinants. Thus, units of data became an individual's perception of experiences as these informed individual fantasies and attributions—data more difficult to generalize across patients and reach consensual agreement about.

Perhaps the clearest statement of this shifting epistemology beginning to distinguish psychoanalysis and developmental psychology came from Anna Freud, who, although respectful of her academic psychology colleagues' careful studies of children's development, maintained a diplomatic but cautious alliance with a tradition she felt had at times misunderstood and misused the psychoanalytic

method (Mayes and Cohen 1996). Although both psychoanalysis and developmental psychology seek to "understand present-day behavior and present day existence as an evolution of possibilities given at some past date" (A. Freud 1951a/1967, p. 118), the analyst is, Anna Freud suggests, involved in "action research" in which findings emerge in the context of the relationship between analyst and child (or adult). Standard tools of measurement that codify objectively specific behaviors or reactions to experimental conditions do not adequately describe a child's response to more usual and complex life situations such as separation and loss, nor in Anna Freud's mind did these techniques give sufficient weight to the unconscious background of conscious behaviors. At the heart of her distinctions was the nature of observational data: how they were gathered, categorized, coded, and interpreted, and what the limits of behavioral observation were. On the one hand, she argued for meticulous, carefully recorded observations of children's moment-to-moment activities and behaviors; on the other, she felt that academic psychology ran the risk of deriving meaning solely from conscious behaviors with little to no understanding that one behavior might have multiple unconscious determinants:

> [T]he observation of manifest, overt behavior marks a step which is not undertaken without misgivings. We ask ourselves whether observational work outside of the analytic setting can ever lead to new discoveries about underlying trends and processes, and can thereby supplement the data gathered through the analyses of adults and children. (A. Freud 1951b/1967, p. 144)

While this may have been a partial misinterpretation, based perhaps on misinformation about how the most creative of academic psychologists working with children were approaching their field, Anna Freud's cautions mark an important, and quiet, shift in basic psychoanalytic observational emphasis and a sign of the gradually more divergent epistemologies. As psychoanalysis moved toward more emphasis on individual experience and meaning, academic psychology started to focus on explaining across groups of individuals and on breaking complex developmental abilities such as imagination, social relationships and attachment, and learning and remembering into modular components (Trop et al. 2002). To be sure, many academic psychologists (Emde et al. 1991; Sander 1987) remain committed to psychoanalysis and study phenomena of interest and relevance to the material emerging in both adult and child analyses, including social referencing, affect regulation, early prosocial behaviors, and the impact of early parental deprivation and loss. Findings from studies of these domains have provided useful metaphors for thinking about analytic material from both children and adults, as discussed at length in the many debates about the relevance of infant research for adult (and child) analysis (Lachmann 2003; Stern 2000; Wolff 1996). However, these studies often take place in the laboratory far from either the consulting room or natural settings such as nurseries, schools, or home. Indeed, current developmental theories have become increasingly modular and function-specific.

To be sure, most of the developmental psychological sciences, until very recently, remained more closely allied with the basic tenets of nineteenth-century empiricism: behavioral observation, consensus among observers, and an emphasis on linear prediction of developmental stages. Most notable is the idea that complex processes are best understood if broken into their component parts. This economy of effort and thought permits a detailed understanding of individual processes and mechanisms of action. Developmental psychology is based on the discovery of regularities in manifest behavior observed across many individuals. In contrast, psychoanalysis shifted to a more individualistic perspective centered on a single patient and analyst. Clinical listening moved away from a primary focus on a theory of development and pathogenesis with an objective observer of the patient's inner life to an appreciation of the subjective experience of the observer and the mutual interactive nature of the psychoanalytic process. The patient's patterns of self-organization and of constructing meaning in the analytic experience are key. In the most extreme form of psychoanalytic subjectivity, linear continuities from past to present are not sought; patient and analyst focus on present-day experiences and forces, particularly in the context of their own dyadic relationship. In child psychoanalysis, these changes in epistemology were reflected in an increasing emphasis on the child's fantasy life in the context of the session with the analyst, paralleled by less involvement by child analysts with parents or in consultative and observational work outside the analytic situation.

In other words, psychoanalysts seek consistencies *within* an individual's life story, whereas practitioners in the developmental sciences seek consistencies *across* individuals. These different epistemologies lead to different kinds of inquiries. For example, psychoanalysts are cautious about generalizations based on exposure to a given set of events such as early abuse, whereas developmental investigators focus on the expectable or most likely consequences of such early events. Although psychoanalysts do not deny that such exposures are life-altering and that there are consistencies among some patients, they tend to gather data patient by patient and thus understand the diverse range of maladaptive and adaptive responses, while the basic investigative developmental epistemology is painstakingly to look for patterns and regularities.

Bringing the Two Epistemologies Together: A Developmental Psychoanalytic Epistemology

The brief review of shifting epistemologies in the previous section does not do full justice to the individual details in the evolution of both fields or to the remaining common ground. Nor does it make clear that in either field these changes were not monolithic. Indeed, with these shifts from a more authoritative faith in the objective observer to an emphasis on meaning and subjectivity, psychoanalysis became more pluralistic and fractionated—no one epistemology prevailed—making it even more difficult in some ways to find common grounds with other fields. But the contrast is for now sufficient to make the point that with such a divergence, the types of questions and methods most central to inquiry in psychoanalysis and developmental psychology also developed along different trajectories.

These differences in questions and methods are a crucial issue for nurturing an empirical tradition within psychoanalysis. It is a matter of learning not simply how to do research in terms of methods of measurement and data analysis (though these are of course important skills), but rather more fundamentally how to think and ask questions in these different epistemologies. These are not inconsistent epistemologies, but they are more readily merged when the differences are made explicit. Consider the following clinical vignette from a research training program in London (Emde and Fonagy 1997; Wallerstein and Fonagy 1999) that brings psychoanalysts interested in empirical research together with established investigators.

A highly motivated psychoanalyst was concerned that so many mothers in a community mental health clinic where she consulted were experiencing the trauma of domestic violence, and she wished to study this phenomenon, with a latent pragmatic goal of refining aspects of her therapeutic interventions with such mothers and their children. Her initial question was how does domestic violence impact a child and parent's development as viewed from a psychoanalytic perspective. What she meant by a psychoanalytic perspective was how a mother understood the meaning of the trauma and how the mother's interpretation of the meaning of the event impacted her ongoing psychological adjustment and response to treatment. The psychoanalyst's goal was to understand the impact of domestic violence not on a group of mothers or their children, but rather on individuals in specific cases, studied one by one. On the basis of this accumulated clinical experience, the psychoanalyst hoped to understand how to inform her therapeutic understanding and interpretations with the next family. In other words, her way of knowing was to accumulate clinical data one case at a time. This method is an important and respectable approach to clinical inquiry, something all clinicians implicitly do in their daily practice, but it is a different epistemology from the one implicit in studying mothers as a group.

When seminar consultants began raising questions about how she would select her sample, such as how she would define domestic violence—Was it first-time or repeated? Was it physical, verbal, or both? Who was the abuser? Were the children witnesses? Were any comorbid conditions present?—the analyst was puzzled by the implicit focus on selecting and defining a sample by external criteria. Equally puzzling were the host of suggestions about assessing maternal functioning that focused on measurable behavior in the parent or child or the parent's response to self-report measures about perceptions, behavior, and emotional responses. The clearest demonstration of different epistemologies was the suggestion that perhaps domestic violence was not a uniquely different type of event, but rather a specific example of an acute trauma, with the attendant hypotheses of how acutely traumatic events impact an adult's ability to function as a parent and a child's emotional development. That is, in addition to domestic violence having unique meaning for the individual, it is also one of a larger category of traumatic events that impact groups of psychological functions by a similar mechanism. The analyst was focusing on understanding individual internal meaning, whereas the developmental investigator was trying to formulate a research question that was generalizable to other similar traumatic phenomena and, hence, mechanisms of effect.

The two perspectives began to come together around reformulating the question as a study of how acute traumatic disruptions in one aspect of perception of self or self-identify (e.g., acutely seeing oneself as a victim who is now vulnerable) impact a mother's self-appraisal across other areas. In this way, the strength of the psychoanalytic focus on an individual and on the individuality of experience and self-definition was brought to bear, while at the same time a model was implicit that required summarizing across individuals and making predictions based on accumulated trends and patterns. An epistemology based on knowing from close process with individuals was integrated with one based on finding patterns across individuals.

Furthermore, once the emphasis is placed on disruption in self-identity as one mechanism for the traumatic impact of domestic violence, it is possible to think across other, similar insults to a person's sense of self and to generate related questions and hypotheses. The methods are then more easily defined and the required measurements clearer. Also, once a model is made clear, it is possible to be open to competing or complementary points of view—maybe not only the disruption in self-identity but rather or additionally the experience of shame, fear, vulnerability, and isolation. The well-conceived question generates

other research questions. How does a change in an adult's self-perception concerning her safety and vulnerability influence her self-perception as a parent, her perception of her children's psychological needs, and in turn her children's perception of and behavior toward her. The question is dynamic in three ways: exploring internal meaning, including relationships to internalized objects; considering change across time; and taking into account the relational context of the event and the impact on other persons. Also implied is a model of therapeutic change: as perception of self-identity changes, internal appraisals also change, and with that, presumably external behavior changes as well. In this kind of rephrasing, analysts and developmentalists are then working at the same table with overlapping investigative epistemologies.

To be more explicit: what features of a developmental psychoanalytic epistemology would permit this kind of collaborative empirical psychoanalytic inquiry? At least four principles must be followed (Cicchetti and Cohen 1995):

1. Recognize that individuals may shift between normal and abnormal modes of functioning as a consequence of differing developmental stressors and environmental conditions.
2. Focus on individual patterns of adaptation and maladaptation as defined by the context of the individual's environment. For example, extraordinary vigilance and preoccupation may be adaptive for some children growing up in the midst of community violence, but it poses problems for their adjustment to a classroom or their ability to feel safe and able to play imaginatively.
3. Examine transactions between biological or genetic factors and external environmental conditions as related to patterns of adaptation and maladaptation.
4. Use naturally occurring events or "experiments of nature," such as trauma, to understand the expected developmental ontogeny of specific functions. These traumatic or stressful events show the interaction between often psychologically and biologically overwhelming events and developmental adaptation.

The emphasis in of these points is on individual change and self-ordering and on nonlinear progression across development; it is on studying the development of the individual in interaction with others. Most questions emerging from this perspective are not ones of linear causality—asking whether early trauma leads to later depression, for example—or linear stability—asking whether early self-regulatory difficulties convey a lifelong vulnerability to anxiety. Rather, the emphasis is on asking how patterns or trajectories of development impact ongoing adaptation, much as clinicians often ask how patterns of interaction between analyst and patient play out across sessions and prevent or facilitate flexibility and change.

One example of this developmental perspective and epistemology comes from studies of children exposed to toxins and/or maternal stress during pregnancy. Often these studies are predicated on a very basic developmental question: Does an adverse early event such as prenatal drug exposure lead to disturbances in later cognitive, emotional, or social development? Asking a question in this way is compatible with the original psychoanalytic developmental epistemology implicit in asking how early constitutional vulnerabilities affect emerging ego capacities (e.g., cognitive functioning, language development, regulation of emotions) or how these vulnerabilities are expressed in children's response to a therapist's interventions. Key in each of these questions is the presumption of the linear impact of an earlier adverse event on later impaired functioning. Indeed, there is growing evidence linking early stress such as maternal anxiety or maternal use of drugs such as cocaine to later childhood problems with emotional regulation, delayed social and language skills, poor impulse control, and impoverished parent-child interactions when children exposed to these conditions are compared with nonexposed children (Mayes 2002; Mayes and Ward 2003).

But simple questions of whether exposure to X leads to Y early or late in development do not address in detail interactions between biological vulnerability and environment and do not prompt study of patterns or trajectories of development across time, the key focus of a developmental psychoanalytic perspective. For example, a mother's capacity to reflect on her own and her child's mental states as separate and distinct from her own serves vital regulatory functions that are central to attenuating the effects of drug use and trauma on a range of child and parent outcomes. Similarly, children's ability to use their imaginary world as a practice ground, a place for emotional solace or pleasure, and a place to protect and nurture their deepest of desires emerges in the context of their parents' making room for their children in their own mental world. It may be that, although prenatal exposure to drugs of abuse conveys vulnerability in stress response systems that in turn have an impact of other areas of functioning, including language and cognitive capacities, these early to later relationships are more or less expressed depending on a mother's psychological reflective capacities vis-à-vis her child. In turn, the better developed are children's capacities for metarepresentation, the less severe is the apparent effect of prenatal exposure on later cognitive, language, and other neuropsychological functions subserving attention and emotional regulation. Maternal reflective capacities and children's metarepresentational abilities may also me-

diate the impact of exposure to the community violence and general environmental poverty so characteristic of drug-using environments (Mayes and Truman 2001). In these models, a perinatal biological risk is only a starting point in a transactional, nonlinear model of development that is compatible with psychoanalytic theories of development and also with the investigative standards of contemporary developmental science.

Assuming an Investigative Mind-set in Psychoanalysis: Models for Collaboration

From the standpoint of other developmental sciences, it is a fertile time to introduce these developmental psychoanalytic points of view. A number of developmental scholars have called for perspectives that move away from emphases on linear models of development and prediction toward nonlinear perspectives (Emde 1994; Mayes 2001; Sameroff 1989; Thelen 1984, 1989; Thelen and Smith 1994). Furthermore, within developmental psychology, there are many examples of investigations that are formulating questions about the multiple factors that mediate the impact of, for example, early trauma that are compatible with psychoanalytic ways of thinking. There is interest in the possibility that in the full organism studied in the context of family, community, and culture, capacities such as emotional regulation function differently than when studied in the laboratory.

The past two decades have brought us dramatic advances in understanding the complexity of brain functioning and brain development. Contemporary working theories of, for example, learning reveal a much more dynamic model of the brain than heretofore understood—a brain in which structure changes at the cellular level in response to both positive and negative events, new connections and networks are formed throughout life, and apparently new neurons are generated in the healing aftermath of stress and trauma (Royo et al. 2003). Neuroimaging techniques allow neural response to be visualized in nearly real time, and functional neuroimaging paradigms are becoming ever more psychologically sophisticated so as to permit studying the interface of emotion and cognition and the responses of a parent to the salient cues of a new infant (Lorberbaum et al. 2002) or of an adult to a romantic partner (Bartels and Zeki 2000). Similar advances in genetics have opened up whole new areas of understanding how experiences turn genes on and off, regulating aspects of neural function (Davis et al. 2003). Notably, while many psychoanalysts are catching on in their conviction of the relevance of neuroscience for psychoanalysis, cognitive and social psychologists have already formed very productive collaborations with the basic neurosciences, particularly around the development of creative neuropsychological paradigms to be used with functional neuroimaging procedures. Partnerships among the psychological and neural sciences are demonstrating the creative possibilities in collaborations across disciplines that have traditionally worked at different levels of discourse. Cognitive neuroscientists have also rekindled interest in subjective experience as a legitimate arena for empirical study (Fuchs 2002). The implicit question is, How can psychoanalysts also create such productive collaborations and join investigative teams?

While the epistemological differences already discussed create one barrier to models of collaborative psychoanalytic research, a second barrier comes from a deeply held concern within psychoanalysis that any attempt to link psychoanalytic concepts to the basic brain, cognitive, or social sciences exposes psychoanalysis to the leveling, homogenizing effects of reductionism (Bickle 1998). In other words, joining in basic research runs the risk of a loss of the clinical richness and vitality that many feel are most valuable about psychoanalysis and make our field unique, especially in the contemporary climate of symptom- and pharmacology-focused mental health care. Among the common fallacies about what it means to be an investigator is the suggestion that to embrace an empirical stance is to give up a certain flexibility and openness. For some psychoanalysts, the act of research distills and desiccates the hot ebb and flow of life into the cold, distant, measured world and changes an individual human being with a story into a research subject and, ultimately, to a lifeless line of data. There is a continuing, and sometimes apparently wide, divide between the analytic practitioner and the analytic scholar working as theoretician, empirical investigator, or both.

While it may be true that the developmental and brain sciences do not have a direct or immediate impact on clinical psychoanalytic practice, there are considerable risks in continuing the divide, real or perceived, between psychoanalytic practitioners and those seeking to advance the interface with the physical, brain sciences—even if these identities sometimes reside in the same individual. Ignoring the need to develop a culture of inquiry and an empirical tradition within psychoanalysis ultimately and tragically will limit the intellectual evolution of psychoanalysis by limiting opportunities to form collaborative partnerships with our colleagues in other disciplines who are interested in similar questions of mind and brain. Once again, making this potential barrier regarding fears of reductionism explicit is a key step in developing viable models of applied psychoanalytic research.

For psychoanalytic inquiries, top-down approaches that relate mental functions to more molecular or neurobiological domains are more compatible than bottom-up approaches that seek to build functions from their molecular elements. There are a number of examples of successful partnerships between psychoanalysts and developmental scientists around these kinds of top-down models that seek to relate, for example, a function such as repression to other biological and psychological domains. It is important to note that these top-down approaches are different from intellectual curiosity about convergences with another field such as neuroscience; the former involve actually studying dynamic constructs in collaboration with scientists from other disciplines such as behavioral neuroscience.

The recent interest in the neurobiology of affiliation provides an example of this kind of psychoanalytic developmental inquiry that involves collaborations among psychoanalysts, developmentalists, neuroscientists, and neuroimagers. A growing body of data from preclinical models reveals that an adult's transition to parenthood involves a complex cascade of genetic and neurobiological conditions and events that change both neural structure and function and are related to very specific caretaking behaviors by the adult toward the infant (Francis et al. 1999, 2002; Leckman and Herman 2002). Thus, the initiation of parental caregiving reflects an individual's genetic endowment, the priming of critical neurobiological circuits, and the early experience of being cared for as a child. These studies are also supporting traditionally held psychoanalytic clinical tenets in the intergenerational transmission of parenting behaviors and the impact of parenting on neural regulatory systems such as stress reactivity and novelty responsiveness (Francis et al. 1999; Ladd et al. 2000).

At the same time, the psychological transition to parenthood has been a phase of great interest to psychoanalysts. Winnicott (1956/1975) captured this psychological transition in his concept of primary maternal preoccupation. Describing the state as "almost an illness," he called attention to the psychological experience that mothers must have and recover from in order to create and sustain an environment that can meet the physical and psychological needs of their infant. In other words, pregnancy and the perinatal period involve an altered mental state characterized by excitement and heightened sensitivity to environmental and emotional cues, especially those from the infant. Although this concept has been incorporated into many clinical formulations of failed or disordered mother-infant interactions, it has received little attention as a normative process. That is, how much do both men and women need to become psychologically preoccupied with their infant-to-be, to make room in their minds, as it were, for a new person, in order to be able to care for that infant and be attentive to all its physical and psychological needs? A further question is, Are there neural and physiological concomitants to this change?

Studies conducted by psychoanalytically informed investigators lend reliable methods to efforts to explore Winnicott's clinical formulations. In humans, the initiation of maternal behavior is associated with intense parental preoccupations (Leckman and Mayes 1999; Leckman et al. 1999, 2004). The content of these preoccupations includes intrusive worries concerning the parents' adequacy as parents and the infant's safety and well-being. Even before the child is born, parents preoccupy themselves with creating a safe and secure environment for the infant. Major cleaning and renovation projects are commonplace as the human form of nest building unfolds. After birth, this same sense of heightened responsibility will compel parents to check on the baby frequently, even at times when they know the baby is fine. Cleaning, grooming, and dressing behaviors also carry a special valence to the degree that they permit the closeness between parent and infant and provide for frequent inspection of the infant's body and appearance.

How these complex mental states of preoccupation are reflected in neural circuitry and how a special neural circuitry prepares adults to be especially sensitive to the needs of their infant is the focus of a series of studies from at least three different laboratories, of which two involve psychoanalysis as members of the research team. Neuroimaging studies from these laboratories have begun to examine human parental response to infant cries and visual cues (Lorberbaum et al. 2002; Swain et al. 2003). In these studies, which show more activity in regions of the brain involved especially with reward pathways (e.g., medial prefrontal, orbitofrontal and cingulate cortices, thalamus, midbrain, hypothalamus, and striatum), considerable attention is also being given to the relation between brain activation and complex psychological constructs such as parental preoccupation and sensitivity to infant cues. This work is an example of the top-down approaches to linking psychoanalytic constructs with more basic biological and neurological levels of analyses that illustrate collaborative research models most conducive to psychoanalysts joining the research team.

The current trend among both the basic and social sciences is to cross disciplines, share methods, and work together on questions of common interests. As a result, traditional disciplines are being reordered as traditional boundaries are broken and redrawn along thematic lines. Thus, the time is especially appropriate for building collaborative programs involving psychoanalysts and, vice versa, to make a place for colleagues from related scientific fields

in psychoanalytic institutes and professional organizations. These interdisciplinary collaborations between developmentalists and psychoanalysts are also facilitated by psychoanalysts actively engaging in discussions with colleagues from other disciplines, co-teaching seminars, and encouraging candidates to be curious about related fields. Similarly, basic developmental research seminars need to be a key component of psychoanalytic education that bring young analysts together with experienced investigators with an interest in developmental issues that are at the interface of psychoanalysis. This model of collaboration is different from intellectual curiosity about convergences with another field such as neuroscience. Instead, in such a model, psychoanalysts are full collaborators—members of the research team engaged furthering discourse, learning and developing methods, and refining questions.

Conclusion

Strengthening an empirical tradition within psychoanalysis raises a number of challenges. Not the least of these is the challenge of coming to terms with divergent epistemologies, one of which focuses on individuals and the other of which focuses on patterns across individuals. Addressing this epistemological divide, as well as attitudes toward empirical methods, is an essential step in developing and nurturing a developmental psychoanalytic research tradition that studies trajectories across time in the most basic and complex of psychological functions, including attachment, internalization, and the building-up of a representational world. It is critical that new models of collaborative psychoanalytic research be encouraged in which psychoanalysts join multidisciplinary research teams. Techniques borrowed from other fields can be fruitfully applied to psychoanalytically relevant developmental questions. While there is no doubt that the psychoanalytic focus on mental representations and meaning constitutes a domain of discourse very different from the neuroscience focus on cellular processes or basic cognitive computations, drawing on the work from the developmental brain sciences is not about finding brain mechanisms to correspond to mental capacities, but instead about defining and studying a psychoanalytic phenomenon from converging and complementary perspectives.

References

Aber JL, Belsky J, Slade A, et al: Stability and change in maternal representations of their relationship with their toddlers. Dev Psychol 35:1038–1048, 1999

Auchincloss EL: The place of psychoanalytic treatments within psychiatry. Arch Gen Psychiatry 59:501–503, 2002

Bartels A, Zeki S: The neural basis of romantic love. Neuroreport 11:3829–3834, 2000

Bellak L: Research in psychoanalysis. Psychoanal Q 30:519–548, 1961

Bickle J: Psychoneural Reduction: The New Wave. Cambridge, MA, MIT Press, 1998

Belsky J: Developmental origins of attachment styles. Attach Hum Dev 4:166–170, 2002

Blatt SJ, Auerbach JS: Psychodynamic measures of therapeutic change. Psychoanal Q 23:268–307, 2003

Blatt SJ, Zuroff DC, Bondi CM, et al: Short- and long-term effects of medication and psychotherapy in the brief treatment of depression: further analyses of data from the NIMH TDCRP. Psychotherapy Research 10:215–234, 2000

Bowlby J: The role of attachment in personality development and psychopathology, in The Course of Life, Vol 1: Infancy. Edited by Greenspan SI, Pollock GH. New York, International Universities Press, 1989, pp 229–270

Cicchetti D, Beeghly M: Symbolic development in maltreated youngsters: an organizational perspective. New Dir Child Dev 36:47–68, 1987

Cicchetti D, Cohen DJ: Perspectives on developmental psychopathology, in Developmental Psychopathology, Vol 1: Theory and Methods. Edited by Cicchetti D, Cohen DJ. Oxford, England, Wiley, 1995, pp 3–20

Clements NA: Evidence-based psychotherapy. Journal of Psychiatric Practice 8:51–53, 2002

Corvin A, Fitzgerald M: Evidence-based medicine, psychoanalysis, and psychotherapy. Psychoanalytic Psychotherapy 14:143–151, 2000

Davis S, Bozon B, Laroche S: How necessary is the activation of the immediate early gene zif268 in synaptic plasticity and learning? Behav Brain Res 142:17–30, 2003

Edelson M: The nature of psychoanalytic theory: implications for psychoanalytic research. Psychoanal Q 9:169–192, 1989

Emde R: Individuality, context, and the search for meaning. Child Dev 65:719–737, 1994

Emde R, Fonagy P: An emerging culture for psychoanalytic research? Int J Psychoanal 78:643–652, 1997

Emde RN, Biringen Z, Clyman RB, et al: The moral self of infancy: affective core and procedural knowledge. Dev Rev 11:251–270, 1991

Erikson EH: A Way of Looking at Things: Selected Papers From 1930 to 1980. New York, WW Norton, 1995

Fajardo B: A new view of developmental research for psychoanalysts. J Am Psychoanal Assoc 46:185–207, 1998

Fonagy P: Points of contact and divergence between psychoanalytic and attachment theories: Is psychoanalytic theory truly different? Psychoanal Q 19:448–480, 1999

Fonagy P: The human genome and the representational world: the role of early mother-infant interaction in creating an interpersonal interpretive mechanism. Bull Menninger Clin 65:427–448, 2001

Fonagy P: Evidence-based medicine and its justification, in Outcomes of Psychoanalytic Treatment: Perspectives for Therapists and Researchers. Edited by Leuzinger-Bohleber M, Target M. London, Whurr Publishers, 2002, pp 53–59

Fonagy P: Attachment theory and psychoanalysis. Journal of Child Psychotherapy 29:109–120, 2003a

Fonagy P: The research agenda: the vital need for empirical research in child psychotherapy. Journal of Child Psychotherapy 29:129–136, 2003b

Fonagy P, Target M: Psychoanalytic Theories: Perspectives From Developmental Psychopathology. London, Whurr Publishers, 2003

Fonagy P, Gergely G, Jurist EL, et al: Affect Regulation, Mentalization, and the Development of the Self. New York, Other Press, 2002a

Fonagy P, Target M, Cottrell D, et al: What Works for Whom? New York, Guilford, 2002b

Francis DD, Champagne FC, Liu D, et al: Maternal care, gene expression, and the development of individual differences in stress reactivity. Ann N Y Acad Sci 896:66–84, 1999

Francis DD, Diorio J, Plotsky PM, et al: Environmental enrichment reverses the effects of maternal separation on stress reactivity. J Neurosci 22:7840–7843, 2002

Freud A: The contribution of psychoanalysis to genetic psychology (1951a). The Writings of Anna Freud, Vol 4. New York, International Universities Press, 1967, pp 107–142

Freud A: Observations on child development (1951b), in The Writings of Anna Freud, Vol 4. New York, International Universities Press, 1967, pp 143–162

Freud S: On the history of the psycho-analytic movement (1914a), in Standard Edition of the Complete Psychological Works of Sigmund Freud, Vol 14. Translated and edited by Strachey J. London, Hogarth Press, 1957, pp 3–66

Freud S: On narcissism: an introduction (1914b), in Standard Edition of the Complete Psychological Works of Sigmund Freud, Vol 14. Translated and edited by Strachey J. London, Hogarth Press, 1957, pp 67–102

Freud S: An autobiographical study (1925[1924]), in Standard Edition of the Complete Psychological Works of Sigmund Freud, Vol 20. Translated and edited by Strachey J. London, Hogarth Press, 1959, pp 1–74

Fuchs T: The challenge of neuroscience: psychiatry and phenomenology today. Psychopathology 35:319–326, 2002

Galatzer-Levy RM, Bachrach H, Skolnikoff A, et al: Does Psychoanalysis Work? New Haven, CT, Yale University Press, 2000

George N, Dolan RJ, Fink GR, et al: Contrast polarity and face recognition in the human fusiform gyrus. Nat Neurosci 2:574–580, 1999

Gill MM, Hoffman IZ: Analysis of transference, II: studies of nine audio-recorded psychoanalytic sessions. Psychol Issues 54:1–236, 1982

Gray SH: Evidence-based psychotherapeutics. J Am Acad Psychoanal 30:3–16, 2002

Haken H: Synergetics: An Introduction. Heidelberg, Germany, Springer-Verlag, 1977

Haken H: Information and Self-Organization. Heidelberg, Germany, Springer-Verlag, 1988

Hesse P, Cicchetti D: Perspectives on an integrated theory of emotional development. New Dir Child Dev 16:3–48, 1982

Jones EE: How will psychoanalysis study itself? in Research in Psychoanalysis. Edited by Shapiro T, Emde RN. Madison, CT, International Universities Press, 1995, pp 91–108

Jones EE, Windholz M: The psychoanalytic case study: toward a method for systematic inquiry. J Am Psychoanal Assoc 38: 985–1015, 1990

Jones EE, Cumming JD, Pulos SM: Tracing clinical themes across phases of treatment by a Q-set, in Psychodynamic Treatment Research: A Handbook for Clinical Practice. Edited by Miller NE, Luborsky L. New York, Basic Books, 1993, pp 14–36

Joseph ED: Psychoanalysis-science and research: twin studies as a paradigm. J Am Psychoanal Assoc 23:3–31, 1975

Kantrowitz JL: The beneficial aspects of the patient analyst match. Int J Psychoanal 76:299–313, 1995

Kantrowitz JL: The triadic match: the interactive effect of supervisor, candidate, and patient. J Am Psychoanal Assoc 50: 939–968, 2002

Kantrowitz JL, Katz AL, Paolitto F: Follow-up of psychoanalysis five to ten years after termination, III: the relation between the resolution of the transference and the patient-analyst match. J Am Psychoanal Assoc 38:655–678, 1990

Lachmann F: Some contributions of empirical infant research to adult psychoanalysis. What have we learned? How can we apply it? J Anal Psychol 48:130–134, 2003

Ladd CO, Huot RL, Thrivikraman KV, et al: Long-term behavioral and neuroendocrine adaptations to adverse early experience, in Progress in Brain Research: The Biological Basis for Mind Body Interactions. Edited by Mayer EA, Saper CB. Amsterdam, Elsevier, 2000, pp 81–103

Leckman JF, Herman A: Maternal behavior and developmental psychopathology. Biol Psychiatry 51:27–43, 2002

Leckman JF, Mayes LC: Preoccupations and behaviors associated with romantic and parental love: perspectives on the origin of OCD. Child Adolesc Clin North America 8:635–65, 1999

Leckman JF, Mayes R, Feldman R, et al: Early parental preoccupations and behaviors. Acta Psychiatr Scand 100:1–26, 1999

Leckman JF, Feldman R, Swain JE, et al: Primary parental preoccupation: circuits, genes, and the crucial role of the environment. J Neural Transm 111:753–771, 2004

Lorberbaum JP, Newman JD, Horwitz AR, et al: A potential role for thalamocingulate circuitry in human maternal behavior. Biol Psychiatry 51:431–445, 2002

Lustman SL: Some issues in contemporary psychoanalytic research. Psychoanal Study Child 18:51–74, 1963

Margolis BD: Research in modern psychoanalysis. Modern Psychoanalysis 14:131–144, 1989

Mayes LC: Clocks, engines, and quarks—love, dreams, and genes: what makes development happen? Psychoanal Study Child 54:169–192, 1999

Mayes LC: The twin poles of order and chaos: development as a dynamic, self-ordering system. Psychoanal Study Child 56:137–170, 2001

Mayes LC: A behavioral teratogenic model of the impact of prenatal cocaine exposure on arousal regulatory systems. Neurotoxicol Teratol 24:385–395, 2002

Mayes LC, Cohen DJ: Anna Freud and developmental psychoanalytic psychology. Psychoanal Study Child 51:117–141, 1996

Mayes LC, Truman S: Substance abuse and parenting, in Handbook of Parenting. Edited by Bornstein M. Hillsdale, NJ, Erlbaum, 2001, pp 329–359

Mayes LC, Ward A: Principles of neurobehavioral teratology, in Neurodevelopmental Mechanisms in Psychopathology. Edited by Cicchetti D, Walker E. New York, Cambridge University Press, 2003, pp 3–33

McCarthy G, Puce A, Gore JC, et al: Face-specific processing in the human fusiform gyrus. J Cogn Neurosci 9:605–610, 1997

Messer SB: The psychoanalytic process: theory, clinical observation, and empirical research. Psychoanalytic Psychology 6:111–114, 1989

Mortimore C: What works for whom? A critical review of treatments for children and adolescents. Br J Clin Psychol 42: 433–434, 2003

Prigogine I, Stengers I: Order Out of Chaos: Man's New Dialogue With Nature. New York, Bantam, 1984

Rosen CS, Schwebel DC, Singer JL: Preschoolers' attributions of mental states in pretense. Child Dev 68:1133–1142, 1997

Rossion B, Schiltz C, Robaye L, et al: How does the brain discriminate familiar and unfamiliar faces? A PET study of face categorical perception. J Cogn Neurosci 13:1019–1034, 2001

Royo NC, Schouten JW, Fulp CT, et al: From cell death to neuronal regeneration: building a new brain after traumatic brain injury. J Neuropathol Exp Neurol 62:801–811, 2003

Sameroff A: Commentary: general systems and the regulation of development, in Systems and Development: The Minnesota Symposia on Child Psychology. Edited by Gunnar M, Thelen E. Hillsdale, NJ, Lawrence Erlbaum, 1989, pp 219–235

Sander L: Awareness of inner experience: a systems perspective on self-regulatory process in early development. Child Abuse Negl 11:339–346, 1987

Slade A: Reflective functioning: a discussion. Journal of Infant Child and Adolescent Psychotherapy 1:43–48, 2001

Sonnenberg SM: Self-analysis, applied analysis, and analytic fieldwork: a discussion of methodology in psychoanalytic interdisciplinary research, in The Psychoanalytic Study of Society, Vol 18: Essays in Honor of Alan Dundes. Edited by Boyer LB, Boyer RM. Hillsdale, NJ, Analytic Press, 1993, pp 443–463

Steele H, Steele M, Croft C, et al: Infant-mother attachment at one year predicts children's understanding of mixed emotions at six years. Social Development 8:161–178, 1999

Stern DN: The relevance of empirical infant research to psychoanalytic theory and practice, in Clinical and Observational Psychoanalytic Research: Roots of a Controversy. Edited by Sandler J, Sandler A-M. Madison, CT, International Universities Press, 2000, pp 73–90

Swain JE, Leckman JF, Mayes LC, et al: The neural circuitry of human parent-infant attachment in the early postpartum (Poster 192). Presented at the 42nd annual meeting of American College of Neuropsychopharmacology, December 7–11, 2003

Taylor M, Carlson SM: The relation between individual differences in fantasy and theory of mind. Child Dev 68:436–455, 1997

Thelen E: Learning to walk: ecological demands and phylogenetic constraints, in Advances in Infancy Research. Edited by Lipsitt LP. Norwood, NJ, Ablex, 1984, pp 213–250

Thelen E: Self-organization in developmental processes: can systems approaches work, in Systems and Development: The Minnesota Symposia on Child Psychology. Edited by Gunnar M, Thelen E. Hillsdale, NJ, Lawrence Erlbaum, 1989, pp 77–117

Thelen E, Smith LB: A Dynamic Systems Approach to the Development of Cognition and Action. Cambridge, MA, MIT Press, 1994

Trop GS, Burke ML, Trop JL: Thinking dynamically in psychoanalytic theory and practice: a review of intersubjectivity theory, in Postmodern Self Psychology: Progress in Self Psychology. Edited by Goldberg A. Hillsdale, NJ, Analytic Press, 2002, pp 129–147

Wallerstein RS: Psychoanalysis, psychoanalytic science, and psychoanalytic research: 1986. J Am Psychoanal Assoc 36:3–30, 1988

Wallerstein RS: Psychoanalysis as science: challenges to the data of psychoanalytic research, in Psychodynamic Treatment Research: A Handbook for Clinical Practice. Edited by Miller NE, Luborsky LE, et al. New York, Basic Books, 1993, pp 97–106

Wallerstein RS: Psychoanalytic research: where do we disagree? in Clinical and Observational Psychoanalytic Research. Edited by Sandler J, Sandler A-M, et al. Madison, CT, International Universities Press, 2000, pp 27–31

Wallerstein RS: Psychoanalytic therapy research: its coming of age. Psychoanal Q 23:375–404, 2003

Wallerstein RS, Fonagy P: Psychoanalytic research and the IPA: history, present status, and future potential. Int J Psychoanal 80:91–109, 1999

Wellman HM, Cross D, Watson J: Meta-analysis of theory-of-mind development: the truth about false belief. Child Dev 72:655–684, 2001

Winnicott DW: Primary maternal preoccupation (1956), in Through Paediatrics to Psycho-Analysis. New York, Basic Books, 1975, pp 300–305

Wolff P: The irrelevance of infant observations for psychoanalysis. J Am Psychoanal Assoc 44:369–392, 1996

10

Attachment Theory and Research

MARY TARGET, Ph.D.

IN THE LAST DECADE, attachment theory has become of increasing interest and appeal to psychoanalysts, and attachment research has partially jumped the general barrier between psychoanalysts and researchers (see Chapter 9, "Integrating the Epistemology of Clinical Psychoanalysis and Developmental Science"). This development is remarkable, given that Bowlby's development of attachment theory initially drew heated criticism from the pioneers of child psychoanalysis in particular and from psychoanalysts in general (Fonagy 2001). However, as I maintain in this chapter, some features that made attachment theory anathema at first have gradually come to be acceptable and are now advantages: the introduction of biological principles in understanding personality and relationships (really a reintroduction because, of course, Freud began with that framework); a linking of empirical and theoretical evidence and, related to that, a building of bridges with a range of neighboring disciplines; and attention to the nonconscious (procedural or implicit) as well as dynamically unconscious determinants of our feelings, thoughts, and actions. These procedural or implicit determinants of personality structure and affect regulation are, in my view, closely relevant to the understanding of character devel-

opment and personality disorder. They are our staple clinical diet now, in contrast to the neurotic conditions that preoccupied Freud and his early followers and the psychotic disorders that interested some—such as Kleinian—analysts, both of which focused on primitive defenses and states of mind.

Perhaps the most important of these reasons for interest in attachment theory among analysts is the extensive empirical base that attachment theory has developed, together with the lively interest in the theory among those in neighboring disciplines, not just psychology but developmental neuroscience and other biological fields as well. Such interest is not so easy for psychoanalysis to come by, and we may wish to consider why it is that attachment theory, rather than other offshoots of psychoanalysis, has attracted continuing and growing respect from other scientists.

Along with a strong empirical base, attachment theory offers a unifying, life-span perspective: a systematic way of understanding (and studying) the impacts of early and later emotional relationships and of traumatic experiences. It is a theory of development that has not only things to say about the infant mind and what makes the "good

This chapter draws on previous work in collaboration with Dr. Peter Fonagy. The author gratefully acknowledges his contributions.

enough mother," but also—increasingly as the theory and its research base grow—new insights into middle childhood, adolescence, sexual partnership, parenthood, aging, and death—about the vicissitudes of love and loss. Hence, it potentially speaks to some of our most profound emotional experiences and to their underlying organization: intimacy, joy, anxiety, loneliness, jealousy, feelings of being safe and accepted with our needs understood, and what we have to do to our minds when that feeling is not there.

Background: Foundations in Bowlby

John Bowlby's thinking about parent-child attachment started at the beginning of his working life, in a home for maladjusted boys. He worked with two boys whose relationships with their mothers had been severely disrupted, and he was convinced that this had had a formative impact. Ten years later, he published a study of the backgrounds of 44 juvenile thieves (Bowlby 1944), consolidating his view that early mother-child separation laid the foundations for social and emotional disturbance. These juveniles, especially those who appeared "affectionless," were much more likely than other referred children to have experienced prolonged separation from parents. In the following years, Bowlby (1951) reviewed evidence on the effects of institutionalization on young children and found that those who had had least maternal care tended to show the same symptoms as the "affectionless" delinquent juveniles.

Bowlby's hypothesis that disturbed behavior was a result of maternal deprivation came under heavy criticism (e.g., Rutter 1971) from those who thought that the empirical evidence was weak or ambiguous and the "mother blaming" simplistic. However, the films of James Robertson, which directly represented the impact on toddlers of separation from their parents when they were admitted to hospital or residential nursery (Robertson 1962), did much to persuade the public and professionals of Bowlby's case, and helped to change entrenched attitudes to the health and social care of children. Christoph Heinicke's research replicated Robertson's findings (see Heinicke and Westheimer 1966).

Bowlby (1969, 1973) later formally described a sequence of reactions to separation: *protest, despair,* and then *detachment.* Protest is shown by crying, anger, attempts to escape, and searching for the parent. The sequence may last a week, and the reactions are worse at night. Despair follows: the child withdraws from contact and activity, cries less but appears sad, and may be hostile to another child or a favorite object brought from home (Bowlby 1973). The final phase, detachment, involves apparent recovery of sociability and the acceptance of care by other adults, but the child behaves very abnormally (with indifference or coldness) if the original caregiver comes back.

Bowlby was interested in and influenced by a number of other disciplines, especially embryology, ethology, control systems theory, and cognitive science (I. Bretherton 1985). He adopted the concept of critical periods in embryology:

> If growth is to proceed smoothly, the tissue must be exposed to the influence of the appropriate organizer at certain critical periods. In the same way, if mental development is to proceed smoothly, it would appear to be necessary for the undifferentiated psyche to be exposed to the influence of the psychic organiser—the mother. (Bowlby 1951, p. 53)

Thus, he suggested that the child's capacity for self-regulation is built on an experience of being regulated by the mother: "She is his ego and his superego. Gradually he learns these arts himself, and as he does, the skilled parent transfers the roles to him" (Bowlby 1951, p. 53). In general, he noted, "The infant and young child should experience a warm, intimate, and continuous relationship with his mother (or permanent mother substitute) in which both find satisfaction and enjoyment" (Bowlby 1951, p. 13). Bowlby thought that the child who did not have this would show partial deprivation—an excessive need to be loved or to punish, self-dislike, or depression—or complete deprivation—listlessness and delayed development, and later on, superficiality, callousness, poor concentration, lying, and compulsive stealing (Bowlby 1951). Later, Bowlby enriched his model in line with the growing evidence of multiple developmental pathways, in which a variety of constitutional, social, and relational factors jointly determine which final pathway is followed (Rutter 1989).

The influence of ethology can be seen in Bowlby's comparison between imprinting as in animals in critical periods and human attachment behavior. Bowlby did not share the psychoanalytic view that attachment was secondary to need satisfaction (feeding). Affectional bonds were seen as primary. So a baby's sucking, clinging, following, and smiling were instinctual responses serving to form a bond between mother and child (Bowlby 1958). These "proximity-seeking signals" prompted corresponding caregiving behavior from the parent. Attachment behavior was conceptualized as a motivational system, distinct from other drives or motivational systems. Developmental psychology has made this point of view seem obvious (e.g., Meltzoff 1995), but for the psychoanalytic orthodoxy at the time it was entirely unacceptable.

Bowlby (1973) distinguished two separate "control systems," one that maintains access to the attachment figure, and another that promotes exploration of the world. Both children and adults try to maintain homeostasis between attachment behavior, prompted when the feeling of security is threatened, and exploratory behavior (play or learning), when this threat is low. Under threat, the child will withdraw to the "secure base" of his or her attachment figure (see also Ainsworth et al. 1971). Observed behavior in small children is thus seen as the outcome of the tension between the attachment and exploratory systems.

Bowlby (1969) described four phases in development of the attachment behavioral system:

1. For the first 2–3 months, the baby does things (such as cry) that elicit attention and concern, but he or she has only a small capacity selectively to direct these appeals to established attachment figures.
2. From months 3 to 6, the baby directs distress signals more specifically to particular familiar individuals.
3. For the second half of the first year, the baby seeks closeness in more differentiated ways; attachment signals to each attachment figure have been shaped by past experience with that person, and the baby can crawl around to maintain physical closeness and more readily "switches off" the attachment behavior once the sense of security is restored.
4. "Goal-corrected partnership" develops, in which the toddler perceives the attachment figure's behavior to be organized around his or her own goals, and these are taken into account in selecting the child's bids for closeness.

By the fourth year, with the newly developed ability to recognize that he and his attachment figure have different perspectives, and that the internal and external situations can differ, the child becomes much less dependent on actual physical proximity and is increasingly able to rely on availability "in principle." (That is, the mother may, for example, have left the child at preschool, but he knows she would come if he were badly hurt, and will in any case be there at lunch time.)

In the second volume of his trilogy, Bowlby established the "set goal" of the attachment system as maintaining the caregiver's accessibility and responsiveness, combined into the term *availability* (Bowlby 1973, p. 202). In the late 1970s, Alan Sroufe and Everett Waters (1977) redefined the set goal of the attachment system as "felt security" rather than regulating physical closeness. So internal states such as mood or tiredness could affect the child's response to separation as well as external events. The search for felt security made sense of attachment behavior and needs

throughout life (Cicchetti et al. 1990). Sroufe (1996) later reframed attachment theory in terms of affect regulation. Securely attached people are seen as having internalized capacities for self-regulation, in contrast to those who either suppress affect (avoidant/dismissing) or escalate it (resistant/preoccupied). Both older children and adults continue to monitor the accessibility and responsiveness of attachment figures, especially when internal capacities for affect regulation have not been well developed or are temporarily under stress (e.g., in illness, under conditions of loss or fear).

Along with the idea of the secure base, one of the most central concepts to attachment theory has been that of *internal working models* (IWMs) (Bowlby 1973). Bowlby saw the attachment behavioral system as organized by a set of cognitive mechanisms, embodying the expectations built through experience; following Craik (1943), these became known as internal working models. Craik (1943) described the idea as follows:

> If the organism carries a small-scale model of external reality and of its own possible actions within its head, it is able to try out various alternatives, conclude which is the best of them, react to future situations before they arise, utilize the knowledge of past events in dealing with the present and future and in every way to react in a much fuller, safer and more competent manner to emergencies which face it. (p. 61)

This idea has been creatively developed by several major contributors in the field (e.g., K. Bretherton and Munholland 1999; Crittenden 1994; Main 1991; Sroufe 1996). Four representational systems are implied in these reformulations: 1) expectations of how caregivers will interact, beginning in the first year of life and later modified; 2) event representations in which general and specific memories of attachment-related experiences are stored; 3) autobiographical memories connected through personal meaning; and 4) understanding of one's own feelings and motives and those of others.

An important reason for the antagonism to Bowlby (1973) was that although he recognized that IWMs involved internal objects and object relationships, he thought these were largely formed through external experience: "The varied expectations of the accessibility and responsiveness of attachment figures that different individuals develop during the years of immaturity are tolerably accurate reflections of the experiences those individuals have actually had" (Bowlby 1973, p. 235). IWMs of the self and of parents are thus first built on early representations of the relationship and then evolve into free-standing yet interlocking images of the self and attachment figures (I. Bretherton 1985). By interlocking, it is meant that a child who has IWMs of attachment figures as unloving and rejecting will in turn hold a model of the self as unlovable, unworthy, boring, and so forth. By contrast, a child who holds IWMs of attachment figures as loving and sensitive to his or her needs will hold a complementary model of the self as deserving their love and care. Presumably when the separate IWMs based in different attachment relationships are similar, the IWM of the self will be relatively consistent and harder to change with subsequent experience.

Clearly, IWMs will only be adaptive for the person holding them if they enable that person to anticipate how people will behave toward him or her in future important situations (Will loved ones protect the person if he or she is sick, injured, in danger or simply feeling bad, or will they not notice, not care, be cruel, or misunderstand?). Accurate anticipation requires that earlier experiences, on which prediction is based, have been perceived fairly realistically. Here, one immediately sees that distorted perceptions (e.g., by the operation of primitive defenses) and cognitive limitations natural at early stages of development may lead a young child to draw wrong conclusions from half-understood interactions. If the underlying distortions are not corrected, they may be reinforced rather than modified in more realistic directions by later experiences. The protective value of IWMs could then be undermined and replaced by self-defeating misattributions and defensive strategies. These can be seen in the organized but "insecure" forms of attachment behavior and representation, described by attachment researchers and summarized later in this chapter, and familiar to psychotherapists.

Reception of Attachment Theory Within Psychoanalysis

Before going on to summarize more recent developments in the attachment field, let us acknowledge the objections to a reconciliation between psychoanalysis and its prodigal child, attachment theory. These objections remain relevant and may be in the minds of readers of this chapter.

The publication of John Bowlby's paper "Grief and Mourning in Infancy and Early Childhood" (Bowlby 1960) led to an immediate hostile reception (A. Freud 1960/1969; Schur 1960; Spitz 1960). In London, where Bowlby had been trained and continued to work at the Tavistock Centre, attachment theory was seen as mechanistic, nondynamic, and thus not psychoanalytic. The Kleinians, who had accepted and taught him, saw him as having failed to understand the primacy of unconscious phantasy and the

relative insignificance of observable, external experiences. He was also, more surprisingly, rejected by the group around Anna Freud, who had themselves done many studies of children exposed to severe external deprivations (e.g., A. Freud 1973) and had made serious contributions to public policy affecting the care of children (Goldstein et al. 1973, 1979). Many further important voices from psychoanalysis joined in criticizing attachment theory (e.g., Engel 1971; Hanly 1978; Kernberg 1976).

The major criticisms that have been leveled at attachment theory are that it

1. Emphasizes evolutionary survival value, which is of less interest in the modern world than are the higher human capacities.
2. Reduces motivation to one basic system and excludes the dynamic unconscious.
3. Focuses only on safety and danger, leaving aside the rest of human emotional life.
4. Ignores biological and social vulnerabilities other than separation and other attachment traumas.
5. Ignores ego development and the later psychosexual phases.

In short, it leaves out everything that makes psychoanalysis interesting and powerful, keeping only a crude and partial biological model. These points were relevant and remain important to keep in mind for analysts. Nevertheless, much of the work that has been done in attachment theory and research over the intervening decades—for instance, Bretherton's work elaborating the concept of internal working models (I. Bretherton 1987, 1995)—has served to redress these shortcomings, which is probably an important reason why this area has become increasingly attractive to psychoanalysts. Several workers from both sides have built bridges between attachment theory and psychoanalysis, with considerable success (see, e.g., I. Bretherton 1987; Fonagy 2001; Holmes 1993, 1997; Lichtenberg 1989).

In the remainder of this chapter, I outline more recent developments in attachment theory and research and summarize the more recent views of psychoanalysts and clinicians who have interested themselves in both fields. I close the chapter by touching on some of the continuing tensions between these two approaches.

Findings of Attachment Theory

In this section I outline the major findings of attachment research that either have advanced theory or are especially relevant to psychoanalysis. Interested readers are referred to *The Handbook of Attachment* (Cassidy and Shaver 1999) for a much fuller presentation and discussion of recent research and current theory in this area.

Much work in attachment research over the last 20 years has been devoted to extending the study of attachment to later development, the most important example being attempts to access the shift to the "level of mental representations" (Main et al. 1985) through the development of an interview-based method for identifying the parent's state of mind with respect to attachment (the Adult Attachment Interview [AAI]; C. George, N. Kaplan, M. Main, unpublished manuscript, 1985; Hesse 1999). The shift from studying behavior to measuring disruptions in discourse processes has resulted in a huge body of literature beginning with but going far beyond the demonstration of concordance between parents' attachment status and their infants' patterns of specific attachment behavior with them. Increasingly, in recent years, interest has been focused on clinical issues and on the measurement of attachment representations and behavior in all the years between babyhood and parenthood.

A related area of interest has been the extent to which infant attachment classification predicts the corresponding later pattern (e.g., "avoidant" baby to "dismissing" adult). The extent to which this longitudinal continuity can be shown is in fact often used as a test of the validity of an attachment measure in childhood or adolescence. The assumption of continuity is, however, one that should be questioned. Crittenden (e.g., Crittenden 1992), drawing on an information processing approach, has developed an alternative, "dynamic maturational" model, in which maturation and experience interact, leading either to change or to continuity in patterns of attachment. She sees patterns of infant and later attachment as reflecting ways of processing attachment information, giving greater weight to either cognition or affect, distorting one or both, or balancing the two. Within this model, whereas secure children (and adults) balance cognitive and affective channels, avoidant ones (dismissing adults) depend heavily on cognition and minimize affect, and ambivalent children (preoccupied adults) use a coercive strategy, amplifying affect and distorting cognition as necessary.

This work has extended the thinking of Bowlby (1977a, 1977b, 1980, 1987) himself, who found an information-processing cognitive model increasingly useful in thinking about attachment patterns. Bowlby suggested that different patterns of attachment reflect differences in access to certain kinds of thoughts, feelings, and memories. For example, avoidant models of attachment restrict access to attachment-related thoughts, feelings, and memories, while ambivalent/resistant ones exaggerate or distort information in the area of attachment.

Categorization of Attachment Behavior in Babies

Mary Ainsworth (e.g., Ainsworth 1969, 1985) paved the way for a vast amount of subsequent research with her systematic observations in the home that were brought into the developmental laboratory in the form of the Strange Situation: a set experimental procedure in which babies of about 1 year of age are separated from their caregiver and left with a friendly stranger in a pleasant but unfamiliar playroom. Four main patterns of behavior are observed between parents and their babies in this situation (from which the baby's attachment classification to his or her parent is coded). *Secure babies* explore the playroom with interest as long as the parent is there, are wary of the stranger, are very upset by their parent's absence, actively seek comfort from her on return, and are quite quickly reassured after which they turn back to the toys (often staying closer to the parent, however, and perhaps involving her more in their play). There are two categories of "insecure" attachment, in which the babies behave very differently: the *anxious/avoidant* and *anxious/resistant* categories. Those in the first category show little emotion or apparent distress in all phases of the situation, and are relatively focused on the play environment. Those in the second are fussy, anxious, and miserable, before and during the separation; difficult to comfort; and little interested in the playroom. A fourth category of attachment behavior (which cuts across the previous three) is known as *disorganized/disoriented* (Main and Solomon 1990). Babies in this category may show odd behavior, such as hand clapping, head-banging, or trying to get away from the parent, at various points in the Strange Situation, or may behave oddly just once, such as freezing when the parent returns after separation (Lyons-Ruth and Jacobovitz 1999; Main and Solomon 1986).

As stated earlier, Sroufe (1979) extended the interpretation of a baby's behavior in the Strange Situation—as an IWM in action—to an exploration of it as indicating the baby's experiences of affect regulation with that caregiver. A secure baby's behavior is seen as showing the capacity to remain emotionally organized and effective under stress, on the basis of the experience of sensitive interactions in which the parent has kept stimulation and anxiety at manageable levels and been able to soothe the baby when necessary. This experience leads the baby to feel less disturbed by his or her anxiety, expecting that its meaning will be recognized by the parent and thence the anxiety will become more manageable (Grossmann et al. 1986; Sroufe 1996). Anxious/avoidant children are assumed to overregulate their distress because the parent has not been able to contain it in past interactions, being either rejecting of the distress or overly intrusive. Anxious/resistant children escalate and prolong their expressions of distress, perhaps because of experiences in which the parent was preoccupied or unpredictable in response to the baby's communications.

The understanding of the origins of disorganized/disoriented behavior has been of particular interest in the last decade and is dealt with further below.

Early Attachment as Predictive of Social Development

Prospective studies have shown that secure children are more likely to become resilient, self-reliant, empathic, and confident and more able to form deep relationships (Kestenbaum et al. 1989; Sroufe et al. 1990; Waters et al. 1979), possibly because IWMs persist. Attachment security has been shown to be fairly stable in longitudinal studies of infants assessed with the Strange Situation and followed up in young adulthood with the AAI.

The AAI is a semistructured research interview that bears a resemblance to a psychotherapy intake interview, covering memories of the early relationships with each parent, separations, illness and injury, punishment, deaths, and abuse. The interview asks for general judgments and descriptions, together with particular memories. The coding is primarily focused on distortions of communication, such as passive, confused speech, uncontrolled anger, derogation of attachment, lack of memory for attachment experiences, and contradictions. These and other aspects of speech are coded along several dimensions and aggregated into a scale of *coherence*, which is used as a sort of barometer of security. The system (M. Main, R. Goldwyn, unpublished manuscript, 1994) then assigns categories that parallel the infant ones with respect to loss or trauma: secure/autonomous, insecure/dismissing, insecure/preoccupied or unresolved. Secure people recognize the importance of attachment relationships and integrate their memories of these (whether good, bad, or mixed) into a plausible and understandable story. Dismissing people avoid thinking and feeling about attachment memories by denying them or by idealizing or denigrating their childhood relationships. Preoccupied individuals are confused, overwhelmed, angry, fearful, or muddled in relation to childhood experiences. Unresolved speakers talk in contradictory or disrupted ways when referring to traumatic experiences; for example, they may speak as though a dead attachment figure were still alive, or lapse into a prolonged silence without apparently being aware of the gap.

Many studies have shown (van IJzendoorn 1995) that the AAI category strongly predicts the child's attachment category with the parent, which is independent of the child category with another caregiver. Arietta Slade and her colleagues have helped us to understand how attachment security is transmitted. They showed that mothers who were judged secure on the basis of the AAI talked about their relationship with their toddlers in a more coherent way, and described more joy and pleasure in the relationship, than did dismissing and preoccupied mothers (Slade et al. 1999). Thus, the mother's picture of the individual child is crucial, which may help to explain why children of the same mother can have different types of attachment to her. It seems likely that the way in which she represents the different children unconsciously communicates to each of them a different place in her mind and a different message about the child's self—one as special or needing protection, another as tough and doing best with space or discipline, another as so like her that the image gets blurred. Certainly some explanation is needed for the remarkably low concordance between the attachment classification of siblings (van IJzendoorn et al. 2000), and the dimension that Slade and colleagues have been exploring may well hold the key.

Since the late 1970s, attachment research has been increasingly concerned with trauma, and to a lesser extent with psychiatric illness and personality disorder, although interest in the latter—fed mainly by clinicians who became interested in and trained in attachment methods and then tried to apply them to psychiatric populations—has so far been hampered by the limited applicability of assessments and coding systems developed for normal populations.

It is likely that attachment disorganization will prove the strongest predictor of later clinical problems (see Solomon and George 1999), but there has also been much work exploring the connection between security and later positive personality development. Thus, preschool children who had been securely attached as babies were judged by teachers (who were unaware of earlier attachment status) as having better self-esteem, emotional adjustment, compliance with social demands, cheerfulness, and sense of effectiveness. These benefits were confirmed at 10 years of age (Elicker et al. 1992) and right into adulthood, with many possibly confounding factors controlled for (Carlson 1998; Weinfield et al. 1999). On the other hand, some studies (e.g., Feiring and Lewis 1996) failed to confirm these results. Across the whole population, the distinction between secure and insecure is not a good predictor of later psychopathology, in contrast to the disorganized/disoriented distinction (e.g., Carlson 1998; Vondra et al. 2001). However, within high-risk samples, security does seem to protect against externalizing problems over many subsequent years (Warren et al. 1997; Weinfield et al. 1999). Perhaps surprisingly, avoidant babies had the highest rate of later disorder (70%); children who had been resistant babies were not at higher risk than children who had been secure as babies.

There is general agreement that attachment security can serve as a protective factor against adult psychopathology and that it is associated with a wide range of good outcomes, such as lower anxiety (Collins and Read 1990), less hostility and greater ego resilience (Kobak and Sceery 1988), and greater ability to regulate affect through interpersonal relatedness (Vaillant 1992). Insecure attachment is associated with more depression (Armsden and Greenberg 1987); anxiety, hostility, and psychosomatic illness (Hazan and Shaver 1990); and less ego resilience (Kobak and Sceery 1988). Five studies have linked insecure attachment, and especially unresolved trauma, with psychiatric illness (Dozier et al. 1999), although specific attachment types and psychiatric conditions do not neatly map onto one another. There is some evidence, for example, that preoccupation with attachment experiences and with trauma may be associated with mental ill health but that dismissing attachment may predict physical symptoms more than psychological complaints (Eagle 1999). A serious problem with such studies to date is the partial confounding of attachment coding with emotional and cognitive disturbance; some investigators, including our group in London, are working on ways to disentangle these influences on interview data.

Mary Dozier's work on attachment and treatability has shown that dismissing adults are difficult to reach in psychotherapy and tend not to seek emotional help (Dozier 1990). Preoccupied people take to therapy more readily but can become highly dependent (Dozier et al. 1991). Sidney Blatt's distinction (e.g., Blatt et al. 1998) between "introjective" and "anaclitic" pathology, respectively, may map onto this contrast between dismissing/self-sufficient and preoccupied/dependent personality types, their reactions to therapy, and their ways of becoming depressed.

Disorganization of Attachment

The most clinically interesting area of attachment research at the moment is the study of disorganized/disoriented attachment behavior. As described earlier, this behavior is marked in the Strange Situation by contradictory features: undirected or interrupted movements, stereotypies, strange postures, freezing, fearful reactions to the parent, or apparent confusion (Main and Solomon 1986). Main and Hesse (1992) advanced the idea that these babies are showing an approach/avoidance conflict, because the parent is and has previously been both the source of fear and the only hope of comfort. Babies would either be afraid of their attachment figure or feel alarming to him or her, and in either case they would not be able to expect reassurance

by getting close to the parent (Main 1995). Disorganized behavior has been shown to be linked to child abuse (e.g., Cicchetti and Barnett 1991), major depressive disorder (Lyons-Ruth et al. 1990), and unresolved trauma in the mother's AAI narrative (van IJzendoorn 1995). It has become clear that the baby does not need to have been openly maltreated to show disorganization of attachment behavior with a particular parent. It can be enough that the mother has been traumatized herself and has been unable to resolve and process that experience; it leaks out when she talks about her history and in her behavior with her child (Schuengel et al. 1999b; van IJzendoorn 1995).

This association must be mediated by parental behavior, and we are beginning to be able to see how. Jacobovitz and colleagues (1997) found a strong association between signs of unresolved trauma in the AAI during pregnancy, and frightened or frightening behavior (e.g., threatening, looming grimaces, or dissociation) toward the baby at 8 months. Trauma during childhood or adolescence seemed to be more likely to lead to this leakage into behavior toward the baby. The unresolved mothers were not, however, more likely to be generally insensitive or unresponsive. Schuengel and colleagues (1999a) confirmed the observations of significantly more frightened or frightening behavior, but also showed that the behavior was most marked in those children classified as having unresolved and insecure attachment (Schuengel et al. 1999a). They also found that dissociated behavior was an even stronger predictor of disorganization than frightened or frightening behavior in general. Lyons-Ruth and colleagues (1999a) added to the emerging picture by showing that frightened and frightening behavior predicted disorganization most strongly when the mother seriously misinterpreted the baby's attachment behavior and when the mother herself gave conflicting attachment cues.

There is considerable evidence, from cross-sectional and longitudinal studies, that disorganized attachment predicts later difficulty in relating: controlling attachment behavior in middle childhood and poorer social and problem-solving skills (Jacobovitz and Hazen 1999; Wartner et al. 1994).

Measurement of Attachment Between the Preschool Years and Early Adulthood

An area of the attachment field that is only now being opened up is addressing the question, What happens to attachment representations in the phase of life between early childhood, when attachment is measured by the infant's observable behavior toward the parent or another attachment figure, and late adolescence and adulthood, when it is measured by distortions and slips in narrative about childhood relationships? The empirical observation is that small children have separate and independent attachment relationships with each caregiver. In adult attachment research, however, it is assumed that adults have formed a unitary organization of attachment representations so that they generally operate according to a single IWM. They are by then designated as having, for example, "secure" or "dismissing" attachment in general and not simply in relation to specific attachment figures. Those with more than one attachment strategy are currently designated "cannot classify" by Main and Hesse (1992), although the Crittenden clinical extension scales for the AAI allow for a bit more differentiation.

Those who have coded many adult attachment interviews, especially from clinical populations (not to mention those who have worked as psychotherapists), may well doubt that adults do in fact develop an integrated stance toward all subsequent attachment relationships. But it is certainly of interest to see how preschool children's different behavior toward their attachment figures may become consolidated into a style of relating based on more generalized expectations of other people. Middle childhood and early adolescence are years when of course close relationships with peers, teachers, and others outside the family become of crucial importance, and parents are not present to regulate distress and other intense feelings most of the time. What templates of self and other does the child bring to his or her school and social experiences, and how well do they serve him or her in the search for safe exploration and expansion of his or her emotional world?

With Peter Fonagy and Yael Shmueli-Goetz, I have been trying to explore attachment in middle childhood, using an interview (the Child Attachment Interview: Target et al. 2003) that draws on not only the AAI (in its form) but also video observation of nonverbal behavior (in its coding scheme). Our results suggest that this interview allows reliable and valid coding of the child's attachment representations and strategies in the age range of 8 to 14 years, and that, as in infancy, children have different actual attachment behavior and relationships with each parent in this age group. At the same time, like adults, they have developed quite a unified emotional and cognitive stance toward attachment experiences, which is reflected in their language, their nonverbal responses, and their capacity to think about and deal with feelings about their attachment relationships. The attachment classifications of these children relate quite strongly to their friendships, cognitive, personality, and clinical characteristics. What we need to find out next is whether, as we expect, attachment patterns change with effective treatment, and especially with psychotherapy or psychoanalysis that is prolonged, intensive, and focused on relationship templates and representations and on the feelings embedded in them.

Psychoanalytic Views of Attachment Theory

A number of major authors in attachment theory have been significantly influenced by psychoanalytic ideas, and vice versa. It is in the writings of authors such as Karlen Lyons-Ruth, Arietta Slade, Morris Eagle, and Peter Fonagy that the fertility of the meeting between attachment theory and psychoanalysis has been most richly explored. Their writings should be read by any interested in this interface (see Fonagy 2001). In this section, I mention some directions these writers have taken in exploring the reintegration of attachment concepts into psychoanalytic theory and technique.

Selma Fraiberg (1980; Fraiberg et al. 1975), while not advocating an attachment framework, was one of the first to show how parent-infant problems could be traced to unresolved conflicts from the parents' own childhoods. Alicia Lieberman (1991) has more recently linked the form of parent-infant therapy pioneered by Fraiberg with attachment theory (Lieberman and Pawl 1993; Pawl and Lieberman 1997), focusing on the feelings within important relationships and on how these feelings may also be being experienced in relation to the baby. Fraiberg observed that the baby is the focus of transference, with the mother identifying with the baby and unconsciously reactivating a past emotional constellation with her own mother (or other attachment figure). The intensity is magnified because the birth of the child triggers maximum caregiving impulses together with powerful current and past attachment feelings. In Lieberman's development of the Fraiberg model, both the mother's and the baby's feelings and expectations are understood in terms of IWMs of relationships.

Arietta Slade is a further example of investigators who have linked psychoanalytic clinical practice and attachment research (see, e.g., Slade 1999). Slade's interest is not in advancing a particular technique compatible with attachment theory, but in showing how awareness of attachment and of its manifestations can enrich clinical thinking (Slade 1996, 1999). Thus, listening to the form of speech, as well as to the words themselves, can illuminate the underlying relationship expectations in a clinical narrative, as in an attachment interview. Changes in narrative style, which may be subtle shifts in emphasis or coherence—for example, from factual to more whimsical or hard to follow, from organized to mildly contradictory or partial in details, from rich to impoverished in memories—could indicate a change in the active working model. The analyst may be able to follow the gaps, slips, and resistant areas of the mental world so that "unmentalized" experience can be worked on. Of course, this might be what the analyst would be doing without an attachment framework; however, such a framework gives systematic suggestions as to the forms of narrative that might indicate unassimilated experience and even to the kinds of experiences that might lie behind the changes in the form of representation.

Slade (1999, 2000), a child therapist as well as an adult therapist, has explored the further dimensions of this perspective for clinical work with children. As Anna Freud stressed, the child patient is still living surrounded by not just his own attachment history but his parents' attachment histories as well. Arietta Slade, in her research, has (as mentioned above) shown that mother's mental representation of the particular child as a person, especially her capacity to understand her relationship with her child in psychological terms, may mediate the transmission of attachment security—or, perhaps, different facets of the mother's working models of attachment relationships—to her different children, depending on what each of them means to her, makes her feel, and reminds her of, and whether she can think about these responses.

Karlen Lyons-Ruth is a significant writer on psychoanalysis and a major contributor to research and thinking on disorganized attachment. She has advanced a psychoanalytically informed model of the data on disorganization, the *relational diathesis model* (Lyons-Ruth et al. 1999b), which helps to explain why and how trauma is likely to be repeated and to continue to be unresolved in an attachment relationship that is already insecure and/or disorganized. The model greatly extends the sophistication of thinking about attachment and trauma, with a focus on the background relational factors (especially the splitting of roles into hostile/intrusive vs. helpless, and situations of dependency in which one person's relationship needs drive out the other's). The vulnerability model has many intriguing links with clinical analytic work, in which, for example, her dichotomy of hostile vs. helpless relating is very reminiscent of a major dimension of personality disturbance. It also has links that could be explored with Crittenden's "dynamic maturational" attachment model, the clinical extension of which has a dimension of attachment preoccupation that similarly hinges on hostile and helpless relating. (In Crittenden's model, every individual who appears to be a passive, helpless type is also shown to have an underlying hostility, and vice versa—a feature of her model that makes a clear link with, for example, Rosenfeld's and Bateman's ideas about types of narcissistic personality functioning, and the way that relating oscillates between the thick-skinned and thin-skinned stances [Bateman 1998].) Lyons-Ruth might be more interested in bringing together more fully her relational attachment model with the psychoanalytic work of the Boston group (of which she is also a part) on change processes in psychoanalysis (e.g., Stern et al. 1998), and this is also a line of work with much potential.

Morris Eagle is another writer who has engaged very seriously with both attachment theory and psychoanalysis and with the implications of each for the other (e.g., Eagle 1998, 1999). He sees the subjective experiences in infancy of "felt security" or of its absence as parallel to the experiences described in object relations theory and the creation of internal objects. Eagle (1997) sees Bowlby, in his development of attachment theory, as having corrected the emphasis in classical analytic theory, both Freudian and Kleinian, on inner forces and phantasies to the neglect of real, historical experiences. However, he does not accept that IWMs reflect these actual interactions directly (e.g., Eagle 1999), emphasizing, rightly, that different babies will be constitutionally disposed to experience the same maternal behavior in different ways. He sees the persistence of infantile attachment-related relationship styles (e.g., avoidance of emotional involvement, leading in adulthood to a retreat into work) as an indication of the failure to negotiate later psychosexual conflicts, especially the oedipal situation. This is part of a valuable focus in these papers on the need to try to bring what we know analytically about sexuality and the search for pleasure into relation to attachment and object relational ideas.

Eagle (1997) describes how the stickiness of the transference—persistent efforts to actualize infantile role relationships, and the tendency toward role responsiveness, in Sandler's terms (Sandler 1976)—reflects efforts to reaffirm and keep alive those earliest relational experiences and suggests that others will tend to play their parts. There is evidence from attachment research to show that, at least in childhood, later relationships (at school) do tend to repeat early patterns (Sroufe et al. 1990), and Eagle explores this way of understanding the repetition compulsion in our patients. Another area of attachment theory that Eagle has helped us to be more critical about is the easy equation (extended from the basis of AAI coding) between security and narrative coherence. Eagle (1997) helpfully challenges the idea that developing a "good story" about one's childhood experiences makes for emotional security in adulthood, although it might help toward a more secure relationship with one's own child.

Peter Fonagy (e.g., Fonagy 2001; Fonagy et al. 2002), has made major contributions to both psychoanalytic theory and attachment research (and to related developmental research on social cognition as well). He has built strong bridges between both areas of theory and between these areas and work in related scientific fields. Drawing both on clinical psychoanalytic work (e.g., Fonagy 1991) and on attachment findings (e.g., Fonagy et al. 1991), Fonagy gradually built a model of the mental processes underlying both personality functioning and disorder, and the intergenerational transmission of attachment and trauma. His best-known contributions to psychoanalytic developmental theory are probably the concept of reflective function, or *mentalization,* as a fundamental component of both personality development and therapeutic change (e.g., Fonagy 1991; Fonagy and Target 1997), and the understanding of psychic reality and its normal and disturbed development (Fonagy and Target 1996, 2000; Target and Fonagy 1996). Recently (see, e.g., Fonagy 2003), he has been developing a much broader and more comprehensive model of early personality development, still rooted in the attachment relationship but now with a much clearer account of the neural underpinnings of a group of related mental processes underlying personality functioning (the "interpersonal interpretative function"). This approach offers the possibility of an eventual close integration of developmental neuroscience, attachment research, and psychoanalytic theory and practice.

How May Psychoanalysis and Attachment Theory Regard Each Other Now?

There are two aspects of the question of how psychoanalysis and attachment theory may regard each other at present: 1) the extent to which attachment theory is research-based (which touches on the relationship between psychoanalysis and empirical research) and 2) the acceptability of the attachment model in relation to psychoanalytic theory.

For a considerable time, the extensive research base of attachment theory, and the involvement in this research of many scientists who were not analysts, probably deepened the sense that attachment was not part of psychoanalysis, particularly outside North America. The common attitude, however, that research could not inform—or even exist at close quarters with—analytic theory and clinical work seems to be changing. Even outcome research is becoming cautiously accepted, and developmental and neuroscientific studies are of interest to an increasing number. This cautious acceptance may be because psychoanalysts have become rightly worried about being marginalized, with a dwindling presence in university clinical faculties and more popular among researchers in the humanities than among those concerned with psy-

chology or psychiatry. In contrast, attachment theory attracted mainstream scientific funding and large numbers of gifted researchers from a range of neighboring disciplines, some of whom then became interested in psychoanalysis. In turn, analysts perhaps began to see in attachment theory a powerful explanatory model of early psychic and social development, which could be tested, was in fact fast becoming accepted as proven, and had some strong clinical implications. These clinical implications were far easier to see and accept given the shift in analytic theory toward object relations and a broadly relational perspective (with a downgrading of sexuality and drive theory) and, perhaps increasingly, an implicit maternal model of the clinical situation. This shift will be the final topic to be touched on in the present chapter.

The rise of object relations theory, focused more on representations of early central emotional relationships than on psychosexuality, and of ego psychology, with its emphasis on the development of positive mental capacities, together with the increasing sophistication of attachment theory in addressing representations (as opposed to assuming attachment behavior simply reflects external interactions), meant that the original objections to attachment theory as part of psychoanalysis lost some of their conviction. In addition, it has become clear that a number of widely accepted aspects of psychoanalytic theory have much in common with basic tenets of attachment theory. The idea of psychic trauma as something that breaches and overwhelms the ego, disorganizing or limiting its functioning and having delayed and far-reaching effects; Erikson's notion of basic trust; Winnicott's and Bion's ideas of mirroring and containment by the mother as laying the basis for the "true" (secure) self, for affect regulation, and thinking; Winnicott's recognition that play and creativity could develop only if fear was defused by the parents; Sandler's ideas of the background of safety and of role-responsiveness—all these are highly consonant with aspects of attachment theory, which indeed binds them together in a coherent framework. This framework connects these psychoanalytic ideas with biology, as Freud intended, and with newer fields of development and cognition, which Freud could not know of, but which have become of central importance to the study of psychology and mental disorder.

In this area, though, lies a continuing problem—or perceived problem—in bridging attachment theory and psychoanalysis. Attachment theory does encompass, with increasing sophistication, formative emotional experience that is outside awareness; however, this experience is largely nonconscious, implicit or procedural rather than dynamically unconscious and the result of (largely sexual) conflict, classically the focus of psychoanalysis. Some would say that without maintaining that primary focus, psychoanalysis loses its heart, its purpose, and its uniqueness. This criticism would be true if allowing for the shaping of personality and emotion regulation through procedural learning necessitated the abandonment of a motivational model based on drives, conflict, and defense. There is, however, no such forced choice, and we now have evidence that both are important aspects of character formation and symptomatology. Some of us are also trying to extend the attachment model to encompass psychosexuality and the patterns of later sexual relating, based in the earliest, attachment relationship (P. Fonagy and M. Target, unpublished manuscript, 2004). This is an integration of perspectives that would help the field of psychoanalysis to achieve greater coherence and communication but that, as of this writing, has barely begun.

As stated at the beginning of this chapter, it may be that character pathologies, now so central to most analytic practices, push us toward extending our theory to allow for the forming of expectations of relationships and interactions, such that templates from the past get superimposed on each opportunity for something new. Some of these expectations may indeed be the result of neurotic conflicts. It seems plausible, however, that some are formed very early, in the first months and years, not just from drive forces but also from the way internal and external threats are met—with protection and attunement or perhaps confusion, panic, or humiliation of the child. Furthermore, attachment theory does not deal only with situations of fear and danger; there is also the child's love and need to be recognized and loved, and the child's curiosity about himself and the other and, later, the wider world. Attachment theory helps to explain why these needs and desires have to be met hierarchically. If the child is physically safe, he stays alive; if he is emotionally safe, he feels secure; if the person who keeps him safe is interested in him and receptive, then he learns about himself through her recognition of him and her response to what she sees. Through these steps and afterward, the child is increasingly free to explore his world, including people's minds and feelings toward him, expecting on the whole to be safe and appreciated.

Conclusion

The early attachment context provides the setting—initially external, but over time becoming mental, outside awareness and taken for granted—for later formative experiences. These experiences will, of course, include conflicts and the need to defend against them, together with many subsequent influential relationships. Attachment theory proposes that the way in which a person rises to these later opportunities and challenges will be crucially shaped by the residue of his or her early experiences of being loved, protected, and understood, or perhaps abandoned, derided, exploited, or in other ways left alone. We often are alone, as older children and adults, in facing the demands of life, but whether we feel alone is—according to attachment theory—a result of the cast of mind left by memories that cannot be retrieved, only ever reenacted, in the transference in analysis and elsewhere. This cast of mind is in turn a product of the way we felt treated by our attachment figures, which we understand to be what we deserved, a measure of the self and its value. It takes a new, powerful attachment relationship, such as with the analyst, to allow such measures to be questioned emotionally as well as cognitively, to be taken less for granted, and perhaps to change.

References

Ainsworth MDS: Object relations, dependency and attachment: a theoretical review of the infant-mother relationship. Child Dev 40:969–1025, 1969

Ainsworth MDS: Attachments across the lifespan. Bull N Y Acad Med 61:792–812, 1985

Ainsworth MDS, Bell SM, Stayton DJ: Attachment and exploratory behavior of one year olds, in The Origins of Human Social Relations. Edited by Schaffer HR. New York, Academy Press, 1971, pp 17–57

Armsden GC, Greenberg MT: The inventory of parent and peer attachment: individual differences and their relationship to psychological well-being in adolescence. J Youth Adolesc 16:427–454, 1987

Bateman AW: Thick- and thin-skinned organizations and enactment in borderline and narcissistic disorders. Int J Psychoanal 79:13–25, 1998

Blatt SJ, Zuroff DC, Bondi CM, et al: When and how perfectionism impedes the brief treatment of depression: further analyses of the National Institute of Mental Health treatment of depression collaborative research program. J Consult Clin Psychol 66:423–428, 1998

Bowlby J: Forty-four juvenile thieves: their characters and home life. Int J Psychoanal 25:19–52, 1944

Bowlby J: Maternal Care and Mental Health: WHO Monograph Series, No 2. Geneva, World Health Organization, 1951

Bowlby J: The nature of the child's tie to his mother. Int J Psychoanal 39:350–373, 1958

Bowlby J: Grief and mourning in infancy and early childhood. Psychoanal Study Child 15:3–39, 1960

Bowlby J: Attachment and Loss, Vol 1: Attachment. New York, Basic Books, 1969

Bowlby J: Attachment and Loss, Vol 2: Separation: Anxiety and Anger. New York, Basic Books, 1973

Bowlby J: The making and breaking of affectional bonds, I: aetiology and psychopathology in the light of attachment theory. An expanded version of the 50th Maudsley Lecture, delivered before the Royal College of Psychiatrists, 19 November 1976. Br J Psychiatry 130:201–210, 1977a

Bowlby J: The making and breaking of affectional bonds, II: some principles of psychotherapy. The 50th Maudsley Lecture. Br J Psychiatry. 130:421–431, 1977b

Bowlby J: Attachment and Loss, Vol 3: Loss: Sadness and Depression. New York, Basic Books, 1980

Bowlby J: Attachment, in The Oxford Companion to the Mind. Edited by Gregory R. Oxford, England, Oxford University Press, 1987, pp 57–58

Bretherton I: Attachment theory: retrospect and prospect. Monogr Soc Res Child Dev 50:3–35, 1985

Bretherton I: New perspectives on attachment relationships: security, communication, and internal working models, in Handbook of Infant Development. Edited by Osofsky JD. New York, Wiley, 1987, pp 1061–1100

Bretherton I: Attachment theory and developmental psychopathology, in Fourth Rochester Symposium on Developmental Psychopathology on "Emotion, Cognition, and Representation." Edited by Cicchetti D, Toth S. Hillsdale, NJ, Lawrence Erlbaum, 1995, pp 231–260

Bretherton K, Munholland KA: Internal working models in attachment relationships: a construct revisited, in Handbook of Attachment: Theory, Research, Clinical Applications. Edited by Cassidy J, Shaver PR. New York, Guilford, 1999, pp 89–114

Carlson EA: A prospective longitudinal study of attachment disorganization/disorientation. Child Dev 69:1107–1128, 1998

Cassidy J, Shaver PR (eds): Handbook of Attachment: Theory, Research, and Clinical Applications. New York, Guilford, 1999

Cicchetti D, Barnett D: Attachment organization in preschool aged maltreated children. Dev Psychopathol 3:397–411, 1991

Cicchetti D, Cummings EM, Greenberg MT, et al: An organizational perspective on attachment beyond infancy, in Attachment in the Preschool Years: Theory, Research, and Intervention. Edited by Greenberg M, Chicchetti D, Cummings EM. Chicago, IL, University of Chicago Press, 1990, pp 3–49

Collins NL, Read SJ: Adult attachment, working models and relationship quality in dating couples. J Pers Soc Psychol 58:644–663, 1990

Craik K: The Nature of Explanation. Cambridge, England, Cambridge University Press, 1943

Crittenden PM: Quality of attachment in the preschool years. Dev Psychopathol 4:209–241, 1992

Crittenden PM: Peering into the black box: an exploratory treatise on the development of self in young children, in Disorders and Dysfunctions of the Self: Rochester Symposium on Developmental Psychopathology, Vol 5. Edited by Cicchetti D, Toth S. Rochester, NY, University of Rochester Press, 1994, pp 79–148

Dozier M: Attachment organization and treatment use for adults with serious psychopathological disorders. Dev Psychopathol 2:47–60, 1990

Dozier M, Stevenson A, Lee SW, et al: Attachment organization and familiar overinvolvement for adults with serious psychopathological disorders. Dev Psychopathol 3:475–489, 1991

Dozier M, Stovall KC, Albus KE: Attachment and psychopathology in adulthood, in Handbook of Attachment: Theory, Research, and Clinical Applications. Edited by Cassidy J, Shaver PR. New York, Guilford, 1999, pp 497–519

Eagle M: Attachment and psychoanalysis. Br J Med Psychol 70:217–229, 1997

Eagle M: Attachment research and theory and psychoanalysis. Paper presented at the annual meeting of the Psychoanalytic Association of New York, November 15, 1999

Elicker J, Egeland M, Sroufe LA: Predicting peer competence and peer relationships in childhood from early parent-child relationships, in Family Peer Relationships: Modes of Linkage. Edited by Parke R, Ladd G. Hillsdale, NJ, Erlbaum, 1992, pp 77–106

Engel GL: Attachment behavior, object relations, and the dynamic point of view: critical review of Bowlby's Attachment and Loss. Int J Psychoanal 52:183–196, 1971

Feiring C, Lewis M: Finality in the eye of the beholder: multiple sources, multiple time points, multiple paths. Dev Psychopathol 8:721–733, 1996

Fonagy P: Thinking about thinking: some clinical and theoretical considerations in the treatment of a borderline patient. Int J Psychoanal 72:1–18, 1991

Fonagy P: Attachment Theory and Psychoanalysis. New York, Other Press, 2001

Fonagy P: Genetics, developmental psychopathology, and psychoanalytic theory: the case for ending our (not so) splendid isolation. Psychoanalytic Inquiry 23:218–247, 2003

Fonagy P, Target M: Playing with reality, I: theory of mind and the normal development of psychic reality. Int J Psychoanal 77:217–233, 1996

Fonagy P, Target M: Attachment and reflective function: their role in self-organization. Dev Psychopathol 9:679–700, 1997

Fonagy P, Target M: Playing with reality, III: the persistence of dual psychic reality in borderline patients. Int J Psychoanal 81:853–874, 2000

Fonagy P, Steele H, Moran G, et al: The capacity for understanding mental states: the reflective self in parent and child and its significance for security of attachment. Infant Ment Health J 13:200–217, 1991

Fonagy P, Gergely G, Jurist E, et al: Affect Regulation, Mentalization, and the Development of the Self. New York, Other Press, 2002

Fraiberg S: Clinical Studies in Infant Mental Health. New York, Basic Books, 1980

Fraiberg SH, Adelson E, Shapiro V: Ghosts in the nursery: a psychoanalytic approach to the problem of impaired infant-mother relationships. Journal of the American Academy Child Psychiatry 14:387–422, 1975

Freud A: The Writings of Anna Freud, Vol 3: Infants Without Families: Reports on the Hampstead Nurseries (1939–1945). New York, International Universities Press, 1973

Freud A: Discussion of Dr. Bowlby's paper (Grief and mourning in infancy and early childhood) (1960), in the Writings of Anna Freud, Vol 1. New York, International Universities Press, 1969, pp 167–186

Goldstein J, Freud A, Solnit AJ: Beyond the Best Interests of the Child. New York, Free Press, 1973

Goldstein J, Freud A, Solnit AJ: Before the Best Interests of the Child. New York, Free Press, 1979

Grossmann KE, Grossmann K, Schwan A: Capturing the wider view of attachment: a reanalysis of Ainsworth's Strange Situation, in Measuring Emotions in Infants and Children, Vol 2. Edited by Izard CE, Read PB. New York, Cambridge University Press, 1986, pp 124–171

Hanly C: A critical consideration of Bowlby's ethological theory of anxiety. Psychoanal Q 47:364–380, 1978

Hazan C, Shaver PR: Love and work: an attachment theoretical perspective. J Pers Soc Psychol 59:270–280, 1990

Heinicke C, Westheimer IJ: Brief Separations. New York, International Universities Press, 1966

Hesse E: The Adult Attachment Interview: historical and current perspectives, in Handbook of Attachment: Theory, Research, and Clinical Applications. Edited by Cassidy J, Shaver PR. New York, Guilford, 1999, pp 395–433

Holmes J: John Bowlby and Attachment Theory. London, Routledge, 1993

Holmes J: Attachment, autonomy, intimacy: some clinical implications of attachment theory. Br J Med Psychol 70:231–248, 1997

Jacobovitz D, Hazen N: Developmental pathways from infant disorganization to childhood peer relationships, in Attachment Disorganization. Edited by Solomon J, George C. New York, Guilford, 1999, pp 127–159

Jacobovitz D, Hazen N, Riggs S: Disorganized mental processes in mothers, frightening/frightened caregiving and disoriented/disorganized behavior in infancy. Paper presented at the Biennial Meeting of the Society for Research in Child Development, Washington, DC, April 1997

Kernberg OF: Object Relations Theory and Clinical Psychoanalysis. New York, Aronson, 1976

Kestenbaum R, Farber E, Sroufe LA: Individual differences in empathy among preschoolers' concurrent and predictive validity, in Empathy and Related Emotional Responses: New Directions for Child Development. Edited by Eisenberg N. San Francisco, CA, Jossey-Bass, 1989, pp 51–56

Kobak R, Sceery A: Attachment in late adolescence: working models, affect regulation and perceptions of self and others. Child Development 59:135–146, 1988

Lichtenberg J: Psychoanalysis and Motivation. Hillsdale, NJ, Analytic Press, 1989

Lieberman AF: Attachment theory and infant-parent psychotherapy: some conceptual, clinical, and research issues, in Rochester Symposium on Developmental Psychopathology, Vol 3: Models and Integrations. Edited by Cicchetti D, Toth S. Hillsdale, NJ, Lawrence Erlbaum, 1991, pp 261–288

Lieberman AF, Pawl J: Infant-parent psychotherapy, in Handbook of Infant Mental Health. Edited by Zeanah CH. New York, Guilford, 1993, pp 427–442

Lyons-Ruth K, Jacobovitz D: Attachment disorganization: unresolved loss, relational violence, and lapses in behavioral and attentional strategies, in Handbook of Attachment Theory and Research. Edited by Cassidy J, Shaver PR. New York, Guilford, 1999, pp 520–554

Lyons-Ruth K, Connell DB, Grunebaum HU: Infants at social risk: maternal depression and family support services as mediators of infant development and security of attachment. Child Development 61:85–98, 1990

Lyons-Ruth K, Bronfman E, Parsons E: Atypical attachment in infancy and early childhood among children at developmental risk, IV: maternal frightened, frightening, or atypical behavior and disorganized infant attachment patterns. Monogr Soc Res Child Dev 64:67–96, 1999a

Lyons-Ruth K, Bronfman E, Atwood G: A relational diathesis model of hostile-helpless states of mind: expressions in mother-infant interaction, in Attachment Disorganization. Edited by Solomon J, George C. New York, Guilford, 1999b, pp 33–70

Main M: Metacognitive knowledge, metacognitive monitoring, and singular (coherent) vs multiple (incoherent) model of attachment, in Attachment Across the Life Cycle. Edited by Parkes CM, Stevenson-Hinde J, Marris P. London, Tavistock/Routledge, 1991, pp 127–159

Main M: Recent studies in attachment: overview, with selected implications for clinical work, in Attachment Theory: Social, Developmental, and Clinical Perspectives. Edited by Goldberg S, Muir R, Kerr J. Hillsdale, NJ, Analytic Press, 1995, pp 407–474

Main M, Hesse E: Disorganized/disoriented infant behavior in the Strange Situation, lapses in the monitoring of reasoning and discourse during the parent's Adult Attachment Interview, and dissociative states, in Attachment and Psychoanalysis. Edited by Ammaniti M, Stern D. Rome, Gius, Latereza, & Figli, 1992, pp 86–140

Main M, Solomon J: Discovery of an insecure-disorganized/disoriented attachment pattern, in Affective Development in Infancy. Edited by Brazelton TB, Yogman MW. Norwood, NJ, Ablex, 1986, pp 95–124

Main M, Solomon J: Procedures for identifying infants as disorganized/disoriented during the Ainsworth Strange Situation, in Attachment During the Preschool Years: Theory, Research, and Intervention. Edited by Greenberg MT, Cicchetti D, Cummings EM. Chicago, IL, University of Chicago Press, 1990, pp 121–160

Main M, Kaplan N, Cassidy J: Security in infancy, childhood, and adulthood: a move to the level of representation. Monogr Soc Res Child Dev 50:66–104, 1985

Meltzoff AN: Understanding the intentions of others: re-enactment of intended acts by 18-month-old children. Developmental Psychology 31:838–850, 1995

Pawl J, Lieberman AF: Infant-parent psychotherapy, in Handbook of Child and Adolescent Psychiatry, Vol 1. Edited by Noshpitz J. New York, Basic Books, 1997, pp 339–351

Robertson J: Hospitals and Children: A Parent's Eye View. New York, Gollancz, 1962

Rutter M: Maternal Deprivation Reassessed. Harmondsworth, England, Penguin, 1971

Rutter M: Epidemiological approaches to developmental psychopathology. Arch Gen Psychiatry 45:486–500, 1989

Sandler J: Countertransference and role-responsiveness. International Review of Psychoanalysis 3:43–47, 1976

Schuengel C, Bakermans-Kranenburg M, van IJzendoorn M: Frightening maternal behavior linking unresolved loss and disorganized infant attachment. J Consult Clin Psychol 67:54–63, 1999a

Schuengel C, Bakermans-Kranenburg MJ, van IJzendoorn MH, et al: Unresolved loss and infant disorganisation: links to frightening maternal behavior, in Attachment Disorganization. Edited by Solomon J, George C. New York, Guilford, 1999b, pp 71–94

Schur M: Discussion of Dr. John Bowlby's paper. Psychoanal Study Child 15:63–84, 1960

Slade A: A view from attachment theory and research. Journal of Clinical Psychoanalysis 5:112–123, 1996

Slade A: Attachment theory and research: implications for the theory and practice of individual psychotherapy with adults, in Handbook of Attachment: Theory, Research, and Clinical Applications. Edited by Cassidy J, Shaver PR. New York, Guilford, 1999, pp 575–594

Slade A: The development and organization of attachment: implications for psychoanalysis. J Am Psychoanal Assoc 48:1147–1174, 2000

Slade A, Belsky J, Aber L, et al: Mothers' representations of their relationships with their toddlers: links to adult attachment and observed mothering. Developmental Psychology 35:611–619, 1999

Solomon J, George C: Attachment Disorganization. New York, Guilford, 1999

Spitz RA: Discussion of Dr. John Bowlby's paper. Psychoanal Study Child 15:85–94, 1960

Sroufe LA: Socioemotional development, in Handbook of Infant Development. Edited by Osofsky J. New York, Wiley, 1979, pp 462–516

Sroufe LA: Emotional Development: The Organization of Emotional Life in the Early Years. New York, Cambridge University Press, 1996

Sroufe LA, Waters E: Attachment as an organizational construct. Child Development 48:1184–1199, 1977

Sroufe LA, Egeland B, Kreutzer T: The fate of early experience following developmental change: longitudinal approaches to individual adaptation in childhood. Child Development 61:1363–1373, 1990

Stern D, Sander L, Nahum J, et al: Non-interpretive mechanisms in psychoanalytic therapy: the "something more" than interpretation. Int J Psychoanal 79:903–921, 1998

Target M, Fonagy P: Playing with reality, II: the development of psychic reality from a theoretical perspective. Int J Psychoanal 77:459–479, 1996

Target M, Shmueli-Goetz Y, Fonagy P: Attachment representations in school-age children: the early development of the Child Attachment Interview (CAI). Journal of Child Psychotherapy 29:171–186, 2003

Vaillant GE: Ego Mechanisms of Defense: A Guide for Clinicians and Researchers. Washington, DC, American Psychiatric Press, 1992

van IJzendoorn MH: Adult attachment representations, parental responsiveness, and infant attachment: a meta-analysis on the predictive validity of the Adult Attachment Interview. Psychol Bull 117:387–403, 1995

van IJzendoorn MH, Moran G, Belsky J, et al: The similarity of siblings attachments to their mothers. Child Dev 71:1086–1098, 2000

Vondra JI, Shaw DS, Swearingen L, et al: Attachment stability and emotional and behavioral regulation from infancy to preschool age. Dev Psychopathol 13:13–33, 2001

Warren SL, Huston L, Egeland B, et al: Child and adolescent anxiety disorders and early attachment. J Am Acad Child Adolesc Psychiatry 36:637–644, 1997

Wartner UG, Grossman K, Fremmer-Bombrik E, et al: Attachment patterns at age six in South Germany: predictability from infancy and implications for pre-school behaviour. Child Dev 65:1014–1027, 1994

Waters E, Wippman J, Sroufe LA: Attachment, positive affect, and competence in the peer group: two studies in construct validation. Child Dev 50:821–829, 1979

Weinfield NS, Sroufe LA, Egeland B, et al: The nature of individual differences in infant-caregiver attachment, in Handbook of Attachment: Theory, Research, and Clinical Applications. Edited by Cassidy J, Shaver PR. New York, Guilford, 1999, pp 68–88

11

The Psychoanalytic Understanding of Mental Disorders

The Developmental Perspective

EFRAIN BLEIBERG, M.D.

A DEVELOPMENTAL PERSPECTIVE HAS been at the core of psychoanalysis from the beginning. Psychopathology was, in fact, conceptualized by Freud (1926/1959) as a recapitulation of earlier modes of functioning to which the person regresses and/or has been fixated. This genetic/developmental point of view—the psychogenetic assumption that all psychopathology originates in an earlier phase of a developmental sequence—gave rise to the most far-reaching psychoanalytic ideas on human functioning: These ideas constitute the belief that development, particularly early development, shapes adult relationships, coping mechanisms, identity, and the overall capacity to work, love, and find gratification in both normality and psychopathology. This perspective is also at the heart of psychoanalytic treatment, an enterprise designed to enable patients to free themselves from maladaptive solutions that are thwarting their development.

Recent epidemiological studies of birth cohorts (e.g., Kim-Cohen et al. 2003) have given dramatic support to this developmental perspective. These studies demonstrated that adult psychopathology is largely preceded by diagnosable childhood disturbance. Most significantly, developmental psychopathology, which investigates em-

pirically the developmental trajectories leading to patterns of adjustment or psychopathology (Cicchetti and Cohen 1995), is emerging as a discipline capable of integrating psychodynamic, developmental, psychosocial, family systems, neurobiological, and cognitive perspectives.

The potential of these integrative efforts to revolutionize our understanding and ability to treat and even prevent psychopathology makes it urgent to examine the status of psychoanalytic models of psychopathology from a developmental perspective. In this chapter, I review the developmental approaches to psychopathology within the major psychoanalytic traditions and argue for a psychoanalytic model that can be supported or revised on the basis of direct observation of children's development and of empirical developmental research. (This examination is carried out in much more detail in Fonagy and Target 2003.)

Classical Freudian Developmental Model of Psychopathology

Freud's developmental model evolved over the course of his career. Initially, he saw symptoms as the direct expression of repressed wishes and feelings. Subsequently, he presented a more complex picture of adaptation and development, encompassing a struggle to balance the following conflicting forces: the surging power of constitutionally based sexual-libidinal and aggressive drives located in the id and seeking discharge without delay; the (internalized) demands of societal norms, moral values, and parental authority embedded in the superego; and the mediating and adaptive functions organized within the ego.

To briefly summarize Freud's well-known formulation: Freud proposed a constitutionally set sequence of psychosexual development in which the main erotogenic mode of gratification shifted from the oral to the anal and then to the phallic-genital mode. All psychopathology, stated Freud, arises from a *fixation* and/or a *regression* to a formerly outgrown mode of drive discharge. Fixations result from the interaction of constitutional predisposition to, for example, increased strength of drives and undue environmental frustration or gratification of these drives—the "complementary series" between constitution and experience. Regressions are seen as the result of internal conflicts that the ego is unable to manage, leading to a retreat to a point of fixation. The resulting revival of infantile urges intensifies the clash with other psychological agencies representing societal norms and values and the striving for adaptation to reality. Psychopathology and symptoms are compromise formations that allow the individual to find an internal equilibrium, albeit an unstable one, made possible by a restriction in functioning and some degree of psychic pain.

In Freud's classic formulation, the adult's neurosis repeats a compromise reached in childhood—the infantile neurosis—which children develop largely to cope with the problems associated with the Oedipus complex. Freud (1924/1961) thought that children feared the same-sex parent's retaliation for their hostile, competitive strivings, which are, in turn, fueled by the children's sexual wishes for the other-sex parent. Children resolve the dilemma of striving for or giving up forbidden satisfactions by internalizing the parent's ban on oedipal gratification and by identifying with the same-sex parent. Identification with the same-sex parent allows children to postpone sexual gratification and provides them with an ideal, a map to guide the development of their identity, their sexual roles, and their sexual choices.

The superego, which Freud referred to as "the heir to the Oedipus complex," is thus established as a psychic system with limit-setting and direction-giving functions (Hartmann and Loewenstein 1962). The superego prompts the ego to block the awareness and expression of oedipal wishes. The ego mobilizes an array of defensive mechanisms, but with repression—which is conceptualized as the ego's taking over the energy of the drives to counter or block their access to consciousness and to expression in action—as the basic mechanism. The "shape" of a neurotic symptom, in turn, depends on the specific compromise between defense mechanisms and drives reflecting particular developmental fixations (e.g., repression and displacement mobilized against predominantly oedipal impulses and wishes leading to phobias or cognitive-emotional isolation; reaction formation and repression seeking to neutralize oedipal and anal-sadistic impulses, generating obsessive-compulsive neurosis). These compromise formations come to life in the relationship with the analyst, thus providing an ideal opportunity to resolve the neurotic compromise via interpretation.

Thus, in the classical Freudian paradigm, the psychoneurosis came to be conceptualized as 1) a compromise formation between forbidden oedipal wishes (and reactivated preoedipal strivings) and defense mechanisms blocking their expression; 2) a category of mental disorder characterized by particular symptoms and underlying structure (i.e., the infantile neurosis); and 3) a treatment indication for psychoanalysis.

Psychoneurosis became central to the generally agreed-on indications for psychoanalysis, particularly in North America. Psychoanalytic writers, however, have noted problems with the concept. As the focus shifted in the literature to preoedipal development, questions were raised about the obligatory link between neurosis and oedipal conflicts. Tyson (1992) questioned such a link and proposed instead that the central factors of the neurosis are 1) a predominance of internalized conflicts producing the symptoms, 2) a capacity for affect regulation, and 3) a capacity for self-responsibility. In addition, as Kernberg (1976) pointed out, neuroses are characterized by a predominance of defenses centered on repression. In Anna Freud's (1946) classic definition, when the forces underlying children's neurosis become rigid, stabilized, and monotonous in their expression, the neurosis is in danger of remaining permanently and treatment is indicated.

Outside of psychoanalysis, the concept of neurosis has been assaulted with much greater ferocity. Derided as vague, unreliable, impossible to verify empirically, over-inclusive, and tied to an obsolete theory, it has been excluded from psychiatry's official diagnostic classifications. Despite these objections, neurosis refuses to disappear. Empirical studies (e.g., Achenbach and Edelbrock 1978) of psychiatric symptoms in children support a dichotomy between internalizing (emotional) disorders and externalizing (conduct) disorders. Obviously an easy differentiation between inner suffering versus outwardly directed misery does not stand up well to close scrutiny. Aggressive, delinquent, and hyperactive children experience much suffering and inner turmoil (e.g., Katz 1992), just as anxious and inhibited youngsters can entrap parents and teachers in a tight web of control and unhappiness. Nonetheless, the internalizing-externalizing dichotomy captures meaningful dimensions of children's psychopathology. Children referred with internalizing disorders resemble the children with anxious, inhibited, and neurotic symptoms that constitute the primary indication for child psychoanalysis according to the child psychoanalytic literature.

Despite this consensus, a notable controversy regarding childhood depression illustrates the problems of child psychoanalysts in dismissing theoretical constructs in the face of conflicting clinical and empirical data. Until the early 1960s, the prevailing view in the child psychoanalytic literature in North America was that depression could not exist in childhood. Rochlin (1959) argued that the child's weak superego led him or her to readily accept substitutes for lost objects rather than engage in the protracted clinging to ambivalent relationship that was considered the key pathogenic factor in depression. Lacking a fully developed and internalized superego, children were deemed incapable of experiencing the guilt, critical self-appraisal, and inwardly turned aggression that result from the superego's disapproval of the person's destructive feelings toward loved ones. Mahler (1961) added, "We know that systematized affective disorders are unknown in childhood. It has been conclusively established that the immature personality structure of the infant or older child is not capable of producing a state of depression. Their ego cannot sustain itself without taking prompt defensive actions against object loss" (p. 342). Rie (1966) agreed with Rochlin and Mahler, noting further that persistently low self-esteem was developmentally impossible before adolescence, given children's unstable self representations and limited ability to evaluate the self. Children, of course, remained capable of sustained misery regardless of theoretical constructs, to the ultimate detriment of the credibility of psychoanalytic developmental formulations.

More serious disorders, on the other hand, were seen as contraindications for psychoanalysis. Freud viewed psychosis and so-called narcissistic neurosis, such as melancholia and hypochondriasis, as representing states of fixation or regression of the ego itself to a state in which drive energy is not discharged into external objects but instead invested in the ego and/or in its own functions. These conditions were seen by Freud as recapitulating the earliest stages of development, the stage of primary narcissism (Freud 1914/1957). This period is, as Greenacre (1953) stated, "at the very dawn of the ego, roughly around 6 months and a little later" (p. 10), when Freud assumed that infants function in a state of perceptual and cognitive undifferentiation—the "oceanic feeling." Freud postulated

that babies were protected from overstimulation by a combination of the parents' interventions and a quasi-physical barrier, the "stimulus barrier" (Freud 1920/1955)—a hypothesized high threshold to environmental stimulation of the infants' sensory receptors and perceptual apparatuses. This "barrier" was thought to prevent stimulation from the outside world from disrupting the infants' homeostasis. Freud thought that infants, existing behind this barrier, had little investment in other people or the outside world. Thus, narcissistic disorders involved a regression to states of basic self-absorption and limited reality testing—or ability to differentiate self from external reality. Lack of investment in others precluded the currents of the person's feelings and conflicts being transferred to the analyst and thus established a contraindication for psychoanalytic treatment.

Classical Model and the Observation of Children

In spite of Freud's keen theoretical interest in children's mental life, he shied away from treating children, preferring instead to *reconstruct* childhood from the analysis of adult patients. The closest Freud came to directly analyzing a child was in the case of little Hans (Freud 1909/1955), in which the analysis of a 5-year-old boy was conducted by the boy's own father, under Freud's supervision.

Freud did not regard the "pedagogic experiment" he undertook with Little Hans as a step toward developing a therapeutic approach to children's mental problems, or even as a particularly significant way to validate or amend his hypotheses about development and pathogenesis. In fact, until otherwise convinced by his daughter Anna, rather late in his career, Freud remained relatively skeptical that children could be amenable to psychoanalysis.

Freud's disregard for the direct study of child development inevitably led to the kind of psychoanalytic circular thinking about development and psychopathology that Peterfreund (1978) characterized as a dual conceptual fallacy: normal infancy and childhood were adultomorphized and pathologized on the basis of the accounts of their childhoods given by adult patients, while early stages of normal development were defined in terms of hypothesis about later states of psychopathology. Such assumptions were not supported by independent evidence of developmental continuities in the trajectories leading to mental disorders.

While there are still objections within psychoanalysis to straying from reconstruction as the path to generate data about development (Green 2000), beginning in the 1930s and 1940s a number of child-analytic pioneers brought a fresh perspective to the psychoanalytic understanding of development and psychopathology based on direct observations of child development. Outstanding examples of such contributions are the perspectives of Anna Freud, René Spitz, and Margaret Mahler.

Anna Freud

Anna Freud was, of course, strongly influenced by her father's intellectual legacy as well as by the elaboration of Freud's ideas by the ego psychologists who developed the North American tradition of ego psychology—a tradition focused on the evolution and deployment of adaptive capacities and coping mechanisms. But perhaps the most significant influences on Anna Freud's thinking were her experiences at the Hampstead nurseries and her clinical practice with children and adolescents. From such experiences, Anna Freud evolved one of the most influential systems of child psychoanalysis.

Anna Freud's studies of children's anxieties are a good example of the value of direct observation of children. In her report of her wartime experience at the Hampstead nurseries (A. Freud and Burlingham 1944), she noted that children differ from adults in their reaction to external—or "objective"—threats. She observed that children's traumatic responses to the bombings inflicted on the English population were mediated by the presence and emotional state of the children's mothers. Children whose mothers remained calm were far less likely to develop prolonged and severe anxiety after the attacks. This early observation, later empirically supported by carefully conducted studies of children's reactions to threats (e.g., Laor et al. 1996), was a step toward the realization of the intersubjective and relational nature of experience and psychopathology.

Anna Freud's study of the link between development and adaptation (A. Freud 1963, 1965/1974) led her to conclude that psychopathology was not invariably the result of conflict. She charted normal development along a series of "developmental lines" that defined the achievement of sequences of developmental tasks, with each person presenting a distinctive developmental profile at any point in the course of their development (see Chapter 8, "Psychoanalytic Developmental Theory").

Anna Freud's vision of psychopathology and adaptation interwoven with the negotiation of developmental tasks is at the heart of the integrative discipline of developmental psychopathology. By defining a multiplicity of developmental profiles—and trajectories—Anna Freud provided an alternative to Sigmund Freud's "developmental fallacy" whereby a single line of development was conceptualized and pathological conditions were seen as regressions and/or fixations to early, normal childhood stages. Last, but not least, her consideration of developmental deficits, arrests, and deviations in narcissism, object relations, and control over aggression provided a framework that helped pave the way for the study and treatment of personality disorders, which have arguably supplanted psychoneurosis as the choice indication for psychoanalytic treatment.

René Spitz

René Spitz (1965) was another major figure within the ego psychological tradition to demonstrate the significance of direct observation of children's development. Spitz proposed that major changes in the development of the infant's mental organization are marked by the emergence of specific behaviors, for example, the social smile or the anxious response to the presence of strangers. Spitz suggested that the social smiling response emerging at age 2 months signals the beginning of differentiation between self and object. Stranger anxiety marks the completed differentiation of self and object and the capacity to distinguish mother from other people.

Spitz's (1965) observation about the role of the infant-mother interaction in the emergence of "psychic organizers" and emotional regulation was a clear precursor to contemporary attachment theory and research (Ainsworth et al. 1978), notwithstanding Spitz's criticism of Bowlby's early contributions (Spitz 1960). This criticism is remarkable given the resonance of Bowlby's discussion of grief and loss in infancy with Spitz's own observations about the devastating impact of early object loss and neglect in clinical manifestations such as "anaclitic depression" and "hospitalism."

Margaret Mahler

The work of Margaret Mahler (Mahler et al. 1975) offers a third example of the potential of direct observation of young children to revolutionize psychoanalytic concepts about development and psychopathology. Mahler served as one of the bridges between the North American tradition of ego psychology and object relations theory. Her description of the separation-individuation process was informed by her detailed observations of toddlers and preschool children. *Separation* refers to children's awareness of being distinct and separate from their mothers. *Individuation*, on the other hand, refers to the progressive achievement of psychological organization necessary for autonomous functioning. This process encompasses the evolution of increasingly effective coping and adaptive skills, such as regulation of affect and arousal, self-soothing, and the capacity to communicate one's internal states and "read" other people's mental states. According to Mahler, infants are able to tolerate the awareness of separation only after they have achieved a state of sufficient structuralization of their internal world to ensure relative intrapsychic autonomy.

Mahler's ideas about the first year of life were *not* informed by direct observation of infants and have been widely challenged by infancy researchers (e.g., Stern 1985). Infancy research musters impressive evidence that normally developing babies are active, organized, and invested in the outside world, and that they are exceptionally biased to seek out and respond to human stimulation and proximity and to evoke protective responses from caregivers who are themselves disposed to interpret and respond to the infant's signals. Such a view, of course, counters Freud's concept of primary narcissism or Mahler's (Mahler et al. 1975) notion of "normal autism."

Mahler postulated a normal state of "symbiosis," between 2 and 4 months of life, during which infants are not yet able to differentiate what belongs to them and what belongs to mother, and experience instead an intrapsychic state of fusion of the mental representations of the self with their primary libidinal object. For Mahler, the developmental task between the fourth and tenth months is for infants to put together in their minds a slowly coalescing core sense of self with clear boundaries, and the pieces of their mother's image, as a separate mental representation: Mahler called this process "hatching."

Mahler linked the phase of "normal autism" to the syndrome of early infantile autism and the symbiotic phase to childhood schizophrenia or "symbiotic psychosis." Contemporary research on early infantile autism (e.g., Baron-Cohen 1995; Gergely et al. 1999), however, demonstrates clear differences in the processing of social and emotional information and multiple abnormalities in brain activity in autistic children. Such empirical evidence exposes again the developmental fallacy of equating normal development with psychopathology.

Mahler's formulation of the separation-individuation process, on the other hand, was observation-based and had a seminal effect and more lasting impact in the burgeoning field of developmental psychopathology, particularly in the study of the developmental trajectories leading to the dramatic personality disorders. According to Mahler, children between 10–12 and 36 months of age go through a series of stages during which they 1) internalize some of the soothing, equilibrium, maintaining, regulating functions performed by the parents, thus acquiring the capacity to carry out these functions with some degree of autonomy; 2) practice ego skills and use them to expand their knowledge of themselves and the world; and 3) integrate the "good" and the "bad" representations of the self and the object. These achievements, in turn, enable children to ac-

cept the reality of their existence as separate individuals and develop object constancy—that is, the ability to maintain an internal connection and to evoke the loving and comforting image of the object in spite of separation and frustration.

Mahler claimed that derailment of these developmental processes leads to borderline and narcissistic psychopathology. Mahler's formulation provided a framework to understand and treat children who have been described in the literature as "atypical" or "borderline." These children fluctuate between a neurotic and a psychotic level of reality contact, object relations, and defensive organization. They present a wide and shifting array of problems, including impulsivity; low frustration tolerance; uneven development; proneness to withdraw into fantasy or to regress into primitive thinking in response to stress, lack of structure, or separation from caregivers; pervasive, intense anxiety and multiple neurotic symptoms, such as phobias, compulsions, or ritualistic behavior; somatic complaints; and sleep problems (Frijling-Schreuder 1969; Rosenfeld and Sprince 1963).

Masterson and Rinsley (1975) exemplify those psychoanalytic authors influenced by Mahler who advanced a developmental formulation of the pathogenesis of borderline disorders. According to Masterson and Rinsley, specific patterns of mother-child interaction thwart the separation-individuation process and generate borderline psychopathology. In their view, the mothers of future borderline individuals take pride in their children's dependency. These mothers, claimed Masterson and Rinsley, reward passive-dependent behavior while withdrawing and punishing in response to active striving for mastery and autonomy. The central message communicated to these children, said Rinsley (1984), is that to grow up is to face "the loss or withdrawal of maternal supplies, coupled with the related injunction that to avoid that calamity the child must remain dependent, inadequate symbiotic" (p. 5).

Such selective maternal attunement splits the maternal representation into two components: one rewarding and gratifying in response to dependency, and the second punitive and withdrawing in response to autonomy, mastery and separation. This representational split and the associated inhibition of autonomy come to the fore at times when developmental and/or psychosocial pressures push toward separation, particularly during adolescence.

Mahler's work has had an enormous influence on clinicians working with children and adults with severe personality disorder. Evidence of low parental care combined with high overprotection in the background of individuals with borderline personality disorder has been documented in empirical studies (e.g., Zweig-Frank and Paris 1991). Research on parent-child relationships in Japan and in the

United States, however, does not support the contention that prolonging the "symbiotic union" between mother and infant undermines the achievement of autonomy (e.g., Rothbaum 2000). Gabbard (1996) cogently pointed out the overemphasis of Mahler's formulation on the separation-individuation process at the expense of other developmental stages, such as the oedipal phase and adolescence. Equally significant is the lack of consideration of neuropsychiatric vulnerabilities to affective dysregulation, hyperarousal and impulsivity, and/or anxiety. Last, but not least, Mahler's model likely exaggerates maternal responsibility—a common pitfall of psychoanalytic formulations of developmental psychopathology—while largely ignoring the role of others, such as uninvolved or abusive fathers (e.g., Goldberg et al. 1985), and other forms of adversity, such as parental loss (e.g., Stone 1990) or physical and sexual abuse (e.g., Herman 1992).

Object Relations Perspective on the Development of Psychopathology

The psychoanalytic model pioneered by Melanie Klein gave rise to the object relations tradition that was to become the dominant psychoanalytic model in Britain and South America. Klein's view of development (Klein 1932, 1946) followed Freud's emphasis on the death instinct (Freud 1920/1955), in what he postulated was a constitutionally based struggle between life (or libidinal) forces, which seek unity and integration, and the opposing forces of the death instinct, which seek fragmentation and the eventual return to an inorganic state.

Klein and her followers (e.g., Bion 1957) believed that projection was the most basic and, if dominant, the most maladaptive mechanism available throughout development for dealing with one's destructiveness, ridding oneself of destructive, fragmenting tendencies by placing them onto others. Projection is at the heart of the earliest mode of functioning postulated by Klein: the paranoid-schizoid position (see Chapter 8). This position describes the state of mind that Klein believed was typical of the first 2 months of life. Projection of the infant's own destructiveness turns the object into a "bad" object that threatens the infant with annihilation and disintegration. Projected destructiveness creates a split in the representation of the object by producing a separation of the maternal object infused with libido and gratification (the "good breast") from the "bad breast" onto which the infant's sadism and frustration have been projected. The reintrojection of the destructive bad breast, in turn, induces a cleavage and fragmentation in the ego. The projection of these fragmented aspects of the ego into the representation of the object leads to terrifying experiences with what Bion (1957) called "bizarre objects."

Ego development—which requires a predominance of libido over sadism and destructiveness—leads, according to Klein, to the depressive position, at about 2 months of age. This position is ushered in by the realization that the loved object (the good breast) and the hated object (the bad breast) are one and the same. The earlier defenses, including projection, introjection, projective identification, omnipotence, splitting, and denial, which are marshaled for protection from annihilating and persecutory anxieties, are replaced by efforts to *repair* the real or fantasized damage inflicted on the object.

The Klein-Bion view of development and of the development of pathology aroused much skepticism, particularly in North America, given its rather extravagant claims for the mental capabilities of very young babies. In this view, psychotic states represent a regression to the earliest months of infancy. Under the sway of the paranoid-schizoid position, psychotic individuals are thought to experience a delusional belief that their minds and/or bodies are under the control of objects imbued with the projections of destructive impulses and split-off parts of the ego. As Hanna Segal (1964), an articulate representative of the Kleinian tradition, stated: "Through a study of the case histories of schizophrenic and schizoid patients, and from observation of infants from birth, we are now increasingly able to diagnose schizoid features in early infancy and foresee future difficulties" (p. 55).

Segal's observation illustrates both the appeal and the limitations embodied in the Klein-Bion model. While Segal fails to specify the "markers" of early development that "foresee future difficulties," contemporary research provides empirical support to the view that neurodevelopmental dysfunction antedates the emergence of the full schizophrenic syndrome (Davidson et al. 1999; Malmberg et al. 1998). Furthermore, recent developmental research has confirmed at least some of Klein's claims regarding infants' capabilities, particularly concerning the perception of causality in early infancy (Bower 1989).

The greatest impact of Kleinian ideas has perhaps been felt in the understanding of the distortions in development and functioning that characterize the severe personality disorders (Klein 1948a, 1948b/1975). The paranoid-schizoid position offers a template with which to conceptualize the functioning of the borderline personality disorder:

1. Predominance of splitting in object relations in which other people are either idealized or denigrated but are not experienced or understood as real people.

2. Absence of genuine sadness, guilt, or feelings of mourning following losses as a depressive position of full appreciation—and integration—of the self and the object representations is avoided.
3. Predominance of projective identification that impedes mutuality and empathy and results in manipulative and coercive efforts to evoke in others the assumption of roles complementary with the borderline individual's personality.

On the other hand, Klein's speculations about infants' mental states and her disregard for environmental factors challenge both common sense and known facts. Such skepticism extends to the direct analogies proposed by Klein and her followers between infancy and psychotic states. The limited self-regulatory capacities of infants may indeed turn intense affects into disorganizing experiences. Yet, as infancy research demonstrates (e.g., Jaffe et al. 2001), beginning during the first few days after birth, infants are engaged in subtle and complex mutual cueing and interacting with their caregivers that belie the suggestion of a paranoid-schizoid mode of functioning dominated by projective mechanisms. Even if a crude analogy could be drawn between the emotional dysregulation present in infancy and that observed in psychotic states, the differences in mental contents are still significant. Psychotic individuals struggle with the multiplicity of experiences, memories, and mental representations acquired and processed over a lifetime. A baby's dysregulation, on the other hand, more likely involves a general state of hyperarousal, only gradually acquiring representational "shape" in the course of intersubjective exchanges with the caregivers (Gergely 2001).

Contemporary Kleinian analysts (O'Shaughnessy 1981; Rosenfeld 1987; Sohn 1985; Spillius 1988a, 1988b; Steiner 1987) pay more attention to defensive and adaptive operations. Among their contributions is the concept of "organization," a relatively stable construction of impulses, anxieties, and defenses that they propose as the central structure underlying borderline, narcissistic, schizoid, and other severe personality disorders. The key feature of these defensive organizations is that they provide relative internal stability and protection from utter chaos by precluding new knowledge and understanding about the self and others. In effect, as Bion (1962) suggested, these organizations represent a disabling of the psychic processes that make understanding possible. This model, as it will be discussed later, has influenced psychoanalytic investigators such as Bollas (1987) and Fonagy (1991).

Contrasting with the naive developmental position of Melanie Klein, which is radically nativistic in its disregard of environmental influences, the British independent group (Balint 1968; Bollas 1987; Fairbairn 1963; Guntrip 1969; Winnicott 1965) advanced a radical environmental stance. Fairbairn (1954) asserted that the basic striving was not for pleasure but for relationships. Fairbairn postulated that failures in intimacy and connection give rise to splits in the ego aspects of self that develop as a schizoid, defensive withdrawal from the traumatic experience of not being intimately known and loved. Fairbairn (1954) regarded the schizoid reaction as a fundamental mechanism underlying all psychopathology. The schizoid or affectionless personality, for example, arose in Fairbairn's view out of the infant's conviction that his or her love can damage or destroy the mother, leading him or her to inhibit all relatedness. Schizophrenia represents for Fairbairn (1954) an even more radical withdrawal from emotional contact with the outer world, leading to a disturbed sense of external reality.

In contrast to Mahler, whose theories were rooted in the North American tradition of ego psychology and emphasize separation, British object relations theorists focused on attachment. As Guntrip (1969) stated, the growth of the self takes place as infants experience themselves as

> becoming a person in meaningful relationships.... Meaningful relationships are those which enable the infant to find himself as a person through experiencing his own significance for other people and their significance for him, thus endowing his existence with those values of human relationship which make life purposeful and worth living. (p. 243)

Donald Winnicott contributed a number of fundamental psychoanalytic notions of normal and pathological development (see also Chapter 8). These notions include the concept of the true self, which he proposed evolves in the relation with a "good enough" mother who provides a holding environment and a mirroring function. These functions allow infants to find *themselves* when looking at their mother's face (Winnicott 1965). A false self, on the other hand, results from mothers whose response to their infant "reflect (their) own mood or, worse still, the rigidity of (their) own defenses. They (babies) look and they do not see themselves....What is seen is the mother's face" (Winnicott 1967, p. 29). According to Winnicott (1965), antisocial behavior is rooted in environmental failure to provide "good enough" holding and mirroring but is sustained by its reparative intent. Winnicott (1965), for example, described an 8-year-old boy whose stealing he interpreted as the boy's hopeful search for his good mother. Winnicott's (1953) seminal idea about transitional objects and experiences, an intermediate area of experience in which children can both accept reality and create an illusory control over the soothing and regulating capacities of the caregivers, influenced psychoanalysts who were seeking to grapple with the processes of self-development, the achievement of self-regulating capacities, and the ability to recognize and share one's subjectivity.

Winnicott's influence is particularly clear, though unacknowledged, in the work of Heinz Kohut (1977). Kohut proposed that the self has its own developmental path, a narcissistic line of development in which caregivers serve as "selfobjects" (or transitional objects, in Winnicott's terminology) that provide cohesion and mirroring to the self (see Chapter 8).

The British independent object relations school shifted the focus to caregiver sensitivity and the mother-infant relationship, thus providing the psychoanalytic roots of attachment theory and research (Bowlby 1969, 1973). Contemporary developmental research, however, raises questions about exclusive role of maternal contributions to difficulties in early relationships, let alone to subsequent psychopathology.

Evidence supports the view that low levels of parental warmth and support, as well as parental rejection, hostility, and family conflicts, are associated with a wide range of psychological problems in children (e.g., Ge et al. 1996). Yet privileging disturbances in the mother-infant relationship as the bedrock of psychopathology flies in the face of accumulating evidence of the importance of genetic factors in most instances of childhood psychopathology (e.g., Rutter et al. 1999a, 1999b). For example, a landmark investigation of genetic and environmental influences in adolescent development (Reiss et al. 2000) demonstrated that of 52 statistically significant associations between family relationship (e.g., parental warmth or sibling relationships) and measures of adjustment (e.g., depression or antisocial behavior), 44 showed genetic influences that accounted for more than half of the variance. In almost half of the 52 items, genetic influence accounted for most of the association. Of the environmental influences, the lion's share appeared to involve nonshared aspects of the environment, while shared aspects, such as measures of parental sensitivity, had limited weight in explaining variance (Plomin 1994). Such data support the notion that while early relationships with caregivers are enormously significant in shaping subsequent development, such relationships depend on contributions from both caregivers and children. Evidence shows that children's own characteristics significantly shape the environment, including the family environment and parenting that are likely to impact their own development (Deater-Deckard et al. 1999).

Thus, there is accumulating evidence that British independent object relations theorists and their followers on both sides of the Atlantic overstated the case for environmental influences on pathological development. Just as surely, evidence points to an equally significant neglect of environmental and interactional factors in the Klein-Bion tradition.

Integrating Models

Daniel Stern

Daniel Stern's (1985, 1995) research and conceptualizing have created a bridge between psychoanalytic and research-based developmental models. Although Stern has studied normative development, his model of self and self-with-other development offers a useful framework to investigate the developmental trajectories leading to psychopathology. Stern is particularly interested in how infants represent and structure their experience of being in relationship with others and come to construct a sense of self out of such intersubjective experiences. He distinguishes four stages in the early development of the self, described in Chapter 8 of this textbook by Peter Fonagy.

Stern proposes that the emerging sense of self is forged in the context of various domains of self-other relatedness. He distinguishes *complementing* self-other relatedness, in which the actions of each member of the interacting dyad complement the other; *sharing* self-other relatedness, which stems from the infants' experience of sharing a common mental state with another person; *transforming* self-other relatedness, in which the actions of the other change the infants internal state; and *verbal* self-other relatedness, brought about by the development of language and symbolic representational capacities.

Stern's (1995) research supports the view that infants have the capacity and the proclivity to schematize the elements of their experiences, particularly of their experiences of "self-with-other," and are strongly biased to link schemas together into "coherent experiences made up of many simultaneously occurring, partially independent parts" (p. 89). Stern (1995) refers to the organizational format that "holds" this integrated set of schemas as the proto-narrative envelope. This "envelope" contains experience organized with the structure of a narrative. But until verbal-representational capabilities emerge during the second year of life, the narrative is a story without words or symbols, a plot visible only through the perceptual, affective, and motoric strategies to which it gives rise.

Stern (1998) refers to the "knowledge" contained within the proto-narrative envelope as *implicit relational knowledge*. This knowledge is about *how* to be with someone—that is, the form and intensity of approach, state of activation, affective quality, and so forth that will be welcomed or rejected at any given moment and that come to life in the performance of perceptual, motoric, and affective strategies.

Stern's (1995) research leads to an investigation of the developmental path leading from protonarrative envelopes to symbolic representational processing. Or as he asks, "What is the process of going from history to narration, from fixed serial order to arranged reorderings, from one pattern of emphasis and stress to a new pattern, from objective events in reality to imaginary events in virtual time?" (p. 94).

Stern's model is based on infant research and is not informed by clinical observation. Yet his work opens a path to examine procedural (i.e., nonverbal and nonconscious) aspects of experience and relationships that appear to be critical elements of psychoanalytic practice and of psychopathology, particularly of the core of the rigid and maladaptive patterns of coping, relating, and experiencing that define the personality disorders (Stern et al. 1998). Other authors (e.g., Bleiberg 2001), coming from a clinical background, have also sought to build integrative links between empirical developmental research, cognitive neuroscience, and the various psychoanalytic traditions that emphasize constitution or environment. Attachment theory and research are a prime example, elaborated in Chapter 10 ("Attachment Theory and Research") of this textbook by Mary Target.

Otto Kernberg

Kernberg, whose psychoanalytic formation in Chile was steeped in the Kleinian tradition, immersed himself in the North American tradition of ego psychology at The Menninger Clinic. In the creative cross-fertilization that ensued, Kernberg was able to bring to bear the ideas of Jacobson, Sandler, Loewald, and Mahler, as well as the Klein-Bion and British object relations models, in a new synthesis (Kernberg 1984, 1992). Kernberg's model focused on the level of personality organization, defined as the integration and coherence achieved by self and object representations linked by particular affect states, especially those organized under the aegis of libidinal or aggressive states.

For Kernberg, the underlying level of personality organization determines the person's ability to function, their degree of disturbance, and the focus of therapeutic intervention. This perspective is at least partially validated by empirical studies (e.g., Reich and Vasile 1993) demonstrating poor outcomes in the treatment of patients with an Axis I diagnosis accompanied by an Axis II diagnosis with either psychotherapy or pharmacotherapy. Unlike many psychoanalysts, however, Kernberg seriously considers empirically validated Axis I diagnostic categories as important indicators of psychopathology and predictors of treatment response.

Kernberg is rightly regarded as a leading contributor to the study and treatment of the severe personality disorders, particularly the borderline and the narcissistic personality disorders. Kernberg (1975) regards a number of Axis I and Axis II disorders, including the narcissistic, schiz-

oid, paranoid, and antisocial personality disorders, as well as low-level forms of histrionic personality disorder, as generally structured at a borderline level, which is a level of organization between the neurotic and the psychotic levels. Kernberg (1975) defines borderline personality organization on the basis of persistent splitting—that is, a defensively generated lack of integration of the partial self representation organized around libidinal experiences with the partial self representation organized around aggression, and the complementary lack of integration of libidinal and aggressive part object representations. The clinical manifestations of the borderline level of personality organization are, according to Kernberg, 1) nonspecific ego weakness manifested in poor impulse control, limited tolerance for affects and restricted capacity to sublimate; 2) primitive defenses centered on splitting and including denial, projection, and introjection; 3) intact reality testing, but with a vulnerability to shift to "dream-like," primary process thinking when under stress; and 4) pathological internalized object relationships characterized by limited empathy and a constant need to control the object. Kernberg postulates that borderline conditions result from excessive aggression overcoming the relative weaknesses of the ego mechanisms available to manage destructiveness. Wisely, however, he leaves open the question of whether such intense aggressiveness is associated with environmental adversity or malevolence, with an inborn predisposition, or with a combination of the two. Thus, his formulation is not challenged by the mounting research evidence of substantial genetic factors predisposing to borderline personality disorder (e.g., Torgersen 2000). Paulina Kernberg's (1990) concept of borderline as a developmental and structural level of personality organization resonates with similar notions evolving among clinicians working with children.

Kernberg's formulation served to illuminate the developmental and clinical continuities between adult personality disorders and patterns of coping, perceiving, thinking, and relating present in children and adolescents. Paulina Kernberg (P. F. Kernberg 1990; P. F. Kernberg et al. 2000) presents evidence that these patterns, including traits such as egocentricity, inhibition, sociability, and activity, endure across time and situation and warrant the designation of personality disorder, regardless of age, when they 1) become inflexible, maladaptive, and chronic; 2) cause significant functional impairment; and 3) produce severe subjective distress.

Kernberg's readiness to test his model empirically is lending support to his approach. A model of psychotherapy, the transference-focused psychotherapy, developed by Clarkin and colleagues (1999), is rigorously described and implemented in a pilot study (Clarkin et al. 2001), in the most systematic psychoanalytically based attempt so far to demonstrate the effectiveness of a treatment program for borderline personality disorder.

The Relational School

An alternative integrating approach is represented by the relational school (Mitchell 1988; Ogden 1994; see also Chapter 8). Relational models reject the classical epistemological and clinical framework of psychoanalysis by conceiving of both development and treatment as co-constructions between active, transacting, mutually influencing subjectivities, parent-child and analyst-patient. Thus, relational approaches replace notions of objective truth with an emphasis on subjectivity, of a focus on the intrapsychic with an intersubjective perspective, and of a reliance on interpretations of content in psychoanalytic treatment with observations about process. This perspective is illustrated by Stolorow and Atwood's (1991) statement that "the concept of an isolated individual mind is a theoretical fiction or myth....The experience of distinctness requires a nexus of intersubjective relatedness that encourages and supports the process of self-delineation throughout the life cycle" (p. 193).

Relational approaches offer a clear link to Bowlby's attachment theory (see Chapter 10). Bowlby identified attachment as the basis of emotional regulation and internal working models not only in infancy but throughout life. As Bowlby (1980) stated, "Intimate attachments to other human beings are the hub around which a person's life revolves, not only when he is an infant or a toddler or a schoolchild but throughout his adolescence an his years of maturity as well, and into old age" (p. 422). Research evidence is consistent with the relational view that emphasizing exclusively early relationships as the basis of psychopathology overlooks the impact of *current* relationships in determining the emergence, course, and severity of psychological disturbance (Lewis 1998) or serving as a protective factor against maladjustment (Laub 1998).

The Menninger Clinic and The Menninger Child and Family Program

A fourth effort to advance an integrating psychoanalytic developmental model is emerging from the studies at The Menninger Clinic and The Menninger Child and Family Program at Baylor College of Medicine concerning the development of personality disorders (Allen 2001; Bleiberg 2001; Bleiberg et al. 1997; Fonagy et al. 2002; Gabbard 2000). This evolving model is closely linked to attachment theory and focuses on the development of self as an agent in attachment relationships underpinned by the capacity to mentalize and regulate affects, arousal and attention.

At the heart of this model is the development of the capacity to mentalize. *Mentalizing* refers to the genetically prepared, experience-expectant capacity to spontaneously, implicitly, *and* explicitly ascribe, interpret, and represent intentionality, meaning, and mental states (e.g., the thoughts, feelings, goals, attitudes, etc., underlying human behavior, both one's own and others'). Mentalizing and other genetically prepared, experience-expectant interpreting, appraising, and regulating functions shape and are shaped by the psychosocial context and mediate gene expression. The focus on mentalizing places the "old wine" of venerable psychoanalytic concepts, such as "empathy," "insight" and "observing ego," in a new bottle that captures the relational, cognitive, and neurobiological aspects of these concepts while placing them in the context of contemporary developmental theory and empirical research. A central hypothesis of this model is that the psychological self and reciprocal, secure, intimate attachments are rooted in the attribution and interpretation of mental states, that is, on the capacity to mentalize (Fonagy et al. 2002).

Empirical research (e.g., Gergely 2001, 2003) supports the view that mentalizing emerges in the context of interactions with caregivers who are disposed to respond and interpret the infant's behavioral signals of distress with protective, regulating responses. Caregivers' responses are effective in promoting mentalizing when they are *contingent*—that is, when they accurately (and procedurally) match the infants' internal states (Stern 1985)—and *marked* (Gergely and Csibra 2003)—that is, when they convey through motoric, perceptual, and affective strategies that the caregivers are *not* expressing their own internal state but reflecting their experience of the infants' internal state. Caregivers' mentalizing allows for the integration of the child prementalizing modes of processing emotional and interpersonal experience: 1) the teleological stance (Gergely and Csibra 2003), which is the infant's biologically "pre-wired" appraisal of human behavior in terms of physical constraints and the physical end state reached; 2) the psychic equivalence mode (Target and Fonagy 1996), in which infants regard mental reality and external reality as equivalent; and 3) the pretend mode, in which prementalizing children regard their mental states as "not only" not real but as having no implications in the external world.

This developmental model suggests that incongruent and/or unmarked mirroring generates distortions in mentalizing that result in enfeebled affect and attentional regulation and affect representation (Arntz et al. 2000). Such enfeeblement appears to be a crucial ingredient in disorganized attachment systems (Main and Solomon 1986), which are characterized by a lack of a coherent attachment strategy. These infants exhibit a mix of approaching, avoiding, clinging, and trancelike behavior during separations and reunions that has been linked to caregivers frightening and/or dissociated behavior (Lyons-Ruth et al. 1999), maltreatment (Cicchetti and Barnett 1991), prolonged or repeated separations (Chisolm 1998), and maternal depression or bipolar disorder (Lyons-Ruth and Jacobovitz 1993).

Incongruent/unmarked parenting establishes within the child's developing self structure an aspect that corresponds, as Winnicott (1965) suggested, to the mother's own predicament, yet is experienced as both part of the self and an alien part of the self (Fonagy and Target 1996). This disorganization of the developing self and attachment systems may account for the controlling and coercive behavior of 5- and 6-year-olds with a history of disorganized attachment in infancy (see Chapter 10), reflecting a teleological stance in which human connections and intentions can be accessed and regulated only through concrete, procedural means.

Coercive, controlling cycles increase the odds of maltreatment that, combined with the legacy of deeply insecure/disorganized early attachments, has profoundly maladaptive consequences in subsequent development: 1) it inhibits playfulness, which is critical for the further development of mentalizing, symbolic processing, mutual empathy, and social reciprocity (Dunn et al. 2000); 2) it directly disrupts affect regulation, impulse control, and attentional and arousal control systems (Arntz et al. 2000); and 3) it can bring about a defensive strategy that appears central to the future development of borderline psychopathology: the inhibition of mentalizing in attachment contexts (Fonagy et al. 2002).

Coercive/controlling behavior becomes the means to externalize and control the alien aspects of the self in developing borderline personality disorder. Relationships are thus essential to stabilize the self but are also the source of greatest vulnerability because the self is destabilized if the other is not present or otherwise escapes from control and coercion.

Self-harm, a frequent outcome of the failure of coercive behavior to compel the other person to provide a "perfect match" that ensures self-coherence (Kemperman et al. 1997), reflects the activation of uncoupled psychic equivalence and pretend modes. In the pretend mode of organizing their subjective experience, patients with borderline personality disorder often believe that they—or their true self—will survive the suicide attempt, attempts that are not felt to be truly "for real," or truly lethal (Stanley et al. 2001), while convinced that the alien part of the self will be destroyed. Such conviction is sustained by the equivalence between the alien aspect of the self and the person's physical self—or a part of the body.

The treatment implications of this developmental model (Bleiberg 2001; Bleiberg et al. 1997) include a concerted and systematic focus on interrupting coercive cycles and promoting mentalizing, particularly under the attachment conditions in which it is regularly inhibited.

Conclusion

Every psychoanalytic tradition is rooted in a developmental framework that provides the conceptual scaffolding supporting the tradition's perspective on psychopathology and on the foci of therapeutic intervention. It is indeed axiomatic within the majority of psychoanalytic schools of thought that the psychic processes underlying development concern the same processes resulting in psychopathology. This brief review makes the case that such assumptions are often poorly supported and at times openly contradicted by empirical evidence and contemporary developmental research. Even when similarities can be drawn between infants' or young children's modes of mental functioning and the adult's mind in distress, evidence points to the impact of subsequent development in modifying earlier structures and mental processes. Thus, psychoanalytic schools have often fallen prey to the circular thinking of a developmental fallacy that undermines their scientific credibility and their potential to assess basic psychoanalytic developmental hypotheses in the context of empirically based disciplines such as the cognitive neurosciences and contemporary developmental research.

In this chapter I advocate a developmental psychoanalytic approach to psychopathology that is evaluated against the background of direct observation of children and is consistent with empirical findings. This developmental psychoanalytic model offers the opportunity to align psychoanalysis with the mainstream of contemporary research in developmental neurobiology and developmental psychopathology by systematically and comprehensively mapping the sequential emergence of constellations of mental capacities and patterns of coping, relating, and experiencing and to adaptive or maladaptive developmental trajectories.

References

Achenbach T, Edelbrock CS: The classification of child psychopathology: a review and analysis of empirical efforts. Psychol Bull 85:1275–1301, 1978

Ainsworth MDS, Blehar MC, Waters E, et al: Patterns of Attachment: A Psychological Study of the Strange Situation. Hillsdale, NJ, Lawrence Erlbaum, 1978

Allen JG: Traumatic Relationships and Serious Mental Disorders. Chichester, NY, Wiley, 2001

Arntz A, Appels C, Sieswerda S: Hypervigilance in borderline disorder: a test with the emotional Stroop paradigm. J Personal Disord 14:366–373, 2000

Balint M: The Basic Fault. London, Tavistock, 1968

Baron-Cohen S: Mindblindness: An Essay on Autism and Theory of Mind. Cambridge, MA, MIT Press, 1995

Bion WR: Differentiation of the psychotic from the non-psychotic personalities. Int J Psychoanal 38:266–275, 1957

Bion WR: Learning From Experience. New York, Basic Books, 1962

Bleiberg E: Treating Personality Disorders in Children and Adolescents: A Relational Approach. New York, Guilford, 2001

Bleiberg E, Fonagy P, Target M: Child psychoanalysis: critical overview and a proposed reconsideration. Psychiatr Clin North Am 6:1–38, 1997

Bollas C: The Shadow of the Object: Psychoanalysis of the Unthought Known. New York, Columbia University Press, 1987

Bower TR: The Rational Infant: Learning in Infancy. New York, WH Freeman, 1989

Bowlby J: Attachment and Loss, Vol 1: Attachment. New York, Basic Books, 1969

Bowlby J: Attachment and Loss, Vol 2: Separation: Anxiety and Anger. New York, Basic Books, 1973

Bowlby J: Attachment and Loss, Vol 3: Loss: Sadness and Depression. New York, Basic Books, 1980

Chisolm K: A three-year follow-up of attachment and indiscriminate friendliness in children adopted from Russian orphanages. Child Dev 69:1092–1106, 1998

Cicchetti D, Barnett D: Attachment organization in preschool aged maltreated children. Dev Psychopathol 3:397–411, 1991

Cicchetti D, Cohen DJ: Developmental Psychopathology, Vols 1 and 2. New York, Wiley, 1995

Clarkin JF, Kernberg OF, Yeomans F: Transference-Focused Psychotherapy for Borderline Personality Disorder Patients. New York, Guilford, 1999

Clarkin JF, Foelsch PA, Levy KN, et al: The development of a psychodynamic treatment for patients with borderline personality disorder: a preliminary study of behavioral change. J Personal Disord 15:487–495, 2001

Davidson M, Reichenberg A, Rabinowitz J, et al: Behavioral and intellectual markers for schizophrenia in apparently healthy male adolescents. Am J Psychiatry 156:1328–1335, 1999

Deater-Deckard K, Fulker DW, Plomin R: A genetic study of the family environment in the transition to early adolescence. J Child Psychol Psychiatry 40:769–795, 1999

Dunn J, Davies LC, O'Connor TG, et al: Parents' and partners' life course and family experiences: links with parent-child relationships in different family settings. J Child Psychol Psychiatry 41:955–968, 2000

Fairbairn R: An Object-Relations Theory of the Personality. New York, Basic Books, 1954

Fairbairn WRD: Synopsis of an object-relations theory of the personality. Int J Psychoanal 44:224–225, 1963

Fonagy P, Target M: Playing with reality, I: theory of mind and the normal development of psychic reality. Int J Psychoanal 77:217–233, 1996

Fonagy P, Target M: Psychoanalytic Theories: Perspectives From Developmental Psychopathology. London, Whurr, 2003

Fonagy P, Gergely G, Jurist E, et al: Affect Regulation, Mentalization, and the Development of the Self. New York, Other Press, 2002

Freud A: The Psychoanalytic Treatment of Children. London, Imago Publishing, 1946

Freud A: The concept of developmental lines. Psychoanal Study Child 18:245–265, 1963

Freud A: Normality and pathology in childhood (1965), in The Writings of Anna Freud, Vol 6. New York, International Universities Press, 1974, pp 25–63

Freud A, Burlingham D: Infants Without Families. New York, International Universities Press, 1944

Freud S: Analysis of a phobia in a five-year-old boy (1909), in Standard Edition of the Complete Psychological Works of Sigmund Freud, Vol 10. Translated and edited by Strachey J. London, Hogarth Press, 1955, pp 1–149

Freud S: On narcissism: an introduction (1914), in Standard Edition of the Complete Psychological Works of Sigmund Freud, Vol 14. Translated and edited by Strachey J. London, Hogarth Press, 1957, pp 67–102

Freud S: Beyond the pleasure principle (1920), in Standard Edition of the Complete Psychological Works of Sigmund Freud, Vol 18. Translated and edited by Strachey J. London, Hogarth Press, 1955, pp 1–64

Freud S: The dissolution of the Oedipus complex (1924), in Standard Edition of the Complete Psychological Works of Sigmund Freud, Vol 19. Translated and edited by Strachey J. London, Hogarth Press, 1961, pp 173–182

Freud S: Inhibitions, symptoms and anxiety (1926), in Standard Edition of the Complete Psychological Works of Sigmund Freud, Vol 20. Translated and edited by Strachey J. London, Hogarth Press, 1959, pp 75–175

Frijling-Schreuder ECM: Borderline states in children. Psychoanal Study Child 24:307–327, 1969

Gabbard GO: Psychodynamic Psychiatry in Clinical Practice: The DSM-IV Edition. Washington, DC, American Psychiatric Press, 1996

Gabbard GO: Psychodynamic Psychiatry in Clinical Practice, Third Edition. Washington, DC, American Psychiatric Press, 2000

Ge X, Conger RD, Simmons RL: Parenting behaviors and the occurrence and co-occurrence of adolescent symptoms and conduct problems. Dev Psychol 32:717–731, 1996

Gergely G: The obscure object of desire: "nearly, but clearly not, like me." Contingency preference in normal children versus children with autism, in Contingency Perception and Attachment in Infancy (Spec Issue Bull Menninger Clin). Edited by Allen J, Fonagy P, Gergely G. New York, Guilford, 2001, pp 411–426

Gergely G, Csibra G: Teleological reasoning in infancy: the naive theory of rational action. Trends Cogn Sci 7:287–292, 2003

Gergely G, Magyar J, Balázs A: Childhood autism as 'blindness' to less-than-perfect contingencies (poster). Paper presented at the biennial conference of the International Society for Research in Childhood and Adolescent Psychopathology, Barcelona, June 16–20, 1999

Goldberg RL, Mann L, Wise T, et al: Parental qualities as perceived by borderline personality disorders. Hillside J Clin Psychiatry 7:134–140, 1985

Green A: What kind of research for psychoanalysis? in Clinical and Observational Psychoanalytic Research: Roots of a Controversy. Edited by Sandler J, Sandler A-M, Davies R. London, Karnac Books, 2000, pp 21–27

Greenacre P (ed): Affective Disorders. New York, International Universities Press, 1953

Guntrip H: Schizoid Phenomena, Object Relations and the Self. New York, International Universities Press, 1969

Hartmann H, Loewenstein R: Notes on the superego. Psychoanal Study Child 18:42–81, 1962

Herman J: Trauma and Recovery. New York, Basic Books, 1992

Jaffe J, Beebe B, Feldstein S, et al: Rhythms of dialogue in infancy. Monogr Soc Res Child Dev 66:i–viii, 2001

Katz C: Aggressive children, in Psychotherapies With Children and Adolescents: Adapting the Psychodynamic Process. Edited by O'Brien J, Pilowsky DJ, Lewis O. Washington, DC, American Psychiatric Press, 1992, pp 91–108

Kemperman I, Russ MJ, Shearin E: Self-injurious behavior and mood regulation in borderline patients. J Personal Disord 11:146–157, 1997

Kernberg OF: Borderline Conditions and Pathological Narcissism. New York, Jason Aronson, 1975

Kernberg OF: Object Relations Theory and Clinical Psychoanalysis. New York, Jason Aronson, 1976

Kernberg OF: Severe Personality Disorders: Psychotherapeutic Strategies. New Haven, CT, Yale University Press, 1984

Kernberg OF: Aggression in Personality Disorders and Perversions. New Haven, CT, Yale University Press, 1992

Kernberg PF: Resolved: borderline personality exists in children under twelve. J Am Acad Child Adolesc Psychiatry 29:478–482, 1990

Kernberg PF, Weiner AS, Bandenstein KK: Personality Disorder in Children and Adolescents. New York, Basic Books, 2000

Kim-Cohen J, Caspi A, Moffitt TE, et al: Prior juvenile diagnoses in adults with mental disorder: developmental followback of a prospective longitudinal cohort. Arch Gen Psychiatry 60:709–717, 2003

Klein M: The Psycho-Analysis of Children. London, Hogarth Press, 1932

Klein M: Notes on some schizoid mechanisms, in Developments in Psychoanalysis. Edited by Klein M, Heimann P, Isaacs S, et al. London, Hogarth Press, 1946, pp 292–320

Klein M: Contributions to Psycho-Analysis, 1921–1945. London, Hogarth Press, 1948a

Klein M: On the theory of anxiety and guilt (1948b), in Envy and Gratitude and Other Works, 1946–1963. New York, Delacorte Press, 1975

Kohut H: The Restoration of the Self. New York, International Universities Press, 1977

Laor N, Wolmer L, Mayes LC, et al: Israeli preschoolers under Scud missile attacks: a developmental perspective on risk modifying factors. Arch Gen Psychiatry 53:416–423, 1996

Laub JH: The interdependence of school violence with neighborhood and family conditions, in Violence in American Schools: A New Perspective. Edited by Elliot DS, Hamburg B, Williams KR. New York, Cambridge University Press, 1998, pp 127–155

Lewis JM: For better or worse: interpersonal relationships and individual outcome. Am J Psychiatry 155:582–589, 1998

Lyons-Ruth K, Jacobovitz DE: Attachment disorganization: unresolved loss, relational violence and lapses in behavioral and attentional strategies, in Handbook of Attachment Theory and Research. Edited by Cassidy J, Shaver PR. New York, Guilford, 1999, pp 520–554

Lyons-Ruth K, Bronfman E, Atwood G: A relational diathesis model of hostile-helpless states of mind: expressions in mother-infant interaction, in Attachment Disorganization. Edited by Solomon J, George C. New York, Guilford, 1999, pp 33–70

Mahler M: On sadness and grief in infancy and childhood: loss and restoration of the symbiotic love object. Psychoanal Study Child 16:332–351, 1961

Mahler MS, Pine F, Bergman A: The Psychological Birth of the Human Infant: Symbiosis and Individuation. New York, Basic Books, 1975

Main M, Solomon J: Discovery of an insecure-disorganized/disoriented attachment pattern, in Affective Development in Infancy. Edited by Brazelton TB, Yogman MW. Norwood, NJ, Ablex, 1986, pp 95–124

Malmberg A, Lewis G, David A, et al: Premorbid adjustment and personality in people with schizophrenia. Br J Psychiatry 172:308–313, 1998

Masterson JF, Rinsley D: The borderline syndrome: the role of the mother in the genesis and psychic structure of the borderline personality. Int J Psychoanal 56:163–177, 1975

Mitchell S: Relational Concepts in Psychoanalysis: An Integration. Cambridge, MA, Harvard University Press, 1988

Ogden T: Subjects of Analysis. Northvale, NJ, Jason Aronson, 1994

O'Shaughnessy E: A clinical study of a defensive organization. Int J Psychoanal 62:359–369, 1981

Peterfreund E: Some critical comments on psychoanalytic conceptualizations of infancy. Int J Psychoanal 59:427–441, 1978

Plomin R: Genetics and Experience: The Interplay Between Nature and Nurture. Thousand Oaks, CA, Sage, 1994

Reich JH, Vasile RG: Effect of personality disorders on the treatment outcome of axis I conditions: an update. J Nerv Ment Dis 181:475–484, 1993

Reiss D, Neiderhiser J, Hetherington EM, et al: The Relationship Code: Deciphering Genetic and Social Patterns in Adolescent Development. Cambridge, MA, Harvard University Press, 2000

Rie HE: Depression in childhood: a survey of some pertinent contributions. J Am Acad Psychiatry 5:653–668, 1966

Rinsley DB: A comparison of borderline and narcissistic personality disorders. Bull Menninger Clin 48:1–9, 1984

Rochlin G: The loss complex: a contribution to the etiology of depression. J Am Psycholanal Assoc 7:299–316, 1959

Rosenfeld H: Impasse and Interpretation: Therapeutic and Antitherapeutic Factors in the Psychoanalytic Treatment of Psychotic, Borderline and Neurotic Patients. London, Tavistock/The Institute of Psycho-Analysis, 1987

Rosenfeld S, Sprince M: An attempt to formulate the meaning of the concept borderline. Psychoanal Study Child 18:603–635, 1963

Rothbaum: The development of close relationships in Japan and the United States: paths of symbiotic harmony and generative tension. Child Dev 71:1121–1142, 2000

Rutter M, Silberg J, O'Connor T, et al. Genetics and child psychiatry, I: advances in quantitative and molecular genetics. J Child Psychol Psychiatry 40:3–18, 1999a

Rutter M, Silberg J, O'Connor T, et al. Genetics and child psychiatry, II: empirical research findings. J Child Psychol Psychiatry 40:19–55, 1999b

Segal H: Introduction to the Work of Melanie Klein. New York, Basic Books, 1964

Sohn L: Narcissistic organization, projective identification, and the formation of the identificate. Int J Psychoanal 66:201–213, 1985

Spillius EB (ed): Melanie Klein Today: Developments in Theory and Practice, Vol 1: Mainly Theory. London, Routledge, 1988a

Spillius EB (ed): Melanie Klein Today: Developments in Theory and Practice, Vol 2: Mainly Practice. London, Routledge, 1988b

Spitz RA: Discussion of Dr. John Bowlby's paper. Psychoanal Study Child 15:85–94, 1960

Spitz R: The First Year of Life: A Psychoanalytic Study of Normal and Deviant Development of Object Relations. New York, International Universities Press, 1965

Spitz R, Wolf R: Anaclitic Depression. Psychoanal Study Child 5:113–117, 1946

Stanley B, Gameroff MJ, Michalsen V, et al: Are suicide attempters who self-mutilate a unique population? Am J Psychiatry 158:427–432, 2001

Steiner J: The interplay between pathological organizations and the paranoid-schizoid and depressive positions. Int J Psychoanal 68:69–80, 1987

Stern DN: The Interpersonal World of the Infant: A View From Psychoanalysis and Developmental Psychology. New York, Basic Books, 1985

Stern DN: The Motherhood Constellation: A Unified View of Parent-Infant Psychotherapy. New York, Basic Books, 1995

Stern DN: The process of therapeutic change involving implicit knowledge: some implications of developmental observations for adult psychotherapy. Infant Ment Health J 19:300–308, 1998

Stern D, Sander L, Nahum J, et al: Non-interpretive mechanisms in psychoanalytic therapy: the "something more" than interpretation. Int J Psychoanal 79:903–921, 1998

Stolorow R, Atwood G: The mind and the body. Psychoanalytic Dialogues 1:190–202, 1991

Stone MH: Abuse and abusiveness in borderline personality disorder, in Family Environment and Borderline Personality Disorder. Edited by Links PS. Washington, DC, American Psychiatric Press, 1990, pp 133–148

Target M, Fonagy P: Playing with reality, II: the development of psychic reality from a theoretical perspective. Int J Psychoanal 77:459–479, 1996

Torgersen S: Genetics of patients with borderline personality disorder. Psychiatr Clin North Am 23:1–9, 2000

Tyson P: Neurosis in childhood and in psychoanalysis. Paper presented at the 145th annual meeting of the American Psychoanalytic Association, Washington, DC, May 2–7, 1992

Winnicott DW: Transitional objects and transitional phenomena. Int J Psychoanal 34:1–9, 1953

Winnicott DW: The Maturational Process and the Facilitating Environment. London, Hogarth Press, 1965

Winnicott DW: Mirror-role of the mother and family in child development, in The Predicament of the Family: A Psycho-Analytical Symposium. Edited by Lomas P. London, Hogarth Press, 1967, pp 26–33

Zweig-Frank H, Paris J: Parents' emotional neglect and overprotection according to the recollections of patients with borderline personality disorder. Am J Psychiatry 148:648–651, 1991

Treatment and Technique

SECTION EDITOR: HENRY F. SMITH, M.D.

12

What Is Psychoanalysis?
What Is a Psychoanalyst?

PAUL WILLIAMS, PH.D.

AS MEMBERS DEPARTED THE scientific evening at a psychoanalytic society in Europe, in which a young analyst had presented an unusually wide-ranging discussion of conceptualizations of disorders of the self, a prominent analyst known for an adherence to a particular school of psychoanalysis took the presenter aside and inquired, "Tell me: just what *are* you?" The young analyst thought for a moment and replied, "I'm a *psychoanalyst.*" This anecdote, which is true, reflects the vicissitudes of pluralism that characterize contemporary psychoanalysis. We live, psychoanalytically, in an age of multiple conceptual systems that have emerged from interpretations and developments of the classical paradigm of the first half of the last century. Some see these competing theoretical systems as so divergent as to be ultimately incompatible. Others argue that there is a good deal that these schools share in common, despite their diversity. One way of approaching the question "What is psychoanalysis?" is to reflect upon this history of pluralism and the principal psychoanalytic approaches that have emerged from it.

What Is Psychoanalysis?

Few people remain unaware that psychoanalysis began with the work of Sigmund Freud; his theories continue to occupy psychoanalysts, and other serious thinkers about the mind, to this day. There are numerous biographies and studies of Freud and the Freudian oeuvre. However, what is fundamental to the psychoanalysis Freud created is the introduction of psychological tenets that permitted unprecedented access to the internal world and to the motives and meanings of mental events. How did Freud accomplish this? Originally an anatomist, he was struck early in his career by the fact that certain physiological symptoms could not be related to the anatomical structures associated with them. These illnesses and symptoms seemed to be connected to psychological processes rather than to anatomical ones, and he formulated a theory of the unconscious to account for these and other unexplained psychological phenomena.

The concept of the unconscious lay at the heart of the new discipline called psychoanalysis and was held to play a significant role in the origins of psychological disturbance as well as in normal mental functioning. Mental processes are regarded as unconscious when the subject is unaware of them. Some of these can be recalled to consciousness without much difficulty (*descriptively* unconscious, or *preconscious);* others, held in repression, cannot (*dynamically* unconscious). As a noun, the term *unconscious* refers to a functioning structure in the mind, which in Freud's early conceptualizations he called the *system Unconscious.* Freud understood the unconscious to constitute the larger part of mental life, following a logic and rules of its own. Freud called these rules the *primary processes* of thought, in contrast to the *secondary processes* of the conscious mind. The concept of the unconscious has been approached more recently from the perspective of mathematical logic as a differentiating and classifying system (Matte-Blanco 1988), whereas Melanie Klein, in her theories, introduced the term *unconscious phantasy* to denote the primary psychic expression of innate libidinal and destructive instincts (Klein 1946, 1984b). For Klein, the unconscious phantasies that have proliferated from the time of birth underlie the individual's mental processes. Unconscious phantasies may be managed by normal defenses or give rise to pathological structures (see below).

The mysterious physical symptoms of the kind Freud witnessed early in his career (and which Charcot had also demonstrated in his Salpêtrière patients) became, as a result of Freud's theory of the unconscious, amenable to investigation by way of a framework hitherto the preserve of poets, anthropologists, and philosophers. Freud did not invent the unconscious, but he was the first to explore its nature and function from a psychological perspective. Freud showed how thinking and behavior are influenced by nonrandom unconscious ideas, thoughts, and feelings that can conflict with one another and with conscious wishes and thoughts, resulting in confusion, symptoms, and even illness. Conflicting feelings and thoughts are familiar to everyone, but Freud drew a radical distinction between conscious and unconscious conflicts that was revolutionary for understanding normality and psychological disturbance and that paved the way for a *psychodynamic* psychology.

Several theoretical and clinical approaches employ the concept of mental forces in dynamic interplay, but what distinguishes the psychoanalytic theoretical system from others is its developmental perspective and fundamental concepts: *instinctual mental life (conscious* and *unconscious), developmental phases, conflicts* and *defenses, internal (psychic) reality,* the *tendency to repeat the past in the present,* the phenomena of *transference* and *countertransference,* and *the dynamic working-through of pathogenic concepts during the course of treatment.* These constitute a psychoanalytic, or psychodynamic, theory and perspective that permit identification of meaning in mental events and of psychic reality.

Instinctual Mental Life

Freud's initial ideas centered around a "trauma-affect" model in which the overflow of dammed-up feelings could give rise to psychological symptoms. The impact of external reality on the production of symptoms was seen as central (hence Freud's concern with incidences of child sexual abuse), whereas the internal world's influence on the way in which reality is construed came to occupy Freud subsequently. The respective roles of external and internal reality, particularly the impact of trauma, are debated by psychoanalysts to this day.

In 1900 Freud conceived of the "topographical" model of the mind, which emphasized a spatial organization of mental functions as they responded to internal reality—to the impact of instincts or drives (Freud 1900/1953). In this theory he divided the mind into three "systems": unconscious, preconscious, and conscious. The *unconscious* comprises repressed material largely inaccessible to the subject. Repression is a mechanism used to reduce conflict and mental pain (e.g., anxiety, guilt) by keeping certain ideas from consciousness. Repressed ideas can, under certain circumstances, generate physical and psychological symptoms. "Above" the unconscious proper lie ideas that are unconscious but accessible in the *preconscious*. Finally, there is *conscious* awareness. Unconscious "primary process thinking" (e.g., dreaming, phantasies) evades rationality and logic, whereas "secondary process thinking" embodies rationality. Instincts—predominantly sexual and aggressive—seek satisfaction through discharge; dealing with this activity is a lifelong psychological task, with important developmental implications in childhood. The construction of flexible defenses is required to manage derivatives of instincts, and if the trajectory of instinct management does not run evenly, or defenses become rigid or overemployed, symptoms can arise.

Freud's views underwent major changes in 1923 with the formulation of his structural theory, which superseded his topographical theory (Freud 1923/1961). During this later period some of his most important papers were written—on narcissism, depression, anxiety, identification and conscience (superego). This phase culminated in Freud's clearest depiction of instinctual mental life: the mind became divided conceptually into three major parts—ego, superego, and id. The *id*, a product of biological endowment, denotes inborn instincts (sexuality and aggression) that strive toward satisfaction. The *ego* is an agency that corresponds to a capacity for rational thought and appraisal of external reality and is charged with managing the competing internal demands such as wishes and needs. When functioning satisfactorily, the ego is capable of taking into account others' needs as well as one's own. In his earlier topographical theory, Freud had conceived of the "ego ideal" as a mental representation or template of a good figure that becomes the internal model for the subject's aspirations and development. This somewhat static concept gave way in the structural theory to the broader, dynamic notion of the *superego*. This development brought into focus the relationship between environmental impact and the structuring effects of phantasy and projection and has proved to be a fertile source of research data and clinical understanding, not least of the roles of unconscious anxiety and guilt in states of persecution. The superego concept is designed to reflect the dialectical nature of relations between subject and object. The young child not only internalizes the values and judgments of caregivers but reshapes and distorts them as a result of the child's immature cognitive function. In contemporary object relations terms, what is internalized is a modified version of the object containing transformations and distortions of the object's characteristics. Like the ego, the superego functions consciously and unconsciously.

Developmental Phases

Freud adhered to a developmental model that is analogous to a physiological model, in that growth is seen as taking place according to identifiable, unfolding stages. The influence on Freud of John Hughlings Jackson was significant in this respect. Hughlings Jackson, a neurologist, had studied the progressive and regressive activities of the nervous system, and his neurological model (together with the anatomical thinking of the day) inspired Freud's view of personality development within which progressive and regressive potentials coexist (Jackson 1932). Development may proceed without undue difficulty or may be impeded by conflicts or, in severe cases, psychological crises. These crises can occur at any stage, but the consequences are especially important for infancy and childhood. The notion of developmental arrest at a particular stage in early life is important for Freud's views on the origins of psychopathology. The earlier the crises, the more potentially damaging the consequences.

In addition to psychological stages, Freud postulated associated "erotogenic zones"—the mouth, anus, and genitals (Freud 1905/1953). The first stage of development is oral and reflects experiences of the infant at the breast. The infant's world is colored by experiences of rooting, sucking, and feeding. For Freud such impulses are biologically determined and form the basis of the drive for human contact. This highly sensitive period is infused with affects, images, and experiences associated with taking in food and care, and ridding oneself of elemental "bad" experiences such as hunger, cold and separateness. Disruption at this stage is held to result in psychological traumas associated with excessive greed and difficulties in differentiating the self from others. The anal stage is located at 2–3 years and reflects the infant's concerns with control of the sphincter and bladder—psychologically speaking, with what remains inside and what is expelled outside. This period is associated with the emergence of increased movement—critically, away from the mother—requiring tolerance of separation anxiety. Disruption is likely to be reflected in symptoms concerned with control, obsessionality, and withholding. The genital stage, at 3–5 years, heralds Freud's best-known theory—the Oedipus complex—during which

awareness of gender and negotiation of sexual identity emerge. Anxieties surrounding castration anxiety and penis envy are paramount at this stage. Put simply, the acceptance by a boy of father's prior authority and the renunciation of infantile phantasies of possessing mother, or vice versa for a girl, represent forms of exclusion that will determine the child's capacity to differentiate himself or herself from the parents and establish a secure sexual identity in later life. The Oedipus complex has, theoretically and practically, stood the test of time, although many aspects of it have been modified by subsequent generations of psychoanalysts (Britton et al. 1989).

The notion of erotogenic zones associated with discrete stages at risk of fixation or arrest tends today to be viewed as oversimplified and unrealistically linear. "Penis envy," though relevant to Freud's epoch, is less plausible a century on. Similarly, the distinction between an "instinctual" infant and a separate impinging environment has been shown by developmentalists and infant researchers to underestimate the intensity with which the newborn infant instigates relationships and brings to bear on these an emerging sense of self. Negotiating trust, suspicion, fear, separateness, shame, and guilt within an object relationship is more likely to reflect the actual complexity of a neonate's life and of character as the child grows up. Although the rise of object relations theory has been inexorable in the study of these inter- and intrapersonal psychic states, attachment theory has undergone a major revival in the past decade as a consequence of its qualitative and quantitative research into infant-caregiver relationship formation. Bowlby's work underlies attachment theory and links psychoanalysis with ethology, sociobiology, psychobiology, cybernetics, and theories of cognitive development (Bowlby 1969, 1973, 1980, 1988). Attachment formation is seen as the expression of a behavioral *system* that underlies and mediates the discrete behavior of the individual. The differences and often unrecognized links between contemporary psychoanalytic concepts and attachment theory have been recently highlighted in the work of, among others, Fonagy (2001).

One important casualty of Freud's theoretical system has been the concept of "primary narcissism" (Freud 1914a/1957): this state of primary, infantile self-absorption that precedes the development of a capacity to love others is seldom referred to today because of its "blank slate" portrayal of infantile experience. A further concept linked to development that arouses controversy is the role of regression. In the face of psychological stress, the individual may regress to an earlier and less mature level of functioning. This can be understood as a defensive retreat to infantile stages that are never completely outgrown, and may at times have the constructive potential of a withdrawal to a safe base where mental forces can be regrouped. Regression may have a beneficial effect (therapeutic regression) or a destructive one (malignant regression), hence its controversial clinical status. Opinion is divided on the question of encouraging this process, particularly in patients with severe personality disorders. In psychotic patients the use of regression is generally considered to be at the very least unwise and at worst dangerous, as the psychotic patient is usually experiencing enough regression and the problem is more one of containing the prevailing regression.

Klein's work on development gave rise to the perspective of psychic "positions" that denote states of greater or lesser integration and maturity. Klein asserted that by the age of 3–6 months, the normally developing infant has reached sufficient mental maturity to be able to integrate split and opposing versions of his or her mother ("good-providing" and "bad-withholding"). Before this, feelings of love and hatred were dealt with by primitive defense mechanisms, principally splitting and projective-introjective procedures. This early developmental stage is the *paranoid-schizoid* position, and the later one is the *depressive* position. The latter can be regarded as a maturational achievement, equivalent to the "stage of concern" (Winnicott 1958). The first stage is accompanied by persecutory guilt, in which the concern is for the survival of the self, and the second is accompanied by depressive guilt, in which the concern is for the object. Attainment of the capacity for depressive anxiety is considered a necessary quality for the forming or maintaining of mature object relationships, as it is the source of generosity, altruistic feelings, reparative wishes, and the capacity to tolerate the object's separateness. It is not a once-and-for-all acquisition in which the paranoid-schizoid mode is left behind, but rather a dialectical (or diachronic) relationship between different levels of integration that continues throughout life. Increasing maturity brings a growing capacity to function at the level of the depressive position. Such growth does not bring an idealized freedom from unhappiness, but rather brings new and different burdens, albeit of a human sort, and a potential for freedom to make responsible choices. It is not the resolution of a dilemma: "one is stuck with it, with all its advantages and disadvantages, unless one regressively flees from it into the refuge and imprisonment of the paranoid-schizoid position or through the use of manic defenses" (Ogden 1992). Klein's view of the development of infantile cognition remains somewhat controversial, having been challenged in the postwar years by Anna Freud and her coworkers and subsequently by some infant researchers. It is one of many models that have proven useful for the practicing psychoanalyst but that do not necessarily reflect the actual experience of the infant, which is, to be sure, ultimately inaccessible.

Closely tied to developmental growth is the significance of reparative impulses. For example, in her analytic work with small children, Klein recognized the distress and guilt that accompanied destructive wishes and observed the growth of feelings of remorse and desire to repair damage done in phantasy to ambivalently loved figures who are the target of hatred and envy. Such reparative desires often take the form of obsessional activity, partly understandable as an attempt to preserve the object or to repair damage by magical means. In the course of analytic therapy with adults, failed attempts at reparation may often be discerned, and manic states may contain similar strivings. Manic reparation does not succeed because the subject is unaware of the damage he unconsciously believes he has done, and also does not know how to go about repairing it. The emergence of depressive guilt and reparative wishes marks a higher level of integration and is a mainspring of true creative processes. The concept of the need to repair *internal* as well as *external* objects permits the possibility of addressing in analysis feelings of regret and mourning, even if the victim of destructive wishes is long dead.

Conflicts and Defenses

The notion of mental conflict is an inherent feature of the human condition and has been central to psychoanalysis from the outset. The existence of *unconscious* wishes that compete with one another and with conscious desires renders subjective experience fraught with complexity. If I am at odds with a wish or impulse—say of a sexual or aggressive nature—I experience anxiety and guilt as I struggle between what I *want* to do and what I *should* do. This conscious conflict must be endured if I am to arrive at a realistic solution, and to reach this solution I need to tolerate painful feelings for which I will need certain defenses. If I have desires that are *unconscious* and these conflict with conscious or other unconscious wishes, the affects involved can be even more powerful and confusing, and anxieties may arise that I can neither fathom nor manage. The defenses that protect me against normal internal conflicts may prove to be inadequate, and if my ego is unable to defend against and address the impact of feelings of loss, humiliation, shame, or other guilt and anxiety-inducing experiences, these defenses may become pathological, compromising my grasp of reality.

While the majority of defenses are normal and adaptive, they can create disturbance if they are applied maladaptively. Maladaptive defensiveness can take many forms, as seen in the following example.

A female patient in her 30s with a history of anorexia became aware in her analysis that when she and her analyst were separated for a few days (at weekends or during holidays), she would become "hard" and overly "adult" in her attitude, as though detached from her feelings and needs. At the same time she dreamed of violent scenes, including of a girl being thrown out of her house or reprimanded for bad behavior, the nature of which was never clear. The patient tended at these times to engage in sadomasochistic forms of relating with her partner. She would become wary of her analyst upon resumption of sessions, as though the analyst might be angry with her. Mention of her unmet emotional needs tended to elicit withering, often self-punishing responses that concealed—including from her—severe reprimands of the analyst.

In this patient's case, *repression* of feelings of need and loss played a main defensive role, but she had gone further by attempting to eradicate awareness of her infantile needs using splitting and projective identification. The combined effect of these maneuvers was to create a threat of persecutory anxiety and fear of collapse into paranoid-schizoid confusion. Repression was considered by Freud to be the primary defense that "pushed" unacceptable feelings and impulses into the unconscious, where they remain concealed or disguised. These concealed impulses press to surface to consciousness, and this pressure generates anxiety. Further defensive activity (such as that described above) can produce symptoms as a result of the distorting impact of successive defenses on internal (psychic) reality.

Other defenses in addition to repression include *denial* (a refusal to acknowledge an aspect of reality by detaching awareness of it from the ego) and *disavowal*. The work of Klein in particular led to further ways of conceptualizing defensive activity in the area of primitive mental functioning. *Projective identification* (a concept developed out of the psychic mechanisms of identification and projection) refers to an unconscious belief that a part of the self or inner world, usually unwanted, can be disposed of by relocation into the mental representation of another object. This is usually regarded as a primitive form of the mental mechanism of *projection*, different in that it may involve behavior by the subject toward the object in a way that will allow her to confirm her omnipotent supposition. The projectively identifying mechanism can be used for purposes of disposing of unwanted elements or of controlling the object or of communication. In the latter case, the therapist is required to attend to his own nonrational responses to the patient's communications—the *counter-transference*—which will constitute an important source of information about the patient's state of mind at that moment. Many psychoanalysts hold that projective identification is a primary form of communication between mother and baby, comparable with the *attunement* described by workers in infant observation research (Stern 1985). *Splitting*

of the object is as important a concept as projective identification: it can give rise to extreme idealization and devaluation of the object (and thus of the self). When the object is split, love and hate of the object are kept apart—as though the object were two different people—and this obviates the need to deal with the anxiety and pain of experiencing both sets of affects towards someone who is all too humanly a mixture of good and bad characteristics.

Contemporary thinking, particularly in Europe, has focused on the systematic organization of defenses that serve to reinforce narcissistic and paranoid states of mind. In the United Kingdom, for example, Rosenfeld (1971, 1987), Steiner (1987, 1994), Britton (2003), and most recently O'Shaughnessy (1999) have emphasized the organized quality of primitive defenses and how this can have the effect of subjugating the individual's depleted ego and sense of self.

Internal (Psychic) Reality

Freud argued that psychic reality is grounded in biological reality and expresses itself psychologically via the lens of repression. The analyst can potentially discern the psychic reality of the subject, and its origins, from the structure and content of the analysand's words. We can see here two conceptualizing attitudes at play with this formulation of internal reality: a process of induction using broad concepts, followed by induction in order to apply the concepts clinically. It is important not to imagine that a concept like "psychic reality" is a concrete reality: it is a heuristic device. In modern psychoanalytic theory, an object refers to a person, part of a person, or a symbol representing the whole or part person, which the subject relates to in order to achieve instinctual satisfaction and fulfill attachment needs.

Today, priority tends to be given to the need for persons and relationships rather than simply the wish to satisfy instinctual drives. Theoretical developments in this area have led to the conceptualization of internal objects and relationships in the unconscious and of psychic reality. Psychic reality today denotes the interplay of mental representations of individuals and relationships, usually unconscious, with external (actual) objects in the outer world, and takes into account the psychic structures that have evolved to mediate this activity. In other words, psychic reality describes the internal world view the subject brings to bear on relationships and onto the external world. Psychic reality is a focus of attention in every analysis, regardless of theoretical persuasion.

One further aspect of psychic reality that has escaped the serious attention of many psychoanalysts is Freud's concept of *Nachträglichkeit*, or, as translated in France (where the concept is used widely), *après-coup*. In the *Dictionnaire International de la Psychanalyse* (de Mijolla 2003), Laplanche offers this definition: "the notion of après-coup is important for the psychoanalytical conception of temporality. It establishes a complex and reciprocal relationship between a significant event and its resignification in 'afterwardsness,' whereby the event acquires new psychic efficiency." Faimberg (2005) comments on après-coup as follows:

> [T]here is no article written by Freud specifically centered on this concept. This may at least partially explain its variable fate....we give credit to Lacan for being the first, in 1953, to underline the importance of this Freudian concept referring exclusively to the Wolf Man case. ...Nachträglichkeit was translated by Strachey as "deferred action." By choosing this term Strachey was trying to convey the idea of a link between two moments. But the word "deferred" suggests, in addition, a linear conception of time. It also expresses the direction of the arrow of time, in a sense opposite to that suggested by "Après-Coup"—which is retroactivity. But the choice of translation involves perhaps a particular way of conceiving temporalization and psychic causality.

As Faimberg puts it, après-coup embodies anticipation and retrospection. It is these two frameworks that allow for temporally progressive and retrospective resignification of past events in the present, and the implications for the ways in which memory functions are, of course, profound.

Transference and Countertransference

These two linked concepts have been the subject of much study and elaboration over many decades since their inception. It is not possible to summarize this literature here. It is, however, useful to identify their essential features and to pose questions regarding their theoretical significance and clinical function. From being a phenomenon first thought by Freud and Breuer to be a source of interference in therapeutic work, transference and countertransference have come to occupy a central place in the analyst's theoretical and technical armamentarium.

Historically, the concept of *transference* denoted the way in which the patient reproduced past relationships and experiences in the context of the relationship with the neutral analyst, with all the misrepresentations of reality this can imply. The task of analysis was to gradually diminish these misreadings of reality (deriving from infantile perceptions and wishes) and replace them with a more mature ego better able to perceive external reality while managing internal impulses. The problem with this conception is that it has been increasingly shown (because of its "one person" emphasis) to underestimate the complexity of the subject's relationship to the analyst, particularly in the manner in which the individual organizes and adapts his or her self representational system to accommodate analytic developments that foster change in the therapeutic relationship.

Contemporary views of transference address multiple axes of communication and the flexibility and evolution of self states that accompany them (Gabbard 2001; Kernberg 1987; Mitrani 2001; Roth 2001). Joseph (1985) has argued for appreciation of a "total transference situation" in which all aspects of the patient's communications can be understood as transference communications. In complete contrast, representatives of the relational, interpersonal, and intersubjective points of view argue that transference as a means of reenacting neurotic strivings that are displaced from the past onto the analyst is an erroneous conception. Transference is instead a phenomenon generated within the intersubjective field, which is in turn the product of the meeting of two distinct subjectivities (Lionells et al. 1995).

That transference actually exists few analysts would dispute; nevertheless, important questions as to its nature and impact are today being asked. For example:

1. What is the contemporary epistemological status of transference and its role in structuring psychic reality?
2. Does transference represent the "truth" of the patient's personality and object-relating capacities?
3. Is transference of necessity a distorted reflection of reality viewed through the lens of neurosis, or even of psychosis?
4. Is "truth" a misapplied notion altogether in the context of transference phenomena? Is transference an aspect of an ever-changing narrative that acts as a here-and-now medium in which to construct meaning from past and present events?
5. Is the traditional model of transference as a distortion of reality (whether in classical or modern guise) an artifact of a hierarchical developmental model that no longer carries the credence it once did?
6. Should we view transference as a form of adaptive intelligence that brings "learning from experience" into every new situation?

In addition to these questions of conceptualization, there are quite specific transference constellations that the psychoanalyst must deal with, such as transference *neurosis*, transference *psychosis*, and the *erotic* transference. These will be discussed in the section "What Is a Psychoanalyst?" later in this chapter.

Countertransference, also thought of initially by Freud as a form of interference in analytic treatment (Freud

1912/1958), has been the subject of more investigation in recent years than perhaps any other psychoanalytic subject. It has become an indispensable clinical resource and is of interest and importance to analysts on all continents. Today, the detached, "surgical" analytic stance of Freud and his immediate followers (with the partial exception of Ferenczi) has given way to an emphasis on the continuous impact of the patient on the analyst's thoughts and feelings. How the patient influences the analyst's mental and emotional states could be said to be pivotal in the construction of interpretations.

It is possible to trace through the twentieth century an increasing emphasis among certain schools in Europe and America on the need to deepen conceptualization of the analytic *relationship* rather than to rely solely on the classical, transference-based perspective. Heimann's 1950 paper is the best known articulation of the way in which the analyst's feelings, often unexpected and maybe difficult to identify, are produced under the influence of the patient's personality and are therefore the creation, to an extent, of the patient. This radical view brings with it the new task of differentiating those aspects of the patient's unconscious mental life from those of the analyst's psychic reality. Conceptually, the concepts of transference and countertransference have become inextricably linked since the work of Heimann. Racker was the first to elaborate this link, but many subsequent theorists, including a number of followers of Klein, made significant contributions (Bion 1959, 1970; Brenman-Pick 1985; Little 1951; Money-Kyrle 1956/1978; Racker 1968; Steiner 1982, 1994). Other groups, such as Independent object relations theorists (Bollas 1987; Coltart 1986; Symington 1986), interpersonalists (Mitchell 1988; Orange et al. 1998), and contemporary Freudians epitomized by Sandler (1976) and others (Kernberg 1987, 1992; Stern 1985), have also contributed heavily to present-day understanding of transference-countertransference communications.

The subject of countertransference lies at the heart of much British Independent thinking, and the influence of Melanie Klein on this emphasis has been decisive. The object relations view is that the psychoanalytic situation is always created and developed from specific and unique interaction between the patient and analyst; the analyst is never an outsider. Michael Balint argued that countertransference comprises the totality of the analyst's attitudes, feelings, and behavior toward his or her patients, although most Independents would not agree with this today. One of the most widely accepted views of the use of countertransference is as a containing and metabolizing function used by the analyst (cf. Bion 1959, 1962) to receive and digest projective identifications that the patient cannot, for the time being, bear. This perspective is particularly relevant to work with severely disturbed individuals but can apply to the primitive mental functioning of all patients. In every use of countertransference today, the analyst is required to empathize and identify with the patient's affective state, while remaining sufficiently separate and psychically available to help transform the patient's communications into a symbolic form usable by the patient's ego.

Working-Through

That psychoanalysis takes time is well known. That the need for time is based on a requirement for a systematic "working-through" of problems in (broadly speaking) a series of stages is less well known. In "Remembering, Repeating and Working-Through," Freud (1914b/1958) noted how individuals are compelled to repeat their experiences and how change in psychoanalysis accrues through repetition and subsequent working-through. It is only when the patient becomes convinced in depth (emotionally) of the authenticity of his or her experiences (as opposed to intellectual awareness) that durable therapeutic change is possible. This is a difficult, often surprising experience for any analysand in a genuine analysis: getting to know the impact of the unconscious can be unnerving, upsetting, stimulating, and transformational. Integrating insights may be pleasurable or painful, but in all cases it takes time.

Working-through takes up most of the work in analysis once the transference is established and self-knowledge has begun to develop. New insights are repeatedly assessed and tested and may be experimented with in the outside world to determine their veracity and effectiveness. As confidence builds in the analytic process, the patient may develop a growing capacity for tolerating many more and different kinds of experiences, leading to intensification of self-knowledge that requires further conscious and unconscious integration. (Dreams not only herald unconscious news; they can be of great importance in working through analytic discoveries and crises.) The patient "uses" the analyst intensively to foster the process of growth (Winnicott 1971b). At a certain point (usually difficult to anticipate or predict), when the patient has truly come to inhabit the "depressive position" (Klein 1984a) or "stage of concern" (Winnicott 1971b) through an acquired capacity to mourn losses and the effects of his or her destructive impulses, and to embrace a creative, reparative approach to relationships, the question of separation from the analyst and termination of the analysis may arise. This point may be reached sooner by some than by others (never usually before 3–5 years).

What Is a Psychoanalyst?

Professionally, the traditional definition of a bona fide psychoanalyst is someone who has completed a lengthy, formally accredited training. This training usually takes the form of a "tripartite" model comprising a thorough personal analysis, clinical and theoretical instruction, and the treatment of several patients in analysis under supervised control conditions. This postgraduate training varies in length from 4 to 10 years depending on cultural and pedagogical traditions on different continents. There is great variation in the type and theoretical stance of the various training programs around the world (reflected in our pluralistic psychoanalytic culture). The term *psychoanalyst* has no legal title, and there are many people who undertake other trainings and some others who do comparatively little training and call themselves "psychoanalysts." It is important for all concerned to ascertain the qualifications and credentials of a psychoanalyst, as the maintenance of agreed-on clinical and ethical standards is the safeguard of the discipline and of patients' welfare.

A psychoanalyst may belong to one (or more) of the different psychoanalytic schools that characterize psychoanalysis today. In the United States, ego psychology (rooted in classical psychoanalytic theory) held sway for many decades, with its emphasis on the growth of ego function through the integration of internal and external experiences (Hartmann 1939/1958; see also Pine 1990). Today, this hegemony is gone: influence of Kleinian and British Independent thinking from abroad and the impact of relational perspectives within the United States have led to a pluralistic situation within American psychoanalysis. The *co-construction* of the analytic relationship is now hotly debated there. The rise of self psychology in the United States in the past 25 years is a response to a growing emphasis on disorders of the self and the pathological impact of narcissism (Kohut 1977; Kohut and Wolf 1978). In Latin America, a complex amalgam of classical, object relations, and Kleinian theory, together with important influences from the United States, has created a psychoanalytic culture unique to the region (see Chapter 28, "Psychoanalysis in Latin America," in this volume).

Object relations theory, including the work of Melanie Klein, is today increasingly being discussed in the United States, having firmly established itself in Europe in the form of Independent thinking and post-Kleinian theory (cf. Bronstein 2001; Spillius 1988). The Independent British psychoanalysts created and developed the theory of *object relations*, a term that, though overused, designates the subject's mode of relation to his or her world. This relation is the entire complex outcome of a particular organization of the personality and apprehension of objects, to some extent phantasized. (Authors who have written on this include Jones, Sharp, Glover, Flugel, Hain, Rickman, Strachey, Brierley, Fairbairn, Winnicott, Balint, Klauber, Kahn, Rycroft, Limentani, Bowlby, Mitchell, Bollas, Kohon, Rayner, Parsons, and Casement). The Independents were the original host group of the British Psychoanalytical Society and took their name from their philosophy of making use of concepts and practices from all schools of psychoanalysis. They have always placed an emphasis on the impact of the external environment on intrapsychic life, as well as on the world of fantasy itself. The Independents facilitated the arrival of many Viennese, German, and other analysts into the United Kingdom prior to World War II, and today the Group coexists equally in the British Society with the Contemporary Freudians and the Klein Group within the framework of the famous "gentleman's agreement" reached by two eminent ladies, Anna Freud and Melanie Klein, during the controversial discussions of the 1940s (King and Steiner 1991).

The contemporary Freudians (predominantly in the United Kingdom) have adapted the classical Freudian tradition in developing a revised body of theory that now attracts a significant following (their representatives include the Sandlers, Fonagy, and Perelberg). Perhaps one of the most striking turns of fate for any body of psychoanalytic theory is the resurgence of interest in attachment theory in recent years. For a long time the "poor relation" of the psychoanalytic canon because of its perceived departure from established psychoanalytic concepts, such as unconscious phantasy and the internal object world, and its links with ethology, attachment theory is now at the forefront of research into infant development and infant-caregiver relations (cf. Fonagy 2001).

The situation in France regarding psychoanalytic theory is interesting and different from that in any other country in the world: most psychoanalysts there have been influenced by Lacan, although there is a division between formal Lacanian psychoanalysis (the Lacanians formed a separate organization many years ago) and, for example, the Paris Society and International Psychoanalytical Association analysts elsewhere in France, where a tradition from Freud onward has been maintained that more closely corresponds to other European schools of psychoanalysis (Irigaray 1985; Kristeva 1982; Lacan 1998; Roudinesco and Lacan 1990; see also Chapter 27, "Psychoanalysis in the French Community," in this volume).

Contemporary psychoanalysis everywhere has been heavily influenced by the explosion of research into neurobiology: rapidly accumulating knowledge regarding brain function, dreaming, memory, and consciousness appears to corroborate many of the central tenets of psychoanalysis from a neuropsychological perspective (Damasio 1999; Edelman and Tononi 2001; Panksepp 1998; Shevrin et al. 1996; Solms 1997; see also Chapter 36, "Neuroscience"). These hitherto inaccessible data place psychoanalysis on the threshold of a new era of development.

While the theoretical orientation of the psychoanalyst may be an intricate matter, links with classical psychoanalysis have not disappeared, and these can be seen clearly in psychoanalysts' technique and clinical work. For example, many psychoanalysts are committed to the free association method and its meaning, although some dispute its usefulness. Freud employed the metaphor of a train to describe free association, inviting patients to reflect on their own thoughts as if they were in a train observing their thoughts as they went on their way. What is revealed by this process is a train of thought, sometimes clear, more often than not obscure, usually requiring time to elicit and occasionally destined to remain elusive. By placing the patient in the unusual position of observer of his or her own thoughts, with the aim of facilitating associations between what is present and what is absent, Freud created a unique form of personal anthropology. We become ethnographer *and* indigenous object of study: there is an unconscious other to whom we relate.

Closely tied to the use of free association is the *therapeutic alliance* that arises within a carefully maintained analytic frame. Therapeutic alliance is not a popular term in some quarters; it is sometimes criticized as an artificial construct. The opposing argument is that when the patient feels understood—that is, when the psychic reality of the patient becomes consciously apparent to both parties in an atmosphere of trust—a bond is created and becomes the foundation of the trajectory of the analysis. It is probable that all analysts and patients seek to establish a therapeutic alliance, whether or not they agree with the term.

The other, fundamental and universal component of every analysis is *interpretation*. The psychoanalyst is trained, by means of the conceptual tools outlined earlier, to interpret the psychic reality of the patient in the context of past and present experiences. More has been written on interpretation than any other psychoanalytic subject. It embodies both the science and the art of the psychoanalyst and is the principal medium of communication that every analyst strives most to deepen and develop in his or her clinical work. It must be added that a focus on transference and countertransference, however defined, also defines a psychoanalyst.

The types of psychological conditions psychoanalysts are asked to help with have changed over the years. It is no longer the case that analysts are seen to be capable of treating only patients with neurotic conditions. Extensive inquiry into personality disorders (particularly borderline personality), perversions, dissociative states, and psychosis has yielded a substantial body of clinical and theoretical knowledge. (A recent, comprehensive electronic source containing virtually all the principal learned papers published by psychoanalysts over the past 75 years is the PEP [Psychoanalytic Electronic Publishing] CD-ROM. Full-text articles reflecting advances not only in understanding severe disturbances but in all key areas of conceptual development are available.) The roots of these enquiries are again traceable to classical psychoanalysis. For example, the early work of Freud on psychosis gave rise to a new epistemology. Thanks to this and subsequent analytic investigations, we today possess compelling and coherent ways of explaining severely disturbed thought processes and otherwise inexplicable, bizarre human behavior. These insights are not merely intellectually satisfying: they make practically possible dynamic engagement with the disturbed mind and the inclusion of a psychotherapeutic component in the management and treatment of severe disorders including psychosis.

The contemporary psychoanalyst is likely to treat a wide range of problems, and patients may be children, adults, or families. The typical setting is the consulting room with its quiet, undisturbed atmosphere conducive to facilitating reflection and communication. However, many psychoanalysts also work in hospitals and other mental health institutions, adapting psychoanalysis to different contexts. In academia, interest in psychoanalysis has never been greater, and many analysts have forged links with universities. Other psychoanalysts undertake interdisciplinary studies, not only on academic subjects but also on socially crucial issues such as terrorism and conflict resolution (cf. Covington et al. 2003; Varvin and Volkan 2003).

Conclusion

An oft-quoted phrase that characterizes the turbulent recent history of psychoanalysis is "The Crisis of Psychoanalysis." This epithet refers to the many scientific challenges to psychoanalytic theory that have arisen in the past 20 years: to the impact of the rise of a postmodern "quick-fix" culture in the West; to the related surge in the use of sophisticated pharmacological products to treat and control patients; to dramatically changed attitudes to sexuality; and to growing social and political inequalities, violence, and war and the implications of these for the role of the psychoanalyst. Psychoanalysts provide a powerful human dimension to the fostering and development of self-understanding; this contribution is evolving and adapting to the enormous social changes ushered in by the twenty-first century.

References

Bion WR: Attacks on linking. Int J Psychoanal 40:308–315, 1959

Bion WR: A theory of thinking. Int J Psychoanal 43:306–310, 1962

Bion WR: Attention and Interpretation. London, Tavistock, 1970

Bollas C: Expressive uses of the counter-transference, in The Shadow of the Object: Psychoanalysis of the Unthought Known. London, Free Association Books, 1987

Bowlby J: Attachment and Loss, Vol 1: Attachment. New York, Basic Books, 1969

Bowlby J: Attachment and Loss, Vol 2: Separation: Anxiety and Anger. New York, Basic Books, 1973

Bowlby J: Attachment and Loss, Vol 3: Loss: Sadness and Depression. New York, Basic Books, 1980

Bowlby J: A Secure Base: Parent-Child Attachment and Healthy Human Development. New York, Basic Books, 1988

Brenman-Pick I: Working through in the countertransference. Int J Psychoanal 66:157–166, 1985

Britton R: Sex, Death, and the Superego: Experiences in Psychoanalysis. London, Karnac Books, 2003

Britton R, Feldman M, O'Shaughnessy E, et al: Oedipus Complex Today. London, Karnac Books, 1989

Bronstein C: Kleinian Theory: A Contemporary Perspective. London, Whurr Books, 2001

Coltart M: Slouching towards Bethlehem...or thinking the unthinkable in psychoanalysis, in The British School of Psychoanalysis: The Independent Tradition. Edited by Kohon G. London, Free Association Books, 1986, pp 185–99

Covington C, Williams P, Knox J, et al: Terrorism and War: Unconscious Dynamics of Political Violence. London, Karnac Books, 2003

Damasio A: The Feeling of What Happens: Body and Emotion in the Making of Consciousness. New York, Harcourt Brace, 1999

de Mijolla A: Dictionnaire International de la Psychanalyse. Paris, Calmann-Lévy, 2003

Edelman G, Tononi G: A Universe of Consciousness: How Matter Becomes Imagination. New York, Basic Books, 2001

Faimberg H: Debate on Après Coup With Ignes Sodre. Int J Psychoanal 86(1), 2005

Fonagy P: Attachment Theory and Psychoanalysis. New York, Other Press, 2001

Freud S: The interpretation of dreams (1900), in Standard Edition of the Complete Psychological Works of Sigmund Freud, Vols 4 & 5. Translated and edited by Strachey J. London, Hogarth Press, 1953

Freud S: Three essays on the theory of sexuality (1905), in Standard Edition of the Complete Psychological Works of Sigmund Freud, Vol 7. Translated and edited by Strachey J. London, Hogarth Press, 1953, pp 130–243

Freud S: The dynamics of transference (1912), in Standard Edition of the Complete Psychological Works of Sigmund Freud, Vol 12. Translated and edited by Strachey J. London, Hogarth Press, 1958, pp 99–108

Freud S: On narcissism: an introduction (1914a), in Standard Edition of the Complete Psychological Works of Sigmund Freud, Vol 14. Translated and edited by Strachey J. London, Hogarth Press, 1957, pp 67–102

Freud S: Remembering, repeating and working-through (further recommendations on the technique of psycho-analysis II) (1914b), in Standard Edition of the Complete Psychological Works of Sigmund Freud, Vol 12. Translated and edited by Strachey J. London, Hogarth Press, 1958, pp 145–156

Freud S: The ego and the id (1923), in Standard Edition of the Complete Psychological Works of Sigmund Freud, Vol 19. Translated and edited by Strachey J. London, Hogarth Press, 1961, pp 12–66

Gabbard G: What can neuroscience teach us about transference? Canadian Journal of Psychoanalysis 9:1–18, 2001

Hartmann H: Ego Psychology and the Problem of Adaptation (1939). Translated by Rapaport D. New York, International Universities Press, 1958

Heimann P: On countertransference. Int J Psychoanal 31:81–84, 1950

Irigaray LI: This Sex Which Is Not One. Translated by Porter C. Ithaca, NY, Cornell University Press, 1985

Jackson JH: Selected Writings of John Hughlings Jackson, Vols 1 & 2. Edited by Taylor J. London, Hodder & Stoughton, 1932

Joseph B: Transference: the total situation. Int J Psychoanal 66:447–454, 1985

Kernberg OF: Ego psychology-object relations theory approach to transference. Psychoanal Q 56:197–221, 1987

Kernberg OF: Psychopathic, paranoid, and depressive transferences. Int J Psychoanal 73:13–28, 1992

King P, Steiner R: The Controversial Discussions: 1941–1946. London, Routledge, 1991

Klein M: Notes on some schizoid mechanisms. Int J Psychoanal 27:99–110, 1946

Klein M: Envy and gratitude and other works: 1946–1963, in The Writings of Melanie Klein, Vol 3. New York, Free Press, 1984a

Klein M: Love, guilt and reparation, and other works: 1921–1945, in The Writings of Melanie Klein, Vol 1, Free Press, 1984b

Kohut H: The Restoration of the Self. New York, International Universities Press, 1977

Kohut H, Wolf ES: The disorders of the self and their treatment: an outline. Int J Psychoanal 59:413–426, 1978

Kristeva J: Powers of Horror: An Essay on Abjection. New York, Columbia University Press, 1982

Lacan J: Encore: The Seminar XX. Translated by Fink B. New York, WW Norton, 1998

Little M: Countertransference and the patient's response to it. Int J Psychoanal 32:32–40, 1951

Lionells M, Fiscalini J, Mann CH, et al: Handbook of Interpersonal Psychoanalysis. Hillsdale, NJ, Analytic Press, 1995

Matte-Blanco I: Thinking Feeling and Being. London, Routledge, 1988

Mitchell S: Relational Concepts in Psychoanalysis: An Integration. Cambridge, MA, Harvard University Press, 1988

Mitrani J: "Taking the transference": implications in three papers by Bion. Int J Psychoanal 82:1085–1104, 2001

Money-Kyrle R: Normal countertransference and some of its deviations (1956), in The Collected Papers of Roger Money-Kyrle. Perthshire, England, Clunie Press, 1978

Ogden T: The Primitive Edge of Experience. London, Karnac Books, 1992

Orange DM, Atwood GE, Stolorow RD: Working Intersubjectively: Contextualism in Psychoanalytic Practice. Psychoanalytic Inquiry Book Series, Vol 17. Hillsdale, NJ, Analytic Press, 1998

O'Shaughnessy E: Relating to the Superego. Int J Psychoanal 80:861–870, 1999

Panksepp J: Affective Neuroscience: The Foundations of Human and Animal Emotions. Oxford, England, Oxford University Press, 1998

Pine F: Drive, Ego, Object, and Self: A Synthesis for Clinical Work. New York, Basic Books, 1990

Racker H: Transference and Countertransference. London, Hogarth Press, 1968

Rosenfeld H: A clinical approach to the psychoanalytic theory of the life and death instincts: an investigation into the aggressive aspects of narcissism. Int J Psychoanal 52:169–78, 1971

Rosenfeld H: Projective identification in clinical practice, in Impasse and Interpretation: Therapeutic and Antitherapeutic Factors in Psychoanalytic Treatment of Psychotic, Borderline, and Neurotic Patients. London, Routledge, 1987, pp 157–190

Roth P: Mapping the landscape: levels of transference interpretation. Int J Psychoanal 82:533–544, 2001

Roudinesco E, Lacan J: A History of Psychoanalysis in France, 1925–1985. Translated by Mehlman J. Chicago, IL, University of Chicago Press, 1990

Sandler J: Countertransference and role-responsiveness. Int Rev Psychoanal 3:43–48, 1976

Shevrin H, Bond JA, Brakel LAW, et al: Conscious and Unconscious Processes: Psychodynamic, Cognitive, and Neurophysiological Convergences. New York, Guilford, 1996

Solms M: The Neuropsychology of Dreams: A Clinico-Anatomical Study. Mahwah, NJ, Lawrence Erlbaum, 1997

Spillius E: Melanie Klein Today, Vols 1 & 2. London, Routledge, 1988

Steiner J: Perverse relationships between parts of the self. Int J Psychoanalysis 63:241–251, 1982

Steiner J: The interplay between pathological organizations and the paranoid-schizoid and depressive positions. Int J Psychoanal 68:69–80, 1987

Steiner J: Psychic Retreats: Pathological Organizations in Psychotic, Neurotic, and Borderline Patients. London, Routledge, 1994

Stern D: The Interpersonal World of the Infant: A View From Psychoanalysis and Developmental Psychology. New York, Basic Books, 1985

Symington N: The Analyst's Act of Freedom as Agent of Therapeutic Change, in The British School of Psychoanalysis: The Independent Tradition. Edited by Kohon G. London, Free Association Books, 1986, pp 253–272

Varvin S, Volkan V (eds): Violence or Dialogue? Psychoanalytic Insights On Terror and Terrorism. London, International Psychoanalytic Association, 2003

Winnicott D: Collected Papers: Through Paediatrics to Psychoanalysis. New York, Basic Books, 1958

Winnicott D: Transitional objects and transitional phenomena, in Playing and Reality, London, Tavistock, 1971, pp 1–25

Winnicott D: The use of an object and relating through identifications, in Playing and Reality, London, Tavistock, 1971, pp 86–94

13

Transference, Countertransference, and the Real Relationship

ADRIENNE HARRIS, PH.D.

"Discovery" of Transference and Countertransference and Early Developments

Transference and countertransference are the defining processes of a psychoanalytic treatment. Inevitably over a century of work, these terms have been subject to wide and quite distinct interpretations and technical uses. Yet amid such difference there is an abiding conviction, among psychoanalysts, that it is primarily in the crucible of the analytic relationship, in which two people talk, that change and freedom from illness can occur.

Transference appears in Freud's essays on technique as a discovery, while countertransference discussions function mostly as cautionary tale (Freud 1911/1958, 1912a/1958, 1912b/1958; 1913/1958, 1914/1958, 1915/1958). In a number of ways, his discovery that patients revive and relive the crucial conflicts of their psychic lives *in* the analytic relationship was remarkable. First, analysis of transference entails a break with earlier powerful and compel-

ling procedures of suggestion and hypnotic induction, techniques thought to reveal and release hidden sources of pathology and pain. Second, almost immediately Freud made a second discovery, namely, that transference is used by the analysand as resistance to change but that this development could be turned quite uniquely toward psychic growth. It is as though Freud's intelligence functioned like a heat-seeking missile, burrowing into the most tender and incendiary aspect of the analytic relationship and finding there both trouble and revolution. Third, Freud was aware, from the beginning, even if incompletely so, of the dangers, the fascination, and the traps that hide in transference and countertransference. Freud grounded his theory of therapeutics in the most unstable, enigmatic, transpersonal, potent aspects of the analytic situation and never looked back.

Finally, it seems worth noting that the discovery of transference is a rather astonishing victory over personal narcissism. To come to the conclusion that a person who makes an intense declaration of love to you does not really love you but loves *someone else* in an act of transference takes considerable self-esteem and reflectivity.

I would like to thank Henry F. Smith, Glen Gabbard, Lewis Aron, and Rita Frankiel for careful readings of this chapter.

To the physician it represents an invaluable explanation and a useful warning against any tendency to countertransference, which may be lurking in his or her own mind. He must recognize that the patient's falling in love is induced by the analytic situation and is not to be ascribed to the charms of his person....And it is always well to be reminded of this. (Freud 1912a/1958, p. 379)

In retrospect, surprising "discoveries" often carry the seeds of many earlier processes and practices. Many have argued that transference is no exception. Mannoni (1971) noted how frequently Freud mentions hypnosis when trying to account for the mechanisms of transference. In many of the ensuing discussions of transference that I will be reviewing, when authors try to account for the mechanics of transference, something like an altered state, in the analyst as well as the analysand, is often being outlined. There is, it seems, some trance in transference. The remnants of magical elements in analytic experience have also been tied to Freud's perhaps ambivalent relation to traditions in Jewish thought, particular its mystical tradition (Bakan 1958/1998).

Freud's reservations about written communication regarding transference and countertransference may join up with concerns regarding confidentiality, and protecting patients, as well as concerns about professional matters. Part of the renewed interest in analytic subjectivity and matters of technique and disclosure might be seen as an aspect of the ongoing question of who knows what and what information has what effect, concerns that are both self-serving to the analyst and preserving of the integrity of treatment. This paradox in intentions and access to knowledge is perhaps irresolvable. Its ongoing presence has a history in the earliest work on technique and continues to be powerful. (See Dupont 1988; Falzeder 1997; Haynal 1997 for extensive discussions on the complex crucible of Freud's relations with Ferenczi as the site for the development of theories of transference and technique.)

In the early papers on technique, Freud's injunctions against note taking, advice, intellectualizing, use of the patient or treatment for scientific enterprise, and offering of analytic writing to the analysand are all proposed in order to enhance transference so as to remove the barriers between speaker and listener. "Evenly hovering attention" was, for Freud, a guard against overworking and a way to keep distinct relations with numbers of patients and to create conditions in the analyst for a kind of receptivity. To a modern ear, these accounts describe a lot of the conditions for meditative practices, for inducing and self-inducing altered states of consciousness, and for the Eastern practices that attempt to dissolve ego and attachment in order to receive input from another.

In the later papers on technique, Freud (1937a/1964, 1937b/1964, 1938/1964) described transference in a quite experience-laden way. A lifetime of doing treatment had educated him to the dangers of compliance by an analysand along with the complexities of power, historical truth, and narrative truth in analyses. "The analyst may shamefacedly admit to himself that he set out on a difficult undertaking without any suspicion of the extraordinary powers that would be at his command" (Freud 1938/1964, p. 175). And in a paragraph counseling the judicious management of transference to eschew either extremes or love or hostility, Freud (1938/1964) comments on the ongoing often permanent impact of the knowledge an analysand can glean from transference experiences: "For a patient never forgets again what he has experienced in the form of transference: it carries a greater force of conviction than anything he can acquire in other ways" (p. 177).

While many of the early generation of analysts thought of their analytic work as a direct application of Freud's programmatic work on technique, Ferenczi, always the complex son, both admired the work and pushed the envelope (Aron and Harris 1993; Bonomi 1999). Ferenczi (1909/1980) took up the ideas and proposals from the technical papers and began to worry them into more provocative and potentially powerful forms. He used and discarded procedures that indulged and procedures that frustrated the patient, guided by his overarching interest in the emotional impact of each person on the other. There are contradictions in Ferenczi's approach. On the one hand, he widened radically the play and province of transference, as the Kleinians would do after him. Transference phenomena were considered to be ubiquitous in the analytic relationship. On the other hand, he held out a separate space for a "real" relationship with the analyst as a "real" person. We shall see how this term *real* transforms over the century of psychoanalytic theory building. Here the term "real" seems to acknowledge the impact of the analyst's psyche (hostile and loving) but also, enigmatically, keeps something out of the transference.

One powerful aspect of Ferenczi's work on transference is his attunement to hostility and hatred in the transference and countertransference.

> The narcissism of the analyst seems suited to create a particularly fruitful source of mistakes; among others the development of a kind of narcissistic countertransference which provokes the person being analyzed into pushing into the foreground certain things which flatter the analyst and, on the other hand, into suppressing remarks and associations of an unpleasant nature in relation to him. (Ferenczi 1909/1980, p. 41)

In this regard he may have fared better as a theorist of hostility than as practitioner. Amid the powerful creativity of his efforts at mutual analysis, one feels the masochism and suffering in his relationship to R.N. (herself a therapist, the American Elizabeth Severn). Amid brilliant, imaginative thoughts and vital work that deeply reveal the analyst's affective presence in the treatment, we see, also, the dangerous erasures of self that can arise in work with severely regressed patients (Ferenczi 1932).

The status of "influence" is an aspect of transference and countertransference experiences that exerts a kind of gravitational pull on efforts in the field to sort out what happens, why, and how it helps. The official version is that transference is the revolutionary break from hypnosis. However, we can see a continuing debate over the power of speech's structural properties (symbolic register, interpretation, reflective functioning) and the power of speech's pragmatic, rhetoric, and object relational properties (cures by love, force of power, *erlebnis*, corrective emotional experience, or procedural "now" moments). The following case vignette suggests the presence of both elements of transference.

> In my work with Laura, a young woman scientist in her mid-30s who came into analysis in the throes of a crisis in her first important relationship, we cycled through many different modes of relating and living within transferential patterns. This woman described her mother as angry and powerfully intrusive, ruling the family with rageful attacks and affect storms before which everyone fled or collapsed. Her father, disabled by alcoholism and attached to his daughter in a too sexualized, desperate way, could not be a trustworthy refuge.
>
> In analysis, an early and quite idyllic calm was broken whenever I became overly anxious about her relationship and its crises. She would be in great agitation, feeling hopeless and trapped, and that feeling would be imaginatively recast in me. I would feel in danger of failing her, worried that my lack of analytic skill was keeping her trapped in a dangerous and hopeless situation (both the analysis and her relationship). I was anxious about her state of mind and often in the grip of a strange sense of a foreshortened future, of a precipice just ahead and no way to manage a sense of ongoingness. In those states, I always made analytic missteps, commenting or interpreting out of our shared states of panic. Over time, as we could capture these experiences, we worked on the triggers, the mistakes in my way of being with her. We worked on the transference implications of what was happening between us. What I disclosed was a clear belief that I had made an error, and we could then trace the impact of my interventions and repair ruptures. We could see that we were passing back and forth between us the affect-storming mother; the incompetent, unboundaried father; and the terrified, uncontained child.

What helped in my work with Laura? The enactment? The disclosure? The interpretations, transferential and genetic? Living through and repairing rupture? I suspect it was all of those things.

The Real Relationship

One quandary that threads through discussions of technique, transference, and countertransference is whether there is, in addition to experiences of transference and countertransference, a "real" relationship. It is as though the term *real* unsettles the field of inquiry. Do not transference and countertransference subsume all the aspects of the relationship? What surplus meaning or what unmanageable aspects of the analytic experience require this category of the "real"? Examining how this idea evolves through the literature on transference, you see that the meaning of the real relationship has altered over our history.

Lipton (1977) makes a good case for the importance and presence of such a distinction in Freud's own thinking, in that he distinguishes what Freud actually did from the idealized picture of Freudian technique in the classical tradition. In fact, Lipton argues that a word like "classical" already idealizes and perhaps fetishizes technique in a way rather different from Freud's own way of practicing. There is a fascinating and illuminating perspective on Freud's technique and the real relationship seen through a recently published collection of the circling correspondence of the symbolist poet H.D. (Hilda Doolittle); Bryher, her lover, who was also an involved member of the psychoanalytic community; and Freud (Friedman 2002). The letters of this fascinating group, written during and after two periods of analysis H.D. had with Freud in Vienna in 1933 and 1934, give a fascinating view of Freud's power as a clinician and the tremendous strength of transference phenomena coexisting with many strands of a "real" relationship. There is some considerable confusion of real and analytic ties. There are instances of dual functioning that professionally we would criticize. Bryher and Freud exchange letters about the financing of various aspects of the psychoanalytic movement during H.D.'s analysis, which was being paid for by Bryher. But there are, throughout the correspondence, equally compelling signs of the early emergence and continuing potency of transference phenomena and their impact on H.D.'s psyche.

Granted that such letters are perhaps a somewhat unorthodox source of clinical information, I want to argue that we have a very interesting entrée into Freud's application of technique, seeing both that he went by the book and that the book could also be thrown away. From H.D.'s (1956) account of her first day in analysis, we learn the following. Freud greets H.D. on her first hour with a command not to pet the dog that is in the consulting room with them. She disobeys. The dog does not bite. We have a meaning-filled enactment to imagine and think about. Later there is quite a long and (to Bryher and H.D., worrying) correspondence about the gift of two puppies, which Freud wished to send to them in Switzerland. Simultaneously we learn that the Freud who undertakes H.D.'s analysis is beloved, clear in his interpretive process, pragmatic in his inhabiting a maternal transference, uninterested in altering her bisexuality, and genuinely helpful in unjamming a work block. His capacity to imaginatively swim in complex multiple experiences of gender and desire is startlingly modern. There seems plenty of transference and countertransference to go around.

Greenson (1967) wrote the definitive midcentury account of the mix of transference and real relationship. He holds a distinction between neurotic and nonneurotic aspects of the analysand's relationship to the analyst. In this, he is contrasting Stone's (1984) ideas, which involve a variety of relational configurations between analyst and analysand and something like a working alliance, with what he sees in the Kleinian approach as a relative indifference to such an ego-based alliance. Greenson goes on to distinguish and hold separate places for a working alliance and a real relationship. The working alliance encompasses many elements: continuity, commitment, ways of being within the hour, and management of time and money—elements that we would think of as aspects of the frame. Greenson, in discussing the real relationship distinct from matters that deepen or hold the therapeutic alliance, speaks about genuineness (including straightforward admission of errors) and an orientation to reality, as well as an appreciation of the extra-analytic reality of the analyst (e.g., family, frailties, contexts). He saw the working alliance as a permanent aspect of an analysis and the emergence of the "real relationship" as an aspect of the later stages of analysis. We shall see that in the 1990s, with a great sea change in the understanding and exploration of countertransference, the "real" relationship was explored and understood in a somewhat different way.

Evolution of Transference and Countertransference Matrices

Classical Psychoanalytic Theory: American Ego Psychology

Over the twentieth century there was a steady attempt at expanding and deepening the concept of transference within mainstream psychoanalytic circles. Transference phenomena could be seen as a kind of growth industry in psychoanalytic writing, while countertransference remained relatively undertheorized until the 1990s. I am going to take three moments in the literature, like freeze frames, when a history is visited and assessed: Orr in 1954; Bird in

1972; and, nearly 30 years later, several key reviews by Gabbard (1995), Jacobs (1999, 2001), and Smith (1999, 2000, 2003b), as well as Jacobs's (1991) own constructions and uses of countertransferences.

Orr's (1954) review shows the field in the 1950s to be deeply engrossed in the workings of unconscious phenomena. There is disagreement with the interpersonal perspective, and the work of Horney in particular, but that perspective is clearly part of the canon. There is scarcely any discussion of countertransference, and what occurs is made a matter of the analyst's unconscious and is treated as an intrusion in the work of transference analysis.

Orr paraphrases Glover's lists of the uses of the transference neurosis as the keystone to analytic work:

1) convincing the patient through his or her actions of the nature of his or her unconscious fantasies and ego resistances; 2) tracking down early identifications and denoting specific superego components; 3) effecting greater conviction in the patient because of the discrepancy between emotion and actual stimulus; 4) effecting the expression of many tendencies and experiences never before conscious; 5) providing a "lever" for recollection; and 6) offering proof of the existence of transference fantasies and their connection with infantile impulses. (Orr 1954, p. 637)

Transference is useful as a ground for interpretation, not for its relational properties. Orr does, however, note some exceptions to this dominant view. Macalpine (1950), for example, thought countertransference was inevitable and was disavowed by analysts because of the strains of hypnotism that must be excised from analytic understanding. Fenichel (1940a, 1940b), Orr notes, was another figure with a worrying glance at countertransference. Interestingly, Fenichel was concerned with the analyst's defenses and anxieties, not the dangers of sexuality. And equally interesting to a modern reader, Orr thought there was really little need to write or discuss these matters, as the management of countertransference was finally dependent on the honesty, self-reflection, and analytic history of the analyst.

Orr's treatment of the elements of the "real" relationship is intriguing. He draws on Balint's (1939, 1950) ideas to consider how the material conditions of the analyst's world impinge on the treatment

in countless ways—the nature and arrangement of his office, the hardness or softness of his couch, his way of covering or not covering the pillow, the frequency, timing, affective emphasis and even diction of his interpretations and, indeed, his whole way of working, some of which in itself is likely to be a carry-over from the transference to his own training analyst—and it is the sum total of these and other, subtle or not so subtle influences—coloring, if not markedly affecting, the patient's experience. (Orr 1954, p. 649)

In the 1970s, Bird (1972) wrote a wide-ranging review in which the domination or ascendancy of ego psychology is quite apparent. Interpersonal perspectives are now quite invisible. In my view, Bird strips away complexity and reduces it to ego function problems, yet his approach at the time was considered groundbreaking.

> Accordingly, wresting transference from its syntonic limbo is not likely to be easy and may be impossible; but doing so, bringing it out into open view where it can be contemplated as a major member of the ego family, is to me an utterly fascinating prospect, one that permits me to see transference not only as the best tool clinical analysis has, but possibly the best tool the ego has. (Bird 1972, p. 301)

One of the most powerful developments in technique following from this focus on ego functioning is the work of Paul Gray (1994). Gray's technical recommendations, called initially "close process monitoring" and later "close process attention," counseled for an approach to transference in which the defensive aspects were the primary sites of work. Carrying on the tradition Bird was describing, Gray's recommendations to keep attuned to the surface in any analytic hour as a way to provide experience-near material for the analysand constitute an approach designed to augment and expand consciousness and ego function.

I am going to approach the contemporary classical consideration of transference and countertransference through the work of Loewald (1975, 1980, 1986) and Schafer (1997). Loewald appreciated the theatricality of transference—its repeating of a repetition and its mimetic nature. He did this without getting mired in the struggles of authenticity versus production/performance. Because his way in was through the theory of rhetoric and performance in theatre, the question of falseness does not exactly arise. Transference enactments or interactions are artistic forms, fueled by primary process, intense affect, and transference phenomena, and their careful handling in analysis took an artist's hand, not the hand of a surgeon or a scientist.

One of the striking aspects of a long look back at theoretical and clinical work on transference and countertransference matrices is the distinct but parallel channels through which ideas evolve and flow, often with little crossover. Loewald, for example, in his quite prescient and forward-looking 1986 essay "Transference-Countertransference" did not reference Racker, yet developed a very integrated picture of these processes.

> I believe it is ill-advised, indeed impossible, to treat transference and countertransference as separate issues. They are the two faces of the same dynamic, rooted in the inextricable intertwining with others in which indi-

vidual life originates and remains throughout the life of the individual in numberless elaborations, derivatives, and transformations. One of these transformations shows itself in the encounter of the psychoanalytic situation. (Loewald 1986, p. 276)

Loewald saw analytic empathy, the emotional investment of the analyst, and the analyst's ability to tolerate extremes of feeling as central elements in the curative potential of psychoanalytic treatment. This approach certainly reflects a modern sensibility, but it is also true that contemporary classical analysts bring the paradox and conflictual approaches more center stage. Schafer (1997) points out the contradictions in Freud's own earliest formulations. There is the startling fact of the discovery of transference and the direction to analysts to override their own narcissism and find the prehistory being parachuted into the analytic relationship. Yet in the earliest use of transference, Schafer argues, Freud is mostly interested in a kind of controlling hygiene. Transference effects, muddying and clouding the analytic waters, should be swept up and away to allow the keen penetration of analytic understanding. Patriarchy and authority in these earliest writing occlude the revolutionary nature of the "discovery" of transference.

Examining the development of Freud's views of transference, Schafer has an interesting perspective. Like a number of feminist critics, Schafer notes that the suturing of transference to father love—to oedipal ties to the father—constricted Freud's clinical and theoretical vision. Schafer also differentiates how Freud got tangled up in the distinctions and relations of transference and resistance (a remnant of that patriarchal stance) but at the same time forged interesting conceptual and clinical insights in linking transference and acting out. Perhaps we might see in this light that when Freud put aside his own resistances (his difficulties in taking up the feminine), he found a different access to the complexity of transference—the mother ties, the bisexuality, the multiplicity of sexual desires.

The current situation within the more classical tradition is one of ongoing debate within and across orientations on the status, function, and limits of countertransference analysis (Gabbard 1995). Jacobs's (1991) original theoretical work on the uses of the analyst's countertransference draws from object relations, from contemporary Freudians (Sandler 1976), and from self psychology. With Jacobs, countertransference emerges in more florid and multiply configured forms, as rich in its own way and as problematic as transference. In Jacobs's work, the analyst's instrument—the creative use of body, mind, fantasy, and interpersonal experience—is crucial for analytic work. Now countertransference is not a problem but a solution, a necessary register for the analyst's work. Built into the suppositions of Jacobs's use of analytic subjectivity is his assumption of the subtle and pervasive communications—meta, conscious, preconscious, and unconscious—that undergird and network through the experiences of all analytic couples. Meaning making, being so richly co-constructed, inevitably requires that the analyst understand and explore very deeply his or her own part in these complex communications.

In the developing debates within the classical tradition, there is a sensitivity to the complex relation of particular theories and particular ways of practicing—a sense that people mostly work in multiple models and at multiple levels of awareness and abstraction (Jacobs 2001; Smith 1999, 2000, 2003a, 2003b). No particular school holds the patent on spontaneity. Most crucially, spontaneity and "authenticity" are not prosthetics against missteps in analytic work, a point made by Aron (1996) and others in the relational tradition often associated with an uncritical valorization of "throwing away the book" (a term from Hoffman 1998). As Smith (2003c) notes,

> I am not taking a stand for or against either self-disclosure or intersubjectivity. Rather, I would suggest that the form of argument linking theory and technique in such a fashion ignores the fact that many aspects of practice—including what we reveal about ourselves, deliberately or not, along with our tone of voice, gestures, affective engagement, and authenticity, not to mention the level of uncertainty we tolerate and our capacity to question our own assumptions—are not the province of any one theoretical position or school of analysis. (p. 7)

For Jacobs and Smith, and for the more object relational analysts such as Ogden (1994, 1995) and Gabbard (1994a, 1994b), even as they differ, the analyst's subjectivity is crucial for the self-analysis that moves analytic work forward. In many instances, more is disclosed to colleagues than to analysands. Countertransference more typically is now thought of as enactment. Analytic subjectivity is seen as inevitable or ubiquitous, if not for everyone "irreducible" (a term coined by Renik [1993] to speak to the dense, ever-present potency of the analytic subject in clinical dyads). Enactments and intersubjectively rich co-constructions are opportunities for psychic movement, although not unambivalently so. This perspective seems relevant for theorists with one-person and with two-person psychologies.

Smith (2003c) proposes that countertransference may be a project that both (even simultaneously) retards analytic progress and enhances it. In a way, Smith is doing for countertransference what Freud was establishing for transference, namely, that it is likely to be both resistance and a necessary engine of change. As with the repetition compulsion, there is simultaneously an impulse for health and for illness. It is important to keep in mind, with regard to countertransference phenomena, that unconscious forces will have their not fully calculable effect regardless of analytic rigor, theoretical orientation, and self-monitoring.

The Kleinian Tradition

Much of the rich understanding of the powerful effect of intersubjective process on analyst, analysand, and treatment is deeply indebted to the evolution in Kleinian thought from Klein, through Bion (1959, 1961), Rosenfeld (1987), and Racker (1968), and into the next two generations. The work of Segal (1962/1981, 1967/1981), Joseph (1989), Spillius (1988a, 1988b, 1993), and O'Shaughnessy (1983), divided in its allegiance to Klein and the increasing influence of Bion, has been followed by the current theoretical and clinical work of Britton (1989), Steiner (1998), and Feldman (1993).

For Bion (1959, 1961), the maternal countertransference reverie was a crucial analog to analytic work. The analytic instruments—mind and heart and body—are aspects of a metabolizing function whereby the patient is held, including held in mind. The stirring of fantasy and disruptive affect and mental states in the analyst is a crucial site of analytic understanding. Analytic instruments are, from this perspective, porous structures through which archaic fantasy, including destructive and aggressive wishes and fantasies, can come to light and become the occasion for interpretive work.

In this evolution, the more alienated, metapsychological treatment of projection and projective identification morphed into a living, breathing, interpersonal process whereby minds, affect states, and bodies are cannibalized, evacuated, altered, and perturbed. The most striking clinical innovations come in the work of Betty Joseph (1989) through whose work Kleinian and post-Kleinian ideas have become very widely influential. What characterizes this work is a careful and systematic appreciation of the presence of powerful unconscious anxieties expressed in the transference. Steiner (1984) makes a good case for the clinical utility of this kind of listening for unconscious phantasy expressed as transference manifestations and subtly pervasive within the analysand's communications.

The Kleinian tradition's attunement to countertransference primarily uses those phenomena as a source of clinical data on the patient's dynamics. In regard to countertransference, the theoretical evolution of the concept of projective identification and Bion's development of the notions of containment and alpha-function (a mental and psychological capacity in the analyst to metabolize and absorb primary process material and re-present it to the analysand) led to a keen appreciation of the infusion of analyst mind and affect and body ego with the analysand's unconscious and preconscious process. Projective identifications of the analyst remain an undertheorized aspect of the thought of Kleinians, with the exception of Alvarez, whose book *Live Company* (1992) describes clinical work with autistic and borderline children that relies a lot on countertransference intuition and is seen in quite deeply interactive terms.

In my work with Laura (see case example in section "'Discovery' of Transference and Countertransference and Early Developments" earlier in this chapter), I try to pay attention both to the co-construction and to my contribution to the scenes of debilitation and anxious passivity. From a Kleinian perspective, however, I also use my countertransference as an index of induced countertransference and projective identifications, unconsciously transmitted from the patient. Laura evacuates pain and fear and hopelessness into me. Our work together involves trying to use not only the metabolized bits of process reproduced in me but also those coming from Laura in order to understand the degree of conflict and anxiety in her mind. In the particular situation of her treatment, her guilt and high anxiety are connected to deep fantasies involving greed, theft, and forbidden pleasures in her love relationship. It is often the case that the transference carries the weight of guilty anguish in regard to these aspects of Laura's internal and interpersonal world.

There is one particular development in Kleinian work on transference that is noteworthy. Transference widens dramatically to include a wide range of experiences and transaction. While the widening perspective on transference occurs through the work of Sandler and in the ego psychological tradition, it is Kleinian influences, via Racker and the work of Betty Joseph, that promote the ubiquitousness of transference and its relevance to the "total situation." It is this acute focus on the pervasiveness of transference phenomena that alters clinical listening—the ability to hear the echoes and strains of archaic relationships and processes in ways of talking, gesture, and nonverbal, enactive, and communicative experiences—that is of such potential use to the beginning clinician.

Because the Kleinian interests have been addressed to early and profound and normal conditions of fantasized destructiveness and aggression, there is a considerable attunement to negative therapeutic reaction and to the power and unconscious presence of negative transference. The Kleinians are wonderfully astute at letting us think and hold reveries about the hostility in compliance—the subtle undoing and demeaning of the analytic project. It is to such endeavors that they mostly give the term "perversion." In Joseph's hands, perversion, while still tied formally and clinically to sexuality, is most deeply tied up with de-

structiveness. Perversion in the analysand encompasses the myriad strategies, conscious and unconscious, aimed at destroying the object of help and helpful experiences as well.

One of the more intriguing Kleinian rivers to follow surfaces and flourishes in Argentina in the work of Heinrich Racker. de Leon de Bernardi (2000), in a review of the Latin American tradition on countertransference phenomena, locates Racker's influences as more Kleinian than Freudian, saying that they draw deeply on ideas of unconscious fantasy and of the mechanisms of projection and introjection as binding aspects in the analytic situation. Racker himself also looks to Ferenczi and to the particular constellation of object relations writing on transference and countertransference done by Heimann (1982) and Little (1981) and by one of the central sources of Ferenczian ideas about the analytic relationship, Michael Balint (1939, 1950).

Racker has been a profound influence on the interpersonal tradition. Racker's work, mostly published versions of lectures, has a wonderfully personal quality. One feels talked to in a Racker paper and invited to think about the astonishingly rich fantasies of patient and analyst that make up analytic work. Interestingly, when Racker talks about the analyst's method of work, "evenly hovering attention," he uses what we would now recognize as a Buddhist parable, described by him as a story by a "Chinese sage." He is imagining that the analyst must work in a kind of altered state, a lifting of ego, a "non-search" attunement.

Racker, most interestingly, developed the idea that manic reactions in the analysts can lead to flooding the patient and to impeding analytic progress with too overwhelming a reactivity to the patient's material. He analyzed the resistance (in the field and in the analyst) as a matter of shame. Racker (1968) concluded his essay on countertransference with the following thoughts:

> Freud once said that his pupils had learnt to bear a part of the truth about themselves. The deepening of our knowledge of countertransference accords with this principle. And I believe we should do well if we learnt to bear this truth about each of us being also known by some other people. (p. 194)

The British Object Relations Tradition

The middle group, or Independent tradition, has (sometimes obscured) historic links to Ferenczi via Balint. It is perhaps for this reason the tradition with the deepest appreciation for the curative aspects of regression. Some of this flavor of regression and rebirth lingers in Winnicott's (1974) and Balint's (1950) ideas of transference to the point of original breakdown.

Winnicott is a crucial figure in the emergence of ideas about countertransference, particularly in his conceptualization of the mutative and necessary role for aggression as an aspect of countertransference, work that casts a long shadow in the Independent group: from Margaret Little (1981), who spoke eloquently of the depth of transference forms of hate and blocked vitality, to, in a later generation, Christopher Bollas (1987), who promoted a careful attunement to countertransference as the bearer of disavowed aspects of the analyst. In his two papers "Aggression in Relation to Emotional Development" (1950/1958) and "Hate in the Countertransference" (1947/1975), Winnicott both identifies the inevitability of aggression and hatred in the analyst and highlights its clinical utility. Hatred is paired with, not opposed to, love and primary maternal preoccupation. It is boundary making and aids in separation and in the ability of the analysand to disentangle fantasy and reality so as to lessen the dangerous experience of omnipotence. In this way, the hating aspect of the analyst, including, as Winnicott brilliantly suggested, the hatred that is in the ending of the hour, is a crucial ingredient in change in the analysand.

I am going to include Paula Heimann in this grouping, although her initial relationships after her flight from Vienna were to the Kleinian group. She herself dates her beginning independence from Klein and her reconnection to the worlds of Ferenczi and Balint with her essay "On Countertransference," written in 1949 (Heimann 1982). That essay has a quite balanced mix of insistence on the rich play of emotional responsiveness in the analyst and caution as to emotional expression. She seems to have considered analytic countertransference as a kind of creation of the patient, useful to the analyst. We might note her nascent ideas that have developed through Bion, Ogden, and others on the use of analytic reverie and the analytic object as a new creation. Interestingly, her clinical vignette includes her sense of the countertransference as both clue and misclue.

There is also in Heimann's writing a caution as to the limits of transference. It is quite poignant to read in this émigré analyst, for whom the war had been a series of traumatic losses, the idea that part of analytic work is to recover some predefensive sense of lost love objects (echoes of Balint) and to mourn them. In that context, the analyst steps back, functioning as guide and observer, and the heat of transference is turned down (temporarily) to afford time for grief at real losses.

In the British middle group tradition, the modern evolution of these ideas has been in the work of Sandler (1976) and Bollas (1979, 1987), which is an interesting bridge between the work of Winnicott and that of Fonagy. Bollas is interested in the use of countertransference reverie as a source of analytic work, but he is more interested in the mutative effect of nonverbal affect states than in interpretation. Analytic work is often, for Bollas, in the preverbal register, providing a holding function as much as insight. Bollas, for example, has the interesting idea that sometimes interpretation pulls for a certain precocity in the analysand who is actually not fully available to symbolic process in a deep sense. There is then the danger of intellectualization.

Fonagy's work on transference and countertransference brings back the tradition of Bowlby on the deep relational patterns in early attachment. These ideas about attachment patterning are joined with a Bion-like attention to the mentalizing function in the analyst's countertransference. If we translated their views into the language of transference phenomena, Fonagy and his colleagues (Fonagy 2001; Fonagy and Target 1996, 2000; Fonagy et al. 2003) see change not via transference interpretation but through the analyst's holding in mind the disavowed process in the patient until the capacity to mentalize is induced in the analysand through the relational transactions.

In Fonagy's clinical vignettes, it is often the case that the analyst is infused, even infested, with patient material, extruded and evacuated by the patient into the analyst in desperate unconscious efforts to keep the mind uncontaminated. Countertransference, in this way, entails extensive amounts of management, without repression or the more usual wish to download the toxic mental products back into the patient. I see many such subtle problems in mentalization with a patient I will call Ellen, who lives in thrall to terrible early losses that remain largely unmetabolizable. Even in the midst of a long treatment, she can be surprised by what I hold in mind of her history. By virtue of my interest in her early history of disruption—indeed my insistence that it matters—we held together some narrative of what occurred. But for a long time, only I remembered or thought about her love for her lost mother, while she had quite subtle but distinguishable difficulties in object constancy with me.

We lived through an incident that made some alteration in this. She made a very rare and desperate call to me on a weekend and then could not be reached. I realized that I was left in a deeply unsettled state, unable to keep the thread of my own day going and unable to help. When we examined this experience and its impact on me, I think it was important that this patient could experience her capacity to damage me, always the fearful thought behind the loss (to illness) of her mother and the catastrophic events that followed. Mentalization that is held and then offered to the patient through transactions must also have to engage some subjective experience of agency and intentionality. Ellen lived what was factually true for her, a life of passive dependence on unreliable others. But she also carried a more hidden fantasy of being dangerous and destructive. This coming to life in an enactment was useful to her own development of reflective functioning.

Lacanian Models of Transference

Having mentioned Lacanian influences on the work in transference developing in Latin America, I want to take up what Lacan and Lacanians have done with these concepts. Lacan (1977), although alienated and repudiated by a considerable portion of mainstream psychoanalysis, has much to offer a consideration of transference and countertransference because he approaches the phenomena as discourse, finding in the analytic dyad a particular form of speech through which analytic work actually goes on. Transference can be mutative when it addresses the unconscious carried in discourse. It is part of resistance when the relational experiences are cast in preoedipal, imaginary, sensory, or narcissistic elements. Lacan was attempting (successfully or not, depending on your point of view) to mine a paradox. Analytic authority was a dangerous illusion. Speech from that perspective was doomed to founder and leave the analysand untouched and unchanged. But regression and merger states were equally problematic (either in the transference or the countertransference).

Authority, Lacan (1977) argues, or rather authoritative knowledge, resides in the unconscious of the analysand, though often projected out into the analyst as "the one who knows." The magisterial qualities of the analyst, so crucial for what Freud was noticing in developing the concept of transference and so fundamental to many ideas about transference, are for Lacan an illusion, an experience lived out in the register of the Imaginary. The analytic task is to be attuned to the signals in the analysand's speech of the workings of unconscious desire and drives, particularly death drives, and for that reason countertransference is simply another one of the resistances (like the analysand's focus on pleasure and projections of authority) to be pared away. For Lacan, there is probably no real relationship, just as in the realm of sexuality there is no sexual rapport. The enigmatic and potently controlling aspects of Otherness, present and interactive between analyst and analysand, make conditions of alienation normative and conditions of attunement and identification merely chimerical.

I consider the cautionary aspects of Lacanian theory a useful guide in my work with Ellen (see subsection "The British Object Relations Tradition" earlier in this chapter). For all the intensity of our relationship and our shared hard work at building representations and capacities to love and hate in Ellen and in me, there is a haunting ele-

ment never far from awareness. What Lacanians term "the real," which is not reality but only the effect on any psyche of unassimilable trauma, provides for the enigma in any character. The gaps in Ellen and in our shared analytic object cannot be filled in, only sutured, and inadequately at that. Aftershocks are a very strong element in her subjective experience and shifting states; massive dissociation and frightening alterations of affect and capacities are a regular part of our work. Transference and countertransference, in other words, are always driven by forces beyond words and beyond full mentalization.

The Interpersonal Tradition: Fromm, Wolstein, Levenson

From the 1920s on, as one sees in Orr (1954), there is some dialogue between classical and interpersonal analysts. These links had pretty much disappeared by the 1970s. Yet this elision is occurring as an alternative, more interpersonally focused approach to transference, initiated by Karen Horney and developed by several generations of interpersonalists, from Sullivan (1953, 1964) through Fromm (1941, 1947), Levenson (1972), Wolstein (1956, 1971), and, more recently, Stern (1997), Ehrenberg (1992), Blechner (1995), and Hirsch (1987, 1996).

The interpersonal tradition was more formally in the United States inaugurated by Sullivan, with crucial contributions by Thompson, drawing on Fromm and Ferenczi. Mitchell in exploring the technical questions of analytic authenticity shows some interesting differences within this tradition. For Mitchell, there is a persistent divide in the analytic writers on transference and countertransference. In one, the more classical position, reaching from Freud to Schafer and then Sullivan, there is an argument for restraint and for a sidelining of analytic "personality." For Mitchell, the breakpoint in the interpersonal tradition comes with Fromm, in whose work authenticity in the analytic situation becomes a therapeutic goal in itself. Certainly Ferenczi would be a powerful influence in this way of thinking and working. The transference situation for Fromm seems to be a hotbed of experienced agency, intentionality, and subjectivity coming into awareness. Transference has become part of the inherent conditions of communication: free expression, honesty, and sincerity.

In the next generation of interpersonalists, I would single out Wolstein and Levenson, each of whom made unique and different contributions to the understanding of transference. Wolstein (1956, 1971) is perhaps the purest exemplar of the "radical interpersonalists." For Wolstein, metapsychology is the inevitable contaminant (Shapiro 2000). This particular interpretation of the interpersonal stance does not so much deny an internal world of objects and identifications as refuse to focus on that world in the transference. The psychic reality of the patient is paramount, and the analyst's work is more in the direction of inventorying the patient's experiences. There is, in the interpersonal tradition, a kind of distaste for regression. For Wolstein, the juice is in the transference as lived scenes. He also pulls for an experience that is not so easy to conceptualize—that is, communication that would go from unconscious to unconscious, an idea from Ferenczi. Wolstein's focus is on the uniqueness of the individual and the core experience of self as lived in the analytic dyad. The contemporary analyst whose work has evolved from Wolstein's is Ehrenberg (1992), who highlights the fresh, affectively tuned, intersubjectively unique, amplified transactions as sites of psychic transformation.

Levenson (1972) also takes this radical interpersonal stance, but his clinical and technical interests are in the analyst's use of countertransference. Levenson views the enmeshment of analyst in transference messes as crucial for analytic change. The patient digs a trap. You must fall into it, and in digging your way out, the patient is helped to find a new understanding of the transactions and to find the analyst as a new object. Levenson would seem to be saying that transference change arises when the analyst is first an old and then a creatively and actively new object.

Contemporary interpersonalists draw on a hermeneutic model of clinical conversations, on truths co-constructed, and on a decentering of analytic authority. Identification with the analyst is quite explicitly discouraged. Hirsch (1987, 1996), in particular, translates the interpersonalist project of shared experience and relational fields into the language of enactments as the inevitably ongoing process in which the psychic life of the analysand emerges and alters. Blechner (1995) is interested in the patient's use of fantasies of the analyst's countertransference (whether or not the accuracy of these fantasies is acknowledged). It is as though, for certain patients, it is important to "borrow" or "inhabit" the analyst's subjectivity in order to explore something not yet emergent and conscious in the patient's psyche. Here countertransference is offered as a transitional space for the analysand.

Self Psychology: Idealizing and Mirroring Transference

Kohutian self psychology and its multiple lines of evolution focus on transference but with a strong emphasis on the beneficial and mutative aspects of positive transference. Transference as a source of conflict is for the most part seen as a countertransference failure. The premium is put on careful, acute, attuned clinical listening, and an attempt to mirror as closely as possible the emotional experience of the analysand. Idealization of the analyst, often seen as a sign of covert hostility or a worrying protection of the analyst in Kleinian terms, is in self psychology a key to psychic change.

Fosshage (1994, 1997) speaks of the shifting listening perspectives in the analyst. Self attunement and attunement to the analysand interweave. One criticism of this perspective is that the idealization in the analytic relationship remains too unexamined. The process seems to require ongoing attunement by the analyst, with errors and misattunement addressable only by the analyst. This epistemologically complex, somewhat unstable situation has its echoes in the self psychological work on intersubjectivity.

Countertransference remained relatively untheorized until the inauguration of interest in intersubjectivity and co-construction, the work of Stolorow and his colleagues (Stolorow 1997; Stolorow et al. 2001). They hold a quite unique perspective on transference and countertransference, seeing a total situation of co-construction in which unconscious aspects are more elements on a horizon than topographically organized underlying features of mind. This project is frankly and self-consciously anti-Cartesian, focusing on a more deeply phenomenological experience of enmeshed self-other interaction.

The Relational Turn

Mitchell worked on matters of technique primarily in two books *Hope and Dread and Influence* (Mitchell 1993) and *Autonomy in Psychoanalysis* (Mitchell 1988). Mitchell, along with Pizer (1998), Bromberg (1998), Aron (1996), and others, opened up the question of analytic subjectivity and co-construction of meaning in the analytic relationship by thinking of two revolutions in psychoanalysis: the revolution in what patients need and the revolution in what the analyst knows. From Renik (1993) and Maroda (1994) and others, we would have to add that there is a revolution in what the analysand knows about the psychic action of the analyst. For all these writers, a seminal influence is Merton Gill (1982).

From Mitchell's clinical writing there is a powerful sense that countertransference affects are the engines for psychic movement. His vignettes often catch the analytic pair in moments of hopeless despair. Without that "felt" experience of hopelessness, the analyst is not impelled to do the work of understanding and identification. The analytic work is to analyze the process by which such impasses take hold. There are then always two speakers with authority. Impasse, improvisation, and the undoing of knots and paradoxes are at the heart of relational work on transference (Bromberg 1998; Davies 2001; Pizer 1998). Many strategies are deployed: creative play, imaginative use of countertransference, and a willingness to be stirred up and disrupted are of central value. One theorist evoked by this work is Harold Searles (1979), for whom the engine of transformation was often to be found in a widening experience in the analyst.

Aron (1996) has developed more theoretical purchases on the questions of mutuality and asymmetry. Aron's work on technique has been both to organize and to summarize the relational and interpersonal turn with regard to these matrices and to develop his own conceptions of analytic pattern and authenticity. His 1996 book *A Meeting of Minds* is to my mind a good alternative to the tendency to equate all relational work with unthoughtful disclosure and limitless relativism. Reading Aron, one can find an alternative perspective to the one amusingly caricatured in Spezzanno's (1998) article title "What Do Relationalists Do Between Disclosure and Enactment?"

Aron (1996), for example, describes a spectrum of experiences that analysands have of their analyst, with the spectrum moving from opacity to translucency to transparency through disclosure, but crucially including experiences in which analysts are more porous to analysands than we like to imagine. He also takes pains to describe another spectrum, along the orthogonal dimensions of symmetry on the one hand and intersubjectivity on the other hand. There can be mutually porous and disclosing relationships—relationships that retain the asymmetry and hierarchy of analytic dyads without refusing some role for analytic subjectivity.

Aron argues that many technical choices can flow from the position that analytic work is always a co-construction. Hoffman (1998) is associated with a strong emphasis on authenticity and the value both of having a book and of throwing it away. Ehrenberg's (1992) clinical and theoretical work stresses the affective links with patients—the mutative power of living and functioning at an affective edge in which the feeling states and subjectivity of the analyst is decidedly present. Maroda (1994) is sensitive both to the perceptual skill of the analysand and to the difficult presence of power. For Maroda, countertransference disclosure often takes on an ethical aspect, a move in the name of honesty as much as spontaneity.

Benjamin's (1995) template of "doer and done to"—the relations of complementarity in which each person in the dyad is held and traumatized through the historical and frozen object relations of their own history—has influenced relational analytic listening. It is important to remember that although Benjamin's work holds out a perhaps utopian goal for analytic growth to conditions of mutual recognition, recognition is not total attunement and empathic links to another. In Benjamin's idea of an object who is also a subject as one outcome of transference

and countertransference, it is the inalienable individuality of that subject that is crucial. Drawing from Ghent (1990) and originally from Winnicott (1974), Benjamin argues that the outcome of analytic transactions is an experience of individuality that is private, recognizable, and appreciated but also inalienable. Ghent's particular interest lies in the defensive vicissitudes in patient's object relations in transference, whereby sustained respectful relatedness could be spoiled and defended against by collapses alternatively into either sadistic object probing or masochistic submission.

Bromberg's (1998) clinical choice is most often to pay close attunement to the surfaces of language and speech practices; the genres, styles, and idiosyncrasies of human performance as the surface registration of internal worlds. These metaphors of "surface" and "inside" do not capture the sense of shifting psychic realities shaping the interpersonal relationship, with each state expressed and elaborated through its own unique experience-near styles of being and talking. Deploying theoretical concepts of dissociation and a strong investment in multiplicity and shifting self states as an inevitable attribute of transference and countertransference, Bromberg draws on his countertransference experiences as a guide to the transforming object relations lived out in the transference.

Davies' (1994, 2001) use of countertransference disclosure has been controversial but also influential. She intentionally uses disclosures of affect states and sexual fantasy in the hopes of opening and altering unresolved sources of unconscious shame and guilt. Regarding the erotic and sexual aspects of countertransference. Davies' clinical choice—either to disclose or not to disclose—is guided by an assumption that sexual secrets can be massively dangerous to patients and iatrogenically reproduced in analyses. Davies views transference and countertransference as a set of interlocking matrices in which the analyst is called on to live out disowned and dissociated aspects of the object world and the self state of analysands. She uses the metaphor of hot potatoes passed back and forth as transference and countertransference phenomena are lived out, processed, and defused.

Much the same process appears in Gabbard's clinical account of work with erotic transference. In a clinical report on erotic transference (Gabbard 2001), the potency of words in writing, in e-mail communications inside and outside the analytic frame, in reading aloud, and in analytic speech was powerfully mobilized in the treatment, and transference and countertransference erotics were both cultivated and defused. Most interestingly, Gabbard seemed to have transformed a charged, driven eroticized transference into a form of transference love through which the analysand grew and changed. And he did so through open talk.

The Real Relationship Revisited

In the turn to countertransference and in the critiques of neutrality and one-person psychology models, the question of reality has arisen again, though now in a way quite unpredicted by Greenson. With influences as various as social constructionism, existentialism, phenomenology, postmodernism, and philosophy of mind, analysts across a spectrum of positions have begun to have an effect on other analysts across a broad theoretical spectrum who began to question technique. Renik (1993, 1996), a theorist with ties to the classical and to the relational world, is perhaps the most powerful and visible spokesperson for allowing analytic subjectivity as an irreducible fact into explicit interpretations and into a wide variety of analytic communications.

With this new interest in countertransference and an opening or ventilating of the intersubjective matrix of the relationship, the question of the analyst's contribution took a new turn. The question of explicit use of countertransference (via disclosure) is perhaps the most hotly debated issue in clinical psychoanalysis at this moment. There are many things to consider. Are all affects, including hatred, sexual interest, erotic excitement, or despair, suitable for disclosure in analyses? And can useful psychoanalytic work be conducted in the wake of these disclosures?

One problem with the distinction between real and performed—authentic and managed—technique is that the categories leak in both directions. Choice, including silence, at any given clinical moment is not always the enactment of false self, even without the postmodern critique that considers all communications and forms of identity aspects of performance. There must be the potential for variation in style, in character, and in modes of relating (Greenberg 1995, 2001; Harris and Gold 2001; Smith 2003a, 2003b). Hoffman (1998) has built one of the most systematic arguments for a dialectical relationship between technique and spontaneity. On the other hand, Greenberg (2001), among others, has pushed for more demanding accountability and judgment about the impact of disclosures and countertransference phenomena.

It is worth noting that the new expansion of thinking about countertransference has been accompanied by a new openness in talking about, addressing, and acting on boundary violations. Spearheaded by Glen Gabbard and others, we now have a discourse about the facts of boundary violations and some of the preconditions (institutional and personal) that can lead to these devastating and destructive misuses of analytic power.

Rough Magic

Why does transference work? How does talk "cure"? How do words work their performative magic? I am going to propose some answers, or further questions on this matter, drawn from the psychoanalytic tradition I feel personally closest to, the relational perspective. Talk cures because of the excess in words, because of words' materiality and their archaic residues of love and loss, and because the constitutive power of speech always depends on the intense object relations hidden within it (Aron and Bushra 1998). Talk cures through the puzzling interdependence of transference and speech's effects. Transference, I am going to argue, is a kind of mimesis that arises and effects its particular magic only because the distinctions between word and act, and self and other, are unstable and dissolving and because this blurring is tied to archaic but potent relational matrices.

My scientist patient, Laura (see section "'Discovery' of Transference and Countertransference and Early Developments"), told me an important memory from quite early in childhood. She is sitting on a bed and her mother has come in, in an angry, stormy state. Her mother sits beside her, looks deeply into Laura's face, and says, "I don't know why you hate me. I don't know why you have turned against me." Laura, listening, had the initial feeling that this was crazy, that she had not turned on her mother, that she did not hate her. Then the more she stayed with the experience, the truer these words became. This was crazy talk; she could feel herself, in the wake of these words, begin to turn away. This experience came to life in the treatment whenever I interpreted anger or hostility in Laura's communication to me. My words had the effect of making something true inside her. If I spoke of hatred or anger, I constituted those feelings in her.

Much of the time in her analysis Laura keeps me good, or at least benign and more ominously irrelevant. Recently, she allowed as how her goal in the treatment was to emerge unscathed—changed but untouched by her experience of me. Our words, with all their embodied, affective charges, of course make this task impossible. When I spoke from a moment of conflict between us with some emotional force, beginning a sentence with "Truthfully, I don't really know what is right here," the effect on Laura was electrifying. She reported she felt she might slide off the couch. My words held actual doom for her. However she likes the reason and calm of our analytic life, there is always lurking in the spaces between us, both in her and in me, this archaic power of speech, the power that transference draws on, the power that prevents change and enables it.

Transference is a doseable form of trance that is dependent on the aspects of speech that constitute its connective tissues, not its separating function. The shifts from empty to full speech, from presymbolic to protosymbolic to symbolic representation, are part of the curative form endowed by language. I have neglected here that more rational feature of speech, the way language comes to aid a patient in making a story, taking responsibility for it, and constructing coherence and nuanced distinctions. This function obviously is also part of the curative power of language. The reasonableness of words must help and can calm and regulate and structure the speaker and the listener. But the power of speech to effect and alter soma and psyche comes not from reason but from its mimetic origins: its tie to an archaic maternal imago and the modes of being and related connected to that imago.

Conclusion

The heart of what makes psychoanalysis *psychoanalysis* is the talking cure. Yet transference and countertransference phenomena are unstable conceptions. One of the crucial dimensions of transference and countertransference experiences is power. In many ways, although the focus of interest has shifted much more to the study of countertransference, a crucial debate remains. Does analysis cure by experience or by interpretation? Are analytic cures cures by love or cures by widening the ego? Does psychic change or mutative action come as a byproduct of enhanced reflection or from the "now" moments of affective link between analyst and analysand? Can these differences become more interdependent?

Because different theoretical groups often work in isolated uncomprehending parallel, there are sometimes antagonisms that hide underlying affinities. When we look at these groups comparatively, one can see some strange bedfellows. Lacanians, interpersonalists, and ego psychologists, working with close process recording, can all sound rather alike in their distaste for regression. Interest in analytic subjectivity crosses Freudian, relational, and self psychological perspectives, although the use of such subjectivity remains both contested and quite differentiated and controversial. There are links between relational and Kleinian perspectives in regard to the importance of regression in the transference

One of the most interesting examples of cross pollinations and hybrid theorizing is in the work of Evelyn Schwaber (1995, 1998), who draws on Kohutian ideas of analytic listening while remaining well rooted in the more classical Freudian canon. Schwaber has been interested in how much the patient's constructions and communications, including transference communications, are shaped by the analyst's way of listening. Patient resistance, Schwaber suggests, has roots in the resistance and defensiveness of the analyst. It is almost as though the analysand's constructions function as a kind of subtle supervision to the analyst, guiding shifts and attunements in a listening stance.

Reviewed across a century, the concept of transference still sets off a certain puzzle of love and hate that impels thought and movement. Psychoanalytic work—at its heart, work in transference and countertransference—is very beautiful, dangerous magic. There is an irreducible intimacy and closeness among great power, great transformative energy, and grievous error. Hence the title of the preceding section, "Rough Magic," the term Prospero gives the magic arts and creativity about which he has become so ambivalent:

> I have bedimm'd
> The noontide sun, called forth the mutinous winds
> And twixt the green sea and the azured vault
> Set roaring war: to the dread rattling thunder
> Have I given fire, and rifted Jove's stout oak
> With his own bolt: …
>   Graves at my command
> Have waked their sleepers, oped and let them forth
> By my so potent art. But this rough magic
> I here abjure. (*The Tempest* V, i, 32–55)

References

Alvarez A: Live Company. London, Routledge, 1992

Aron L: A Meeting of Minds: Mutuality in Psychoanalysis. Hillsdale, NJ, Analytic Press, 1996

Aron L, Bushra A: Mutual regression: altered states in the psychoanalytic situation. J Am Psychoanal Assoc 46:389–412, 1998

Aron L, Harris A (eds): The Legacy of Sandor Ferenczi. Hillsdale, NJ, Analytic Press, 1993

Bakan D: Sigmund Freud and the Jewish Mystical Tradition (1958). Boston, MA, Beacon, 1998

Balint A, Balint M: On transference and counter-transference. Int J Psychoanal 20:223–230, 1939

Balint M: Changing therapeutic aims and techniques in psychoanalysis. Int J Psychoanal 31:117–124, 1950

Benjamin J: Like Objects, Love Subjects. New Haven, CT, Yale University Press, 1995

Bird B: Notes on transference: universal phenomenon and hardest part of analysis. J Am Psychoanal Assoc 20:267–301, 1972

Bion W: Attacks on linking. Int J Psychoanal 40:308–315, 1959

Bion WR: A theory of thinking. Int J Psychoanal 43:306–310, 1961

Blechner M: The patient's dreams and the countertransference. Psychoanalytic Dialogues 5:1–25, 1995

Bollas C: The transformational object. Int J Psychoanal 60:97–107, 1979

Bollas C: The Shadow of the Object: Psychoanalysis of the Unknown Thought. New York, Columbia University Press, 1987

Bonomi C: Flight into sanity: Jones's allegations of Ferenczi's mental deterioration reconsidered. Int J Psychoanal 80:507–542, 1999

Britton R: The missing link: parental sexuality in the Oedipus complex, in The Oedipus Complex Today: Clinical Implications. Edited by Steiner J. London, Karnac Books, 1989, pp 83–102

Bromberg PM: Standing in the Spaces. Hillsdale, NJ, Analytic Press, 1998

Davies JM: Love in the afternoon: a relational reconsideration of desire and dread in the countertransference. Psychoanalytic Dialogues 4:153–170, 1994

Davies JM: Erotic overstimulation and the co-construction of sexual meanings in transference-countertransference experience. Psychoanal Q 70:757–788, 2001

de Leon de Bernardi B: Countertransference: a Latin-American view. Int J Psychoanal 81:331–352, 2000

Dupont J: Ferenczi's madness. Contemporary Psychoanalysis 24:250–261, 1988

Ehrenberg DB: The Intimate Edge: Extending the Reach of Psychoanalytic Interaction. New York, WW Norton, 1992

Falzeder E: Dreaming of Freud: Ferenczi, Freud, and an Analysis Without End. Psychoanalytic Inquiry 17:416–427, 1997

Feldman M: Aspects of Reality, and the Focus of Interpretation. Psychoanalytic Inquiry 13:274–295, 1993

Fenichel O: Criteria for interpretation (book review). Psychoanal Q 9:576, 1940a

Fenichel O: New Ways in Psychoanalysis. Psychoanal Q 9:114–121, 1940b

Ferenczi S: Introjection and transference (1909), in First Contributions to Psychoanalysis. Translated by Balint M. London, Karnac Books, 1980, pp 35–93

Ferenczi S: The Clinical Diary of Sandor Ferenczi. Edited by Dupont J. Translated by Balint M, Jackson NZ. Cambridge, MA, Harvard University Press, 1932

Fonagy P: Attachment Theory and Psychoanalysis. New York, Other Press, 2001

Fonagy P, Target M: Playing with reality, I: theory of mind and the normal development of psychic reality. Int J Psychoanal 77:217–233, 1996

Fonagy P, Target M: Playing with reality, III: the persistence of dual psychic reality in borderline patients. Int J Psychoanal 81:853–874, 2000

Fonagy P, Gergely G, Jurist E, et al: Attachment, Mentalization, and the Regulation of the Self. New York, Other Press, 2003

Fosshage J: Towards reconceptualizing transference: theoretical and clinical considerations. Int J Psychoanal 75:265–280, 1994

Fosshage J: Listening/experiencing perspectives and the quest for a facilitative responsiveness, in Conversations in Self Psychology: Progress in Self Psychology. Edited by Goldberg A. Hillsdale, NJ, Analytic Press, 1997, pp 33–55

Freud S: The handling of dream interpretation in psychoanalysis (1911), in Standard Edition of the Complete Psychological Works of Sigmund Freud, Vol 12. Translated and edited by Strachey J. London, Hogarth Press, 1958, pp 89–96

Freud S: The dynamics of transference (1912a), in Standard Edition of the Complete Psychological Works of Sigmund Freud, Vol 12. Translated and edited by Strachey J. London, Hogarth Press, 1958, pp 99–108

Freud S: Recommendations to physicians practising psycho-analysis (1912b), in Standard Edition of the Complete Psychological Works of Sigmund Freud, Vol 12. Translated and edited by Strachey J. London, Hogarth Press, 1958, pp 109–120

Freud S: On beginning the treatment (further recommendations on the technique of psycho-analysis I) (1913), in Standard Edition of the Complete Psychological Works of Sigmund Freud, Vol 12. Translated and edited by Strachey J. London, Hogarth Press, 1958, pp 121–144

Freud S: Remembering, repeating and working-through (further recommendations on the technique of psycho-analysis II) (1914), in Standard Edition of the Complete Psychological Works of Sigmund Freud, Vol 12. Translated and edited by Strachey J. London, Hogarth Press, 1958, pp 145–156

Freud S: Observations on transference love: further recommendations in the technique of psycho-analysis (1915), in Standard Edition of the Complete Psychological Works of Sigmund Freud, Vol 12. Translated and edited by Strachey J. London, Hogarth Press, 1958, pp 157–171

Freud S: Analysis terminable and interminable (1937a), in Standard Edition of the Complete Psychological Works of Sigmund Freud, Vol 23. Translated and edited by Strachey J. London, Hogarth Press, 1964, pp 209–253

Freud S: Constructions in analysis (1937b), in Standard Edition of the Complete Psychological Works of Sigmund Freud, Vol 23. Translated and edited by Strachey J. London, Hogarth Press, 1964, pp 255–269

Freud S: An outline of psycho-analysis (1940), in The Standard Edition of the Complete Psychological works of Sigmund Freud, Vol 23. Translated and edited by Strachey J. London, Hogarth Press, 1964, pp 144–207

Friedman S: Analyzing Freud: Letters of HD, Bryher, and Their Circle. New York, New Directions, 2002

Fromm E: Escape From Freedom. New York, Avon, 1941

Fromm E: Man for Himself. New York, Fawcett, 1947

Gabbard GO: On love and lust in erotic transference. J Am Psychoanal Assoc 42:385–403, 1994a

Gabbard GO: Sexual excitement and countertransference love in the analyst. J Am Psychoanal Assoc 42:1083–1106, 1994b

Gabbard GO: Countertransference: the emerging common ground. Int J Psychoanal 76:475–485, 1995

Gabbard GO: Cyberpassion: e-rotic transference on the Internet. Psychoanal Q 70:719–738, 2001

Ghent E: Masochism, submission, surrender: masochism as a perversion of surrender. Contemporary Psychoanalysis 26:108–136, 1990

Gill M: The Analysis of Transference, Vols 1 and 2. New York, International Universities Press, 1982

Gray P: The Ego and Analysis of Defense. New York, Jason Aronson, 1994

Greenberg J: Psychoanalytic technique and the interactive matrix. Psychoanal Q 64:1–22, 1995

Greenberg J: The analyst's participation: a new look. J Am Psychoanal Assoc 49:359–380, 2001

Greenson R: The Technique and Practice of Psychoanalysis. New York, International Universities Press, 1967

H.D. [Hilda Doolittle]: Tribute to Freud. Boston, MA, David R. Godine, 1956

Harris A, Gold B: The fog rolled in: induced dissociative states. Psychoanalytic Dialogues 11:357–384, 2001

Haynal A: For a metapsychology of the psychoanalyst: Sándor Ferenczi's quest. Psychoanalytic Inquiry 17:437–458, 1997

Heimann P: About Children and Children-No-Longer: Collected Papers 1942–1980. London, Routledge, 1982

Hirsch I: Varying modes of analytic participation. J Am Psychoanal Assoc 15:205–222, 1987

Hirsch I: Observing-participation, mutual enactment, and the new classical models. Contemporary Psychoanalysis 32:359–383, 1996

Hoffman IZ: Ritual and Spontaneity in the Psychoanalytic Process: A Dialectical-Constructivist View. Hillsdale, NJ, Analytic Press, 1998

Jacobs T: The Use of the Self: Countertransference and Communication in the Analytic Situation. Madison, CT, International Universities Press, 1991

Jacobs T: Countertransference past and present: A review of the concept. Int J Psychoanal 80:575–594, 1999

Jacobs T: On misreading and misleading patients: some reflections on communications, miscommunications and countertransference enactments. Int J Psychoanal 82:653–659, 2001

Joseph B: Psychic Equilibrium and Psychic Change. London, Tavistock, 1989

Lacan J: Ecrits: A Selection. Translated by Sheridan A. New York, WW Norton, 1977

Levenson E: The Fallacy of Understanding. New York, Basic Books, 1972

Lipton SD: The advantages of Freud's technique as shown in his analysis of the rat man. Int J Psychoanal 58:255–273, 1977

Little M: Transference Neurosis and Transference Psychosis. New York, Jason Aronson, 1981

Loewald H: Psychoanalysis as art and the phantasy character of the psychoanalytic situation. J Am Psychoanal Assoc 23:277–299, 1975

Loewald H: The transference neurosis: comments on the concept and the phenomenon, in Papers on Psychoanalysis. New Haven, CT, Yale University Press, 1980, pp 302–314

Loewald H: Transference-countertransference. J Am Psychoanal Assoc 34:275–287, 1986

Macalpine I: The development of the transference. Psychoanal Q 19:501–519, 1950

Mannoni O: Freud. New York, Pantheon, 1971

Maroda K: The Power of Countertransference. Northvale, NJ, Jason Aronson, 1994

Mitchell S: Hope and Dread in Psychoanalysis. New York, Basic Books, 1993

Mitchell S: Influence and Autonomy in Psychoanalysis. Hillsdale, NJ, Analytic Press, 1997

Ogden T: Subjects of Analysis. London, Karnac Books, 1994

Ogden T: Analyzing forms of aliveness and deadness of transference-countertransference. Int J Psychoanal 76:695–709, 1995

Orr DW: Transference and countertransference: a historical survey. J Am Psychoanal Assoc 2:621–670, 1954

O'Shaughnessy E: Words and working through. Int J Psychoanal 63:281–289, 1983

Pizer S: Building Bridges: The Negotiation of Paradox in Psychoanalysis. Hillsdale, NJ, Analytic Press, 1998

Racker H: Transference and Countertransference. London, Hogarth Press, 1968

Renik O: Analytic interaction: conceptualizing technique in light of the analyst's irreducible subjectivity. Psychoanal Q 62:553–571, 1993

Renik O: The perils of neutrality. Psychoanal Q 65:495–517, 1996

Rosenfeld H: Impasse and Interpretation: Therapeutic and Antitherapeutic Factors in Psychoanalytic Treatment of Psychotic, Borderline, and Neurotic Patients. London, Routledge, 1987

Sandler J: Countertransference and role-responsiveness. Int Rev Psychoanal 3:43–47, 1976

Schafer R: Tradition and Change in Psychoanalysis. Madison, CT, International Universities Press, 1997

Schwaber E: The psychoanalyst's mind: from listening to interpretation—a clinical report. Int J Psychoanal 76:271–281, 1995

Schwaber E: From whose point of view: the neglected question in psychoanalytic listening. Psychoanal Q 67:645–681, 1998

Searles H: Countertransference and Related Subjects. New York, International Universities Press, 1979

Segal H: The curative factors in psycho-analysis (1962), in The Work of Hanna Segal. New York, Jason Aronson, 1981, pp 69–80

Segal H: Melanie Klein's technique (1967), in The Work of Hanna Segal. New York, Jason Aronson, 1981, pp 3–24

Shapiro S: The unique Benjamin Wolstein as experienced and read. Contemporary Psychoanalysis 36:301–341, 2000

Smith H: Subjectivity and objectivity in analytic listening. J Am Psychoanal Assoc 47:465–484, 1999

Smith H: Countertransference, conflictual listening and the analytic object relationship. J Am Psychoanal Assoc 48:95–128, 2000

Smith H: Analysis of transference: a North American perspective. Int J Psychoanal 84:1017–1041, 2003a

Smith H: Conceptions of conflict in psychoanalytic theory and practice. Psychoanal Q 72:49–96, 2003b

Smith H: Theory and practice: intimate partnership or false connection. Psychoanal Q 72:1–12, 2003c

Spezzanno C: Listening and interpreting: how relational analysts kill time between disclosures and enactments (commentary on papers by Bromberg and by Greenberg). Psychoanalytic Dialogues 8:237–246, 1998

Spillius EB (ed): Melanie Klein Today, Vol 1: Mostly Theory. London, Routledge, 1988a

Spillius EB (ed): Melanie Klein Today, Vol 2: Mostly Practice. London, Routledge, 1988b

Spillius EB: Varieties of envious experiences. Int J Psychoanal 74:1199–1212, 1993

Steiner J: Some Reflections on the Analysis of Transference: A Kleinian View. Psychoanalytic Inquiry 4:443–463, 1984

Steiner J: The Oedipus Complex Today. London, Karnac Books, 1998

Stern D: Unformulated Experience. Hillsdale, NJ, Analytic Press, 1997

Stolorow R: Dynamc, dyadic, and intersubjective systems. Psychoanalytic Psychology 14:337–346, 1997

Stolorow R, Orange D, Atwood G: World horizon: a postcartesian alternative to the Freudian unconscious. Contemporary Psychoanalysis 37:43–61, 2001

Stone L: Transference and Its Context: Selected Papers on Psychoanalysis. New York, Jason Aronson, 1984

Sullivan HS: The Interpersonal Theory of Psychiatry. Edited by Perry HS, Gawel ML. New York, WW Norton, 1953

Sullivan HS: The Fusions of Psychiatry and Social Science. New York, WW Norton, 1964

Winnicott DW: Hate in the countertransference (1947), in Collected Papers: Through Paediatrics to Psychoanalysis. New York, Basic Books, 1975, pp 194–203

Winnicott DW: Aggression in relation to emotional development (1950), in Collected Papers: Through Paediatrics to Psychoanalysis. New York, Basic Books, 1958, pp 204–218

Winnicott DW: The fear of breakdown. Int Rev Psychoanal 1:103–107, 1974

Wolstein B: Countertransference. New York, Grune & Stratton, 1956

Wolstein B: Human Psyche in Psychoanalysis. Springfield, IL, Charles C Thomas, 1971

14

Theories of Therapeutic Action and Their Technical Consequences

JAY GREENBERG, PH.D

IN 1931, EDWARD GLOVER published his provocatively titled paper "The Therapeutic Effect of Inexact Interpretations." The paper is remarkable both because Glover identified a crucial, previously unnoticed paradox in traditional psychoanalytic accounts of the mechanism of therapeutic action and because his argument introduced and authorized an illogical resolution of the paradox, a resolution that has haunted psychoanalysis for decades.

The paradox that Glover noticed hinged on the idea that since its beginnings, psychoanalysis had been claiming to cure neurotic symptoms by interpretation—that is, by making the unconscious conscious. Moreover, since *Studies on Hysteria* (Breuer and Freud 1893–1895/1955), analysts had insisted that cure was possible only if patients became fully aware of the repressed mental contents that were driving the symptoms. Some improvement might be possible along the way, of course, but stable cure depended on the full and precise identification of the relevant unconscious material. And, unlike all other treatment modalities, psychoanalytic cure required *only* that the patient become aware of what had previously been banished from consciousness. The experience of treatment itself, the bond with the doctor that had always been recognized as

a weighty force in nonanalytic approaches, played a facilitative but ultimately reducible role in psychoanalytic cures. This ruled out mechanisms of therapeutic action that might characterize other methods; Glover (1931, p. 397) specifically addressed the impact of suggestion and of relying on "fresh discoveries [to provide] more convenient or rapid access to affective reactions" (i.e., catharsis).

The other side of the paradox lay in the rapid changes (or, as Glover would have it, advances) in psychoanalytic theorizing in the 36 years between the publication of the *Studies on Hysteria* and the appearance of his paper. To mention a few: the seduction hypothesis had come and gone; the dual-instinct theory had been introduced and modified; the theory of anxiety had undergone profound revisions; the topographic model of the mind had been introduced and superceded by the tripartite structural model. The upshot of this, especially relevant for clinical work and for theorizing about therapeutic action, was what Glover characterized as "the discovery of fresh phantasy systems" (Glover 1931, p. 397). In other words, by 1931 analysts knew that they needed to uncover repressed mental contents that their predecessors could not have found because they were unaware of their existence.

How to account for decades of claimed cures—cures by interpretation—when the analysts claiming those cures did not even know what they were supposed to be looking for? Glover found his solution at the heart of the declared difference between psychoanalysis and other therapies: the effects of suggestion. Cleverly and elaborately applying then-current metapsychological principles, he argued that *inexact* interpretations (those that were reasonably close to the mark but that did not precisely capture the essence of the repressed fantasies) could have the same effects as suggestions; by serving as a displacement object, they could alleviate anxiety and thus contribute to symptom reduction.

Historically, then, analysts had unwittingly trafficked in suggestion; they had provided therapeutic cure but not analytic cure. The latter depended on complete knowledge of the nature and contents of the unconscious. But this, of course, is where Glover's illogic entered the picture and created a paradox more vexing than the one he had set out to resolve. Because if analytic cure requires that we know the unconscious completely and exactly, then cure is possible only when psychoanalysis has nothing more to learn! That is, analytic discovery and analytic cure are incompatible with each other.

Freud never directly responded to Glover's argument, despite being its implicit target. Most likely this reflects his relative disinterest in the problem of therapeutic action, especially late in his career. He put it quite strikingly in "Analysis Terminable and Interminable," suggesting that the problem of "how a cure by analysis comes about" is "a matter which I think has been sufficiently elucidated" (Freud 1937a/1964, p. 221).

But despite this dismissiveness, he responded to Glover implicitly in the paper "Constructions in Analysis" (Freud 1937b/1964). The analyst is bound to make mistakes (inexact interpretations, inaccurate constructions, and the like), he admitted, but if these are relatively rare, no harm will be done other than wasting time. He comes closest to addressing Glover directly when he asserts that in the face of the analyst's error, "the patient remains as though he were untouched by what has been said" (p. 261). Not only will there be no analytic movement, but suggestive effects are unlikely. "The danger of our leading a patient astray by suggestion, by persuading him to accept things which we ourselves believe but which he ought not to, has certainly been enormously exaggerated" (p. 262). By Glover, presumably. And then, in what may reflect his reaction to a personal affront, Freud added, "I can assert without boasting that such an abuse of 'suggestion' has never occurred in my practice" (p. 262)—this in the face of Glover's idea that any therapeutic change prior to the "discovery" of the death instinct and the revision of the theory of anxiety must prima facie indicate that suggestive influence was at work.

But Freud's argument in the "Constructions" paper did not stop there; it very quickly took an ambiguous turn that reflects a tension in psychoanalytic thinking about therapeutic action that runs throughout the history of the discipline. Shortly after asserting that only a correct construction will lead to psychic change and then denying that he had participated in any "abuse of suggestion," Freud seems to have reversed his field entirely. Quite often, he said, we do not actually succeed in getting the patient to remember what has been repressed. But treatment can still be effective if we "produce in [the patient] an assured conviction of the truth of the construction, which achieves the same therapeutic result as a recaptured memory" (Freud 1937b/1964, pp. 263–264). How this differs from suggestion seems, from a contemporary perspective, obscure at best. Indeed, Freud signaled perplexity, if not great interest, maintaining that "how it is possible that what appears to be an incomplete substitute should nevertheless produce a complete result…is a matter for a later enquiry" (p. 264). This is a strange comment considering Freud's declaration, 6 months earlier, that the problem of how cure comes about had been resolved.

These two attempts to think about therapeutic action—one ending in logical incoherence, the other in internal contradiction and abandonment of the problem—reflect a dilemma that has faced psychoanalysis since its beginnings. In its simplest form, elaborated in but continuing to shape contemporary discourse, the question involves the relative importance attributed to the workings of interpretation (i.e., expansion of self-awareness) versus the importance attributed to the relationship created between analysand and analyst. At different times in the history of psychoanalysis the latter has been understood in terms of suggestion, of the importance of the affective experience (in the analysis generally and with the analyst in particular), of recapitulations and rectification of relationships with the parents, of the analyst's empathic presence and/or willingness to recognize the analysand, and so on.

However these relational effects have been specified in the work of different theorists, all attempts elaborate an apparently simple alternative to Freud's views that was expressed almost as soon as he first proposed them. In *Studies on Hysteria*, Freud declared that cure depended on recovering repressed memories of lived experience. These were memories of moments that were traumatic for his patients, although he considered unbearable inner conflict to be traumatic, thus avoiding the dichotomous distinction between intrapsychic and interpersonal experience that plagues us today. In *The Interpretation of Dreams* (Freud 1900/1953), Freud shifted the emphasis, if not the essence, of this formulation, narrowing his vision of unconscious mental contents and insisting that it is invariably forbidden wishes that need to be retrieved. He further, in *Three Essays on the Theory of Sexuality* (Freud 1905/1953), narrowed his ideas about what needed to be uncovered, declaring that interpretation must focus on repressed sexual desires and the fantasies to which they had given rise.

Like so many of Freud's radical, provocative ideas, his assertion that self-awareness was not only an ethical and aesthetic value but also a cure for disease quickly aroused alternative hypotheses. As early as 1906, in an admiring letter expressing interest in joining the emerging psychoanalytic movement, Jung risked one minor protest: "Your therapy seems to me to depend not merely on the affects released by abreaction but also on certain personal rapports" (quoted in McGuire 1974, p. 4). Within 15 years, this small quibble had burgeoned into the Freud-Ferenczi debate, focused on whether interpretation alone was responsible for change or whether the new experience with the analyst was curative in its own right (Ferenczi and Rank 1924). By the time of the Marienbad conference in 1936, there were so many competing viewpoints on the workings of therapeutic action that Glover himself warned against overemphasizing the importance of any one factor in the analytic situation. Referring to interpretation on the one hand and to the analyst's endurance, humaneness, and even his or her unconscious attitude toward the patient on the other, Glover worried that our theories of therapeutic action are at risk of degenerating into what he criticized as "mere special pleading" (Glover 1937, p. 131).

But despite Glover's wise if somewhat perplexing warning (perplexing in light of his own special pleading only 6 years earlier), analysts continued to claim that they could isolate and identify *the* element of the psychoanalytic situation that was responsible for therapeutic change. Twenty-five years after Marienbad, at the 1961 Edinburgh conference on therapeutic action, several of the presenters took the position that interpretation is the only carrier of analytic change and that the analyst must resist the impulse to offer anything else to the analysand. The Kleinian analyst Hannah Segal (1962) expressed this view most clearly, arguing that "insight is a precondition of any lasting personality change achieved in analysis.... To be of therapeutic value, it must be correct and it must be deep enough" (p. 211). And in a summary review another quarter-century later, Blatt and Behrends (1987) found that "interpretation leading to understanding is assumed by most analysts to be the primary mutative force in psychoanalysis" (p. 279).

The insistence on the primacy or even the exclusivity of interpretation, bound as it is to the avoidance of what Valenstein (1979) called "interpersonally promoted experiential effects" (p. 117), entails a peculiar assumption that

has remained central to many approaches to the problem of therapeutic action: it suggests that most of what we know about ordinary human involvements does not apply to the analyst-analysand relationship. Indeed, Freud (1915/1958) wrote that "the course the analyst must pursue...is one for which there is no model in real life" (p. 166; cf. King 1962, p. 224). What analysts do with and for patients is unlike what anybody else (parent, friend, doctor) does. Thus, we need not—and cannot—look for the therapeutic action of psychoanalysis in the relational effects that it offers. The analytic relationship is, uniquely, one in which personal influence can be—indeed must be—reduced to a vanishing point if the objectives of the treatment are to be achieved.

Wishful thinking must have shaped this formulation; it reflects Freud's hope that defining the psychoanalytic relationship as sui generis—perhaps even defining the relationship out of the psychoanalytic situation entirely—would concentrate attention on the workings of "correct" and "deep enough" interpretations. The importance of this to Freud and to other analysts (including many contemporary theorists) cannot be overestimated, because it appears to solve two problems simultaneously. First, it establishes the uniqueness of psychoanalysis as a treatment compared with all other therapies, which historically trade on relational effects. Second, in a kind of circular reasoning, therapeutic success can be taken as a validation of the findings and the hypotheses of psychoanalytic science; if cure depends on correctness, then cure demonstrates truth.

But, predictably, Freud's vision of the uniqueness of the analyst's role generated alternatives. Theorists following the lead of Jung and Ferenczi looked at the psychoanalytic situation and found not only "interpersonally promoted experiential effects" but a relationship that might have analogs in human development. Although initially there was no direct challenge to Freud's claim that the analytic relationship was unique, the implication of their argument is that his claim grew out of a failure to look in the right direction. If we pay attention, we will see that even analysts who scrupulously followed standard technique were participating with their analysands in ways that not only exert personal influence but can be understood as revisiting particular sorts of early experience. Along with the information that their interpretations conveyed, analysts have always been implicitly and perhaps even inadvertently repairing some of the damage that had been done as a result of the analysand's faulty early object relations. This relationally based reparation could not be avoided even if the analyst wished to do so; it was inherent in the nature of analytic engagement itself.

The first to point out a salient parallel and its healing potential was James Strachey (1934). Strachey noted that the analyst, in the course of applying standard technique, was behaving like and was bound to be experienced as a gentler, more accepting father than the patient had known in the course of growing up. As a result, the analyst would be taken into the patient's inner world in ways that are bound to soften a harsh and punitive superego. Although Strachey ultimately emphasized the centrality of what he termed "mutative interpretations," his ideas about the way in which the analyst will be perceived and introjected imply that psychic structure itself can be modified purely on the basis of the experienced relationship. He thus opened the understanding of therapeutic action to include the direct impact of developmentally based relational effects.

Strachey was writing in a time during which psychoanalytic thinking was still dominated by Freud's phallocentric emphasis on the role of the oedipal father in child development; thus, he stressed the relationship with the analyst as benign father and its implications in terms of superego modification. Some 25 years later, as interest shifted to earlier developmental stages and to the importance of mother-child relations, Hans Loewald proposed a new analog that highlighted different implications of the analyst-analysand relationship. For Loewald, the analyst behaves like and is experienced as a mother who can hold the tension between her child's current level of development and his or her potential in the future. Loewald's (1960) analyst is not simply a more permissive and resilient figure, as Strachey believed. Rather, the analyst is "a person who can feel with the patient what the patient experiences and how he experiences it, and who understands it as something more than it has been for the patient" (p. 26). Because the analyst is this sort of person, the patient will be able to claim his or her potential at a higher or more mature level of organization and integration.

Most recently, the strategy of seeking developmental analogies to explain relational contributions to therapeutic action has pushed even further back into the analysand's past. Daniel Stern and the Boston Change Process Study Group find their analog in the parent-infant dyad (Stern et al. 1998). As analyst and analysand work together to give shape to their analytic project, they re-create early connections between the infant and his or her caregiver:

> Unlike the largely nonverbal behaviours that make up the background of the parent-infant environment, the verbal content usually occupies the foreground in the consciousness of both partners. In the background, however, the movement is towards intersubjective sharing and understanding. The verbal content should not blind us to the parallel process of moving along towards an implicit intersubjective goal. (Stern et al. 1998, p. 909)

It is this jointly created experience that brings about the crucial "something more than interpretation" that lies at the core of therapeutic action (Stern et al. 1998, p. 903).

Note that Stern and colleagues, like Strachey and Loewald, emphasize that the necessary "something more" happens as an intrinsic aspect of psychoanalytic engagement (although more than the earlier authors they do eventually argue for significant modifications of standard technique). Similarly, over the years other theorists have suggested ways in which the interpreting analyst provides mutative relational experience in the course of conducting a traditional treatment. To mention a few, consider Winnicott's vision of the analyst as the resilient target of murderous aggression, Bion's idea that the analyst is a container of toxic projections, and Weiss and Sampson's concept of the neutral analyst disconfirming the patient's archaic pathogenic beliefs. Similarly, many of the concepts most frequently used in the current literature direct our attention to ways in which interpretations (and all other ways in which the analyst intervenes) exert relational effects. Role-responsiveness, enactment, the analyst as self-object, transference as a total situation, and countertransference both as source of information and as a determinant of analytic ambience come to mind in this regard.

Persistence and Impenetrability of the Debate

So for almost a century now, the issue has been joined. Some analysts believe that analytic change, by definition, depends on interpretation alone. Others insist that even the analyst operating in accord with the most narrowly construed version of standard technique inevitably provides a quality of relational experience (in some versions analogous to earlier developmental experience, in others unique and unprecedented) that directly contributes to therapeutic action. There have been many attempts to resolve or at least to influence the debate: large-scale studies have been undertaken, volumes of anecdotal evidence have been offered, and elegant arguments have been proposed in support of all positions. Recently, Gabbard and Westen (2003) suggested that interest in the "interpretation versus relationship" debate has waned, and indeed it seems that there is little more to say about it. But this is not because we have moved closer to an answer, or even toward any consensus. Rather, it is because it is seeming increasingly improbable that we will ever reach a satisfying conclusion.

History suggests that there is something about the psychoanalytic process that makes it more likely that we will come up with interesting questions than that we will arrive at convincing answers. In this sense psychoanalysis may be different from other "treatments," despite having its own claims to therapeutic efficacy. Raising questions about this difference is intriguing; it will open a perspective on our conversations about therapeutic action that is likely to be illuminating.

Consider the problem of what must happen to make it possible for a patient to participate in a treatment as rigorous as psychoanalysis. This is a problem that seems amenable to some resolution, because it is apparently accessible to investigation on the basis of empirical evidence. Virtually all analysts agree that participating in and benefiting from analysis are difficult for the patient. The difficulty is imposed by the nature of the analytic project itself: modifying ways of being in and of experiencing the world that have seemed, from the patients' perspective, effective and even essential for their entire lives. Analysis has always required that patients think the unthinkable and take terrifying risks.

But this observation, deceptively simple, raises a question that touches directly on the problem of therapeutic action: What can the analyst offer to the analysand (beyond what is bound to be a vague and often elusive suggestion that life could be better) that will facilitate the analysand's ability to participate in—and at times endure—the treatment?—what, in Roy Schafer's (1983) words, constitutes an optimal "analytic attitude"?

Perhaps surprisingly, there is little consensus about this question; each analytic school of thought (e.g., Kleinian, relational, interpersonal, contemporary conflict theory, Lacanian, self psychological) comes complete with a prescribed analytic stance that is passionately promoted even if, as Joseph Sandler (1983) noted, it might be honored in the breach by individual practitioners. Why can't the disagreement be resolved?

The reason for this lack of resolution may become clear if we consider one facet of the problem that has been widely discussed although never directly debated: is the analysis best facilitated by the analyst's steady presence—his or her persistent adherence to a way of being with the analysand regardless of pressures in the transference-countertransference, and regardless of the feelings that either participant may experience in response to this persistence? Or is some measure of technical flexibility—some adaptation to the character, needs, and even wishes of the analysand—crucial?

Even a cursory consideration of this question should reveal that any thoughtful, experienced psychoanalyst is likely to be able to argue either side. Indeed, both sides have been argued vigorously. Sometimes, the arguments focus on specific technical issues: frame flexibility, gratifi-

cations, the analyst's spontaneous affective participation, self-disclosure, and so on; sometimes the issue is taken up in more general terms. A clear example that argues the general point is the comment of Paula Heimann (1962), who, during the 1961 Edinburgh Symposium on "The Curative Factors in Psychoanalysis," wrote,

> [I]f the analyst's technique changes decisively in the course of the analysis, I fear that this is bound to introduce an element of inconsistency into the analytic situation which is only too reminiscent of experiences which the patient as a child inevitably had with his parents, and which is not compatible with the atmosphere of steadiness and stability which the analytic situation aims at creating. (p. 229) (cf. a similar argument in Casement 1982, 1990)

Note that this statement is couched in terms that suggest a conclusion drawn from Heimann's experience as an analyst; much like the advice in Freud's (1911–1915/1958) "Papers on Technique," it is apparently based in empirical observation, not theory. But the observation is hardly universal; unlike Heimann, Daniel Stern and colleagues (1998) in the Process of Change Study Group see flexibility as crucial. They stress the centrality to therapeutic action of

> communications that reveal a personal aspect of the self that has been evoked in an affective response to another. In turn, it reveals to the other a personal signature, so as to create a new dyadic state specific to the two participants. ...*It is marked by a sense of departure from the habitual way of proceeding in the therapy. It is a novel happening that the ongoing framework can neither account for nor encompass. It is the opposite of business as usual.* (p. 916; emphasis added)

These two formulations, each putatively reflecting a *need of the analysand that can be discerned by an observant analyst*, are each intuitively appealing, yet they are irreconcilably at odds with each other. Heimann and, years later, Casement believe that "steadiness" is reassuring and "inconsistency" is terrifying. Stern and his colleagues insist that conducting "business as usual" is rejecting and stultifying, while creating "a new dyadic state" will free the analysand from bondage to familiar yet pathogenic ways of being in relationship. Offering a somewhat different explanation of the importance of a flexible stance, Irwin Hoffman (1994) notes, "When the patient senses that the analyst, in becoming more personally expressive and involved, is departing from an internalized convention of some kind, the patient has reason to feel recognized in a special way" (p. 188).

The question is posed: Do our analysands *need* steadiness to ease them through the rigors of doing analytic work, or do they *need* flexibility? Or, to put it another way, is inconsistency or rigidity more frightening?

Put so boldly, the question appears strange. It is difficult to imagine any psychoanalyst—indeed anybody who spends a great deal of time engaged with and thinking about the emotional lives of other people—who could not adduce considerable evidence that both steadiness and flexibility are facilitative and that both inconsistency and rigidity are frightening.

We are left with a strong suspicion that theory is at work, silently influencing the reported observations. And, broadly speaking, the observations and their attendant technical recommendations have come (predictably, although not without exceptions) from opposing theoretical traditions: consistency has been promoted by classical Freudians and Kleinians, and flexibility has been promoted by analysts working within the relational and intersubjective traditions. In addition, the opposing sensibilities developed at different times, both in the history of psychoanalysis and in society at large. This amplifies the role of theory, because the different times contribute to the shaping of observation by imposing different demands and constraints on the observer. At the beginning, Freud (despite the famous leeway he allowed himself) was at particular pains to warn practitioners of his new, dangerously intimate method that they must constantly fight their temptation to succumb to the countertransference. Succumbing can take many forms, Freud knew, of which overt boundary violations were only the most egregious tip of the iceberg. Thus, there arose the idea—hinted at by Freud and developed more explicitly by many of his followers—that countertransference, especially the sort that goes unnoticed by the analyst, always lurks behind the analyst's inclination to modify technique.

Prescriptions of technical flexibility are especially appealing today, when authority is so broadly questioned throughout our culture and when, in the eyes of many, technical consistency has hardened into authoritarian rigidity. There is, accordingly, a corrective aspect of these recommendations; they address a pendulum that is thought to have swung too far. But these prescriptions also have a long history, dating back at least to Ferenczi and reaching a peak of notoriety in Franz Alexander's suggestion that analysts should provide a "corrective emotional experience" tailored to the developmental history of each analysand (Alexander 1950, 1954). Recently, reflecting both clinical experience with the more diverse group of patients who are considered "analyzable" and broad social changes in attitudes toward authority, flexibility has become a mainstream technical recommendation. In addition to its prominence in the work of analysts operating within the relational tradition (Hoffman 1998; Mitchell 1997; Pizer 1998), it is echoed through the writings of Kleinians (Steiner 1994), contemporary conflict theorists (Smith 2000, 2001), and self psychologists (Goldberg 1999).

It is tempting, of course, to view change as evidence of progress, as a sign that we are moving toward more effective technique and toward a deeper understanding of therapeutic action. But despite historical ebbs and flows, there is still no consensus on the issue among contemporary analysts. In any case, to assume that we are simply improving on the work of our predecessors discounts the influence both of our personal theories and of the constraints imposed on psychoanalytic practice (and even on analytic thinking) by cultural trends. When we fail to distinguish change from progress, we lose touch with insights that may have arisen at a different time and under the sway of different premises.

Consider, as a cautionary tale, a paper by Sander Abend (1979) that stands clearly in opposition to the mainstream of contemporary thinking about flexible technique in particular and to "revisionist" theories of therapeutic action in general. Abend suggests that it is crucial that we explore and understand our analysands' personal theories of what contributes to and results from analytic "cure." His idea is that in many cases these theories reflect wishes to rectify childhood experiences and/or to gratify infantile fantasies.

But then, boldly and provocatively, Abend asserts that analysts who believe that departures from "standard technique" are often necessary may be giving expression to their own, similar fantasies. Analysts who suggest modifying technique (and Abend's targets are not marginal characters; they include Winnicott, Nacht, and Gitelson, as well as the easily debunked though easily misunderstood Alexander) are inadequately aware of themselves. According to Abend (1979), their "less rational and realistic desires seem to be undetected as they ride along below the surface,…attached to the consciously acceptable, readily understandable, appealing 'legitimate' needs of the suffering patient" (p. 595; see also his similar argument in Abend 1982).

Abend's argument, a product of its time and one that his more recent work retracts at least implicitly, falters as a consequence of his failure to recognize that *all* theories of analytic cure—including, of course, his own—reflect the workings of the theorist's unconscious fantasies. Certainly holding fast to any received technique as a matter of principle is no less likely to be an expression of such fantasies as is modifying technique. The analyst's personal motives—unconscious as well as conscious, fantastic as well as realistic—shape every clinical decision and even every observation. No prescription can immunize us from expressing our own unconscious wishes in our technical choices.

But we have much to learn from Abend's perspective, despite the logical shortfall that limits its scope and that has kept it far outside the contemporary psychoanalytic mainstream. Today, as discourse about therapeutic action has moved in a very different direction, analysts—mercifully—do not talk about the unconscious fantasies of their theoretical opponents. But, sadly, they do not talk very much about the analyst's unconscious at all. Instead, they are likely to discuss technical modifications in terms of patient needs rather than in terms of the analyst's fantasies (see, e.g., Gabbard and Westen 2003; Hoffman 1998; Pine 2001; Stern et al. 1998, and, from a very different perspective, Steiner 1994; for an exception, see Smith 2004).

Clinical practice has benefited significantly from this shift in focus; we have learned that many patients previously considered "unanalyzable" can participate effectively in psychoanalytic treatment if their analysts can find ways of helping them to do so. Technical flexibility not only extends our capacity to work analytically to previously unreachable patients but also, more generally, teaches us a great deal about what different people need to help them use psychological treatment. And even more broadly, it has enhanced our understanding of what it takes for people to live effectively in a world of other people.

We lose something crucial, something that Abend reminds us of, when we explain our analytic choices exclusively in terms of patient needs. What we lose (and this is not quite Abend's language) is the idea that as analysts we are personally motivated to do whatever we do, that these motivations may be deeply unconscious, and that accordingly we can easily mislead ourselves when we explain our choices to ourselves or to others.

Returning to the question with which I began this section, we see why it is so difficult to decide whether technical consistency or technical flexibility is more "therapeutic," even after a century of observational experience. If we reject technical flexibility out of hand, we are unlikely to learn very much about possible ways of helping patients to work that are not included in our received technique. But if we embrace flexibility (even if we demand that we reflect on our choices, which is always good advice but which is always subject to self-deception), we are unlikely to look inside ourselves as deeply as we must to discover personal motivations for whatever changes we initiate. It is not enough to advise analysts to keep both possibilities in mind, despite the patent wisdom of the suggestion. Beyond this, examination of and conversations about the implications of various choices are necessary, and these will be best served by the investigations of analysts who are committed to the alternative perspectives and by conversations among them.

Multiple Models, Multiple Unconscious Registers

The difficulty of resolving what appear on the surface to be straightforward questions, the range of observations that suggest contradictory answers, and the dichotomously alternative technical recommendations that follow from them have led many contemporary theorists to the idea of multiple models of therapeutic action. On this view, there is no one way of structuring an analytic relationship that works across the board, and no one aspect of the psychoanalytic situation that accounts for therapeutic action in all cases (Gabbard and Westen 2003; Pine 2001). Different analysands require different modes of engagement—a point that has been stressed especially by Pine—and different analysands benefit from different aspects of the analytic experience—the particular emphasis of Gabbard and Westen.

The introduction of multiple models appears to create an inclusiveness that encompasses and endorses a range of clinical observations. Along with this turn in clinical theory, many analysts have been impressed with ideas they have taken from recent developments in cognitive neuroscience. In light of these developments, theorists suggest, our ideas about therapeutic action no longer have to rest on mere clinical impressions or on more or less broadly drawn developmental analogies. There is a *structural* basis, even more structural than Freud's, because it is anchored in dazzling new methods and findings from the laboratory that support new approaches to the problem of therapeutic action.

The ideas that many have found particularly appealing relate to the hypothesis that the unconscious is not a unitary "place" or structure within the mind that operates in a singular way, as Freud's topographic model and, to a lesser extent, the tripartite structural model suggested. There are, according to this hypothesis, any number of unconscious registers in which memories are stored, and they behave quite differently from one another. Traditionally, according to this view, psychoanalysis has dealt with what is now referred to as "declarative" or "autobiographical" memory. Experiences that are capable of verbal expression are stored in the declarative system; these experiences vary in their accessibility to conscious recall and are thus the target of traditional psychoanalytic interpretations. When an interpretation succeeds in "making the unconscious conscious," whatever change is effected occurs within the declarative register.

But the declarative system (which is usually assumed to contain ideas and experiences that have been repressed) constitutes a relatively small proportion of the unconscious mind. More extensive by far is the procedural unconscious, which consists of nonverbal aspects of experience that were never repressed, because they were shaped outside of awareness from the beginning, and are inaccessible to introspection and thus to interpretation. The representations encoded in procedural memory decisively influence how we behave in the world; skills learned and practiced without conscious reflection—such as riding a bicycle—are examples of the kinds of information involved. These unconscious but never repressed, probably nonverbal, memories were recognized but marginalized by the American ego psychologists. Heinz Hartmann, in particular, wrote about what he called the "pre-conscious automatisms" that make it possible for us to perform any number of routine tasks (Hartmann 1939/1958). But these representations (Hartmann did not use this more contemporary word to describe the automatisms) were of interest mainly to the extent that psychoanalysis aspired to become a "general psychology"; they had little impact on either the dynamics of neurotic psychopathology or the theory of therapeutic action.

The idea of a procedural unconscious has recently taken center stage in clinical and theoretical discourse. Unconscious representations, many theorists suggest, do much more than make the performance of physical tasks efficient, as Hartmann thought they did. Beyond this, they guide our engagement with the interpersonal world, what we have learned to expect from other people, and how we have learned to behave with them. These representations, often referred to under the broad heading of "implicit relational knowing" (Gabbard and Westen 2003; Lyons-Ruth 1998; Stern et. al. 1998), are not, by their nature, conducive to verbal expression; think of how difficult it would be to describe in words what we must do to ride a bicycle. They are, however, subject to modification on the basis of lived, nonverbal experience, especially the sort of experience that patients have in an intense, complex relationship such as the relationship with their analyst. These changes, regardless of how accessible to verbal expression they are, will alter the nature of the analysand's way of seeing the world and their behavioral responses to it.

The hypothesis that different interventions an analyst might make would touch different neural systems is tantalizing, especially since the concepts of declarative and procedural memory seem to map so neatly on to the distinction between interpretive and relational effects. This allows for a new theoretical strategy: the priority of one or another mechanism of therapeutic action can be asserted not simply on the basis of anecdotal clinical experience but on the basis of changes that are believed to occur at one or another neural level. Gabbard and Westen (2003), for example, use the distinction between declarative and procedural memory to anchor their idea that we must forgo theories that favor any unitary therapeutic action in favor of those that embrace multiple actions.

For some theorists, the concept of procedural memory decisively redefines the problem of therapeutic action. Perhaps the most radical exponent of this strategy is Peter

Fonagy (1999), who claims that "[m]emories of past experience can no longer be considered relevant to therapeutic action....Change occurs in implicit memory leading to a change of the procedures the person uses in living with himself and with others" (p. 17). Somewhat less drastically (from a conceptual point of view), Daniel Stern and colleagues (1998) believe that the procedural unconscious provides a structural scaffolding that supports the clinically based idea that "something more" than interpretation is essential to the workings of therapeutic action.

It can almost seem that developments in contemporary neuroscience provide the key to solving the dilemma of therapeutic action: perhaps we no longer must tie ourselves to theoretically biased "special pleading." If there are multiple unconscious registers that are touched by psychoanalytic interventions, we need no longer be bound by our preconceptions. Our observations that different analysands benefit from different events in treatment are grounded, and the idea of multiple therapeutic actions (Gabbard and Westen 2003; Pine 2001) is strongly supported.

But things are not so simple. The different ways in which theorists wield the concept of a procedural unconscious create familiar difficulties. The problem begins with the presumed nature of the procedural unconscious, which is by definition made up of patterns that are nonverbal. Because of this, any attempt to translate these patterns into the language of psychoanalysis (or into any other language) is bound to involve the biases of the translator; translation is creation, and our theories come into play as soon as we attempt to translate.

Consider where we are left when we decline to translate. Edgar Levenson (2001), who appreciates the importance of implicit changes in patterns of behavior and experience but who is unwilling to put words to what he considers an ineffable process, is content to say, "We do not cure; we do our work and cure happens" (p. 241). Ironically distancing himself from the translation project that so many analysts eagerly undertake, Levenson concludes that "[w]e may spend the next millennium happily figuring out how that might happen" (p. 241). But few analysts are as comfortable with (or as gleeful about) this kind of uncertainty as Levenson is. And, if we examine the thinking of those who base their theorizing on the new neuroscientific models, we find that we are left with the familiar conceptual divides.

For example, both Peter Fonagy and Daniel Stern's group believe that therapeutic change involves shifts in "implicit relational knowing." But Fonagy (1999), despite his insistence that recovery of memories plays no part in therapeutic action, describes any number of complex interpretations of current relational patterns that he considers central. Consider, for example, the following: "infantile grandiosity defensively activated in the face of maltreatment may generate an image of the self as responsible for neglectful or cruel behavior. Although an illusion of control and predictability may be acquired in this way, the self will also be seen as guilty and deserving of punishment" (Fonagy 1999, p. 17).

Note the number and quality of the words that are being used to capture an experience that has been defined as nonverbal: "defensively distorted," "grandiosity," "maltreatment," "self," "responsible," "neglectful," "cruel," "control," "guilty." And Fonagy believes that it is essential that the analysand be helped to translate his or her nonverbal experience into words that are similar to the analyst's translation. Thus, describing his clinical work with a male analysand, he writes: "It took some time for me to be able to make him aware of this strategy he had....He became aware of how he was doing this with his mother, and we finally understood it as a way he had of coping with anyone who he felt was intrusive" (Fonagy 1999, p. 19). In other words, change in implicit memory depends on interpretation, although the target of the interpretation (Friedman 2001) is contemporary experience and behavior, not history.

Fonagy thus makes very different use of the idea of a procedural unconscious than Stern and colleagues (1998). For them, change in implicit relational knowing depends on a particular quality of interpersonal experience, one that does not need to be interpreted or otherwise verbalized:

> When we speak of an "authentic" meeting, we mean communications that reveal a personal aspect of the self that has been evoked in an affective response to another. In turn, it reveals to the other a personal signature, so as to create a new dyadic state specific to the two participants. (Stern et al. 1998, p. 916)

And, unlike Fonagy, in his emphasis on the interpretation of patterns that emerge in the course of analysis, they insist that

> [w]hereas interpretation is traditionally viewed as the nodal event acting within and upon the transferential relationship, and changing it by altering the intrapsychic environment, we view "moments of meeting" as the nodal event acting within and upon the "shared implicit relationship" and changing it by altering implicit knowledge that is both intrapsychic and interpersonal. (p. 916)

If Freud and Ferenczi had been focusing their debate on how to facilitate changes in implicit memory, their competing emphases on interpretation and experience would have sounded virtually identical to the differences between Fonagy and the Stern group. Developments in cognitive neuroscience do not and cannot dissolve these fundamental differences in clinical sensibility.

Why Does the Debate Matter?

Throughout this chapter, we have seen that what appear to be even the simplest formulations about the meaning or the efficacy of particular psychoanalytic interventions invite opposing assertions. Attempts to engage the larger questions, such as the relative effects of interpretation and relationship, become shrouded in the fog of theoretical bias and eventually sound very much like Glover's "special pleading."

In light of this, is there any value in talking about therapeutic action at all? Are we better served by giving up on the problem, as Freud seemed to do in the "Constructions" paper, or declaring it solved, as he did in "Analysis Terminable and Interminable"? Or should we dismiss the problem as irrelevant and even inimical to the analytic process, as many French psychoanalysts do (see Laplanche 1992)?

Embracing these conclusions, after almost a century of debates that have convinced only the already committed, is tempting. But to do so risks impoverishing psychoanalytic discourse by curtailing detailed investigation of the problems involved. Accordingly, in contrast to the French perspective, I suggest that our concern with the problem remains central not only because our analysands come to us with therapeutic goals in mind, but also because studying therapeutic action provides a window into what happens in the course of analysis and what changes as a result of the unique interpersonal encounter that we offer. Unlike Freud, I believe that nothing about therapeutic action has been or ever can be "sufficiently elucidated." Despite, or perhaps because of, the chaos that has characterized decades of debate, our conversations about the nature of therapeutic action are not only valuable but essential. We do, however, have to look carefully at what we are hoping to achieve when we take up the problem.

In considering the goal of such questioning, we must rethink why we need to keep talking about therapeutic action. We must also entertain the possibility that we have been misguided in looking to our discussions about it as a way of *solving* a problem—that is, the problem of which facet of the clinical encounter is responsible for change. Instead, we might imagine that these conversations have been and will continue to be vital because they are likely to *create* a problem—namely, the problem that no matter what any particular theorist has observed about what has gone on in the course of treatment, there is something else that could be observed but that has not been attended to, and that has consequences that have not been sufficiently noticed.

This approach will work especially well in the pluralistic world of contemporary psychoanalysis, where conversations are carried out among analysts who represent different theoretical traditions. Fortunately, the situation today contrasts dramatically with the circumstances that prevailed for many years. During those years, analysts talked almost exclusively to colleagues committed to the same fundamental assumptions that they were, and they typically heard their own observations reiterated. The uncontradicted repetition of anecdotal data can easily be taken as evidence of the truth of the idea that is being promoted, and it is easy to see how analysts' attention was directed to only those aspects of the workings of treatment that were deemed salient within their own tradition. This overly narrow focus led not only to vehement forms of Glover's "special pleading" but to theory-bound, unidimensional descriptions of analytic process. Description, as is well known, rests upon the narrator's underlying assumptions about what matters. In psychoanalysis, the framework that determines what we believe is worth describing is our theory. What is not described cannot be theorized, so our accounts and the conclusions we draw from them tend to be circular (see Greenberg 1981; Pine 2001).

In the first and probably still the most famous recorded example of a psychoanalyst choosing not to report some of what happened in an analysis, Freud neglected to describe having fed herring to the Rat Man in his formal account of the case. In his private record, he laconically noted that his patient "was hungry and was fed" a meal that included the herring, which the Rat Man disliked and left untouched (Freud 1909/1955, pp. 303, 308). Although in less than a week the patient reported a dramatic anal erotic fantasy involving herring (pp. 307–308), Freud did not mention the meal publicly, nor did he seem—even privately—to place much weight on the connection between what he did and the fantasy (see Lipton 1977, 1988, for a full discussion of this event). This elision of detail is by no means unique to Freud or even to "orthodox Freudians." Consider Guntrip's (1975) account of his analysis with Fairbairn. Guntrip stressed the austerity of Fairbairn's presence and his reliance on formal, oedipal interpretations. But strikingly, his description of his analytic experience does not include what he considered extra-analytic contact, the time after each session during which he and Fairbairn would drink tea together and talk about psychoanalytic theory and other matters of mutual interest. This slanting of description does not reflect a failure of narrative skill. Rather, it reflects what it is inherent in description itself: completeness and coherence are at odds with each other, and coherence is achieved by the application of prejudices that dictate what needs to be included and what can be omitted.

This is where, perhaps surprisingly, there is a place for a contemporary version of "special pleading" in our new psychoanalytic conversation, assuming that analysts who represent a range of theoretical perspectives will be in-

vited to plead their cases. Pluralistic conversations will always highlight aspects of the psychoanalytic situation that have gone untheorized or even unattended to in the work of any given observer. It would be unthinkable in today's climate that Freud's account of the Rat Man case could stand without questions being raised about the therapeutic implications of the meal or about the assumption that hungry analysands (or this particular hungry analysand) must be fed. And, of course, far more subtle omissions will be noted and highlighted and new narratives of the familiar event will be erected on the foundation created out of the new observations.

The therapeutic action debate, despite its resistance to resolution, remains an important one. Because it invites observers to speculate not only about what *works* but—before that—about what *happens* in the course of an analysis, the debate provides us with a crucial platform from which to view the various events that, taken together and in their intricate interconnections, constitute the psychoanalytic process.

References

Abend S: Unconscious fantasies and theories of cure. J Am Psychoanal Assoc 27:579–596, 1979

Abend S: Serious illness in the analyst: countertransference considerations. J Am Psychoanal Assoc 30:365–379, 1982

Alexander F: Analysis of the therapeutic Factors in Psychoanalytic treatment. Psychoanal Q 19:482–500, 1950

Alexander F: Some quantitative aspects of psychoanalytic technique. J Am Psychoanal Assoc 2:685–701, 1954

Blatt S, Behrends R: Internalization, separation-individuation, and the nature of therapeutic action. Int J Psychoanal 68: 279–297, 1987

Breuer J, Freud S: Studies on hysteria (1893–1895), in Standard Edition of the Complete Psychological Works of Sigmund Freud, Vol 2. Translated and edited by Strachey J. London, Hogarth Press, 1955, pp 1–319

Casement P: Some pressures on the analyst for physical contact during the re-living of an early trauma. Int J Psychoanal 9:279–286, 1982

Casement P: Learning From the Patient. New York, Guilford, 1990

Ferenczi S, Rank O: The Development of Psychoanalysis. Madison, CT, International Universities Press, 1924

Fonagy P: The process of change and the change of process: what can change in a "good analysis"? Keynote address presented at the spring meeting, division 39, American Psychological Association, New York, April 1999

Freud S: The interpretation of dreams (1900), in Standard Edition of the Complete Psychological Works of Sigmund Freud, Vols 4 and 5. Translated and edited by Strachey J. London, Hogarth Press, 1953

Freud S: Three essays on the theory of sexuality, I: the sexual aberrations (1905), in Standard Edition of the Complete Psychological Works of Sigmund Freud, Vol 7. Translated and edited by Strachey J. London, Hogarth Press, 1953, pp 135–172

Freud S: Notes upon a case of obsessional neurosis (1909), in Standard Edition of the Complete Psychological Works of Sigmund Freud, Vol 10. Translated and edited by Strachey J. London, Hogarth Press, 1955, pp 151–318

Freud S: Papers on technique (1911–1915), in Standard Edition of the Complete Psychological Works of Sigmund Freud, Vol 12. Translated and edited by Strachey J. London, Hogarth Press, 1958

Freud S: Observations on transference love: further recommendations in the technique of psycho-analysis (1915), in Standard Edition of the Complete Psychological Works of Sigmund Freud, Vol 12. Translated and edited by Strachey J. London, Hogarth Press, 1958, pp 157–152

Freud S: Analysis terminable and interminable (1937a), in Standard Edition of the Complete Psychological Works of Sigmund Freud, Vol 23. Translated and edited by Strachey J. London, Hogarth Press, 1964, pp 209–253

Freud S: Constructions in analysis (1937b), in Standard Edition of the Complete Psychological Works of Sigmund Freud, Vol 23. Translated and edited by Strachey J. London, Hogarth Press, 1964, pp 255–269

Friedman L: Interpretation. Keynote address presented at the Conference of the Journals of the PEP [Psychoanalytic Electronic Publishing], 2001

Gabbard G, Westen D: Rethinking therapeutic action. Int J Psychoanal 84:823–841, 2003

Glover E: The therapeutic effect of inexact interpretation: a contribution to the theory of suggestion. Int J Psychoanal 12:397–411, 1931

Glover E: Symposium on the theory of the therapeutic results of psycho-analysis. Int J Psychoanal 18:125–131, 1937

Goldberg A: Between empathy and judgment. J Am Psychoanal Assoc 47:351–365, 1999

Greenberg J: Prescription or description: the therapeutic action of psychoanalysis. Contemporary Psychoanalysis 17:239–257, 1981

Guntrip H: My experience of analysis with Fairbairn and Winnicott (how complete a result does psycho-analytic therapy achieve?). Int J Psychoanal 2:145–156, 1975

Hartmann H: Ego Psychology and the Problem of Adaptation (1939). Translated by Rapaport D. New York, International Universities Press, 1958

Heimann P: The curative factors in psychoanalysis: contributions to discussion. Int J Psychoanal 43:228–231, 1962

Hoffman I: Dialectical thinking and therapeutic action in the psychoanalytic process. Psychoanal Q 63:187–218, 1994

Hoffman I: Ritual and spontaneity in the psychoanalytic process. Hillsdale, NJ, Analytic Press, 1998

King P: The curative factors in psychoanalysis: contributions to discussion. Int J Psychoanal 43:225–227, 1962

Laplanche J: Seduction, Translation, Drives. London, Institute of Contemporary Arts, 1992

Levenson E: The enigma of the unconscious. Contemporary Psychoanalysis 37:239–252, 2001

Lipton S: The advantages of Freud's technique as shown in his analysis of the Rat Man. Int J Psychoanal 58:255–273, 1977

Lipton S: Further observations on the advantages of Freud's technique. Annual of Psychoanalysis 16:19–32, 1988

Loewald H: On the therapeutic action of psychoanalysis. Int J Psychoanal 41:16–33, 1960

Lyons-Ruth K: Implicit relational knowing: its role in development and psychoanalytic treatment. Infant Ment Health J 19:282–289, 1998

McGuire W (ed): The Freud/Jung Letters. Princeton, NJ, Princeton University Press, 1974

Mitchell S: Influence and Autonomy in Psychoanalysis. Hillsdale, NJ, Analytic Press, 1997

Pine F: Listening and speaking psychoanalytically—with what in mind? Int J Psychoanal 82:901–916, 2001

Pizer S: Building Bridges: The Negotiation of Paradox in Psychoanalysis. Hillsdale, NJ, Analytic Press, 1998

Sandler J: Reflections on some relations between psychoanalytic concepts and psychoanalytic practice. Int J Psychoanal 64:35–45, 1983

Schafer R: The Analytic Attitude. New York, Basic Books, 1983

Segal H: The curative factors in psychoanalysis: contributions to discussion. Int J Psychoanal 43:212–217, 1962

Smith H: Countertransference, conflictual listening, and the analytic object relationship. J Am Psychoanal Assoc 48:95–128, 2000

Smith H: Hearing voices: the fate of the analyst's identifications. J Am Psychoanal Assoc 49:781–812, 2001

Smith H: The analyst's fantasy of the ideal patient. Psychoanal Q 73:627–658, 2004

Steiner J: Patient-centered and analyst-centered interpretations: some implications of containment and countertransference. Psychoanalytic Inquiry 14:406–422, 1994

Stern D, Sander L, Nahum J, et al: Noninterpretive mechanisms in psychoanalytic therapy: the "something more" than interpretation. Int J Psychoanal 79:903–921, 1998

Strachey J: The nature of the therapeutic action of psychoanalysis. Int J Psychoanal 15:127–159, 1934

Valenstein A: The concept of "classical" psychoanalysis. J Am Psychoanal Assoc 27 (suppl):113–136, 1979

15

Process, Resistance, and Interpretation

ESLEE SAMBERG, M.D.

ERIC R. MARCUS, M.D.

PROCESS, RESISTANCE, interpretation, and trans-ference are the basic descriptive terms of psychoanalytic treatment. These four are linked. *Process*, the ongoing un-folding of the analysis, is facilitated by the *interpretation* of resistance and transference. In this chapter, we define and describe three of the four terms: process, resistance, and interpretation (see Chapter 13, "Transference, Counter-tranference, and the Real Relationship," for a discussion of transference). We explore their interrelationships, de-scribe our contemporary understanding of these con-cepts, and discuss how different theories have viewed and continue to view these terms.

Our own perspective reflects a view of mental function based on unconscious conflict and compromise, organized both within fantasies of the self in its relationship to oth-ers and by the associated structuring processes. The cen-tral task of a psychoanalytic treatment is the elaboration of the patient's intrapsychic experience and its organiza-tion, motivated by the patient's suffering and facilitated by the analyst's educated and trained attempts to under-stand. The ultimate goal of the treatment is to improve the patient's capacity to adapt to the demands and gratifica-tions of internal and external reality.

Technique is the method by which the analyst achieves the goals of a therapeutic analysis. It reflects not only the

analyst's fundamental theory of the mind but also those aspects of the theory he or she chooses to emphasize with a particular patient. A technique reflects the analyst's as-sessment of the particulars of each patient and the nature of each patient's participation in the therapeutic process. A technique also reflects the particulars of the analyst's disposition and experience. All aspects of this description of technique operate both consciously and unconsciously in the minds of both patient and analyst.

Process

Definitions

Process refers to the progressive unfolding of the psycho-analytic treatment in which more and more of the patient's unconscious, dynamic psychology and its organization are revealed, elaborated, and explicated. *Dynamic*—the contin-ual ebb and flow of affect intensity, its quantities and qual-ities, and associated ideational and fantasy contents—refers to the interplay of mental motivations in a conflict-compromise model of the mind.

The term *process* is used because there are certain com-monalities to the progression of all analyses regardless of content: organizations, relationships, and their predictable, stable patterns. Because a successful analysis progresses according to these patterns, there can be a describable psychoanalytic process.

Process is what happens in an analysis and how what happens comes to happen. It is not only the patient's story but also the story as it comes to be told. It is the dramatization of the story—the dynamic organization and the nature of unfolding; the structure of the story and of its telling; and most especially, the how, when, and why the story becomes apparent. The how and when require technique.

Psychoanalytic process is the sine qua non of psychoanalytic work. It is used to describe a level of intensity and depth of psychological engagement that is less commonly achieved in other forms of psychotherapy, even dynamic ones. Conceptualizations of process reflect a theory of mind and the dynamic fulcrum of how and why a patient gets better through the course of a psychoanalytic treatment. Process encompasses the overall course of a treatment, from its beginning and working-through to its end. If and when a psychoanalytic process has been established, the patient is said to be "in analysis."

Process, according to Abrams (1987), is the infrastructure of analytic work. It is a conceptual as well as a descriptive term that includes impetus, sequence, organization, intervention, and direction. Process and therapeutic action are inseparable, since the psychoanalytic process is the route by which neurotic mechanisms are overcome. Boesky's (1990) focus, too, is the relationship between process and therapeutic change or outcome.

Various analysts, schools, views, diagnostic groups, and individual patient analyses emphasize various parts of this definition in the actual analysis. Smith (2002) attempts to parse the essential elements of process from the presentations of several analysts, each representing a different theoretical orientation. All conceptualize quite differently their manner of listening, their foci of interest within the emotional experience of their patients and themselves, and how these relate to each other, their theories of the mind, and how analysis works.

Requirements

A dynamic description of process engages the capacities of both patient and analyst, individually as well as combined into an analytic dyad. All three are crucial determinants of whether an analytic process can be established and, ultimately, whether a psychoanalytic treatment provides a therapeutic outcome. We examine here the capacities of the patient and of the analyst that facilitate this process, and we also consider the complex relationship between process and the analytic dyad.

Patient Capacities

Patient factors—single functions, groups of functions, and how they work together—are capacities necessary for the establishment of an analytic process that can be used by the patient for growth.

The most important function is reality testing: the ability of the mind to experience emotional material without losing the capacity for an uncontaminated reality experience. The patient must be able to experience and reexperience warded-off, emotionally intense memories and fantasies, sometimes focusing on the analyst, without losing a parallel experience of the analyst as a real person. This dual capacity, for fantasy and reality simultaneously, is the crucial element in being able to experience yet use psychoanalysis.

Two categorical examples are love/sex and aggression. Will the patient be able to experience loving and sexual feelings for the analyst without needing to enact them in reality? Will the patient be able to experience anger at the analyst without breaking the real therapeutic relationship? These two categories are the frequent transference feelings that allow for the exploration of the patient's feelings and attitudes toward important people in their lives, historically and in the present.

Similarly, it is helpful, even crucial, for the patient to have the ability to observe self-experience, not just feel or behave. The ability to self-observe is helpful in engaging reality testing and in separating the experience of others from self-experience. It is also helpful in triggering processes of change and growth.

The patient must also have the capacity to shift back and forth from a self-observing perspective to an experiential one. This facility requires the capacity for dissociation in the ego, described by Sterba (1934), in which the ego is able to both experience and take itself as its own object for the purposes of self-observation. Such dissociation is a capacity for controlled regression, or regression in the service of the ego. The emotionally intense experiences of the transference relationship often involve regressions to wishes, expectations, and fears of earlier times. The patient's ability both to experience these feelings and then to reflect on them is necessary for the attainment of greater insight combined with a sense of emotional conviction. Often this ability reflects the patient's relative capacity to tolerate, without recrimination, his or her own fantasy life, especially as it is progressively revealed within the transference relationship.

The patient's capacity to free-associate (Seidenberg 1971)—that is, say what comes to mind—typically develops over time and is similarly facilitated by a capacity for controlled regression. Early in the history of psychoanalysis, free association was regarded as a method of facilitating the lifting of repressions. With the advent of ego psychology, free association was understood to provide the best field for observing defensive processes in action. The patient must have the capacity to tolerate the regressive aspects of the free-associative process and then shift to a self-reflective stance. This involves a dynamic shifting of attention between primary and secondary process modes of thinking. *Primary process* modes of thinking refer to all emotionally laden experience as well as to their symbolic representations, as in dreams and fantasies. *Secondary process* modes of thinking refer to all more linear logic–based modes of reality-experience thinking. It is the patient's capacity for mobility between the two that is most critical. Processes of change and growth also depend on capacities to integrate, synthesize, and apply new information. These capacities are needed in order to organize new emotional experience.

The capacity for change depends on the relative plasticity of defenses guarding against new emotional experience. Crucial are the plasticity and modulation capacity of responses that are triggered as defenses against attitudes, fantasies, wishes, fears, and affect intensities, content, and qualities. Defenses that are too rigid or too brittle, sensitive, or eruptive make for a deadlocked and stormy analysis that may be of little use for change. These capacities are part of the dynamic-structural considerations the analyst tries to test when considering a patient for analysis.

Motivation and commitment are also crucial variables affecting the ability of a patient to endure the rigors and length of psychoanalysis. Often dependent on the other capacities described above, motivation and commitment may also be separate capacities. Will power and determination are helpful in all areas of achievement, including the quest for growth and mental health.

It should be understood that ego capacities are not static phenomena. Patients' capacity to participate in the analytic process evolves over time as their emotional experience deepens and their understanding of the task broadens. In addition, ego capacities inevitably reflect anxiety levels, mood states, and conflict intensities and in such cases may therefore rapidly improve in psychoanalytic treatment.

Patients may present for treatment without one or another of these capacities but with the need for help—even the need for psychoanalysis. The analyst may then elect to help in a psychological and/or psychiatric treatment to address the ego capacity problems so that a patient might then be able to participate at a later time in a psychoanalytic process with therapeutic outcome. A psychotherapeutic treatment preparatory to analysis would have the goal of stabilizing or expanding the ego functions already described that are crucial to a patient's capacity to participate in a psychoanalytic treatment.

Nonetheless, it should be understood that a rigidly dichotomous view of ego function is not accurate. Previous categorizations of patients as suffering from either conflict or deficit, oedipal or preoedipal pathology, or constitutional or environmental conflicts (the former treatable by psychoanalysis and the latter not) are no longer maintained. Most patients present for treatment with a complex interplay of some or all of these contributing factors.

Analyst Capacities

The analyst plays a crucial role in catalyzing the analytic process. The analyst must know when to be silent and when to speak, when to question, when to confront, and when to interpret. The analyst must be well trained enough to be able to tolerate the self-discipline required, and well analyzed enough to ensure that his or her neurosis will not interfere. Only then can the analyst use countertransference as a guide to the analysis of the patient's transference. It helps, of course, if the analyst is empathic and kind as well as fearless and clear.

The analyst's capacity to participate in a psychoanalytic process may be taken as a given based on adequate competence attained through training and personal analysis. However, more subtle issues involve countertransference reactions evoked by patients whose psychological conflicts interdigitate with those of the analyst's in significant and meaningful ways. Current views of countertransference recognize the ubiquity and utility of the analyst's psychological and emotional experience within the treatment situation, rather than viewing it only as an intermittent obstruction (Abend 1989; Blum 1986; Smith 2000). Nonetheless, the analyst must be able to recognize the presence of countertransference intrusions that significantly obstruct understanding and empathy.

Analysts of diverse theoretical orientations view countertransference as valuable data about the patient. Gabbard (1995) views countertransference from an interpersonal and intrapsychic perspective. Countertransference is both evoked by the patient and shaped by the analyst's psyche; it may be viewed as co-created. When countertransference is conceptualized in this way, projective identification (modern Kleinian), enactment (ego psychology/object relations), the analytic third (Ogden 1994), and role responsiveness (Sandler 1976) all describe similar entities. The intersubjective experience of both analyst and patient is acknowledged and understood. In each of these constructs, the patient evokes something in the analyst of sufficient intensity to capture the emotional and psychological experience of both participants. The conscious exploration, explication, and working-through of this experience describe an important aspect of process.

The Analytic Dyad

Considerations of the relationship of the analytic dyad to psychoanalytic process include the question of where the psychoanalytic process is located: primarily within the patient but facilitated by the analyst's interventions or located within the interaction between patient and analyst? In our view, the answer to this question need not be conceptualized as either/or.

From the moment Freud (1912a/1958) discovered that the transference represented not only the greatest obstacle to treatment but also the most powerful vehicle for cure, he recognized the necessary and peculiar manner in which psychoanalytic process occurs: that the patient's earliest mental and emotional experience of object relatedness would be re-evoked within the analytic situation not only in memory but by repetition. For that fantasy to come alive within the present, it would necessarily be modified in certain ways by the specificities of the current situation ("revised editions"; Freud 1905[1901]/1953), just as it had been previously modified by the process of development. Psychoanalysis was from the beginning a relationship process. Subsequent perspectives and understandings have all elaborated on that fundamental point, although moving in different directions and with different emphases.

Arlow and Brenner (1990) define process as the dynamic interplay between patient and analyst. To the extent that they view the analyst as the agent of change, process and technique are indistinguishable.

Boesky (1990) views psychoanalytic process as interactional but from an intrapsychic perspective. Both the patient and the analyst analogously participate in the complex creation of transference resistances as each attempts to perform his or her own task within the psychoanalytic endeavor. Boesky is clear that he is not shifting to a view of the relationship as mutative. He is instead attempting to explain the complexity of the psychoanalytic process, especially the aspect that involves the analyst's attempts to formulate interventions to help the patient. Resistance, too, in Boesky's view, is inevitably and productively a unique and specific creation by each patient-analyst pair.

The Ornsteins, writing from a self psychological perspective, describe the analytic process as a developmental process in which the analyst provides functions (self-object functions) that may be ultimately relinquished by the patient once they have become internalized (through transmuting internalizations). In their view, the analytic relationship and a technique based on empathic-reconstructive interpretation provides the optimal environment for the patient's recovery (Ornstein and Ornstein 1980).

Loewald (1979) understands psychoanalytic process to be similar to the mother-child relationship and views therapeutic change as similar to developmental processes that occur throughout life. He describes the internalization of dynamic interactions (i.e., between mother and child or analyst and patient) that serve to build or rebuild psychic structure. Loewald's idea of therapeutic action shifted the emphasis to the object matrix provided by the analyst/mother.

Loewald's (1971) process-oriented view of the transference neurosis further defines his perspective on how analysis works. He sees the transference neurosis as a product of the patient's and analyst's mutual participation in the analytic process. Through interpretation, the patient's repetitive stereotyped transference fantasy becomes a new, reenacted version, which then offers the potential for change and growth. Loewald's views in many respects bridge several current theoretical perspectives—self psychological, object relational, and intersubjective—yet originate from an ego psychological and drive conflict model of the mind.

The significance of the relationship between analyst and patient in determining the therapeutic outcome of any analysis is a subject of accelerating interest and debate. The complexity of this topic is in part attributable to the increasing delinkage of theory from practice (Smith 2003). How one understands the relationship and how one uses that relationship in a technical sense may vary quite independently. For example, a conflict/compromise theory of the mind easily encompasses considerations of the subjectivity of both participants and a complex conceptualization of transference and countertransference as analogously derived. Yet, what is done with such considerations from a technical standpoint may be quite different from what may be done by a self psychologist or an intersubjectivist or a Kleinian. The emphasis will remain the elucidation of the patient's mental and emotional experience in terms of conflict and compromise. But the analyst's interpretive function in all schools will be informed by his or her capacity to listen for unconscious meaning, to empathically identify with the patient's experience, and to perceive as much as possible the ongoing countertransference dimensions of his or her experience and use these as much as possible for the benefit of the patient.

Gabbard and Westen (2003) assert that the "interpretation versus relationship" debate has waned and that a multiplicity of mutative factors in a therapeutic analysis is a generally accepted premise. They describe a broadening conceptualization of what is mutative and include those factors that foster insight, such as interpretation, and those that use the relationship for a variety of purposes, ranging from corrective emotional experience to internalizations of the analyst's function or affective attitudes.

Resistance

Resistance is the name given to all those mental processes, fantasies, memories, reactions, and mechanisms that serve to defend against the progress of the analytic process—both its deepening and its emotional impact. Because patients resist in characteristic ways, resistance is often a demonstration of basic character and its reaction patterns and defenses. Progress in the process of the analysis therefore requires interpretation of resistance in order to change static, repetitive, stereotyped emotional reactions into a progressive, changing process. Resistance to change is a ubiquitous phenomenon in all psychological treatments, because despite the patient's conscious desire for change, unconscious fears and wishes and associated character defenses oppose it. The definition of resistance is thus linked to analytic process. Because resistance is inevitable, there is no psychoanalytic process unimpeded by it. One could therefore look at resistance as an integral part of the analytic process rather than an episodic intrusion.

Resistance is a crucial part of the psychoanalytic process because of the basic character defenses that articulate it. Resistance analysis requires the recognition and interpretation of these defenses. These defensive patterns often are object relations compromise formations of basic conflicts that are crucial organizers of both symptoms and character. The analysis of resistance thereby allows entrée into the structure of the neurosis, and the analysis thus proceeds into the unconscious conflicts central to a successful treatment.

The resistance to the process often focuses on and organizes an intense transference, capturing the transference in the service of resistance. The transference is then referred to as *transference resistance.* The advantage of this common occurrence is the emotional intensity of the experience. Then, with interpretation of the transference, the patient is able to experience an intense validity to the interpretation. In its effect, interpretation of the transference resistance may provide the most crucial emotional and, therefore, therapeutic leverage within a psychoanalytic treatment. The emotional intensity of the transference experience also serves to orient the analyst to its importance both developmentally and in the here and now.

The complex and essential link between transference and resistance highlights its expression of an unconscious object relations fantasy in which the analyst becomes the object of wishes and fears and the object by which compromise satisfaction may be obtained. The derivation of this fantasy from the past, and its expression within the present context of the treatment, are the essential elements of the transference resistance.

Much current discussion is focused on how much the transference is influenced or modified by specific attributes of the analyst or other aspects of the here and now. These differences in view are often, but not always, linked to differences in the technical approach to interpretation of the transference.

Resistance is a dynamic intrapsychic concept. However, because it may be expressed with the most emotional intensity within the transference relationship, resistance has both interpersonal and behavioral manifestations. As a result of defensive operations such as displacement and projection, the intrapsychic sources of resistance are shifted to the analytic dyad in their expression. Since resistance may have an oppositional aspect to it (i.e., opposition to intrapsychic change), the conflict may take on the form of opposition to the analyst.

Schafer (1973) warns against a countertransference view of resistance in which the patient's "oppositional stance" evokes a negative attitude toward the patient. The analyst must attempt to understand the affirmative reasons for the patient to oppose change—for example, to protect relationships, to remain faithful to ideals, to maintain pride and autonomy, and to achieve mastery. In addition, the patient's defiance toward the analyst may serve the objective of differentiation and growth and oppose the patient's own unconscious wish to regress or merge.

Conceptualizing the interpretation of transference resistance as the most important catalyst for change distinguishes psychoanalysis from other forms of treatment. Freud's (1911–1915/1958) understanding that the analysis of resistance is the psychoanalytic method rather than its obstacle had profound implications for theory and technique. Initially defining resistance broadly in terms of anything that interfered with the process of free association, Freud recognized that resistance was something to be interpreted rather than overcome through suggestion or injunction.

Identifying the unconscious nature of resistance ultimately led Freud (1937/1964) to an increasingly sophisticated understanding of the multiple sources of resistance, including resistances originating in id, ego, and superego. He attributed resistance to dynamic developmental factors, biological-constitutional factors, and traumatic experiential factors. These considerations were related to the question of why analysis takes so long. Freud recognized that very intense and rigid resistances might even be beyond the scope of psychoanalytic cure.

Perhaps most complex in all of his considerations about resistance was the issue of the relationship between transference and resistance. While Freud recognized that transference could serve as resistance, he also understood that transference provided the "most important vehicle for cure." Friedman (1991) describes this complex dialectic in his discussion of Freud's "Papers on Technique." In Freud's earlier theory that focused on the recovery of memories, resistance could be looked at simply as the patient's opposition to remembering. Yet Freud came to recognize that the patient is not so much opposed to remembering as he or she is opposed to relinquishing the chance for gratification of childhood wishes and avoidances of childhood fears. The analyst through his or her method both encourages the patient to reexperience those desires in relation to the analyst and requires the patient to subject them to scrutiny, dissect them, examine them, and ultimately relinquish them. The patient's transference includes both a willing participation in the analytic process and an opposition to it. The patient's resistance is an opposition to the requirement by the analyst that he or she participate in this unusual and highly difficult "double-track" experience, of feeling on the one hand and reflecting and integrating on the other.

The ascendance of ego psychology placed increasing emphasis on the analysis of resistance as the central technical tool of the analyst but focused on its relationship to mental structure and character. Wilhelm Reich (1945) and Anna Freud (1936/1966) provided divergent approaches to the technique of analyzing these character resistances. Reich emphasized the analyst's attack on character resistance that led to an unfortunate link between the technique of resistance analysis and a view of the analyst as authoritarian. Anna Freud, on the other hand, emphasized the analyst's neutral and balanced stance toward the analysis of ego, id, and superego resistances, never focusing on one at the expense of the others.

The persistence of an almost exclusive focus on resistance analysis as the optimal therapeutic technique is demonstrated by the work of Gray (1996) and Busch (1992), two contemporary ego psychologists. Both emphasize a method of close process monitoring in which the analyst intervenes at the moment of associative break to demonstrate to the patient the defensive activity that just occurred in response to unconscious danger. Gray acknowledged that this very disciplined technique deprives the analyst of the more aesthetically gratifying aspects of a less focused approach and also exposes the analyst more consistently to the patient's aggression. For these reasons, the analyst's own resistance to this technique is mobilized. Busch (2000, 2001) has expanded his view of resistance analysis to include the interpretation of "active resistances" that require confrontation and "inhibiting resistances" that require close process monitoring.

Most other contemporary perspectives on resistance (Samberg 2004), whatever their theoretical underpinning, tend to emphasize the relationship of resistance to the analytic dyad. These perspectives recognize as well that the patient's resistance may be a trigger for the analyst's countertransference and may challenge the analyst's capacity to interpret from a position of therapeutic neutrality. Freud (1912b/1958) recognized early on the contribution of the analyst's unconscious resistance to the course of treatment, and he understood that this countertransference serves as a crucial source of data rather than an obstacle to the progress of analysis. Contemporary perspectives on resistance also consider a more complex set of ideas pertaining to the difficulties in bringing about change. These include the understanding that interpretation may elicit narcissistic injury and multiple anxieties about change and loss.

The therapeutic technique of self psychologists (Kohut 1977; Stolorow et al. 1987) depends on the analyst's empathic immersion within the patient's psychological experience. Self psychologists empathize with both the conflict and the adaptive aspects of the compromise in a way that affirms the patient. They describe the inevitability of repetitive subtle trauma evoked by the analyst's interventions that threaten the patient's self structure and evoke defenses manifested as transference resistance. The meaning of resistance is therefore understood within the analytic dyad as a co-constructed transference/countertransference resistance. The self psychologist's empathy includes both arms of the transference and countertransference. The interpretive focus is shaped with this understanding in mind.

Interpersonalists such as Gill (1982) view transference as co-constructed by patient and analyst. All relationships are transferential, and both participants have a valid view of that relationship. The central task of the analyst is the active interpretation of the transference and the resistances to it, which may take the form of resistance to awareness of the transference, resistance to its resolution, or resistance to involvement in it.

Modern Kleinians (Schafer 1994) emphasize the meaning of the total transference and countertransference situation in its relationship to the patient's specific anxieties and fantasies. Interpretive work focuses on understanding the enactment of complex transference-countertransference fantasies in the here and now and tracing their meaning to their genetic antecedents.

In all contemporary approaches to the analysis of resistance, the fundamental issue is the analyst's view of what analysis is and how it works.

Interpretation

Both broad and more specific definitions of interpretation have been offered. A broad conceptualization of interpretation is all that the analyst says to facilitate the process of the analysis. This general definition involves the psychoanalyst's conceptualization of what he is doing with the patient, what he says or does not say to the patient, and the atmosphere he creates to facilitate the work of analysis. The goal of interpretation is the patient's increasing capacity for insight and, most importantly, the effective application of that insight for change.

Interpretation is the psychoanalyst's descriptions to the patient of his or her unconscious experiences and their function. These mental functions include the patient's defenses, conflicts and compromises, drive derivatives, superego and ego ideal functions, integrative and dissociative self states, and the object relations fantasies that articulate these mental functions, especially within the transference. It is the analyst's task to facilitate the patient's affectively meaningful understanding of their motivated present state with emphasis on what, how, and why.

The interpretation of preconscious experience and function, with a goal of facilitating the analytic process, often focuses on resistances. Resistances often contain within them the conflicts and compromises that underlie mental symptoms. They are defenses against affects, drive derivatives, superego pressures, reality frustrations and challenges, and the conflicts evoked. The analysis of resistance and the descriptive analysis of mental functions and states are therefore synchronous.

Because psychoanalytic processes catalyze transference reactions, and because transference reactions are often resistances to the deepening of the analysis, the interpretation of transference and transference resistance is central to analytic technique. Again, because transference resistance and intensity of analysis occur synchronously, and because transference resistance involves basic defenses, conflicts, and compromises, the analysis of transference resistance and the description of mental functions are synchronous.

A more specific definition distinguishes interpretation from other technical interventions, such as clarification, confrontation, explanation, suggestion, and technical manipulation. Bibring (1954) distinguished psychoanalysis from other psychotherapies by its relative emphasis on interpretation proper, especially as the analysis progresses. While these other interventions may facilitate the early stages of the process, interpretation becomes the predominant mode of intervention by the analyst. It is the hallmark of psychoanalytic work.

A full interpretation aims to make the unconscious conscious—especially affect and its representation elaborated within unconscious fantasy—and, in its completeness, attempts to link past to the present. Full interpretation describes what has happened and is happening and how someone felt and feels about it, linked to how they now suffer with symptoms and character attitudes.

Interpretation is a process that is often accomplished in piecemeal fashion and assembled gradually over an extensive period of time. Unconscious fantasy, memories, affects and their symbolic representations, object relations, and reality evokers and adaptations are progressively made more conscious and placed within a present-day reality and past developmental context. Often this synthesis occurs within the interpretation of the transference.

The analyst's decision to make a particular interpretation is based on his or her perception of the patient's capacity to utilize the interpretation effectively at that time. This decision-making process is referred to as *analytic tact*. However it does not follow that the analyst's interpretive activity is always a preconceived strategy. In fact, much of the analyst's interpretive work proceeds on a preconscious level and may be assimilated after the fact (Kris 1950).

Loewenstein (1951) described a sequence of preparation for the full interpretation but regarded the entire process as part of interpretive work. He included first the linking by the analyst of similar events, then the description to the patient of the similarity of his behavior within those events, then the dynamic meaning of that behavior, then the defensive aspects within those dynamics, and finally the origins of those dynamics. Such a sharp delineation of sequence is neither attainable nor even desirable, but it does give a clear sense of the nature of the task.

The interpretive process has multiple goals that reflect the multiple goals of any psychoanalytic treatment. All goals of psychoanalytic treatment express in somewhat different ways the effort to broaden capacities. One goal of interpretation is to make the unconscious conscious, with the ultimate aim of achieving insight and change. This process involves past and present, id, superego, reality, and their unconscious fantasy syntheses. Another goal is to strengthen the ego, especially its affect tolerance and capacity for more nuanced affect experience, fantasy tolerance, flexibility, adaptability, and synthetic ability. Still another goal is to facilitate more adaptive compromise formations, especially as they relate to the ability to establish and maintain less-conflicted external object relationships. This often involves the integration and tolerance of aggressive strivings and conflicts. All of these goals contribute to the ultimate goal of increasing the patient's capacity for intimacy and sublimation, or, as expressed by Abend (2001), his or her "freedom of choice."

Most analysts, regardless of theoretical orientation, agree that the attainment of insight without meaningful change in a person's life does not constitute a satisfactory outcome to a therapeutic analysis. The method of arriving at meaningful change may certainly vary, but not, for the most part, the ultimate goal. Most analysts no longer distinguish between life goals and treatment goals (Ticho 1972), nor do they distinguish between symptomatic improvement and character change. A therapeutic analysis hopes to achieve growth in all areas. These modifications in conceptualization of the goals of a therapeutic analysis narrow the gap between the analyst's goals and the patient's goals, a distinction of historical significance.

Within the history of our psychoanalytic literature, there have been different interpretive loci that have been identified as the most mutative. Kris (1951) described changes in analytic technique as a function of changes in theory. He contrasted the emphasis on the interpretation of drive with the later emphasis on the interpretation of defense, which changes the strategy and tactics of interpretation.

Arlow (1987) traced the relationship of interpretation to therapeutic goal from an historical perspective. The early aim of interpretation was narrowly defined as the recovery of repressed memories. Now the recovery of memories is regarded as a product of effective analytic work rather than the mutative factor. In doing interpretive work, the analyst has shifted his or her emphasis from content factors to the dynamic aspects of how the process unfolds in response to the specific impact of interpretation. Additionally, it is understood that an interpretation may have different meanings to the patient than to the analyst and that those meanings may change over time. Finally, the analyst as interpreter is also regarded as a participant-observer in the analytic situation.

Loewald (1960) too presented a process view of interpretation. He saw the analyst's interpretations as enabling the patient's understanding by creating links between the psyche of the patient and the analyst and by creating links within the patient's mind to layers of understanding not previously connected or reestablishing connections that had been lost. Such linking might involve the connecting of primary process to secondary process experience. Loewald viewed interpretation as a therapeutic step and a dialectic process between patient and analyst. It is only when the patient feels understood that the analyst can feel he or she has understood him.

Strachey (1934) is perhaps best remembered for his view of what constitutes the mutative interpretation. Although incorrectly credited with advocating transference interpretation exclusively, he believed that the therapeutic effect of analysis derives from qualitative modification in the patient's superego brought about by interpretation of specific distortions in the patient's transference relationship. Because the analyst becomes the object of the patient's id impulses as well as the patient's auxiliary superego, interpretation of superego distortions has the emotional urgency and immediacy necessary to produce change. Change in the structure of the superego allows for change within the full scope of the patient's internalized object relations.

Viewed more broadly, mutative factors (of interpretation of the past, of transference, of real relationship, of drive, or of behavior) vary with patients and with their illnesses. What is crucially helpful for one patient may not be for another, and what is crucially helpful at one phase of the analysis may not be helpful at another phase. Psychoanalysis is first and foremost a technique based on uniqueness and the discovery of the rules of mental organization that define individual patients' experience, processes, and the singularities of their mental organization.

A current discussion/argument in our psychoanalytic literature is the relative importance of interpretation versus relationship in effecting change. Greenberg (1981, 1995; see also Chapter 14, "Theories of Therapeutic Action and Their Technical Consequences") presents a relational view in which the relationship between analyst and patient, conceptualized as "the interactional matrix," contributes significantly to therapeutic effect. Our perspective is that the relationship between analyst and patient necessarily includes and is shaped by what the analyst says to the patient. From this perspective, both polarities are part of the psychoanalytic process and both polarities need each other.

Much has been made in the history of psychoanalysis of the inner stance of the analyst in interpretation. It is said that the analyst is neutral. Rather, the analyst always has a positive investment and therapeutic stance. Although she did not use the term *neutrality*, Anna Freud (1936/1966, p. 28) described a therapeutic stance in which the analyst places himself or herself equidistant in interpretive focus among the agencies and reality, facilitating the emergence and exploration of all components of conflict. Neutrality, however, does not mean that the analyst is neutral about the illness, the outcome, the patient as a person, or the treatment.

Levy and Inderbitzen (1992) similarly define neutrality as a therapeutic stance whose goal is the emergence of all of the multiple determinants of mental conflict. A modern ego psychology would view interpretation as always pointing toward the ego, with the goal of increasing the autonomous integrative function of that agency (Marcus 1999). However, when reality ego, or superego, is so damaged as to be health- and life-threatening, then therapeutic attention must shift toward the damaged agency.

Of great concern to psychoanalysts is the issue of validity of interpretation. How do we know when an interpretation is "correct"? The crucial indicator is not whether the patient agrees or disagrees, but rather whether the psychoanalytic process advances. This advancing of the psychoanalytic process is the goal of interpretation and may be indicated by any or all of the following: liberation of new material or a new affect experience of old material, a shift in dominant affect, new memories, a dream recalled, a greater elaboration of a core unconscious fantasy, and a shift in symptom or behavior that is part of why the patient has sought treatment.

The issue of validity must be separated from the issue of reliability. Reliability means that several observers can agree on what is observed. Validity means that the observation is properly reflective of the unique patient at the unique moment. Psychoanalytic practitioners, like other medical clinicians, are more concerned about validity and helping the patient than they are about reliability. For researchers, the opposite is true.

In the present practice of psychoanalysis, different theoretical schools emphasize different interpretive foci. More classical ego psychologists will focus on conflict and compromise. Contemporary ego psychologists will include autonomous ego function. Object relations theorists will look particularly for core unconscious fantasies that reveal object relations contents and scenarios. The more Kleinian of the object relations theorists will look for drive derivatives that are articulated in these object relations fantasies, especially aggression and its derivatives. Self psychologists will look especially at overall integrations of conflict material into compromise formations contained in self experience, especially in regard to self-esteem and its systematic organization and dissociations. Analysts in the interpersonal school will look at the relationship in the present between the analyst and the patient as the most enlightening and affect-meaningful illustration of unconscious fantasy and object relations. Intersubjective analysts will focus on the emotional experience of the relationship in the here and now between the doctor and the patient for the same reasons as the interpersonal psychoanalyst.

All of these schools have in common a making of the unconscious conscious. All attempt to help the ego tolerate and understand the patient's own dynamic psychology and reach a better compromise integration than the neurotic compromise with which the patient came. All use interpretation of transference, although with different understandings of what constitutes transference and with different understandings of what effects optimal therapeutic outcome. Each attempts to enter the dynamic unconscious of the patient from a different vantage point or surface. Although each of them looks at a different organizational level of entry, the overall goals are probably the same.

Case Example

A 37-year-old man begins psychotherapy suffering from anxiety and depression after his steady girlfriend, with whom he shares a warm and intimate friendship, gives him a marriage ultimatum as she nears her 35th birthday. If he doesn't propose to her, she will break off the relationship. It would be an easy choice to marry her, but what to do with the simultaneous secret love affair of 10 years with a woman he finds irresistibly exciting sexually although emotionally demanding and immature?

The patient feels that his problem is not psychological but, rather, reality based in that he feels he is being forced to choose. He wants the analyst to tell him which of the two women he should choose.

The analyst sees the problem as trying to help the patient understand that the dilemma is not of two but of any one, and that it is an internal problem. The two is a resistance to the one—a precarious compromise in reality that now isn't working. The analyst confronts both aspects, first the dissociation in reality and then the inability to see the internal conflict. The analyst says, "If only the two women could be put together as one." "Yes!" says the patient, "I have often thought that! But I have never found such a woman." The analyst now responds, "Perhaps such a woman doesn't exist, but perhaps you have trouble putting the two types of relationships together into one." "What am I to do?" asks the patient. The patient thus indicates he understands the dissociation problem but still sees it as something to do with reality.

The analyst therefore stays with the reality and tries to work with the conflict there before another attempt to deal with reality as a defense against inner conflict. The analyst says, "Have you ever tried being more sexual with the girlfriend or tried to get to know the lover?" The patient says, "I have tried," but he is relatively impotent with the friendship woman and is soon bored after wild sex with the lover. The analyst asks, "Has this always been true in your relationships with women?" The patient acknowledges that it has always been true; each of his past relationships was one or the other but never both. The analyst, by clarifying and confronting each side of the dissociation, reveals the neurotic inhibitions against which the dissociation tries to defend by the compromise of two women.

Further exploration reveals that the patient apparently feels his sexuality is too intense, dirty, and aggressive. He cannot respect any woman who likes such intense sexuality, and with any woman he respects, he cannot feel free sexually. He feels his sexuality would ruin the relationship with the friendship woman and that friendship with the lover would be impossible because of the sex.

The analyst clarifies the enactments into reality of a defensive dissociation of the intimate object from the sexual object, a classic Madonna-and-Whore complex. The analyst attempts to clarify the resistance to seeing the intrapsychic dissociation by confronting the story and its enacted dissociation in reality.

Rapid progress is made, and the patient recognizes a psychological problem of long-standing—his sexual inhibition—which has stalemated his growth and development in the area of a committed relationship. He is now able to recognize his need for a psychological treatment. Psychoanalysis is recommended after a treatment history reveals many failed psychotherapies.

The analysis proper begins. The patient reveals that he has started a simultaneous consultation with a woman psychoanalyst to see if perhaps he should work with a woman, rather than his current male analyst, because his problem is with women. The male analyst sees this as an enacted transference—now the two, instead of the one, are affecting the analytic relationship—expressing a resistance to deeper transference experience. The analyst asks the patient what comes to mind about this? The patient tells a story about his car in which he keeps two spare tires, because, after all, it could be that on a lonely road at night, the car might go over glass and get two flat tires. Then where would he be with two flat tires and only one spare?

The analyst says, "It sounds like an issue of safety. Perhaps it isn't that the other analyst is female, but that with two analysts you could feel safe." The analyst again confronts a dissociation by interpreting the theme in common that bridges the two. The patient says, "I don't know about two analysts, but yes, the issue of two tires is one of safety. I feel more secure traveling when I don't have to depend on only one tire!"

The analyst says, "Not wanting to depend on only one is a profound point and might apply to women and to analysts as well." The patient says he does feel that way about women, in that in his situation he can't rely on his friendship woman for his intense sexual needs or on his lover for a friendship. The analyst says, "And the two analysts?" The patient responds, "Maybe there, too, each would have a different thing to give." The patient is indicating great resistance to bringing the two together, so the analyst tries to get a deeper theme to bridge the two.

"What comes to mind about that?" the analyst inquires. "Well," said the patient, "perhaps the woman analyst could teach me what the male analyst couldn't and vice versa." The analyst said, "Perhaps it is difficult for you to imagine and to accept that one person could give you both a man's and a woman's view of sex and friendship."

The analyst's interpretation once again brings both sides of both dissociations, women and analysts, together. At this point, the patient stops seeing the female analyst, committing himself to analysis with his male analyst. He thereby seems to indicate in his choice that interpretation is helping him put two sides of a central conflict together.

The patient then starts to miss sessions, and when this is pointed out, he enters a depressive transference. He feels he might have chosen the wrong analyst and that now it's too late; the male analyst doesn't like him because he hurt the male analyst's pride by his need to choose, and he offended and alienated the woman analyst by not choosing her. The problem is again two and still in reality, only now, instead of idealization, there is depressive despair.

Thus began a long sequence in the analysis that elaborated the patient's despair that he had nothing completely good in his relationships, no one perfect woman, and no one perfect analyst. He had ruined his relationship with the analyst and was about to ruin it with both women, because if he had to depend on either one alone, the relationship could not last.

The analytic process could be described as follows: The interpretation of the dissociation resistance led to the patient's feelings about safety and then to depression about failure. With the exploration of failure came the material about his intense longing for perfection. Because these dynamic paradigms also applied to his feelings within the analysis, they were not only important contents in the structure of his dissociated symptom compromise but also defenses and resistances in the transference. Interpretation helped the analysis progress to the conflicts in layers of dynamic material and within the transference.

With each new transference paradigm, the analyst first helped the patient explore the dynamics being expressed and, later, their relevance to the dissociations. At this point in the treatment, it was understood that he dissociated relationships with women because he never felt safe enough with any one of them to express both his friendship and his sexuality. He feared that they would not like him or he would not like them because they or he would be revealed to be less than perfect. This lack of perfection was connected with a profound despair about their worth and his own. The same was true with his analytic transference.

As the analysis progressed, the focus was increasingly centered on the transference. The patient began to idealize the analyst and worried that any anger might destroy the relationship. The analyst said, "Anger might not destroy the relationship but rather the idealization of it. This is in many ways parallel to your feeling that sex would destroy friendship. But the real issue is your worry that your sexual feelings will destroy your friendship feelings because of guilt and despair about your sexual feelings which you feel are dirty and bad and aggressive."

Now the interpretation was more complete in its descriptive linking of the parts of the conflict, its latent content, and the conflict in the latent content that the manifest dissociation defended against. This insight was gained by analyzing the split transference and its latent content against which the split transference defended. The analysis went on the explore the childhood history of the judgmental attitude to sex and its relationship to the perfection fantasies that were defending his low self-esteem and the origins of that.

The analysis helped him to be able to finally get to know the lover, to be sexual with the friend, and to allow him to choose the one, the other, or a third woman with aspects of both friendship and sexuality.

Conclusion

Certain elements are present in psychoanalytic treatment. Three of these elements—process, resistence, and interpretation—have been described in this chapter. Although analysts of different theoretical orientations may conceptualize these elements somewhat differently, there are also fundamental aspects that seem universal and essential. However, the relationship between theoretical orientation and technique is not always so firmly linked.

Analytic treatment is a dynamic process that requires the active participation of both patient and analyst. Intrapsychic change that occurs over time within the mind of the patient requires the analyst's active role as interpreter. The analyst must help the patient to find meaning, and the patient must be able to integrate this knowledge and move forward. The patient's conscious desire for change and unconscious need to preserve the status quo, understood as resistance, are expressed in complex ways within a transference that provides the focus and fulcrum of much of the analytic work. This process occurs within the context of an unusual and compelling human relationship between the analyst and the patient. The significance of that relationship to therapeutic outcome is a matter that we have explored.

References

Abend SM: Countertransference and psychoanalytic technique. Psychoanal Q 58:374–395, 1989

Abend SM: Expanding psychological possibilities. Psychoanal Q 70:3–14, 2001

Abrams S: The psychoanalytic process: a schematic model. Int J Psychoanal 68:441–452, 1987

Arlow JA: The dynamics of interpretation. Psychoanal Q 56:68–87, 1987

Arlow JA, Brenner C: The psychoanalytic process. Psychoanal Q 59:678–692, 1990

Bibring E: Psychoanalysis and the dynamic psychotherapies. J Am Psychoanal Assoc 2:745–770, 1954

Blum H: Countertransference and the theory of technique: discussion. J Am Psychoanal Assoc 34:309–328, 1986

Boesky D: The psychoanalytic process and its components. Psychoanal Q 59:550–584, 1990

Busch F: Recurring thoughts on unconscious ego resistances. J Am Psychoanal Assoc 40:1089–1115, 1992

Busch F: What is a deep interpretation? J Am Psychoanal Assoc 48:237–254, 2000

Busch F: Are we losing our minds? J Am Psychoanal Assoc 49:739–779, 2001

Freud A: The ego and the mechanisms of defense (1936), in The Writings of Anna Freud, Vol 2. New York, International Universities Press, 1966, pp 28–41

Freud S: Fragment of an analysis of a case of hysteria (1905 [1901]), in Standard Edition of the Complete Psychological Works of Sigmund Freud, Vol 7. Translated and edited by Strachey J. London, Hogarth Press, 1953, pp 1–122

Freud S: The dynamics of transference (1912a), in Standard Edition of the Complete Psychological Works of Sigmund Freud, Vol 12. Translated and edited by Strachey J. London, Hogarth Press, 1958, pp 99–108

Freud S: Recommendations to physicians practising psycho-analysis (1912b), in Standard Edition of the Complete Psychological Works of Sigmund Freud, Vol 12. Translated and edited by Strachey J. London, Hogarth Press, 1958, pp 109–120

Freud S: Papers on technique (1911–1915), in Standard Edition of the Complete Psychological Works of Sigmund Freud, Vol 12. Translated and edited by Strachey J. London, Hogarth Press, 1958, pp 85–173

Freud S: Analysis terminable and interminable (1937), in Standard Edition of the Complete Psychological Works of Sigmund Freud, Vol 23. Translated and edited by Strachey J. London, Hogarth Press, 1964, pp 209–253

Friedman L: A reading of Freud's papers on technique. Psychoanal Q 60:564–595, 1991

Gabbard G: Countertransference: the emerging common ground. Int J Psychoanal 76:475–486, 1995

Gabbard G, Westen D: Rethinking therapeutic action. Int J Psychoanal 84:823–841, 2003

Gill MM: Analysis of Technique, Vol 1: Theory and Technique. New York, International Universities Press, 1982

Gray P: Undoing the lag in the technique of conflict and defense analysis. Psychoanal Study Child 51:87–101, 1996

Greenberg JR: Prescription or description: the therapeutic action of psychoanalysis. Contemporary Psychoanalysis 17:239–257, 1981

Greenberg J: Psychoanalytic technique and the interactive matrix. Psychoanal Q 64:1–22, 1995

Kohut H: The Restoration of the Self. New York, International Universities Press, 1977

Kris E: On preconscious mental processes. Psychoanal Q 19:540–560, 1950

Kris E: Ego psychology and interpretation in psychoanalytic therapy. Psychoanal Q 20:15–30, 1951

Levy AT, Inderbitzen LB: Neutrality, interpretation, and therapeutic intent. J Am Psychoanal Assoc 40:989–1011, 1992

Loewald HW: On the therapeutic action of psychoanalysis. Int J Psychoanal 41:16–33, 1960

Loewald HW: The transference neurosis: comments on the concept and the phenomenon. J Am Psychoanal Assoc 19:54–66, 1971

Loewald HW: Reflections on the psychoanalytic process and its therapeutic potential. Psychoanal Study Child 34:155–167, 1979

Loewenstein RM: The problem of interpretation. Psychoanal Q 20:1–14, 1951

Marcus ER: Modern ego psychology. J Am Psychoanal Assoc 47:843–871, 1999

Ogden TH: The analytic third: working with intersubjective clinical facts. Int J Psychoanal 75:3–19, 1994

Ornstein PH, Ornstein A: Formulating interpretations in clinical psychoanalysis. Int J Psychoanal 61:203–211, 1980

Reich W: Character Analysis. New York, Touchstone Press, 1945

Samberg E: Resistance: how do we think of it in the twenty-first century? J Am Psychoanal Assoc 52:243–254, 2004

Sandler J: Countertransference and role responsiveness. Int Rev Psychoanal 3:43–47, 1976

Schafer R: The idea of resistance. Int J Psychoanal 54:259–285, 1973

Schafer R: The contemporary Kleinians of London. Psychoanal Q 63:409–432, 1994

Seidenberg H: The basic rule: free association—a reconsideration. J Am Psychoanal Assoc 19:98–109, 1971

Smith HF: Countertransference, conflictual listening, and the analytic object relationship. J Am Psychoanal Assoc 48:95–128, 2000

Smith HF: Creating the psychoanalytical process. Int J Psychoanal 83:211–228, 2002

Smith HF: Theory and practice: intimate partnership of false connection? Psychoanal Q 72:1–12, 2003

Sterba R: The fate of the ego in analytic therapy. Int J Psychoanal 15:117–126, 1934

Stolorow RD, Brandchaft B, Atwood GE: Psychoanalytic Treatment: An Intersubjective Approach. Hillsdale, NJ, Analytic Press, 1987

Strachey J: The nature of the therapeutic action of psychoanalysis. Int J Psychoanal 15:127–159, 1934

Ticho E: Termination of psychoanalysis: treatment goals, life goals. Psychoanal Q 41:318–333, 1972

16

Termination and Reanalysis

MARTIN S. BERGMANN, PH.D.

SOCIOLOGICAL AND DEVELOPMENTAL events within the history of psychoanalysis have conspired to give the problems of termination and reanalysis a new urgency. To address the sociological aspect, we first have to face the fact that there is a substantial subgroup within the population that requires continued professional assistance just to keep functioning. It is no longer rare that one is consulted by a patient who is now middle aged or older and has been in continuous treatment since early adulthood or even childhood. It is even conceivable that in the future, mental health practitioners will be trained as auxiliary figures whose job will be to assist those who cannot function on their own. In the language that Kohut created, these will be professionals willing and able to function as an auxiliary selfobject to severely impaired patients. The other group will be trained, as most psychoanalysts are today, to bring the treatment to conclusion, with greater attention to termination than is customary in the current training.

Today all analysts have among their patients a mixture of the two groups. The professional training of the psychoanalyst today is geared to the second group. Thus, when psychoanalysts have to deal with the first group—those needing ongoing assistance—their own professional commitment and self-esteem suffer, since they are dealing with patients whose treatment is either interminable or very prolonged. To put it into technical psychoanalytic language, if the superego of the therapist demands a cure within a number of years and the patient is in need of life-

long assistance, the match will not be a good one. In this chapter, I deal primarily with the historical culture of psychoanalysis, but the sociological pressures should always be kept in mind.

In two earlier papers on the subject of termination (Bergmann 1988, 1997), I did not have the courage, as I see it now, to think the matter through to the end. What prevented me from doing so was a sense of guilt toward Freud for understanding the history of psychoanalysis in a way he could not, and which, now that I am past my 90th birthday, I feel I can do. This reluctance was not unique to me but characterized a whole generation of orthodox Freudian psychoanalysts. The internal structure of psychoanalysis is such that it does not allow us, Freud's disciples, to go easily beyond what Freud achieved. For me it was a relief to discover that a paradigm on termination does not exist, for now I am free to think about the issue and even encourage the readers of this chapter to reflect on how the decision to end the treatment is arrived at, and what is the nature of the pressure exerted on the two parties to bring termination about.

In 1997 I published a paper titled "Termination: the Achilles Heal of Psychoanalytic Technique" with the following opening statement:

> In retrospect, we should have been more surprised than we were that Freud's papers on technique never included one on termination. Had we idealized Freud less,

we would have realized earlier that psychoanalytic technique lacks anything like a "royal road" toward termination. (p. 163)

Continuing to reflect on this subject, I found that this failure on Freud's part was not an accident and that we have to face the historical fact that Freud did not develop a consistent technique to bring a psychoanalysis to a satisfactory conclusion. This was indeed an Achilles "heal" that Freud had difficulty admitting publicly until 1937. Somewhere in the back of our minds, we have known this all the time, but not facing the problem squarely has handicapped our work.

Harold Blum (1989) may well have been the first psychoanalyst to point out that psychoanalysis lacks the paradigm for its own termination: "During Freud's lifetime there was an opening and middle phase of clinical analysis. There was no description of a concluding or terminating phase in an otherwise open-ended, timeless analytic process" (p. 275). He went on to note: "Termination had not been taught or supervised in analytic training. Prior to 1950 it had been assumed that anyone who could conduct analysis properly could terminate it correctly. A terminated case was not required for institute graduation, nor for certification in the American Psychoanalytic Association" (p. 283).

It is precisely now that psychoanalysis is facing new criticism that we have to examine termination problems with renewed efforts. My first task will be to demonstrate that, indeed, Freud had no technique for termination at his disposal. As the first "witness," I will ask my readers to remember the Wolf Man's difficulties in termination (Freud 1918/1961).

Freud and the Problem of Termination

In that case history, Freud described "peculiarities of the patient's mentality which were revealed by the psychoanalytic treatment but not further elucidated and were accordingly not susceptible to direct influence." Among those were "tenacity of fixation," "propensity to ambivalence," and "contradictory libidinal attachments" capable of functioning at the same time (Freud 1918/1961, pp. 118–119). The special difficulties of this case made Freud resort to a new technical procedure.

> I determined—but not until trustworthy signs had led me to judge that the right moment had come—that the treatment must be brought to an end at a particular fixed date; and eventually the patient came to see that I was in

earnest. Under the inexorable pressure of this fixed limit his resistance and his fixation to the illness gave way, and now in a disproportionately short time the analysis produced all the material which made it possible to clear up his inhibitions and remove his symptoms. (p. 11)

With the Wolf Man, the concept of "forced termination" became part of the psychoanalytic technique. The use of the term "trustworthy signs" should make us pause. Instead of instructing us as to when this point is reached in treatment, Freud relied on his own intuition, and as subsequent events showed, he was mistaken in believing that the Wolf Man was close to termination. Because the Wolf Man remained in contact with psychoanalysis for the rest of his life, we know that he was not cured either by Freud or by his subsequent analysts (Gardiner 1971).

In 1926, when Freud reevaluated his anxiety theory, he returned to the Wolf Man and explained his failure to cure him by the instinctual regression of the Wolf Man to the oral stage and, hence, his fear of being eaten by the seven wolves. Freud also reconstructed that two opposed instinctual impulses, sadistic aggressiveness toward the father and a tender passive love for him, were repressed. Thus, repression attacked almost all the components of the Oedipus complex and, by implication, made a satisfactory termination impossible (Freud 1926/1959, p. 108).

In the last few years André Green (1980) has made us aware of the pivotal role that the Wolf Man played in the history of psychoanalysis. As he put it, "After 1915 the wolf man haunts theory ceaselessly" (p. 231). Green locates the main reason for Freud's inability to cure the Wolf Man in "the patient's power of maintaining simultaneously the most various and contradictory libidinal cathexes, all of them capable of functioning side by side" (p. 229).

The Wolf Man was in reanalysis with Ruth Mack Brunswick between October 1926 and February 1927. The prewar rich Russian aristocrat was now a destitute refugee in Vienna. We are told without any comment by the therapist that Freud collected money for his former patient, "who had served the theoretical ends of psychoanalysis so well." From a humanitarian point of view, this offering of help was on Freud's part an act of generosity, but from a psychoanalytic point of view it was a disaster, for it made this very passive man even more passive and a permanent patient of psychoanalysis. Without a word of criticism of Freud, Mack Brunswick said that the Wolf Man became greedy, wondering every year how large the next year's gift would be. I myself recall Paul Federn saying that the Wolf Man complained that he could not get anything published under his real name but that everything he writes is published when he writes as the Wolf Man. He was discharged as being "well and relatively productive." During the second treatment, the Wolf Man was suffering from a "hypochondriacal idée fixe" that he was a victim of a nasal injury. The supposed injury compelled him to stare for long periods into the mirror. Mack Brunswick attributed the source of the new illness to an unresolved remnant of the transference, but when she describes the current illness of the Wolf Man, she leaves little doubt in the mind of the reader that the Wolf Man was a seriously ill, paranoid man.

It is relevant for my discussion of termination that the Wolf Man had developed an ambivalent attitude toward Freud. He blamed Freud for the loss of his fortune, and this blame justified Freud collecting money for him, but at the same time he claimed to be Freud's favorite patient. It seems that Mack Brunswick did not analyze the meaning of Freud's financial subsidy, but rigorously attacked the belief that he was Freud's favorite. She pointed out that his was not the only published case and therefore had no right to be proud. What I believe Mack Brunswick did not realize was that instead of a cure, psychoanalysis had given the Wolf Man a permanent new sense of identity as Freud's famous patient. Once, detained by Russian authorities in Vienna, he announced, "I am the Wolf Man." The whole analysis with Freud was transformed into a new myth, resulting in a new identity. Deutsch (1957) reported that something similar happened to Dora, who was proud of having been Freud's famous case. Mack Brunswick does not explain why she felt compelled to attack the Wolf Man's feeling that he was a special case. Was it sibling rivalry? In any case the fact that analysis can give a patient a new identity was not subjected to psychoanalytic scrutiny. By reconstructing the past along new lines, every analysis effects the sense of identity of the analysand, but for the Wolf Man the analysis represented a new birth fantasy, forcing us to accept the fact that an analysis can itself be transformed by the irrational forces of the unconscious.

As my next example of Freud's inability to terminate an analysis, I cite the case of the poet Hilda Doolittle, known as H.D. Precisely because her book *Tribute to Freud* (H.D. 1956) is so positive in the expression of love toward Freud, it is useful to illustrate that Freud could not bring his analyses to a termination. Fortunately for the history of psychoanalysis, H.D.'s book can be supplemented by a more recently published book edited by Susan and Stanford Friedman (2002). There we learn that in 1932 Freud was corresponding with Bryher, H.D.'s financial supporter, about the possibility of her "cousin" H.D. entering analysis with Freud. In fact, Bryher and H.D. had been lovers and later were part of a ménage à trois with Bryher's second husband until the latter abandoned them both to become a homosexual. On the 13th of November Freud wrote

to Bryher the following astonishing letter from which I am quoting in part:

> With me things are no longer the way they used to be. I am old, often ill, and only work for 5 hours with students or patients. There isn't a long waiting list anymore, clients in need of help prefer younger people. But material circumstances force me to keep on earning money. Until recently my fee was $25 per hour; as a result of the general impoverishment I have lowered this to $20 or $15. I donate one of my five hours free of charge, something which I would like to be able to do in general anyway. But I can't do that. Some of my adult children are out of work and have to be assisted or supported.
>
> If you designate £100 for your cousin's analysis, I calculate that this sum won't last beyond one month, and I am worried that this time frame and number of hours will not be sufficient to achieve anything for her. With such a limitation it seems more ethical not to begin anything at all. We consider three months the shortest possible time limit for a trial period. (Friedman and Friedman 2002, pp. 7–8)

Freud was clearly not concerned with anonymity toward his future patients. He apologizes for his fees and describes himself as old and exhausted. In later times the phrase "trial period" acquired the meaning of a period in which the analyst determines whether the patient is analyzable or not, but that is not what Freud meant. He felt that 3 months was the minimum time the patient must allot if the patient wishes to benefit from the analysis. As late as 1932 Freud still believed that 3 months might suffice and that, only if necessary, the patient could return for further analysis.

H.D. (1956) reported the following outburst by Freud from her analysis.

> The Professor himself is uncanonical enough; he is beating with his hand, with his fist, on the head-piece of the old-fashioned horsehair sofa that had heard more secrets than the confession box of any popular Roman Catholic father-confessor in his heyday....*Consciously*, I was not aware of having said anything that might account for the Professor's outburst. And even as I veered around, facing him, my mind was detached enough to wonder if this was some idea of *his* for speeding up the analytic content of redirecting the flow of associated images. The Professor said, "The trouble is—I am an old man— *you do not think it worth your while to love me*." (p. 21)

Later, H.D. will show the Professor that he is worth loving by coming to an hour of therapy when the civil war raging in Vienna made this visit a life-threatening one. An enactment by the analyst leads to a dangerous acting-out by the patient. In my view, Freud stepped out of his role as interpreter to act as a rejected lover; by doing so he forged with the patient a real bond that remained unanalyzable, and therefore the analysis could not be brought to a satisfactory termination.

Every psychoanalytic cure contains a mixture of two components. The first consists of the insights gained by the recovery of what was repressed, a new understanding of a more realistic picture of the self and the major love objects in the patient's life. The other consists of what is called the "corrective emotional experience." This second type of cure comes about when the therapist behaves in a way different from what the analysand expected and different from the way the early parental figures behaved. The more disturbed the patient is, the more important is the corrective emotional experience. To the extent that the first predominates, termination can be reached; if the second predominates, ending treatment is more difficult. To put it in psychoanalytic language, to the extent that the analyst is a transference figure either as a result of displacement from parental figures or as a projection of unacceptable aspects of the self, the end of the analysis can be reached. But to the extent that the psychoanalyst is a new object and the treatment a "corrective emotional experience," the therapist becomes a primary object like the parent and termination becomes uncertain. If the analyst, as a result of the patient's traumatic past, becomes the first reliable object the patient ever had, termination is in danger of becoming another traumatic event. Only a transference relationship has a termination point; a primary relationship cannot be terminated.

The patient who preceded H.D. in therapy with Freud was J.J. van der Leeuw, a now-forgotten but at the time well-known explorer and popular writer. H.D. developed the type of fantasies about him that analysands create in such situations. When van der Leeuw's plane crashed in Africa, H.D. (1956) returned to Freud and said:

> I know there is the great body of the Psycho-Analytical Association, research workers, doctors, trained analysts and so on! But Dr. van der Leeuw was different. I know that you have felt this very deeply. I came back to Vienna to tell you how sorry I am. The Professor said, "You have come to take his place." (p. 6)

It is hard to read this encounter without feeling that Freud's sense of timing was not always right. He may have guessed the patient's unconscious correctly, but the interpretation was premature. The patient had been away; the analyst did not know what changes had occurred in the patient over the months of separation. To say that she had come back to replace the dead rival may have had a kernel of truth but was needlessly wounding. The encounter raises the question of what kind of termination can be expected if the analyst's interpretations disregard timing and are wounding.

If we examine H.D.'s book carefully, we come to the conclusion that what H.D. felt for Freud was more than transference. He is "real" to her, and what she develops toward him is something akin to real love.

In 1977 Samuel Lipton created a minor storm within psychoanalysis when he published his paper "The Advantages of Freud's Technique as Shown in His Analysis of the Rat Man." In the analysis of the Rat Man, Freud could not get the analysand to utter the forbidden words "into the anus," and Freud himself verbalized them for the patient. Lipton cites a literature that criticized Freud for uttering those words. Lipton went on to defend Freud's "spontaneity" against the attack of later psychoanalysts, indicating that the restriction imposed on the analyst to be only an interpreter took place after Freud's death. The case of the Rat Man remained ambiguous in the history of psychoanalysis. Sherwood (1969) praised it as a specimen of psychoanalysis, and Eissler (1953) used this case to show that an obsessive neurosis could be relieved by interpretation only. Kris (1951) and Jones (1955) criticized it as excessive in indoctrination. Zetzel (1966) criticized Freud for feeding the hungry patient by giving him herring to eat. Lipton's paper is relevant in the current context because it makes clear that the psychoanalytic technique in what I called the Hartmann era (Bergmann 2000) was a different technique than the one that Freud created and envisioned.

There are other aspects of Freud's technique, which I can mention only briefly, that have militated against termination. In the "New Introductory Lectures" (Freud 1933[1932]/1964, p. 78), Freud mentions that he forbade one of his patients to telephone the girl the patient was in love with. As a result the patient made the parapraxis and called the girl instead of calling Freud. What matters in our context is that Freud forbade the patient to call his lover. Freud at that time could not have understood the strictly symbolic or metaphorical nature of the analytic relationship. But when an analyst actually forbids a patient to see his girlfriend, he or she steps out of the symbolic role of the interpreter and into an actual role of a father. When an analyst forbids a patient to gamble, masturbate, or smoke, he or she is behaving like a real father. Whatever the reaction, positive or negative, the transference cannot be based purely on displacement or projection but on some aspects of the real analyst. A transference based on real behavior of the analyst tends to blur the difference between parental figures and analyst.

When the topographic model dominated Freud's thinking, termination was relatively easy to conceptualize. The immature ego of the child must resort to repression; repression pushes upward to return to consciousness in relatively harmless ways, as in parapraxis and dreams, and in more detrimental ways, as in neurotic symptoms. An analyst, by enabling the analysand to know the repressed unconscious, liberates wishes and ideas that had to be repressed from their imprisonment in the unconscious. The stronger ego of the adult can face the ideas that were too much for the immature child to handle without resort to repression. The basic assumption was that what has become repressed is limited in content and primarily connected with derivatives of the Oedipus complex, which can become conscious, and when that happens termination can take place. Repression was often compared to a secret police force that requires a large part of the national budget. Once analysis makes repression less necessary, a great deal of new energy should become available for new life goals and creative endeavors.

The topographic point of view, with its greater optimism, was closer to the optimism of the Enlightenment. The greater emphasis on aggression and the death instinct—as well as the clearer awareness of intrapsychic conflict of the structural point of view, with its differentiation between ego, id, and superego—confronted psychoanalysis with the recognition that insight may or may not result in change. For example, a single woman in treatment has a relationship with her boss, a married man. She feels guilty about the relationship but cannot break it off. The analysis will show her that the relationship is based on her Oedipus complex; however, the insight may lead to a diminishing of the superego pressure and continuation of the relationship or to a breakup. To add another complication, let us assume that the therapist, a woman, is in the same situation, or in the opposite situation, that of the married woman. In either case, the therapist will have difficulty in remaining neutral, which may prolong the analysis. The question of when insight leads to change and when this cannot happen is a very urgent one, raised by Freud's 1937 paper "Analysis Terminable and Interminable" (Freud 1937/1964), that still awaits exploration.

As long as the topographic point of view prevailed, the unwritten contract between analyst and patient was that by examining dreams, free associations, and transference resolution, patients would reveal to analysts what they had to repress and that making conscious the unconscious would cure them. When the structural point of view gained dominance after 1920, the unwritten contract was changed; making the unconscious conscious was no longer the cure but only the way the intrapsychic conflict between id, ego, and superego became clear. Changing the relationship between the three structures in favor of the ego had become the new goal.

> Our aim will not be to rub off every peculiarity of the human character for the sake of schematic "normality," nor yet to demand that the person who has been thoroughly analyzed shall feel no passion and develop no in-

ternal conflicts. The business of analysis is to secure the best possible psychological conditions for the function of the ego; with that it has discharged its task. (Freud 1937/1964, p. 250)

The definition reflects Freud's commitment at that time to ego psychology. The ego should at the end of the analysis be stronger than both the id and the superego, but when this optimal strength has been reached—particularly since future internal conflicts are visualized—is not easy to determine.

> The work of analysis proceeds best if the patient's pathogenic experiences belong to the past, so that his ego can stand at a distance from them. In states of acute crisis analysis is to all intents and purposes unusable. (Freud 1937/1964, p. 232)

To this remark of Freud's we can say that neurosis for which treatment is sought is rarely entirely in the past. Most patients come in acute crisis.

> The patients cannot themselves bring all their conflicts into the transference; nor is the analyst able to call out all their possible instinctual conflicts from the transference situation. (Freud 1937/1964, p. 233)

The passage above gave rise to the famous controversy as to whether only transference interpretations are mutative. If Freud was right and only part of the inner conflict is reflected in the transference, what will be the fate of the conflicts that never enter the transference?

> The defensive mechanisms directed against former danger recur in the treatment as resistances against recovery. It follows from this that the ego treats recovery itself as a new danger. (Freud 1937/1964, p. 238)

Even though it was not recognized at that time, the publication of "Analysis Terminable and Interminable" was a major event in the history of psychoanalytic technique, for as Shapiro (2003) shows, it marked the end of a cherished illusion of the "complete psychoanalysis." The logic of that paper demanded either a continuous capacity for self-analysis after termination, the periodic return to analysis with the same analyst, or a series of analyses with different psychoanalysts. Fenichel's (1974) opposition to Freud's paper is of historical interest because it shows what a blow that paper was to the next generation. The prolonged analysis that followed during "the Hartmann era" can be read as another response to that paper: a prolonged attempt to demonstrate that a complete analysis is possible.

Freud went on to add that "the sense of guilt and need for punishment" is a force "absolutely resolved to hold on to illness and suffering" (Freud 1937/1964, p. 242). Freud coined the interesting term "psychical enthropy." He then added "masochism" and "the negative therapeutic reaction," phenomena that are "unmistakable indications of the presence of the instinct of aggression...which we trace back to the original death instinct of living matter" (Freud 1937/1964, p. 243). And finally the famous passages:

> The ego ceases to support our efforts at uncovering the id; it opposes them, disobeys the fundamental rule of psychoanalysis (free association) and allows no further derivatives of the repressed to emerge. (Freud 1937/1964, p. 239)

> We often have the impression that with the wish for a penis and the masculine protest we have penetrated through all the psychological strata and have reached bedrock, and that thus our activities are at an end. (Freud 1937/1964, p. 252)

Perhaps the most controversial assertion was Freud's rejoinder to Ferenczi's criticism that his analysis had been incomplete: it is impossible and needlessly painful for the analysand to try to analyze latent conflicts. After 1937 psychoanalysts came close to the position of Goethe's sorcerer apprentice, who could command a broomstick to fetch water but could not stop the broom once the work was done.

The death instinct as a concept may well be one of the concepts that in a recent paper Fonagy (2003) called "overspecifying the theory." Overspecifying takes place when psychoanalysts create new concepts to which the psychoanalytic interview can offer no clear answers. It is at these points that dissidence and controversy develop (Bergmann 2004). The introduction of the death instinct had a major impact on the question of termination. Since in the course of treatment the impact of the death instinct can be diminished in favor of the life instinct but never eliminated, it becomes difficult to decide when termination is to be reached. Even after termination, aging, illness, bereavement, and other traumatic events can change the balance of forces once more in favor of the death instinct and its manifestation in depressive illnesses.

Post-Freudian Concepts of Termination

What Freud failed to do, other psychoanalysts attempted to do. But since they too shied away from facing the problem, their contribution remained limited. As I summarized elsewhere:

The first psychoanalysts to address difficulties in termination were Ferenczi and Rank (1924). In keeping with Freud's (1914) idea that during psychoanalysis the infantile neurosis is transformed into a transference neurosis, they advocated that the analyst should set the termination date the moment this transformation occurs. They believed that only then could a repetition of clinging to the early object be avoided. The termination date must be set this early if fixation on the mother is not to give way to transference fixation. They advocated that analysis must end before it can become a vehicle for the repetition-compulsion. (Bergmann 1997, p. 164)

The innovation forced by Ferenczi and Rank showed how already in 1924 termination had become a problem. Ferenczi's paper of 1927 was the first paper to address the problem of termination:

> The proper ending of an analysis is when neither the physician nor the patient put and end to it, but when it dies of exhaustion....A truly cured patient frees himself from analysis slowly but surely; so long as he wishes to come to analysis he should continue to do so....The patient finally becomes convinced that he is continuing analysis only because he is treating it as a new but still a fantasy source of gratification, which in terms of reality yields him nothing. (Ferenczi 1927/1955, p. 85)

All subsequent efforts to address the problem of termination (Firestein 1964; Glover 1955; Waelder 1960) came to the same conclusion: that there is no royal road to termination. Glover (1955) devoted two chapters to the terminal phase, in which he speaks of "transference weaning and ego readaption" (p. 139). Glover took it for granted that it is the analyst's task to give the notice of termination. The analysand will frequently react to the danger of termination by a return of the symptoms that have already been overcome, and a new period of working-through will then take place. The termination phase can take months and even years. Glover was well aware that many analyses that are terminated end because a stalemate has been reached. What Glover called stalemate I see as a new equilibrium that the two parties collaborated in establishing, and like other states of equilibrium, this equilibrium is apt to last at least until the analyst, perhaps after some consultation, understands the role she or he played in establishing the equilibrium. A stalemated analysis is not fundamentally different from a stalemated marriage or nonproductive relationship between parent and offspring. In all such relations, unconscious destructive needs are met.

Freud's dual-instinct theory gave rise to the Kleinian point of view, which assumes that the child comes into the world in the paranoid position, where destructive wishes projected on the mother hold sway. Only later, by the infusion of the mother's libido, does the child reach the depressive position, where he or she is willing to make restitution for these aggressive wishes. In the Kleinian model, treatment takes place between the paranoid and the depressive position, but even if the depressive position is in the ascendancy, the victory is never certain and never permanent, and termination is always to some extent arbitrary.

We know now that the conclusions reached by Freud in 1937 were not acceptable to many psychoanalysts, and one of the sharpest criticisms came from Otto Fenichel. The culture of psychoanalysis before World War II was such, however, that Fenichel's paper was written only for the circular letters and not meant to be published. It was published posthumously in 1974 (or, as the editors euphemistically put it, the paper "was recently discovered in Mrs. Frances Deri's estate").

Fenichel (1974/1998) criticized Freud's assumption that the ego is naturally always hostile to the instincts and instead postulated that if the ego can control undesirable instincts, it can guide the person to a realistically possible gratification of instinctual demands (p. 111). Against Freud's claim that it is neither possible nor desirable to analyze latent conflicts, Fenichel argued that in the analytic process latent conflicts are always mobilized and analyzed and are never completely latent (p. 112). Here I believe the difficulty was terminological. Fenichel is right: latent conflicts are continuously brought up in analysis. But that does not mean that in the analysis of a single, childless woman one can analyze a future conflict between mothering and wishes for career advancement. Some latent problems do emerge in psychoanalytic treatment, but others do not.

More could be said about Fenichel's criticism of Freud's 1937 paper, but ultimately the greatest difference in the two men's views centered on Freud's death instinct theory. Fenichel's opposition to Freud's theory was shared by most psychoanalysts committed to social revolution. Freud's death instinct theory was unacceptable not only to Fenichel (1935) but to a whole generation of psychoanalysts who believed that war was an aspect of capitalism and would disappear under socialism. The death instinct, to the extent that it became a belief rather than a mere hypothesis, set limits on the possibility of any termination that was not a compromise formation between the two antagonists: libido and aggression, or libido and the death instinct.

After World War II something fundamental happened to the culture of psychoanalysis that increased the lengths of analyses from months to years and from terminable analyses into interminable ones. During the same period, under the influence of Loewald in the United States and Winnicott in England, the aim of analysis slowly changed from relief from painful symptoms and neurotic character traits to resumption of growth and development. Whereas Freud and Abraham recognized only arrest in the development of the sexual drive manifesting itself in fixation on pregenital stages of the libido, Loewald and Winnicott set new goals for psychoanalysis. They saw neurosis as impeding the whole development of the person and psychoanalysis as the technique that enables the former analysand to keep growing after termination.

One of Freud's important contributions to the understanding of human nature was his realization that reality allows gratification of only a small part of our libidinal and aggressive wishes. Many of these wishes remain ungratified. The transference to the psychoanalyst is the result of the mobilization of many of the wishes left ungratified. What precisely these wishes are becomes the subject matter of the analysis, but to the extent that these aroused wishes have no outlet in reality, the ending of treatment reestablishes the preanalytic state of lack of gratification and makes the termination difficult. However, as long as the patient can verbalize these wishes within the safe confines of the treatment, some relief is obtained. In opposition to this idea it will be argued that in the analysis these wishes are experienced and verbalized for the first time and therefore lose the tyrannical power they have. That may well be so, but the question remains as to whether they lose most or only some of their power, and if so, whether termination once more will be experienced as an unwelcome and forced weaning process.

Glover (1955) touched on, but did not adequately deal with, the differences between those analysands who end on a positive transference, praise the analyst to their friends, and send new patients and those who end on a negative transference. The latter are apt to seek a reanalysis because their analysis ended without resolution. If the relationship is strongly negative, an analyst of a different school may be sought. Now the patient and the new analyst will tend to ascribe the limitations of the analysis to the particular school to which the previous analyst belonged until a new equilibrium in the form of a second stalemate sets in.

The weak point in Glover's book is his inability to tell the analyst at what point to give the notice of termination and to differentiate between a stalemate of analysis and a genuine termination point. In my own supervisory teaching, I have found that the less experienced therapist reaches the stalemate position much earlier than the experienced therapist and that a major task of the supervisor or control analyst is to point out to the student how to break out of the stalemated position. Because of the barrier between unconscious and preconscious, and because of the power of the repetition compulsion, all but the few very gifted analysands soon begin to go in circles and repeat rather than discover new data. It is the therapist's task to break through the repetition and point out derivatives of new unconscious thoughts in the material or even draw attention to the fact that the border between conscious and unconscious has been shut.

Waelder's (1960, pp. 242–243) discussion of the completion of analysis is much shorter than Glover's but contains a similar difficulty. Waelder accepted that a complete analysis in the sense of complete understanding of a person's psychic life is beyond our capacity to achieve. However, from a therapeutic point of view, an analysis is complete "if the pathological structures have been fully understood both dynamically and structurally...and if the psychopathology has thereby disappeared or has been rendered comfortable." But like Glover, he also noted that "an analysis should be terminated when we have reached the point of diminishing returns." Waelder did not comment on the contradiction between a complete termination and a stalemated one.

Waelder assumed a prolonged postpsychoanalysis truce between superego, ego, and id and the repetition compulsion. The ego, the most mature part of the personality and the agency closest to the reality principle, may well favor such a truce, but will the other agencies abide it? It seems that when discussing termination, many psychoanalysts forget what they know about id, superego, and the repetition compulsion.

Ella Sharpe (1937) ended her book on dream analysis with a chapter titled "Analyzed Persons and Their Dreams." She delineated an analyzed person "as one in which direct instinct gratification and sublimation is accompanied by zest and a feeling of well being" (p. 192). She noted that in the dreams of analyzed and unanalyzed individuals, the difference is mainly that dreams that used to evoke painful affects can now be dreamt with greater ease. Furthermore, she felt that the need to disguise is not as great and that the capacity of dreams to affect the mood of the next day is less pronounced. These analyzed people also had the capacity to analyze their dreams without resistance. The ego of the analyzed person is capable of accepting the primitive wishes better, and the punishment of the superego is greatly diminished. Sharpe also felt that prolific dreaming indicates faulty working of the psychic apparatus. According to Sharpe, repetitive dreams are not experienced by analyzed people, and absence of dreams indicates that there is something wrong intrapsychically. These ideas were written before studies of rapid eye movements showed that we all dream about 20%–25% of our sleeping time. Sharpe's book, in contrast to Freud's "Analysis Terminable and Interminable" (Freud 1937/1964) (written in the same year), is an optimistic appraisal of what an analysis can achieve. Sharpe's data are impressionistic, and to my knowledge no systematic study has either confirmed or disconfirmed her hypothesis that psychoanalysis does in fact alter the dreaming process.

Internalization of the Psychoanalyst

How is the analyst to be internalized? In his classic paper in 1934, Strachey argued that the analyst becomes internalized as a more rational superego imposed on or supplementing the harsher superego of the analysand. By contrast, Sterba (1934), in a paper written in the same year, laid more stress on identification with the psychoanalyst and, in contrast to Strachey, stressed the therapeutic alliance based on the capacity of the patient's ego for disassociation. In 1936, 3 years after Hitler claimed power, an important symposium took place in Marienbad, Czechoslovakia. There, for the first time, ego psychoanalysts, those who absorbed some of the implications of the new view adopted by Freud, faced the older generation, who still adhered to the topographic point of view. At that moment, two kinds of analysis were conceivable. The first and more authoritarian kind would aim to replace the excessively condemnatory superego of the analysand by a more reasonable superego of the internalized psychoanalyst. The other kind, recognizing the supposed fact that only changes in the ego structure are enduring, would work toward modifying the ego. Depending on the point of view, different terminations will be reached.

A truly optimistic termination is found in Menninger's (1958) conclusions, in which a terminating patient is quoted as saying:

> I have gotten what I paid for; I can do for myself. I can assume a mature role in preference to one of expectant pleading; I can substitute hoping for despairing, enjoying for expecting, giving for taking. I can endure foregoing what must be foregone and accept and enjoy without guilt such pleasures as are accessible to me. (p. 159)

But even Menninger does not tell us how often in treatment analysands get to this point and if this state of feeling endures over the years and becomes a permanent acquisition of the analysand.

> If, for instance, the patient could be made less frightened of his super-ego or introjected object, he would project less terrifying imagos on to the outer object and would therefore have less need to feel hostility towards it; the object which he then introjected would in turn be less savage in its pressure upon the id-impulses, which would be able to lose something of their primitive ferocity. (Menninger 1958, p. 341)

In an earlier paper (Bergmann 1988), I pointed out that in real life there is no analogue to the experience of termination of an analysis. Children grow up and leave home, but they return for holidays. Couples separate but continue to meet at certain special occasions. Psychoanalysis is unique in demanding a radical separation not based on hate or death; psychoanalysis makes a heavier demand on internalization than is generally demanded in life.

Since termination of treatment is in opposition to basic human needs for continuity, we should not be surprised that it frequently fails to reach the desired aims. It runs counter to the natural needs of many analysands and many analysts. Furthermore, since most wishes to "do it alone" are based on early disappointments, and these wishes are in the course of an analysis systematically exposed as resistances, they leave as residue early wishes for union rather than wishes for independence. In most cases, the wish for merger, unity, and continuity is stronger than the wish for independence.

When the analysis is still in progress, the voice of the analyst is slowly internalized; for the time being it is often heard by the patient. Eduardo Weiss (1960) called this stage "psychic presence." To cite a clinical example, a young woman was so anxious on her first date that the man would not call her again that she felt obliged to end every date in a sexual relationship. As the analysis progressed, she "heard" the voice of her analyst telling her that she did not have to end every date in a sexual relationship. This "psychic presence" should in time become internalized; her own self-esteem should replace the voice of the analyst. This internalization process will be impeded if the symbolic nature of the analytic relationship is allowed to become a real relationship.

In a paper published in 1967 but available in English only since 2003, titled "Diachrony in Psychoanalysis," André Green pointed out that "what is created by the unsatisfied need is not cancelled out by satisfying the need" and furthermore that what is created by satisfying the need is not cancelled out by removing the unsatisfied need. Green did not have termination of treatment in mind when he postulated these psychic states. They are, however, relevant to termination. Even a successful analysis cannot cancel out the unhappiness and suffering that preceded it. Psychic life is so constructed that nothing that once existed can cease to exist; our past is always with us.

In a recent historical study of dissidence (Bergmann 2004), I found a third possibility: the analysand, dissatisfied with the results of the analysis or in competition with the analyst, embarks on a self-analysis that may lead to reformulation of the conclusions reached in the analysis. This postanalytic self-analysis often leads to dissidence and a new school of psychoanalysis. In the symposium mentioned earlier, André Green reformulated Freud's "rock bottom" (Freud 1937/1954) to mean the "psychotic core" that many or all analysands have. Many people who live more or less normal lives nevertheless have psychotic lacunae at various parts of their psychological structure. The analysis comes to a stop when these lacunae, or this "psychotic core," is reached. Green pointed out that in the early years of psychoanalysis, the other side of neurosis was thought to be perversion. Perversion in turn was conceptualized as a pregenital fixation. After the two papers of 1924 on neurosis and psychosis (Freud 1924[1923]/1961, 1924/1961), Freud no longer compared neuroses with perversion but with psychosis. These observations of Green are relevant to termination. In the older view, the reaching of full genitality with orgasm was a sign that the patient was no longer fixated on an earlier pregenital phase of the libido that Abraham (1924) had postulated; thus, reaching genitality could be seen as a termination point. When neurosis was compared with psychosis, and particularly when a large number of analysands, if not all of them, were seen as having a psychotic core, the point of termination became more difficult to determine.

This brings me to another unsettled controversy in psychoanalysis. Under the leadership of Margaret Mahler (1968), American ego psychology during the Hartmann era emphasized that under favorable conditions, the child develops genuine wishes for separation-individuation from the mother. This separation and individuation is conflict-free if the mother does not retaliate or herself separate prematurely from the child. By contrast, French psychoanalysis under Lacan's influence developed a different model in which neither mother nor child desires separation; the separation is imposed upon the dyad by the will of the father, who is the unwelcome separator. Readers of Proust will recall how the boy sent to bed longs for mother's goodnight kiss and how the mother wishes to give this kiss but the father is opposed to it as an indulgence of the child. Mahler's model is friendly to the idea favored by Ferenczi that the analysand separates when she or he is ready; the Lacanian view favors Freud's (1918/1961) forced separation.

Most people seeking psychoanalytic help are not fortunate enough to have gone through the good separation-individuation that Mahler outlined. It is also likely that most therapists also are not so fortunate and that, for both analyst and analysand, termination is brought about by the invisible father—namely, the superego—not always by the consent of the ego and almost never by the wishes of the id. In every analysis, the analyst is both a transference object and a new object never encountered before. For many analysands, the analyst becomes a primary object, healing severe shortcomings of the original primary objects. One of the questions awaiting further study is whether termination is more difficult to achieve when the analyst is primarily a new object and the analysis functions as a corrective emotional experience.

The psychoanalytic situation is also unique in another respect. Nowhere else in life has anyone been privileged to say everything that occurs to them. Once the analysis is terminated, this privilege is forever withdrawn. This also works against termination. I am familiar with the case of a woman who, after termination of treatment, felt compelled to confess to her husband her marital infidelities, with serious results. Alarmed by the results, the patient asked for a postanalysis consultation. It became evident that she wished to transfer to the husband some of the feelings she had for her analyst and wanted to create a relationship in which "everything can be said," but this turned out to be more than the husband could bear.

Bringing the analysis to a truly satisfactory conclusion, if my assumptions are correct, demands a great deal from therapist and patient. Brenner (1982) has called attention to the fact that relationships and life in general consist from a psychoanalytic point of view of a series of equilibria. An equilibrium can be upset if life conditions change, such as occurs when economic conditions change, when retirement takes place, or when death or divorce changes our lives. If the psychoanalysis is prolonged, the analyst inevitably gets absorbed in the life equilibrium of the patient and the patient in the equilibrium of the therapist. Breaks in equilibrium are usually painful and therefore avoided. For example, a patient's tendency for extramarital relationship diminished during the analysis since the patient could complain about the partner in the analysis. This change improved the couple's relationship, but after termination, with no outlet for the aggression against the partner, the tendency reasserted itself. Both patient and therapist did not realize that the analysis fulfilled a need that could not be met as well by the outside world. The therapist may also develop a need for the patient not only as a source of income but also as a child substitute, source of prestige, and many other functions, all of which work against successful termination.

The Terminal Phase

Psychoanalysis owes to Glover (1955) the concept that termination demands a phase of its own. The Wolf Man (Freud 1918/1961) showed Freud that certain issues do not emerge until the analysand is convinced that termination will indeed take place. It has been generally accepted that this phase should be given full scope to develop. Narcissistic wishes for perfection, as well as wishes for a perfect analyst or a perfect analysis, should be allowed to emerge and have their day in the treatment situation. Tyson (1995) particularly emphasized that

sometimes a patient may withhold the full intensity of rage associated with infantile loss of impotence and helplessness in order to preserve the relationship with the analyst, maintaining unconscious hopes of ultimate fulfillment of grandiose infantile wishes. When the patient finally recognizes the futility of such hopes, he or she may feel there is nothing in the relationship with the analyst to preserve. (p. 504)

In other cases, all this may not take place. When the center of the analytic process is reliving of the Oedipus conflict, the conflict will appear once more. When during infancy the separation-individuation process was incomplete or derailed by premature separation by the mother, the pain of individuation will have to be relived. Adolescent conflicts will also reemerge, because adolescence is a kind of second separation-individuation phase. On the other hand, feelings of love and gratitude hitherto not expressed may find expression for the first time. Therapists who themselves fear separation may be tempted to cut this phase short.

It took Freud until close to the end of his life to face the limitations of the method of treatment he discovered. It took psychoanalysis much longer to face the fact that a complete analysis is not reachable and may even be a contradiction in terms. When, because a stalemate has been reached or because all that needed to be analyzed has in the opinion of the analysand and analyst been accomplished, the analysis is terminated, four possible conclusions can be reached:

1. *The analysand decides to live with the limitation of the analysis.* This decision may be based on a sense of well-being and a productive life or on the feeling that nothing further can be achieved. One has to accept in good grace what cannot be changed. This piece of wisdom is expressed in the line from the opera *Die Fledermaus:* "Happy is he who forgets what cannot be changed."
2. *Analyst and analysand believe that self-analysis can now replace the analyst.* A well-known quip of Bernfeld is often quoted against this solution: "Question: What is wrong with self-analysis? Answer: Countertransference." Beyond the quip, self-analysis is often useful in solving problems associated with the psychopathology of everyday life, such as finding a lost key or remembering a forgotten name, but it is seldom up to the task of solving a serious crisis.
3. *The analysand stays in prolonged analysis or undertakes a series of reanalyses.* This solution may be the only one available in cases of serious mental pathologies, and it deserves a legitimacy of its own. However, apart from being often unproductive and repetitive, it has the difficulty of denying analysands the opportunity that they may become adults and masters in their own houses.

4. *Analysand and analyst find their own termination point.* Since we have not found a royal road to termination, every psychoanalytic couple must find their own termination point. Both the limitations of the therapist and those of the patient play a role. It may happen that during the termination phase new insights open new doors; in that situation we need not fear to say that what seemed like termination turned out to be a deepening of the analysis.

There is a time-honored tradition in psychoanalysis that the analysis should be continued to the very last moment, and indeed many authors have shown that very important new psychoanalytically significant material does emerge in the last hour. Nevertheless, in my opinion, it may well be indicated in certain cases to devote the last few hours to the evaluation of the analytic work. When this approach is followed, the patient should be asked to sit up and not necessarily free-associate but rather discuss his or her own understanding of the whole analytic procedure, what has been achieved, and what further work there still is for him or her to do after the analysis is finished. The analyst should feel free to participate in the discussion. During this time, the two partners are speaking to each other more as equals than they did during the analysis itself.

Reanalysis

A future historian of psychoanalysis may be surprised to discover how many panels of the American Psychoanalytic Association and articles were devoted to the question of reanalysis. In a recent paper, Meyer and Debbink (2003) noted that between 1959 and 1994, six panels and many more papers were published on this topic alone. To read this literature in succession is an interesting but also sobering experience. One is struck both by the changing climate in organized psychoanalysis through the years and by the steady recurrence of the same problems that resist resolution.

I found the first 1959 symposium (McLaughlin 1959) to be of special interest. One gets the impression that the panel could not cope with the many problems of reanalysis. There was first the lingering and disturbing impact of the two analyses of the Wolf Man. Viennese analysts who by then were in the United States had many memories to tell. Jenny Waelder-Hall stressed that the underlying pathology of the Wolf Man, with his "deeply passive and feminine orientation" and his megalomania, was not appreciated at the time. Grete Bibring stressed how Mack

Brunswick's own transference to Freud complicated the picture. By contrast, in another panel on reanalysis, chaired by McLaughlin and reported by Johan in 1985 (Panel Report 1985), Ruth Eissler stressed Brunswick's capacity in the reanalysis to penetrate the grandiose fantasies the Wolf Man used against the feelings of his infantile helplessness. The Wolf Man's legacy to psychoanalysis was the realization that an analysis that fails can nevertheless be powerful enough to serve as the basis for a new psychopathology, which only a reanalysis can discover.

The relationship of the new therapist to the previous one poses the danger of an alliance between the patient and analyst against the first analyst, who exists only in the recollections of the patient, and this recollection is conducive to a collusion between new analyst and patient. Cases in which an analysis ended successfully and the reanalysis takes place because life has radically changed are the least problematic for the next analyst, while the opposite is true if the first analysis failed or ended in a negative transference. In the latter case, it is the most problematic for the second analyst, because the first analysis ended traumatically, increasing resistance to the second. One of the surprises to me was the recognition that many former patients returned to analysis not because new problems arose but because the superego could not tolerate a significant prize or a major promotion; they represent the type Freud (1916/1957) described as "wrecked by success." The very fact that analysis enabled the former analysand to succeed beyond expectations may make another analysis necessary.

What is difficult to accept for analysts who were attracted to psychoanalysis precisely because it offered such high hopes is that a perfect solution is beyond our reach. A good termination is more likely if the analyst does not become emotionally or financially dependent on the patient. Throughout this chapter, I have stressed the advantage of the new internalization of the analyst that a good analysis should achieve. This precludes social contacts after the termination. Former patients, such as powerful politicians, can do us psychoanalysts many favors. However, a good analysis demands that the former analysand remain free from such obligations. In a training analysis, when the former analyst and the former patient continue to meet socially and professionally, such a termination is not possible. I do not wish to imply that, therefore, training analyses cannot end well, but merely to point out that when social contact replaces analytic contact, the analysand has the added task of reconciling the image of the analyst created during the analysis with the image that emerges in postanalytic contact. Many analysands are intensely curious about what the real analyst is like: her or his political views, how he or she spends vacations, and how well he or she plays tennis. The analytic process demands that imagination, and not facts, be the center of attention. If the analysis was good enough, the postanalytic experience need not play a significant role, but here too the results are not easily predictable, especially if analyst and former patient do not see eye to eye on important issues. It may be useful to anticipate such a possibility during the last phase of analysis, to prepare the candidate for postanalytic encounters.

Conclusion

A survey of the history of psychoanalysis has shown that a fully satisfactory termination of a psychoanalysis—and, by implication, a psychotherapy—occurs only rarely. The disappearance of the original symptoms is not a reliable test, since symptoms can be exchanged for other symptoms or for a character neurosis. Real life offers no paradigm for termination, since human relationships usually end in lack of gratification, hostility, or death.

Typically the therapist becomes included in the life equilibrium of the patient, and the analysand becomes part of the life equilibrium of the therapist. Such equilibria resist termination. Most active wishes in psychoanalysis tend to be reaction formations to earlier and deeper passive yearnings. When the active wishes are analyzed, these passive wishes are left over. Most psychoanalyses come to an end when a therapeutic standstill is reached. However, the standstill only reflects the limitation of the therapist. A consultation with a senior colleague can often reopen the clogged channels. A therapist aware of these pitfalls can conduct a better and deeper analysis for the greater benefit of the analysand.

References

Abraham K: A short study of the development of the libido in the light of mental disorders, in Selected Papers of Karl Abraham. London, Hogarth Press, 1924, pp 418–501

Bergmann MS: On the fate of the intrapsychic image of the psychoanalyst after termination of the analysis. Psychoanal Study Child 43:137–153, 1988

Bergmann MS: Termination: the Achilles heal of psychoanalytic technique. Psychoanalytic Psychology 14:163–174, 1997

Bergmann MS (ed): The Hartmann Era. New York, Other Press, 2000

Bergmann MS: Understanding Dissidence and Controversy in the History of Psychoanalysis. New York, Other Press, 2004

Blum HP: The concept of termination and the evolution of psychoanalytic technique. J Am Psychoanal Assoc 37:275–295, 1989

Brenner C: The Mind in Conflict. New York, International Universities Press, 1982

Deutsch F: A footnote to Freud's analysis of a case of hysteria. Psychoanal Q 26:159–167, 1957

Eissler KR: The effect of the structure of the ego on psychoanalytic technique. J Am Psychoanal Assoc 1:104–143, 1953

Fenichel O: A critique of the death instinct, in The Collected Papers of Otto Fenichel. New York, WW Norton, 1935, pp 363–371

Fenichel O: A review of Freud's analysis terminable and interminable. Int Rev Psychoanal 1:109–116, 1974

Ferenczi S: The problem of termination of the analysis (1927), in Final Contributions to the Problems and Methods of Psychoanalysis. London, Hogarth Press, 1955, pp 77–86

Fenichel S: Rundbriefe, Vols 1 and 2. Edited by Ghl;itner EM, Reichmayr J. Frankfurt, Germany, Stromfeld, 1998

Ferenczi S, Rank O: The Development of Psycho-analysis (1924). New York, Nervous & Mental Disease Publishing, 1925

Firestein S: Termination in Psychoanalysis. New York, International Universities Press, 1964

Fonagy P: Some complexities in the relationship of psychoanalytic theory and practice. Psychoanal Q 72:13–47, 2003

Freud S: Remembering, repeating, and working-through (1914), in Standard Edition of the Complete Psychological Works of Sigmund Freud, Vol 12. Translated and edited by Strachey J. London, Hogarth Press, 1958, pp 145–156

Freud S: Some character types met with in psychoanalytic work, I: the exceptions (1916), in Standard Edition of the Complete Psychological Works of Sigmund Freud, Vol 14. Translated and edited by Strachey J. London, Hogarth Press, 1957, pp 309–315

Freud S: From the history of an infantile neurosis (1918), in Standard Edition of the Complete Psychological Works of Sigmund Freud, Vol 17. Translated and edited by Strachey J. London, Hogarth Press, 1961, pp 1–122

Freud S: Neurosis and psychosis (1924[1923]), in Standard Edition of the Complete Psychological Works of Sigmund Freud, Vol 19. Translated and edited by Strachey J. London, Hogarth Press, 1961, pp 147–153

Freud S: The loss of reality in neurosis and psychosis (1924), in Standard Edition of the Complete Psychological Works of Sigmund Freud, Vol 19. Translated and edited by Strachey J. London, Hogarth Press, 1961, pp 181–187

Freud S: Inhibitions, symptoms and anxiety (1926), in Standard Edition of the Complete Psychological Works of Sigmund Freud, Vol 20. Translated and edited by Strachey J. London, Hogarth Press, 1959, pp 75–175

Freud S: New introductory lectures on psycho-analysis (1933 [1932]) (Lectures XXIX–XXXV), in Standard Edition of the Complete Psychological Works of Sigmund Freud, Vol 22. Translated and edited by Strachey J. London, Hogarth Press, 1964, pp 1–182

Freud S: Analysis terminable and interminable (1937), in Standard Edition of the Complete Psychological Works of Sigmund Freud, Vol 23. Translated and edited by Strachey J. London, Hogarth Press, 1964, pp 209–253

Friedman S, Friedman S (eds): Analyzing Freud: Letters of HD, Bryher, and Their Circle. New York, New Directions, 2002

Gardiner M (ed): The Wolf-Man. New York, Basic Books, 1971

Glover E: The Technique of Psychoanalysis. New York, International Universities Press, 1955

Green A: Passions and their vicissitudes, in On Private Madness. Madison, CT, International Universities Press, 1980, pp 214–253

Green A: Diachrony in Psychoanalysis (1967). New York, Free Association Books, 2003

HD [Hilda Doolittle]: Tribute to Freud. Boston, MA, David R. Godine, 1956

Jones E: The Life and Work of Sigmund Freud, Vol 2: The Years of Maturity, 1901–1919. New York, Basic Books, 1955

Kris E: Ego psychology and interpretation in psychoanalytic therapy. Psychoanal Q 20:15–20, 1951

Lipton S: The advantages of Freud's technique as shown in his analysis of the Rat Man. Int J Psychoanal 58:255–273, 1977

Mahler MS: On Human Symbiosis and the Vicissitudes of Individuals. New York, International Universities Press, 1968

McLaughlin F: Problems of reanalysis. J Am Psychoanal Assoc 7:537–547, 1959

Menninger KA: Theory of Psychoanalytic Technique. New York, Basic Books, 1958

Meyer JK, Debbink NL: Reanalysis in the career of the analyst. Journal of Clinical Psychoanalysis 12:55–71, 2003

Panel Report: Reanalysis. J Am Psychoanal Assoc 33:187–200, 1985

Shapiro T: Reanalysis and twentieth century psychiatry. Journal of Clinical Psychoanalysis 12:19–29, 2003

Sharpe E: Dream Analysis. London, Hogarth Press, 1937

Sherwood M: The Logic of Explanation in Psychoanalysis. New York, Academic Press, 1969

Sterba R: The fate of the ego in analytic therapy. Int J Psychoanal 15:117–126, 1934

Strachey J: The nature of the therapeutic action of psychoanalysis. Int J Psychoanal 15:127–153, 1934

Tyson P: Termination of psychoanalysis and psychotherapy, in Textbook of Psychoanalysis. Edited by Nersessian E, Kopff RG Jr. Washington, DC, American Psychiatric Press, 1995, pp 501–524

Waelder R: The Basic Theory of Psychoanalysis. New York, International Universities Press, 1960

Weiss E: The Structure and Dynamics of the Human Mind. New York, Grune & Stratton, 1960

Zetzel ER: Additional notes upon a case of obsession neurosis: Freud 1909. Int J Psychoanal 47:123–129, 1966

17

Psychoanalysis and Psychopharmacology

STEVEN P. ROOSE, M.D.

DEBORAH L. CABANISS, M.D.

WHEN PSYCHOTROPIC MEDICATIONS were first introduced in the late 1950s, primarily for the treatment of schizophrenia and depression, the initial reaction of the psychoanalytic community ranged from skepticism to outright rejection. In general, psychoanalysts considered psychotropic medication to be a "superficial" treatment that addressed symptoms but did not affect the underlying psychic conflicts presumed to be the etiology of psychological illness (Sarwer-Foner 1960). Nonetheless, embedded within the rejection of psychotropic medication was the recognition that the use of medication to reduce florid symptoms could control behavior that interfered with the development of the analytic situation and that, therefore, at times medication could be useful and even necessary. Even if effective, however, medications were considered at best a necessary but undesirable adjunctive treatment, and it was thought that, if possible, the psychoanalytic situation should be left undisturbed (Ostow 1962). For example, in 1986 Normand and Bluestone wrote the following about the indication for adjunct use of medication in psychoanalysis:

> Analytic therapy in general does not aim primarily at elimination of symptoms, but at improvement of uncon-scious conflicts, which produce unsatisfactory behavior, including symptoms. Most [psychoanalysts] who use drugs do so only if the symptoms are so severe that they threaten the patient or the analysis, and do not respond to analysis. In short drugs are not a substitute for but an adjunct to the analytic process. (p. 220)

Over the subsequent two decades, many psychoanalysts have reconsidered the initial resistance to the use of psychotropic medication. In his reconsideration of the psychoanalysis of a patient with masochistic personality who also met diagnostic criteria for dysthymia and panic disorder, Arnold Cooper (1985) concluded that "retrospectively, pharmacological assistance earlier might have provided a much clearer focus on her content-related psychodynamic problems and would have made it more difficult for her to use her symptoms masochistically as proof that she was an innocent victim of endless emotional pain" (p. 1400).

The conflictual origins of many syndromes, including some considered to be paradigmatic of psychoanalytic theory such as obsessional neurosis, have been questioned, and the lack of therapeutic efficacy of psychoanalysis in these conditions has been noted (Esman 1989). It has been argued that one-dimensional theoretical models are no longer tenable and that combining multiple modalities of treatment is not only conceptually more sophisticated but therapeutically advantageous. Unfortunately, constructive re-evaluation of psychoanalytic theories of etiology and therapeutic efficacy in certain conditions has led some clinicians to artificially divide psychopathology into two groups. According to this construct, Axis I disorders are biological (i.e., not derived from intrapsychic conflict), and therefore somatic rather than psychological treatments are necessary. In contrast, Axis II disorders are the result of intrapsychic conflict, and the primary modality of treatment should be a psychoanalytic approach (see Roose 1995). If both Axis I and II disorders are present, medication should be combined with psychoanalysis because "there is an analysis being conducted simultaneously with the management of a medical illness" (Finkel 1986). Although acknowledging the therapeutic effect of medication, this approach is problematic for two reasons: 1) there is no empirical or theoretical basis for this division, and 2) artificially dividing the etiologies of Axis I and Axis II disorders reflects a discredited mind-body dichotomy.

Despite these theoretical debates, clinical pragmatism has ultimately led not only to an appreciation of the therapeutic effects of psychotropic medication but also to the relatively widespread use of medication in combination with psychoanalytic treatment. Studies indicate that approximately 20%–35% of patients in analysis are also taking psychotropic medication (Caligor et al. 2003; Donovan and Roose 1995; Roose and Stern 1995; Yang et al. 2003). Although psychoanalysis and psychotropic medication are now commonly used concurrently, these two treatments, based on different models of the mind and requiring divergent styles of intervention on the part of the clinician, have not been technically or theoretically integrated. Currently, the critical clinical issue is no longer whether analytic patients should be prescribed psychotropic medication, but rather how to combine these treatments most effectively. Specific questions include the following:

1. How does the analyst decide when to prescribe or to refer the patient for a medication consultation?
2. Can a psychoanalyst practice optimal psychopharmacology in the psychoanalytic situation?
3. What is the impact of psychotropic medication prescription on the analyst, the patient, and the treatment itself?

In this chapter, we consider these questions and review data from the relevant empirical studies.

Empirical Studies: Rates of Combined Treatment With Medication and Psychoanalysis

The rate of psychotropic medication use in the psychoanalytic setting has been documented in a number of studies surveying candidates, graduate analysts, and training analysts. The first systematic assessment of the combination treatment of psychotropic medication and psychoanalysis was a study of control case patients being treated by candidates at the Center for Psychoanalytic Training and Research at Columbia University. In this study, 89% of candidates returned a survey inquiring about psychotropic medication use, and they reported that 29% (16/56) of patients currently in analysis were also being prescribed medication (Roose and Stern 1995). This practice was not restricted to a few candidates; 46% (11/24) of candidates returning the survey had at least one patient in analysis who was also taking psychotropic medication.

It could be hypothesized that the results of this study are based on a skewed sample and do not reflect general practice in psychoanalysis—that is, the rate of medication prescription by a cohort of candidates trained in clinical psychiatry after the use of psychotropic medication became standard treatment for mood and psychotic disorder might be significantly greater than the rate in a group of more senior analysts trained in a previous era. However, a subsequent study of training and supervising analysts at Columbia produced strikingly similar results (Donovan and Roose 1995). In this study, 76% (34/45) of the training analysts returned the survey. The group had a mean age of 60±8 years; that is, they were considerably older than the candidate cohort in the previous study.

The training analyst group reported on 277 patients who had been in analysis within the past 5 years, 18% (51/277) of whom had been prescribed psychotropic medication. Again, this was not a practice restricted to just a few: 62% (21/34) of training analysts reported having had at least one patient who was taking medication. The training and supervising analysts also reported that of the 51 psychoanalytic patients taking medication, 43 (84%) were diagnosed by the treating analyst as having either major depressive disorder or dysthymia. Not surprisingly, antidepressants were the most common class of medication prescribed. The psychoanalysts were also asked to assess the impact of medication on the mood disorder and on the analytic process. In 84% (36/43) of the patients with a current mood disorder who were prescribed medication, the psychoanalysts reported that the mood disorder improved and that the analytic process deepened.

Recently, studies at two psychoanalytic institutes (Columbia and Cincinnati) reported the rates of psychotropic medication use in current psychoanalytic cases among graduate analysts (Yang et al. 2003). In the Columbia study, 87 analysts reported on 241 patients in psychoanalysis, 31% (75/241) of whom were being prescribed psychotropic medication. In the Cincinnati study, of 69 patients in psychoanalysis reported on by 23 analysts, 36% (25/69) were being prescribed psychotropic medication. These studies, conducted in 2002, document that the prescription of psychotropic medication, once considered the quintessential anti-analytic intervention, is now the most accepted and prevalent significant change in the practice of psychoanalysis during the last 30 years. The rates of prescribing psychotropic medication, primarily antidepressants, appear appropriate given studies that have shown that 30%–50% of patients currently entering psychoanalysis have an Axis I mood and/or anxiety disorder (Vaughan et al. 2000).

The Decision to Prescribe Medication

The nature of the information necessary for a clinician to make an informed recommendation about medication requires an evaluation approach that may be a significant departure from standard technique for many psychoanalysts. Patients presenting to a psychoanalyst often do so with the intent of entering into a psychodynamic psychotherapy or psychoanalysis. The standard psychoanalytic evaluation focuses on developing a dynamic case formulation and an assessment of whether the patient has qualities, such as psychological mindedness or the capacity to contain intense affect states, considered necessary to engage in a long-term psychodynamic treatment. The initial evaluation is more an assessment of the "analyzability" of the patient than a diagnostic evaluation.

There is no consensus among psychoanalysts on either the validity of a phenomenologically based diagnostic system, such as DSM-IV (American Psychiatric Association 2000) or the relevance of psychiatric diagnoses to the recommendation for psychoanalysis. Indeed, some psychoanalysts believe the initial evaluation of a patient is so limited by the patient's defenses and the absence of a therapeutic alliance that the information necessary for an accurate diagnosis of character structure, defenses, and core psychic conflicts can emerge only through the analytic process itself. Thus, the goal of the initial consultation is not to gather information but rather to see if the patient can engage in the process that is unique to psychodynamic treatment.

Clinical Example

Ms. A presented to Dr. Z, a psychoanalyst, with the complaint that she seemed to have lost some of her "drive for life." A 52-year-old businesswoman, Ms. A had continued to work effectively but complained that she came home every night and collapsed on the couch while watching television. In response to Dr. Z's question about what was happening at this point in her life, Ms. A noted that she had been divorced for 5 years and that her son, with whom she felt quite close, had just started college 2 months ago. When Dr. Z made the connection between the onset of her decreased energy and her son's departure, Ms. A became tearful and said that she felt alone and empty without him. Dr. Z made a mental note of Ms. A's capacity to reflect on her circumstances in an affectively connected way, and thought that this boded well for her ability to work in psychotherapy or analysis. However, Dr. Z failed to ask Ms. A other questions about her symptoms and general emotional state (e.g., questions about sleep, appetite, concentration problems, self-esteem), did not ascertain how long these symptoms had persisted, and thus was not able to make a diagnosis.

Though such an approach to consultation may be effective for assessment of character pathology and appropriate for psychodynamic psychotherapy or analysis, it is not an optimal approach for the diagnosis of affective and anxiety disorders. The issue of diagnosis is particularly critical with respect to the recommendation of medication; data on the efficacy and side effects of psychotropic medications come from studies that diagnose patients on the basis of phenomenologically based diagnostic systems such as DSM-IV. The primary goal of the consultation in clinical psychiatry, in contrast to the psychoanalytic consultation, is to make a diagnosis. Although such a consultation should include the assessment of the patient's core conflicts, level of personality organization, family structure and dynamics, occupational functioning, and socioeconomic status, an accurate clinical diagnosis is always a goal of the consultation, and this diagnosis will feature prominently in the clinician's treatment recommendations.

Currently, clinical diagnosis is based on the phenomenological diagnostic system outlined in the DSM series. The phenomenological approach was brought into prominence by DSM-III (American Psychiatric Association 1980), which itself was based on the Research Diagnostic Criteria (RDC; Spitzer et al. 1978) developed to facilitate clinical trials in patients with mood disorders and schizophrenia. Psychoanalysts have had strong disagreements with the conceptual and clinical approach used in DSM-III and DSM-IV to define and diagnose Axis II (personality) disorders, and perhaps with good reason. However, this has led many psychoanalysts to reject DSM Axis I disorders, despite the fact that the diagnostic system for these disorders is evidence-based, supported by extensive field trials, and proven to be quite useful. Data on the efficacy and side effects of psychotropic medications come from studies that include patients selected on the basis of phenomenologically based diagnostic systems such as DSM-IV. This is not to say that the only patients who should be treated with psychotropic medications are those who meet the full criteria for Axis I mood or anxiety disorders. Indeed, patients with subsyndromal conditions and syndromes included in the research appendix of DSM-IV but not the main body (e.g., mixed anxiety-depression states) are also commonly prescribed psychotropic medications in clinical practice.

The very act of making a clinical psychiatric diagnosis may conflict with many psychoanalysts' approach to initial evaluation in which they attempt 1) to engage the patient, 2) to evaluate the patient's capacity for psychodynamic treatment, and 3) to judge the appropriateness of the patient for analysis with respect to certain kinds of psychopathology. The specifics of diagnosis are less important to the psychoanalyst who may believe that all the information will come out in the course of time and that how that information is revealed is as important as the information itself. However, the decision regarding whether to recommend medication treatment starts with the presence or absence of an Axis I disorder, and making that determination may require an approach unfamiliar to many psychoanalysts. For example, the diagnosis of major depressive disorder is based on whether a patient has a certain number of specific symptoms, the determination of which requires a more active interview approach that may be unusual or even uncomfortable for many psychoanalysts. Many psychoanalysts contend that in the hands of a skilled clinician, an unstructured, open-ended interview that focuses on process and unconscious content will gather all of the information necessary to make a phenomenological diagnosis. However, this has not been supported by a number of studies, which showed that psychoanalysts frequently had missed the diagnosis of Axis I mood, anxiety, or substance abuse disorders that were subsequently diagnosed on the basis of a structured diagnostic interview (Vaughan et al. 2000). To ensure the most informed treatment recommendations, a psychoanalyst must do a complete clinical assessment that includes both a case formulation and a diagnostic assessment. Though psychoanalysts may not need to administer a structured interview to gather the information necessary to make a diagnosis, they must recognize that their traditional technique is inadequate for making an accurate Axis I diagnosis.

The goals of the traditional psychoanalytic evaluation and the clinical psychiatric evaluation are different but not necessarily competitive or contradictory. On the contrary, they can be complementary and are certainly both necessary. Thus, from the very first time that a psychoanalyst meets a patient, the analyst must be cognizant of the different models of the mind, theories of illness, and clinical techniques that must be equally applied and respected in order to decide on optimal treatment interventions—and the evaluation should reflect this paradigm.

Thus, the decision regarding whether to recommend treatment with psychotropic medication for a patient in psychoanalysis should depend on the psychoanalyst's acquisition and use of appropriate data necessary to make an informed clinical recommendation. However, many other factors, beyond the clinical data, may influence the analyst's decision. For candidates in psychoanalytic training these influences include the pressures of training, such as fears that prescription of medication for a control case might impede a candidate's progression, supervisors who disagree with the use of medication in psychoanalysis, and a supervisor's interpretation that the candidate's wish to medicate represents countertransference issues (Abel-Horowitz 1998).

Clinical Example

Dr. B, a third-year candidate, had been treating Mr. Y in psychoanalysis for 1 year when Mr. Y began to complain of severe anxiety attacks. The onset of these attacks coincided with Mr. Y's graduation from law school and his preparation for taking the bar exam. Dr. B explored the meaning of graduation to Mr. Y, whose father was the managing partner in a large law firm, and interpreted Mr. Y's conflicts about studying law. Despite these interventions, Mr. Y's anxiety attacks worsened. Mr. Y complained to Dr. B that he was having palpitations that woke him from sleep, and said that he feared that he was having a heart attack. Dr. B wondered whether Mr. Y might be suffering from panic disorder but also was confused about the extent to which the psychodynamic issues might be producing the anxiety. He was afraid to approach his supervisor with this issue, fearing that his supervisor might think that he was not "thinking like a psychoanalyst" and worrying that treating the patient with medication might jeopardize his "getting credit for the case."

There are some data that illuminate the influence of the psychoanalytic situation on the candidate's decision to prescribe medication. A study conducted at the Columbia University Center for Psychoanalytic Training and Research compared candidate-training cases in which patients that applied directly to the Psychoanalytic Clinic for treatment with training cases in which patients had been converted from psychotherapy to analysis from the candidates' private practices (Caligor et al. 2003). The clinic and converted case patients did not differ significantly in mean age, sex distribution, or whether or not the candidate received credit for the case. The rates of Axis I mood and anxiety disorders were comparable in both the clinic and converted cases (53% and 58%, respectively), and 9% of both samples had current substance abuse related to drugs other than nicotine. However, despite comparable rates of Axis I disorders, there was a striking difference in the rates of antidepressant medication prescription; 56% of the converted case patients vs. 6% of the clinic case patients were prescribed medication ($\chi^2_1 = 21.2$, $P<0.0001$). If one considers medication prescription only in patients with current Axis I mood disorder, then 0% of the clinic case patients vs. 81% of the converted case patients with the same diagnosis were prescribed medication ($\chi^2_1 = 12.2$, $P<0.0001$). Thus, the same psychoanalytic candidate recommending treatment for diagnostically comparable patients prescribed antidepressant medication for analytic patients in the private practice setting but not for patients entering psychoanalysis through the psychoanalytic clinic. There are many possible explanations for this finding—for example, the desire to have a "pure" analytic case or the influence of the supervisor—and a better understanding of the results of the study awaits further empirical research. However, at the very least, it can be said that the setting affected the decision to prescribe medication.

The influence of factors other than diagnosis on the analyst's decision to recommend medication is not restricted to candidates. Graduate analysts wanting to conduct "ideal" or "standard" psychoanalysis may aspire to adhere to an "abstinent model" that would preclude the use of medication (Kelly 1998). Others have written about their concern that the recommendation of medication might affect the patient's feelings of self-esteem or be a confirmation of the patient's self-representation as defective (Swoiskin 2001).

Treatment Recommendations and Informed Consent

Originally, the process of informed consent was restricted to invasive procedures or participation in research. However, the concept of informed consent has been extended and is now expected to be an explicit part of the interaction between a doctor and patient whenever treatment is recommended. The principles of informed consent mandate that it is the clinician's responsibility to discuss the rationale for the recommended treatment and to inform the patient of all reasonable treatment options including the evidence that supports their efficacy. Therefore, if a psychoanalyst makes a diagnosis of major depressive dis-

order in a patient for whom he or she is recommending psychoanalysis, the psychoanalyst is ethically bound to discuss antidepressant medication as a treatment option, as well as cognitive-behavioral therapy and interpersonal psychotherapy, which have also been demonstrated to have efficacy in treating major depressive disorder.

Since there are treatments with proven efficacy for many Axis I diagnoses, the discussion of these efficacious treatments is mandatory. If there is no Axis I diagnosis, the rationale for the recommendation of psychoanalysis and possible alternative treatments must still be discussed. The process of informed consent is the responsibility of the psychoanalyst regardless of professional background. Therefore, this issue raises the educational responsibility of psychoanalytic institutes with respect to the training of candidates with little or no experience in psychiatric diagnosis and/or the DSM-IV diagnostic criteria, as well as the ethical obligations of non-M.D. psychoanalysts to discuss treatment options that might have to be provided by another practitioner.

To the psychoanalyst, the process of conducting a diagnostic interview to elicit phenomenology and making treatment recommendations according to the concept of informed consent might feel intrusive, awkward, distinctly nonanalytic, and certainly replete with theoretical and technical conflicts with the psychoanalytic attitude. Though cognizant of the therapeutic effectiveness of psychotropic medications and willing to prescribe them for some patients, a psychoanalyst may still feel that the phenomenological diagnostic approach and attention to brain physiology, though necessary, not only are at odds with but threaten the psychoanalytic framework. Such a belief may lead to a perpetuation of the old treatment hierarchy in which psychoanalysis is always the preferred treatment and medication should be recommended only in the most severe circumstances or when there are therapeutic stalemates.

Such a framework may actually work against engaging many depressed patients in a psychoanalytic treatment. Studies have documented that there is an inverse correlation between severity of depression and the capacity for psychological mindedness (Vaughan et al. 2000). Thus, a depressed patient has a reduced capacity to participate in a psychodynamic process. Rather than perpetuate the belief that medication and psychoanalysis are treatments in conflict, psychoanalysts should consider them compatible, synergistic, and even at times mutually dependent. For example, some depressed or anxious patients may benefit from psychopharmacological treatment before entering psychotherapy or psychoanalysis (Roose 1995). With a depressed or very anxious patient, the sequencing of treatments may significantly benefit the induction phase and the development of analytic process.

Clinical Example

Mr. S consulted Dr. J, a psychoanalyst, with the chief complaint that he was having difficulty with public speaking that was interfering with his job performance. Mr. S. gave a history of lifelong shyness in public, which led him, over the years, to avoid courses, and later jobs, that required this of him. Now, however, he had advanced to the point in his company when he could no longer avoid public speaking. In the course of his evaluation with Dr. J, Mr. S explained that when he spoke in public, he sweated profusely, often had palpitations, and had a quivering voice. He also described his mother as quite ambitious for him, particulary in the realm of music, in which he had shown some talent. He recalled that his mother forced him to play in public despite his anxiety and pushed him into music competitions at a very young age. Dr. J asked him about symptoms of other anxiety disorders, which he denied. After two sessions, Dr. J explained to Mr. S that he might suffer from performance anxiety, for which many people took medication but that this might also be treated in psychotherapy. Mr. S said that while he appreciated that there might be a medication for his difficulty, he preferred to try to work on his problems by talking. Dr. J suggested to Mr. S that they begin psychotherapy but that the option for using medication could be revisited at any time.

The Psychoanalyst as Pharmacologist and Issues of Split Treatment

The treatment combination of psychoanalysis and medication can be delivered in two different ways. In the first, referred to as "split treatment," the psychoanalysis and medication treatments are administered by different clinicians. In the second, the psychoanalyst both conducts the analysis and acts as psychopharmacologist.

Split Treatment

Originally, the procedure of split treatment was developed because it was believed that psychoanalysts could not maintain analytic neutrality if they participated in the more active doctor-patient relationship necessary for the effective and safe administration of psychotropic medication. As a way to preserve technical neutrality and avoid the development of iatrogenic transference paradigms, the analysis was separated from the medication treatment, often to the point where the psychoanalyst and psychopharmacologist did not communicate. Obviously, the relationship between the psychoanalyst and patient regarding medication will differ depending on whether the treatment is split or not. In a split treatment, the effective administration of combined psychoanalysis and psychopharmacological treat-

ments requires the establishment of multiple therapeutic alliances: between the analyst and patient, between the patient and psychopharmacologist, and, perhaps most importantly, between the psychoanalyst and psychopharmacologist (Kahn 1991; Roose 1990; Vaughan et al. 1997). This last relationship is often unexplored, is certainly unstudied, and may generate profound theoretical conflicts and professional rivalries that negatively impact the treatment and the way the patient experiences the treatment. If a split treatment is failing, attention to the relationship between the psychoanalyst and psychopharmacologist may be the critical intervention (Roose 1990).

Clinical Example

Ms. R had been in psychoanalysis with Dr. S for 3 years when she developed symptoms of major depression, characterized by anhedonia, depressed mood, and sleep and appetite disturbance. Dr. S, a psychologist, explored Ms. R's symptoms in the context of the transference, which recently had been dominated by Ms. R's rage at the analyst for having taken a 4-week vacation at a time of year that he did not usually go away. Despite his conviction that Ms. R was depressed because of her ambivalently held feelings for him, after a few weeks of hearing Ms. R's symptoms, Dr. S suggested to Ms. R that she have a consultation with a psychopharmacologist. The consultant diagnosed Ms. R with major depression and prescribed an antidepressant. Ms. R, relieved by this decision, returned to Dr. S further enraged that Dr. S had taken a few weeks to send her for a medication consultation. Dr. S was glad that the patient had received the medication treatment but still wondered if Ms. R's symptoms would have remitted with psychoanalysis alone.

Perhaps because of this lingering doubt, Dr. S failed to explore Ms. R's feelings about his inability to prescribe the medication and did not communicate directly with the pharmacologist after receiving his consultation note. In the next few weeks, when Ms. R felt depressed, she called the psychopharmacologist to see whether her medication should be increased, rather than continuing to discuss both aspects of her treatment with Dr. S. Although Dr. S interpreted this split to Ms. R, he did not attempt to discuss this with the consultant. In addition, Dr. S interpreted Ms. R's fantasy that the increase in medication would solve the problems she had with trusting him. Approximately 1 month after Ms. R's depression remitted, she abruptly stopped her analysis, citing Dr. S's lack of conviction about the effectiveness of the medication as her reason for terminating prematurely.

Currently most medically trained psychoanalysts choose not to split treatments. The recent surveys of medication use by graduate psychoanalysts at the Columbia and Cincinnati institutes indicate that it is a relatively rare occurrence for medically trained psychoanalysts not to prescribe medication for their own patients (Yang et al. 2003).

Possible explanations for this change in practice include the increasing recognition that the transference and countertransference paradigms encountered when the analyst prescribes medication can be interpreted as part of the analysis (Cabaniss 1998; Kelly 1998; Roose 1990), as well as the introduction of antidepressant medications (e.g., the selective serotonin reuptake inhibitors, or SSRIs) that appear, perhaps deceptively, easier to dose and are associated with fewer problematic side effects.

Sometimes, however, it may become necessary or prudent for the physician/analyst to suggest that an analysand see a psychopharmacologist for medication. This may occur when the medication management takes up a disproportionate amount of time in the analytic hours, or when an increasingly complex medication regimen exceeds the analyst's pharmacological expertise. This situation may have ramifications for both the transference and the countertransference. It may be difficult for the psychiatrist/analyst to acknowledge the need for help in this area. The psychiatrist practicing pharmacology with his or her analysands may fear that patients will no longer see value in analysis if they are sent to an outside pharmacologist. When present in the analyst, these fantasies need to be explored in self-analysis or with the help of supervisor; when present in the patient, the unearthing of such fantasies is an essential part of a full analysis. An analysand may devalue the analyst who feels the need to have a pharmacologist help with the medication; if interpreted, this response may become part of the necessary understanding of the analyst's limitations.

Clinical Example

Mr. W, a 60-year-old man with a history of heart disease and major depression, was in his third year of analysis. Mr. W had originally presented to the analyst, Dr. I, in the midst of a major depressive episode. The analyst, who was a psychiatrist, had treated Mr. W with fluoxetine, which he had continued to take throughout the analysis. Now Mr. W was having a relapse that was not responding to increasing doses of fluoxetine. Concomitantly, Mr. W was having more difficulties with his underlying cardiac illness, leading to sporadic arrhythmias. Dr. I tried different augmentation strategies, with some success. Mr. W became hopeless, fearing that his cardiologists would not be able to handle his medical condition and that he would have a fatal arrhythmia.

Over the next few weeks, Dr. I became increasingly anxious in sessions with Mr. W. At one point, Mr. W dreamed that he lived in a house with Dr. I and that Dr. I was cooking a meal for him. Dr. I felt unable to listen carefully to the dream and was unable to formulate an interpretation. Usually confident of his formulation of Mr. W's case, Dr. I now sought supervision with a peer, who suggested that Dr. I might be anxious about prescribing increasingly complex antidepressants in the face of Mr. W's underlying medical condition.

Following this supervision, Dr. I suggested to the patient that the dream of the meal might reflect feelings that the patient had about the medication that the analyst was prescribing for the patient. Mr. W said that he had a wish that Dr. I could prescribe all of his medications, including his cardiac medications. Dr. I linked this wish to the dream and told Mr. W that because of his worsening depression and cardiac condition, he felt that Mr. W should consult a pharmacologist with expertise in treatment of depression and arrhythmia. Initially, Mr. W felt angry at Dr. I, stating that he had sought out an analyst who was also a psychiatrist in order to avoid a split treatment. Over the ensuing weeks, Dr. I interpreted the patient's feelings of rejection and their relationship to wishes that Mr. W had about feeling perfectly cared for by the analyst. Eventually, Mr. W agreed to the consultation, and with the new psychopharmacological regimen his depression gradually lifted. Over the next year, this episode became linked to the patient's growing understanding of the analyst's limitations and contributed to his conceptualization of the analyst as a separate, three-dimensional person.

This vignette demonstrates the ways in which the patient's fantasies about the analyst can become intertwined with the pharmacological management. In this way, attending to the vicissitudes of the pharmacology and the roles that both patient and analyst/pharmacologist play in the pharmacological aspect of the treatment can yield important information about the transference/countertransference paradigms that are dominant in the treatment.

Adding a third person to the analytic setting in which the analyst had conducted the pharmacology may reveal new fantasies and enactments. Patients and analysts may value the "secrecy" of the dyadic relationship; thus, the advent of splitting the treatment can bring up interesting fantasies for both patient and analyst. Analysts may have secret fears of being found to be lacking, while patients may seek to protect or attack their analysts with the new member of the team. Once an analysand has consulted with the pharmacologist, the patient may cease to talk about mood problems with the analyst. Rather than approach these potentialities as problematic, they can be seen as adding richness to the analysis in the way that they may unearth unconscious fantasies in analyst and analysand that might have otherwise remained unexplored.

It is a different situation when split treatment is necessary rather than optional—a scenario that occurs with increasing frequency as the number of non–medically trained psychoanalysts grows. The issues raised by split treatment between a nonmedical psychoanalyst and a psychopharmacologist extend beyond the administration of medication and include the process of diagnostic assessment. Given the rates of mood and anxiety disorders in patients currently presenting for psychoanalytic treatment, the psychoanalyst who is not trained in clinical psychiatric diagnosis must nonetheless be able to conduct a diagnostic screening that can adequately identify patients who require a more complete diagnostic and medication evaluation. The issue of diagnosis and prescription of medication is perhaps the most obvious, but not the only, area in which psychoanalytic institutes must consider the educational needs of the non–medically trained psychoanalyst.

The Psychoanalyst-Psychopharmacologist

If a psychoanalyst is also prescribing the medication, the preeminent concern has traditionally been whether the role of pharmacologist will interfere with analytic neutrality or the conduct of the analysis. Specific concerns that have been voiced are whether the use of medication and the subsequent reduction in depression and/or anxiety would undermine the patient's motivation for and commitment to a long-term treatment or whether the quality and quantity of interaction necessary to effectively administer medication would interfere with the development of transference paradigms (Roose 1990). As cited previously, the admittedly few systematically collected data available suggest that the use of medication does not endanger the analytic situation; to the contrary, training analysts have reported that the effective use of antidepressant medication resulted in a deepening of the analytic process (Donovan and Roose 1995). This finding is consistent with data that psychological mindedness and depression severity are inversely correlated and that improvement in depression results in a greater engagement in a psychoanalytic treatment (Vaughan et al. 2000).

However, the impact of being a psychopharmacologist on the role of the analyst and on the analysis may well have dimensions that are not apparent if one looks only within the analysis itself. For example, a study of posttermination contact documented striking and unexpected findings (Yang et al. 2003). In this study, 87 graduate analysts (35% of the sample were training analysts) reported on 241 cases that represented their three most recently terminated psychoanalytic patients. In this sample, 31% (75/241) of patients were taking psychotropic medication during analysis. After termination, 22% (20/87) of the analysts continued to function as psychopharmacologists for at least one of their now terminated psychoanalytic patients. Given that there was full knowledge before the termination that the patient and the analyst would continue to see each other in some professional capacity, this expectation must have affected the termination phase. Thus, the analyst's assuming the role of psychopharmacologist has an impact on all aspects of the psychoanalysis, including the evaluation of the patient, the induction into analysis,

the analytic process, the termination phase, and the posttermination period. This does not mean that the analyst-pharmacologist cannot function well in the analytic role, but rather that all of the ramifications of this dual role need to be more fully studied in order to understand and teach about the impact of this special situation on the analyst, the patient, and the analysis.

To date, the primary concern about an analyst who serves two functions has been whether the role of pharmacologist interferes with the role of psychoanalyst. There has been little consideration of whether a psychoanalyst who prescribes medication and practices psychoanalysis can deliver optimal psychopharmacological treatment—that is, Does the role of psychoanalyst interfere with the conduct of psychopharmacology? This question involves two dimensions, one of knowledge and one of technique. With respect to knowledge, the more frequent prescription of antidepressant medications by psychoanalysts may have resulted not simply from a theoretical reconsideration of the compatibility of the two treatments or the clinical pragmatism to use what works, but also in large part from the introduction of the SSRIs. The first antidepressant medications introduced, the tricyclic antidepressants (TCAs) and monoamine oxidase inhibitors (MAOIs), were complex to use with respect to dosing and the necessity of plasma level measurements, had many poorly tolerated side effects, and were associated with significant safety issues such as cardiovascular effects, a high overdose mortality rate, and the potential for fatal hypertensive crises. The introduction of the SSRIs made available a class of antidepressants with a more benign side-effect profile, fewer safety issues, and greater ease in dosing. Furthermore, the efficacy of the SSRIs in both mood and anxiety disorders may have made precise diagnosis seem less critical.

In reality, while the introduction of the SSRIs may have made antidepressant treatments more accessible to the general clinician, it has in no way made the optimal treatment of depression less complicated. Within the past decade, the cumulative evidence strongly indicates that the goal of the treatment of depression should no longer be symptom reduction, generally referred to as "response" and defined as a 50% reduction in baseline symptoms, but rather "remission" of the illness, which is generally defined as the absence of symptoms and return to premorbid baseline functioning (Frank et al. 1991). Patients who have symptomatic reduction but do not achieve remission have a significantly higher rate of relapse, develop chronic depressive symptoms, and remain at risk for the increased rate of cardiovascular and cerebrovascular disease that is associated with depressive illness (Frasure-Smith et al. 1993; Judd et al. 2000; Paykel et al. 1995).

The designation that attaining remission status represents optimal treatment for depression has two significant implications for clinicians treating this illness. First, fewer than half of patients will achieve remission with the first antidepressant treatment prescribed; most patients require a switch in class of medication or augmentation of the initial antidepressant with a second medication (Thase et al. 2001). Psychopharmacologists understand that treating a depressed patient with medication often requires a series of antidepressant medications or a combination of medications given at an adequate dose for adequate duration. The implication for the psychoanalyst prescribing an antidepressant medication is that residual depressive symptoms present after the first antidepressant trial signify partial response and should not be labeled as character structure until a complete pharmacological strategy has been executed.

Second, clinicians need a method of assessing whether a patient has achieved remission; they cannot simply rely exclusively on their own estimation of symptom reduction. In most studies, remission is defined as a final Hamilton Depression Rating Scale score of 7 or lower (usual score for a depressed patient is from 20 to 30). This rating scale is not usually used by psychiatric clinicians and is certainly out of place in a psychoanalytic treatment. Fortunately, a less intrusive and easier-to-use rating scale, the Clinical Global Impression (CGI) Improvement Scale, has a good correlation with the Hamilton scale. The CGI Improvement Scale combines the clinician's and patient's assessments of improvement from baseline. A score of 1, which corresponds to an 85% improvement, signifies remission. The psychoanalyst who prescribes medication needs to use techniques that are standard in pharmacological practice in order to evaluate effect of medication.

Although rating scales may represent the gold standard for determining presence or absence of the affective disorders described in DSM-IV, clinicians may be unschooled in their use or feel they are awkward to use in the clinical situation. These clinicians may choose to familiarize themselves with the items on the rating scales so that they can seamlessly incorporate them into their evaluation interviews and extract them, if possible, from the analytic material. Whether or not the scales themselves are used, it is important to include phenomenological diagnostic considerations in the evaluation of every patient, even when the patient has presented for psychoanalysis or psychoanalytic psychotherapy, and to rely on phenomenological data when making decisions about medication in the course of treatment.

Clinical Example

When Mr. T presented for evaluation with Dr. W, he described a lifelong history of low mood and poor self-esteem that had not interfered with academic or work

function but that had markedly impaired his object relationships. Upon further exploration of this and other symptoms, Dr. W suggested to Mr. T that he enter psychoanalysis in order to further understand the roots of his low self-esteem and difficulties in his relationships with others. In psychoanalysis, Mr. T quickly developed a masochistic transference to the analyst, characterized by willingness to make any and all schedule changes and an inability to recognize any angry feelings toward the analyst. Dr. W did not think that he was hearing other symptoms of affective disorder and did not prescribe medication. However, 2 weeks prior to Dr. W's 4-week August vacation, Mr. T again brought up his low mood, and Dr. W decided to prescribe medication, since Mr. T wouldn't be seeing the analyst for 4 weeks.

In this example, the analyst made the decision to prescribe medication *not* on the basis of the presence or absence of symptoms that would constitute major depression, but rather because of his anxiety that the patient needed "something" in his absence.

The Practice of Psychopharmacology in an Ongoing Analysis

The information needed to evaluate medication effect and decide if treatment changes are needed will not necessarily just emerge in the course of free association. Even if psychoanalysts employ a phenomenological as well as a dynamic theoretical approach in the initial evaluation, thereby allowing for an informed recommendation about medication, it does not necessarily follow that they will be able to maintain a phenomenological perspective during the course of the analysis and thereby access the information necessary to practice optimal pharmacology.

Psychoanalysts are explicitly trained to look for multiple meanings beyond the manifest content of the patient's verbal associations, affect states, and behaviors. Thus, when a patient reports persistently low mood, anhedonia, hopelessness, worthlessness, and other symptoms of a mood or anxiety disorder, the psychoanalyst will consider this material in the context of the current transference/countertransference paradigm and the unconscious meaning and motivation of the depressive symptoms. For example, the analyst would consider, separate from the therapeutic effect, what meaning and impact the act of prescribing medication could have in the context of the transference. Furthermore, the symbolic meanings of medication to the analysand, such as the fantasy of being fed by the analyst or the medication as transitional object, have been extensively discussed in the literature (Adelman 1985; Cabaniss 2001; Gutheil 1982; Hausner 1985; Levy 1977). Though the analyst must consider the meaning of both the act of taking medication and the act of prescribing, phenomenological data, not dynamic data, are the determinants of medication management. The analyst must temporarily abandon analytic metapsychology and technique in order to practice psychopharmacology and then return to the analytic position. Such transitions, which may need to be done frequently, are difficult.

The only study of the practice of psychopharmacology by psychoanalysts during the course of an analysis is one that included all training cases begun by candidates at the Columbia University Center for Psychoanalytic Training and Research between September 1992 through September 1995 in which the patient either had a diagnosis of an Axis I mood or anxiety disorder at the point of initial evaluation or was prescribed psychotropic medication at some point during the analysis (N. Gwynn, S. Roose: "Medication Management During Psychoanalysis," unpublished manuscript, 2003). All the material in the charts was reviewed, including the initial evaluation by the candidate and supervisor and detailed narrative summaries of the treatment after 3 months and yearly thereafter. All references to diagnosis or to medication were noted, and summaries of the relevant chart material were developed. The case patients were separated into three groups: 1) patients taking medication prior to analysis or patients who started taking medication at the time of beginning analysis, 2) patients who were prescribed and began taking medication during the analysis, and 3) patients diagnosed with mood or anxiety disorder who were not taking medication during analysis.

In this study, 52% (40/77) of the patients had a current mood or anxiety disorder, and 39% (30/77) of the patients were taking medication at some point during the analysis. Of the 30 patients taking psychotropic medication during analysis, two charts were unavailable for review. Of the remaining 28 patients, 9 had started taking medication prior to analysis with no change during the analysis; 8 patients had been taking medication prior to analysis and changes in medication were made during the course of the analysis; and 8 patients entered analysis taking medication, which was discontinued. (In 4 of the last-mentioned cases, there was a significant recrudescence of symptoms and medication was reinstituted.) Only 3 patients started taking medication during the analysis.

A review of the charts led to the following conclusions:

1. Documentation of medication treatment, including assessment of response and side effects, was inadequate in the overwhelming number of charts and absent in many.
2. In many cases, medication was changed in response to either the patient's or the analyst's reaction to an upcoming separation, most notably changes in medica-

tion or initiation of medication within 3 weeks of the summer vacation.
3. In a number of cases there was no evidence in the chart that medication was ever discussed or that the current treatment was reviewed by the analyst.
4. In most cases, the candidate did not make medication decisions on the basis of appropriate data and effectively differentiate this information from the analytic process.

In contrast to the inadequate documentation about medication decisions, the charts included thoughtful documentation of the analytic process, revisions of the initial dynamic formulation, and discussions of transference and countertransference paradigms, some related specifically to the medication.

The results of the study suggest that in this cohort of patients, the analyst did not adequately fulfill the role of psychopharmacologist. Why did this occur? One possible explanation is that in the psychoanalytic setting, the role of psychopharmacologist is considered secondary to being a psychoanalyst, just as the psychotropic medication is considered adjunctive or secondary to the analytic treatment. Another is that there is inadequate didactic and supervisory teaching about the impact the role of psychopharmacologist or the addition of a psychopharmacological consultant will have on all aspects of the psychoanalysis. The impact on the analyst of assuming the responsibilities of psychopharmacologist in the analytic situation has not been sufficiently appreciated, and further study is needed to determine whether a single practitioner can optimally administer both forms of treatment and, if so, what this practice requires. Inquiry of this nature is likely to suggest that psychoanalytic educators need to provide focused teaching—for M.D. analysts and non–medically trained analysts—about the use of phenomenological data in assessing affective disorders in their analytic patients, and about the particular challenges of being both the analyst and the prescriber of medications for the same patient.

Training psychoanalysts about conducting good pharmacology with their analytic patients seems to be an obvious goal. However, it is worth wondering and potentially studying whether psychoanalysts are in fact able to conduct optimal pharmacology with their psychoanalytic patients, even if they possess outstanding pharmacological skills and knowledge. It is possible that the intense pressures of the psychoanalytic situation and the omnipresent vicissitudes and enactments of the transference and countertransference preclude even the most knowledgable pharmacologist from conducting optimal pharmacology while also analyzing a patient. It may behoove pharmacologist-analysts to at least consider this possibility and to acknowledge their limitations when and if they arise.

Conclusion

Although pharmacology still has little place in the theory of psychoanalysis, studies of clinical practice indicate that from 20% to 36% of patients in psychoanalysis are concomitantly being treated with psychotropic medication. The use of medication affects every aspect of the psychoanalysis. The efficacy of these psychotropic medications has been demonstrated in clinical trials based on the phenomenological diagnoses outlined in the DSM series. Therefore, all psychoanalysts must be trained to make Axis I diagnoses, understand the treatment implications of these diagnoses, and discuss alternative treatment options with their potential psychoanalytic patients. They must also be able to continue to evaluate symptoms of depression and to make appropriate treatment recommendations in the context of an ongoing psychoanalysis. Most of all, psychoanalysts must be cognizant that we are only beginning to appreciate the many ways in which the prescription of medication impacts the analytic situation, and they must remain alert to these potential effects in their practice of psychoanalysis and pharmacotherapy.

References

Abel-Horowitz J: Psychopharmacotherapy during an analysis. Psychoanalytic Inquiry 18:673–701, 1998

Adelman SA: Pills as transitional objects: a dynamic understanding of the use of medication in psychotherapy. Psychiatry 48:246–253, 1985

American Psychiatric Association: Diagnostic and Statistical Manual of Mental Disorders, 3rd Edition. Washington, DC, American Psychiatric Association, 1980

American Psychiatric Association: Diagnostic and Statistical Manual of Mental Disorders, 4th Edition, Text Revision. Washington, DC, American Psychiatric Association, 2000

Cabaniss D: Shifting gears: the challenge to teach students to think psychodynamically and psychopharmacologically at the same time. Psychoanalytic Inquiry 18:639–656, 1998

Cabaniss DL: Beyond dualism: psychoanalysis and medication in the 21st century. Bull Menninger Clin 65:160–170, 2001

Caligor E, Hamilton M, Schneier H, et al: Converted patients and clinic patients as control cases: a comparison with implications for psychoanalytic training. J Am Psychoanal Assoc 51:201–220, 2003

Cooper AM: Will neurobiology influence psychoanalysis? Am J Psychiatry 142:1395–1402, 1985

Donovan SJ, Roose SP: Medication use during psychoanalysis: a survey. J Clin Psychiatry 56:177–179, 1995

Esman AH: Psychoanalysis and general psychiatry: obsessive-compulsive disorder as paradigm. J Am Psychoanal Assoc 37:319–335, 1989

Finkel J: Discussion. Contemporary Psychoanalysis 22:234–240, 1986

Frank E, Prien RF, Jarrett RB, et al: Conceptualization and rationale for consensus definitions of terms in major depressive disorder: remission, recovery, relapse, and recurrence. Arch Gen Psychiatry 48:851–855, 1991

Frasure-Smith N, Lesperance F, Talajic M: Depression following myocardial infarction: impact on 6-month survival. JAMA 270:1819–1825, 1993

Gutheil TG: The psychology of psychopharmacology. Bull Menninger Clin 46:321–330, 1982

Hausner R: Medication and transitional phenomena. Int J Psychoanal Psychother 11:375–398, 1985

Judd LL, Paulus MJ, Schettler PJ, et al: : Does incomplete recovery from first lifetime major depressive episode herald a chronic course of illness? Am J Psychiatry 157:1501–1504, 2000

Kahn DA: Medication consultation and split treatment during psychotherapy. J Am Acad Psychoanal 19:84–98, 1991

Kelly K: Principles, pragmatics, and parameters in clinical analysis: the dilemma of pharmacotherapy. Psychoanalytic Inquiry 18:716–729, 1998

Levy ST: Countertransference aspects of pharmacotherapy in the treatment of schizophrenia. Int J Psychoanal Psychother 6:15–30, 1977

Normand W, Bluestone H: The use of pharmacotherapy in psychoanalytic treatment. Contemporary Psychoanalysis 22:218–234, 1986

Ostow M: Drugs in Psychoanalysis and Psychotherapy. New York, Basic Books, 1962

Paykel ES, Ramana R, Cooper Z, et al: Residual symptoms after partial remission: an important outcome in depression. Psychol Med 25:1171–1180, 1995

Roose SP: The use of medication in combination with psychoanalytic psychotherapy or psychoanalysis (Chapter 13), in Psychiatry, Vol 1–8. Edited by Michels R. Philadelphia, PA, JB Lippincott, 1990

Roose SP: Does anxiety obstruct or motivate treatment? When to talk, when to prescribe, and when to do both, in Anxiety: Symptoms and Signals. Edited by Roose SP, Glick RA. Hillsdale, NJ, Analytic Press, 1995, pp 155–169

Roose SP, Stern RH: Medication use in training cases: a survey. J Am Psychoanal Assoc 43:163–170, 1995

Sarwer-Foner GJ: The Dynamics of Psychiatric Drug Therapy. Springfield, IL, Charles C Thomas, 1960

Spitzer RL, Endicott J, Robins E: Research Diagnostic Criteria: rationale and reliability. Arch Gen Psychiatry 35:773–785, 1978

Swoiskin MH: Psychoanalysis and medication: is real integration possible? Bull Menninger Clin 65:143–159, 2001

Thase ME, Entsuah AR, Rudolph RL: Remission rates during treatment with venlafaxine or selective serotonin reuptake inhibitors. Br J Psychiatry 178:234–241, 2001

Vaughan SC, Spitzer R, Davies M, et al: The definition and assessment of analytic process: can analysts agree? Int J Psychoanal 78:959–973, 1997

Vaughan SC, Marshall RD, MacKinnon RA, et al: Can we do psychoanalytic outcome research? A feasibility study. Int J Psychoanal 81:513–527, 2000

Yang S, Caligor E, Cabaniss D, et al: Posttermination contact: a survey of prevalence, characteristics, and analytic attitudes. Poster presented at the annual meeting of the American Psychoanalytic Association, New York City, December 2003

18

Technique in Child Analysis

JUDITH A. YANOF, M.D.

THE CHILD ANALYST AND the adult analyst have the same goals in doing analysis with their patients, and they rely on many of the same general principles. For both, the analytic engagement is about establishing a relationship in which analyst and patient, together, make meaning of what happens between them, with a particular focus on how it is experienced in the mind of the patient. This unusual engagement involves creating conditions of both safety and freedom for the elaboration and exploration of internal thoughts and external behavior. The nature of this engagement usually has to be affective and experiential to be successful. It involves establishing a clear, bounded, but negotiable "frame" in which imagination is enhanced. The purpose of this venture, of course, is to improve the patient's quality of life.

For many years child analysts were preoccupied with how much their technique matched, or differed from, the technique prescribed for adult patients by adult analysts, and for many years adult analysts questioned whether or not child analysis was "real" analysis. Today this question has receded in importance. Contemporary psychoanalysis is marked by a diversity of perspectives. There is not one psychoanalytic technique, but many. This is no less true for child psychoanalysis.

In a recent article on therapeutic action, Gabbard and Westen (2003) draw attention to three major trends in current psychoanalytic discourse that influence technique: 1) increasing recognition that there are *multiple* modes of therapeutic action (no longer the polarized, either/or debate between interpretation and relationship), 2) a shift in

emphasis from reconstruction to a focus on in-the-moment interactions in the relationship between patient and analyst, and 3) a movement toward flexibility and negotiation in defining the boundaries, frame, and "rules" of the analytic endeavor (pp. 823–824).

Child analysts found themselves moving in all of these directions long before their adult analyst counterparts, because working with children forced them to recognize the limitations of a "standard" adult psychoanalytic technique (Kris 2001). For example, child analysts appreciated and accepted the pivotal place of action long before "enactment" was an everyday concept. They long acknowledged that the relationship with the analyst was a crucial part of the therapeutic action, and recognized that at different times and with different children the analyst was used in different ways. Child analysts often worked without relying on reconstruction, self-reflection, or verbal interpretation because many children have not yet developed the cognitive capacities to use these techniques.

A major difference between child and adult analysis is that children are in the midst of a developmental process at the same time that they are participating in the analytic process. The child's cognitive abilities, as well as his or her developmental tasks and conflicts, become important factors in how one understands the child and conceptualizes the analytic relationship, and how the analyst chooses to communicate with the child. Children do not free-associate, and the analyst must rely heavily on action and nonverbal forms of communication to have a dialogue with the child. In particular, using play or relying on the *play process* becomes an important technical avenue. (In using the term *play* in this chapter, I am referring to children's imaginative play, which may also include drawings and stories.)

Another important difference in analyzing children is that children's conflicts are part of a family system. Children cannot participate in treatment without their parents, so the family becomes crucial to every treatment in which a child is involved. Moreover, a child's way of seeing himself or herself and the world is profoundly influenced by the family culture, a culture that is communicated explicitly and implicitly.

The Role of Play

In the past, child analysts looked at play primarily in terms of its themes and content. Having historically conceptualized their work with children from the perspective of adult analysis, child analysts viewed play as a way of gaining access to the child's dynamically unconscious thoughts, wishes, and troubling conflicts. In addition, psychoanalysis has long recognized that play in children is a natural tool for mastering and integrating difficult and traumatic experience by turning passive into active (S. Freud 1920/ 1955; Waelder 1933).

Developmentalists have historically taken a different tack, focusing on the structure of imaginative play in young children and how it unfolds cognitively (Scarlett 1994). In recent years there have been attempts to integrate these two traditions (Slade and Wolff 1994). Many child analysts have begun to write about play as valuable and therapeutic in its own right (Cohen and Solnit 1993; Frankel 1998; Neubauer 1994; Solnit et al. 1993; Winnicott 1986). Many have wondered if helping the child to develop and engage in the play process is just as important as verbalizing the meaning of the play content. Many analysts propose that helping the child play promotes development, not by *uncovering* meaning but by helping the child to *make* meaning (Ferro 1999; Fonagy et al. 2002; Neubauer 2001; Slade 1994).

Imaginative play is symbolic and uses conceptual metaphor, as does language. Lakoff and Johnson (1980, 1999; Lakoff 1987) define *metaphor* not as figure of speech, but as a fundamental aspect of human thinking: the way humans categorize their experience. Metaphors transfer meaning from one domain to another: from a domain that is more concrete and known to a domain that is more complex and more difficult to define. Lakoff and Johnson hypothesize that metaphors are conceptual and occur largely outside of awareness.

Play is used by children to think, imagine, and construct meaning in the way language is used by adults. Therefore, play is one of the most valuable tools that the child analyst has in engaging a child in the psychoanalytic process of meaning-making and communication. When a child and an analyst play together, they talk to each other in a nonverbal language, even though they may use words as dialogue in the play.

Play is a highly effective way of accessing and communicating affect. Affects are communicated in facial expressions, body language, and tone of voice, but they are difficult to describe in words, especially for children. People often use conceptual metaphors to communicate feelings (Lakoff 1987; Lakoff and Johnson 1980, 1999), both in language and in play. Moreover, because there is often a narrative structure embedded in imaginative play, children share affects in a much more sophisticated and nuanced way through play than when they use words alone. If you ask a child how he or she feels, the child often says, "I am happy" or "I am sad." If you ask a child, instead, "What happened then?" you get a narrative story that conveys much more emotional complexity (Siegel 1999).

For children, the fact that play is "pretend" allows them to elaborate wished for, forbidden, or disavowed aspects of themselves more freely and with less conflict. For example, they are not the dinosaurs, aliens, or monsters that unleash aggression, nor are they the helpless, small creatures that can be hurt. In play, children can "try on" particular ideas or roles without being committed to them. They can "remember" experience that is too difficult to remember or has never been laid down in verbal, semantic memory systems (Schacter 1996). Children can regulate affect incrementally by changing the story or disrupting the play (see also Erikson 1940 for discussion of play disruptions).

Although there is nothing in adult analysis that truly corresponds to engaging in pretend play, the use of free association is probably most closely analogous. Like free association in adult analysis, the use of play provides a structure in which ordinary constraints are let go and there is an attempt to express what cannot be expressed in ordinary discourse. It is the oscillation between intense affective engagement with the analyst (engagement that feels and is emotionally "authentic") and the simultaneous sense that what is being expressed is "pretend," "as if," and can be disavowed (or reflected upon) that is paradoxical. This oscillation characterizes both child and adult analysis. Adults do not consider their associations "pretend," but neither do they consider what they say bound by intent. In adult analysis, this oscillation is also part of the complex state of transference (Modell 1990). In psychoanalysis when things are going well, both play and free association create a paradoxical state of being in two realms at once, the real world and the world of the imagination.

A child is not born with the ability to play. Play is built on a series of cognitive maturational developments that are achieved sequentially over the first 3 years of life (Mayes and Cohen 1996). Fonagy and colleagues (2002) write convincingly about the intimate relationship between the caregiver's early attitude toward the infant as an intentional being, the ability of the dyad to "mark" certain communications as pretend, and the subsequent ability of the child to mentalize—that is, to understand that he and others can hold different ideas about external reality. Very young children behave as if their thoughts and others' thoughts accurately mirror the external world. Fonagy and colleagues (2002) call this mode of thinking "psychic equivalence." Young children at a certain age come to be able to use another kind of thought in play, "pretend mode." In play, ideas are represented that the child knows are not accurate representations of the real world; ideas are freed from their real-world referents. Fonagy and colleagues (2002) hypothesize that a child's ability to mentalize and develop a reflective stance is a developmental achievement that is the result of an integration of these dual modes of thought: psychic equivalence mode and pretend mode.

What is significant in this theory for the child analyst's work is that in play the child may be working with a more flexible mode of thought than might otherwise be available to him developmentally. It has been shown in research experiments that children are often able to comprehend complex relationships (such as false belief) in play before they can do so in real life. (There are many experiments that show that a young child [approximately] under 4 years of age does not cognitively understand that another person may have different beliefs from himself or herself or that some beliefs are false; see Fonagy et al. 2002; Perner et al. 1987.)

Let us take a clinical example:

Four-year-old Emily enacted the following compelling story. She took two dolls and called one Mother and one Child. In her story Mother was taking Child ice skating. Emily made Child fall down again and again, while Mother repeated in a saccharine voice, "Oh, how beautifully you skate, my darling!" completely oblivious to Child's difficulty maintaining her equilibrium.

This ice-skating interaction might or might not have occurred in real life. In either case, the play vividly represented Emily's feelings through the use of a conceptual metaphor. The child's slipping on ice conveyed Emily's vulnerable emotional state through a universal and concrete physical experience, falling down. In Emily's meta-

phor, Child was off-balance. In contrast, well-being is typically conveyed metaphorically in terms of verticality (Lakoff 1987; Lakoff and Johnson 1980, 1999) (hence, expressions such as "I'm feeling up," "I'm on a high," "I'm sinking"). Beyond the primary conceptual metaphor referring to self state, however, Emily's play also used a rich and unique individual metaphor. She communicated something very nuanced and very specific about what it was like for her to be with her mother. In this metaphor, she experienced her mother as unable or unwilling to recognize that she needed help and, therefore, unable to respond to her needs. In her play the concrete ice-skating incident stood for the more general emotional gestalt of the relationship. The play sequence conveyed in a simple way a much more abstract conceptualization: the striking disconnect between two worldviews—mother's and child's—the mother's lack of response to the child's psychic reality, and the child's experience of the mother's supportive words as contextually meaningless because she felt unrecognized.

As a result of Emily's articulate communication in her play metaphor, I intuited immediately that she also must have been telling me something about her current experience with me. I remembered that this precocious little girl had walked into my office as if she were in total command of the situation, separating easily from her mother, although she hardly knew me. I had seen her as quite firmly grounded. However, underneath her self-sufficient veneer was someone smaller, more frightened, and feeling shaky.

Certainly Emily would not have been able to say in words what she experienced with her mother or what she was feeling with me. As a young child, she did not have conceptual language for these ideas. By playing with the dolls, she was able to convey her experience by acting out the narrative with its attendant affective component. However, the act of playing was not simply the communication of a previously developed, unshared thought, although it was probably motivated by Emily's wish to be known. The frame of pretend play optimized the use of her imaginative and metaphorical capacities and helped her to organize what had been inchoate experience. In making meaning through play, Emily likely discovered something about herself, as an adult patient can discover new meaning in the narrative act of telling his or her story.

Therefore, the benefit of playing with a child in child analysis derives not simply from being in a relationship, having fun, being met affectively, or negotiating particular kinds of transactions, although it may include all of these beneficial factors. I believe that the analytic encounter, when it works at its best, requires an analyst to be engaged with the child in the process of making meaning and in recognizing that meaning is being made.

Working Within the Play

Although the content of a child's play may seem to have obvious meaning to the analyst, it is important not to treat this material as if the child is communicating directly about his or her inner thoughts. Such a stance ignores the child's fundamental assumption that play is "pretend." The young child may have no cognitive awareness that play and internal thoughts are connected (Mayes and Cohen 1993), while the latency-age child may need to use play defensively without being intruded upon. As in adult analysis, timing is important, and the analyst must direct his or her interventions to the child's cognitive level and state of emotional receptivity.

There are many ways Emily's material could have been engaged. Suppose the analyst had said to Emily, "You are like the little girl in your play. You feel like you are falling down inside and your mommy doesn't see how much help you need." While this intervention stays close to the child's metaphor, this translation makes an explicit link between Child doll and the patient. Making play and reality equivalent tends to confuse young children and tends to shut down the play in older children, if they are not ready to acknowledge the feelings that they are only "trying on." If the analyst were to disregard defenses and say, "You are angry at your mother because she doesn't know what you are feeling," the child might feel frightened and guilty for letting out something that she was not yet ready to say.

Hence, there is some wisdom in making one's interventions from inside the play first, a technique a number of child analysts have recommended (Ritvo 1978). Using such a technique and staying at the surface, the analyst might simply say, "Child has a falling-down feeling and the Mother doesn't notice." This is not likely to be intrusive because the analyst stays in pretend mode and yet conveys that she has recognized the child's communication. Of course, for one child any verbalization might be jarring, whereas another child might say openly, "That's what happened to me."

What one chooses to say depends on what one feels is most salient in the moment. If the analyst substitutes "grown-up" for "mommy," saying, "Child has a falling-down feeling, and the grown-ups don't notice," this opens up the communication to include the analytic situation. If the analyst discerns that the child is very anxious in the moment and needs active support, she might say directly, "Sometimes it's really confusing to be in a new place and not know what is going to happen."

If the analyst were less concerned about Emily's anxiety, she might pick up the Child doll and expand the play elaboration herself. She might give it an emotional dimen-sion, such as irritation, by complaining, "Look, Mother, I'm falling down!" By accenting the affect, one communicates understanding as well as gives permission for negative, disavowed feelings to become part of the exchange.

One can listen to play material at many different levels. I first heard Emily's play metaphor as a communication about her experience, her history, and her view of the relationship with her mother. On another level, the ice-skating metaphor was also a communication about how she was experiencing being with me in the moment, the transference. At still another level, Emily's play sequence could be understood as a metaphor for her internal landscape: the disconnect between the falling-down part of herself and her need to put on a happy face. Ideally, the analyst wants to hear the child's material on as many levels as possible.

The Play Process

The child analyst comes to appreciate that children have variable capacities to engage in the play process. Children who can play readily engage in pretend play that is pleasurable and has a momentum. Their play involves the creation of new metaphors and associated narratives in the context of a relationship in which both child and analyst have a space to have a voice. Although both recognize that the child's story is salient, it is impossible to differentiate what is strictly the child's and what emerges as part of the interaction. During play the analyst helps the child to create a meaningful story that would not be created in precisely the same way outside of that relationship.

In playing with a child like Emily who has achieved the capacity to play, one can participate in a variety of ways. The analyst can show interest by asking questions about the story. She can focus on the feelings of the play by resonating with its affective rhythms or appreciating the dilemmas of its main characters. The analyst can add interesting ideas or insights about the play from a vantage point inside the play via a character or from outside of the play, so long as this facilitates, rather than disrupts, the play process. Eventually, one hopes that, at times, analyst and child will be able to reflect on the play process together, although this is not a sine qua non of child analysis.

While many analysts are uncomfortable about "just playing," participating in the play as a player also can be an important way of deepening the play process. To do this, one takes as many cues as possible from the child about whom one's character is supposed to be and how this character is supposed to respond. The cues come from the child's direction and from everything that is known about the child: his or her history, family life, areas of interest, favorite stories, and from the past experience of playing together. Cues also come from the child's immediate affective response to the analyst's presence. One need not be afraid to introduce something new, particularly when one marks it as "pretend," if one attends to how it is being metabolized by the child. When things are going well, the child's story deepens and becomes more elaborated, and the analyst feels more emotionally involved with the child.

Take the following example from the play of a 4-year-old child, seen twice a week, who had an excellent capacity to engage in the play process:

> Randy was consumed with a story that he had been read about a pirate. He had me make a sword out of cardboard, and he carried it around with him to fight off a variety of dangers in his imaginary world. He pretended that it was night and that my couch was his bed. He placed his sword under the couch. I was his male sidekick and had to sleep on the floor. My role was to inform him that his sword had been stolen in the middle of the night. We played this game many times in various versions and permutations. Sometimes this story was "just a dream," and sometimes it was "real." Sometimes at night I became his mother and tucked him in. Sometimes I was his mother and he protected me from a dangerous intruder and I was rescued. Sometimes I hid his sword and we pretended that it was stolen. I generally followed his lead and waited to see what would emerge.
>
> One day when the game seemed to lose its momentum, I added something to the story. As the sidekick, I became more shocked and distressed in my announcement that the sword was indeed missing. I exaggerated the pretend. This stirred a more lively engagement in the story, in which Randy told me for the first time that his sister had taken the sword. He then became involved in counterattacks. He yelled at her and warned her that he would shrink her and put her in the computer mouse and that he would gouge out her eyes. However, quite suddenly he became excited and silly, throwing himself off the couch in a dangerous way. Every time he imagined doing something to the sister, he wound up doing something hurtful to himself. He pretended to hurt his leg, he started to break his sword, and he impulsively threw away all his precious treasures, which became missiles flung across my room.
>
> I had to move in quickly and use my real voice to reinstate the play frame. I told him that I liked his pirate story but that we had to keep everything in pretend because somebody might *really* get hurt while we were playing out these big feelings. If he really hurt himself or me, then he would be too frightened to play with me. Only when Randy was back in physical control, did I ask, "Who was that boy who just came into the room and was throwing himself away?" tentatively inviting a reengagement in the play. He told me that the boy was Wild Guy, a wild boy who had no parents and no rules to live by. I showed him how he could *pretend* to be wild. He shook his head "no" and told me that we had to get rid of the out-of-control Wild Guy for good. I said, "I think Wild Guy is scary because he gets so out of control that he scares himself. But we can't get rid of him until we get to know him and his secrets and what makes him do the things he does, because everybody has a Wild Guy in them and we need to be able to figure out what he is trying to tell us." Tentatively he took his sword, saying, "Follow me then. Stay very close to me. We have to look for him." However, although we tried to find him, Wild Guy had safely disappeared for the rest of the hour.
>
> Several days later, however, the play involved some action figures who were throwing furniture out of the dollhouse and scaring the family. It was the end of the hour, and when I said, "It's time to go," Randy escalated, "I won't and you can't make me! I won't! I won't! And I won't!" And then with a mixture of fear and delight he whispered, "Because *I* am a Wild Guy boy!" and left the session with no further ado.

Children, particularly young children, move in and out of the play frame often with little warning. The process of this play sequence is a good example of this in a typical young child's play. Randy goes from playing pretend pirate, in very good control of his impulses, to throwing himself off the couch dangerously. Here pretend and real suddenly collapse into each other. Older children with trouble regulating affect also display this lack of regulation during play, and any child in treatment under the pressure of certain affects at times will be unable to maintain the pretend state.

There is a great deal going on in this short vignette. In his play Randy moves in and out of different characters quite fluidly but quite coherently. He goes from positions of strength to positions of vulnerability and back again. He is a fearless pirate with a big sword, a brave hero who saves his mother from intrusion, a small boy who needs to be tucked in, an unsuspecting pirate who is tricked and has his sword stolen, a vengeful boy who gouges out his sister's eyes, a boy who breaks his own sword in a silly frenzy, and a Wild Guy who lives without rules and has to be banished. Certainly the content of the play touches on some of the commonplace developmental conflicts of an oedipal-age boy. Is he big or little? Does he have a big sword or a little one? Would his mother love him better if he were big and strong, or does she want him to stay small? If he wants what the big man has, will he have to steal it from him? If he has such big, aggressive wishes, will he expose himself to retaliation and danger? Is he good or is he bad? Is he the hero or the intruder? Will he live by the rules or not?

What is most significant to the child analyst about the play is the degree of conflict that the child experiences about being big, which is associated with being aggressive—a common concern. In play Randy spends most of the time waiting apprehensively for his sword to get stolen. When he does move into a more aggressive position in fantasy, briefly shrinking someone and gouging out eyes, he begins to get overexcited and silly. He turns the hurting impulses on himself by throwing himself off the couch, not just in fantasy but in reality, while symbolically throwing away his treasures and destroying his sword. The play frame is disrupted. The feelings are very charged. One might wish to share the idea with Randy that he needs to "throw himself away" shortly after he thinks about hurting someone. Yet, this probably is not the time to take up this defense because Randy needs to be in a state receptive enough to hear such a complicated thought. Later on, the analyst might introduce a character who "throws himself away" following an aggressive act.

Randy is using play as a way to work out conflicts that he has about growing up, being phallic, being aggressive, being a competitive force, and finding his place in the family. He is using play to communicate his fears about affectively getting out of control, being defiant, and keeping his body intact. The play demonstrates that when he throws away his sword, he feels momentarily protected from the danger of his aggressive conflicts. What the play does not yet reveal is why he feels so anxious.

Different child analysts will have different ways of working with this material. My own goal was to help Randy continue and deepen the elaboration of his story in play, during which issues could be reworked in conceptual metaphors. Therefore, I scaffolded his play by setting limits, keeping the frame, reminding him of pretend, and helping him return to the play after it was disrupted. I was also a player in the play. I was often assigned the role of partner, a Robin to his Batman. In this role reversal, I took orders from Randy and admired his competence. This infused our play with a meaningful, affectionate bond that was paradoxically pretend and authentic at the same time.

My own addition to the play was to intensify the affect around the missing sword. In retrospect, I think I was trying to communicate affectively that I understood that whenever we talked about the sword, we were talking about something very significant—we were symbolically representing some kind of calamity. This might be equivalent to commenting to an adult patient that he or she was telling me something terribly sad but had taken all the sadness out of the story in the telling. My intervention *did* increase the affect in the room, as well as the story's elaboration, but perhaps it also overwhelmed Randy's capacity to stay in pretend mode.

Putting into words what we were trying to do together gave Randy not only information about the frame but also permission to play with certain dangerous ideas. Telling him that we had to find Wild Guy was a way of talking to him in a language that he could understand at his stage of development through the use of his own play-metaphor. This intervention seemed fruitful when 2 days later he was willing to acknowledge that he, too, was a Wild Guy boy. His ability to name and talk about his Wild Guy feelings helped him to leave the session under control. Work on affect regulation was an important side effect of a process that I had initiated in order to make meaning.

Children Who Cannot Play

Children between the ages of 3 and 6 years are developmentally at a prime time to enjoy imaginative play. However, a child's age is not the sole factor in whether or not he or she will be able to engage in pretend play. Young children who need to be too "grown up" in their behavior or are afraid to be "bad" have great difficulty "letting go" enough to play. On the other hand, children in latency may have begun to put aside playing imaginatively with their friends, as part of their developmental process. They may think that play is babyish or fear its regressive pull. Learning the rules of sports and board games gives latency-age children a sense of mastery in the real world, but it also can be used as a retreat from the expression of more conflicted, unacceptable feelings in analysis. Children in latency may begin treatment by turning to more structured games, but they often learn to have a great investment in imaginative play if their analysts help them play. The play of latency-age children allows them to revisit past themes and old ways of thinking in the presence of their more mature cognitive functioning—this promotes integration.

There are many reasons why children have difficulty engaging in a play process. There are children who cannot play imaginatively on a biological basis. These children fall into the spectrum of children with autism and pervasive developmental disorder (PDD) (Cohen and Volkmar 1997). They also exhibit disturbances on false belief tests and do not develop a robust theory of mind.

Other children cannot play because they have not developed a way of coherently organizing their experience. This may be due to failures in their emotional development and/or failures in their caregivers' ability to provide experiences conducive to making sense of the world, such as by regulating stimulation, naming, and teaching them to pretend (Greenspan and Lieberman 1994; Slade 1994).

There are also children who have difficulty in engaging in the play process secondary to conflict. For some children play threatens to liberate into action impulses that are barely contained. For others there is an avoidance of a process in which unacceptable feelings and thoughts might more easily be revealed. Whenever children cannot engage in the play process, it is the analyst's task to help them to do so (Winnicott 1986).

One 7-year-old boy refused to play pretend for many months of his two-times-per-week treatment. After we introduced psychoanalysis, with its increased frequency of sessions, this youngster allowed himself a freedom of thought and expression unprecedented in our previous meetings. When he finally allowed himself to play, he presented a rich fantasy world, populated with many different characters that we remained engaged with for many years. The world he created was like a complex novel. He was unwillingly to play early on because he was too frightened of his own disavowed inner world—to know or to share it. This seemed to be a play inhibition brought about by conflict. Even as his play process evolved more deeply, he did not talk about it with reference to his own situation or dilemmas.

Some children begin to play but have difficulty in engaging in a play process. These children frequently develop a theme that does not go anywhere or seems to get locked into a stereotyped, unchanging configuration. Such children may take up the action figures and fight, shooting and killing in a rote way, only to begin all over again when everyone is dead. The characters are often interchangeable, the story undeveloped, and the affective range narrow. There may be a resistance to letting the analyst have an autonomous voice in the play, refusing the introduction of anything new. The play may provide a motoric outlet for the child or be a concrete expression of an impulse like aggression. What is significant is that the play does not seem to function in a *metaphorical* way. A true play process, on the other hand, is characterized by open-endedness, an increasing range of affect, and a shifting experimentation with new metaphors, narratives, and compromise formations.

Sometimes stereotyped play has defensive functions. For example, the expression of aggression may become too disorganizing for the child, so that he or she shuts down the play or simply repeats it, robotlike. Progress may occur incrementally via play as the analyst helps the child to tolerate increased affect without disorganization, or progress may be facilitated by the analyst's ability to address the defensive function of the play.

At other times such stereotyped play may function as an enactment that demands negotiation between the analyst and the child. Defense and enactment are not mutually exclusive. For example, one 9-year-old girl, who at times had trouble engaging in the play process, invented a story in which I was a slave and she was a queen. Although we used dolls, the story was that I had to submit to all her demands and humiliations. Not only would she dictate how my doll had to look and what it had to wear, but anything I added had to be undone. She would make a mess of the office and insist that my slave doll clean it up. The line between real and pretend collapsed. Over time this play became rigid and concrete, losing its metaphorical capacity.

At times her stereotyped play had a compulsive quality that seemed to be used to manage anxiety that might result from a more open-ended play situation. At times her control over me seemed to gratify her. The queen/slave play configuration also represented a transference paradigm that had historical significance; she turned passive into active. However, this play paradigm was not very useful to the analysis because it could not be reflected on, modified, or "played with." I tried many ways of addressing this impasse both from within the play and by interpreting the enactment directly. Finally, when I refused to play this game by her rules, she turned her fury on me. We were then able to talk more fruitfully about her disappointment and anger at me. There are times when there seems no way to work with such rigid play. These children who cannot play may be quite similar to the adults, whom Smith (2003) describes, who have great difficulty entering into a full-fledged transference relationship.

For children who cannot play, the analyst tries to help them enter a play process. Asking questions about a story may help children to learn what the ingredients of a narrative are. The analyst can provide the structure herself, suggesting, "Let's write a story about what happened in the waiting room. I'll draw the picture. What do you want to be doing?" Or the analyst can make a puppet show for the child, choosing a theme that she knows will be appealing and putting it into displaced form. If the child is playing a board game, the analyst can become the voice of one of the pieces, elaborating a story about how it feels to be losing or winning or being jumped. Or the analyst can put on a puppet and do something silly or act vulnerable. The analyst can model a way of being free in using pretend.

Interpretation and Insight

Child analysts disagree about the place of interpretation and insight in the play process, including 1) what understandings need to be decoded from the play, applied to the real world, and interpreted directly to the child; 2) what understandings need to be verbalized but can be articulated as part of the play displacement; and 3) what understandings can or should go unsaid. Clearly some of this controversy has to do with theoretical disagreements about how psychoanalysis brings about change. When interpretation was considered to be the primary agent of change in adult psychoanalysis, there was a tendency to apply the same thinking to child analysis. Therefore, there was an expectation that in order to do "real analysis," the child analyst should decode the conflicts uncovered in the play material and relate them directly to the child's actual circumstances for acknowledgement (Fraiberg 1965, 1966). Unfortunately, this often shut down the play process.

Developmental theory tells us that older children have a greater capacity to appreciate that the stories they are playing emerge from their own thoughts and fantasies (Mayes and Cohen 1993). Under favorable environmental circumstances, children gradually achieve a self-reflective capacity by late latency. However, despite the fact that one might expect the capacity to verbalize feelings to increase with age, age is not always an indicator of who will be able to self-reflect. Some children of all ages have difficulty acknowledging their feelings, while some very young children can talk about their feelings directly and easily.

As a result of increased data from the neurosciences, we now know that implicit associational memory systems operate and are influenced outside conscious awareness (Gabbard and Westen 2003). Change can occur in different systems—conscious systems and nonconscious systems, with and without words. Implicit change is possible during play not only because procedural schemas of interacting with another (Stern et al. 1998) can shift but also because conceptual (symbolic) ideas can be "played with" metaphorically without being brought to awareness.

Furthermore, conscious and implicit change is not an either/or matter; they often enhance each other (Gabbard and Westen 2003). For example, we assume that the degree and stability of therapeutic change may be facilitated in children, as in adults, by making them aware of factors initially outside of awareness, such as how they relate to others. Moreover, verbalizing what happens in play is helpful to children because words are powerful tools. By naming things, words give permission for certain ideas and feelings to exist, and they can put a space between thought and action.

For insight to work with children, however, it is important that the analyst put his or her ideas in a language that a child can understand. It is helpful to use the child's own metaphors in interpreting—metaphors that have been developed in the process of playing. With children, conscious awareness and self-reflection are more apt to occur toward the end of and as a result of the analysis.

Transference in Child Analysis

Anna Freud (1927/1969) initially believed that children did not form transferences because their parents contin-ued to be present in their lives as primary objects and, therefore, they enacted their conflicts with their parents and did not "transfer" them to the person of the analyst. Later (A. Freud 1965/1974) she reversed this position, agreeing that children do, indeed, develop transferences during their analytic treatment and that these transferences can be similar, but not equal, to the "transference neurosis" of the adult. The absence or presence of a transference neurosis in child analysis comparable to the adult's became a subject of scrutiny and controversy for many years (Fraiberg 1965, 1966; Harley 1967; Sandler et al. 1980; Scharfman 1978; Tyson 1978) until the concept "transference neurosis" lost its prominence in adult analysis (Brenner 1982; Smith 2003).

Chused wrote a seminal paper in 1988, making the point that contemporary child analysts often do not observe as much transference in child analysis because their technique hinders the development of a full-blown transference. Chused believed that child analysts often gave up a neutral position and took on the traditional (and more gratifying) role of adult with a child. In this way Chused's view echoed the earlier position of Melanie Klein (1932/1975, 1955), who believed that children could be analyzed by classical adult technique through the analysis of their play. Klein felt that as long as the child analyst systematically interpreted the child's negative impulses, especially those directed at the analyst, and avoided educative methods, a transference neurosis analogous to the adult variety would develop.

Other authors, however, believed that transference is less observable in children because the child analyst is used by the child in different ways more of the time—not simply as a transference object, but as a new, real, or developmental object or as an object of externalization (Abrams 1996; Furman 1980; Lilleskov 1971; Sandler et al. 1980; Tyson 1978). These uses of the child analyst were recognized, differentiated from transfer proper, and credited with contributing to the therapeutic action in child analysis.

Despite differences of opinion, work in the transference continues to have a central place in child analysis, as it does in adult analysis. In the broadest sense, transference includes all the child's feelings and attitudes toward the analyst. In analysis, the repetition of the past always occurs in the context of a new relationship in which there is an attempt to negotiate a different outcome. At the same time, the current analytic situation is always framed by past paradigms. While it may be theoretically useful to differentiate these feelings, operationally they occur as part of the same package. This position recognizes the ubiquity of transference (Joseph 1985): whatever the child chooses to play or do with the analyst during the session has relevance to the transference.

Children, and especially young children, however, are not readily able to experience the intensity of their transference feelings, and simultaneously recognize its "as if" nature (Yanof 1996). Reconstructions do not often have the same appeal for children that they do for adults (Yanof 1996). One of our goals with adult patients is for them to achieve an appreciation of the paradoxical nature of the transference. Perceptions of the analyst are simultaneously "real" and "illusory" (Smith 2003)—illusory in that they are partially determined by what is projected onto the person of the analyst. It is often at the point when this paradox is recognized that the adult patient is able to gain a sense of mastery in separating present from past. Because the child has limited understanding of transference conceptually (i.e., its "as if" nature), transference work must be done with children "in the moment."

Transference in children is most likely played out or enacted. Children rarely talk about how they experience the analyst, rarely report dreams that are explicitly about the analyst, and rarely speculate about the analyst in undisguised fantasy. However, transference should be thought of whenever the child expresses direct curiosity about the analyst. Sometimes children ask the analyst questions about his age, his family configuration, or other patients. It is difficult for a child to understand why a familiar and intimate adult would not answer a simple question. Asking a child to fantasize about an answer withheld is generally misunderstood and counterproductive. It is most fruitful to try to address the reasons behind the child's curiosity, whether or not a direct answer is provided. "You are wondering what I do with the other children who come to see me and how I feel about them." "You are wondering if I am a mother and what kind of mother I would be."

Sometimes the transference is revealed in the play displacement, as in the example of Emily, who played about falling down on the ice. Although it was not explicit, she was talking about her experience in the moment with her analyst as well as her experience at home. It is useful for the analyst to ask herself why the child is telling this story at this time. The transference may also come up in play in a more explicit way through characters who are "feelings-doctors" who enter the play to do brain surgery, kidnap children, marry them, or send them to someone else to treat.

When work in the transference is most mutative, as with adults, it is affectively alive in the interaction between the child and the analyst. Often the analytic frame provides intense moments at which it is particularly effective to take up the transference. Beginnings and endings of sessions, or vacations, are such opportunities. The child may fear coming into the session or refuse to leave, or demand to take home a toy he or she has been playing

with. Each of these situations can be used to articulate feelings toward the analyst or defenses against allowing such feelings to emerge. When child and analyst are deeply engaged in the play process, affects become more intense, and the transference/countertransference paradigms also become more transparent. This is another place when transference can be taken up "in the moment," either from within or outside of the play. As with adults, transference often feels less cohesive and consolidated in the beginning than it does later in the treatment. The following clinical example (first presented in Yanof 1996), involves Jeremy, a selectively mute boy whom I analyzed from ages 4 to 7.

> At the beginning of treatment, Jeremy played for many hours with action figures in my dollhouse, his back turned toward me, in complete and utter silence. He responded to nothing that I said and nothing that I interpreted about the feelings in the room. There was an important turning point in the treatment when I abandoned words altogether and limited myself to making noises that accompanied his action-play as closely as possible. Later, Jeremy began to use words, yet the paradigm of an interrupted dialogue repeated itself again and again in the interaction that we developed.
>
> At first I thought of Jeremy's silence as a resistance to treatment, a symptom or obstacle we had to eliminate. Later I began to understand the silence or the disrupted dialogue as a metaphor and a transference: a repetition of an earlier way of being with the other. At first we negotiated our relationship through action: How much silence, excitement, or control would I tolerate before I set limits, disengaged, talked, or stopped talking? As the transference became more coherent and consolidated, I began to verbalize what felt affectively alive and available between us. Sometimes I did this indirectly through the voices of the characters in the stories we wrote together. However, over time I was increasingly able to speak to Jeremy in my own voice.
>
> One day Jeremy turned his back to me in silence in a way that was quite reminiscent of the past. I said during the course of the session, "You are a different kind of Jeremy today. I feel like I have lost you." He acknowledged that he knew what I meant when I talked about losing him. I went on, "Today I think you stopped talking to me because you felt like you had lost me when you saw that I had been playing with another child." He didn't respond. Later I added, "I think when your mommy is worried about your sick sister, you feel like you have lost her too." Jeremy responded to this affirmatively, with a nod. In a poignant way he then associated to death. He asked: "Is your mother alive?" "How can you live without a mother?"

Silent disengagement was a way of being with me in which Jeremy abandoned me and simultaneously avoided being abandoned by me. In the session Jeremy could straddle two realities at once: he felt as if I had left him, but he could also reconnect with me to talk about it. This is very close to an adult version of working in the transference, although Jeremy would not have been able to conceptualize this idea as an adult would have.

Development

Child analysts have long recognized that the analyst is not simply a transference figure but serves multiple functions to the child in analysis. This serving of multiple functions is necessitated in part because children are in the midst of the developmental process at the same time that they are engaged in the psychoanalytic process. Anna Freud (1965/1974), in writing about the differences between children and adults in analysis, said, "The adult's tendency to *repeat*, which is important for creating transference, is complicated in the child by his hunger for *new experience* and new objects..." (p. 27). The assumption behind this thinking is that childhood experience is internalized in a more comprehensive and influential way during the developmental process than after development has been completed. Identifications made in early life are more enduring (Sandler et al. 1980).

A number of child analysts have tried to distinguish between the use of the "real relationship" in adult and child analysis and the more specific *developmental* use of the analyst as a "new object" in child analysis (Abrams 1996; Abrams and Solnit 1998; Neubauer 2001). These authors define development as a time-limited process *in a child* that is sequential; yields hierarchical, discontinuous changes; and leads to *new psychological organizations*. Children, in search of interactive relationships to complete their developmental program, will seek out new experience with their analysts, whom they use as "new objects." Adults, on the other hand, change by integrating new experience into existing psychological organizations, but not by making new, discontinuous psychological organizations (Abrams and Solnit 1998). A developmental object, therefore, describes an analyst who fulfills a current developmental need during a particular window in time.

Not all analysts agree that the use of the analyst as a new object is qualitatively different in children and adults. A number of analysts believe that psychological development continues beyond adolescence and that adults continue to make phase-specific reorganizations and structural changes throughout the life cycle (Colarusso 1990, 2000; Emde 1985; Erikson 1963).

It is often difficult to sort out how one is being used by a child at any given moment. As with adults, there are some child patients who seem to use the analyst along one dimension more than along another. These differences cut across age groups and diagnostic categories. The use of the analyst may change during particular periods of a child's analysis. For instance, some children, at times, need developmental assistance if they are going to use the play process or interpretation in analysis, as in the following clinical example:

> Robert was a 7-year-old boy who came for psychoanalysis because he had problems with self-esteem and impulse control. Earlier in the treatment, he had used imaginary play as a vehicle to express his anger and his fears that his rage made him unlovable. Although he was extremely bright and creative, difficulty in learning to read compromised his success in school. He lacked the perseverance and frustration tolerance necessary to stick to a task in order to overcome his learning difficulties. At school his teachers became frustrated with his lack of effort. He seemed to be caught up in a vicious cycle of feeling bad about himself and refusing to try.
>
> During the analytic sessions, Robert began to use Legos for the first time. He wanted to make some complicated objects that he saw in a Lego construction manual. These objects were difficult to build because the directions were hard to follow. Whenever Robert came to something difficult, he began to complain that he could not do it—that he was not smart enough to do it. He immediately demanded that I do it for him. I made a technical decision not to do it for him but to support his plan to build the object. I did not interpret conflict, but I told him that learning how to do things was hard work and it made everyone feel like giving up. At times I gave him strategies. Much of the time he was angry at me for not doing enough. However, when he finally finished the project, he was elated. I gave him lots of credit for persevering. He made many models, each increasingly difficult. Each time he fumed and cried in the beginning but succeeded in completing what he was building.

I understood that there were psychological issues that we did not directly address during these sessions. He was tied to his parents by being the baby, and felt that the only way to get his needs met was to stay little. To Robert being a baby meant not being too independent or too powerful with all his pent-up anger—things that (in his mind) would lead his parents to abandon him. At the same time, being incompetent was a way of punishing his achievement-oriented parents and himself. Most of all, he was self-defeating.

There were other dynamic factors operating as well. My summer vacation was coming up. Robert used an old defensive solution—"being baby"—to avoid his powerful anger and sadness at the interruption. He tried to provoke helpless, angry feelings in me by being so demanding, but he also communicated in the displacement of building Lego projects his feeling that he could not manage alone.

Because Robert was beginning latency, there were many developmental pressures on him to join and function competently in the world of his peers, to achieve more psychological separation from his parents, and to tolerate "not knowing" so that he could learn. I made the decision to support Robert's development by helping him increase his frustration tolerance so that he could become more competent. I believe I was functioning in the capacity of a new object during much of this time. Although I felt that this approach furthered the long-term goals of the analysis, most of my interventions in the moment were not directed at working with conflict or the making of meaning. While I did address his feelings about our separation, I had to postpone analyzing how he dealt with these feelings. I believe that many child analysts use noninterpretive ego-building techniques of this kind during the course of a child analysis. It is always difficult to assess exactly how these decisions affect the long-range course of the analysis.

Work With Parents

Perhaps the most difficult part of doing child analysis is balancing the work with the child and the work with parents. While most child analysts agree that work with parents is an essential part of the treatment, historically parent work has been ignored in writing about child analysis (Novick and Novick 2001). In Fonagy and Target's (1996) retrospective outcome study of child analysis, the treatment and guidance of parents alongside the child's treatment was a factor that improved outcome.

While the child analyst is committed to creating a protected private space for the child, he or she must also create a "holding environment (Modell 1976; Winnicott 1965)" for the parents so that they can support the analytic endeavor. Parents affect the child in a greater way, qualitatively and quantitatively, than family members in an adult patient's life. The child's daily sessions, for instance, will be more influenced by what has just happened at home than will the adult's. In addition, as Anna Freud said, "Full internalization of conflict does not occur for many years, and the child may need help with the environment. Therefore, in child analysis, assistance from both sides is needed—internal help for the method of coping, but external help for undue pressures on the child" (quoted in Sandler et al. 1980, p. 268).

Working with children means understanding how their problems fit into the dynamics of the family system. When parents bring their child for treatment, they bring the child because he or she is suffering and because they are suffering. They see the child as the designated patient, but

they also see themselves as inadequate parents. One of the most important assessments that the child analyst can make in proposing psychoanalysis for a child is whether the family can support the analysis emotionally over the course of time. This means that the parents have to have enough commitment to the venture to continue treatment when the child no longer appears to be suffering, when they are no longer suffering, and at those difficult periods when the treatment seems to be the *cause* of the suffering. The commitment of the parents to the analytic treatment requires an accurate initial picture of the psychoanalytic process, including its approximate length and its potential difficulties.

Psychoanalytic treatment is difficult for parents to choose for many of the same reasons that make it hard for adults to choose. In addition, parents are very concerned about the attachment and influence that the child analyst will have in the life of their child. Parents often bring their child to a therapist when their relationship with their child is at a low point. It is a difficult time to entrust a child to someone who will have a very important role in the child's life and will often become a beloved figure. Despite this, parents will rarely voice this common fear; yet, child analysts must be sensitive to it.

While parents have to feel that they are in a partnership with the analyst, children simultaneously need to feel that the analysis remains a private place in which they can say or play whatever they want. Young children often imagine that their parents know everything that happens to them, even when they are not with them. If the analyst's style is very different from the parents'—more permissive, let us say—this can stir fears or conflicts of loyalty in the child. On the other hand, older children are very aware of what they keep separate or hidden from their parents. Adolescents may need to have the analyst completely out of contact with their parents in order to feel that the analysis is truly theirs and to use it successfully.

The analyst needs to be honest with child patients about meetings with parents and their purpose. The analyst needs to translate the child's inner world to the parents without giving details of the child's confidential communications. The analyst's understanding of the child's inner struggles helps parents to be more empathic (Ornstein 1977) and make better-informed parenting decisions. What one shares with a parent has much to do with the age of the child and the capacity of the parent to respect the child's privacy, as well as the need of the parent to feel included. Deciding how much to disclose can be quite a balancing act, and obviously the decision has to be different with each patient and family.

The sense of trust a parent has comes from how the analyst talks about the child to the parent—her knowledge and appreciation of, and affection for, the child; her respect for the parents' struggles; and her lack of blaming them. On the other hand, the child's trust can be severely compromised if the analyst brings to the child's attention the information and concerns that the parents convey to the analyst. The analysis must be the child's analysis—to develop at his or her own pace without the interference of the parents' agenda. However, since the child and his family are in an intricate pattern of interaction with each other, it is often difficult not to be drawn into the family's dance.

There have been many different technical approaches to working with the families. For example, some child analysts, particularly in past decades, advocate that the analyst limit his or her contact with the family. While I do not advocate this approach, it is based on an appreciation that seeing a child multiple times a week can be very effective treatment by itself. As a portal of entry into the family system, changes within the child can often lead to broader changes within the family.

Limited contact, however, if it means lack of involvement with parents, carries its own serious risks. It may make parents feel excluded from the child's treatment, stimulating resistance to its support. Parents can subtly undermine a treatment by making a child feel guilty for his or her involvement with the therapist or by making the child feel solely responsible for the family's troubles. Moreover, to the degree that the child's difficulties inevitably are intertwined with the parents' issues, the parents may contribute to the child's troubles without being aware of it. Nor are parents always pleased when a child gets better, if getting better means a psychological separation that feels threatening to them (Novick and Novick 2002).

There are some child analysts who, after evaluating the child, work for a substantial period with the parents in parent guidance before taking the child into psychoanalysis (J. Chused, personal communication, 2004; Novick and Novick 2001; Rosenbaum 1994). This allows parents to see what gains can be made in improving family interactions prior to their child receiving treatment. Such an experience often provides parents with conviction about the necessity for the analysis and helps them feel more strongly aligned with the analyst before the treatment begins. After an initial examination, some child analysts preferentially work via the parents when treating young children (under age 5), believing that the input from the environment is always a factor of greater significance for the young child (Furman 1957).

Some analysts treat a child individually from the outset, while working with the parents alongside the child's treatment. This decision is often made when the child is suffering significantly, when development is derailed, when the child's issues appear to be largely internalized, and/or

when the child needs a place apart from the family setting to express his or her feelings. However, child analysis should be undertaken only if parents are likely to support the treatment until its completion. Assessing this commitment may require a prolonged evaluation.

When a child analytic patient is preadolescent or younger, I generally see the parents separately from the child. Ideally, I work with parents weekly or biweekly in the beginning of an analysis and less frequently later on. When working with adolescents, it is much more variable how and when I see the parents. In all circumstances I consider the alliance with parents to be a top priority. If parents need comprehensive child guidance at the same time that the child's analytic privacy needs more protection, I may recommend that the parents work with another therapist. This therapist is preferably another child analyst but someone with whom I can communicate frequently and freely. On the other hand, I have occasionally found it necessary to see a parent regularly for a given period to discuss rather deep-seated issues, related, for example, to a parent's feelings about the child or about me. I have undertaken this when the analysis seemed in danger of being disrupted.

When things go well, the child's analysis is supported by the family and the family will feel supported by the child's treatment. At some time during the treatment, however, transference/countertransference issues with one or both parents inevitably heat up, and they must be dealt with flexibly, thoughtfully, and at times innovatively. Interestingly, this is true whether or not parents are in their own individual treatments. In fact, it is often the case that parents in treatment may not talk about their parenting issues to their own therapists, no matter how much turmoil these issues may be causing. Although the child analyst is often an object of transference to parents, parents do not often consider themselves to be the child analyst's "patient." Therefore, parents do not have the same commitment and motivation to communicate feelings, as opposed to enacting them. It stands to reason that a good relationship with parents and their inclusion in the process from the beginning through regular contact make the situation easier when thorny issues do emerge, as they inevitably will.

Other Theoretical Models

The technical ideas I have proposed in this chapter reflect my own way of working with children. There are many analysts who do not work in the play displacement as extensively and consistently as I do. Many do not use developmental assistance. Other child analysts use other theoretical models, and I want to mention a few of them. Of course, I do not have the space to really do justice to any of these theories.

Antonino Ferro (1999) has presented a model of child analysis that leans heavily on Bion's idea that the work of analysis is not primarily about making the unconscious conscious, but rather about increasing the mind's capacity to "think" and to "contain" certain raw, indigestible experiences that could not otherwise be integrated. Ferro feels that the analyst's goal is not to decode meaning, but to use interpretation and play to help the analytic dyad rearrange and re-create meanings in a way that facilitates the expansion of what is thinkable. This is actually quite close to my own view about play. Like Kleinian analysts, Ferro uses his countertransference and the concept of projective identification to understand, interpret, and respond to the child's state. He is particularly attentive to the moment-to-moment feelings between child and analyst.

Spillius (1999) notes that, like Ferro, modern Kleinians accept and use much of Bion's thinking, believe that the analyst is influenced by the patient's projections, and believe that the analytic relationship is the main object for analytic study. Both Ferro and the modern Kleinians appear to make many more direct and explicit verbal interpretations of the transference during a child analysis than their American counterparts, including myself.

Such a dominant focus on the moment-to-moment relationship between analyst and patient has similarities to the relational school of psychoanalysis in the United States. Relational theorists have written about child psychotherapy, but rarely about child psychoanalysis (Altman et. al 2002). The primary focus of change for the relational child therapists is not interpretation, but the particular transactions that occur between patient and analyst: the negotiation of a new kind of relating. While play is important, it is not privileged, and there is a value placed on the ability of children to make direct declarative statements about their feelings and their own lives.

Conclusion

The technique described in this chapter privileges play process because it provides a more flexible mode of thought for the child, taking into account defenses, as well as the developmental and cognitive capacities of the child. Moreover, play uses conceptual metaphor, making it particularly useful to convey affect and ideas that are difficult for a child to express in language. When a child cannot play, I believe it is the analyst's job to help the child join the analyst in a play process. This may mean giving the child developmental assistance. Using the play process enhances the value of using countertransference, working in the transference, and making interpretations in forms that a child can understand.

References

Abrams S: Differentiation and integration. Psychoanal Study Child 51:25–34, 1996

Abrams S, Solnit AJ: Coordinating developmental and psychoanalytic processes: conceptualizing technique. J Am Psychoanal Assoc 46:85–103, 1998

Altman N, Briggs R, Frankel J, et al: Relational Child Psychotherapy. New York, Other Press, 2002

Brenner C: The Mind in Conflict. New York, International Universities Press, 1982

Chused JF: The transference neurosis in child analysis. Psychoanal Study Child 43:51–81, 1988

Cohen DJ, Volkmar FR: Handbook of Autism and Pervasive Developmental Disorders. New York, Wiley, 1997

Cohen PM, Solnit AJ: Play and therapeutic action. Psychoanal Study Child 48:49–63, 1993

Colarusso CA: The third individuation: the effects of biological parenthood on separation-individuation processes in adulthood. Psychoanal Study Child 45:170–194, 1990

Colarusso CA: Separation-individuation phenomena in adulthood: general concepts and the fifth individuation. J Am Psychoanal Assoc 48:1467–1489, 2000

Emde RN: From adolescence to midlife: remodeling the structure of adult development. J Am Psychoanal Assoc 33:59–112, 1985

Erikson E: Studies in interpretation of play, I: clinical observations of play disruption in young children. Genet Psychology Monogr 22:557–671, 1940

Erikson E: Childhood and Society. New York, WW Norton, 1963

Ferro A: The Bi-Personal Field: Experiences in Child Analysis. London, Routledge, 1999

Fonagy P, Target M: Outcome predictors in child analysis. J Am Psychoanal Assoc 44:27–77, 1996

Fonagy P, Gergely G, Jurist EL, et al: Affect Regulation, Mentalization, and the Development of Self. New York, Other Press, 2002

Fraiberg S: A comparison of the analytic method in two stages of a child. J Am Acad Child Psychiatry 4:9–48, 1965

Fraiberg S: Further considerations of the role of transference in the child. Psychoanal Study Child 21:213–236, 1966

Frankel JB: The play's the thing: how the essential processes of therapy are most clearly seen in child therapy. Psychoanalytic Dialogues 8:149–182, 1998

Freud A: Four lectures in psychoanalysis (1927), in The Writings of Anna Freud, Vol 1. New York, International Universities Press, 1969, p 3–69

Freud A: Normality and pathology in childhood (1965), in The Writings of Anna Freud, Vol 6. New York, International Universities Press, 1974, pp 25–63

Freud S: Beyond the pleasure principle (1920), in Standard Edition of the Complete Psychological Works of Sigmund Freud, Vol 18. Translated and edited by Strachey J. London, Hogarth Press, 1955, pp 1–64

Furman E: Treatment of under-fives by way of parents. Psychoanal Study Child 12:250–262, 1957

Furman E: Transference and externalization in latency. Psychoanal Study Child 35:267–284, 1980

Gabbard GO, Westen D: Rethinking therapeutic action. Int J Psychoanal 84:823–841, 2003

Greenspan SI, Lieberman AF: Representational elaboration and differentiation: a clinical-quantitative approach to the assessment of 2- to 4-year-olds, in Children at Play. Edited by Slade A, Wolff D. New York, Oxford University Press, 1994, pp 3–32

Harley M: Transference developments in a five-year-old child, in The Child Analyst at Work. Edited by Geleerd ER. New York, International Universities Press, 1967, pp 115–141

Joseph B: Transference: the total situation. Int J Psychoanal 66:447–454, 1985

Klein M: The Psychoanalysis of Children (1932). New York, Delacorte Press/Seymour Lawrence, 1975, pp xv–xvi

Klein M: The psychoanalytic play technique. Am J Orthopsychiatry 25:223–237, 1955

Kris AO: Discussion of "Anna Freud and the evolution of psychoanalytic technique." Psychoanal Study Child 56:96–100, 2001

Lakoff G: Women, Fire, and Dangerous Things. Chicago, IL, University of Chicago Press, 1987

Lakoff G, Johnson M: Metaphors We Live By. Chicago, IL, University of Chicago Press, 1980

Lakoff G, Johnson M: Philosophy in the Flesh: The Embodied Mind and Its Challenge to Western Thought. New York, Basic Books, 1999

Lilleskov RK: Transference and transference neurosis, in The Unconscious Today. Edited by Kanzer M. New York, International Universities Press, 1971, pp 400–408

Mayes LC, Cohen DJ: Playing and therapeutic action in child analysis. Int J Psychoanal 74:1235–1244, 1993

Mayes LC, Cohen DJ: Children's developing theory of mind. J Am Psychoanal Assoc 44:117–142, 1996

Modell A: "The holding environment" and the therapeutic action of psychoanalysis. J Am Psychoanal Assoc 24:285–307, 1976

Modell A: Other Times, Other Realities. Cambridge, MA, Harvard University Press, 1990

Neubauer PB: The role of displacement in psychoanalysis. Psychoanal Study Child 49:107–119, 1994

Neubauer PB: Emerging issues: some observations about changes in technique in psychoanalysis. Psychoanal Study Child 56:16–38, 2001

Novick J, Novick KK: Parent work in analysis: children, adolescents, and adults, Part 1: evaluation. Journal of Infant, Child, and Adolescent Psychotherapy 1:55–77, 2001

Novick J, Novick KK: Parent work in analysis: children, adolescents, and adults, Part 3: middle and pretermination phases of treatment. Journal of Infant, Child, Adolescent Psychotherapy 2:17–41, 2002

Ornstein A: Making contact with the inner world of the child: towards a theory of psychoanalytic psychotherapy with children. Compr Psychiatry 17:3–26, 1977

Perner J, Leekam SR, Wimmer H: Three-year-olds' difficulty in understanding false belief: cognitive limitation, lack of knowledge, or pragmatic misunderstanding. British Journal of Developmental Psychology 5:125–137, 1987

Ritvo S: The psychoanalytic process in childhood. Psychoanal Study Child 33:295–305, 1978

Rosenbaum AL: The assessment of parental functioning: a critical process in the evaluation of children for psychoanalysis. Psychoanal Q 63:466–490, 1994

Sandler J, Kennedy H, Tyson R: The Technique of Child Analysis. Cambridge, MA, Harvard University Press, 1980

Scarlett WG: Play, cure, and development: perspective on the psychoanalytic treatment of young children, in Children at Play. Edited by Slade A, Wolff DP. New York, Oxford University Press, 1994, pp 48–61

Schacter DL: Searching for Memory. New York, Basic Books, 1996

Scharfman MA: Transference and the transference neurosis in child analysis, in Child Analysis and Therapy. Edited by Glenn J. New York, Jason Aronson, 1978, pp 275–307

Siegel DJ: The Developing Mind: How Relationships and the Brain Interact to Shape Who We Are. New York, Guilford, 1999

Slade A: Making meaning and making believe: their role in the clinical process, in Children at Play. Edited by Slade A, Wolff DP. New York, Oxford University Press, 1994, pp 81–107

Slade A, Wolff DP (eds): Children at Play. New York, Oxford University Press, 1994

Smith H: Analysis of transference: a North American perspective. Int J Psychoanal 84:1017–1041, 2003

Solnit AJ, Cohen DJ, Neubauer PB: The Many Meanings of Play. New Haven, CT, Yale University Press, 1993

Spillius EB: Introduction to The Bi-Personal Field: Experiences in Child Analysis by Ferro A. London, Routledge, 1999, pp ix–xviii

Stern DN, Sander LW, Nahum JP, et al: Noninterpretive mechanisms in psychoanalytic therapy. Int J Psychoanal 79:903–921, 1998

Tyson P: Transference and developmental issues in the analysis of a prelatency child. Psychoanal Study Child 33:213–236, 1978

Waelder A: The psychoanalytic theory of play. Psychoanal Q 2:208–224, 1933

Winnicott D: The Maturational Process and the Facilitating Environment. New York, International Universities Press, 1965

Winnicott D: Playing and Reality. London, Tavistock, 1986

Yanof JA: Language, communication, and transference in child analysis. J Am Psychoanal Assoc 44:79–116, 1996

19

Ethics in Psychoanalysis

ERNEST WALLWORK, Ph.D.

PSYCHOANALYSIS HAS A LONG history of deep ambivalence about *ethics*, defined as critical reflection about "right" and "wrong" actions and "good" and "bad" character traits and other states of affairs. Ethics differs from *morality* in providing arguments on behalf of our most basic normative standards, whereas morality is a more descriptive concept referring to how people do in fact think and behave within particular cultural contexts.

Many of Freud's interpreters have concluded that classical psychoanalytic theory makes ethical reflection and discourse pointless, since genuine moral conduct is simply not possible, given what metapsychology holds about determinism, the pleasure principle, and the superego (see Gregory 1975; Hospers 1950; Wallwork 1991; Yankelovich and Barrett 1970). Freud's comments on "the determination of mental life" (Freud 1910/1957, p. 38) appear to undermine both freedom of choice and moral responsibility. The pleasure principle's governance of the psychic apparatus seems to entail an egoistic hedonism of a sort that precludes genuine concern for others for their own sake. And Freud's explanation of morality in terms of the superego ostensibly embraces an ethical relativism inconsistent with any rational way of adjudicating among rival moral standards, which apparently vary systematically with the vicissitudes of child development, personality type, and sociocultural context (see Hartmann 1960). The body blow to traditional ethics wrought by the cumulative effect of these and other psychoanalytic doctrines is seen by contemporary cultural critics as partially responsible for the culture of narcissism and privatism that pervades modern Western societies (see Bellah et

al. 1985; Lasch 1979; Rieff 1961, 1968; Wallwork 1991). This is one reason why today many potential patients are so profoundly suspicious of psychoanalysis.

Yet, as I argue in my book *Psychoanalysis and Ethics* (Wallwork 1991), psychoanalytic practice is constituted by what Freud calls a moral "pact" involving implicit reciprocal duties of both analysand and analyst (Freud 1940[1938]/1964, p. 173). The analysand is expected to speak as truthfully as possible, even about the most shameful matters, and to keep his or her promises, minimally, by showing up on time for appointments and paying the bill by the agreed date. The patient must also begin to assume "moral responsibility" for disavowed motivations, fantasies, and behaviors (Freud 1925/1961, p. 133). The analyst, in turn, is guided by such standards as *primum non nocere* ("above all [or first] do no harm"), respect for the patient (Breuer and Freud 1893–1895/1955, p. 282), truthfulness (Freud 1926/1959, p. 207), protection of confidentiality (Freud 1913/1958, p. 129), and the therapeutic goals of relieving suffering and restoring the patient's autonomy (see Freud 1926/1959, p. 207, 1915a/1958, p. 164, 1940[1938]/1964, p. 176). These are not trivial moral standards of concern only to a few analysts. They constitute the conditions of the possibility of psychoanalytic treatment.

Serious analytic thinking about the contradiction between the anti-moral implications of classical psychoanalytic theory and the moral aspects of analytic practice has been astonishingly scant (Hartmann 1960, p. 13; Wallwork 1991). Why this should be merits study. Answers found in such a study would help explain how the moral aspects of psychoanalysis have been obscured for so long. What is clear is that the failure of Freud's followers to find an adequate approach to ethics has served as a major impetus for many of those, like Alfred Adler and Erich Fromm, who have broken ranks with the classical tradition, as well as those, such as Erik Erikson, Heinz Kohut, and Irwin Hoffman, who have revised psychoanalysis substantially from within, partly in order to find an ethic in psychoanalysis (see Erikson 1963, 1964; Fromm 1941, 1947, 1956; Hoffman 1998). The widespread skepticism toward ethics among psychoanalysts has undoubtedly contributed to the sad history of boundary violations by experienced clinicians, who have falsely imagined themselves blessedly liberated from morals by a value-free, "a-moral" profession.

The first generation of analysts after Freud eschewed ethical reflection, in part because they were convinced that psychoanalysis was, or should aim at being, a value-neutral science, free of the distorting effects of moral values (Hartmann 1960, p. 160). Psychoanalysis, it was asserted, describes and explains the facts of mental life and behavior, including moral conduct, without passing judgment on them, whereas ethics belongs to another (suspect) discipline about how we "ought" to think and act (see Flugel 1945, p. 11). This fact-value dichotomy held sway during the heyday of positivism and its chief ethical corollary, emotivism, which stretched from the 1930s through the 1950s (see Hudson 1970, pp. 107–154; Stevenson 1944). One result was that moral judgments came to be seen as little more than an unjustifiable expression of an individual's private affects and biases. In contrast with factual propositions, which were in principle verifiable, it was thought that moral claims could not be empirically or rationally supported. Had not Freud himself declared: "There are no sources of knowledge of the universe other than the intellectual working-over of carefully scrutinized observations—in other words, what we call research—and alongside of it no knowledge derived from revelation, intuition or divination" (Freud 1933[1932]/1964, p. 159)? Forgotten, for the time being, was that Freud also often approvingly quoted F.T. Vischer's statement, "What is moral is self-evident." Not only did Freud require psychoanalysts to honor traditional normative standards, he demanded that the analyst's "own character must be irreproachable" (Freud 1905/1953, p. 267).

The clinical consequence of the construal of psychoanalysis as a value-free science by Freud's immediate followers was that the analyst was expected to practice a neutrality, anonymity, and abstinence that mirrored the natural scientist's detachment from the world of investigation. Leading figures like Ernest Jones and Heinz Hartmann admonished colleagues to keep their "scientific work free from the interference of value judgments" (Hartmann 1960,

p. 54). Freud's depiction of the analyst as a mirror and surgeon and his "The Question of a Weltanschauung" (Freud 1933[1932]/1964, pp. 158–182) were (and are) much cited in support of a concept of neutrality requiring freedom from morals, as if Hartmann was right to attribute to Freud Max Weber's epistemological skepticism about ethics, as part of a value-free methodology (Hartmann 1960, pp. 78–79), even though Freud's own technical writings make it clear that clinical work must be guided by moral standards (see Breuer and Freud 1893–1895/1955, p. 265; Freud 1913/1958, p. 129, 1926/1959, p. 227, 1940[1938]/1964, pp. 172–174; Wallwork 1991). The pejorative attitude toward ethics was so prevalent in the 1950s that the single mention of "ethics" by the then president of the American Psychoanalytic Association, Ives Hendrick, in his 1955 presidential address on professional standards, was to the self-serving "basic principle…[that] it is unethical" to teach psychotherapy in any organization not directly affiliated with the association (Hendrick 1955, p. 576)!

The primary goal of psychoanalysis as a scientific undertaking became restricted to discovering psychological truths, with the result that other values, such as the therapeutic aims enshrined in the Hippocratic tradition and the patient's expectations for enhanced freedom of thought and action, were eclipsed—at least as explicit treatment goals (see Grinberg 1988, p. 132; Joan Riviere, cited in Phillips 1988, pp. 43–44). Freud was again cited, out of context, to the effect that therapeutic goals inevitably interfere with the analyst's primary aim, interpreting unconscious truths (Freud 1912/1958, p. 119, 1937/1964, p. 251). That Freud scarcely imagined that his warnings against *excessive* "therapeutic ambition" *(furor sanandi)* and "passion for curing people" implied goallessness is evident in the following key passage:

> [T]he doctor should hold himself in check, and take the patient's capacities rather than his own desires as guide. Not every neurotic has a high talent for sublimation; one can assume of many of them that they would not have fallen ill at all if they had possessed the art of sublimating their instincts. If we press them unduly towards sublimation and cut them off from the most accessible and convenient instinctual satisfactions, we shall usually make life even harder for them than they feel it in any case. As a doctor, one must above all be *tolerant* to the weakness of a patient, and must be content if one has won back some degree of *capacity for work and enjoyment for a person*.…[I]n those who have a capacity for sublimation the process usually takes place of itself as soon as their inhibitions have been overcome by analysis. In my opinion, therefore, efforts invariably to make use of the analytic treatment to bring about sublimation of instinct are, though no doubt always laudable, far from being in every case advisable. (Freud 1912/1958, p. 119; emphasis added)

Freud's advice about tempering therapeutic ambition is here set in a broader conception of an ethics of practice in which less grandiose ambitions are seen as the best means toward the moral aim of providing optimal patient benefit at the least harm. The analyst's temporary goallessness is *ethically* justified, because in the long run it is deemed most likely to benefit the patient by discovering the true meaning of his or her symptoms and helping the patient work them through. "The removal of the symptoms of the illness is not especially aimed at, but is achieved, as it were, as a by-product if the analysis is properly carried through" (Freud 1921/1955, p. 251). For Freud, truth is a leading goal but never the sole aim of analytic work, because the therapist has a broad set of "duties towards the individual patient" beyond the pursuit of knowledge (Freud 1905 [1901]/1953, p. 8; see Wallwork 1991).

One problem with the post-Freudian claim that psychoanalysis is singularly focused on pursuing emotional truth, whatever the cost, is that it de-legitimizes other ethical questions and concerns—for example, whether unrelenting pursuit of the truth with a patient might be a form of coercion, aiming at compliance, rather than authentic analytic exploration. This was one of Kohut's concerns: "the primacy of the [classical psychoanalytic] value system that it is 'good' to know…that it is 'bad not to know'" may lead to a cognitive penetration that overtaxes the resilience of the analysand (Kohut 1977, p. 176; Lichtenberg 1983, pp. 647–664; see also Schafer 1997, p. 196).

It was commonly believed, and still is in some circles, that taking a value-free stance enables therapists to be non-biased toward all of the patient's communications. However, as feminists and cultural historians such as Michel Foucault (1990) have pointed out, the neutral scientific discourse of medicine is no guarantor of the moral innocuousness of theories and practices, especially regarding gender and sexual behavior. To the contrary, claims of scientific objectivity about these topics are apt to be all the more dangerous morally for pretending to be value-free (see Wallwork 1995). The psychoanalytic bias against homosexuality during most of the last half century is one example of an injustice perpetuated in the name of presumptions about scientific objectivity. Until recently, these biases could not be subjected to ethical interrogation for their "unfairness" and lack of "respect" for the homosexual patient, because they were thought to be based on objective, value-neutral findings.

The narrowing of ethics to the value of scientific truth failed because the suppressed question kept returning: How is the analyst to account for the other values, particularly therapeutic standards, that are part and parcel of the analytic relationship? One popular answer was found in the old adage that "the truth will set you free," to which it was often added that the truth also, fortunately, tends to reduce suffering and to unlock optimal possible internal conditions for autonomy and happiness. The singular focus on scientific truth was thus quietly expanded to include such central moral goals as increasing the patient's freedom and autonomy, reducing pain and suffering, and improving the patient's capacity for experiencing pleasure and happiness. Yet analysts continued to assert that even if these desirable byproducts of the search for truth did not occur, a good analysis had occurred nonetheless. And some, including Hartmann, contended that therapeutic values were not really moral values and so analysis could continue to be construed as truly value-free.

One problem with treating therapeutic aims as non-moral health values is that the concept of mental health cannot be separated from moral and ethical considerations. Mental health is neither a statistical norm nor the absence of psychic discomfort. A patient with an "average" state of depression scarcely represents the psychoanalytic idea of the mentally healthy person. A "happy" narcissist is not free of psychopathology because he or she is not experiencing discomfort. Most formulations of mental illness have to do with some failure to understand oneself or to guide one's own actions, not with departures from a statistical average or pleasurable mental state (see Daly 1991). Diminished or impaired mental functioning not only cannot be measured against a natural norm but also cannot be articulated without the help of implicit moral standards like authenticity, self-knowledge, and autonomy that together constitute what we mean by agency. When someone's authentic self-guidance is impaired by irrational underlying motives or inexplicable behavior to such an extent that the agent is no longer the author of her or his actions, we consider the person mentally ill (see Feinberg 1970).

Hartmann notwithstanding, the presence of moral values in our concepts of mental illness and health, as well as in our beliefs about efficacious technique, does not constitute an undesirable interference with psychoanalysis. Rather, moral evaluations are a necessary condition for having standards of health and illness and therapeutic practices to treat them. Just as there are no facts without theories, there are no mental illnesses and states of well-being without some implicit moral evaluations. Psychoanalysts may not often think consciously about moral evaluations in their daily work, but all aspects of psychoanalysis can be examined for their ethical dimensions (see Schafer 1997, p. 213). Moral standards like truthfulness, confidentiality, beneficence, nonmaleficence, and promise keeping, as well as the role-specific virtues and treatment goals discussed in this chapter, set the context within which analysis takes place. Many ordinary interpretations presuppose the analysand's concurrence about the moral harm of, say, projective identification, irrational rage, or self-defeating conduct. Thus, the issue is not whether value-freedom is a desirable state of affairs, since it is not possible to attain such a mental condition; the issue is how we think ethically of the standards that we do hold (or should hold) about the work that we do.

Ethical Aspects of Neutrality

Since Hartmann's era, the concept of *neutrality* has given rise to considerable controversy about both its meaning and its usefulness. If the term today less often signifies an amoral value-free posture, it continues to be used in writings on technique for a desirable mental state consisting of a combination of benignly attentive and tolerant attitudes and dispositions that are constitutive of analytic listening (see Laplanche and Pontalis 1973, pp. 271–272; Moore and Fine 1990, p. 127).

The term *neutrality*, which Strachey introduced as a translation of Freud's *indifferenz* (see Freud 1915a/1958, p. 164), comes from the Latin *neuter*, meaning "neither one nor the other." Unlike "abstinence," which involves not doing something, such as revealing personal information, neutrality is a state of mind. The term attempts to capture Freud's recommendation that the analyst listen with "evenly suspended attention" (Freud 1912/1958, p. 111), which Anna Freud characterized in structural terms as taking up a mental position equidistant from the demands of the id, ego, and superego (A. Freud 1936/1966, p. 28; Smith 1999, pp. 469–470, 2003, pp. 1020–1021). To the Freuds, to be neutral in the sense of free-floating attention was not to be value-free, because the rationale for this listening mode was that it would benefit the patient by enabling the analyst to hear the full range of meanings in the patient's communications with minimal distortion and interference from the analyst's subjective opinions. "We will suspend our judgment and give our impartial attention to everything that is there to observe," Freud advised in the Little Hans case (cited in Balsam 1997, p. 5). The analyst was cautioned not to lend a special ear to particular parts of the patient's discourse or "read particular meanings into it, according to…theoretical or moral preconceptions" (Laplanche and Pontalis 1973, p. 271). The idea was to foster "reverie" in the analyst, enabling him or her to be receptive to what Bollas calls "unthought knowns," but also to create a mood essential for the analysand's freedom to speak without fear of being encroached upon by the analyst's personal biases, opinions, and judgments (see Bollas 1999, pp. 5–26).

However, this temporary suspension of the analyst's narcissistic investment in favored theories, moral judgments about the patient's conduct, and particular life goals for the patient does not extend to the moral framework that makes analysis possible or to the analyst's moral character or to the long-term moral goals toward which the analysis is directed. For instance, neutral attention does not suspend the principle of respect for the patient as a person or the general obligation to avoid gratuitous harm. Rather than dispensing with moral character, neutrality actually requires it, in that the analyst cultivates the moral attitude of attentive tolerance, even toward the most extraordinarily provocative behavior.

If neutrality is conceived as a technical stance involving evenly suspended attentiveness, it characterizes the way the analyst is present (not absent, as some relational critics contend) in the analytic situation. This way of being present creates an ambiance that fosters both the analysand's freedom to speak and the analyst's ability simultaneously to hear the multiple meanings of the patient's verbal and nonverbal communications, without either party being pressured by the constraints of theories, morals, or goals. This analytic attitude/disposition is in turn warranted by such moral considerations as respect for the patient and benefiting him or her optimally by facilitating freedom of expression, self-understanding, and autonomy. The patient is respected both as the conscious not-yet-analyzed self-determining subject who chooses to speak at any given moment and as the more fully self-aware agent he or she might become with the advent of fuller, more authentic and richer speech (for discussion of these two notions of respect for the analysand, see Blass 2003). Freud described the respect-for-the-patient's-autonomy aspects of neutrality this way: "We refused most emphatically to turn a patient who puts himself in our hands in search of help into our private property, to decide his fate for him, to force our own ideals upon him, and with the pride of a Creator to form him in our own image and to see that it is good" (Freud 1919/1955, p. 164).

That neutrality has been imagined as value-free rather than intertwined with these and other moral considerations reveals the crimped, duty-oriented ("deontological") construal of morality that has been at work in psychoanalysis. It is a picture that has hindered ethical thinking among psychoanalysts by portraying ethics as always imposing impossibly demanding moral duties and unachievable ideals. Fortunately, ethical reasoning requires neither absolute, universal principles nor deductive procedures imposed without regard for the unique particulars of a moral situation. Today, ethicists no longer subordinate moral reasoning to a single metaprinciple or decision procedure. Instead, ethical thinking is seen as involving a plurality of nonabsolute prima facie moral standards that, because they often conflict in practice, require the agent to weigh and balance standards against one another in light of their significance for the main stakeholders in some specific moral situation. The term *prima facie moral standards* comes from the writings of Sir David Ross (1930, 1939), who proposed a decision-making model that weighed a plurality of often conflicting standards as an alternative to both Kantian deontological absolutism and utilitarianism.

Beyond prima facie guidelines for dealing with right and wrong actions ("act-ethics"), ethics is also concerned with such questions as What is the best way to live one's life? and How should we go about trying to handle complex moral dilemmas? The clarifications and distinctions ethicists have elaborated in treating these issues can help analysts differentiate ethical aspects from technical considerations in controversial issues such as (in addition to neutrality) empathy, treatment goals, termination criteria, self-disclosure, and the value of interpersonal mutuality. Analytic thinking about these contentious issues today is often muddled by failure to distinguish ethical disagreements from technical ones.

Acknowledging that neutrality, as a mental state, is supported by moral standards carries with it the implication that the analyst's evenly suspended attentiveness may be—indeed, should be—modified if the weight of ethical and technical considerations warrants a more engaged style that better facilitates analytic listening (possibly through retrospective interpretation of enactments) as well as a particular patient's freedom of expression, expanded self-understanding, and autonomy. The differentiation of ethical considerations thus supports one of the chief contentions of relational critics of neutrality (Aron 1996). At the same time, awareness of the ethical aspects of neutrality highlights the relational critic's need for an equivalent analytic stance, both to listen attentively without undue inner static and to intervene without interfering excessively in the patient's unfolding self-understanding Relational critics of neutrality commonly object to the emotionally distant, cool, and aloof attitude they associate with neutrality, as if the concept endorses the authoritative style that became the stereotype of some schools of analysis in the 1940s and 1950s (see Stone 1961). However, neutrality in the sense of benign attentiveness is certainly not incompatible with either personal warmth or empathy. In fact, neutrality is intended to facilitate empathy, so that if it does not, some adjustments in its practice are ethically desirable.

Freud's Ethics

The ethics of clinical practice for psychoanalysis do not stand or fall with what Freud or his disciples thought, but it is instructive to look at the deep ethic that informs classical psychoanalytic theory and practice. This ethic, which

I explore at length in *Psychoanalysis and Ethics* (Wallwork 1991), has not been widely appreciated by psychoanalysts, largely because the prevailing value-neutral, "scientistic" (Habermas 1971) bias against ethics has led to the distortion of Freud's thought on a number of issues central to moral philosophy. However, the deep ethic that informs Freud's work persists to this day as one of the unacknowledged factors that unite psychoanalysts, despite theoretical and technical differences among contemporary schools.

Determinism

One widely shared misperception is the assumption that Freud embraced the hard determinist thesis that the individual could not have acted otherwise. For example, Arlow and Brenner (1964) echo Ernest Jones (1953, pp. 365–366) when they write, "[Mental processes] follow the same general laws of cause and effect which we customarily assume to operate in the physical world. Psychoanalysis postulates that psychic determinism is as strict as physical determinism" (p. 7).

However contrary to the suppositions of Jones, Arlow and Brenner, and Yankelovich and Barrett, among others, none of the few brief references to determinism in Freud's writings actually advocate the metaphysical determinist thesis that all human actions are causally necessitated by antecedent conditions and universal laws (Wallwork 1991, pp. 49–100). Freud writes only about "*psychic* determinism," and he is careful to confine the concept to "motives" as "causes" that affect the occurrence of an outcome, without actually requiring it. In the main, Freud employs "psychic determinism" to signal that some particular kinds of behavior (e.g., dreams, symptoms, parapraxes, and free associations) do not occur accidentally or fortuitously, as his predecessors had thought, but are traceable to the influence of repressed unconscious motives that function as "causes" in the realm of mental life. Thus, when Freud states that "psychoanalysts are marked by a particularly strict belief in the determination of mental life," he goes on to explain: "For them there is nothing trivial, nothing arbitrary or haphazard. They expect in every case to find sufficient *motives* where, as a rule, no such expectation is raised" (Freud 1910/1957, p. 38, emphasis added).

For Freud, "psychic determinism" does not imply an absence of choice so much as the claim that all behavior is motivated and, as such, may fall under conscious voluntary control (Wallwork 1991, 1997). Choice is made possible in the structural theory by the "I" or the "ego," which has "voluntary movement at its command" (Freud 1940[1938]/1964, p. 145). Thus, it is not inconsistent with "psychic determinism" for Freud to claim that the goal of psychoanalysis is to expand the range of "conscious will-power" and "freedom" *(Freiheit)* (Freud 1905/1953, p. 266, 1915a/1958, p. 170). In fact, the ultimate goal of psychoanalysis is "to give the patient's ego *freedom* to decide one way or the other" among the motives or reasons for action available to consciousness (Freud 1923/1961, pp. 50–51).

Psychoanalysis is well known for shrinking the domain of moral responsibility by bringing to light new excusing circumstances that explain that an individual acted in a given way in some situation because of unconscious motivations. But psychoanalysis, paradoxically, also expands the realm of moral responsibility by encouraging owning one's own disavowed motivations. The analysand is expected to assume responsibility for not only conscious intentions and conduct, as the Western ethical tradition advises, but also unconscious motivations. In his remarkable 1925 essay on "Moral Responsibility for the Content of Dreams," Freud (1925/1961) states:

> I must assume responsibility for both [conscious and unconscious motives]; and if, in defence, I say that what is unknown, unconscious and repressed in me is not my "ego," then I shall not be basing my position upon psycho-analysis, I shall not have accepted its conclusions—and I shall perhaps have to be taught better by the criticisms of my fellow-men, by the disturbances in my actions and the confusion of my feelings. I shall perhaps learn that what I am disavowing not only "is" in me but sometimes "acts" from out of me as well. (p. 133; see my discussion of Freud's views on moral responsibility in Wallwork 1991, pp. 75–100)

Egoistic Hedonism

A second commonplace misreading of Freud that undermines both the possibility of morality and the point of ethical reflection attributes psychological egoistic hedonism to the pleasure principle (see Asch 1952, p. 9; Fromm 1973, p. 52; Gregory 1975, p. 102; Hoffmann 1976, p. 124; Wallwork 1991, pp. 103–190). Certainly, Freud sometimes writes as if he subscribes to the psychological hedonist thesis that human desire and volition are "always determined by pleasures or pains, actual or prospective" (Sidgwick 1962, p. 40).

But the key ethical issue at stake is whether Freud's hedonism always directs the agent egoistically, so that all seemingly disinterested behavior, such as pursuit of the truth, can be reduced ultimately to a desire for pleasure for oneself alone. That Freud tried to stake out a place for nonegoistic motives is obvious. Writing against egoism, he declares that it is both possible and desirable to pursue knowledge, even though it offers "no compensation for… [those] who suffer grievously from life" (Freud 1927/1957,

p. 54). He makes a similar point about the possibility of loving others for their own sake *("ihnen zu Liebe")* (Freud 1921/1955, p. 92). In Freud's early work, disinterested motives are attributed to the reality principle's opposition to unrestrained libidinal pleasure seeking. In 1915, Freud adds that nonegoistic motivations are a result of the developmental "transformation of egoistic into altruistic inclinations" (1915b/1957, pp. 283–284). There is an enormous difference, Freud argues, between the egoist (or narcissist) who "acts morally" only for egoistic reasons—that is, because "such cultural behaviour is advantageous for his selfish purposes"—and the person who acts morally "because his instinctual inclinations compel him to" (1915b/1957, p. 284). The latter individual has undergone "the transformation of instinct *[Triebumbildung]* that differentiates the 'truly civilized' from 'cultural hypo-crites.'" The civilized moral agent finds "satisfaction" in acting benevolently for another, but the basis of this is no more egoistic than it is in the writings of those many Western moralists since Aristotle who have emphasized the pleasurable aspects of acting morally.

Ethical Relativism

A third common misinterpretation of Freud that affects current attitudes toward ethics derives from the potentially relativistic implications of the concept of the superego (see Wallwork 1991, pp. 221–259). If the superego is synonymous with morality, as Freud sometimes indicates (Brenner 1982, p. 123; Freud 1933[1932]/1964, pp. 61, 66–67; Kafka 1990, pp. 249–249), and if the superego is nothing more than a set of purely arbitrary standards that the individual has internalized by introjecting the prohibitions and ideals of his or her parents and other authority figures, then nothing can be said in defense of moral standards other than that they are the standards one happens to have. There is no principled basis for choosing one set of ethical norms over another as guides for action—no grounds for reasoning that might persuade in the presence of conflict—other than egoistic strategies for obtaining rewards and avoiding external punishments and internal guilt or shame.

This is not Freud's position, however. Freud resists the pull of ethical relativism by arguing that there are certain reasonable moral guidelines that can be rationally defended (Wallwork 1991, pp. 230–243). This side of Freud's work has not been appreciated because it occurs as the subtext of Freud's all-out attack on religion in *Future of an Illusion*. Here, Freud's sub rosa point is that weakening the religious grounds for morality poses dangers to society and requires new rational justifications—the main task of ethics. Against ethical relativism, Freud declares that the time has come to "put forward rational grounds for the precepts of civilization" (1927/1957, p. 44). The challenge to contemporary analysts is to locate these grounds.

The Deep Ethical Theory Informing the Practice of Psychoanalysis

Although Freud never directly addressed the "rational bases" for morality, much can be adduced about the deep ethic in his work from what he says about happiness as the goal of life, the primacy of love of and respect for others as natural dispositions, the good of community, and the value of shared rules (see Wallwork 1991). This deep ethic continues to inform psychoanalysis today.

Freud's alternative ethic to superego moralism is often missed because it is drowned out by the negativity of his critique of religious and duty-oriented—particularly Kantian—ethics. Readers are unprepared for the Aristotelian form of ethics (oriented toward achieving personal happiness) that informs Freud's thinking, including his critique of superego moralism. Instead of viewing ethics as seeking an ahistorical, perspectiveless set of universal principles legitimated by reason alone, without reference to local commitments or particular experiences and affects, Freud sees ethics (at least when he is thinking constructively) primarily as dealing with the question of how it is best to live our lives. Here ethical deliberation is not about finding and applying a meta-decision-making procedure, such as Kant's categorical imperative or Bentham's utilitarian calculus, to resolve moral dilemmas. Rather, ethics is a matter of negotiating or straddling multiple incommensurate conscious and unconscious responsibilities and values that emerge out of "thick" reasoning, supportive of the most fitting moral judgment for the agent(s) in some specific context.

As for the paramount moral standard, Freud is quite explicit that the good that humans universally seek is "happiness" (*eudeamonia* in Greek, *beatitude* in Latin):

[W]hat [do] men themselves show by their behaviour to be the purpose and intention of their lives…? The answer to this can hardly be in doubt. They strive after happiness; they want to become happy and to remain so. (Freud 1930/1957, p. 76)

In identifying "happiness" as the *summum bonum*, Freud is in agreement with the mainstream of the Western moral tradition stretching from Aristotle through Augustine, Thomas Aquinas, and J.S. Mill. Like them, Freud does not leave the constituents of the intrinsic good of happiness for an individual to arbitrary personal preference (as

it is in current formulations of utilitarianism). Nor does he think that subjectively pleasurable mental states alone determine happiness (see Freud 1930/1957, pp. 76–84). Happiness for Freud, as for Aristotle, is more a matter of *functioning well* than feeling good. The mentally healthy person's happiness consists in the well-being that comes with certain forms of sublimation: loving and being loved, creative work, the pursuit of knowledge, freedom, and aesthetic appreciation. These goods of life that make happiness possible are not instrumental means to functioning well, but constituent aspects of happiness. It is by means of love and work (*lieben* and *arbeiten)*, for example, that we are as happy as human beings are capable of being (Freud 1912/1958, p. 119; 1930/1957, pp. 80–82).

Love is privileged by Freud as a constituent of happiness partly because the qualitatively unique "union of mental and bodily satisfaction in the enjoyment of love is one of its [life's] culminating peaks" (1915a/1958, p. 169). Mutual love ("loving and being loved") is universally recognized as one of the chief means for finding "a positive fulfillment of happiness" (Freud 1930/1957, p. 82). Freud also accords love pride of place because it underlies so many other nonegoistic values: love of family, friendship, love of others in a community (which provide Freud's rationale for acceptance of a community's rules and regulations), and love of humankind. Indeed, Freud (1930/1957) defines "civilization" as a "process in the service of Eros, whose purpose is to combine single…individuals, and after that… peoples and nations, into one great unity" (p. 122). By means of libidinal ties to the community, the individual feels concern for the welfare of others and can be motivated to "conform to the standards of morality and refrain from brutal and arbitrary conduct" (Freud 1915b/1957, p. 280), even when it is "disadvantageous" in terms of the agent's short-range self-interest. Of course, Freud never forgets that "man's natural aggressive instinct, the hostility of each against all and of all against each, opposes this programme of civilization" (Freud 1930/1957, p. 122). With characteristic realism, he cautions that few get beyond common human unhappiness.

Freud is well known, of course, for his sharp criticism of the love commandment ("Thou shalt love thy neighbor as thyself") in *Civilizaiton and Its Discontents*. Less widely appreciated is that this critique is directed only against the *excessive* demands for self-abnegation and self-sacrifice of the Christian version of the commandment, and that Freud actually reinterprets the love commandment along more modest, broadly humanistic lines. "I myself have always advocated the love of mankind," Freud wrote to Romain Rolland, whose humanism he respected (letter 218, in E.L.Freud 1975, p. 374). In 1933, 3 years after his harsh criticism in *Civilization and Its Discontents*, Freud himself explicitly embraced "the love commandment" as the antidote to human aggression.

> If willingness to engage in war is an effect of the destructive instinct, the most obvious plan will be to bring Eros, its antagonist, into play against it. Anything that encourages the growth of emotional ties between men must operate against war.... There is no need for psychoanalysis to be ashamed to speak of love in this connection, for religion itself uses the same words: "thou shalt love thy neighbour as thyself." (Freud 1933/1964, p. 212)

Ever the realist, Freud adds, "This, however, is more easily said than done."

Unlike Kantians, who justify moral duties like promise keeping and justice by appealing to the dictates of unmotivated practical reason, guided by the categorical imperative, Freud grounds social principles and rules in love of the community that the rules help constitute and maintain. By means of libidinous ties to the community, the individual feels concern for the welfare of others and is motivated to "conform to the standards of morality and refrain from brutal and arbitrary conduct" (Freud 1915b/1957, p. 280). According to Freud (1925/1961), "Social [and moral] feelings rest on identification with other people" (p. 37). This in turn is rooted in "aim-inhibited libido" that "strengthen[s] the communal bond by relations of friendship" and citizenship (Freud 1930/1957, p. 109; see also Freud 1930/1957, p. 112; Freud 1933[1932]/1964, p. 208).

Of course, Freud diverges from the received ethical tradition in disavowing the possibility of pure moral motivations. For psychoanalysis, the morally good act is always mixed with less honorable motivations. For instance, altruistic acts are motivated in part by unconscious aggressive and narcissistic motives that compromise the consciously intended conduct. That actual conduct is always a product of mixed motivations, however, does not detract from the fact that genuine moral motives are possible as components of compromise formations. These moral components may be strengthened, clinical experience testifies, if the agent acknowledges and takes responsibility for the unseemly motivations that are part of the mixture. This complex picture of moral conduct lies behind the following declaration by Freud:

> It is not our intention to dispute the noble endeavours of human nature, nor have we ever done anything to detract from their value.... We lay a stronger emphasis on what is evil in men only because other people disavow it and thereby make the human mind, not better, but incomprehensible. If now we give up this one-sided ethical valuation, we shall undoubtedly find a more correct formula for the relation between good and evil in human nature. (Freud 1915–1916/1961, pp. 146–147)

Clinical Ethics Today

Ethical considerations enter into psychoanalytic practice in four different ways that standard philosophical distinctions help identify and clarify: 1) as *guidelines or principles* that constitute the manifest or latent expectations of both parties to the relationship; 2) as the *virtues* psychoanalysts cultivate as constituents of the analytic role; 3) as the *goals* of the work; and 4) as the *moral decisions* analysts and analysands must make about serious dilemmas.

Principles, Rules, and Guidelines

As noted earlier in this chapter, the conduct of each of the parties to the analytic relationship is guided by implicit and explicit normative standards without which analysis could not occur. On the patient's side, truthfulness and promise keeping are particularly salient. The patient who violates these norms is not blamed or punished, but is expected to appreciate that a departure from a normative expectation has occurred that is worthy of exploration. Interpretations that show, for example, that the analysand wants to hurt his analyst, perhaps by subverting her effectiveness or tarnishing her professional reputation, typically presuppose that the patient is capable of understanding that his wish to harm in these circumstances is not morally warranted. For some analysts, interpretations are made with the expectation that the patient seeks not only to understand the obscure motivations behind the desire to harm but also to change the behavior once the hidden motivations are uncovered. Other analysts hold that it is perfectly ethical to make these interpretations with the goal of giving the patient a rational choice, but that taking up a mental stance that the patient "should" then do the right thing is coercive and clinically counterproductive. Nonetheless, interpretations commonly rely on the silent doings of moral agreement for their effectiveness in that the patient needs to "own" formerly unconscious harmful motives in such a way as to diminish their strength. If an analysand were defiantly unwilling to try to be truthful about such conduct or were to remain recalcitrant about engaging in a mutual understanding of that resistance, the analysis would be endangered unless the analyst were able to find some way of reactivating the analysand's moral engagement in the work.

On the analyst's side, duties include the set of general principles enunciated in the revised Principles and Standards of the American Psychoanalytic Association (Dewald et al. 2001). At the most general level, these include duties to 1) provide competent service; 2) respect patients, their family members, colleagues, and students without regard to age, disability, gender, sexual orientation, race, or religion; 3) inform the patient fully about psychoanalysis beforehand and to obtain consent to treatment; 4) maintain the confidentiality of the patient's communications; 5) deal honestly and forthrightly; 6) avoid all forms of exploitation of current or former patients; 7) conform to scientific principles in research, for example, by communicating truthfully with colleagues; 8) strive to protect patients or potential patients from impaired colleagues; 9) comply with the law, unless it is unethical; and 10) be thoughtful, considerate, and fair in all professional relationships.

Since these "principles" are too abstract and vague to guide conduct very precisely, their implications are explicated more fully in a longer "Standards" section of the American Psychoanalytic Association code that sets forth more concretely current thinking about what these principles mean for the analyst's conduct in problematic areas. For example, the principle "Avoidance of Exploitation" is interpreted in the Standards section as prohibiting all financial dealings with current or former patients, including solicitations of financial contributions to psychoanalytic groups. The analyst is expected to recuse himself or herself from any influence over the use of funds donated by a patient or former patient to a psychoanalytic organization to which he or she belongs. Here, as in the other standards, such as the absolute prohibition on sexual relations with present or former patients, the aim is to minimize any exploitation of the inequality of power inherent in the transference relationship.

Despite its duty-oriented, or "deontological," structure (*deon* in Greek means "duty"), the new code is not meant to encourage analysts to think primarily in terms of rules in resolving moral dilemmas. Explicit rules are necessary but of limited usefulness. They serve mainly to provide an explicit framework within which the free play of analysis can occur safely for both parties. But rules alone, no matter how well formulated, fail to provide sufficient moral guidance to the morally perplexed analyst. For one thing, rules conflict. For another, they are constructed at a level of generality that seldom does justice to the complexities of real moral dilemmas. Good moral decision making is usually about balancing conflicting rules, values, and responsibilities in relationship to the particular facts and dynamics of specific situations.

Consider the new American Psychoanalytic Association confidentiality guidelines. The Standards specify that patient privacy must be protected in presentations by disguising the patient and/or obtaining his or her informed consent (Dewald et al. 2001, pp. iv, viii–x). There are myriad variables to consider: the patient's character structure and views about confidentiality; the adequacy of the disguise in preventing identification; the potential that the

treatment will suffer as a consequence of the analyst's request for consent; the likelihood of identification despite the disguise and its probable effects on the patient, as well as his or her friends or relatives; the likelihood that the disguise will mislead colleagues in ways that undermine the goals of the professional communication; the varying risks to the patient of different settings for the analyst's presentation (e.g., consultation, small group discussion, lecture, publication); the audience (whether clinicians governed by confidentiality, or the public). No currently available ethical decision-making procedure, whether a contemporary version of Kant's categorical imperative or some form of utilitarianism, even if it could be justified as the definitive ethical approach, is capable of adjudicating among these and other complexities that need to be taken into account in arriving at a reasonably good decision about using case material. The morally responsible analyst has to sort through conflicting considerations to arrive at the best judgment under the circumstances, which might not be the best judgment for a different patient under similar circumstances, the famed "universalizability" criterion in ethics notwithstanding. The code of the American Psychoanalytic Association states that "no code of ethics can be encyclopedic in providing answers to all ethical questions that may arise in the practice of…psychoanalysis," partly because many moral cases outstrip the explicit standards that govern them.

Virtues

In addition to general moral principles and rules, psychoanalysts are expected to cultivate certain attitudes and dispositions toward analysands. These dispositional traits—for example, patience, benign tolerance, honesty with self and others, and respect—are seldom identified explicitly as "virtues" in the psychoanalytic literature, presumably because the self-righteous connotations of the term *virtue* make analysts squeamish. Nonetheless, these traits certainly are virtues in the traditional sense of dispositions or habits that are valued and cultivated as the (moral) qualities exhibited by the reasonably "good enough" analyst. A trait like the suspension of moralistic criticism is desirable in an analyst because it advances goods—such as self-exploration—internal to the practice of psychoanalysis.

The idea that virtues are indispensable to realizing the goods internal to a practice such as psychoanalysis comes from Alasdair MacIntyre (1984). Following MacIntyre, a "practice" is "any coherent and complex form of socially established cooperative human activity through which goods internal to that form of activity are realized in the course of trying to achieve those standards of excellence which are appropriate to, and partially definitive of, that form of activity…" (MacIntyre 1984, p. 187). Tennis and chess are examples of practices, as is psychoanalysis. To enjoy the goods internal to the practice of tennis, one has to play according to the rules and standards of excellence of the game. Enjoyment of a game of tennis or of a good analytic hour comes not from contingent extrinsic rewards, such as fame or riches, but from actualizing the standards of excellence for that kind of activity. A virtue, according to MacIntyre (1984) is *an acquired human quality the possession and exercise of which tends to enable us to achieve those goods which are internal to practices and the lack of which effectively prevents us from achieving any such goods"* (p. 191, emphasis in the original).

The analytic attitudes and dispositions (virtues) that advance the goods of analysis are taught by the example of training analysts, supervisors, and exemplary clinical accounts of how the analyst comports herself or himself, especially when pressured by the patient to act differently. These attitudes and dispositions enable the analyst to see and act correctly with patients—for example, in tolerating being "used" by the patient, as Winnicott depicts it in his paper "The Use of an Object" (Winnicott 1982, pp. 86–94). To be virtuous in the context of analyzing is not only to be disposed to act in a certain way when tempted to do otherwise, but to do so with the appropriate affects. For example, a good analyst is able to restrain a momentary countertransference desire to retaliate against a provocative patient by tapping stronger professional attitudes that help to contain his or her own and the patient's destructive affects, without rattling the patient with excessive traces of the analyst's hostility. If an unintentional enactment occurs, additional traits are called forth from the analyst, such as the courage to probe what has transpired and the honesty to admit one's own contribution, even when doing so is humiliating, if this facilitates the analytic relationship and work.

Analysts typically rely more on attitudes and traits (i.e., "virtues") than on professional principles and rules for guidance in ordinary interactions with patients. Freud said as much when he wrote in 1927 that psychoanalytic "tact," under which he said he subsumed "everything positive that…[the psychoanalyst] should do," was ultimately more important than rules, which are often too "inelastic" to guide actions well (quoted in Jones 1955, p. 241). Elsewhere, Freud observed that learning analytic technique is like learning to play chess: the rules of the game are less important than the example of master players.

Most of the character traits associated with the analyst's role are variants on familiar virtues in the Western moral tradition. The analyst is expected to be prudent, patient, honest, kind, curious, discreet, tolerant, spontaneous, humorous, courageous, and wise, to mention only a few of the most obvious traits (see Friedman 1996, p. 260; Grinberg 1980, p. 25; Jaffe and Pulver 1978, p. 630; Schafer 1983). Conversely, narratives of psychoanalytic misconduct depict familiar moral "vices," such as egotism and hostility, under the rubrics of "narcissism," "masochism/sadism," and "sadism" (see Gabbard and Lester 1995). However, the distinctive ways analysts comport themselves are sufficiently unique to require a specialized terminology, such as the one formulated below.

What, then, are the virtues of psychoanalysts? The answers vary somewhat among postclassical psychoanalytic schools, but some traits are shared across schools because they are so basic to the analyst's role. These virtues facilitate an intrapsychic and interpersonal environment conducive to the analytic process. These "process virtues" are very different from the idealized "virtues" of the Western moral tradition and the hypocritical ego ideals that many patients bring to treatment. They foster, rather than oppose, the patient's self-reflective capacities by making a virtue out of not being virtuous in the conventional senses of denying deplorable motives. In place of moral grandiosity, analysts cultivate the courage to accept narcissistic deflation in the arduous process of pushing the boundaries of self-knowledge while tolerating not knowing what cannot yet be grasped.

Empathic Respect

Empathic respect for the patient as a unique individual—evident from the outset of the relationship in the tone, affect, and rhetorical quality of the psychoanalyst's verbal and nonverbal responsiveness to the particulars of the patient's life, difficulties, affects and choices—is an all-important virtue critical to the success or failure of an analysis. Patients come into analysis suffering from self-punitive mental states, and the analyst's ability to recognize this and empathize with what the patient is feeling, while continuing to respect the person who is always more than a bundle of symptoms or a diagnosis, is essential in order for the therapeutic alliance to take hold. "Respect" insufficiently captures this analytic attitude, however, because respect can be cold and distant, whereas the analyst's affective responsiveness makes genuine empathic contact with what the patient is experiencing consciously and unconsciously. Similarly, empathy alone, without respect, is too close to sympathy, which involves compassionate identification with the other's plight in a way that can feel false or even arrogant and presumptuous to the recipient, evoking suspicion of inauthenticity. Sympathy also connotes agreement with the sufferer's explanation of his or her problems, which the analyst rebuffs. When genuine empathy with the patient's actual unconscious experience in the here and now is joined with genuine respect, the patient is free to continue to explore obscure affective states independently of the analyst's presumptions, wishes, and desires (see Freud 1919/1955, pp. 164–165; Freud 1940 [1938]/1964, p. 175).

Benign and Tolerant Curiosity

The analyst's attitude of benign and tolerant curiosity—"the most sympathetic spirit of inquiry," in Freud's (1905/1953, p. 16) discourse—is clearly as important as empathic respect in creating an environment that fosters analysis (see Grinberg 1980, p. 25). The analyst's curiosity bypasses normal critical reactions, reaching for a tolerance that makes it safe for the patient to acknowledge and verbalize the most troublesome intrapsychic disturbance. The analyst's nonthreatening exploratory wish to know how things are and how they have arisen helps counter the powerful defenses aligned against knowledge on both sides of the couch. Tolerance of the infantile, the perverse, the dangerous, and the ridiculous creates an atmosphere that the patient can use to explore what he or she wishes not to know and actively defends against knowing. If things go well, the patient will eventually be able to incorporate benign and tolerant curiosity into his own attitude toward herself or himself.

Emotional Honesty

The fundamental emotional honesty of the analyst, conveyed by his or her truthful speech and interest in the analysand's (and his or her own) emotional truth, is another important virtue in the analyst's repertoire. As Heinrich Racker (1966) noted, "Psychoanalysis'…highest value—'the good' that rules it—resid[es] in the knowledge of [emotional] truth, or more precisely, in the search for and discovery of truth…" (p. 62). The patient's experience of the analyst's unrelenting honesty, involving a commitment to noticing and saying what is understandable and pursuing subtle clues wherever they might lead, is indispensable to the patient's willingness to adhere to the process of revealing what he or she has spent a lifetime concealing, even from internal recognition. As one new analytic patient put it when I acknowledged an error that I thought I could have concealed, "Even though I didn't know for sure, I figured it was your fault, and if you hadn't 'fessed up, I would have been out of here. How could I tell you my deepest secrets if I couldn't trust you absolutely to level with me?" In contrast with traditional ideals of truthfulness, part of the analyst's honesty involves bearing "not knowing" and not being able to help a patient for long periods.

Openness and Humility

The analyst's role also requires a combination of openness and humility. Analytic openness involves suspending the effort of conventionally virtuous people to smother differences by eliminating the unexpected, obstreperous, and uncontrolled. To be open, in the sense required by analysis, is to be able to suspend self-defensiveness and self-interest sufficiently to be willingly surprised by countertransference responses and to make an effort to understand what is strange and unexpected. It is to be nondefensively attentive to the unknown and unknowable, allowing the novel and the disturbing to challenge one's usual ways of seeing and doing things. As Grotstein puts it, "One learns by listening to oneself listening!" (personal communication to Eigen 1998, p. 184). To do this, one must not be too attached to familiar ways of perceiving, thinking, and acting. Humility, in the form of a willingness to examine one's motivations unflinchingly and to learn about one's shortcomings from one's patients and from one's mistakes, is required. The result of such humble openness is the freedom to know one's own thoughts.

Restraint or Self-Control

The restraint or self-control with which the analyst listens and responds represents yet another psychoanalytic virtue. Like the cardinal virtue of temperance in Western moral philosophy, restraint keeps in check the analyst's spontaneous instinctual reactions to seductive and aggressive provocations, without the analyst losing affective contact with the patient. This is best done by scanning internally for the ubiquitous signals of human temptation that emerge subtly and unexpectedly. As Freud warned, the analyst deals with hazardous materials that require special precautions, lest the handler be gravely injured (see Freud 1937/1964, p. 249). Winnicott's evocative discussion of the "use of an object" conveys the importance of the analyst surviving, without retaliation, the patient's destructive desires:

> The subject says to the object: "I destroyed you," and the object is there to receive the communication. From now on the subject says; "Hullo object!" "I destroyed you." "I love you." "You have value for me because of your survival of my destruction of you." "While I am loving you I am all the time destroying you in (unconscious) fantasy." (Winnicott 1982, p. 90)

In this process, the subject places the object outside the area of its imagined omnipotent control, acknowledging the object's autonomy as substantial enough to survive his or her attempts to destroy it. This opens the way for a new realness of self-feeling, because the other is now experienced as really Other, outside the subject's boundaries, and capable of sustaining a genuine encounter (Eigen 1999).

■ ■ ■

Each of the contemporary schools of psychoanalysis tilts toward a different configuration of these and allied virtues. Whereas classical and ego psychoanalysts emphasize respect for the individual patient and a studied neutrality/abstinence believed to enhance ego strength and autonomy, self psychologists, intersubjectivists, and relational therapists stress interpersonal virtues like empathy, egalitarianism, and mutuality. The classical analyst's authoritative stance is replaced in postclassical theory by respect for the analysand as an equal with whom can be realized a mutual relationship of divided functions, one in which the analyst may muster the courage to use self-disclosure judiciously.

Since the traits that enable the analyst to function well are specific to this particular professional role, analytic virtues do not necessarily make the analyst a person of high moral character outside the consulting room (see Schafer 1983). The analyst's virtues make the practice of psychoanalysis possible. However, while some continuity of behavior is to be expected between the consulting room and the rest of the analyst's life, a considerable body of empirical research shows that virtues are more context-specific than ordinary opinion supposes.

My aim in highlighting the virtues that constitute the analyst's role is not to make a case for using virtue language regularly to describe the way we work. Rather, it is to sharpen awareness of this underacknowledged moral dimension of psychoanalytic practice and its importance in striving to live up to professional standards. The profound effect of role-specific virtues on the analyst's behavior helps us appreciate how central morality is to everything that we do, as contrasted with boundary ethics, which confines morals to the edges or borders of our practices. Awareness of the role of virtues is essential in designing training programs and continuing education activities.

For all its usefulness, the problem with virtue language lies with its potential for enflaming narcissistic self-satisfaction and complacency about the goodness of one's strivings, to the exclusion of more complex motivations. To describe an analyst as virtuous seems counterintuitive, even hypocritical, to the extent that virtues derive from mixed motivations. Still, virtues can be acknowledged as indispensable to good conduct, even if they are in need of constant scrutiny for their nonvirtuous aspects. The analyst's recognition of virtues here rests not with the traditional moralist's intension of isolating purely good traits, but with the realist's awareness that we are capable of cultivating attitudes and dispositions that facilitate what we do, even if our best traits are inevitably mixed with less praiseworthy motivations. We cannot assume unitary and consistent virtues. Overdetermination means that conscious virtues mask other motives that find expression in seemingly "good" attitudes and behaviors. The taboo on virtue language among analysts derives partly from dissatisfaction with the Western moral tradition's failure to acknowledge the mind-in-conflict, but this taboo has not been good for the profession. Appreciation of the role-specific virtues of psychoanalysts is needed to bring ethics to center stage, from its isolation at the boundaries where it guards against boundary violations. While a conception of unitary and consistent virtues is foreign to analytic thinking, it is not what is called for here.

Goals

On the rare occasions when analysts invoke the term *ethics* in conjunction with treatment goals, it is usually to criticize overly ambitious ideals, such as "self-realization." To David Shapiro (1989, pp. 115–139), "ethical aims" are "inspirational" rather than descriptive; to Charles Brenner (1976, pp. 167–169), they refer to ideals of self-actualization beyond the analyst's concerns. But in truth, ethical standards are embedded on all sides in the enduring controversies over the goals of analysis (see the 2001 issue of *The Psychoanalytic Quarterly* on "The Goals of Clinical Psychoanalysis"). Those who oppose all therapeutic goals in favor of insight do so in part because they prioritize the value of emotional "truth" as the polestar of analysis, but they usually also see therapeutic goals like the modification of symptoms as the unintended by-product of understanding. Those who embrace therapeutic goals in addition to self-understanding imply that they have a stronger case ethically, because "other things being equal" a broader set of good consequences is preferable to a narrower set, and therapeutic aims include not only self-knowledge but reduced suffering, increased mental freedom, and augmented autonomy. Gabbard (2001, p. 294) is undoubtedly right that analysts who claim not to be interested in symptomatic changes are disingenuous, because "of course we want to help our patients with distressing symptoms." But the debate continues over whether we should focus directly on treatment goals and, if so, how and with what degree of commitment.

Ethical issues arise in connection with treatment goals chiefly in terms of 1) who chooses the goals and 2) on what basis. With regard to the first, the analyst's role in setting treatment goals was privileged until roughly the middle of the last century, when the Hippocratic tradition's preference for paternalistic decisions informed by the physician's beliefs about the patient's best interests (under the moral principle of beneficence) began to give way, following the civil rights and feminist movements, to the moral principle of respect for the individual patient's autonomy. Owen Renik recently put the implications of this ethical shift boldly when he proposed that the patient has "the last word" regarding both "the definition of the goals of a particular analysis, and judgments concerning progress towards those goals" (Renik 2001, p. 239). The ethical idea behind Renik's position is not only that the patient has the right, under the moral principle of autonomy, to make an informed decision about what outcomes to pursue, but that he or she alone possesses the comprehensive information about, and full perspective on, his or her own life to decide what goals are worth pursuing at what cost in terms of time, money, and effort. In other words, the patient is better suited than the physician to decide what is or is not compatible with his or her prudential interests.

While Renik's position captures respect for the patient as a person in deciding on goals, it needs to be balanced by an understanding of the role of collaboration and negotiation between patient and the analyst in arriving at a mutually agreed-on set of realizable aims for their joint undertaking. Ethically, it seems best to view the goals of an analysis as a joint product, unique to each analytic dyad. The result of respectful negotiation and mutual agreement between the parties at the outset of treatment, goals should be repeatedly renegotiated over the course of the analysis as the relationship between the parties changes. The patient can be expected to alter treatment goals as he or she becomes aware of the role of unrealistic unconscious fantasies in initial expectations and arrives, as the analysis unfolds, at more realistic treatment goals and, in turn, life goals.

Ethical considerations enter latently into most efforts to clarify the proper goals of psychoanalysis. Consider, for example, Ernst Ticho's (1972) familiar distinction between therapeutic goals and life goals. For Ticho, life goals are the personal goals (e.g., a better job, marriage, artistic creativity) that the patient would seek, were she or he to overcome inhibiting intrapsychic obstacles. Treatment goals, on the other hand, concern "removal of obstacles to the patient's discovery of what his/her potentialities are" (Ticho 1972, p. 315). Unlike the attainment of treatment goals, the realization of life goals depends on favorable conditions beyond the influence of the analysis, such as the reaction of others in the outside world, material resources, or just plain luck. Although some interpreters of Ticho have linked ethics with life goals, therapeutic goals are no less ethical. They differ simply in being the *moral*

goals—such as reduction of suffering and increased freedom of thought—sought in treatment, as contrasted with the prudential and moral aims toward which the patient's life is directed.

Ticho's formulation correctly focuses attention on therapeutic goals as the primary moral aims of analysis. But it is far too vague about the complex conceptual issue of what it means to be mentally ill and to participate in a "treatment" or "therapy" for it. The conceptual door is thus left wide open by Ticho for analysts of varying schools to smuggle high moral ideals, such as Kohut's transmutation of narcissism, into analytic treatment as "therapeutic" goals, rather than clearly identifying them as "moral" aims. Put in terms derived from various theoretical systems (or lexicons), these allegedly therapeutic goals include the following (see Berman 2001, p. 36; Kohut 1980):

- Making unconscious affects and fantasies conscious
- Encouraging greater flexibility of thought
- Making the superego less persecutory and more subtle
- Facilitating the transition from the paranoid-schizoid position to the depressive position
- Moderating and modifying perfectionist fantasies
- Expanding freedom to know one's own mind, including unwelcome as well as welcome and bad as well as good thoughts
- Improving accuracy in testing the validity of external or internal realities
- Helping one to unflinchingly confront the emotional truth of one's own experience
- Increasing tolerance and curiosity about oneself and others
- Unrolling the life plan or curve of life laid down in each human being's nuclear self
- Remobilizing deep emotional capacities for genuine empathy and love
- Introjecting the analyst's analyzing function as a form of self-examination

Some of these goals are clearly therapeutic, but others are moral ideals, particularly those having to do with releasing empathic capacities and living the kind of examined life urged by Western moralists since antiquity (see Wallwork 1999).

Whatever the moral goals of the analytic enterprise, however, they are best kept in the background as distant aims as the analysis proceeds. Gabbard (2001) is rightly concerned that "the analyst who is too concerned with achieving certain goals may paradoxically promote a transference-countertransference enactment in which the patient defeats the analyst's efforts, thereby winning by losing" (p. 292).

Moral Decision Making

Moral decision making is a fourth way ethical considerations enter into psychoanalytic practice, around such issues as boundary crossings, self-disclosures, financial relations, breaches of confidentiality, a patient's threat to seriously harm another, damaging rumors about colleagues, and analyst impairment. These topics raise moral dilemmas requiring unique decisions, because an action must be chosen among alternatives, each of which is supported by good principles and values. For example, a pregnant analyst may feel morally conflicted about disclosing her pregnancy, because she wants, on the one hand, to advance the patient's self-understanding by waiting for him to notice her pregnancy so that they can understand together the meaning of the patient's denial, and, on the other hand, to make sure the patient has sufficient time to process the meaning of the pregnancy before the due date and to make plans for the time they will not be meeting. Ethical conundrums like this may be complicated by unconscious motivations that may interfere with finding a timely resolution of the dilemma, such as the analyst's guilt about how she imagines her patient will react to news of the pregnancy. A common feature of unethical conduct by analysts lies with failure to fully understand the potential harm to the patient—in this case, perhaps, the patient's painful humiliation upon belated discovery of his denial, reinforced by feelings of being toyed with and betrayed by his analyst during the long period she chose to keep him ignorant.

Sometimes the ethical action is transparently obvious, such as whether or not to sleep with a lovesick patient. Yet very distinguished analysts have rationalized sexual contact at odds with clear ethical standards against exploiting the asymmetric power of the transference, with profoundly damaging consequences for patients who trusted themselves to their care. Gabbard and Lester's work in their book *Boundaries and Boundary Violations in Psychoanalysis* humanizes boundary violators by bringing out some typical vulnerabilities. These include a history of abuse, thin defenses, and narcissistic features such as desperate need for validation from patients, a hunger to be loved and idealized, a tendency to use others to regulate self-esteem, superego, and ego lacunae. Boundary violators demonstrate in the extreme the unconscious dynamics often at work in analysts who prove unable to think clearly about lesser ethical issues.

Sometimes analysts face seemingly unresolvable conundrums. Consider the case of a therapist, such as Amy Morrison, who finds herself confronting the difficult problem of how to handle a diagnosis of cancer with her patients (Morrison 1990). In addition to the usual difficulties of the psychodynamic work, the gravely ill therapist is torn in different directions by her wish to help her patients, concerns about her own well-being, and the impact of her illness on both of them. She may be committed to being open and telling the truth, but not all patients can handle the truth, or at least not all of it at once, and there are issues not only of whether but how and when to disclose, and, then, whether and how to go on together. As Judith Chused (1997) points out in a thoughtful review of how Amy Morrison handled her life-threatening illness with her patients, these ethical/technical issues have to be worked through anew with each patient. The sick therapist has the obligation we all have to hear the patient's reactions verbally and nonverbally, with their multiple conscious and unconscious meanings, and to listen to how we receive these messages and how our own subjectivity colors our reactions, and to find a way of using this information in framing fresh interpretations and real choices that will be heard by the particular patient, even as they help the therapist help herself. Here again, the therapist must be honest with herself about her "therapeutic ambitions, about those goals which are specific for an individual patient and those that the therapist holds dear and would like to achieve with all patients" (Chused 1997).

Historically, analysts have not shown much interest in the problem of thinking ethically about moral dilemmas. Rather, analysts have tended to assume that colleagues who act unethically need more analysis, and so additional analytic work or supervision has been considered an apt punishment of and rehabilitation for ethical violators. But additional analysis does not necessarily help someone who is at sea about how to think about the moral conflicts that create genuine dilemmas.

To think ethically, the moral analyst needs both a stock of traditional rules and their justifying principles, such as those contained in the American Psychoanalytic Association's Principles and Standards, and virtuous attitudes and dispositions, without which there is little motivation to be moral. But rules and virtues provide inadequate guidance in the absence of "wise judgment" (*phronesis*, in Aristotle), which involves the developed capacity to balance conflicting values and responsibilities in relation to the particular facts and dynamics of specific situations. From the perspective of wise judgment, rules and principles set forth a form of boundary ethics that help identify the moral aspects of a situation. But because often rules conflict in practice, the "good enough" moral analyst must creatively adapt the meaning of moral standards to the particular circumstances. The boundary metaphor for ethics that has taken root recently in psychoanalysis fails to do justice to wise moral judgment, which is more aptly captured by "playing the game well within the court" (see Wallwork 2003).

The case method supplies a particularly apt pedagogical approach for the development of wise judgment, because it engages the reader in actively thinking about typical situations of moral conflict, as contrasted with complying passively with rules. Good cases have no "solutions." Their value lies in stimulating a type of role-playing that entails struggling with difficult moral problems by interrogating feelings, biases, selective misperceptions, value preferences, and ethical standards before arriving at a creative decision appropriate to unique circumstances. For psychoanalysts, joining with colleagues to grapple with morally difficult cases is particularly relevant, because ethical problems for us are intertwined with technical considerations, which also entail moral issues, to the extent that technique aims at optimally benefiting the patient (Wallwork 2003). Case discussions also prepare analysts to consult colleagues about perplexing moral problems when they arise.

References

Arlow JA, Brenner C: Psychoanalytic Concepts and the Structural Theory. New York, International Universities Press, 1964

Aron L: A Meeting of Minds: Mutuality in Psychoanalysis. Hillsdale, NJ, Analytic Press, 1996

Asch SE: Social Psychology. Englewood Cliffs, NJ, Prentice-Hall, 1952

Balsam R: Active neutrality and Loewald's metaphor of theater. Psychoanal Study Child 52:3–16, 1997

Bellah RN, Madsen R, Sullivan WM, et al: Habits of the Heart: Individualism and Commitment in American Life. Los Angeles, University of California Press, 1985

Berman E: Psychoanalysis and life. Psychoanal Q 70:35–66, 2001

Blass R: On ethical issues at the foundation of the debate over the goals of psychoanalysis. Int J Psychoanal 84:929–944, 2003

Bollas C: The Mystery of Things. New York, Routledge, 1999

Brenner C: Psychoanalytic Technique and Psychic Conflict. New York, International Universities Press, 1976

Brenner C: The Mind in Conflict. New York, International Universities Press, 1982

Breuer J, Freud S: Studies on hysteria (1893–1895), in Standard Edition of the Complete Psychological Works of Sigmund Freud, Vol 2. Translated and edited by Strachey J. London, Hogarth Press, 1955, pp 1–319

Chused J: The patient's perception of the analyst's self-disclosure: commentary on Amy Lichtblau Morrison's paper. Psychoanalytic Dialogues 7:243–256, 1997

Daly RW: A theory of madness. Psychiatry 54:368–385, 1991

Dewald P, Rita C, Clark R (eds): Ethics Case Book of the American Psychoanalytic Association. New York, American Psychoanalytic Association, 2001

Eigen M: Wilfred R. Bion: infinite surfaces, explosiveness, faith, in Psychoanalytic Versions of the Human Condition. Edited by Marcus P, Rosenberg A. New York, New York University Press, 1998, pp 183–205

Eigen M: The area of faith in Winnicott, Lacan, and Bion, in Relational Psychoanalysis: The Emergence of a Tradition. Edited by Mitchell SA, Aron L. Hillsdale, NJ, Analytic Press, 1999, pp 1–37

Erikson EH: Childhood and Society, 2nd Edition. New York, WW Norton, 1963

Erikson EH: Insight and Responsibility. New York, Norton, 1964

Feinberg J: Doing and Deserving: Essays in the Theory of Responsibility. Princeton, NJ, Princeton University Press, 1970

Flugel JC: Man, Morals, and Society: A Psychoanalytical Study. New York, International Universities Press, 1945

Foucault M: The History of Sexuality. Translated by Hurley R. New York, Vintage Books, 1990

Freud A: The ego and the mechanisms of defense (1936), in The Writings of Anna Freud, Vol 2. New York, International Universities Press, 1966, pp 3–191

Freud EL (ed): The Letters of Sigmund Freud. New York, Basic Books, 1975

Freud S: On psychotherapy (1905), in Standard Edition of the Complete Psychological Works of Sigmund Freud, Vol 7. Translated and edited by Strachey J. London, Hogarth Press, 1953, pp 257–268

Freud S: Fragment of an analysis of a case of hysteria (1905 [1901]), in Standard Edition of the Complete Psychological Works of Sigmund Freud, Vol 7. Translated and edited by Strachey J. London, Hogarth Press, 1953, pp 1–122

Freud S: Five lectures on psycho-analysis (1910), in Standard Edition of the Complete Psychological Works of Sigmund Freud, Vol 11. Translated and edited by Strachey J. London, Hogarth Press, 1957, pp 9–55

Freud S: Recommendations to physicians practising psycho-analysis (1912), in Standard Edition of the Complete Psychological Works of Sigmund Freud, Vol 12. Translated and edited by Strachey J. London, Hogarth Press, 1958, pp 109–120

Freud S: On beginning the treatment (further recommendations on the technique of psycho-analysis I) (1913), in Standard Edition of the Complete Psychological Works of Sigmund Freud, Vol 12. Translated and edited by Strachey J. London, Hogarth Press, 1958, pp 121–144

Freud S: Observations on transference love: further recommendations in the technique of psycho-analysis (1915a), in Standard Edition of the Complete Psychological Works of Sigmund Freud, Vol 12. Translated and edited by Strachey J. London, Hogarth Press, 1958, pp 157–172

Freud S: Thoughts for the times on war and death (1915b), in Standard Edition of the Complete Psychological Works of Sigmund Freud, Vol 14. Translated and edited by Strachey J. London, Hogarth Press, 1957, pp 275–300

Freud S: Introductory lectures on psycho-analysis (1915–1916), in Standard Edition of the Complete Psychological Works of Sigmund Freud, Vol 15. Translated and edited by Strachey J. London, Hogarth Press, 1961, pp 9–239

Freud S: Lines of advance in psycho-analytic therapy (1919), in Standard Edition of the Complete Psychological Works of Sigmund Freud, Vol 17. Translated and edited by Strachey J. London, Hogarth Press, 1955, pp 159–168

Freud S: Group psychology and the analysis of the ego (1921), in Standard Edition of the Complete Psychological Works of Sigmund Freud, Vol 18. Translated and edited by Strachey J. London, Hogarth Press, 1955, pp 65–143

Freud S: The ego and the id (1923), in Standard Edition of the Complete Psychological Works of Sigmund Freud, Vol 19. Translated and edited by Strachey J. London, Hogarth Press, 1961, pp 12–66

Freud S: Some additional notes on dream-interpretation as a whole (1925), in Standard Edition of the Complete Psychological Works of Sigmund Freud, Vol 19. Translated and edited by Strachey J. London, Hogarth Press, 1961, pp 127–138

Freud S: The question of lay analysis (1926), in Standard Edition of the Complete Psychological Works of Sigmund Freud, Vol 20. Translated and edited by Strachey J. London, Hogarth Press, 1959, pp 183–258

Freud S: Future of an illusion (1927), in The Standard Edition of the Complete Psychological Works of Sigmund Freud, Vol 21. Translated and edited by Strachey J. London, Hogarth Press, 1957, pp 5–56

Freud S: Civilization and its discontents (1930), in Standard Edition of the Complete Psychological Works of Sigmund Freud, Vol 21. Translated and edited by Strachey J. London, Hogarth Press, 1957, pp 57–145

Freud S: New introductory lectures on psycho-analysis (1933 [1932]) (Lectures XXIX–XXXV), in Standard Edition of the Complete Psychological Works of Sigmund Freud, Vol 22. Translated and edited by Strachey J. London, Hogarth Press, 1964, pp 1–182

Freud S: Why war? (1933), in Standard Edition of the Complete Psychological Works of Sigmund Freud, Vol 22. Translated and edited by Strachey J. London, Hogarth Press, 1964, pp 199–215

Freud S: Analysis terminable and interminable (1937), in Standard Edition of the Complete Psychological Works of Sigmund Freud, Vol 23. Translated and edited by Strachey J. London, Hogarth Press, 1964, pp 209–253

Freud S: An outline of psycho-analysis (1940[1938]), in Standard Edition of the Complete Psychological Works of Sigmund Freud, Vol 23. Translated and edited by Strachey J. London, Hogarth Press, 1964, pp 139–207

Friedman L: Overview: knowledge and authority in the psychoanalytic relationship. Psychoanal Q 65:154–265, 1996

Fromm E: Escape From Freedom. New York, Holt, Rinehart & Winston, 1941

Fromm E: Man for Himself. New York, Holt, Rinehart & Winston, 1947

Fromm E: The Art of Loving. New York, Harper & Row, 1956

Fromm E: Freud's model of man and its social determinants, in Sigmund Freud. Edited by Roazen P. Engelwood Cliffs, NJ, Prentice-Hall, 1973, pp 45–58

Gabbard GO: Overview and commentary. Psychoanal Q 70: 287–296, 2001

Gabbard GO, Lester EP: Boundaries and Boundary Violations in Psychoanalysis. New York, Basic Books, 1995

Gregory I: Psycho-analysis, human nature, and human conduct, in Nature and Conduct. Edited by Peters RS. New York, St Martin's Press, 1975, pp 99–120

Grinberg L: The closing phase of the psychoanalytic treatment of adults and the goals of psychoanalysis: the search for truth about one's self. Int J Psychoanal 61:25–37, 1980

Grinberg L: Los fundamentos de la técnica psicoanalítica. Int J Psychoanal 69:132–135, 1988

Habermas J: Knowledge and Human Interests. Translated by Shapiro J. Boston, MA, Beacon Press, 1971

Hartmann H: Psychoanalysis and Moral Values. New York, International Universities Press, 1960

Hendrick I: Presidential address: professional standards of the American Psychoanalytic Association. J Am Psychoanal Assoc 3:561–599, 1955

Hoffman IZ: Ritual and Spontaneity in the Psychoanalytic Process: A Dialectical-Constructivist View. Hillsdale, NJ, Analytic Press, 1998

Hoffmann ML: Empathy, role taking, guilt, and development of altruistic motives, in Moral Development. Edited by Lickona T. New York, Holt, Rinehart, & Winston, 1976, pp 124–143

Hospers J: Meaning and free will. Philos Phenomenol Res 10: 313–330, 1950

Hudson WD: Modern Moral Philosophy. Garden City, NY, Doubleday/Anchor Books, 1970

Jaffe D, Pulver S: Survey of psychoanalytic practice 1976: some trends and implications. J Am Psychoanal Assoc 26:615–631, 1978

Jones E: The Life and Work of Sigmund Freud, Vol 1: The Formative Years and the Great Discoveries. New York, Basic Books, 1953

Jones E: The Life and Work of Sigmund Freud, Vol 2: The Years of Maturity, 1901–1919. New York, Basic Books, 1955

Kafka E: The uses of moral ideas in the mastery of trauma and in adaptation, and the concept of superego severity. Psychoanal Q 59:249–269, 1990

Kohut H: The Restoration of the Self. New York, International Universities Press, 1977

Kohut H: Reflections on advances in self psychology, in Advances in Self Psychology. Edited by Goldberg A. New York, International Universities Press, 1980, pp 473–554

Laplanche J, Pontalis J-B: The Language of Psycho-Analysis. Translated by Nicholson-Smith D. New York, WW Norton, 1973

Lasch C: The Culture of Narcissism. New York, WW Norton, 1979

Lichtenberg JD: The influence of values and value judgments on the psychoanalytic encounter. Psychoanalytic Inquiry 3: 647–664, 1983

MacIntyre A: After Virtue, 2nd Edition. Notre Dame, IN, University of Notre Dame Press, 1984

Moore BE, Fine BD (eds): Psychoanalytic Terms and Concepts. New Haven, CT, Yale University Press, 1990

Morrison A: Doing psychotherapy while living with a life threatening illness, in Illness in the Analyst: Implications for the Treatment. Edited by Schwartz H, Silver A. New York, International Universities Press, 1990

Phillips A: Winnicott. Cambridge, MA, Harvard University Press, 1988

Racker H: Ethics and psychoanalysis and the psychoanalysis of ethics. Int J Psychoanal 47:62–80, 1966

Renik O: The patient's experience of therapeutic benefit. Psychoanal Q 70:231–242, 2001

Rieff P: Freud: The Mind of the Moralist. Garden City, NY, Doubleday, 1961

Rieff P: The Triumph of the Therapeutic. New York, Harper & Row, 1968

Ross WD: The Right and the Good. Oxford, England, Clarendon Press, 1930

Ross WD: The Foundation of Ethics. Oxford, England, Clarendon Press, 1939

Schafer R: The Analytic Attitude. New York, Basic Books, 1983

Schafer R: Tradition and Change in Psychoanalysis. Madison, CT, International Universities Press, 1997

Shapiro D: Psychotherapy of Neurotic Character. New York, Basic Books, 1989

Sidgwick H: The Method of Ethics, 7th Edition. Chicago, IL, University of Chicago Press, 1962

Smith HF: Subjectivity and objectivity in analysis. J Am Psychoanal Assoc 47:465–484, 1999

Smith HF: Analysis of transference: a North American perspective. Int J Psychoanal 84:1017–1041, 2003

Stevenson CL: Ethics and Language. New Haven, CT, Yale University Press, 1944

Stone L: The Psychoanalytic Situation. New York, International Universities Press, 1961

Ticho E: Termination of psychoanalysis: treatment goals, life goals. Psychoanal Q 41:315–333, 1972

Wallwork E: Psychoanlaysis and Ethics. New Haven, CT, Yale University Press, 1991

Wallwork E: Social control of sexual behavior, in Encyclopedia of Bioethics, 2nd Edition, Vol 5. Edited by Reich W. New York, Macmillan, 1995, pp 2386–2392

Wallwork E: Determinism, free will, compatibilism. J Am Psychoanal Assoc 45:307–314, 1997

Wallwork E: Psychodynamic contributions to religious ethics: toward reconfiguring askesis. Annual of the Society of Christian Ethics 19:167–189, 1999

Wallwork E: Thinking ethically with the new ethics code. The American Psychoanalyst 37:23, 2003

Winnicott D: Playing and Reality. New York, Tavistock, 1982

Yankelovich D, William B: Ego and Instinct. New York, Random House, 1970

PART IV

Research

SECTION EDITOR: JUDITH KANTROWITZ, M.D.

20

Outcome Research

ROBERT S. WALLERSTEIN, M.D.

IN THIS CHAPTER, I present an overview of the field of psychoanalytic therapy outcome research, tracing its history and development from origins as close to the start of the past century as 1917, through the current exponential burgeoning and worldwide geographical spread, as described in a 1999 article by Peter Fonagy and myself. This exposition is carried out within an organizing framework of successive "generations" of psychotherapy outcome research, with each new generation marked by increasing methodological sophistication and technological enhancement.

My presentation will be somewhat unduly weighted toward contributions within the American scene, because of the priority and the primacy of this research development fostered within the pragmatic empiricism of our Anglo-American intellectual tradition. But, of course, psychoanalytic therapy outcome research has never been an exclusively American enterprise. Across the span of my own research career, starting in the early 1950s, there have been parallel developments in both Great Britain and Germany. In fact, Fonagy and colleagues (1999) discussed and categorized some 50 established and currently ongoing psychotherapy research projects worldwide, only 19 of which are in the United States.

Central Psychoanalytic Research Questions in Outcome Studies

The central research questions in psychoanalysis and in expressive and supportive psychoanalytic psychotherapies qua therapy are 1) *What* changes take place during and as a consequence of therapy? (i.e., the outcome question), and 2) *How* do those changes come about, or how are they brought about?—that is, through the interaction of what factors in the patient, in the therapy and the therapist, and in the patient's evolving life situation (i.e., the process question). In theory, process and outcome are necessarily interlocked. Any study of outcome, even if it counts only the percentage of cases in which "improvement" occurred, must establish some criteria for improvement, and these criteria, in turn, must derive from some conception of the nature of the illness and the process of change, regardless of whether such a conceptualization is explicitly formulated. Similarly, any study of process, in delineating patterns of change among variables, makes cross-sectional assessments at varying points in time, which, if compared with one another, provide measures of short- or longer-term outcome.

This chapter is an updated version of three previous reviews of outcome research (Wallerstein 1995, 1996, 2001) (each written from a somewhat different perspective), with, additionally, completely new material on the exciting current development of a range of instruments specifically designed to measure "structure" and "structural change."

On practical grounds, however, outcome studies and process studies are usually separated. Although the two are not conceptually separable, methods that yield the best judgments in the one area are often operationally opposed to those that yield the best judgments in the other. For example, judgments of outcome will be scientifically most convincing if bias is minimized and freedom from contamination maintained by keeping those who make the "after" judgments unaware of the "before" judgments and predictions. From the point of view of process judgments about the *same therapy*, such care to minimize cross-knowledge would be not only unnecessary but counter to the whole spirit of inquiry into process, in which maximum knowledge of all the known determinants, as they have varied over time, is essential in order to best understand the changes that occur. Given this situation, I focus here on the explicitly outcome studies, indicating as well, however, those ("third generation") studies that have endeavored to pursue both outcome and process aims.

First, however, I need to mention some of the considerations related to the topic of research in psychoanalytic therapies—issues that, although beyond the scope of this chapter, are nonetheless germane to its central argument and significant determinants of the complexity of therapy research:

1. *Goals* of these treatment modalities, both ideal and practical (realizable)
2. Issues of suitability or *treatability*, as compared with *analyzability*, which is not the same thing, though the two are easily confounded
3. *Indications* and *contraindications* for this array of treatment possibilities, as it has evolved over time with increasing experience and expanding theoretical and technical knowledge
4. Role of the initial *diagnostic* and *evaluation* procedures in differential treatment planning, as against the view that only a trial of treatment can lead to proper case formulation and prognostication
5. Place of *prediction* in relation to issues of change, of expectable reach, and of limitation
6. *Theory of technique*, or how treatment works and achieves its goals (the relationship of means to ends)
7. *Similarities* and *differences* between psychoanalysis and the dynamic psychotherapies, compared from the perspective of different goals projected for different kinds of patients, from which one determines the specifically appropriate technical approaches from within the available spectrum
8. *Criteria* for satisfactory treatment termination
9. *Evaluation of results* (process and outcome changes, therapeutic benefit, and analytic completeness)

10. Conception of the *ideal state of mental health*, and the unavoidable impingements on its empirical assessment by value judgments, including those from the vantage point and partisan interests of the judge
11. Place of *follow-up study* as a desirable, feasible, and appropriate activity (or not) in relation to psychoanalytic work for research purposes, clinical purposes, or both
12. Place of the continuing accretion of knowledge in relation to all these areas by the traditional *case study method* innovated by Freud, as against the desirability or necessity for more *formal systematic clinical research* into these issues, by methods that are responsive to the subtlety and complexity of the subjectivistic clinical phenomena, while simultaneously remaining loyal to the canons of empirical science

First-Generation Research: Early Statistical Studies

As early as 1917, within the first decade of psychoanalysis in America, Coriat (1917) reported on the therapeutic results achieved in 93 cases, of whom 73% were declared either recovered or much improved; these rates were nearly equal across all his diagnostic categories. As with all the early statistical studies reported here, the judgments of improvement were made by the treating clinician on the basis of (usually) unspecified criteria and without individual clinical detail or supporting evidence.

In the decade of the 1930s, several comparable but larger-scale reports emerged from the collective experiences of the psychoanalytic treatment centers of some of the world's pioneering psychoanalytic institutes. In 1930, Fenichel reported results from the initial decade of the Berlin Institute, the first formally organized psychoanalytic institute in the world. Of 1,955 consultations conducted, 721 patients were accepted for analysis; 60% of the neurotic patients, but only 23% of those who were labeled psychotic, were judged to have received substantial benefit. Ernest Jones (1936) reported on 738 applicants to the London Psychoanalytic Clinic, of whom 74 were taken into analysis; 28 of the 59 (47%) neurotic patients, but only 1 of the 15 (7%) so-called psychotic patients, were judged to have benefited substantially. And a year later, Alexander (1937) reported on 157 cases from the Chicago Psychoanalytic Clinic, with 63% of the neurotic patients, 40% of the psychotic patients, and 77% of those designated "psychosomatic" judged to have received substantial benefit from their treatment. During the same period, Kessel and Hyman (1933), two internists in New York, in following up on 29 patients referred for psychoanalysis, reported that almost all the neurotic patients benefited from the treatment and that all the psychotic patients were found to be either unchanged or worse.

In a review article evaluating the overall results of psychoanalysis, Knight (1941) combined the findings of all these studies (except the first, by Coriat) and added 100 patients treated at The Menninger Clinic in Topeka, Kansas, where the results were judged to be completely comparable with those of the other studies in the observed outcomes with neurotic and psychotic patients. The overall composite tabulation comprised 952 patients, with the therapeutic benefit rate approximately 60% for the neurotic patients, close to 80% for the psychosomatic patients, and only 25% for the psychotic patients. Knight made particular reference to the pitfalls of these simple statistical summaries: the absence of consensually agreed-on definitions and criteria, the crudeness of nomenclature and diagnostic classification, and the failure to address issues of therapeutic skill in relation to cases of varying difficulty.

The most ambitious study of this first-generation genre was the report of the Central Fact-Gathering Committee of the American Psychoanalytic Association (Hamburg et al. 1967). (Although the span from Coriat's [1917] study to this study [Hamburg et al. 1967] is a half-century, I call all of these studies "first generation" in terms of their degree of conceptual and methodological sophistication, rather than in temporal terms, although, of course, each "generation" started at a later point in time, or spanned a later period of time, than its predecessor.) Data were collected over a 5-year period, beginning in 1952; altogether, some 10,000 initial responses to questionnaires were submitted by some 800 analysts and candidates, with some 3,000 termination questionnaires submitted on treatment completion. As with the other studies cited thus far, criteria for diagnosis and improvement were unspecified, and these and other flaws and ambiguities resulted ultimately in a report that was declared to be simply an "experience survey" consisting of 1) facts abut the demographics of analysts' practices, 2) analysts' opinions about their patients' diagnoses, and 3) analysts' opinions abut the therapeutic results achieved. Not unexpectedly, the great majority of patients were declared to be substantially improved.

Finally, in the very next year, Feldman (1968) reported on the results of psychoanalysis in 120 patients (selected from 960 evaluations) treated at the clinic of the Southern California Psychoanalytic Institute over its 11-year history. Again, the reported improvement rates were comparable to those of all the preceding studies, with two-thirds of the outcomes being in the "good" or "very good" categories; and once more, difficulties were experienced because of the lack of clear and agreed-on criteria, concepts,

and language for diagnostic assessment, analyzability, and analytic results.

Altogether, this sequence of so-called first-generation outcome studies of psychoanalysis, spanning a half-century, from 1917 to 1968, was scientifically simplistic and failed to command much interest in the psychoanalytic clinical world. Most practitioners agreed with Glover's (1954) dour assessment: "Like most psycho-therapists, the psychoanalyst is a reluctant and inexpert statistician" (p. 393)—and, it could be added, researcher. It was such conclusions that spurred what I call the "second generation" studies, the efforts at more formal and systematic outcome research, geared toward overcoming the glaring methodological simplicity that marked each of the studies described to this point.

Second-Generation Research: Formal and Systematic Studies

The methodological flaws in the first-generation statistical enumerations of psychoanalytic outcomes have already been indicated. As noted earlier, there was a lack of consensually agreed-on criteria at almost every step—from initial assessments to outcome judgments of therapeutic benefit and analytic results—and these judgments (built on unspecified, and even unformulated, criteria) by the (necessarily biased) therapist, were (usually) the sole evidential primary database. These studies also posed a methodological difficulty, in that they were all retrospective, with all the potential therein for bias, confounding, and contamination of judgments, *post hoc, ergo propter hoc* reasoning, and so forth. Efforts to address these issues, including the introduction of prospective inquiry and even the fashioning of predictions to be confirmed or refuted by subsequent assessment, began in earnest in America in the 1950s and 1960s and have spread worldwide in the subsequent decades.

I very briefly describe six major American projects from this second-generation research approach, three based on group-aggregated studies of clinic cases from the Boston, Columbia, and New York Psychoanalytic Institutes, and three based on individually focused studies in New York, San Francisco, and Chicago. I also mention here, out of the many currently ongoing programs elsewhere in the world, three major programs, although not all three live up to all the second-generation criteria here specified. (One of them is retrospective, albeit with outcome judgments made more objectively, not by the therapists with unspecified criteria, but by independent researchers with carefully worked-out outcome measures.) The three quite large European projects of this kind that I want to mention are 1) the Anna Freud Centre chart review of 765 cases in which patients were treated over a four-decade span with psychoanalysis or psychotherapy (Fonagy and Target 1994, 1996; Target and Fonagy 1994a, 1994b); 2) the German Psychoanalytical Association (DPV) study of the long-term effects of psychoanalysis and the psychoanalytic psychotherapies, involving study by 207 cooperating psychoanalysts of 1,384 completed treatments (Leuzinger-Bohleber et al. 2003); and 3) the European multicenter collaborative study of long-term intensive psychoanalytic treatment involving analysts from Holland, Finland, Norway, Sweden, and Italy (Szecsody et al. 1997).

American Second-Generation Studies

Group-Aggregated Studies

Boston Psychoanalytic Institute.   In 1960, Knapp and his colleagues reported on 100 supervised psychoanalytic patients from the Boston Psychoanalytic Institute, rated initially for suitability for analysis, of whom 27 were followed up a year later with questionnaires addressed to the treating analysts to ascertain just how suitable the patients had indeed turned out to be. Those who made the "after" judgments were blind to the "before" evaluations. There was a fair, but limited, success in this assessment of suitability for analysis from the initial evaluation. However, two significant limitations of this study should be mentioned. First, the testing of the predictions took place only at the 1-year mark, rather than more suitably on treatment termination; clearly much can change in this regard—in both directions—at later points in treatment. Second, and this is a problem with all research on this model, the patients selected by the psychoanalytic committees had already been carefully screened, with obviously unsuitable cases already rejected. The range of variability in the accepted cases was thus considerably narrowed, making differential predictions within that group inherently more difficult and less reliable.

Sashin and colleagues (1975), inspired by this work, studied 183 patients treated at the same institute from 1959 to 1966. Final data were collected on 130 (72%) of these patients after an average of 675 treatment hours, and at a point averaging 6 years after treatment termination. Predictor variables were assessed with a 103-item evaluation questionnaire directed toward six major outcome criteria: 1) restriction of functioning by symptoms, 2) subjective discomfort, 3) work productivity, 4) sexual adjustment, 5) interpersonal relations, and 6) availability of insight. Only 10 of the 103 predictor items demonstrated some predictive value in relation to assessed outcomes, and those

showed only modest (albeit statistically significant) success. As a group, however, these predictor variables "made little clinical sense."

Overall, the Boston Psychoanalytic Institute studies yielded only fair predictions to judgments of analyzability as assessed at the 1-year mark in treatment, and no effective prediction at all regarding treatment outcomes from the patients' characteristics as judged at initial evaluation.

Columbia Psychoanalytic Center.   The Columbia Psychoanalytic Center project, contemporaneous with the Boston studies, was written up in final accounting in a sequence of published reports in 1985 (Bachrach et al. 1985; Weber et al. 1985a, 1985b, 1985c). This project consisted of prospective studies of a large number of patients (1,348 in sample 1, and 237 in the later sample 2), all treated by the same body of therapists. Data were collected over time (initially and at termination) from multiple perspectives, with opportunities to compare findings in psychoanalysis (about 40% of the total) with those in psychoanalytic psychotherapy (the other 60%). The authors stated that all previous studies had been limited in at least one of the following ways: small sample size, inadequate range of information about outcomes, data not based on terminated cases, or study restricted to retrospective data. Further, no other studies had permitted comparison between large numbers of terminated analyses and psychotherapies conducted by the same therapist group. In addition, criteria for therapeutic benefit were established so as to be distinct from the criteria for the evolution of a psychoanalytic process.

The most striking finding from this project was that across every category of patient, the therapeutic benefit measures always substantially exceeded the measures of an evolved analytic process. For example, only 40% of those who finished analyses with good therapeutic benefit were characterized, on the basis of the project criteria, as having been "analyzed." An equally striking finding was that the outcomes of these treatments, in terms of both therapeutic benefit and analyzability, were only marginally predictable from the perspective of the initial evaluation. This finding was, of course, in keeping with the comparable finding from the Boston studies just cited—and for the same reasons. As noted by the authors (Weber et al. 1985a), "The prudent conclusion…is not that therapeutic benefit or analyzability are *per se* unpredictable, but that once a case has been carefully selected as suitable for analysis by a candidate, its eventual fate remains relatively indeterminate" (p. 135).

Expectedly, those selected for psychoanalysis were assessed initially as functioning at higher levels than those selected for psychotherapy, and those in psychoanalysis achieved greater therapeutic benefits than those in psychotherapy. In conclusion, the authors stated that sample 1 was three times larger than in any previously published study and that the project was the first to have a psychotherapy comparison group and one of the first to make a conceptual distinction between analyzability and therapeutic benefit. Sample 2 was smaller, assembled a decade later, with some refinements in methods of data collection and some differences in observational vantage points. In almost every particular, however, all the findings of sample 1 were replicated. From both studies, the authors drew the following conclusion:

> A substantially greater proportion of analysands derive therapeutic benefit than develop an analytic process, and...the development of an analytic process is associated with the highest levels of therapeutic benefit. Yet, what we do not yet know precisely is the nature and quality of benefit associated with the development of an analytic process and without its development. (Weber et al. 1985b, p. 261)

The final article in this series (Bachrach et al. 1985) was devoted to a review of clinical and methodological considerations. The authors stressed the advantages of their project over other comparable studies: the project 1) had a total sample size that was very large; 2) was a prospective study with predictive evaluations performed before outcomes were known; 3) used (mainly) clinically meaningful measures; 4) used independent judges (aside from evaluations by patients and therapists); and 5) compared psychoanalysis and psychotherapy.

(More than a quarter century later, a successor group of psychotherapy researchers in the same treatment center added a study, employing a quite similar methodology, comparing the psychoanalytic treatment courses of patients [clinic patients] who came seeking psychoanalysis and were selected for it, with patients who came as private patients to the same therapists [still candidates in training] and were taken initially into a psychoanalytic psychotherapy but subsequently—with the approval of the designated supervisor and the clinic committee—were "converted" to psychoanalysis [Caligor et al. 2003]. In the demographic characteristics of the two patient cohorts, and in the assessed characteristics of their treatment courses, there were only two significant differences between the two groups: 1) the private patients had better socioeconomic status and paid significantly higher fees (though not up to established private practice levels); and 2) of those patients with diagnosed mood and anxiety disorders, a much high percentage of the privately secured patients were on prescribed psychoactive medication. The authors offer some tentative thoughts about the possible origin and meaning of this distinction.)

New York Psychoanalytic Institute.   The third of these group-aggregated studies, the New York Psychoanalytic Institute studies (Erle 1979; Erle and Goldberg 1979, 1984), were similar in design to the Boston and Columbia studies, although with more of a focus on the study of treatments carried out by more experienced analysts. There were two samples. The first (Erle 1979) consisted of 40 supervised analytic patients selected from 870 applicants to the Treatment Center of the New York Psychoanalytic Institute. The results were completely comparable with those at the Boston and Columbia centers. Twenty-five of the patients terminated satisfactorily, but of these, only 11 were considered to have completed their treatment; 24 of the patients were judged to have benefited substantially, but only 17 were judged to have been involved in a proper psychoanalytic process. A group of 42 private patients, from seven analyst colleagues of the author, who had begun their treatments in the same period and were assessed in the same manner as the Treatment Center patients, showed substantially comparable results. The second sample (Erle and Goldberg 1984) extended the work to a group of 160 private patients gathered over a subsequent 5-year span from 16 cooperating experienced analysts. The outcomes from these experienced analysts were completely comparable to the results of their own and of all the other earlier studies of clinic patients treated by candidates.

(Almost two decades after these reports, the same authors [Erle and Goldberg 2003], following their same methods, presented two further studies, both of these the clinical work of a cadre of experienced psychoanalysts—not candidates in training. Their first study was a retrospective study of all of the analytic work of 16 analysts [161 patients] from the period 1973 to 1977, the time period of the work covered in the earlier reports. Their second study was a prospective study of all the patients started in analyses by a group of 20 analysts [92 patients] between 1984 and 1989, and followed to termination with evaluative reports. Their very detailed findings were completely in keeping with the work they had reported some two decades earlier, which had, of course, focused on the work of neophyte analysts still in formal training.)

Individually Focused Studies

Over a time span parallel to that of these relatively large-scale outcome studies of psychoanalytic clinic patient populations (as well as some comparison private patients), which assessed the patients with pre- and posttreatment rating scales and grouped them statistically, Pfeffer, at the New York Psychoanalytic Institute Treatment Center, initiated a wholly other kind of outcome and follow-up study of terminated psychoanalyses, through intensive individual case studies of a research-procured population (Pfeffer 1959, 1961, 1963). He first reported on nine patients who had completed analyses under Treatment Center auspices and had agreed to a series of follow-up interviews by a "follow-up analyst" who had not conducted the treatment. The interviews were open-ended, once a week, and "analytic" in character, ranging from two to seven in number before the participants agreed on a natural close. The chief finding that occurred in all instances consisted of the rapid reactivation of characteristic analytic transferences, including even transitory symptom flare-ups, as if in relation to the original treating analyst, with subsequent rapid subsidence, at times ended by pertinent interpretations, and in a manner that included the new ways of management of neurotic conflicts that had been achieved in the analysis.

In the last of this sequence of three reports, Pfeffer (1963) attempted a metapsychological explanation of these "follow-up study transference phenomena" (p. 230). His overall conclusion was as follows:

> The recurrence in the follow-up study of the major pre-analytic symptomatology in the context of a revived transference neurosis as well as the quick subsidence of symptoms appear to support the idea that conflicts underlying symptoms are not actually shattered or obliterated by analysis but rather are only better mastered with new and more adequate solutions. (p. 234)

The neurotic conflicts thus "lose their poignancy" (p. 237).

Two other research groups, one in San Francisco (Norman et al. 1976; Oremland et al. 1975) and one in Chicago (Schlessinger and Robbins 1974, 1975, 1983), replicated Pfeffer's studies, with some slight alterations in method, and in both instances confirmed what has come to be called the "Pfeffer phenomenon." The San Francisco group concluded that "the infantile neurosis had not disappeared. What had changed was the degree to which it affected [the patient's] everyday life" (Norman et al. 1976, p. 492). The Chicago group concluded that "psychic conflicts were not eliminated in the analytic process....The more significant outcome of the analysis appeared to be the development of a preconsciously active self-analytic function, in identification with the analyzing function of the analyst, as a learned mode of coping with conflicts" (Schlessinger and Robbins 1983, p. 9).

This overall finding from all three research groups—that even in analyses considered highly successful, neurotic conflicts are not obliterated or shattered, as was once believed, but rather are tamed, muted, or lose their poignancy—is echoed in the well-known analytic quip that we all still recognize our good friends after their analyses.

I note one final consideration: A shared characteristic of these second-generation studies—whether the group-aggregated broad statistical accountings (Boston, Columbia, New York) or the individually focused in-depth research studies (New York [Pfeffer], San Francisco, Chicago)—was the failure to segregate outcome results discerned at treatment termination from the issue of the stability (or not) of these results as revealed at some established follow-up point subsequent to termination, with all the different possibilities—for consolidation and further enhancement of treatment gains, for the simple maintenance of treatment achievements, or for actual regression back toward the pretreatment state.

Conceptually, this was a failure to accord specific theoretical status to what Rangell (1966/1990) called the "postanalytic phase." Rangell described a variety of possible courses that can characterize this phase and concluded that "the desired goal should be a transition to a normal interchange in which the analyst can be seen and reacted to as a normal figure and no longer as an object for continued transference displacement" (p. 722). In the third-generation studies, next to be described, the distinction between results at the termination study point and those at a subsequent prearranged follow-up study point (anywhere from 2 to 10 years later) becomes a clearly demarcated research focus; this is among the advances over the second-generation studies.

Third-Generation Research: Combined Process and Outcome Studies

What I am calling the third-generation studies of the outcomes of psychoanalysis have actually been contemporaneous in time with the second-generation studies just described. These third-generation studies are systematic and formal psychoanalytic therapy research programs that have attempted both to assess analytic outcomes across a significant array of cases and to examine the processes through which these outcomes have been reached via the intensive longitudinal study of each of the individual cases.

The third-generation projects have combined the methodological approaches of the second-generation group-aggregated studies with those of the second-generation individually focused studies. Like the best of the second-generation studies, they have carefully defined their terms, constructed rating scales, and tried to operationalize their criteria at each assessment point. The third-generation studies have been constructed prospectively, starting with the pretreatment assessment of the patients.

Unlike the second-generation studies, they have carefully separated outcomes at termination from functioning at a specified subsequent follow-up point; they also have attempted to account for the further changes, in either direction, that took place during this "postanalytic phase." Bachrach et al. (1991), in their comprehensive survey of research on the efficacy of psychoanalysis, singled out the newer Boston Psychoanalytic Institute studies (Kantrowitz 1986, 1996; Kantrowitz et al. 1986, 1987a, 1987b, 1989, 1990a, 1990b, 1990c) and the Psychotherapy Research Project (PRP) of The Menninger Foundation (Wallerstein 1986, 1988a) as the only ones to fully meet their array of state-of-the-art specifications for outcome studies. The two that I review here are exemplars of this third-generation research.

Newer Boston Psychoanalytic Institute Studies

The Boston studies were undertaken in the 1970s and came to publication in the following decade. Twenty-two supervised analytic cases at the Boston Psychoanalytic Institute were selected for prospective study, with the initial assessment based on a projective psychological test battery used to yield measures of 1) affect availability and modulation, 2) quality of object relations, 3) adequacy of reality testing, and 4) motivation for change. Approximately a year after treatment termination, the initial test battery was repeated, and both the patient and the treating analyst were interviewed.

A series of three articles (Kantrowitz et al. 1986, 1987a, 1987b) described the results. Of the 22 patients, 9 were judged to have had a successful analytic outcome; 5, to have had a limited outcome; and 8, to have been essentially unanalyzed. Nonetheless, the greater number achieved therapeutic benefits along each of the change and outcome dimensions, and along each dimension the therapeutic benefit exceeded the analytic result in terms of the degree of successfully completed analytic work. That is, a consistent and important finding was that therapeutic benefit was achieved by the majority of the patients and was regularly in excess of what could be accounted for by the evocation and the interpretive resolution (as well as possible) of the transference neurosis. However, although most patients derived significant therapeutic benefit from their analytic experience, successful outcome could not be predicted from any of the predictor variables (again, as in the second-generation studies).

This finding led these investigators to speculate that "a particularly important omission (from the predictor variables) might have been consideration of the effect of the [therapist-patient] match in shaping the two-person psychoanalytic interaction" (Kantrowitz et al. 1989, p. 899). By "match" they meant "an interactional concept"—one that "refers to a spectrum of compatibility and incompatibility of the patient and analyst which is relevant to the analytic work" (p. 894). They further noted that although "this mesh of the analyst's personal qualities with those of the patient has rarely been a special focus of [research] attention…most analysts when making referrals do consider it; few assume that equally well-trained analysts are completely interchangeable" (Kantrowitz 1986, p. 273).

This same team then returned for follow-up interviews with the same patient cohort in 1987, now 5–10 years after the treatment terminations. This time the researchers included the retrospective assessment of the goodness of the analyst-patient match as one of the variables contributing to the patient outcomes (Kantrowitz et al. 1990a, 1990b, 1990c). Nineteen of the original 22 patients could be located, and of these, 18 agreed to be interviewed. Again, a variety of change measures were used: global improvement ratings, affect management, quality of object relations, adequacy of reality testing, work accomplishment, and overall self-esteem. Overall results at the follow-up point were as follows: 3 of the 18 were further improved, 4 were stable, 6 had deteriorated but were restored with additional treatment, 4 had deteriorated despite additional treatment, and 1 had returned to the original analyst and was still in treatment and therefore was not counted.

The most striking finding, however, was that, again, the stability of the achieved results in the follow-up period could not be predicted from the assessments at termination. That is, according to Kantrowitz and colleagues (1990a), "psychological changes were no more stable over time for the group of patients assessed as having achieved a successful analytic outcome concomitant with considerable therapeutic benefit than for the other group of patients assessed as having achieved therapeutic benefit alone" (p. 493). In focusing on the assessment of analyst-patient match (Kantrowitz et al. 1990c), the authors concluded that with 12 of the 17 patients, the kind of match (impeding or facilitating) did play a role in the outcome achieved. They gave examples of facilitating matches with good outcomes, impeding matches with poor outcomes, and more complex situations in which the kind of match was at first facilitating to the unfolding of the analytic process but later seemed to have an influence in preventing the completion of the analytic work.

Psychotherapy Research Project of The Menninger Foundation

The other so-called third-generation psychoanalytic therapy research study to be described here is the Psychotherapy Research Project (PRP) of The Menninger Foundation. Of this project, Bachrach et al. (1991) noted:

> Systematic, methodologically informed research about psychoanalytic outcomes began with The Menninger Foundation Psychotherapy Research Project....[It] is by far the most comprehensive formal study of psychoanalyses yet undertaken and remains the only study of outcomes that spans almost the entire life cycle of many of its patients. (p. 878)

Bachrach et al. concluded that the study "stands in a class by itself among psychoanalytic research efforts" (p. 884).

Certainly the PRP was the most ambitious such research program ever carried out (Wallerstein 1986, 1988a; Wallerstein et al. 1956). Its intent was to follow the treatment careers and the subsequent life careers of a cohort of patients (ultimately 42 in number), half in psychoanalysis, and the other half in other psychoanalytic psychotherapies—and each in the modality deemed clinically indicated. The cohort was to be followed from the initial pretreatment comprehensive psychiatric evaluation, through the entire natural span of their treatments (for however many years that entailed), and then into formal follow-up inquiries several years after the treatment terminations, and with as much of an open-ended follow-up thereafter as circumstance might make possible and as the span of interested observation might last. The patients entered into their treatments over the span of the mid-1950s (contemporaneously with the bulk of the second-generation studies); their periods of treatment ranged from 6 months to a full 12 years. All patients were reached—100%—for formal follow-up study at the 2- to 3-year mark, and more than one-third could be followed for periods ranging from 12 to 24 years beyond their treatment terminations (with four still in ongoing treatment when my book *Forty-Two Lives in Treatment*, the overall clinical accounting of this project, was published at the 30-year mark in 1986).

The aim of the PRP was to learn as much as possible about 1) *what* changes actually take place in psychoanalysis and other psychoanalytic psychotherapies (the outcome question) and 2) *how* these changes come about, through the interactions over time of *what variables* in the patient, in the therapy and the therapist, and in the patient's evolving life situation, as they together codetermine those changes (the process question). (On the basis of my statement at the beginning of this chapter that, in theory, process and outcome are necessarily interlocked, the PRP was conceived as an inquiry into both the outcomes and the processes of psychoanalytic therapies. However, as also stated there, operationally the methods appropriate to the two realms of inquiry are often in opposition to each other, and as it turned out, the PRP was indeed much more an out-

come study; the light thrown there on the treatment process was more inferential and based primarily on clinical, not research-specifiable, judgments.) Three overall treatment groups were set up—psychoanalysis, expressive psychoanalytic psychotherapy, and supportive psychoanalytic psychotherapy—in accord with the then (1950s) consensus in the psychoanalytic literature regarding the defining characteristics of these three therapeutic modes, together with differential indications for their deployment derived from the dynamic formulations of the nature of the patients' lives, histories, characters, and illness structures.

The project goals within this framework were to specify in detail the particular reach and limitation of the therapeutic outcome for each kind of patient, appropriately treated within each of the proffered therapeutic approaches. There was a special interest in the more empirical elaboration of the psychological change mechanisms operative within both the uncovering (expressive) and the "ego-strengthening" (supportive) therapeutic modes. My book *Forty-Two Lives in Treatment* represents the full statement of the project's findings and conclusions (Wallerstein 1986). For a summary of the main highlights here, I can best report by paraphrasing (and sharply condensing) a several-page segment from the concluding part of an overview paper about the project (Wallerstein 1988a, pp. 144–149).

The overall project conclusions, as of 1986, can be brought together as a series of sequential propositions regarding the appropriateness, efficacy, reach, and limitations of psychoanalysis and of psychoanalytic psychotherapies (varyingly expressive and supportive)—always, of course, with the caveat that this sample of the overall patient population (i.e., those usually "sicker" individuals who are brought to or who seek their intensive analytic treatment within a psychoanalytic sanatorium setting) are not necessarily representative of the usual outpatient psychoanalytic therapy population:

1. *The changes reached in the more supportive therapies seemed often enough to represent just as much structural change as the changes reached in the most expressive analytic cases.* A distinction is regularly made between true "structural change" (presumably based on the interpretive resolution, within the transference-countertransference matrix, of unconscious intrapsychic conflicts) and "behavioral change" (based on "just altered techniques of adjustment," and presumably all that can come out of the other, non-interpretive, non-insight-aiming change mechanisms). The PRP experience clearly questioned the continued usefulness of this effort to link so tightly the kinds of change achieved with

the intervention mode—expressive or supportive—by which they were brought about.

2. *Therapeutic change was at least proportional to the degree of achieved conflict resolution* (the so-called conventional proportionality argument). Put this way, this proposition is almost unexceptionable, as it is clear that there can be significantly more change than there is true conflict resolution. Change can occur via all the varying supportive bases through which it can be brought about, as well as properly proportionately on the basis of conflict resolution with accompanying insight.

3. *Effective conflict resolution was a necessary condition for at least certain kinds of change* (the so-called necessity argument). This proposition, though often linked to the proportionality argument, is much more debatable and clearly separate from it. The PRP repeatedly demonstrated that a substantial range of changes—in symptoms, in life-functioning, in personality dispositions—were brought about via the more supportive therapeutic modes, cutting across the gamut of declared supportive and expressive (even analytic) therapies.

4. *Supportive therapeutic approaches often achieved far more than was expected of them.* As a counterpart to the previous proposition (i.e., the tendency to overestimate the necessity of the expressive, or analytic, treatment mode's operation via conflict resolution in order to effect therapeutically desired change), the PEP found that the supportive therapeutic approaches often achieved far more than was expected of them. Indeed, they often enough reached the kinds of changes expected to depend on more expressive and insightful conflict resolutions—and did so in ways that represented indistinguishably "structural changes," not overall less stable or less enduring or less proof against subsequent environmental vicissitude.

5. *Psychoanalysis, as the quintessentially expressive therapeutic mode, often achieved less than had been anticipated or predicted.* Considering these PRP treatments from the point of view of psychoanalysis as a treatment modality, just as more was often accomplished than expected with psychotherapy, especially in its more supportive modes, so psychoanalysis often achieved less—at least with these "sicker" patients—than had been anticipated or predicted. This more limited success in part reflected the ethos of the psychoanalytic sanatorium and the psychoanalytic treatment opportunities such a setting is intended to make possible—that is, the protection and life management of those temporarily disorganized individuals who presumably cannot be helped sufficiently with any other or lesser treatment approach than psychoanalysis but who cannot tolerate the rigors of psychoanalytic treatment within the usual outpatient setting.

The shift proposed here is in the departure from the effort at psychoanalysis per se (even "modified" analysis) as the treatment of choice for these "sicker" patients. On this basis, we can speak of the failing of the so-called heroic indications for psychoanalysis and can invite a repositioning of the pendulum in its swings over time around this issue, more in the direction of "narrowing indications" for (proper) psychoanalysis.

6. *Psychoanalysis and the expressive psychotherapies often accomplished less, and supportive psychotherapies often accomplished more, than expected.* The predictions made for prospective courses and outcomes tended to be for more substantial and enduring change (more "structural change") when the treatment was to be more expressive-analytic; pari passu, the more supportive the treatment was intended to be (had to be), the more limited and inherently unstable the anticipated changes were expected to be. All of this presumption was consistently tempered and altered in the actual implementation in the treatment courses. Psychoanalysis and the expressive psychotherapies were systematically modified to introduce more supportive components, and they often enough accomplished less than anticipated. The supportive psychotherapies, on the other hand, often accomplished more—sometimes a great deal more—than initially expected, again, with much of the change on the basis of more supportive techniques than originally specified.

These overall results can be generalized as follows:

1. The treatment results in psychoanalysis and in varying mixes of expressive-supportive psychotherapies tended to converge, rather than diverge, in outcome.

2. Across the whole spectrum of treatment courses, from the most purely analytic-expressive to the most singlemindedly supportive, the treatments carried more supportive elements than originally projected, and these elements accounted for substantially more of the changes achieved than had been originally anticipated.

3. The supportive aspects of psychotherapy, as conceptualized within a psychoanalytic theoretical framework, deserve far more respectful specification than they have usually been accorded in the psychoanalytic literature.

4. From the study of the kinds of changes achieved by this patient cohort, partly on an uncovering insight-aiming basis, and partly on the basis of the opposed covering-up varieties of supportive techniques, the changes themselves—divorced from how they were brought about—often seemed quite indistinguishable from each other in terms of being so-called real or structural changes in personality functioning.

Fourth-Generation Research: Divergence of Directions

Psychoanalytic therapy research in the current, fourth generation has developed along a number of divergent paths. The single most important development—though not within the purview of this chapter—is the current, almost explosive burgeoning of process research (i.e., research into *how* change takes place or is brought about) (see Chapter 21, "Process Research," for further discussion). This dramatic increase has been rendered feasible on a significant scale by the development over the past two decades of suitable technology—namely, the possibility for, and growing acceptance of, (reasonably) unobtrusive audio and video recording of therapeutic sessions, and of computerization with programs for high-speed computer word or situation searches of these recorded sessions. This advance in technology has enabled microscopic study of moment-to-moment psychoanalytic interaction processes, in single hours or in small segments of hours, as well as across multiple hours, in the same, or with other, patients.

It is beyond my designated scope here to indicate anything of this process research development except to mention that the potentially most rewarding direction in this domain would be in the combined study of the most conceptually sophisticated and technologically advanced process measures *and* outcome measures, employed in conjunction with each other on the same therapies, as at an earlier time The Menninger Foundation PRP attempted to do in terms of the then state of the art (the decade of the 1950s). This would be in fulfillment of the principle enunciated by Strupp and colleagues (1988) in the initial chapter of a book devoted to process research: "the description and representation, theoretically and operationally, of a *patient's conflicts*, of the *patient's treatment*, and of the *assessment of the outcome* must be congruent, which is to say, must be represented in comparable, if not identical terms" (Dahl et al. 1988, p. ix). This fundamental integrative principle—proposed to subsume conceptually the entire array of process and outcome researches, however seemingly disparate their concepts and their instruments—is termed the principle of "Problem-Treatment-Outcome Congruence," or PTO Congruence for short (see Strupp et al. 1988, p. 7). A major presentation of the range of modern-day empirical psychoanalytic process studies is contained in the 1988 book *Psychoanalytic Process Research Strategies* (Dahl et al. 1988), the proceedings of a major workshop of American and German psychoanalytic therapy researchers held in Ulm, Germany, in 1985.

A second fourth-generation direction is in enhanced focus in both clinical and research studies on the "postanalytic phase" and therefore the encouragement of systematic follow-up study of psychoanalytic and psychotherapeutic endeavors both in clinic settings, where it can be more easily incorporated (and where it is an established tradition in somatic medicine), and, to the extent of the clinical community's (hopefully growing) willingness, in private practice. I have recounted such efforts briefly elsewhere (Wallerstein 1996, pp. 566–570).

A third direction is in what is called "offset" research, the large-scale statistical study—for example, built on the database of several years of health insurance claims of the Blue Cross/Blue Shield Federal Employees Program (FEP)—of the impact of mental health care (i.e., psychotherapy of varying intensity and duration) on the claims for general medical and surgical care (i.e., to what extent the costs of insurance-covered mental health care are "offset" by reductions in claims for somatic health care). I have also briefly recounted this direction of research elsewhere (Wallerstein 1995, pp. 450–452).

What is specific to the scope of this chapter is still another, fourth, vibrant direction of specifically outcome research: the effort to create scales that go beyond the various measures of targeted symptoms, of general well-being, and of particular behavioral patterns and dispositions (e.g., job absence, medical visits, delinquent infractions or other legal difficulties), and to develop measures of underlying personality structure and structural change. These measures assess the kinds of changes that psychoanalytically based therapies have claimed to be uniquely able to bring about—as contrasted with the claims of behavioral therapies, for example, which are directed (only) at specific symptom removal or specific behavior change.

(The concepts of structure and structural change are not universally embraced within the worldwide psychoanalytic community. For a spirited and sophisticated challenge, see the paper by Rolf Sandell [2002], himself a major psychoanalytic therapy researcher in Sweden and the principal investigator in the Stockholm Outcome of Psychoanalysis and Psychotherapy Project [STOPPP]. Basically, his argument is that these concepts of structure and structural change, however widespread their acceptance and use, are still basically undefined, or circularly defined, and are unnecessary as mediators between phenomena and their explanations [i.e., they are redundant and unnecessary to our efforts at explanation of psychological change]. Whether they are indeed useful, and therefore properly usable concepts in defining distinctions between kinds of changes, will not be properly settled either by fiat or by the weight of conviction. Their usefulness is itself an empirical issue to be settled ultimately by just the kind of research described in this chapter and implicitly being called for as its underlying subtext. Meanwhile, the widespread, even if not universal, support these concepts have gives me [at least temporary] warrant to employ them as I do in this chapter—until the weight of empirical evidence decrees otherwise.)

There are currently several such measures, or scales, of personality structure and of structural change, in various stages of establishing proper psychometric qualities, stability, reliability, and the various kinds of validity (e.g., content validity, "ecological validity," construct validity with both discriminant and convergent validation). Such psychometric properties must be established before these measures can be put to widespread use in studying ongoing therapies before, after, and at predetermined follow-up times. Such studies are necessary to study more definitively questions such as what kinds of changes, structural and/or other, do (or do not) come about in what kinds of patients, treated within what kinds of therapeutic modalities, or whether it is true, and to what extent it is true, that psychoanalytically based therapies can indeed bring about structural changes in the personality functioning that are beyond the merely symptom or manifest behavior changes that all therapeutic approaches claim.

Here I very briefly describe several extant structural change measures in this highly promising and rapidly developing realm of fourth-generation psychoanalytic outcome research. Our research group in San Francisco, referred to as PRP-II, used The Menninger Foundation PRP as its taking-off point. A major focus of the goals of PRP and its findings was the centrality of the conceptions of structure and structural change to the understanding of the putative benefits of psychoanalytically based therapies. A significant limitation of this work, however, was that we had no established metric for these conceptions of structure and structural change, but based these judgments solely on the expertise of experienced clinical judges, with all their inherent possibilities for bias and contamination.

PRP-II was therefore designed to create a valid measure of structure and structural change that would have established psychometric properties. Since the several metapsychologies that represent the diversity, or pluralism, that characterizes the current psychoanalytic theoretical landscape all have different languages—and possibly different meanings—for what constitutes underlying personality structure, and no consensual agreement exists at this time about the nature and scope of these conceptions at the level of experience-distant theorizing (our various metapsychologies), our research group decided to focus our inquiry on experience-near personality attributes. By doing so, we aimed to secure general agreement across our varying theoretical perspectives to ensure

that 1) the measure we created—Scales of Psychological Capacities (SPC)—would encompass the range of personality attributes that, in ensemble, constitute a comprehensive assessment of personality functioning; and 2) change, assessed by the altered patterning of the components of the SPC, would reflect underlying structural changes in personality functioning as agreed on by prominent representatives of each of the diversity of theoretical perspectives, whatever idiosyncratic language these representatives might use to describe those structural changes. Ultimately, these efforts led to an array of 17 scales (usually with 2 subscales each), indicating different directions of deviation from normal or optimal functioning, that together constitute the SPC (which has now been translated and is in use in five different language areas). The whole process of creation and deployment of the SPC as a before-and-after outcome measure of structural change has been described in detail elsewhere (DeWitt et al. 1991; Wallerstein 1988b; Zilberg et al. 1991).

Over these same two decades, a goodly number of other groups worldwide have undertaken—all independently and initially without knowledge of one another—this same task of creating reliable and valid scales of underlying personality structure and of structural change. All these scales are to be used in the same manner, as crucial outcome measures of expectable changes in psychoanalytic therapies. (Some are now being used in comparison with one another in the same study or in conjunction with process measures in order to fulfill the requirements of the principle of PTO Congruence.) Most of these new measures (or scales) have been created along conceptual lines identical to those followed in developing the SPC, an array of (usually experience-near) scales designed to comprehensively encompass the major dimensions of personality functioning, changes in the patterning of which, consequent to therapy, would constitute achieved structural change.

The following scales of underlying personality structure and of structural change have been those developed concurrently with the SPC:

1. *Karolinska Psychodynamic Profile (KAPP).* This set of 18 component scales, some of which are actually identical with some of the SPC 17 (though created totally independently), was devised by a group in Sweden and has already been widely deployed in a succession of studies of personality functioning and as predictor measures in relation to psychotherapeutic and somatic (surgical) intervention processes (Weinryb et al. 1991a, 1991b).

2. *Operationalisierte Psychodynamische Diagnostik (OPD).* A quite comparable creation by German psychoanalytic collaborators across several universities (Kassel,

Hamburg, and Giessen) (Rudolf et al. 1996), this instrument is currently in use in conjunction with the SPC in comprehensive studies of long-term psychoanalytic treatments (Leuzinger-Bohleber et al. 2003; Rudolf and Grande 2001).

3. *Structured Interview of Personality Organization (STIPO).* This interview, created by a group at Cornell, comprises 94 areas of inquiry, divided into 6 major domains of personality functioning (identity, object relations, defenses, aggression, moral functioning, and reality testing) and built around the theoretical conceptualizations of personality functioning of Otto Kernberg (Clarkin et al. 2002). In contrast to the SPC and KAPP, which are scales assessed through studies of audio- or video-recorded regular clinical interview material, the STIPO is itself a specially devised semistructured interview.

4. *McGlashan Semistructured Interview (MSI).* This semistructured interview, created at Chestnut Lodge, assesses 32 areas of personality functioning. It is being used in outcome studies of both hospital inpatient and clinic outpatient psychoanalytic psychotherapies (Goin et al. 1995; McGlashan 1984).

5. *Analytic Process Scales (APS).* Like the SPC and the KAPP, the APS is based on the intensive study of recorded therapeutic hours. Designed by a New York group to assess the ongoing therapeutic process, the APS can be deployed early and late, or before and after, as a measure of change over time, and therefore of outcome. It is being used in conjunction with the SPC as a comparative measure (Waldron et al. 2002).

6. *Psychotherapy Process Q-Set (PQS).* The PQS, developed by Enrico Jones in Berkeley, California, to study psychotherapy process, is based on a 100-item Q-set designed to capture the characteristic features of the patient's and the therapist's involvement in the exchanges of recorded therapeutic hours (in a manner that allows ready comparison with other hours of the same therapy or other therapies). Like the APS, the PQS is usable also as a measure of change over time, and therefore of outcome, with the additional advantage of allowing readily quantifiable comparative study with other cases (Jones 2000; Jones and Windholz 1990).

7. *Object Relations Inventory (ORI).* The ORI is used to assess structural organization and thematic content of an individual's self and object representations via two separate rating scales: a) Qualitative and Structural Dimensions of Parental Descriptions, which rates 12 traits or personal characteristics, and b) Differentiation-Relatedness Scale of Self and Object Representations, a 10-point rating scale for each of these two main factors (Blatt et al. 1988; see also Blatt and Ford 1994).

8. *Shedler-Westen Assessment Procedure (SWAP).* A Q-sort measure, like the PQS (though differently designed than the PQS, but with the same kinds of advantages of cross-hour and cross-case quantifiable comparisons), SWAP was designed specifically to refine and revise DSM-IV categories of personality dysfunction (the Axis II disorders) on the basis of diagnostic clinical interviews (Shedler and Westen 1998; Westen and Shedler 1999).

Of course, there may be other similarly conceptualized measures created to assess personality structure and structural change that have not yet come to my attention.

It is this array of measures that represents the fourth (current and not yet consolidated) generation of psychotherapy outcome research: measures designed to get beyond scales and assessments of symptoms, or of manifest behaviors, to create, rather, measures and scales of personality structure and structural change that will truly be able to assess what kinds of changes (structural or merely in symptoms or manifest behaviors) can be brought about, in what kinds of patients (across the whole psychopathological spectrum), by what kinds of therapeutic modalities (psychoanalysis proper, the array of psychoanalytic psychotherapies, and the array as well of non–psychoanalytically guided therapies). Clearly this research is now poised at a new level—one that holds the possibilities for truly accelerating breakthroughs, not only methodological but also substantive, as these currently conceived fourth-generation studies actually do get carried out through their natural cycle.

Conclusion

I have presented a historical overview of psychoanalytic therapy outcome research divided into four successive generations, both in time of temporal onset and in degree of conceptual and methodological sophistication and complexity. They are as follows: 1) first generation, from 1917 into the 1960s, consisting of simple statistical counts of judged outcomes in different patient categories; 2) second generation, from the 1950s into the 1980s, employing constructed measures and scales, before and after judgments, and predictions to expected outcomes; 3) third generation, from the 1950s into the 1980s (contemporaneous with the second generation), adding process to outcome measures and follow-up studies of the "postanalytic" phase; and 4) fourth generation, from the 1980s into the present, involving new outcome measures specifically geared to the assessment of psychological structure and structural change, coordinated with similarly enhanced more sophisticated process measures. This research is now poised at a new level of possibilities, one that promises accelerated substantive breakthroughs of new and more precise knowledge of mechanisms of change in psychoanalytic therapies that can in turn help guide treatment more precisely and effectively.

References

Alexander F: Five-Year Report of the Chicago Institute for Psychoanalysis, 1932–1937. Chicago, IL, Chicago Institute for Psychoanalysis, 1937

Bachrach HM, Weber JL, Solomon M: Factors associated with the outcome of psychoanalysis (clinical and methodological considerations): report of the Columbia Psychoanalytic Center Research Project (IV). Int Rev Psychoanal 12:379–388, 1985

Bachrach HM, Galatzer-Levy R, Skolnikoff AZ, et al: On the efficacy of psychoanalysis. J Am Psychoanal Assoc 39:871–916, 1991

Blatt SJ, Ford RQ: Therapeutic Change: An Object Relations Perspective. New York, Plenum, 1994

Blatt SJ, Chevron ES, Quinlan DM, et al: The Assessment of Qualitative and Structural Dimensions of Object Representations, Revised Edition. Unpublished research manual. New Haven, CT, Yale University, 1988

Caligor E, Hamilton M, Schachter H, et al: Converted patients and clinic patients as control cases: a comparison with implications for psychoanalytic training. J Am Psychoanal Assoc 51:201–220, 2003

Clarkin JF, Caligor E, Stern BL, Kernberg OF: Unpublished manual, 2002

Coriat I: Some structural results of the psychoanalytical treatment of the psychoneuroses. Psychoanal Rev 4:209–216, 1917

Dahl H, Kächele H, Thomä H: Psychoanalytic Process Research Strategies. New York, Springer-Verlag, 1988, p 334

DeWitt KN, Hartley D, Rosenberg SE, et al: Scales of psychological capacities: development of an assessment approach. Psychoanalysis and Contemporary Thought 14:343–361, 1991

Erle JB: An approach to the study of analyzability and analysis: the course of 40 consecutive cases selected for supervised analysis. Psychoanal Q 48:198–228, 1979

Erle JB, Goldberg DA: Problems in the assessment of analyzability. Psychoanal Q 48:48–84, 1979

Erle JB, Goldberg DA: Observations on assessment of analyzability by experienced analysts. J Am Psychoanal Assoc 32:715–737, 1984

Erle JB, Goldberg DA: The course of 253 analyses from selection to outcome. J Am Psychoanal Assoc 51:257–293, 2003

Feldman F: Results of psychoanalysis in clinic case assignments. J Am Psychoanal Assoc 16:274–300, 1968

Fenichel O: Statistischer Bericht über die therapeutische Tätigkeit, 1920–1930. Internazionale Psychoanalytischer Verlag, 1930, pp 13–19

Fonagy P, Target M: The efficacy of psychoanalysis for children with disruptive disorders. J Am Acad Child Adolesc Psychiatry 33:45–55, 1994

Fonagy P, Target M: Predictors of outcome in child psychoanalysis: a retrospective study of 763 cases at the Anna Freud Centre. J Am Psychoanal Assoc 44:27–77, 1996

Fonagy P, Kächele H, Krause R, et al: An Open Door Review of Outcome Studies in Psychoanalysis: Report Prepared by the Research Committee of the IPA at the Request of the President. London, University College London, 1999, p 330

Glover E: The indications for psychoanalysis. J Ment Sci 100:393–401, 1954

Goin MK, Strauss GD, Martin R: A change measure for psychodynamic psychotherapy outcome research. J Psychother Pract Res 4:319–328, 1995

Hamburg DA, Bibring GL, Fisher C, et al: Report of ad hoc Committee on Central Fact-Gathering Data of the American Psychoanalytic Association. J Am Psychoanal Assoc 15:841–861, 1967

Jones E[nrico]: Therapeutic Action: A Guide to Psychoanalytic Therapy. Northvale, NJ, Jason Aronson, 2000, p 381

Jones E[nrico], Windholz M: The psychoanalytic case study: a method for systematic inquiry. J Am Psychoanal Assoc 38:985–1015, 1990

Jones E[rnest]: Decannual report of the London Clinic of Psychoanalysis, 1926–1937. London, London Clinic of Psychoanalysis, 1936

Kantrowitz JL: The role of the patient-analyst "match" in the outcome of psychoanalysis. Annual of Psychoanalysis 14:273–297, 1986

Kantrowitz JL: The Patient's Impact on the Analyst. Hillsdale, NJ, Analytic Press, 1996, p 283

Kantrowitz JL, Paolitto F, Sashin J, et al: Affect availability, tolerance, complexity, and modulation in psychoanalysis: follow-up of a longitudinal, prospective study. J Am Psychoanal Assoc 34:529–559, 1986

Kantrowitz JL, Katz AL, Paolitto F, et al: Changes in the level and quality of object relations in psychoanalysis: follow-up of a longitudinal prospective study. J Am Psychoanal Assoc 35:23–46, 1987a

Kantrowitz JL, Katz AL, Paolitto F, et al: The role of reality testing in psychoanalysis: follow-up of 22 cases. J Am Psychoanal Assoc 35:367–385, 1987b

Kantrowitz JL, Katz AL, Greenman DA, et al: The patient-analyst match and the outcome of psychoanalysis: a pilot study. J Am Psychoanal Assoc 37:893–919, 1989

Kantrowitz JL, Katz AL, Paolitto F: Follow-up of psychoanalysis 5–10 years after termination, I: stability of change. J Am Psychoanal Assoc 38:471–496, 1990a

Kantrowitz JL, Katz AL, Paolitto F: Follow-up of psychoanalysis 5–10 years after termination, II: development of the self-analytic function. J Am Psychoanal Assoc 38:637–654, 1990b

Kantrowitz JL, Katz AL, Paolitto F: Follow-up of psychoanalysis 5–10 years after termination, III: the relation between the resolution of the transference and the patient-analyst match. J Am Psychoanal Assoc 38:655–678, 1990c

Kessel L, Hyman H: The value of psychoanalysis as a therapeutic procedure. JAMA 101:1612–1615, 1933

Knapp PH, Levin S, McCarter RH, et al: Suitability for psychoanalysis: a review of one hundred supervised analytic cases. Psychoanal Q 29:459–477, 1960

Knight RP: Evaluation of the results of psychoanalytic therapy. Am J Psychiatry 98:434–446, 1941

Leuzinger-Bohleber M, Stuhr U, Rüger B, et al: How to study the "quality of psychoanalytic treatments" and their long-term effects on patients' well-being: a representative, multi-perspective follow-up study. Int J Psychoanal 84:263–290, 2003

McGlashan TH: The Chestnut Lodge follow-up study: follow-up methodology and study sample. Arch Gen Psychiatry 41:573–585, 1984

Norman HF, Blacker KH, Oremland JD, et al: The fate of the transference neurosis after termination of a satisfactory psychoanalysis. J Am Psychoanal Assoc 24:471–498, 1976

Oremland JD, Blacker KH, Norman HF: Incompleteness in "successful" psychoanalyses: a follow-up study. J Am Psychoanal Assoc 23:819–844, 1975

Pfeffer AZ: A procedure for evaluating the results of psychoanalysis: a preliminary report. J Am Psychoanal Assoc 7: 418–444, 1959

Pfeffer AZ: Follow-up study of a satisfactory analysis. J Am Psychoanal Assoc 9:698–718, 1961

Pfeffer AZ: The meaning of the analyst after analysis: a contribution to the theory of therapeutic results. J Am Psychoanal Assoc 11:229–244, 1963

Rangell L: An overview of the ending of an analysis (1966), in The Human Core: The Intrapsychic Base of Behavior, Vol 2. Madison, CT, International Universities Press, 1990, pp 703–725

Rudolf G, Grande T: Comparison and validation of two instruments for rating structure and structural change: the Scales of Psychological Capacities (R.S. Wallerstein) and the Operationalized Psychodynamic Diagnosis (Arbeits gruppe Operationalisierte Psychodynamische Diagnostik). Unpublished manuscript, 2001

Rudolf G, Grande T, Uberbrachs C, et al: Erste empirische Untersuchungen zu einem diagnostischen System. Die Operationalisierte Psychodynamische Diagnostik (OPD). Z Psychosom Med Psychoanal 42:343–357, 1996

Sandell R: The problematic concept of structural change. Presentation at the International Psychoanalytical Association's Joseph Sandler Memorial Research Conference, University College of London, London, 2002

Sashin JI, Eldred SH, van Amerongen ST: A search for predictive factors in institute supervised cases: a retrospective study of 183 cases from 1959 to 1966 at the Boston Psychoanalytic Society and Institute. Int J Psychoanal 56:343–359, 1975

Schlessinger N, Robbins FP: Assessment and follow-up in psychoanalysis. J Am Psychoanal Assoc 22:542–567, 1974

Schlessinger N, Robbins FP: The psychoanalytic process: recurrent patterns of conflict and changes in ego functions. J Am Psychoanal Assoc 23:761–782, 1975

Schlessinger N, Robbins FP: A Developmental View of the Psychoanalytic Process: Follow-up Studies and Their Consequences. New York, International Universities Press, 1983, p 228

Shedler J, Westen D: Refining the measurement of Axis II: a Q-sort procedure for assessing personality pathology. Assessment 5:333–353, 1998

Strupp HH, Schacht TE, Henry WP: Problem-treatment-outcome congruence: a principle whose time has come, in Psychoanalytic Process Research Strategies. Edited by Dahl H, Kächele H, Thomä H. New York, Springer-Verlag, 1988, pp 1–14

Szecsody I, Varvin S, Amadei G, et al: The European Multi-Site Collaborative Study of Psychoanalyses (Sweden, Finland, Norway, Holland, and Italy). Article presented at the Symposium on Outcome Research, International Psychoanalytical Association Congress, Barcelona, Spain, 1997

Target M, Fonagy P: The efficacy of psychoanalysis for children with emotional disorders. J Am Acad Child Adolesc Psychiatry 33:361–371, 1994a

Target M, Fonagy P: The efficacy of psychoanalysis for children: prediction of outcome in a developmental context. J Am Acad Child Adolesc Psychiatry 33:1134–1144, 1994b

Waldron S Jr, Lundin J, Shedler J: Within session measures to assess outcome in psychoanalysis: determination of convergent validity with the Shedler-Westen Assessment Procedure (SWAP), the Scales for Psychological Capacities (SPC), and the Analytic Process Scales (APS), unpublished manuscript, 2002

Wallerstein RS: Forty-Two Lives in Treatment: A Study of Psychoanalysis and Psychotherapy. New York, Guilford, 1986, p 784

Wallerstein RS: Psychoanalysis and psychotherapy: relative roles reconsidered. Annual of Psychoanalysis 16:129–151, 1988a

Wallerstein RS: Assessment of structural change in psychoanalytic therapy and research. J Am Psychoanal Assoc 36(suppl):241–261, 1988b

Wallerstein RS: Research in psychodynamic therapy, in Psychodynamic Concepts in General Psychiatry. Edited by Schwartz HJ, Bleiberg E, Weissman SH. Washington, DC, American Psychiatric Press, 1995, pp 431–456

Wallerstein RS: Outcomes of psychoanalysis and psychotherapy at termination and at follow-up, in Textbook of Psychoanalysis. Edited by Nersessian E, Kopff RG Jr. Washington, DC, American Psychiatric Press, 1996, pp 531–573

Wallerstein RS: The generations of psychotherapy research: an overview. Psychoanalytic Psychology 18:243–267, 2001

Wallerstein RS, Fonagy P: Psychoanalytic research and the IPA: history, present status, and future potential. Int J Psychoanal 80:91–109, 1999

Wallerstein RS, Robbins LL, Sargent HD, et al: The Psychotherapy Research Project of The Menninger Foundation. Bull Menninger Clin 20:221–278, 1956

Weber JJ, Bachrach HM, Solomon M: Factors associated with the outcome of psychoanalysis: report of the Columbia Psychoanalytic Center Research Project (II). Int Rev Psychoanal 12:127–141, 1985a

Weber JJ, Bachrach HM, Solomon M: Factors associated with the outcome of psychoanalysis: report of the Columbia Psychoanalytic Center Research Project (III). Int Rev Psychoanal 12: 251–262, 1985b

Weber JJ, Solomon M, Bachrach HM: Characteristics of psychoanalytic clinic patients: report of the Columbia Psychoanalytic Center Research Project (I). Int Rev Psychoanal 12:13–26, 1985c

Weinryb RM, Rössel RJ, Asberg M: The Karolinska Psychodynamic Profile, I: validity and dimensionality. Acta Psychiatr Scand 83:64–72, 1991a

Weinryb RM, Rössel RJ, Asberg M: The Karolinska Psychodynamic Profile, II: interdisciplinary and cross-cultural reliability. Acta Psychiatr Scand 83:73–76, 1991b

Westen D, Shedler J: Revising and assessing Axis II, I: developing a clinically and empirically valid assessment method, II: toward an empirically based and clinically useful classification of personality disorders. Am J Psychiatry 156:258–272, 1999

Zilberg NJ, Wallerstein RS, DeWitt KN, et al: A conceptual analysis and strategy for assessing structural change. Psychoanalysis and Contemporary Thought 14:317–342, 1991

21

Process Research

WILMA BUCCI, Ph.D.

THE PSYCHOANALYTIC PROCESS IS a unique means of systematic investigation of human experience in an interpersonal context, perhaps the most effective means of such investigation that has ever been devised. In his paper "The Enduring Scientific Contributions of Sigmund Freud," published in relation to the Library of Congress Freud Exhibition, Gedo (2001) stated:

> In my judgment Freud's most lasting and valuable scientific contribution was not conceptual; hence it tends to be overlooked by nonspecialist historians. This achievement was the development of a novel observational method through which it became possible for the first time to gain reliable data about man's inner life. From about 1890, when he began to practice the "talking cure" invented by Breuer, it took Freud roughly twenty years to standardize a "psychoanalytic method" that permitted independent observers to collect such data. It is these unprecedented observations about mental functions and the control of human behavior that have defined the boundaries of psychoanalysis as a scientific domain. In other words, Freud accomplished a methodological breakthrough whereby, single-handedly, he founded a new discipline. (pp. 106–107)

The field of psychoanalytic process research has evolved to carry forward this "new discipline." In this chapter, I discuss the progress that has been made in this work, from the initial method of the case report through the several phases of empirical process research.

Defining the Knowledge Base for Process Research

Research on the psychoanalytic process has been central to psychoanalysis from its beginnings. Freud (1905[1901]/

1953, p. 8; quoted in Kantrowitz 2004a) viewed psychoanalysis as "a theory of mind and a method of research as well as a clinical intervention" and saw the study of treatment, rather than experimental investigation, as the appropriate venue for psychoanalytic research. The traditional database of process research has been the case report; this method is still seen as necessary and sufficient by many analysts. During the past several decades, however, there has been increasing recognition of scientific and clinical problems associated with the case report as a knowledge source. These include problems of potential bias and loss of information resulting from limitation of the observations to the single perspective of the treating analyst; and a wide range of clinical issues, such as the difficulty of balancing patient privacy with clinical validity in published reports, as well as the complex effects on treatment of the analyst's intent to write about a patient. A field of empirical process research—one based on application of objective measures to tape recordings or verbatim transcripts of therapy sessions—has emerged that is responsive to these problems.

The methods of case report and empirical research remain largely dissociated, following separate tracks. According to Wallerstein and Sampson (1971), as recently reviewed by Wallerstein (2001), the major arguments in favor of empirical process research based on audio recording were "the greater completeness, verbatim accuracy, permanence, and public character of the database, as well as the facilitation of the separation of the therapeutic from the research responsibility, with the possibility of thus bypassing the inevitable biases of the analyst as a contaminant of the data filter" (p. 261). According to the traditional position, research on psychoanalytic treatment should be restricted to the clinical method, which "was used by Freud to create and develop psychoanalysis" and which follows "the traditional model of case studies in medicine" (Perron 2002a, p. 3). In a report representing an extensive inquiry among French-speaking analysts who are International Psychoanalytical Association (IPA) members, Perron (2002a) noted that

> any attempt to submit the data of the sessions to the "hard sciences" criteria, and treat them by derived techniques, is likely to destroy the very object of the research, and moreover could not be accepted as proof by the sceptics. Recordings (audio- or video-) are then banned, not only for ethical reasons (due to confidentiality), but also because such a situation, even with the explicit agreement of the patient, disturbs gravely the transference-countertransference relationship. (pp. 7–8)

Controversies Concerning Process Research

The objections to empirical process research, as represented in Perron's report, are largely based on two sets of assumptions: 1) research negatively impacts clinical work and 2) psychoanalytic "facts" are inherently subjective.

Impact on the Treatment

The issues concerning interference with clinical work include the intrusion of the recording device; more general concerns as to conflict between research and therapeutic goals; and ethical issues of patient privacy.

Intrusion of the recording device.   The field of empirical process research depends ultimately on recordings of sessions, usually limited to audio recording. This reliance on recordings has been seen as an insurmountable obstacle by some clinicians. As Perron (2002b) notes, "I know, on the basis of all my analytic experience, that between me and my patients this would interfere, in a way I could not properly analyse. All my French colleagues think that way. If one of my trainees told me that he intended to tape a patient, I would tell him not to do so" (p. 33).

This view is still widely shared, explicitly or implicitly, by many clinicians. Even analysts who are supportive of empirical research are likely to take a NIMP (not in my practice) position. Over the past several decades, however, a small but increasing number of analysts who have carried out recorded analyses have argued that issues raised by tape recording can be handled effectively within the treatment, and that the difficulties of a recorded analysis are not of a different order from the problems of an ordinary analysis (Gill et al. 1968, 1970; Szecsody 2000; Thomä and Kächele 1973; Wallerstein 2001; Wallerstein and Sampson 1971).

The capacity to deal with recording in the treatment will, of course, depend on the procedures used and the attitude of the treating analyst. Recording as a constant presence, set up before the session begins, becomes part of the background; intermittent recording is more likely to be experienced as special and intrusive. The effect of recording is likely to be at least as salient for the analyst as for the patient; analysts need to recognize their own attitudes toward the recording device, including concerns about possible negative evaluations by outsiders of their analytic work.

We should note that objections have also been raised to note taking—after as well as during the session—as interfering with the treatment process; these concerns have been cited as one reason for the infrequency of case histories in the literature (see Michels 2000; Tuckett 2000). It is also widely recognized that a supervisor is a powerful "third presence" in the treatment. Yet this is not seen as precluding the establishment of an analytic process. A major difference between recording for research versus the intrusion of note taking and supervision is that research procedures require recording to be dealt with explicitly as an issue in the analysis, whereas the effects of note taking and supervision may in some cases remain unanalyzed—not confronted by either analyst or patient.

General impact of a research perspective.   The potential intrusion of research, which is explicit in tape-recorded treatments, is implicit in all treatments in which the analyst writes or intends to write and publish case reports. In a series of interviews with 30 American analysts who were authors of papers including clinical illustrations, Kantrowitz (2004a) uncovered a broad range of therapeutic implications of an analyst's intent to write about a patient. Some analysts reported intrapsychic conflicts about the intrusion of a research perspective, motivated by their own professional agendas and ambitions, into a situation that, apart from financial payment, is meant to be solely for the patient's benefit. Considerable concern was reported about whether to ask for patient consent for publication, and when and how to do this, and the possible effects of this request on the relationship. The meaning of a patient's manifest consent in the context of the relationship is complex, as Kantrowitz points out, as is the analyst's motivation to accept this consent without further exploration. In a more specific sense, the theme of the paper that the analyst is developing is likely to influence the analyst's focus in listening and responding to the patient. Thus, the traditional dual role of analyst-writer carries its own set of difficulties for the treatment, which generally remain unexplored.

Threats to patient privacy.   The potential impact on patient privacy has been cited as a major objection to recording for research purposes. The issue of confidentiality has been recognized as central in empirical process research. Patient informed consent is required for all recording, identifying data are removed from tapes and transcripts, and signed confidentiality agreements are required for researchers using treatment data. Research instruments are designed to extract data at a level of abstraction that is clinically and theoretically meaningful, without presentation of specific clinical detail. The use of computerized procedures, and reporting of aggregate rather than individual results, further protect the privacy of the patient.

In contrast to the systematic protection of patient privacy that is in place for empirical research, there are no consistent and established procedures for publishing clinical material in the psychological, psychiatric, or psychoanalytic journals, and no standard requirements for patient consent. The American Psychological Association's "fifteen page enforceable code of ethics does not refer to clinical writing" and its "journal does not have ethical guidelines for authors" (Scharff 2000, p. 430). The psychiatric journals follow ethical guidelines regarding safeguarding of patient confidences through adequate disguise, as stated in the American Psychiatric Association's *Principles of Medical Ethics*, with specific guidelines within each medical journal. The *Principles of Ethics for Psychoanalysts* of the American Psychoanalytic Association carries similar provisions. None of the psychoanalytic journals surveyed by Scharff require patient consent, with the exception of *Contemporary Psychoanalysis*, which requires both disguise and permission (Scharff 2000, pp. 430–431). (The instructions to authors of *Contemporary Psychoanalysis* state, "It is the author's responsibility to disguise the identity of patients when presenting case material and to obtain their written permission to do so.")

The ethical and scientific issues surrounding publication of case material were addressed in depth by the International Committee of Medical Journal Editors (1995), who argued that clinical accounts of patients should not be disguised in any way and suggested that informed consent must always be obtained from the patient who is the subject of a clinical report. The editors of the *International Journal of Psychoanalysis* (IJP) have challenged this position as rigid and unsuitable for psychoanalytic writing (Gabbard 2000; Gabbard and Williams 2001; Tuckett 2000). The conflict between the ethical need to protect a patient and the scientific need to maintain the integrity of clinical reporting in published material was addressed in an IJP editorial (see Gabbard and Williams 2001). The authors of the editorial provided guidelines concerning appropriate methods of preserving confidentiality, and methods of handling this in the treatment (and even after termination), but imposed no specific or standardized requirements and left the decision to the individual analyst, as determined by clinical considerations, tailored to the individual case. Possible approaches suggested in the editorial included disguise of superficial details; request for patient consent; use of case material that is a composite of several patients; presentation of dialogue between analyst and patient in play script form without background biographical information; and conveying clinical material through a colleague as author. Each of these approaches is considered to be ethical, according to IJP policy, but each has its own set of problems, as also discussed in detail by Gabbard (2000). In submitting manuscripts to the IJP, authors featuring clinical material in their papers are required to describe the method of protecting the patient's privacy that was used.

The management of this problem varies among individual analyst-writers. Of the 30 analysts interviewed by Kantrowitz (2004a), only 8 regularly asked their patients for permission to use their clinical material in published work, and only 18 had ever asked a patient's permission. All analysts interviewed by Kantrowitz disguised the clinical material, and did so in a variety of ways, compatible with preserving the dynamics.

Regardless of disguise, the probability of patients' reading about and recognizing themselves remains high. It is essentially impossible to disguise the clinical material of an individual case sufficiently to prevent recognition by a patient, or by others who know the patient, while adequately representing the clinical features. The probability of recognition is increased by the publication appearing under the authorship of the treating analyst (contrasting with the distance provided by authorship of findings by researchers unknown to the patient). The probability is increased further given the large proportion of analytic patients in the mental health field. Eight of the thirty analysts interviewed by Kantrowitz had patients who had read about themselves or heard themselves presented when their analysts had *not* requested their permission to use this material. While the effects on treatment were more obvious and acute in such instances, complex issues emerged whenever patients read their analysts' views of them, as Kantrowitz (2004b) has described.

Status of Psychoanalytic "Facts"

Beyond the clinical issues, many writers, such as Ricoeur (1970), Viderman (1979), and Perron (2002a), have argued that the "facts" of the psychoanalytic process reside in the subjective experience of the participants and are intrinsically unable to be represented by objective measures. Only the case report, as written by one of the participants, has the capability of presenting these facts. Tuckett (1993) generally agrees with this position, but also speaks to the danger of a story that is too well told and too coherent as leaving little space for the reader "to notice alternative patterns and to elaborate alternative narratives" (p. 1183). Thus, he argues in favor of a reasonably detailed clinical account, intended to describe what has gone on in the session and also including the analyst's own experience; this approach potentially provides information that readers can use to infer what the author has not said or even noticed.

Tuckett's argument may be carried further. It is precisely because of the reality of subjectivity—because perception and memory are active and constructive processes rather than passive and reproductive ones, and because an account by any one observer will represent one subjective construction—that it is necessary to preserve a verbatim record for reference. If there are as many versions of an event as there are perceivers, can we afford to be restricted in our records to only one?

Approaches to treatment change over time and place. Some material might not reach the "observing instrument" of "the analyst's subjectivity" because it does not register as significant from his or her theoretical perspective; yet might be seen as meaningful from alternative points of view and in different time periods. There is a tendency, documented by Bernardi (2002), for analysts to report observations supporting their positions and to fail to note disconfirming instances. As shown in a study by Bailey and colleagues comparing verbatim tape recordings with what the analyst intended as exhaustive process notes, only about a third of the material of a session was recorded, and the proportion of unrecorded material was higher for the analyst's than for the patient's speech (K.E. Bailey, J. Greer, W. Bucci, et al.: "What Do Process Notes Contain?" unpublished manuscript, 2004). These findings were replicated in several other studies, to the surprise of participating analysts, who had been convinced their notes were comprehensive. In addition, nonverbal aspects of vocalization, including pausing, vocal tone, and modulation, that figure in unconscious emotional communication would be lost in notes but are preserved in tape recordings.

It should also be emphasized that the case report is limited to material of which *the analyst is aware*. The analyst's unconscious experience or unconscious communication (perhaps including material that the analyst has warded off or defended against) will be missing from the report. This seems a particularly crucial gap for a field that focuses on experience outside of awareness. Perhaps most crucially, the *patient's subjectivity will be present in the report only as filtered through the analyst's*; should not the patient be allowed to speak for himself or herself, and should not

the reader—or the researcher—have the opportunity to make inferences about the patient's subjective experience on the basis of the patient's own material, including experience of which the analyst as well as the patient may be unaware?

On the basis of the information provided by Kantrowitz (2004a), we may also claim that the subjectivity of an analyst who intends to write about a patient is different in basic ways from that of an analyst who is focused entirely on therapeutic goals; this makes these reports intrinsically nonrepresentative of treatment as generally carried out.

Need for Multiple Perspectives

Considering the many threats to patient privacy and to the relationship that are inherent in the traditional dual practitioner-writer role, it seems relevant to raise the question (as has been raised for tape recording) of the extent to which a psychoanalytic process can go on in a treatment in which the analyst has the intent to write for publication. As Kantrowitz (2004a) has argued, the problems for treatment are real, but the complexity of the treatment issues does not argue against the use of patient material in publication: "Writing about patients is like walking in a minefield. There are no good solutions.... The solution is not to stop writing about patients, but to face and struggle with the conflict it creates as directly and honestly as possible" (p. 98). The same may be said for the use of tape recording for purposes of research. In both cases there are questions concerning the representative nature of observed treatments; in both cases issues arise that need to be addressed in the treatment. The solution is not to exclude recording, but to work through the difficulties it may create.

The controversy concerning data sources is of course unnecessary. The database for process research should include both recorded material and subjective reports. If there are issues concerning distortions resulting from either mode of observation, it seems even more crucial to incorporate both.

Evolution of Empirical Process Research

In the remainder of this chapter, I focus on the development of the field of empirical process research: its roots, current state, and future directions. (*Empirical process re*search, should of course be distinguished from *experimental* research on psychoanalytic concepts. The former may be seen as the psychoanalytic method in modern dress, using the basic rule of free association in the context of the relationship as providing a naturalistic context for the systematic study of inner life; the latter borrows from controlled laboratory designs, which have been seen as problematic in application to functions in which interpersonal context plays a crucial role [Thomä and Kächele 1987].)

Wallerstein (2001) has traced the evolution of psychotherapy research through three generations of outcome studies, leading to a fourth generation of research that focuses on process. The three generations of outcome studies address, at increasing levels of precision and depth, the question of *what* changes take place, from relatively simple retrospective counts of improved outcomes, with outcome judgments made by therapists, beginning as early as 1917, to the most elaborate prospective studies, with pretreatment assessment, objective assessment of change, and longitudinal follow-up.

Process studies figure in Wallerstein's outline as the "fourth generation of psychotherapy research" (see Chapter 20, "Outcome Research"), addressing the question of *how* change occurs. The questions of outcome and process are necessarily interlocked in many ways, as Wallerstein points out. Some third-generation outcome studies, such as The Menninger Foundation's Psychotherapy Research Project (Wallerstein 1986), were designed as an inquiry into both outcome and process, including examination of the nature of the intervention modality by which changes were brought about. The generational shift to the modern field of process research came about primarily through the emphasis on recording of session material, which made possible the fine-grained study of therapeutic interaction, and inspired the development of a wide range of measures for such research.

In his review, Wallerstein (2001) did not view generational progression as having developed in process research, largely because of its great conceptual and methodological complexity, coupled with lack of institutional support. While progress has certainly been painfully slow and limited, I would argue that generational progression can be identified during the several decades of work in this field:

1. A first generation, focusing on development of objective measures applied to session material by individual researchers
2. A second generation, characterized by collaborative application of several basic measures to shared data sets of sessions, and in some cases incorporating outcome assessment
3. A third generation, just emerging now, incorporating the subjective experience of the analyst and emphasizing the interaction of research and clinical work

First Generation of Process Research: Development of Objective Measures

The first generation involved development by individual researchers of objective measures of particular aspects of the treatment process, and establishment of their reliability and validity. Most measures require verbatim transcripts; some approaches use coding schemes applied to audiotaped or videotaped materials. Two major categories of measures may be identified: measures of problematic themes, as expressed in the patient's speech; and measures of therapeutic interaction. Several of the more widely used and well-known measures in each of these categories are discussed briefly here. More information on these and other measures may be found in the IPA Open Door Review (Fonagy et al. 2002) and in volumes edited by Dahl and colleagues (1988), Miller and colleagues (1993), and Shapiro and Emde (1995), as well as in the publications of the individual researchers.

Characterization of Problematic Themes

Within the context of process research, the patient's issues are characterized in terms of psychic structure rather than symptoms and behaviors. The primary focus for characterization of psychic structure has been the development of measures of relational patterns: psychological structures of perceptions, expectations, and beliefs about other people that emerged for adaptive purposes in response to the relationships of early life but that have become maladaptive in relation to an individual's current interpersonal world (Bucci 1997; Dahl 1988; Luborsky and Crits-Christoph 1998).

A number of measures have been developed with the goal of identifying such basic relationship patterns. These include the Core Conflictual Relationship Theme (CCRT) method introduced by Luborsky (1977); the method of identifying Fundamental Repetitive and Maladaptive Emotion Structures (FRAMES) developed by Dahl and Teller (1994); the Plan Formulation method of Weiss and Sampson and their colleagues (Weiss et al. 1986); and the Role Relationship Model configurational method of Horowitz and his colleagues (Horowitz et al. 1995). The general relationship pattern identified with these approaches is widely seen as constituting an operational definition of the transference (Luborsky and Crits-Christoph 1998). The convergence of measures of relationship patterns with measures of transference is seen directly in the assessment method represented by the Patient's Experience of the Relationship with the Therapist (PERT) developed by Gill and Hoffman (1982).

Core Conflictual Relationship Theme (CCRT).   The CCRT, initially introduced by Luborsky (1977), is the longest established and most widely used empirical method for deriving central relationship patterns (including transference patterns) from a patient's clinical material. The CCRT may be scored reliably by judges with little or no clinical training. The basic unit of analysis is the *relationship episode* (RE), usually a narrative about the self in relation to another person. Within the RE narrative, judges then identify the *wish*, *response of other* (RO), and *response of self* (RS). The strength of the CCRT lies in its ease of scoring, its reliability, and its capacity to represent, simply and elegantly, the essential components of interpersonal structures: what one desires, how one expects others to respond, and how one expects to feel. The simple structure of the CCRT has also been seen as a limitation with respect to capturing clinical nuances.

FRAMES (Fundamental Repetitive and Maladaptive Emotion Structures).   A contrasting approach to assessing relationship patterns is the method of identifying FRAMES, developed by Dahl and Teller (1994). FRAMES are systematic descriptions of sequences of events in narratives that patients tell in the free association. Events of the narrative plot are classified by means of the empirical classification of emotions developed by Dahl and Stengel (1978), based on the emotion theory developed by Dahl (1979). The FRAMES system differs from the CCRT approach in its method of tracking the specific structure of each narrative. It has the potential to provide a nuanced account of a patient's emotion structures and changes in them but has proven more difficult to score reliably and is less widely used. A promising reliability study was carried out by Siegel (2001); additional reliability studies are needed, as Dahl (2002) has pointed out.

Plan Formulation method.   The Plan Formulation method was developed in the context of a specific clinical theory, the Control-Mastery theory (Weiss 1993; Weiss et al. 1986). This method has generally been characterized as a cognitively oriented approach derived from ego psychology, and more recently as cognitive-relational. The theory holds that patients come to therapy with *unconscious plans* to disprove debilitating *pathogenic beliefs* acquired during childhood that prevent them from pursuing appropriate life goals. The plan formulation covers the patient's goals for therapy, the pathogenic beliefs, the insights that will help the patient achieve therapy goals, and the manner in which the patient will work in therapy to disconfirm the beliefs by testing them in the relationship with the therapist. The strength of this approach is its clear and immediate clinical relevance and its capability of testing alternative clinical hypotheses. However, the method of generating a plan formulation requires trained clinical judges who are familiar with the theory, and the method has had little application outside of the Control-Mastery investigative group itself.

Configurational analysis and the Role Relationship Model.   The central construct in the Role Relationship Model (RRM) configurational method is the person schema, defined as "'structures of meaning' that affect thinking, planning and action concerning the self and others" (Horowitz 2002, p. 189). RRMs provide an organizing framework for identifying person schemas and presenting them diagrammatically. The analysis is carried out by means of videotapes or transcripts. This approach has been utilized by Horowitz and his colleagues to provide a method for systematic individual case formulation that may be used as a basis for effective treatment. Horowitz (2002) has described the symptomatology of personality disorders and their underlying motivation using the full system of configurational analysis, including analysis of developmental level as well as RRM configurations. The approach has the strength and weaknesses of its complexity; Horowitz and his colleagues have shown its direct value for therapeutic work, but the method has not as yet been developed in a way to be readily applied by other researchers.

Other empirical measures of psychopathology.   In addition to measures of central relational themes, other measures have been developed that examine various aspects of personality structure, as expressed in the material of the session. Among the most widely used of these are the Defense Mechanism Rating Scales (DMRS), developed by Perry and Cooper (1989; Perry 2001) as an extension of work done by Vaillant and his colleagues (Vaillant 1977; Vaillant and Drake 1985), and a measure of social cognition and object relations (SCORS) developed by Westen (1991).

Measures of Therapeutic Interaction

In contrast to measures that assess aspects of psychic structure, other approaches look directly at therapeutic interactions and their effects. These include comprehensive process scales; measures of therapeutic discourse employing scales and computerized procedures; classifications of therapeutic interventions; and assessment of intervention effects.

Process scales.   The Psychotherapy Process Q-Set (PQS) (Jones 2000) is a 100-item instrument designed for rating patterns of patient-therapist interactions and other aspects of the treatment process. Judges rate entire hours (audiotaped or videotaped), following definitions and rules provided in a coding manual and using the Q-sort method, a special type of forced-choice procedure based on an assumed normal distribution of variables. High levels of interrater reliability, item reliability, and discriminant and predictive validity have been obtained (Jones and Pulos 1993). The PQS rating method is embedded in an overall project with the goal of studying causal relationships and mechanisms of change. The project focuses primarily on single-case designs and looks at patterns of interaction in relation to both process indicators within the session material and more traditional symptom-based measures of outcome.

The method also provides a common language for description of process that may be applied to different treatment forms. In a comparison of samples drawn from archival data sets, using the PQS, Jones and Pulos (1993) found psychodynamic treatments to be characterized by emphasis on evocation of affect, bringing troublesome feelings into awareness, and integrating current difficulties with previous life experience, using the therapist-patient relationship as a change agent. This emphasis contrasted with focus on control of negative affect through the use of intellect and rationality combined with vigourous encouragement, support, and reassurance from therapists in cognitive-behavioral treatments.

Ablon and Jones (1998) developed prototypes of the contrasting treatments, based on PQS coding by expert panels of therapists. Their findings indicate that analysts can agree on a general definition of analytic process that can be operationalized and quantitatively assessed. Their main point, however, is that there is not just one ideal analytic process; rather, each analytic pair has a unique interaction pattern that is linked to therapy outcome. The experience, recognition, and comprehension of the meaning of such repetitive interactions appear to be a fundamental component of therapeutic action.

A new measure of psychotherapy process, the Comparative Psychotherapy Process Scale (CPPS), developed by Blagys and colleagues (M.D. Blagys, S.J Ackerman, D. Bonge, et al.: "Measuring Psychodynamic-Interpersonal and Cognitive-Behavioral Therapist Activity: Development of the Comparative Psychotherapy Process Scale," unpublished manuscript, 2003), includes items representing key features of both psychodynamic-interpersonal (PI) and cognitive-behavioral (CB) treatment models, derived from empirical studies contrasting these approaches. The PI items include focus on affect and the expression of emotion, identification of central themes, emphasis on past experiences, focus on interpersonal experience, emphasis on the relationship, exploration of dreams and fantasies, and exploration of avoidance or resistance. The CB items include emphasis on thought patterns and belief systems, teaching skills, assigning homework, providing information, and direction of session activity. The CPPS is scored by judges who independently view videotapes of entire sessions. Excellent interrater and inter-item reliability values have been obtained for both subscales.

The analytic process scales (APS) constitutes another research approach that looks directly at patient-analyst interactions and their effects (Waldron et al. 2002, 2004). The instrument includes variables assessing the analyst's and patient's contributions and interactional features of the emerging relationship. All variables were chosen as central, unambiguous, experience-near process features, defined in the language of the clinical surface. Good reliability has been achieved by senior analysts after brief training; the reliability of scoring by nonanalyst judges is being investigated.

Computer-assisted measures. The labor-intensive nature of many of the measures described above limits the number of sessions that can be studied. Computer-assisted procedures have been developed that permit expansion of process investigations to larger samples of sessions and treatments. The computerized measures also serve to identify significant phases within treatments or within sessions. Clinical content measures can then focus on these critical phases.

Dahl (1972, 1974) and Spence (1970) were pioneers in the application of computer-assisted content analysis to psychoanalytic transcripts. Dahl (1974) showed linguistic differences between "work" and "resistance" sessions in a psychoanalytic treatment using categories from the General Inquirer system developed by Stone and colleagues (1966).

The Text Analysis System (TAS) developed by Mergenthaler (1985, 1993) enables microanalytic studies of fluctuations within sessions as well as examination of complete sessions and treatments. Using this approach, Mergenthaler (1996, 2002) developed a Therapeutic Cycles Model (TCM), based on computer-assisted measures of two change agents, Affective Experiencing (measured as "Emotion Tone") and Cognitive Mastery (measured as "Abstraction"). Application of these measures to the verbal expressions of patient and therapist in verbatim transcripts allows for differentiation of what Mergenthaler terms "Emotion-Abstraction" patterns, developed as combinations of varying levels of the two basic measures.

There is an important caveat to be noted in the application of computerized procedures. The very efficiency and power of these methods and their capability of bypassing the problem of interrater reliability may lead to neglect of the problem of their validity. If we are to count words in categories, we require evidence as to what these categories represent. This issue has been carefully addressed by the researchers described above and has also been examined in depth by Bucci (1997).

Measures of the referential process.   Several linguistic measures of the treatment process have been developed within the framework of Bucci's theory of multiple coding and the referential process (Bucci 1997). The referential process concerns the general function of connecting subjective, nonverbal experience, including emotional experience, to the shared verbal code. The integrative work of psychoanalytic treatment is defined as occurring through the phases of the referential process as these play out repeatedly in the associative process and the therapeutic relationship. The phases include 1) arousal of an emotion schema; 2) retrieval of imagery, fantasy, or memory and its telling in narrative form; and 3) emotional reflection, explicating the emotional meaning of the narrative. The last phase is likely to be interactive and to incorporate events of the relationship. Optimally, the words that are spoken, by analyst and patient, connect to components of the emotion schema that have previously been dissociated, leading potentially to the reconstruction of the schema that we characterize psychoanalytically as *structural change.*

Measures have been developed that track the phases of the referential process as these recur in different forms and with different contents throughout a session (Bucci 2002b, 2002c). The basic indicators are measures of Referential Activity (RA), which assess the degree to which language reflects connection to nonverbal experience, including imagery and bodily and emotional experience. High RA language is vivid and immediate, indicating that the speaker (or writer) is immersed in reliving an experience; and tends to evoke corresponding experience in a listener (or reader). Low RA language is general, abstract, and vague, indicating lack of emotional connection in the speaker; and generally fails to make such connections to the listener. Measures of RA, including both scales scored by judges and computerized measures, have been used in a wide range of psycholinguistic and clinical studies (Bucci 2002b, 2002c; Bucci et al. 1992). The first computerized RA measure, the CRA, was developed by Mergenthaler and Bucci (1999); a new computerized RA measure, the WRAD (Weighted Referential Activity Dictionary) developed by Bucci and Maskit (in press), is now in use. Measures of RA reach their peak levels in the narrative phase of the referential process. Other linguistic indicators, representing other phases of the referential process, include measures of affect, reflectivity, and disfluency, and a number of derived measures based on these. The computerized measures are applied with a new text analysis system—the Discourse Attributes Analysis System (DAAP) (B. Maskit, W. Bucci, A.J. Roussos, "Capturing the Flow of Verbal Interaction: The Discourse Attributes Analysis Program, unpublished manuscript, 2004)— which provides a precise scan of the therapeutic interactions.

Classification of therapeutic interventions.   The multidimensional system for analyzing interventions developed by Strupp (1957) provided a basic approach, with demonstrated reliability and validity, that informs most classification systems in use today. The initial system consisted of seven major categories: facilitating communication with minimal activity; exploratory operations; clarification with minimal interpretation; interpretive operations; structuring; direct guidance; interchange that is not directly therapeutic; and a category of unclassifiable interventions. Subdivisions were also identified within each of the major categories. The standard categories have been revised and reconfigured by researchers for application in a broad range of studies requiring systematic quantitative assessment of the therapist's verbal communications.

Other researchers have developed specialized systems of classification focused on specific research questions. Piper et al. (1987) developed the Therapist Intervention Rating System (TIRS), which focuses on distinguishing among types of interpretations and differentiating these from other interventions. From a different perspective, Elliott et al. (1987) compared six rating systems in order to identify a set of primary therapist response modes applying across a range of therapeutic orientations. The six systems were applied by their developers to sessions representing numerous treatments, including behavioral, rational-emotive, time-limited, relationship-insight-oriented, and a Jungian dream analysis, among others. While each approach was characterized by a unique response-mode profile, a set of fundamental categories could be identified as underlying these systems; these included questions, information, advisement, reflection, interpretation, and self-disclosure.

Effects of interventions.   Every process measure carries within it an explicit or implicit change component. Change in a measure in the course of a session constitutes a mini-outcome that may be examined to assess the effects of interventions. The measures differ in the degree to which this change component has been developed. Changes in FRAMES may be traced both within sessions following critical interventions and across treatments; positive outcome would be indicated by change or disappearance of particular recurrent maladaptive structures (Dahl 1998, 2002). Other indicators of mini-outcomes include changes in Emotion-Abstraction patterns (Mergenthaler 1996); measures of experiencing (Klein et al. 1970); patient productivity (Waldron et al. 2002); "associative freedom," based on personal pronoun use (Spence et al. 1993); and fluctuations in RA and other linguistic measures that indicate systematic progression through the phases of the referential process (Bucci 2002b, 2002c).

The implications of the CCRT concerning how patients change are unclear. A patient's CCRT has generally been found to be consistent over time; only moderate changes in CCRT have been found in the course of treatment. In particular, successful outcome is associated with small but significant decreases in the pervasiveness of the negative responses of others and of oneself and increases in positive responses (Crits-Christoph and Luborsky 1990).

Looking at overall treatment outcome rather than within-session effects, Hilsenroth and colleagues (2003) found that techniques directed toward achieving and maintaining focus on expression and exploration of painful affect were most closely related to improvement in depressive symptomatology in relatively short (unfixed term) psychodynamic treatments, lasting generally a year or less. The results concerning effectiveness of psychodynamic techniques in treatment of depression are consistent with findings by Barber et al. (1996) and Gaston et al. (1998).

Second Generation of Process Research: Collaborative Studies

The first phase of process research yielded a broad range of empirical measures of the treatment process, representing central problematic relational structures, therapeutic interactions, and structural change. The second phase focused on application of these measures to shared data sets of sessions in collaborative studies, in some cases including outcome assessment. The development of instruments continued and expanded in new ways in this second generation. The collaborative approach enabled researchers to build the construct validity of the measures in several ways: to demonstrate to what extent a) different methods that claim to measure the same underlying variables converge; b) the measures are assessing what they claim to measure; and c) the mini-outcomes defined with process measures are associated with treatment effects defined in traditional behavioral and symptomatic terms.

Major Collaborative Studies

A workshop of process researchers in Ulm, Germany, in 1985 initiated the second-generation approach. Researchers applied a wide range of empirical measures, including the CCRT, FRAMES, PERT (Gill and Hoffman 1982), and RA, to the same treatment material, a single session from a fully recorded psychoanalysis of a young married woman (Dahl et al. 1988). The Program on Conscious and Unconscious Mental Processes, directed by Mardi Horowitz at the University of California at San Francisco, incorporated a

wide range of the process measures that have been described here as well as videotaped material and physiological measures (Horowitz 1988, 1997, 1998a, 1998b). The Collaborative Analytic Multi-Site Program (CAMP), organized by Wallerstein in 1989 under the auspices of the American Psychoanalytic Association, brought together many active psychoanalytic process research groups to apply their measures to a shared set of psychoanalytic sessions from treatment archives provided by the Psychoanalytic Research Consortium (PRC) (Wallerstein, in press). To provide some indication of treatment outcome as a framework for the study of process, two independent judges evaluated a cohort of these cases in a retrospective manner (by applying measures of psychological health and psychiatric severity to early and late sessions) (Luborsky et al. 2001).

Coordination of Results: The Segmentation Problem

A crucial issue that emerged in these collaborative studies concerns the coordination of scores for different research measures that depend on different units of analysis. Each approach described above uses a different procedure to identify the segments of a session transcript to which the measure will be applied. The boundaries of the REs used to score the CCRT, for example, are generally not equivalent to the units used to score FRAMES or defenses or APS interactions, so that systematic cross-validation cannot be directly carried out. This methodological problem, which may appear mundane and technical, has been a central challenge for collaborative research. At present, the field relies mainly on either segmentation by idea units (Stinson et al. 1994), which requires agreement on boundaries by judges prior to scoring and is thus relatively labor intensive; or arbitrary computerized segmentation by word blocks, which cut across unit boundaries and do not adequately reflect the actual patterns of the clinical interaction.

Narrative as a Unifying Feature

A promising approach to segmentation that is theory based and that applies computerized procedures in a nonarbitrary way involves the use of natural discourse features, in particular the use of narratives, as providing a common structure for collaborative research (Bucci 1995, 1997, 2002b; B. Maskit, W. Bucci, A.J. Roussos, "Capturing the Flow of Verbal Interaction: The Discourse Attributes Analysis Program, unpublished manuscript, 2004). Narratives about interactions with other people constitute the basic unit used for scoring the CCRT, FRAMES, and other widely used measures of relationship patterns and transference themes (Luborsky 1988; Luborsky et al. 1993). From a psychoanalytic perspective, the narratives that patients tell in the free association, including dreams, fantasies, and memories of events from the recent or distant past, are basic vehicles for representation of unconscious experience. In the context of multiple code theory, these narratives are understood as representing the structure of an emotion schema that has been dissociated or warded off, or some component of this schema (Bucci 1997). Narrative segments are indicated by high levels of RA, as measured by the scales or computerized measures (Bucci 2002c; Bucci and Maskit, in press). Several studies have found that both Relationship Episodes (REs) on which the CCRT is based and prototypes or instantiations of Dahl and Teller's (1994) FRAMES are likely to be located in high-RA narrative phases of a session (Doyle 1999; Sammons and Siegel 1998). Changes in emotion schemas are reflected in changes in the thematic contents represented in these narrative peaks.

In contrast to the high-RA narrative phases, phases of low RA indicate parts of the session when work of several different types may be taking place, including processes of arousal, destabilization, and struggle on the one hand, and periods of reflection and insight on the other (Pessier and Stuart 2000; Sammons and Siegel 1998). New computerized measures and other procedures have been developed to represent and distinguish the process in these phases (Bucci 2002b, 2002c; B. Maskit, W. Bucci, A.J. Roussos, "Capturing the Flow of Verbal Interaction: The Discourse Attributes Analysis Program," unpublished manuscript, 2004).

Third Generation of Process Research: Broadening the Scope of Observation

While the second wave of process research addressed the need for multiple indicators from which inference may be made to the constructs of inner experience, the work remained largely limited to one level of observation: that of objective measures applied to transcribed session material. A third generation of process research has begun to broaden the scope of observation and build the connections between research and clinical work. Here I briefly mention two studies, both ongoing, that are in the vanguard of this third generation; these studies are described in more detail elsewhere (Bucci, in press).

Multiple Perspectives on the Analytic Interaction: The IPTAR Single-Case Study

An intensive single-case study of an ongoing treatment, now being carried out by the Research Group of the Insti-

tute for Psychoanalytic Training and Research (IPTAR) (Freedman et al. 2003), is unique in incorporating multiple perspectives on the therapeutic interaction. The patient, a married woman in her 30s, is seen on the couch four times a week by an experienced female analyst. In introducing the research, the analyst explained the research objectives to the patient and obtained her written consent. Immediately after each session, with the tape recorder still on, the analyst dictates her impressions (for 3–5 minutes) of the session just ended. She describes her subjective experience of the session freely and spontaneously without following any preimposed structure or outline. As Freedman et al. (2003) describe it, the analyst's clinical scan captures the immediacy of the session, "the kinds of thoughts and feelings that may permeate an analyst's consciousness just after the patient has left the room" (p. 209). Aside from her role in recording the sessions, and providing her impressions as described below, the analyst has no interaction with the research team.

Senior analysts serving as clinical consultants then listen to and evaluate the session material as filtered through the analyst's scans. On the basis of these evaluations, a subset of sessions are selected, representing variations in treatment effectiveness, for more intensive study. The clinical consultants, using verbatim transcripts, then evaluate the subset of sessions directly. Other clinicians provide detailed examination of the event structure of selected sessions, moment by moment. Objective measures are also applied to the transcripts; these include computerized linguistic measures of the referential process (Bucci 2002c; Bucci and Maskit, in press), measures of defenses (Perry 2001), and the CCRT (Luborsky and Crits-Christoph 1998), as well as measures of psychoanalytic symbolization developed by Freedman and colleagues (2001).

The design has several features that may serve as models for this new generation of research: including the treating analyst as participant and observer; comparing the observations of the analyst with those of clinical consultants; applying objective process measures; and using these measures to examine the differences between analyst and consultant views. Each set of measures serves to build construct validity for the others in an interactive way; the design places the research measures in partnership with clinical observations, as a source of new discoveries, not only as evidence for what clinicians already know.

Direct Clinical Applications of Process Research in the Supervision Process

A study carried out in Buenos Aires at the Psychoanalytic Association of Argentina in collaboration with Belgrano University represents another approach to integrating empirical research methods with clinical work (Lopez Moreno et al. 1999). The study is presented in more detail by Bucci (in press). A wide range of clinical and empirical research measures were applied to treatments of six young women seen by candidates at the reduced-fee psychoanalytic therapy clinic of the Association. Candidate-therapists were supervised by senior analysts, members of the Association. The study was unique in using research results directly in supervision in innovative ways. For example, computerized language measures, in graphic form, pointed to salient moments in a session and served to stimulate the candidate to further exploration of her own feelings at such points. Both supervisors and candidates found these and other research measures useful in providing an additional vision of the session that served to identify potentially significant aspects of process that might not otherwise have been noted by them, and did this in a nonjudgmental way. As in the IPTAR study, the several perspectives are seen as supplementing and complementing one another, rather than privileging the subjective or objective perspectives as holding the actual "facts."

Problems and Goals in Process Research

Considerable growth and development have occurred in the field of empirical process research, as shown in the generational progression outlined in the previous subsections. Nevertheless the field is perhaps still best characterized by its problems, its potential, and its hopes.

Four major sets of problems may be distinguished: clinical, methodological, institutional, and conceptual.

Clinical Issues

The problems concerning dangers of interference with clinical work have already been discussed in detail in this chapter. They may be seen as different but not more critical than the problems that arise in treatments in which the analyst intends to write about a patient, the traditional context of process research as case report.

Methodological Issues

The labor-intensive and costly nature of the microanalytic process work is being addressed, to some degree, through development of more sophisticated computerized procedures and statistical techniques. Transcribing remains a time-consuming roadblock for process research, and voice recognition programs have not as yet proven successful in

expediting this process (K.E. Bailey, J. Greer, W. Bucci, et al.: "What Do Process Notes Contain?" unpublished manuscript, 2004). For measures scored by raters, there remains a trade-off between ease and reliability of scoring and the capacity of a measure to capture clinical nuances. Although considerable progress is being made, this research remains costly in both time and money. This leads directly to the institutional problems facing the field that need to be further addressed.

Institutional Issues

Need for Financial Support

The history of the search for funding for process research has been outlined by Wallerstein (in press). Attempts to obtain government or agency funding have generally failed, in part because the work has unique and nonstandard features and in part because the field has not had sufficient resources to demonstrate its scientific potential to the non-psychoanalytic mental health community. The escape from this catch-22 situation will depend on the continuing dedication of the small band of process researchers, who find ways to keep building their research programs, with some support from psychoanalytic organizations and other private agencies, potentially leading to broader funding opportunities.

Organization and Management of the Database

A fundamental need for advancement of the field is an organized archive that will enable sharing of clinical data and coordination of research results, while maintaining the highest level of safeguards for the confidentiality of the material. A number of treatment archives have been developed, including the Psychoanalytic Research Consortium, the Penn Psychoanalytic Treatment Collection (Luborsky et al. 2001), and the Ulm Textbank. However, sufficient resources have not been available to support the administration of these archives (Roussos et al., in press), and this has severely limited the possibilities of collaborative work. Collaborative studies such as the CAMP projects have thus far largely been limited to a small set of treatments for which few outcome and auxiliary clinical data are available, while new programs with rich contextual material, such as the IPTAR study, lack mechanisms for monitoring the use of their materials by outside researchers.

Training and Support of Psychoanalytic Researchers

The field requires a continuing influx of researchers who are trained in research concepts and methods. The issue of adequate training for research needs to be addressed most immediately in clinical psychology doctoral programs, and psychoanalytic institutes, and in the relation between the institutes and universities. At present, there remain only a very few psychoanalytically oriented clinical psychology doctoral programs, with no dedicated courses in process research at any of these; and the research presence at the institutes remains minimal (Schacter and Luborsky 1998).

Conceptual Issues

The strategy of inference from the patient's words and behavior to his or her inner experience, and, most crucially, from gaps in the patient's associations to unconscious or dissociated experience, was the seminal vision of the psychoanalytic process. This is the strategy of the "psychoanalytic method" as applied in clinical work. This strategy is also, in a basic sense, the epistemological approach of all science, as Freud (1940[1938]/1964) understood. Just as a physicist makes inferences from readings on a meter to the movements of particles that cannot be observed, so the analyst makes inference from the language and behavior of the patient (and the analyst's own experience) to the patient's inner experience, both conscious and unconscious—and so the psychoanalytic researcher makes inference from the language and behavior that are preserved on recordings to the emotional meanings of events for the patient—and for the analyst.

Such inferences provide the means by which we all negotiate our interpersonal worlds; each individual uses observations of others as well as his or her own subjective experience to form inferences—usually implicit—concerning the other's inner state. In contrast to the interpersonal inferences in everyday life, inference in the psychoanalytic situation, as in scientific work, has customarily occurred within an explicit theoretical framework. In this respect, as in many others, Freud's vision presaged the approach of modern science; systematic inferences to unobservable events depend on a theoretical framework within which the concepts of the theory are defined, in terms of one another and in terms of observable events. In well-developed networks, as in physics, the definitions are formal and the relationships are quantified; such formal structures are beginning to be developed in some areas of psychology but have never been developed for psychoanalysis.

In psychoanalytic clinical work today, the framework is mixed, diverse, and often implicit, including both whatever version of psychoanalytic theory guides the analyst's understanding, and also including the analyst's individual schemas based on experience with patients and life experience

(Bernardi 2002; Bucci 1997, 2001a; Sandler 1983; Wallerstein 1998). Many clinicians today, in fact, rely more on their individual schemas of subjective response than on a specific psychoanalytic theory. This emphasis on individual schemas is a function of, on the one hand, the failure of the metapsychology as a coherent framework (Holt 1985) and the ensuing theoretical vacuum in modern psychoanalysis (Thomä and Kächele 1987) and, on the other, the new psychological understanding of the psychoanalytic process, intrinsically involving the experience of the analyst as a source of inference concerning the patient.

Reflecting the lack of a systematic general theory, as well as the modern clinical stance, most process researchers (many of whom are themselves analysts) have focused largely on the surface of therapeutic interaction. This was a successful interim strategy for development of individual research measures, but emerged as a problem with the attempts to carry out collaborative research. Without a coherent theoretical framework, there is no systematic way to develop the operational meanings and interconnections of concepts or to determine the degree to which individual measures may be expected to converge or diverge. We cannot know, for example, to what extent the constructs of transference or conflict or structural change, as measured by the various methods described in the preceding section, correspond to one another, or to the concepts that clinicians understand and use. Although some researchers may focus on the surface, for pragmatic reasons, they of course do not limit their conclusions to quantification of observations, but use their observations as a basis for inferences to internal mental and emotional events. Ultimately, researchers must rely on some theoretical framework to make such inferences; there needs to be movement from reliance on implicit theories to development of systematic and shared theoretical frameworks, as part of the research goals.

A general theory is needed for clinical work as well. It is possible that many of the current controversies in the field reflect vague and shifting definitions of theoretical terms rather than actual differences in how to work with patients. The concepts of projective identification and intersubjectivity are among many examples of such misunderstanding (see Bucci 2001a).

The theory that is needed must be a psychological theory—one not limited to psychoanalytic concepts—and not a neuropsychological theory. The psychological level is needed to provide an interface between psychoanalytic concepts and neurological ones, as neuroscientists also argue (Panksepp 1999). The multiple code theory (Bucci 1997) provides one such theoretical framework; alternative theories may be developed.

Implications for Clinical Work

As noted earlier, the process research field is, at this early stage, characterized more fully by its potential and its problems than by its results. Nevertheless, some findings have emerged from this survey of the field that have importance for clinical work.

The research provides strong and converging support for the role of narratives as vehicles for expression of emotional experience and as vehicles for change. It is not only the dream that provides the "royal road" to experience that has been warded off, but also fantasies, memories, and stories of all sorts. Central conflictual and maladaptive emotion schemas are most likely to be expressed in narratives that represent the self in relation to other people (Bucci 1995, 2002b; Dahl 1988, 1998; Horowitz 1998b; Luborsky and Crits-Christoph 1998). Although the content of the stories is likely to appear trivial and irrelevant, as Freud emphasized—this is particularly the case for narratives representing components of schemas that are dissociated or warded off—their emotional meaning remains to be explicated in the work of the analysis.

These central narratives are likely to be marked in the session material by language that is vivid and immediate, as indicated by high levels of Referential Activity, without abstract reflection (Bucci 2002b, in press). In effective working sessions, the analyst tends to listen without interruption to such narratives and to intervene at their close, often with an interpretation. The themes that are expressed have parallel patterns for the relationship with others and the relationship with the therapist, as Luborsky's studies have shown. There is some evidence that accuracy of interpretation of the themes expressed in these narratives is linked to outcome (L. Luborsky, E. Luborsky, "Supportive-Expressive Dynamic Psychotherapy: Clinical Principles and Research Discoveries," unpublished manuscript, 2004).

Another important finding for which there is converging evidence concerns the importance of focus on emotional experience, including painful experience, in the context of the relationship. Using different instruments for description of process, Jones and his colleagues and Hilsenroth and his colleagues have found similar results. Psychodynamic treatments are characterized by their emphasis on expression and exploration of feelings; the capacity to tolerate such exploration requires the environment of the treatment relationship. This contrasts with the emphasis on thought patterns and beliefs, and focus on control of negative affect through the use of intellect and rationality, in cognitive-behavioral treatments. In several process-outcome studies by these authors, specific therapist techniques directed toward achieving and main-taining focus on affect were found to be most closely related to later positive changes in depressive symptoms.

Studies of the effects of specific interventions on therapeutic outcome in psychoanalytic treatment remain relatively rare. The finding of Ablon and Jones (1998) that each analytic pair has a unique interaction pattern linked to therapy outcome is likely to remain a basic principle in this complex field. Nevertheless, some consistency has been found concerning the relationship of specific techniques to outcome, and the field will continue to search for such relationships to guide clinical work.

Current work outside the field of psychoanalytic research, in fields such as cognitive psychology, psycholinguistics, and neuroscience, provides new areas of support for the findings concerning focus on emotional experience and the telling and explication of narratives that have been outlined here. As discussed by Bucci (1997, 2002d), these processes of arousal, retrieval, and narration in the context of the relationship appear to be ideally designed to provide the basis for entry of components of warded off experience into *working memory*, the arena in which change in psychic organization may occur.

Conclusion and Future Directions

The fundamental goal of process research may be stated as identification and validation of the factors leading to change in maladaptive emotion schemas (defined psychoanalytically as structural change). Optimally, this information should then be used to assess and support the continuing innovation that is going on in clinical psychoanalysis; to develop more effective techniques for a broader range of patients, including those who are at present not well served by psychoanalytic techniques (Bucci 2002a), as well as to develop the psychoanalytic theory; and in a broader sense, to enhance the contributions of psychoanalysis to other disciplines. On the basis of the survey of the field outlined here, we can define the following features that should be incorporated in programs of process research to achieve such goals:

1. Include a wide range of empirical process measures with established reliability and validity, applied on both micro- and macroanalytic levels, and covering the major themes and structures of the patient material, the therapeutic interaction, and the process of change, as attempted in the first and second generations of process research.
2. Include the subjective impressions of the treating analyst, both as recording instrument and as data to be studied by consulting clinicians, as in the IPTAR and Buenos Aires studies.

3. Incorporate systematic assessment of the session material by consulting clinicians, also as in the IPTAR and Buenos Aires studies, and, on a more macroanalytic level, in work by Jones, Hilsenroth and their colleagues.

4. Make the empirical and clinical assessment available as information for the treating clinician, particularly in the supervisory process, as in the Buenos Aires study; this will contribute to validating the measures as well as building the interface between research and clinical work.

5. Set the project within a psychological theoretical framework within which the concepts of psychoanalytic theory may be operationally defined.

6. Provide an investigative context for process research that meets the criteria of the third generation *outcome* studies outlined by Wallerstein (2001), to demonstrate that the analytic (or structural) change that is identified is associated with enduring change in symptoms and behavior. This would require prospective designs with systematic and objective pre- and posttreatment assessment and separate longitudinal follow-up.

No study has been carried out that incorporates more than a few of these features, but there is increasing recognition from scientific and clinical perspectives of the need to develop such research. The assumption in the early phases of the process research field was that the information exchange was essentially a one-way street; new knowledge emerged from clinical work, and research, at best, might serve to validate what clinicians already know. This survey has suggested that the field is entering a new phase in partnership with clinical work—drawing on multifaceted clinical and research perspectives to expand our understanding of the analytic situation. The unique design of Freud's "method"—the basic rule operating in the context of the relationship—gives process research its potential as a source of new scientific knowledge, available in no other way, that has importance for clinical work and also for a wide range of disciplines.

References

Ablon JS, Jones EE: How expert clinicians' prototypes of an ideal treatment correlate with outcome in psychodynamic and cognitive-behavioral therapy. Psychotherapy Research 8:71–83, 1998

Barber J, Crits-Christoph P, Luborsky L: Effects of therapist adherence and competence on patient outcome in brief dynamic therapy. J Consult Clin Psychol 64:619–622, 1996

Bernardi R: The need for true controversies in psychoanalysis: the debates on Melanie Klein and Jacques Lacan in the Rio de la Plata. Int J Psychoanal 83:851–873, 2002

Bucci W: The power of the narrative: a multiple code account, in Emotion, Disclosure, and Health. Edited by Pennebaker J. Washington, DC, American Psychological Association Books, 1995, pp 93–122

Bucci W: Psychoanalysis and Cognitive Science: A Multiple Code Theory. New York, Guilford, 1997

Bucci W: The need for a "psychoanalytic psychology" in the cognitive science field. Psychoanalytic Psychology 17:203–224, 2000

Bucci W: Pathways of emotional communication. Psychoanalytic Inquiry 20:40–70, 2001a

Bucci W: Toward a "psychodynamic science": the state of current research. J Am Psychoanal Assoc 49:57–68, 2001b

Bucci W: The challenge of diversity in modern psychoanalysis. Psychoanalytic Psychology 19:216–226, 2002a

Bucci W: Multiple code theory and the referential process: applications to process research, in An Open Door Review of Outcome Studies in Psychoanalysis, 2nd Edition. Edited by Fonagy P, Kächele H, Kräuse R, et al. London, International Psychoanalytical Association, 2002b, pp 192–195

Bucci W: Referential activity (RA): scales and computer procedures in An Open Door Review of Outcome Studies in Psychoanalysis, 2nd Edition. Edited by Fonagy P, Kächele H, Kräuse R, et al. London, International Psychoanalytical Association, 2002c, pp 286–288

Bucci W: The Referential Process, Consciousness, and the Sense of Self. Psychoanalytic Inquiry 22:766–793, 2002d

Bucci W: Building the interface of research and practice: achievements and unresolved questions, in The Interface of Empirical Research and Analytic Thought: The Vision of Robert Wallerstein. Psychological Issues Monograph Series. Edited by Bucci W, Freedman N. New York, International Universities Press (in press)

Bucci W, Maskit B: Building a weighted dictionary for Referential Activity, in Exploring Attitudes and Affect in Text: Theories and Applications. Edited by Qu Y, Shanahan JG, Wiebe J. New York, AAAI Press (in press)

Bucci W, Kabasakalian R, and the Referential Activity Research Group: Instructions for Scoring Referential Activity (RA) in Transcripts of Spoken Narrative Texts. Ulm, Germany, Ulmer Textbank, 1992

Crits-Christoph P, Luborsky L: Changes in CCRT pervasiveness during psychotherapy, in Understanding Transference: The Core Conflictual Relationship Theme Method, 2nd Edition. Edited by Luborsky L, Crits-Christoph P. Washington, DC, American Psychological Association, 1990, pp 133–146

Dahl H: A quantitative study of a psychoanalysis, in Psychoanalysis and Contemporary Science. Edited by Holt RR, Peterfreund E. New York, Macmillan, 1972, pp 237–257

Dahl H: The measurement of meaning in psychoanalysis by computer analysis of verbal context. J Am Psychoanal Assoc 22:37–57, 1974

Dahl H: The appetite hypothesis of emotions: a new psychoanalytic model of motivation, in Emotions in Personality and Psychopathology. Edited by Izard C. New York, Plenum, 1979, pp 201–225

Dahl H: Frames of mind, in Psychoanalytic Process Research Strategies. Edited by Dahl H, Kächele H, Thomä H. New York, Springer-Verlag, 1988, pp 51–66

Dahl H: The voyage of el Rubaiyat and the discovery of FRAMES, in Empirical Studies of the Therapeutic Hour. Edited by Bornstein R, Masling J. Washington, DC, American Psychological Association, 1998, pp 179–227

Dahl H: FRAMES (FRMS), in An Open Door Review of Outcome Studies in Psychoanalysis, 2nd Edition. Edited by Fonagy P, Kächele H, Kräuse R, et al. London, International Psychoanalytical Association, 2002, pp 179–181

Dahl H, Stengel B: A classification of emotion words: a modification and partial test of de Rivera's decision theory of emotions. Psychoanalysis and Contemporary Thought 1:252–274, 1978

Dahl H, Teller V: The characteristics, identification, and application of FRAMES. Psychotherapy Research 4:252–274, 1994

Dahl H, Kächele H, Thomä H (eds): Psychoanalytic Process Research Strategies. New York, Springer, 1988

Doyle L: The Referential Cycle of the Multiple Code Theory and the CCRT: A Validation Study. A Dissertation of the Gordon F. Derner Institute of Advanced Psychological Studies. Garden City, NY, Adelphi University, 1999

Elliott R, Hill C, Stiles W, et al: Primary therapist response modes: comparison of six rating systems. J Consult Clin Psychol 55:218-223, 1987

Fonagy P, Kächele H, Kräuse R, et al (eds): An Open Door Review of Outcome Studies in Psychoanalysis, 2nd Edition. London, International Psychoanalytical Association, 2002

Freedman N, Kagan D, Russell J, et al: Scales of Incremental Symbolization: Manuals 1–4. New York, Institute for Psychoanalytic Research, Research Division, 2001

Freedman N, Lasky R, Hurvich M: Two pathways towards knowing psychoanalytic process, in Pluralism and Unity? Methods of Research in Psychoanalysis. Edited by Leuzinger-Bohleber M, Dreher AU, Canestri J. London, International Psychoanalytical Association, 2003

Freud S: Fragment of an analysis of a case of hysteria (1905[1901]), in Standard Edition of the Complete Psychological Works of Sigmund Freud, Vol 7. Translated and edited by Strachey J. London, Hogarth Press, 1953, pp 1–122

Freud S: An outline of psycho-analysis (1940[1938]), in Standard Edition of the Complete Psychological Works of Sigmund Freud, Vol 23. Translated and edited by Strachey J. London, Hogarth Press, 1964, pp 139–207

Gabbard GO: Disguise or consent: problems and recommendations concerning the publication and presentation of clinical material. Int J Psychoanal 81:1071–1086, 2000

Gabbard GO, Williams P: Preserving confidentiality in the writing of case reports. Int J Psychoanal 82:1067–1068, 2001

Gaston L, Thompson L, Gallagher D, et al: Alliance, technique, and their interactions in predicting outcome of behavioral, cognitive, and brief dynamic therapy. Psychotherapy Research 8:190-209, 1998

Gedo JE: The enduring scientific contributions of Sigmund Freud. Annual of Psychoanalysis 29:105–115, 2001

Gill MM, Hoffman IZ: A method for studying the analysis of aspects of the patient's experience of the relationship in psychoanalysis and psychotherapy. J Am Psychoanal Assoc 30:137–168, 1982

Gill MM, Simon J, Fink G, et al: Studies in audio-recorded psychoanalysis, I: general considerations. J Am Psychoanal Assoc 16:230–244, 1968

Gill MM, Simon J, Fink G, et al: Studies in audio-recorded psychoanalysis, II: the effect of recording upon the analyst. J Am Psychoanal Assoc 18:86–101, 1970

Hilsenroth MJ, Ackerman SJ, Blagys MD, et al: Short-term psychodynamic psychotherapy for depression: an examination of statistical, clinically significant, and technique-specific change. J Nerv Ment Dis 191:349–357, 2003

Holt RR: The current status of psychoanalytic theory. Psychoanalytic Psychology 2:289–315, 1985

Horowitz MJ (ed): Psychodynamics and Cognition. Chicago, IL, University of Chicago Press, 1988

Horowitz MJ: Formulation as a Basis for Planning Psychotherapy Treatment. Washington, DC, American Psychiatric Press, 1997

Horowitz MJ: Cognitive Psychodynamics: From Conflict to Character. New York, Wiley, 1998a

Horowitz MJ (ed): Person Schemas and Maladaptive Interpersonal Patterns. Chicago, IL, University of Chicago Press, 1998b

Horowitz MJ: Configurational analysis and role-relationship models, in An Open Door Review of Outcome Studies in Psychoanalysis, 2nd Edition. Edited by Fonagy P, Kächele H, Kräuse R, et al. London, International Psychoanalytical Association, 2002, pp 189–191

Horowitz MJ, Eells T, Singer J, et al: Role-relationship models for case formulation. Arch Gen Psychiatry 52:625–632, 1995

International Committee of Medical Journal Editors: Protection of patients' rights to privacy. BMJ 311:1272, 1995

Jones EE: Therapeutic Action: A Guide to Psychoanalytic Research. Northvale, NJ, Jason Aronson, 2000

Jones EE, Pulos SM: Comparing the process in psychodynamic and cognitive-behavioral therapies. J Consult Clin Psychol 61:306–316, 1993

Kantrowitz JL: Writing about patients, I: ways of protecting confidentiality and analyst's conflicts over choice of method. J Am Psychoanal Assoc 52:69–99, 2004a

Kantrowitz JL: Writing about patients, II: patients' reading about themselves and their analysts' perceptions of its effect. J Am Psychoanal Assoc 52:101–123, 2004b

Klein MH, Mathieu PL, Gendlin ET, et al: The Experiencing Scale: A Research and Training Manual. Madison, Bureau of Audio-Visual Instruction, University of Wisconsin, 1970

Lopez Moreno C, Dorfman Lerner B, Schalayeff C, et al: Investigacion empirica en Psicoanálisis. Revista de Psicoanálisis 56:677–693, 1999

Luborsky L: Measuring a pervasive psychic structure in psychotherapy: the core conflictual relationship theme, in Communicative Structures and Psychic Structures. Edited by Freedman N, Grand S. New York, Plenum, 1977

Luborsky L: A comparison of three transference related measures applied to the specimen hour, in Psychoanalytic Process Research Strategies. Edited by Dahl H, Kächele H, Thomä H. New York, Springer-Verlag, 1988, pp 109–115

Luborsky L, Crits-Christoph P: Understanding Transference: The Core Conflictual Relationship Theme Method, 2nd Edition. Washington, DC, American Psychological Association Press, 1998

Luborsky L, Barber J, Diguer J: The meanings of the narratives told during psychotherapy: the fruits of a new operational unit. Psychotherapy Research 2:277–290, 1993

Luborsky L, Stuart J, Friedman S: The Penn Psychoanalytic Treatment Collection: a set of complete and recorded psychoanalyses as a research resource. J Am Psychoanal Assoc 49:217–234, 2001

Mergenthaler E: Textbank Systems: Computer Science Applied in the Field of Psychoanalysis. New York, Springer, 1985

Mergenthaler E: TAS/C User Manual. Ulm, Germany, Ulmer Textbank, 1993

Mergenthaler E: Emotion-Abstraction Patterns in verbatim protocols: a new way of describing psychotherapeutic processes. J Consult Clin Psychol 64:1306–1318, 1996

Mergenthaler E: The therapeutic cycles model (TCM) in psychotherapy research: theory and measurement, in An Open Door Review of Outcome Studies in Psychoanalysis, 2nd Edition. Edited by Fonagy P, Kächele H, Kräuse R, et al. International Psychoanalytical Association, 2002, pp 205–207

Mergenthaler E, Bucci W: Linking verbal and nonverbal representations: computer analysis of referential activity. Br J Med Psychol 72:339–354, 1999

Michels R: The case history. J Am Psychoanal Assoc 48:355–420, 2000

Miller N, Luborsky L, Barber J (eds): Handbook of Dynamic Psychotherapy Research and Practice. New York, Basic Books, 1993

Panksepp J: Emotions as viewed by psychoanalysis and neuroscience: an exercise in consilience. Neuropsychoanalysis 1:15–38, 1999

Perron R: Reflections on psychoanalytic research problems: a French-speaking view, in An Open Door Review of Outcome Studies in Psychoanalysis, 2nd Edition. Edited by Fonagy P, Kächele H, Kräuse R, et al. International Psychoanalytical Association, 2002a, pp 3–9

Perron R: Response to Peter Fonagy, in An Open Door Review of Outcome Studies in Psychoanalysis, 2nd Edition. Edited by Fonagy P, Kächele H, Kräuse R, et al. International Psychoanalytical Association, 2002b, pp 30–33

Perry JC: A pilot study of defenses in psychotherapy of personality disorders entering psychotherapy. J Nerv Ment Dis 189:651–660, 2001

Perry JC, Cooper SH: An empirical study of defense mechanisms, 1: clinical interview and life vignette ratings. Arch Gen Psychiatry 46: 444–452, 1989

Pessier J, Stuart J: A new approach to the study of therapeutic work in the transference. Psychotherapy Research 10:169–180, 2000

Piper WE, Debbane EG, deCarufel FL, et al: A system for differentiating therapist interpretations and other interventions. Bull Menninger Clin 51:532–550, 1987

Ricoeur P: Freud and Philosophy. New Haven, CT, Yale University Press, 1970

Roussos AJ, Bucci W, Maskit B: A second-generation clinical library: first steps, in The Interface of Empirical Research and Analytic Thought: The Vision of Robert Wallerstein (Psychological Issues Monograph Series). Edited by Bucci W, Freedman N. New York, International Universities Press (in press)

Sammons M, Siegel P: Una comparacion de FRAMES con el CCRT y la CRA. Revista Argentina de Clínica Psicológica 7:131–145, 1998

Sandler J: Reflections on some relations between psychoanalytic concepts and psychoanalytic practice. Int J Psychoanal 64:35–45, 1983

Schacter J, Luborsky L: Who's afraid of psychoanalytic research? Analysts' attitudes towards reading clinical versus empirical research papers. Int J Psychoanal 79:965–969, 1998

Scharff JS: On writing from clinical experience. J Am Psychoanal Assoc 48:421–447, 2000

Shapiro T, Emde RN (eds): Research in Psychoanalysis: Process, Development, Outcome. Madison, CT, International Universities Press, 1995

Siegel P: Reliability, identification, and evolution of FRAMES in the case of Mrs. C. A Dissertation of the Gordon F. Derner Institute of Advanced Studies. Garden City, NY, Adelphi University, 2001

Spence DP: Human and computer attempts to decode symptom language. Psychosom Med 32:615–625, 1970

Spence DP, Dahl H, Jones EE: Impact of interpretation on associative freedom. J Consult Clin Psychol 61:395–402, 1993

Stinson CH, Milbrath C, Reidbord S, et al: Thematic segmentation of psychotherapy transcripts for convergent analysis. Psychotherapy 31:36–48, 1994

Stone PJ, Dunphy DC, Smith MS, et al: The General Inquirer: A Computer Approach to Content Analysis. Cambridge, MA, MIT Press, 1966

Strupp H: A multidimensional system for analyzing psychotherapeutic techniques. Psychiatry 20:293–306, 1957

Szecsody I: Commentary on Michels's "the case history." J Am Psychoanal Assoc 48:397–403, 2000

Thomä H, Kächele H: Problems of metascience and methodology in clinical psychoanalytic research. Annual of Psychoanalysis 3:49–119, 1973

Thomä H, Kächele H: Psychoanalytic Practice. New York, Springer, 1987

Tuckett D: Some thoughts on the presentation and discussion of the clinical material of psychoanalysis. Int J Psychoanal 74: 1175–1188, 1993

Tuckett D: Reporting clinical events in the Journal: towards the constructing of a special case. Int J Psychoanal 81:1065–1069, 2000

Vaillant GE: Adaptation to Life. Boston, MA, Little Brown, 1977

Vaillant G, Drake R: Maturity of ego defenses in relation to DSM-III axis II disorders. Arch Gen Psychiatry 42:597–601, 1985

Viderman S: The analytic space: meaning and problems. Psychoanal Q 48: 257–291, 1979

Waldron S, Scharf RD, Firestein SK, et al: Analytic process scales (APS) study of 3 audiotaped psychoanalyses, in An Open Door Review of Outcome Studies in Psychoanalysis, 2nd Edition. Edited by Fonagy P, Kächele H, Kräuse R, et al. International Psychoanalytical Association, 2002, pp 224–227

Waldron S, Scharf RD, Hurst D, et al: What happens in a psychoanalysis? A view through the lens of the Analytic Process Scales (APS). Int J Psychoanal 85:443–466, 2004

Wallerstein RS: Forty-Two Lives in Treatment: A Study of Psychoanalysis and Psychotherapy. New York, Guilford, 1986

Wallerstein RS: The new American psychoanalysis. J Am Psychoanal Assoc 46:1021–1043, 1998

Wallerstein RS: The generations of psychotherapy research: an overview. Psychoanalytic Psychology 18:243–267, 2001

Wallerstein RS: My life as a psychoanalytic therapy researcher and in CAMP, in The Interface of Empirical Research and Analytic Thought: The Vision of Robert Wallerstein. Psychological Issues Monograph Series. Edited by Bucci W, Freedman N. New York, International Universities Press (in press)

Wallerstein RS, Sampson H: Issues in research in the psychoanalytic process. Int J Psychoanal 52:11–50, 1971

Weiss J: How Psychotherapy Works. New York, Guilford, 1993

Weiss J, Sampson H, the Mount Zion Psychotherapy Research Group: The Psychoanalytic Process: Theory, Clinical Observation, and Empirical Research. New York, Guilford, 1986

Westen D: Social cognition and object relations. Psychol Bull 109:429–455, 1991

22

Developmental Research

STANLEY I. GREENSPAN, M.D.
STUART G. SHANKER, D.PHIL.

IT WAS NOT UNTIL LATE in the twentieth century that a true developmental perspective began to emerge in psychology. Prior to this time, any interest in the question "How does the mind develop?" was ultimately concerned with some variant of the question "How does one produce an upright or productive member of our society?" This utilitarian perspective remained prominent until well into the twentieth century, as can be seen, for example, in Watson's (1925) famous boast: "Give me a dozen healthy infants, well-formed, and my own specified world to bring them up in and I'll guarantee to take any one at random and train him to become any type of specialist I might select—doctor, lawyer, artist, merchant, chief, and yes, even beggerman and thief, regardless of his talents, penchants, tendencies, abilities, vocations and race of his ancestors" (p. 104). This behaviorist leitmotif can be traced back to the Romans, if not beyond (see Greenspan and Shanker 2004, Chapter 13). But the psychological question of how the *mind* develops—how a child begins to regulate her affects, how she begins to act purposefully and recognize others as intentional agents with minds of their own, how she learns how to speak and reason and form abstract concepts—only emerged as a *scientific* concern in the latter part of the twentieth century.

In the early days of psychoanalysis, psychoanalytic theorists explored this issue by attempting to reconstruct what early development was like from their research on older children and adults. Margaret Mahler and Anna Freud were among the first to conduct observational studies on preverbal infants, in which the focus remained that of inferring what the internal life of the child must be like from his or her external behaviors. Independent of this line of research, the twentieth century saw the enormous growth of developmental psychology as an academic discipline. It is difficult to summarize the full extent of the important findings that have been made in these studies (Bremmer and Fogel 2001).

Depth psychology concerns itself with levels of the mind that influence mental health and mental illness but are often not manifested directly in surface behaviors and in nonclinical settings. For example, depth psychology concerns itself with the deepest levels of intimacy and sexuality, anger and fear, the tendency to split our inner worlds into polar opposites, and the tendency to project our own wishes and thoughts onto others as well as incorporate the wishes and thoughts of others into ourselves. It concerns itself with the formation of our sense of self and others and the way these are internalized at different levels of differentiation and integration. It also concerns itself with the differentiation of our affects and emotions, their transformation from discharge modes to signals to symbolized feelings, the formation of defenses and coping strategies, and the development of personality patterns and personality disorders, such as obsessive-compulsive, depressive, hysterical, narcissistic, and antisocial. As can be seen, depth psychology concerns itself with some of the most critical and yet perplexing dimensions of human functioning.

Developmental psychology is concerned with the empirical study of physical development (e.g., motor skills, growth, the psychological effect of hormonal changes); neurophysiological patterns (e.g., cortical organization, neural plasticity, the relationship between neural and cognitive development); perceptual development (e.g., visual, auditory, tactile, olfactory); and cognitive (e.g., attention, learning, memory, problem-solving, causal reasoning), communicative (e.g., gesturing, vocalizations, eye gaze), linguistic (e.g., comprehension, production, morphology, pragmatics, reading), social (e.g., attachment, peer relationships, theory of mind), emotional (e.g., how emotions develop; how they influence behavior, perception, and cognition; how they influence the growth of the mind), personality (e.g., temperament and behavior, genetic and environmental influences on temperament), and moral development (e.g., prosocial attitudes, empathy, moral reasoning).

Developmental psychologists use a number of formal techniques to study these domains, such as high-amplitude sucking, habituation, and preferential looking; naturalistic, laboratory, and psychophysiological studies; and ethnographic research. But they have been constrained to look at children's behaviors in situations that involve relatively little affective challenge, rather than in clinical settings. To develop a developmental framework for depth psychology, therefore, we need not only to integrate these important bodies of research, which have hitherto operated in relative isolation from one another, but also to add in clinical work in which we can see children operating in situations of affective challenge in which their mind is stretched, leading to another critical source of information about the normal and pathological growth of the mind.

There now exists an impressive literature seeking to relate the work being done in depth psychology to findings from developmental psychology. The missing piece in this literature, however, is the formulation of a theory that explains the developmental pathways to the essential depth psychological capacities, including capacities for effecting self-regulation, forming relationships, engaging in co-regulated affect signaling, constructing internalized

self and object representations, and forming differentiated and integrated self and object representational structures at successively higher levels of organization. This formulation also needs to explain the development of derivative ego functions, including reality testing, defense and coping capacities, and various levels of reflective or observing ego capacities. As part of the formulation of the developmental pathways leading to these critical human capacities, it is essential not only to look at the observations from each of these fields but also to articulate the strengths and the limitations of their respective findings and weave them together with fresh clinical observations of developing infants and children into a cohesive theory that explains the pathways to these capacities that define our humanity.

A developmental model that would prove useful to the field of psychoanalysis would need to meet the following four criteria:

1. Consider both adaptive or healthy as well as psychopathologic human mental functioning
2. Address the deeper levels of the mind
3. Be based on a confluence of empirical, observable, and clinical studies
4. Be relevant to clinical work by providing an understanding of developmental pathways toward adaptive and pathologic development

Thus, as we construct a developmental framework for depth psychology, we need to take into account the levels of the mind that explain clinically relevant healthy and disordered functioning. At the same time, we need to attend to the enormous number of empirical studies on cognitive, perceptual, motor, social, and emotional development in the past half-century. The challenge to depth psychoanalytic approaches is to make sense of or interpret these findings for our understanding of the deepest levels of the mind.

Distinction Between Depth and Surface Approaches

Depth psychological understanding of the mind has, for the most part, emerged from clinical studies in which the mind's capacities are stretched to deal with such challenges as conflict, anxiety, overwhelming affects, trauma, unusual family patterns, and biological differences. Developmental psychology has largely followed a normative model in which age-related averages are computed from measures of behavior taken on large numbers of children. Most of the latter studies focus on the capacities or behavior of infants and young children in nonclinical contexts—that is, in situations that are relatively familiar to the child and involve minimal stress. Even the experiments that challenge infants and children do so within the expectable range of healthy experiences; for to do otherwise is unethical and not permissible.

The observations of infants and young children under extreme clinical challenges represent landmark studies. Examples are Bowlby's studies of prolonged separation from caregivers (Bowlby 1951), Spitz's studies of institutionalized infants (Spitz 1965), Anna Freud's and Dorothy Burlingham's observations of children in war situations (Burlingham and Freud 1942), Wayne Dennis's research on children in impoverished orphanages (Dennis 1960), as well as more recent work on children exposed to trauma or responding to various types of extreme stress (see Ullmann and Hilweg 1999; La Greca et al. 2002). However, these studies are relatively few compared with the countless studies of emotional, social, and cognitive development in normative contexts that have contributed to the current field of developmental psychology. While many of the results of normative studies are highly important, they often represent findings that have been made on *surface* phenomena.

Such studies would be akin to observations one might make of undergraduate students in familiar situations in which their behavior, emotional expressions, and cognitive operations are operating in a fairly narrow range. Even in situations where undergraduates are exposed to a stress, such as watching a horror movie or undergoing a difficult job interview, they are still operating in a relatively safe and secure environment. But, as indicated earlier, clinical situations often reveal very different levels of functioning, precisely because they occur in much more stressful and often traumatic situations. We are certainly no longer surprised to hear of a student who functions very well in his or her studies and exams but who is deeply anxious or depressed in his or her private life.

To amplify the significance of this fundamental distinction between *depth* and *surface* phenomena and the tendency to mix these two realms of experience together uncritically, we might consider the case of attachment research. These studies have obvious implications for depth psychology, given the importance of caregiver-infant relationships in the development of the mind (Fonagy et al. 2002). The original paradigm in attachment research involved the Strange Situation, typically conducted with children between the ages of 1 and 2 years (Ainsworth et al. 1978). A parent and baby are playing in a room with toys when a stranger enters, sits down, and talks to the parent; the parent leaves the room and the stranger remains, responding to the infant if she is upset. The parent returns and greets her baby, comforting her if necessary, and the

stranger leaves the room; the parent leaves the room again and the stranger reenters, again offering comfort to the baby if necessary. Finally, the parent returns and, if necessary, comforts her child and endeavors to get her reinterested in the toys. Different infant and toddler patterns have been observed using this paradigm, including secure, avoidant, and disorganized patterns. But does this situation allow for the full range and intensity of affects or emotion that would reveal an infant's or young child's defenses and coping strategies, or their depth psychological make-up? Does it reveal the depth of their intimacy, the degree of pleasure they experience in their relationships, their capacity to cope with anger or fear, and so forth? In other words, do the observed patterns in such studies reveal the full range of functioning that children might show in relationship to their capacity for attachment?

Perhaps all that can be said definitively about the significance of the findings that have been made using the Strange Situation for depth psychology is that these studies confirm that short-term, even seemingly minor, disruptions in children's primary relationships lead to some interesting feelings and consequences. Furthermore, some very interesting predictions can be made on the basis of these findings—for example, about personality characteristics (e.g., self-esteem, self-knowledge, enthusiasm, resilience); peer relationships (e.g., sociability, friendliness, cooperativeness, empathy, popularity); relationships with adults (e.g., independence, confidence with strangers, compliance); frustration tolerance and impulse control; persistence in problem-solving, curiosity, and attention span; adjustment (e.g., antisocial behavior, psychopathy); and attitudes toward childrearing.

When we assess toddlers clinically, however, we use a much broader construct of attachment. We look to see how children deal with challenges, and more important, we try to ascertain the depth and range of their affects; the subtlety of the pleasure they experience in their relationships; their warmth, openness, assertiveness, and curiosity; the way they cope with anger; and so on. We look for the richness of the nonverbal communicative behavior with which they negotiate their affects and the degree of differentiation in their co-regulated affect signaling about different sorts of affects. For example, some toddlers excel at negotiating their feelings of assertiveness or aggression but have trouble engaging in co-regulated affect signaling about their feelings of dependency, or one might see the exact reverse pattern.

The basic problem with attachment research, therefore, is that, often, it is used to say a great deal more than is warranted. That is, it has been used to define attachment per se. The assumption here is that a narrow, experimental situation captures the full range of human relationships and intimacy characterized by the word "attachment," or that the few different responses observed are an adequate representation of the full range of a child's functioning vis-à-vis attachment. While in a general sense this research supports an important perspective on the vital nature of relationships in depth psychology, it is often taken beyond its value because of the confusion between *surface approaches* and *depth approaches*. Data from surface approaches thus need to be interpreted within an overall depth psychological framework.

The underlying problem here, when we contrast surface with depth approaches, is the tendency of the former to narrow the conditions in which a phenomenon is studied in such a way as to narrow one's understanding of the very phenomenon one is seeking to understand. Indeed, there could be no better example of this tendency than attachment research. For as has been widely documented, Bowlby's original studies on attachment were informed by his readings in ethology, which led him to formulate his famous hypothesis that attachment behaviors (in both infants and caregivers) were naturally selected in order to protect the infant from predation. (To this day, Bowlby's relatively narrow picture of the evolutionary origins of attachment behavior has continued to inform research in the area, as can be seen, for example, in the numerous attempts to reduce attachment to a psychobiological phenomenon—see, for example, Polan and Hofer 1999.) Even more profound than its role in negotiating security, however, is the role that attachment plays in the co-regulated affect signaling that takes place between infants and caregivers.

As we explained in Chapter 1 of *The First Idea* (Greenspan and Shanker 2004), by the time we come to test infants in the Strange Situation, they have already undergone a considerable amount of development. It is through these early attachment behaviors that babies begin to learn to tame their catastrophic reactions and transform them into interactive signals. For example, a mother smiles and the baby smiles back. She coos and the baby coos back. The baby smiles, raises his arms as if to say, "Hey!" and vocalizes emotionally needy sounds that convey "Look at me!" The mother looks his way. Baby then smiles and flirts, and the mother flirts back. For this type of emotional signaling to occur, a baby needs to have been wooed into a warm pleasurable relationship with one or a few caregivers so that there is another being toward whom he experiences deep emotions, and, therefore, with whom he wants to communicate.

Herein lies a critical deeper function of attachment: the baby needs opportunities to be "intentional"—to express an emotion or need by making a sound, use a facial expression, or make a gesture with his arm, and to have his efforts confirmed by being responded to. Attachment thus provides continuous opportunities to learn and fine-tune the skills of emotional signaling that are used to communicate and negotiate emotional states. By no means, then, is attachment confined to the sort of intense, even catastrophic, emotions that we observe in infants when they are exposed to stressful situations. Even in terms of survival, however, the role of attachment is more complex than is suggested by Bowlby's narrow ethological point of view. For in order for humans to survive, they not only had to protect their infants from predators: more fundamentally, they had to develop the capacity to live in groups. And, as we explained in *The First Idea*, the very growth of this capacity, and thus human survival itself, is derived from the same formative emotional processes that underlie various levels of affective synchrony and in turn lead to symbol formation and logical problem solving. That is, it is through attachment with their caregivers that babies come to learn their group's distinctive manner of communication.

The upshot of this argument, therefore, is that the full depth of attachment cannot be gleaned from conditions that simply stress an infant's sense of security. Bowlby's attachment paradigm was based on the assumption that such conditions must have prevailed in our evolutionary past and that attachment developed as an adaptation to this challenge. To the degree that these situations prevailed, Bowlby's ideas represented a truly pioneering contribution to our understanding one of the foundations of human relationships. However, modern studies of primates in the wild suggest that the original paradigm, as important as it was, is too narrow: nonhuman primate dyads operate in a broad range of environmental contexts and ecologies, and under less threatening conditions we observe a broad array of relationship-type behaviors underlying complex affective signaling and interactions similar to those described above (see Greenspan and Shanker 2004, Chapter 13; see also Falk 2000; Small 1998).

In other words, even nonhuman primates are able to transform emotions from the catastrophic level, which would be operative under conditions of threat, to more differentiated affective expressions in a variety of patterns of co-regulation that typically permit the complex social negotiation of subtle affects dealing with themes of dependency, independence, assertiveness, curiosity, and a variety of problem-solving capacities. What we glean from a more depth-oriented approach to the study of attachment, therefore, is that, in the evolutionary sense, attachment had to serve other purposes besides simply that of survival (i.e., of being able to deal with catastrophic or threatening conditions). Attachment also had to serve as the foundation for co-regulated affect signaling, leading both to higher cognitive and communicative functions and to the formation and coherence of groups.

Constructing a Developmental Framework for Depth Psychology

As indicated in the previous section, in order for the valuable findings from normative experimental studies to contribute to depth psychology (and they should), these findings cannot be translated directly and have to be interpreted within the framework of a depth developmental psychology. To make such an interpretation, we need a clinically relevant developmental model that looks at the broad range of experiences in clinical and nonclinical contexts.

Constructing a developmental framework for depth psychology is important for a number of reasons. Most important, it will serve to define the development of a person (i.e., what it means to be a human being). It will help us avoid the tendency to define a person based on a few narrow capacities, such as this or that cognitive capacity (e.g., IQ). Any developmental framework of human functioning must use a model that captures the full range and depth of what it means to be human. From developmental studies of children forming their minds, we can now systematize the stages whereby children

- Perceive, attend and regulate, and move.
- Form relationships and develop the capacity for sustained intimacy.
- Learn to interact, read social/emotional cues, and express a wide range of emotions.
- Form a sense of self that involves many different emotional feelings, expressions, and interaction patterns.
- Construct a sense of self that integrates different emotional polarities (e.g., love and hate).
- Regulate mood, behavior, and impulses, and engage in ongoing social co-regulation.
- Create internal representations of a sense of self, feelings, and wishes, as well as impersonal ideas.
- Categorize internal representations in terms of reality versus fantasy (as a basis for reality testing), sense of self and others (self and object representations), different wishes and feelings, modification of wishes and feelings (defenses and coping capacities), and use these for judgment, peer relationships, and a range of higher-level self-observing and reflective capacities.

These capacities, as well as others, have adaptive developmental sequences and are compromised to varying degrees in different types of psychopathology. In fact, we will see that our definition of a human being and our framework for a depth psychology will be based on these core capacities. In the remainder of this chapter, we construct a developmental model that addresses the deeper levels of the mind and review the literature supporting this model.

The Stages of Mental (Ego) Development

The psychoanalytic literature is characterized by a long history of developmental observations illustrated by the work of such pioneers as Bowlby (1969), Spitz (1945), Mahler and colleagues (1975), Escalona (1968), Anna Freud (1965), Kohut (1971), and Kernberg (1975). More recent infant and early childhood observers and theoreticians have built on this foundation and discussed preverbal interaction patterns and their psychotherapeutic implications (e.g., Beebe et al. 1992; Emde et al. 1976; Fonagy and Target 1997; Greenspan 1979, 1981, 1989b, 1992, 1997b; Stern 1974b). For example, Beebe has described the implications of dyadic interactions for the psychotherapeutic process (Beebe and Lachman 2002).

Over the past 30 years, we have been able to add to this work and formulate a developmental framework for depth psychology from our clinical work with infants, young children, and their families with a variety of challenges, including severe environmental risks and biological risks.

In an attempt to understand early emotional development, we conducted a number of clinical, observational, and intervention studies on emotional development in infants, young children, and their families. These included multirisk infants and families; infants and children with biologically based developmental problems, such as autism; and infants and families without challenges or problems (Greenspan 1981, 1992; Greenspan and Wieder 1998; Greenspan et al. 1987; Interdisciplinary Council on Developmental and Learning Disorders 2000). Interestingly, it was the clinical work with infants, young children, and their families with both environmental and biological risks that led to an understanding of how different aspects of development work together. This understanding in turn led to the formulation of the Developmental Structuralist Theory and the Developmental, Individual-Difference, Relationship-Based Model (DIRtm) (Greenspan 1979, 1989b, 1992, 1997a; Greenspan and Lourie 1981).

On the basis of this theory and model, we formulated the Functional Emotional Developmental Approach (Greenspan 1992, 1997a), which describes the critical emotional capacities that characterize development. These capacities, such as the ability for effecting regulation, forming relationships, using emotions to signal intentions, and engaging in problem-solving interactions, are broader than the expression of specific affects, such as pleasure or anger. As will be seen, they also serve as the foundations for adaptive development.

In this framework, affect and affective interaction are responsible not only for emotional development and the formation of intrapsychic capacities but for cognitive capacities as well. As we have shown elsewhere (Greenspan 1979, 1997b), Piaget focused on impersonal cognition and the role of motor explorations of the environment in constructing the child's intelligence. He missed the fact that affective interactions actually lead the way. At each stage of intelligence, they construct both emotional and cognitive capacities (Greenspan 1979, 1997b). For example, by 3–4 months of age, infants are learning about preverbal causality ("means-end" relationships) when their smile leads to a caregiver's smile back (way before they can pull a string to ring a bell). The functional emotional developmental framework also serves as an organizing construct for the other aspects of development, including motor, sensory, language, and cognitive functioning. For example, when we describe the child's capacity for two-way interactive, emotional communication at around 8 months (reciprocal affect-cueing) in addition to the emotional features of affect-cueing, we take into account the cognitive component (discerning cause and effect interaction), the motor component (reaching), the language component (exchanging vocalizations that convey affect), and the sensory component (using sight, touch, and perception of sound as part of a co-regulated, reciprocal emotional interaction). Therefore, the Functional Emotional Developmental Approach provides both a way of characterizing emotional functioning and a way of looking at how all the components of development (cognition, language, and motor skills) work together (as a mental team), organized by the designated emotional goals. It enables us to observe not only emotional capacities that are present, including emotional challenges, but also emotional capacities that are missing that should be present (e.g., the capacity for pleasure and intimacy). In this model, emotional capacities enable the full range of expected developmental abilities to work together in a functional manner (Greenspan 1997b).

Developmental Levels of Emotional Functioning

There are six early, basic organizational levels of emotional experience and a number of subsequent ones. For each of these developmental levels, we discuss the relevant research, clinical observations, and implications for mental (ego) functioning.

Self-Regulation and Interest in the World (Homeostasis): 0–3 Months

The first level of development involves regulation and shared attention—that is, self-regulation and emerging interest in the world through sight, sound, smell, touch, and taste. Children and adults build on this early developing set of capacities when they act to maintain a calm, alert, focused state and organize behavior, affect, and thoughts. The infant is capable at birth or shortly thereafter of initial states of regulation to organize experience in an adaptive fashion. The infant's ability for regulation is suggested by a number of basic abilities involving forming cycles and establishing basic rhythms, perceiving and processing information, and exploring and responding to the world (Berlyne 1960; Deci 1977; Harlow 1953; Hendrick 1939; Hunt 1965; Meltzoff and Moore 1977; Sander 1962; White 1963).

Early regulation of arousal and physiological states is critical for successful adaptation to the environment. It is important in the modulation of physiological states, including sleep-wake cycles and hunger and satiety. It is needed for mastery of sensory functions and for learning self-calming and emotional responsivity, and it is also important for regulation of attentional capacities (Als et al. 1982; Brazelton et al. 1974; Field 1981; Sroufe 1979; Tronick 1989). It is generally recognized that self-regulatory mechanisms are complex and develop as a result of physiological maturation, caregiver responsivity, and the infant's adaptation to environmental demands (Lachman and Beebe 1997; Lyons-Ruth and Zeanah 1993; Rothbart and Derryberry 1981; Tronick 1989).

In the early stages of development, the caregiver normally provides sensory input through play and caregiving experiences, such as dressing and bathing, and soothes the young infant when distressed to facilitate state organization (Als 1982). It is an interactive process of mutual co-regulation whereby the infant uses the parent's physical and emotional state to organize himself or herself (Feldman et al. 1999; Sroufe 1996). This synchronization of states that occurs between parent and child is the basis for affect attunement and is the precursor to social referencing and preverbal communication.

During this early stage, the infant learns to tolerate the intensity of arousal and to regulate his or her internal states so that he or she can maintain the interaction while gaining pleasure from it (Sroufe 1979). This process, described as "affective tolerance," involves the ability to maintain an optimal level of internal arousal while remaining engaged in the stimulation (Fogel 1982). The parent first acts to help regulate this arousal and then works to facilitate the infant's responses once the infant can regulate himself or herself. If the infant does not develop affective tolerance, withdrawal from arousing stimuli may occur with resulting challenges to the formation and stability of relationships. Brazelton and colleagues (1974) observed how the mother attempts to adjust her behavior to be timed with the infant's natural cycles. For example, the mother generally reduces her facial expressiveness when the infant gazes away but maintains her expressiveness when the infant looks at her (Kaye and Fogel 1980).

Clinical Observations

As indicated, the infant's first task in the developmental structuralist approach sequence is simultaneously to take an interest in the world and regulate himself or herself. In comparing the ability of certain infants to simultaneously regulate and take an interest in the world with the inability of others to do so, it has been clinically useful to examine each sensory pathway individually as well as the range of sensory modalities available for phase-specific challenges (Greenspan 1992).

Each sensory pathway may be characterized in one of the following ways:

1. Hyperarousable (e.g., the baby who overreacts to normal levels of sound, touch, or brightness)
2. Hypoarousable (e.g., the baby who hears and sees but evidences no behavioral or observable affective response to routine sights and sounds—often described as the "floppy" baby with poor muscle tone who is unresponsive and seemingly looks inward)
3. Neither hypo- nor hyperarousable but having a subtle type of early processing disorder (hypo- or hyperarousable babies may also have a processing difficulty)

It is important to note that the differences in sensory reactivity and processing were noted many years ago and continue to be discussed in the occupational therapy literature (Ayres 1964). If an individual sensory pathway is not functioning optimally, the range of sensory experience available to the infant is limited. This limitation determines, in part, the options or strategies the infant can employ and the type of sensory experience that will be organized. Some babies can employ the full range of sensory capacities. At the stage of regulation and interest in the world (i.e., homeostasis), for example, one can observe that such babies look at mother's face or an interesting object and follow it. When the baby is upset, the opportunity to look at mother helps him or her become calm and happy (i.e., a calm smile). Similarly, a soothing voice, a gentle touch, rhythmic rocking, or a shift in position (offering vestibular and proprioceptive stimulation) can also help such a baby relax, organize, and self-regulate.

There are also babies who functionally employ only one or two sensory modalities. We have observed babies who brighten up and become alert and calm to visual experience but who either are relatively unresponsive, become hyperexcitable, or appear to become "confused" with auditory stimuli. (A 2-month-old baby may be operationally defined as confused when instead of looking toward a normal high-pitched maternal voice and alerting, he or she makes some random motor movements—suggesting that the stimulus has been taken in—looks past the object repeatedly, and continues his or her random movements.) Other babies appear to use vision and hearing to self-regulate and take an interest in the world but have a more difficult time with touch and movement. They often become irritable even with gentle stroking and are calm only when held horizontally (they become hyperaroused when held upright). Still other babies calm down only when rocked to their own heart rate, respiratory rate, or mother's heart rate. The roles of vestibular and proprioceptive pathways in psychopathology in infancy are very important areas for future research.

As babies use a range of sensory pathways, they also integrate experiences across the senses (Spelke and Owsley 1979). Yet there are babies who are able to use each sensory pathway but have difficulty, for example, integrating vision and hearing. They can alert to a sound or a visual cue but are not able to turn and look at a stimulus that offers visual and auditory information at the same time. Instead, they appear confused and may even have active gaze aversion or go into a pattern of extensor rigidity and avoidance.

The sensory pathways are usually observed in the context of sensorimotor patterns: for example, turning toward the stimulus or brightening and becoming alert involve motor "outputs." Some babies have difficulties in the way they integrate their sensory experience with motor output. The most obvious case is a baby with severe motor difficulties. At a subtle level, it is possible to observe compromises in such basic abilities as self-consoling or nuzzling in the corner of mother's neck or relaxing to rhythmic rocking. In this context, Escalona's (1968) classic descriptions of babies with multiple sensory hypersensitivities require further study as part of a broader approach to assessing subtle difficulties in each sensory pathway, as well as associated master patterns.

In this first stage, there are babies who cannot organize their affective-thematic proclivities in terms of the phase-specific tasks. Babies who are uncomfortable with dependency often evidence specific sensory hypersensitivities or higher-level integrating problems, as well as maladaptive infant-caregiver interactions. Babies with a tendency toward hyper- or hypoarousal may not be able to organize the affective-thematic domains of joy, pleasure, and exploration. Instead, they may evidence apathy and withdrawal or a total disregard for certain sensory realms while overfocusing on others (e.g., babies who stare at an inanimate object while ignoring the human world).

Children with sensorimotor dysfunction typically have difficulty using the range of sensory experiences available to them for learning, and as a result they may be unable to organize purposeful, goal-directed movement as well as socially adaptive behaviors. These children oftentimes have maladaptive responses in forming affective relationships or attachments. For instance, an infant who is hypersensitive to touch, sound, and movement may avoid tactile contact and being held and moved in space, and may avert gaze to avoid face-to-face interactions. A child may be unable to play with peers because of problems sequencing actions, a high need for physical contact, or inappropriate affect during interactions because of low muscle tone or poor sensorimotor feedback. Both are examples of how sensorimotor dysfunction may affect emotional behaviors.

In addition, difficulties with muscle tone or coordination can affect the infant's ability to signal interest in the world. For example, the young infant who arches away from the mother's breast during feeding will affect the level of engagement that occurs during a normal feeding experience. In turn, these problems affect the caregiver's ability to respond consistently or inconsistently to their infant's signal: particularly when the caregiver does not understand what the baby's responses mean. The mother whose baby arches away every time he is held may feel that she is a less capable mother, particularly if the baby's tactile hypersensitivities or increased muscle tone are not identified.

Some investigators explore sensory, motor, and affective differences in terms of temperament, which tends to look at overall patterns of behavior. Temperamental differences have been shown to influence the organization and regulation of inter/intrapersonal processes (Campos et al. 1989). Temperamental qualities characterizing the child as "difficult," for example, have been linked to later psychopathology (Thomas and Chess 1984). The difficult temperament might create challenges in self-regulatory processes and potentially affect infant-caregiver interaction adversely. Of course, neither sensory nor temperamental characteristics alone necessarily predict pathology. As a transactional perspective indicates, the effects of particular sensory or temperamental characteristics can be mediated by the attention of a sensitive, responsive caregiver. Because temperament looks at the overall patterns of behavior and the sensory processing pathways described above look at specific capacities, which in many respects underlie temperament and explain temperament,

it is especially important to understand the individual's particular sensory processing ability. For example, a sensory-overreactive infant is very likely to be temperamentally difficult to comfort.

Even when the infant is quite competent from a regulatory standpoint, a caregiver might fail to draw a baby into a regulating relationship. For example, dysregulation may occur with a caregiver who is exceedingly depressed or who is so self-absorbed that there is no soothing wooing of the new infant. A caregiver who is impatient with or threatened by the infant's manifestation of sensory or temperamental sensitivity and who reacts with abuse, withdrawal, or other maladaptive means, may encourage infant reliance on ineffective patterns of behavior and further contribute to the infant's inability to achieve self-regulation.

Implications for Mental (Ego) Functioning

It may be postulated that there are adapted sensorimotor patterns that are part of the "autonomous" ego functions present shortly after birth. It is then useful to consider how these capacities (e.g., the autonomous ego functions of perception and discrimination) are used to construct an emerging organization of an experiential world, including drive derivatives, early affects, and emerging organizations of self and object(s). It would be a logical error to assume that these seemingly innate capacities are themselves a product of early interactional learning or structure building, even though secondarily they are influenced by experiences.

One cannot yet postulate differentiated self-object experiential organizations, because the infant's main goals appear to be involved in a type of sensory awakening and interest and regulation without evidence of clear intentional object seeking or self-initiated differentiated affective interactions. In our observations of both at-risk and normal infants, it was observed that they responded to the overall stimulus qualities of the environments, especially human handling. Likewise, there is little evidence for a notion that the infant is impervious to his or her emotional surroundings. In fact, in our studies of multirisk families (Greenspan et al. 1987), the quality of self-regulation, attention, and sensory-affective interest in the world in the first 1–2 months of life was influenced to a great degree by the physical and emotional qualities of the infant-caregiver patterns (i.e., soothing and interesting caregiving patterns rather than hyper- or hypo-stimulating ones).

But this does not mean that those who, like Mahler and colleagues (1975), suggest a qualitative difference in this early stage (i.e., the autistic phase) may not have an important insight. Even though mother's voice can be discriminated from other sounds, this does not mean there is a caregiver–physical world (e.g., sound of a car) differentiation in terms of abstracting and organizing types of experiences according to general characteristics. In other words, one must distinguish what the infant is capable of (e.g., complex discriminations) from how the infant is functionally involved in phase specific tasks and goals. For example, a 3-year-old with separation anxiety associated with fear of loss of the affective object may have excellent capacities for conserving her impersonal objects. A 6-year-old may be capable of advanced logic in math or science but lag considerably in the logic of reality testing and confuse fantasy and reality. A cognitive capacity may or may not be used for organizing in-depth emotional experience. Our clinical observations suggest that early in life the capacities the infant uses to organize in-depth emotional experience lag behind the capacities he or she uses to process relatively impersonal experience or affective experience lacking in psychological depth.

One may consider a preintentional stage of object relatedness (i.e., prewired patterns gradually coming under interactive control) and a stage in the organization of experience in which the sense of self and the sense of object are not yet organized as distinct entities. At this stage, the experience of "self" and "other" is closely intertwined and unlikely to be separate from other sensory experiences involving the physical world. It is worth repeating that differential infant responses do not necessarily mean differentiated internal experiences, because responses or behaviors can simply be constitutional, reflexive (such as to heat or cold), and/or conditioned responses according to respondent (Pavlovian) or operant learning.

Therefore, the concept of an experiential organization of a *world object*, including what later will become a self–other–physical world, may prove useful. This state of ego organization may be considered to be characterized by two central tendencies: to experience sensory and affective information through each sensory (motor) channel, and to form patterns of regulation. Furthermore, these tendencies may be further characterized by the level of sensory pathway arousal (i.e., sensory hyper- and hypoarousal) in each sensory (motor) pathway and by emerging sensory (motor) discrimination and integration capacities. Under optimal conditions, the early sensory and affective processing, discrimination, and integration capacities—the early functions of the ego—are being used for the gradual organization of experience. Under unfavorable conditions these early ego functions evidence undifferentiated sensory hyperarousal, undifferentiated sensory hypoarousal, and lack of discrimination and integration in all or any of the sensory-affective (motor) pathways. Therefore, the early stage of global undifferentiated self-object worlds may remain or progress to higher levels of organization depending on innate maturational patterns and early experiences

as together they influence each sensory-affective (motor) pathway in terms of arousal, discrimination, and integration.

In addition, as early drive-affect organizations are now being harnessed and integrated by the emerging ego functions of sensory-affect (motor) processing, differentiation, and integration, it is useful to consider drive-affect development from the perspective of the ego. From this perspective, the concept of the oral phase may be considered more broadly as part of a system of "sensory-affective" pleasure that involves all the sensory-affective (motor) pathways, of which the mouth is certainly dominant (in terms of tactile, deep pressure, temperature, pain, and motor, especially smooth muscle, patterns). The mouth's dominance is due to the highly developed nature of its sensory-affective and motor pathways. From the perspective of the ego, however, drive-affect derivatives are elaborated throughout the "sensory surface" of the body.

Forming Relationships, Attachment, and Engagement: 2–7 Months

Another early level concerns engagement, or a sense of relatedness, a lifelong capacity. Once the infant has achieved some capacity for regulation and interest in the world between 2 and 4 months of age, he or she becomes more engaged in social and emotional interactions. There is greater ability to respond to the external environment and to form a special relationship with significant primary caregivers. The infant's capacity for engagement is supported by early maturational abilities for selectively focusing on the human face and voice and for processing and organizing information from his or her senses (Meltzoff 1985; Papousek 1981; Papousek and Papousek 1979; Stern 1985). A sense of shared humanity, a type of synchrony of relating, is evident in the way both infant and parent use their senses, motor systems, and affects to resonate with each other (Butterworth and Jarrett 1980; Scaife and Bruner 1975).

As we saw in the previous subsection, the early quality of engagement has implications for later attachment patterns and behavior (Ainsworth et al. 1974; Bates et al. 1985; Belsky et al. 1984; Grossmann et al. 1985; Lewis and Feiring 1987; Miyake et al. 1985; Pederson et al. 1990). Attachment or relating with the caregiver is important not only because it represents the capacity to form human relationships but also because atypical attachment patterns have been shown to have a negative impact on developmental outcomes (Carew 1980). Longitudinal studies have found that securely attached children tend to have better emotional adaptability, social skills, and cognitive functioning (Cassidy and Shaver 1999). During the school-age and adolescent years, children who had been securely attached as infants were more likely to be accepted by their peers and were better able to form intimate relationships with peers (Sroufe et al. 1999). In addition, a secure attachment seems to provide a protective mechanism for children whose families experience a high level of stress (Egeland and Kreutzer 1991). The key element that underlies a secure attachment is sensitive and responsive caregiving (Ainsworth et al. 1978; De Wolff and van IJzendoorn 1997).

Attachment has a specific research meaning in terms of the studies cited above as well as others. As we emphasized, however, in a clinical as well as normative developmental context, it is useful to consider a broader framework for relationships involving the overall pattern of relating between an infant and caregiver. As we will discuss, this involves the depth of pleasure, range of feelings, and meanings given to relationships. The processes that define relationships go significantly beyond definitions used in various research paradigms (Greenspan 1997a).

Clinical Observations

In the stage of engagement, which involves a growing intimacy with the primary caregiver(s), one can observe babies who are adaptively able to employ all their senses to orchestrate highly pleasurable affect in their relationship with their primary caregiver(s). The baby with a beautiful smile, looking at and listening to mother, experiencing her gentle touch and rhythmic movement, and responding to her voice with synchronous mouth and arm and leg movements, is perhaps the most vivid example. Clinically, however, we observe babies who are not able to employ their senses to form an affective relationship with the human world. The most extreme case is that in which a baby actively avoids sensory and, therefore, affective contact with the human world. Human sounds, touch, and even scents are avoided either with chronic gaze aversion, recoiling, flat affect, or random or nonsynchronous patterns of brightening and alerting. We also observe babies who use one or another sensory pathway in the context of a pleasurable relationship with the human world but cannot orchestrate the full range and depth of sensory experience. The baby who listens to mother's voice with a smile but gaze averts and looks pained at the sight of her face is such an example.

Forming an attachment or relationship organizes a number of discrete affective proclivities—comfort, dependency, pleasure, and joy, as well as assertiveness and curiosity—in the context of a pleasurable caregiver-infant relationship. In the adaptive pattern, protest and anger are organized, along with the expected positive affects, as part of a baby's emotional interest in the primary caregiver. A healthy 4-month-old can, as part of his or her repertoire, become negative but then can also quickly return to mother's beautiful smiles, loving glances, and comforting. Relationship patterns, once formed, continue and further develop throughout the course of life.

Infants and children can already have major limitations in certain affect proclivities. Rather than evidencing joy, enthusiasm, or pleasure with their caregivers, they may instead evidence a flat affect. Similarly, rather than evidencing (periodic) assertive, curious, protesting, or angry behavior in relationship to their primary caregiver, they may only look very compliant and give shallow smiles. In addition to being constricted in their affective range, babies may also evidence a limitation in their organizational stability. An example is a baby who, after hearing a loud noise, cannot return to his earlier interests in the primary caregiver. When environmental circumstances are unfavorable, or when for other reasons development continues to be disordered, early attachment or relationship difficulties may occur. If these difficulties are severe enough, they may form the basis for an ongoing deficit in the baby's capacity to form affective human relationships and to form the basic personality structures and functions that depend on the internal organization of human experience.

Implications for Mental (Ego) Functioning

The pleasurable preference for the human world suggests interactive object seeking. Apathy in reaction to caregiver withdrawal, preference for the physical world, and chronic active aversion in clinically disturbed populations also suggest emerging organized object-related patterns, albeit in maladaptive directions.

Yet there is no evidence of the infant's ability to abstract all the features of the object in terms of an organization of the whole object. Infants seek the voice, smiling mouth, twinkly eyes, or rhythmic movements alone or in some combinations, but not yet as a whole. In addition, the tendency toward global withdrawal, rejection, or avoidance suggests global undifferentiated reaction patterns compared with differentiated patterns in which the influence of a "me" or a "you" is occurring. The 4-month-old does not evidence the repertoire of the 8-month-old in "wooing" a caregiver into a pleasurable interaction. The 4-month-old under optimal conditions evidences synchronous interactive patterns, smiling, and vocalizing in rhythm with the caregiver. When under clinical distress, he or she evidences global reactivity; in comparison, the 8-month-old can explore alternative ways of having an impact on his or her caregiver. These findings suggest that not until this next stage is there a full behavioral (prerepresentational) comprehension of cause and effect or part self-object differentiation. Representational comprehension does not occur until late in the second year of life.

Most likely, during this stage the infant progresses from the earlier stage of a self-other-world object (where both human and not-human worlds are not yet distinct, and the human self and nonself are not distinct) to a stage of intentional undifferentiated human self-object organization. There is the sense of synchrony and connectedness to a human object which suggests that the infant's experiential organization differentiates the human object from physical objects. Even at the behavioral level, there is not yet evidence of a self-object differentiation. In this sense, the concept of symbiosis (Mahler et al. 1975) is not at odds with the clinical observation of a lack of self-object differentiation.

The functioning of the ego at this stage is characterized by intentional object seeking, differentiated organizations of experience (physical from human but not-human, self from human object), and global patterns of reactivity to the human object. These patterns of reactivity include seeking pleasure, protest, withdrawal, rejection (with a preference for the physical world that is based on what appears to be a clear discrimination), hyperaffectivity (diffuse discharge of affects), and active avoidance.

To the degree that later self and object organization are undifferentiated, aspects of experience may combine or seemingly organize in different ways, because of a lack of structure formation, and this is perhaps a precursor to condensations, displacements, and projective and incorporative-introjective mechanisms. Projection, incorporation, and introjection in a differentiated sense, in which distinct images are transferred across boundaries, are not yet in evidence. We therefore see a progression from a stage of undifferentiated world self-object to one of undifferentiated human self-object.

Two-Way, Purposeful Communication (Somatopsychological Differentiation): 3–10 Months

The next stage involves purposeful communication: intentional, nonverbal communications or gestures. These gestures include affective communication, facial expressions, arm and leg movements, vocalizations, and spinal posture. From the middle of the first year of life onward, individuals rely on gestures to communicate. Initially during the stage of purposeful communication, simple reciprocal gestures, such as head nods, smiles or other affective expressions, and movement patterns, serve a boundary-defining role. The "me" communicates a wish or intention, and

the "other" or "you" communicates back some confirmation, acknowledgment, or elaboration on that wish or intention.

The stage of two-way, causal, intentional communication indicates processes occurring at the somatic (sensorimotor) and emerging psychological levels. It is evidenced in the infant's growing ability to discriminate primary caregivers from others and differentiate his or her own actions from their consequences—affectively, somatically, behaviorally, and interpersonally.

These capacities are first seen as the infant develops complex patterns of communication in the context of his or her primary human relationship. Parallel with development of the infant's relationship to the inanimate world, in which basic schemes of causality (Piaget 1962) are being developed, the infant becomes capable of complicated human emotional communication (Brazelton et al. 1974; Charlesworth 1969; Stern 1974a; Tennes et al. 1972). There is both a historic and a newly emerging consensus among clinicians, developmental observers, and researchers that affects are used for intentional communication (Bowlby 1973; Brazelton and Cramer 1990; Mahler et al. 1975; Osofsky and Eberhart-Wright 1988; Spitz 1965; Stern 1985; Winnicott 1960) and that these affective patterns—for happiness, anger, fear, surprise, disgust, and so forth—are similar in different cultures and in both children and adults (Campos et al. 1983; Darwin 1872/1965; Ekman et al. 1972; Izard 1971). Intentional communication, which involves both intuiting and responding to the caregiver's emotional cues, gradually takes on qualities that are particular to relationships, family, and culture (Brazelton and Als 1979; Bruner 1982; Feinman and Lewis 1983; Kaye 1982; Kimmert et al. 1983; Kleinman 1986; Markus and Kitayama 1990; Schweder et al. 1987; Stern 1977; Trevarthen 1979; Tronick 1980).

Clinical Observations

When there are distortions in the emotional communication process—as occurs when a mother responds in a mechanical, remote manner or projects some of her own dependent feelings onto her infant—the infant may not learn to appreciate causal relationships between people at the level of compassionate and intimate feelings. This situation can occur even though causality seems to be developing in terms of the inanimate world and the impersonal human world.

Some babies do not possess the capacity to orchestrate their sensory experiences in an interactive cause-and-effect pattern. A look and a smile on mother's part do not lead to a consequent look, smile, vocalization, or gross motor movement on baby's part. This baby may perceive the sensory experiences mother is making available but seems unable to organize these experiences and either looks past mother or evidences random motor patterns.

We also observe babies who can operate in a cause-and-effect manner in one sensory pathway but not another. For example, when presented with an object, they may clearly look at the object in a purposeful way and then examine it. However, when presented with an interesting auditory stimulus, instead of responding vocally or reaching toward the person or the object, the infant behaves chaotically with increased motor activity and discharge-type behavior, such as banging and flailing. Similarly, with tactile experience, some babies, instead of touching mother's hand when she is stroking their abdomen, begin evidencing seemingly random or chaotic motor responses that appear unrelated to the gentle stimulus.

We observe even more profoundly the differential use of the senses as infants are now also learning to process information in each sensory mode and between modes, in terms of seeing relations between elements in a pattern. For example, some babies learn quickly and some slowly that a sound leads to a sound or a look to a look. The implications for later learning problems of certain sensory pathways not fully becoming incorporated into a cause-and-effect level of behavioral organization (e.g., the differences between children with auditory-verbal abstracting and sequencing problems and those with visual-spatial problems) are intriguing to consider. Motor differences, such as high or low muscle tone or lags in motor development or in motor planning, will also obviously influence the infant's ability to signal his or her wishes. In organizing cause-and-effect–type communications, therefore, a compromise in a sensory or motor pathway not only limits the strategies available for tackling this new challenge but also may restrict the sensory and motor modalities that become organized at this new developmental level and, as will be discussed, the associated drive affect patterns as well.

As babies learn to orchestrate their senses in the context of cause-and-effect–type interactions, we observe an interesting clinical phenomenon in relationship to what have been described in the early neurological literature as "proximal" and "distal" modes. At this time, we may begin seeing a shift toward distal rather than proximal modes of communication. *Proximal modes* of communication may be thought of as direct physical contact, such as holding, rocking, and touching. *Distal modes* may be thought of as involving communication that occurs through vision, auditory cueing, and affect signaling. The distal modes can obviously occur across space, whereas the proximal modes require, as the word implies, physical closeness. The crawling 8-month-old can remain in emotional communication with his primary caregiver through various reciprocal glances, vocalizations, and affect gestures. Some babies, however, seem to rely on proximal modes for a sense of security. Early limitations in negotiating space will be seen later on to affect the capacity to construct internal representations.

If one divides the emotional terrain into its parts, one can see cause-and-effect signaling with the full range of emotions. In terms of dependency, the 8-month-old can make overtures to be cuddled or held. The child shows pleasure with beatific smiles and love of touching (if he or she does not have a tactile sensitivity). There is curiosity and assertiveness as the 8-month-old reaches for a rattle in Mom's hand. There is also anger and protest as he throws his food on the floor in a deliberate, intentional manner and looks at his or her caregiver as if to say, "What are you gonna do now?" There is protest, even defiance (e.g., biting, banging, and sometimes butting as an expression of anger, because at 8 months children have better motor control of their mouths, heads, and necks than of their arms and hands).

Where the caregiver does not respond to the baby's signal, such as returning a smile or a glance, we have observed that the baby's affective-thematic inclinations may not evidence this differentiated organization. Instead, he or she may remain either synchronous, as in the attachment phase, or shift from synchrony to a more random quality. The expected range may be present but not subordinated into a cause-and-effect interchange.

There are also many babies who, because of a lack of reciprocal responses from their caregiver, seemingly evidence affective dampening or flatness and a hint of despondency or sadness. This may occur even after they have shown a joyfulness and an adaptive attachment. In some cases at least, it seems as though when not offered the phase-specific "experiential nutriments" (the cause-and-effect interactions the baby is now capable of), but only the earlier forms of relatedness, the baby begins a pattern of withdrawal and affective flattening. It is as though the baby needs to be met at his or her own level to maintain his affective-thematic range. Most interesting are the subtle cases in which the baby can reciprocate certain affects and themes, such as pleasure and dependency, but not others, such as assertiveness, curiosity, and protest. Depending on the baby's own maturational tendencies and the specificity of the consequences in the caregiving environment, one can imagine how this uneven development occurs. For example, caregivers who are uncomfortable with dependency and closeness may not afford opportunities for purposeful reciprocal interactions in this domain, but may, on the other hand, be quite "causal" in less intimate domains of assertion and protest.

Implications for Mental (Ego) Functioning

It is useful to think of this stage of development as a first step in reality testing. At this time, prerepresentational causality is established. The intentionality of the infant in both adaptive (e.g., reaching out, protesting) and maladaptive (rejecting) modes suggests at least a behavioral comprehension of a "self" influencing an "other." It also suggests self-object differentiation at the behavioral level. Behavioral level in this context means the organization of behavioral patterns or tendencies rather than the later organization of symbols. Only late in the second year does a child begin to have the ability to create mental representations through higher-level abstractions. At this time, however, the "I" is likely an "I" of behavior ("If I do this it causes that") rather than the "I" of a mental representation ("If I feel or think or *am* a certain way, it will have this or that impact"). The capacity to construct mental representations will allow the growing child to organize and even rearrange different elements of the "self" or "other" into mental images. Because there is behavioral cause and effect or differentiated interaction, one can think of a behavioral or prerepresentational type of reality testing.

There is no evidence yet for the child's having the ability to abstract all aspects of the "self" or "other." Experiences are still in fragmented pieces. Temporal and spatial continuity, while rapidly developing, are not yet fully established. The "I" is a physical and behavioral "I"; an "I" that can make things happen in the behavior pattern of the "other." The "I" and the "other" are not yet an "I" and "other" that represent or organize all the aspects of the self or other, however, so it is possible to consider this stage as characterized by somatic and behavioral part self-object differentiation. The ego is characterized now by a capacity to differentiate aspects of experience in both the impersonal and drive-affect domains. It is worth emphasizing again that only at this stage are differentiated internal relationships possible. But even at this stage, what is likely to be differentiated are part-object schemes of behavior, not whole-objects in a representational form. This view differs from other interpretations of infant behavior that are based on normative samples of infants in experimental situations.

Behavioral Organization, Problem Solving, and Internalization: 9–18 Months

The next stage involves the child's capacity for engaging in a continuous flow of complex organized problem-solving interactions (e.g., taking mother to the refrigerator and pointing to the juice) and the formation of a presymbolic sense of self. With appropriate reading of cues and differ- ential responses, the infant's or toddler's behavioral repertoire becomes complicated, and communications take on more organized, meaningful configurations. By 12 months of age, the infant is connecting behavioral units into larger organizations as he or she exhibits complex emotional responses such as affiliation, wariness, and fear (Ainsworth et al. 1974, 1978; Bowlby 1969; Sroufe and Waters 1977). As the toddler approaches the second year of life, in the context of the practicing subphase of the development of individuation (Mahler et al. 1975), there is an increased capacity for forming original behavioral schemes (Piaget 1962), imitative activity and intentionality, and behavior suggesting functional understanding of objects (Werner and Kaplan 1963).

It is recognized that at this stage, the toddler takes a more active role in developing and maintaining the reciprocal relationship with his or her parent (Bell 1977; Goldberg 1977; Rheingold 1969). In addition, much has been written about the growing complexity of the reciprocal dyadic interaction (Cicchetti and Schneider-Rosen 1984; Greenspan and Porges 1984; Talberg et al. 1988; Tronick and Gianino Jr. 1986). These types of complex interactions enable the child to utilize and respond to social cues and eventually achieve a sense of competence as an autonomous being in relationship with a significant other (Brazelton and Als 1979; Lester et al. 1985).

There is now in evidence, therefore, a stage of behavioral organization or a complex sense of self as interactions become more complex and social patterns involve many circles of intentional communication that negotiate intimacy exploration, aggression, and limit setting (e.g., using emotional signals to figure out if a behavior is acceptable or not) (Dunn 1988; Emde et al. 1988; Kagan 1981; Radke-Yarrow et al. 1983; Zahn-Waxler and Radke-Yarrow 1982).

Clinical Observations

This stage involves a baby's ability to sequence together many cause-and-effect units into a chain or an organized behavioral pattern (e.g., the 14-month-old who can take mother's hand, walk her to the refrigerator, bang on the door, and, when the door is opened, point to the desired food). Wish and intention are organized under a complex behavioral pattern. This organized behavioral pattern can be viewed as a task that involves coordinated and orchestrated use of the senses. Here, the toddler who is capable of using vision and hearing to perceive various vocal and facial gestures, postural cues, and complex affect signals is able to extract relevant information from his or her objects and organize this information at new levels of cognitive and affective integration. A toddler who is not able to incorporate certain sensory experiences as part of his or her early cognitive and affective abstracting abilities (Werner et al. 1963) may evidence a very early restriction in how the senses process information.

Balanced reliance on proximal and distal modes of communication becomes even more important during this phase of development. The mobile toddler enjoying his or her freedom in space presumably can feel secure through distal communication modes (e.g., looking and listening across space). It is interesting in this context to examine traditional notions of separation anxiety and the conflicts that some toddlers have over separation and individuation (Mahler et al. 1975). With the use of the distal modes, the toddler can "have his cake and eat it too." If he can bring the caregiving object with him through the use of distal contact with her, he does not have to tolerate a great deal of insecurity. He can "refuel" distally by looking at mother or listening to her voice and signal her back with vocalizations or arm gestures. He can use proximal contact, such as coming over for a cuddle when necessary. The youngster who has difficulty in using his distal modes to remain in contact with the primary caregiver may need more proximal contact. While this reliance on proximal contact can occur because of feelings of insecurity generated by an ambivalent primary caregiver, the limitations of a child's own sensory organization may also be an important factor in this pattern.

From a motor and sensory perspective, therefore, to master this stage, the toddler needs to be able to process sounds and sights, employ reciprocal motor gestures, and comprehend spatial relationships.

The piecing together of many smaller cause-and-effect units of experience involves a range of types of experience, such as pleasure, assertiveness, curiosity, and dependency, into an organized pattern. For instance, it is not unlikely for a healthy toddler to start with a dependent tone of cuddling and kissing her parents, shift to a pleasurable, giggly interchange with them, and then get off their laps and invite them to engage in an assertive chase game in which she runs to a room that is off-limits, such as the living room. When the parents say, "No, you can't go in there," protest and negativism may emerge. Under optimal circumstances, the interaction may come to a relative closure with the toddler back in the playroom, sitting on her parent's lap, pleasurably exploring pictures in her favorite book. Here the child has gone full circle, suggesting that she has connected the many affective-thematic areas.

Around 18 months, as children begin to abstract the meaning of objects, their understanding of the functions of the telephone or brush may have its counterpart in their experiencing the caregiver as a "functional" being invested with many affective-thematic proclivities. Between 12 and 18 months, although children are able to integrate many behavioral units, they do not seem to be able to fully integrate intense emotions. For the moment at least, they do not fully realize that person they are mad at is the same person they love and experience pleasure with. By 18–24 months, the sense of split-off fury seems, at least in clinical observations, to be modified at some level by an awareness of love and dependency.

Implications for Mental (Ego) Functioning

The new capacities for behavioral organization, affective integration, and behavioral sense of self and object in functional terms (a conceptual stand toward the world) characterize this stage of ego development. We can observe three levels:

- Fragmented (little islands of intentional problem-solving behavior)
- Polarized (organized patterns of behavior expressing only one or another feeling states, e.g., organized aggression and impulsivity; organized clinging, needy, dependent behavior; or organized fearful patterns)
- Integrated (different emotional patterns—dependency, assertiveness, pleasure, etc.—organized into integrated, problem-solving affective interactions such as flirting, seeking closeness, and then getting help to find a needed object)

Now there is what may be thought of as a conceptual self-object relationship, because different self behaviors and object behaviors not only are differentiated from one another (as in the earlier stage) but also are viewed as part of a whole. Teasing behavior, jokes, anticipation of emotional reactions, and awareness of how to get others to evidence different emotional proclivities all point to this new conceptual affective ability. But even more important is how the toddler uses his or her ability to organize in all dimensions of life. This is illustrated by the toddler's tendency, under stress, to organize his or her negativism, or to become sophisticated in his or her clinging dependency, develop intricate aggressive patterns, or exploit or manipulate peers and adults in new interpersonal patterns. In worrisome situations one also observes the toddler regress from organized behavioral patterns to highly fragmented patterns, or become withdrawn or rejecting.

The ego can now organize experience in terms of functional expectancies. This capacity of the ego also facilitates integrated functional identifications. Instead of simply copying a behavior, a child can copy or identify with a functional interpersonal pattern. These functional patterns can also be projected or incorporated. Now not simply an isolated behavior (e.g., hitting) but a "behavioral attitude" (e.g., being controlling) can be projected or incorporated. Perhaps most defenses exist on a hierarchy related to stages in the functioning of the ego.

During this stage ego structure formation is undergoing rapid progress. Both deficits of experience and conflicts between behavioral-affective tendencies will likely undermine structure formation. One therefore does not need to postulate either deficit models or conflict models of the mind. Rather, the two tendencies can be seen as working together.

For example, Kohut (1971) would suggest that lack of parental empathy leads the toddler to experience a deficit in terms of his or her self-esteem regulation (an early affective self-object pattern). Kernberg (1975) would suggest that the unadmiring, overcontrolling, or intrusive caregiver increases a condition in which the toddler experiences rage and conflict and then resorts to primitive splitting defenses in order to cope with this situation. It is suggested here that, on the basis of clinical work with and observations of toddlers, both tendencies are operative. A lack of empathy and intrusive overcontrol lead to painful humiliation, rage, and fear of object loss as well as deficits in self-object experiences and the formation of structures regulating self-esteem. For example, the 18-month-old experiencing rage and fear, without therapy, usually resorts to passive compliance, indifferent impulsivity, and avoidance. This regressive way of dealing with conflict during this phase leads to a structural deficit because the ability to abstract affective polarities is not learned. Likewise, a lack of empathic admiration and unavailability seems to leave the toddler feeling too uncertain about his or her objects to experiment with his or her behavioral and affective polarities. In addition, toddlers who evidence overreactivity to sensory and affective experience are likely to experience loss and fear more readily than sensory-craving, assertive, and sometimes aggressive toddlers, who will more readily experience rage. Reconstructive work with older children and adults must deal with both the reality of the early object relationship and the rage, humiliation, fear, and conflict, and the primitive strategies employed at the time and subsequently repeated. At this age, conflict leads to deficits, and deficits (e.g., a lack of capacity to abstract behavioral polarities and to deal with ambivalence) create the increased probability of unresolvable conflicts. Which comes first becomes a chicken-or-egg question, because appropriate structure is necessary to resolve conflict, and conflicts at an early age often lead to structural deficits.

This stage of ego development is characterized by many new capacities and is transitional to the next stages, where mental representations and differentiated self-object representational structures are possible.

Representational Capacity: 18–30 Months

The next level involves the creation, elaboration, and sharing of symbols and meanings. The individual's ability to represent or symbolize experience is illustrated in the pretend play, the verbal labeling of feelings ("I feel happy"), and the functional use of language.

This level begins as the toddler approaches the end of the second year. Internal sensations and unstable images become organized as multisensory, affective images or representations that can be evoked and are somewhat stable (Bell 1970; Fenson and Ramsay 1980; Gouin-Decarie 1965; Piaget 1962). Although this capacity is fragile between 16 and 24 months, it soon becomes a dominant mode in organizing the child's behavior.

Related to the ability to create representations is the capacity for "object permanence." This capacity, which is relative and goes through a series of stages, refers to the toddler's ability to search for hidden inanimate objects (Gouin-Decarie 1965).

Infants progress from engaging in actions with themselves (e.g., feeding self) to using themselves as the agents to act upon others (e.g., toddler uses a doll to feed another doll). The development of language and the capacity to share meanings with others facilitate children's capacity to describe themselves and to understand the difference between themselves and others. This development of perspective coincides with the early stages of empathy and prosocial behavior (Butterworth 1990; DesRosiers and Busch-Rossnagel 1997; Meltzoff 1990; Pipp-Siegel and Pressman 1996; Stern 1983).

The elaboration of ideas or representations gradually becomes more complex, as does the sense of self that now involves symbols, not just behaviors (e.g., use of words for intent and descriptions, use of personal pronouns, improved recognition of self in mirror) (Fein and Apfel 1979; Fenson et al. 1976; Inhelder et al. 1972; Pipp et al. 1987; Rubin et al. 1983). Pretend play and intentional interpersonal use of language illustrate these new capacities (Erikson 1940; Fein 1975; Kraus and Glucksberg 1969; Lowe 1975; Nelson 1973; Peller 1954; Waelder 1933).

Over time, causal schemes are developed at a representational level (McCune-Nicholich 1977; Sinclair 1970), leading to thinking capacities. In addition, as ideas and behaviors are being elaborated, they reflect not only ongoing relationships but prior negotiations as well. A large number of studies on early attachment patterns and later behavior illustrate the importance of early patterns as well as later relationships (Aber and Baker 1990; Arend et al. 1979; Cassidy 1990; Cassidy et al. 1988; Easterbrooks and Goldberg 1990; Egeland and Farber 1984; Goldberg and Easterbrooks 1984; Main et al. 1985; Marvin and

Stewart 1991; Maslin-Cole and Spieker 1990; Matas et al. 1978; Pastor 1981; Sroufe 1983; Sroufe et al. 1983; Waters et al. 1979). As children elaborate their ideas, they use them to make more sense of their experiences and themselves (Bretherton and Beeghly 1982; Dore 1989; Dunn 1988; Dunn et al. 1987; Nelson and Gruendel 1981; Schank and Abelson 1977).

Clinical Observations

A mental representation or idea is a multisensory image that involves the construction of objects from the perspective of all the objects' properties. When the range, depth, and integration of sensory experiences are limited, the very construction of the object and representation will obviously be limited in either sensory range and depth or affective investment and meaning.

As the child learns to construct his own multisensory, affective-thematic image of his experiential world, he organizes affective-thematic patterns at a level of meanings. This new level of organization can be thought of as operating in two ways. The youngster with a representational capacity now has the tool to interpret and label feelings rather than simply act them out. A verbal 2½-year-old can evidence this interpretive process by saying "me mad" or "me happy." Pretend play is, perhaps, an even more reliable indicator than language of the child's ability to interpret and label. Pretend play is an especially important indicator because many children have language delays. For example, a child soon provides a picture of her representational world as she plays out dramas in different thematic realms—for example, dependency (e.g., two dolls feeding or hugging each other).

The representational capacity also provides a higher-level organization with which to integrate affective-thematic domains. Therefore, we observe new experiences as the child develops from 2 to 5 years of age. These include empathy, more consistent love (including object constancy, a love for self and others that is stable over time and survives separations and affect storms such as anger) (Mahler et al. 1975), and later on the ability to experience loss, sadness, and guilt.

Because of the complexities of representational elaboration, the conceptualization of this stage may be aided by subdividing the representational capacity into three levels or subcategories. The first level is the descriptive use of the representational mode (the child labels pictures and describes objects). The second level is the limited interactive use of the representational mode (the child elaborates one or two episodes of thematic-affective interactions, such as statements of "give me candy," "me hungry," or a play scene with two dolls feeding, fighting, or nuzzling). The third level is elaboration of representational, affective-thematic interactions.

Implications for Mental (Ego) Functioning

This stage of ego organization is characterized by the capacity to elevate experiences to the representational level. Current experience can be organized into multisensory, affective "images," and these images are mobile in time and space (e.g., children imagine images of objects in the absence of the object). The representational system can also construct multisensory images of sensations or patterns from within the organism that may have occurred in the past. These earlier patterns of somatic sensation and simple and complex chains of behavior and interaction will now be "interpreted" via representation. How well formed, accurate, or distorted these representations of earlier prerepresentational experience will be will depends on the character of the early patterns, their repetition in the present, the abstracting ability of the ego, and the emerging dynamic character of the ego—that is, its ability to represent some areas of experience better than others.

To the degree there is a less-than-optimal interactive experience available (the caregiver is concrete or ignores or distorts certain representational themes), we observe a series of mental (ego) operations, which include the following:

1. Concretization of experience (Access to representation is never achieved.)
2. Behavioral-representational splitting (Some areas gain access, but core areas remain at behavioral level.)
3. Representational constriction (Global dynamically relevant areas remain outside of the representational system.)
4. Representational encapsulation (Limited dynamically relevant areas remain in more concrete form.)
5. Representational exaggeration or lability (Domains of experience that are ignored or distorted become exaggerated or labile, their opposites become exaggerated or labile, or other "displaced" dynamically related thoughts, affects, or behaviors become exaggerated or labile.)

During this stage, as self and object relationships are being organized at a representational level, they are not differentiated, even though the early prerepresentational behavioral and somatic organizations are differentiated. There is a paradox: differentiation at an earlier level alongside emerging differentiation at the new higher level. At this time we can postulate an undifferentiated representational self-object built on a foundation of somatic and behavioral differentiated self-objects.

Often, at this stage of development, representational elaboration is associated with primary process thinking. Because behavioral and somatic differentiation is already occurring, and representational differentiation occurs simultaneously with representational elaboration, it may prove best to rethink our notions of primary process thinking.

Representational Differentiation: 30–48 Months

The next level involves creating logical bridges between ideas. Shared meanings are used both to elaborate wishes and feelings and to categorize meanings and solve problems. The child elaborates and eventually differentiates those feelings, thoughts, and events that emanate from within and those that emanate from others. The child begins to differentiate the actions of others from his or her own. This process gradually forms the basis for the differentiation of self representations from representations of the external world, animate and inanimate. It also provides the basis for such crucial personality functions as knowing what is real from unreal, impulse and mood regulation, and the capacity to focus attention and concentrate in order to learn and interact.

As logical bridges between ideas are established, reasoning and an appreciation of reality grow, including distinguishing what is pretend from what is believed to be real and dealing with conflicts and finding prosocial outcomes (Dunn and Kendrick 1982; Flavell et al. 1986; Harris and Kavanaugh 1993; Harris et al. 1991; Wolf et al. 1984; Wooley and Wellman 1990). As children become capable of emotional thinking, they begin to understand relationships between their own and others' experiences and feelings. They also illustrate these relationships in their narratives. Emotional thinking also enables children to begin to reason about right and wrong (Buchsbaum and Emde 1990; Emde and Buchsbaum 1990; Harris 1989; Nelson 1986; Smetana 1985; Stewart and Marvin 1984; Wolf 1990). As children move into subsequent stages (e.g., latency) and become more concerned with peers, they begin to appreciate emotional complexity such as mixed feelings (Donaldson and Westerman 1986; Harter and Whitesell 1989).

The capacity for differentiating internal representations becomes consolidated as object constancy is established (Mahler et al. 1975). As the child moves into the oedipal stage, both reality and fantasy become more complex (Bruner 1986, 1990; Dore 1989; Fivush 1991; Greenspan 1993; Singer and Singer 1990). In middle childhood, representational capacity becomes reinforced with the child's ability to develop derivative representational systems tied to the original representation and to transform them in accordance with adaptive and defensive goals. This permits greater flexibility in dealing with perceptions, feelings, thoughts, and emerging ideals. Substages for these capacities include representational differentiation, the consolidation of representational capacity, and the capacity for forming limited derivative representational systems and multiple derivative representational systems (structural learning) (Greenspan 1979). Throughout these stages, but especially in the formation of complex behavior patterns and rituals, in the elaboration of ideas, and in creating bridges between ideas, one observes cultural influences—for example, in the way girls and boys construct aspects of their inner worlds (Reiss 1989). The now well-known finding that in Western cultures men tend to be more assertive and competitive and women more caring and relationship-oriented (Gilligan 1982) is evident during development—with, for example, greater early signs of empathy in girls and parents' inclinations to talk more to boys about anger and girls about sadness (Zahn-Waxler et al. 1992).

At the level of building bridges between ideas, the child can make connections between different ideas and feelings ("I am mad because you took my toy") and balance fantasy and reality. An adult using capacities begun during this stage can similarly hold logical conversations about wishes and feelings and make connections ("I feel lonely and needy, and I get helpless when I feel that way; sometimes I get mad because I can't stand being so vulnerable").

Clinical Observations

For children to meet the challenges of organizing and differentiating their internal world according to "self" and "other," "inside" and "outside," and dimensions of time and space and affective valence, they are, in part, dependent on the integrity of the sensory organization that underlies their experiential world. Now, as earlier, the capacity to process sensory information is critical, including sequencing auditory-verbal and visual-spatial patterns according to physical, temporal, and spatial qualities in the context of abstracting emerging cognitive and affective meanings. The child is now challenged to understand what he or she hears, sees, touches, and feels, not only in terms of ideas but also in terms of what is me and not-me; what is past, present, and future; what is close and far; and so forth. These learning tasks depend on the ability to sequence and categorize information through each of the sensory systems and through all of them working together. Therefore, if anywhere along the pathway of sensory processing there are difficulties, the subsequent ability to organize impersonal or affective information will likely be compromised.

For example, if sounds are confused, words will not be easily understood. Similarly, if spatial images are confused, spatial configurations will not be easily negotiated. If short-term memory for either verbal or spatial symbols is vulnerable, information will be lost before it can be combined with, and compared with, other information in order to abstract meanings. And if higher level auditory-verbal symbolic or visual-spatial symbolic abstracting capacities are less than age-appropriate, the very capacity to categorize experience will be limited. When one considers that the challenge is now to process and organize not only impersonal, cognitive experiences but also highly emotional, interpersonal experiences (which keep moving, so to speak), this challenge to the sensory system is formidable. Furthermore, categories such as "me," "not me," "real," and "make-believe" are high-level constructs that depend on organizing sensory information.

The child appears to use his or her new representational capacity to simultaneously elaborate and differentiate experience, in contrast to earlier views by Freud (1900/1953) and Mahler et al. (1975). There does not appear to be a period of magical representational thinking followed by one of reality thinking. The child continually differentiates affective-thematic organizations along lines that pertain to self and other, inner-outer, time, space, and so forth. This differentiation is based on the child's capacity to experience the representational consequences of his or her representational elaborations with the emotionally relevant people in his world, usually parents, family, and friends. The parent who interacts with the child, using emotionally meaningful words and gestures, and engages in pretend play in a contingent manner (offering, in other words, logical representational feedback) provides the child with consequences that help him or her differentiate his or her representational world. In this view, reality testing—the capacity to separate magical from realistic thought—appears to be a gradual process beginning with the onset of the representational capacity proper and reaching some degree of selective stabilization prior to the child's formal entry into school.

One observes the child's elaborate representational themes along two dimensions. In the horizontal dimension, the child broadens the range of his or her themes to eventually include a range of emotional domains or drive-affect realms, including closeness or dependency, pleasure and excitement, assertiveness, curiosity, aggression, self-limit-setting, the beginnings of empathy, and consistent love. For example, not infrequently one observes repetitive pretend play of a feeding or hugging scene, suggesting nurturance and dependency. Over time, however, the dramas the child may initiate (with parental interactive support) will expand to include scenes of separation (one

doll going off on a trip and leaving the other behind), competition, assertiveness, aggression, injury, death, recovery (the doctor doll trying to fix the wounded soldier), and so forth. At the same time, the logical infrastructure of the child's pretend play and functional use of language becomes more complex and causally connected. The "he-man" doll is hurt by the "bad guys" and therefore "gets them." After the tea party, the little girl doll goes to the "potty" and then decides it is time to begin cooking dinner. In discussions, the 3½-year-old sounds more and more like a lawyer, with "buts" and "becauses" ("I don't like that food because it looks yucky and will make me sick"). There is, therefore, both thematic elaboration and differentiation. Even though the themes may be pretend and phantasmagoric, the structure of the drama becomes more and more logical. The rocket ship to the land of "he-man" uses NASA rocket fuel.

As indicated, representational differentiation depends on a child's not only being representationally engaged in affective-thematic areas but also experiencing cause-and-effect feedback at the representational level. Parents have to be able not only to engage but also to interpret experiences correctly. The parents who react to play with a gun as aggression one day, as sexuality another day, and as dependency on a third day, or who keep shifting meanings within the same thematic play session, will confuse the child. This child may not develop meanings with a reality orientation. Parents who confuse their own feelings with the child's feelings, or cannot set limits, may also compromise the formation of a reality orientation.

Implications for Mental (Ego) Functioning

During this stage one may postulate a self-object relationship characterized by a differentiated, integrated representational self-object. Ego organization, differentiation, and integration are characterized by an abstraction of self-object representations and drive-affect dispositions into a higher-level representational organization, differentiated along dimensions of self-other, time, and space.

Mental (ego) functioning during this stage and the prior stage can be divided up into a number of patterns. These include patterns of the following characteristics:

- Using words and actions together (Ideas are acted out in action, but words are also used to signify the action.)
- Using somatic or physical words to convey feeling states ("My muscles are exploding"; "Head is aching.")
- Using action words instead of actions to convey intent ("Hit you!")
- Conveying feelings as real rather than as signals ("I'm mad," "Hungry," or "Need a hug" compared with "I feel mad," "I feel hungry," or "I feel like I need a hug.")

(In the first instance, the feeling state demands action and is very close to action; in the second one, it is more a signal for something going on inside that leads to a consideration of many possible thoughts and/or actions.)

- Expressing global feeling states ("I feel awful"; "I feel OK.")
- Showing polarized feeling states (Feelings tend to be characterized as all good or all bad.)
- Showing evidence of differentiated feelings (Gradually there are more and more subtle descriptions of feeling states, such as loneliness, sadness, annoyance, anger, delight, and happiness.)
- Creating connections between differentiated feeling states ("I feel angry when you are mad at me.")

What operations are now available to the ego to deal with anxiety and conflict? The ego now has new approaches in addition to the primitive mechanisms described earlier. Observations of both normally developing and disturbed young children suggest that the approaches available to the ego include the following:

1. Global lack of differentiation (Reality and the object ties that provide reality feedback are too disruptive or "scary.")
2. Selective dedifferentiation (Blurring of boundaries and changing meanings, as with "my anger won't make mother leave because we are the same person.")
3. Thought-drive-affect dedifferentiations ("I can think anything, but I won't have feelings so I won't be scared.")
4. Thought-behavior (impulse) dedifferentiation ("If I do it, it's not me. Only when I think and plan it is it me.")
5. Selective constrictions of drive-affect-thematic realms (Areas such as anger or sexual curiosity are avoided and may remain relatively undifferentiated, often because they are associated with disorganizing interactive experience such as withdrawal and overstimulation.)
6. Affect, behavioral, or thought intensification ("If I exaggerate it or its opposite, it can't scare me")
7. Differentiated representational distortions (Meanings are changed along lines of drive-affect dispositions ["I am supergirl, the strongest"], but basic reality testing is maintained ["It is only pretend."])
8. Encapsulated distortions (Dynamically based conflict driven, highly selective shifts of meanings ["I am the cause of mother's anger"].)
9. Transformed differentiational linkages (This is an early form of rationalization. As the child's capacity to connect representational units is forming, he or she can elaborate ["I like mommy because she is home all the time, and I'm mad at daddy because he travels a lot"]. These logical links can undergo subtle shifts to change meanings for defensive purposes ["I like daddy to travel a lot because he brings me presents. I am mad at mommy].)
10. Compromises in representational integration and representational identity (The integration of somatic, behavioral [and representational self-object organizations], and associated drive-affect proclivities is not fully maintained, as evidenced by the irritable-looking 3-year-old who "feels fine" or the hitting 3-year-old who "loves everyone.")

Higher Levels of Mental (Ego) Functioning

The six basic foundations of emotional experience discussed in the previous section create the opportunity to master higher levels of mental (ego) functioning. These later levels build on the basic ones and include *multicause and triangular reasoning about emotions* (e.g., a child can figure out several reasons why she has a feeling and comprehend emotional relationships among three people). They also include *gray-area, differentiated, reflective thinking* about one's own and others' feelings (a child can weigh the relative way in which different feelings contribute to his or others' behavior or the relative impact of different reasons for the way he feels). They further include reflective thinking from a growing internal sense of self and internal standard (the child now has a growing, affectively integrated sense of self that she can use to form an opinion about experiences, i.e., make judgments such as "I usually don't get this angry in this situation"). Once these advanced stages are in place, they enable an individual to increase his or her range and depth of affective experience and negotiate a series of additional stages during adolescence and adulthood (Greenspan 1997b; Greenspan and Shanker 2004).

From Affects to Symbols: The Developmental Pathway to the Formation of Internal Representations

How symbols and internal representations emerge from earlier infant behavior is one of the most important unsolved mysteries in modern psychology. The developmental framework for depth psychology described earlier suggests some answers.

We have observed that two goals need to be met for children to progress to creating meaningful internal representations and symbols. The first is that relevant affective or emotional experiences invest symbols as they form (Greenspan 1997b). Affectively meaningful symbols of self and others become the basis for internal representations. Images without affect can lead to memories without meaning. We see this phenomenon in some children with autism: they may repeat words rather than conveying what the words mean.

The second condition for creating meaningful internal representations and symbols—that *a representation or symbol emerges when perception is separated from its action*—was a dramatic new insight for us and yet so basic in its simplicity that it surprised us. The developmental process that enables a child to separate perception from action provides the missing link in understanding symbol formation, construction of internal representations, and higher levels of consciousness, thinking, and self-reflection (Greenspan and Shanker 2004).

Why does perception have to be separated from action to create symbols or internal representations? In animals, very young infants, and impulsive humans, perception is tied closely to action. One perceives something (an animal perceives a food source or an enemy) and then attacks, moves toward it, runs away, and so forth. The perception triggers an action. There is a closely linked perceptual/motor pattern, with little pause or delay in carrying out the action.

To understand what perception is like when it is not tied to one or a few predetermined actions, first consider that a perception usually involves a multisensory "picture" of the world. Next, imagine forming such a multisensory "picture" and not taking an immediate action. Such a multisensory picture is a "perception" or "image" in its own right (i.e., a freestanding image).

Once a person can form a free-standing image, he or she can accumulate more affective experience with this perception or image. For example, over time, an image or perception of mother can be imbued with many experiences with her, such as emotional interactions in play, eating, and comforting. In this way, the image of mother gradually acquires more and more emotional experience.

As images or perceptions become seasoned with more and more emotional experiences, they gradually form into an affectively meaningful symbol or internal representation. A symbol for something as complex and important as mother will eventually involve many complex meanings, such as love, devotion, control, annoyance, and sacrifice. Over time, meaningful symbols can coalesce into integrated internal representations of "self" and "other" with greater and greater degrees of integration and differentiation (Greenspan 1988, 1989a, 1989b).

Individuals who remain tied to global perceptual motor patterns (e.g., "catastrophic" affects or emotions tied to global, fixed perceptual motor actions such as the fight-flight reaction or massive avoidance) often do not progress to a stage at which they can use internal representations to deal with affective experience. They tend to remain in an action mode.

To separate perception from action, one has to go beyond catastrophic emotions that are part of a primitive perceptual motor (i.e., perceptual action) level. To go beyond or to "tame" catastrophic emotions involves a developmental process through which emotions become transformed into regulated affect signals. In the prior section, we described a number of different levels or stages of affect signaling. Of particular importance for the formation of symbols is the stage at which affects are used intentionally and then progress in the next stage to being used in co-regulated problem-solving affective interactions. During these two stages—the stages of two-way purposeful communication and behavioral organization, problem solving and internalization—there is a dramatic transition or transformation from catastrophic affect to co-regulated affect signaling. As affects are transformed from catastrophic patterns to co-regulated signals, they change from pressing for action to being used for communication, negotiation, and regulation. This transformation frees perceptions from their fixed actions and enables perceptions to operate as free-standing images that can then acquire a variety of affective meaning.

As affect signals are used to communicate and negotiate, they come to govern (i.e., orchestrate) cognitive, social, emotional, motor, and sensory functioning. Also, importantly, as affects become transformed into regulated signals, they integrate prerepresentational (subsymbolic) and representational (symbolic) systems. They remain separate only in pathologic development (Greenspan and Shanker 2004).

This transformation of affects from catastrophic states to co-regulated affect signals occurs over a long period of time. Human beings are somewhat unique, compared with most mammals, in having a long period during which an infant or toddler is dependent on his or her caregivers. During this time, the child can learn to use and to rely on nonverbal, gestural, emotional signals, which he or she shares with many other mammals but has developed to a greater degree to meet basic needs, interact, negotiate, and communicate.

Conclusion

The model presented in this chapter provides a framework for understanding mental health, mental disorders, and psychotherapeutic approaches (see Greenspan and Shanker 2004 and Greenspan 1997a, 1997b for further discussion). Each level in early development identifies a realm of experience and basic capacities that define mental health and are relatively impaired in mental disorders. Examples include the capacity to develop relationships; to express, comprehend, and signal with a broad range of emotions; to construct internal representations and progress to differentiating them as a basis for reality testing; and for higher levels of reflective thinking and social interaction. For each of these realms of experience and capacities, we can observe deficits or varying degrees of constriction (limitations).

In addition, we can also observe the related defenses, character patterns, and associated use of affects. For example, at early levels of catastrophic affect expression, we can observe global defense patterns, such as massive avoidance, passivity, or aggression. At levels of prerepresentational affect signaling, we can observe more differentiated defense patterns, such as negativism, selective aggression, and compulsive rituals. At representational levels, we can observe affects being used as internal signals to mobilize defenses that alter internal experience. These range from condensations and displacements to reaction formations, rationalizations, and sublimations.

A developmental framework for depth psychology also informs understanding of the psychotherapeutic process. It suggests that in addition to clarifying and interpreting internal experience, the therapeutic process must focus on constructing experiences with the patient that enable the mastery of the basic capacities associated with each developmental level (i.e., relationships, affect signaling, a range of affective expression, and the representation differentiation and integration of affective experience). It also suggests that the therapeutic process must concern itself with both the prerepresentational and representational levels of experience. It must deal with the patient's unique way of processing experience (i.e., her unique sensory-affective processing profile) and enable the patient to cope with the full range of experiences, from dependency and sexuality to assertiveness and aggression.

Therefore, a developmental framework for depth psychology informs a distinctly psychoanalytic way of defining mental health and mental health disorders and the therapeutic process. In addition to an absence of symptoms and specific behaviors or maladaptive patterns, mental health must be defined by the realms of experience and capacities that arise and define human development during the course of life.

References

Aber J, Baker AJ: Security of attachment in toddlerhood: modifying assessment procedures for joint clinical and research purposes, in Attachment in the Preschool Years: Theory, Research, Intervention. Edited by Greenberg M, Cicchetti D, Cummings E. Chicago, IL, University of Chicago Press, 1990, pp 427–463

Ainsworth MDS, Bell SM, Stayton D: Infant-mother attachment and social development: socialization as a product of reciprocal responsiveness to signals, in The Integration of the Child Into a Social World. Edited by Richards M. Cambridge, England, Cambridge University Press, 1974, pp 99–135

Ainsworth MDS, Blehar MC, Waters E, et al: Patterns of Attachment: A Psychological Study of the Strange Situation. New York, Lawrence Erlbaum, 1978

Als H: Patterns of infant behavior: analogs of later organizational difficulties? in Dyslexia: A Neuroscientific Approach to Clinical Evaluation. Edited by Duffy FH, Geschwind N. Boston, MA, Little, Brown, 1982, pp 67–92

Als H, Lester BM, Tronick E, et al: Towards a research instrument for the assessment of preterm infants' behavior (APIB), in Theory and Research in Behavioral Pediatrics. Edited by Fitzgerald H, Yogman MW. New York, Plenum, 1982, pp 35–132

Arend R, Gove FL, Sroufe LA: Continuity of individual adaptation from infancy to kindergarten: a predictive study of ego-resiliency and curiosity in preschoolers. Child Dev 50:950–959, 1979

Ayres J: Tactile functions: their relation to hyperactive and perceptual motor behavior. Am J Occup Ther 18:6–11, 1964

Bates JE, Maslin LA, Frankel KA: Attachment, security, mother-child interaction, and temperament as predictors of problem behavior ratings at age three years. Monogr Soc Res Child Dev 50:167–193, 1985

Beebe B, Lachman F: Infant Research and Adult Treatment: Co-Constructing Interactions. Hillsdale, NJ, Analytic Press, 2002

Beebe B, Jaffe J, Lachman F: A dyadic systems view of communication, in Relational Perspectives in Psychoanalysis. Edited by Skolnik N, Waters E. Hillsdale, NJ, Analytic Press, 1992, pp 61–81

Bell R: Socialization findings re-examined, in Child Effects on Adults. Edited by Bell R, Harper L. New York, Wiley, 1977, pp 53–85

Bell SM: The development of the concept of the object as related to infant-mother attachment. Child Dev 41:219–311, 1970

Belsky J, Rovine M, Taylor DG: The Pennsylvania Infant and Family Development Project, III: the origins of individual differences in infant-mother attachment: maternal and infant contributions. Child Dev 55:718–728, 1984

Berlyne DE: Conflict, Arousal, and Curiosity. New York, McGraw-Hill, 1960

Bowlby J: Maternal Care and Mental Health: WHO Monograph Series, No 2. Geneva, World Health Organization, 1951

Bowlby J: Attachment and Loss, Vol 1: Attachment. New York, Basic Books, 1969

Bowlby J: Attachment and Loss, Vol 2: Separation: Anxiety and Anger. New York, Basic Books, 1973

Brazelton TB, Als H: Four early stages in the development of mother-infant interaction. Psychoanal Study Child 34:349–369, 1979

Brazelton TB, Cramer B: The Earliest Relationship: Parents, Infants, and the Drama of Early Attachment. Reading, MA, Addison-Wesley Publishing, 1990

Brazelton TB, Koslowski B, Main M: The origins of reciprocity; the early mother-infant interaction, in The Effect of the Infant on Its Caregiver. Edited by Lewis M, Rosenblum L. New York, Wiley, 1974, pp 61–63

Bremmer R, Fogel A: Handbook of Infant Development. London, Blackwell, 2001

Bretherton I, Beeghly M: Talking about inner states: the acquisition of an explicit theory of mind. Dev Psychol 18:906–921, 1982

Bruner JS: Child's Talk: Learning to Use Language. New York, WW Norton, 1982

Bruner JS: Actual Minds, Possible Worlds. Cambridge, MA, Harvard University Press, 1986

Bruner JS: Acts of Meaning. Cambridge, MA, Harvard University Press, 1990

Buchsbaum HK, Emde RN: Play narratives in 36-month-old children: early moral development and family relationships. Psychoanal Study Child 45:129–155, 1990

Burlingham D, Freud A: Young Children in Wartime: A Year's Work in a Residential War Nursery. London, Allen & Unwin, 1942

Butterworth G: Self perception in infancy, in The Self in Transition: Infancy to Childhood. Edited by Cicchetti D, Beeghly M. Chicago, IL, Chicago University Press, 1990

Butterworth G, Jarrett N: The Geometry of Preverbal Communication. Edinburgh, Scotland, 1980

Campos JJ, Barrett KC, Lamb ME, et al: Socioemotional development, in Handbook of Child Psychology, Vol 2. Edited by Mussen PH (Haith MM, Campos J, vol eds). New York, Wiley, 1983, pp 785–915

Campos JJ, Campos R, Barrett K: Emergent themes in the study of emotional development and emotion regulation. Dev Psychol 25:394–402, 1989

Carew JV: Experience and the development of intelligence in young children at home and in day care. Monogr Soc Res Child Dev 45:1–115, 1980

Cassidy JA: Theoretical and methodological considerations in the study of attachment and self in young children, in Attachment in the Preschool Years: Theory, Research, and Intervention. Edited by Greenberg MT, Cicchetti D. Chicago, IL, Chicago University Press, 1990, pp 87–120

Cassidy JA, Shaver PR (eds): Handbook of Attachment: Theory, Research, and Clinical Applications. New York, Guilford, 1999

Cassidy JA, Marvin RS, with the MacArthur Working Group on Attachment: Attachment Organization in Three- and Four-Year-Olds: Procedures and Coding Manual. Seattle, WA, unpublished coding manual, 1988

Charlesworth WR: The role of surprise in cognitive development, in Studies in Cognitive Development: Essays. Edited by Elkind D, Flavell JH. London, Oxford University Press, 1969, pp 257–314

Cicchetti D, Schneider-Rosen K: Toward a transactional model of childhood depression. New Dir Child Dev 26:5–27, 1984

Darwin C: The Expression of Emotions in Man and Animals (1872). Chicago, IL, University of Chicago Press, 1965

De Wolff MS, van Ijzendoorn MH: Sensitivity and attachment: a meta-analysis on parental antecedents of infant attachment. Child Dev 68:571–591, 1997

Deci E: Intrinsic Motivation. New York, Plenum, 1977

Dennis W: Causes of retardation among institutionalized children: Iran. Journal of Genetic Psychology 96:47–59, 1960

DesRosiers FS, Busch-Rossnagel NA: Self-concept in toddlers. Infants Young Child 10:15–26, 1997

Donaldson S, Westerman M: Development of children's understanding of ambivalence and causal theories of emotions. Dev Psychol 22:655–662, 1986

Dore J: Monologue as reenvoicement of dialogue, in Narratives From the Crib. Edited by Nelson K. Cambridge, MA, Harvard University Press, 1989, pp 27–73

Dunn J: The Beginnings of Social Understanding. Cambridge, MA, Harvard University Press, 1988

Dunn J, Kendrick C: Siblings. Cambridge, MA, Harvard University Press, 1982

Dunn J, Bretherton I, Munn P: Conversations about feeling states between mothers and their young children, in Symbolic Play: The Development of Social Understanding. Edited by Bretherton I. New York, Academic Press, 1987, pp 132–139

Easterbrooks MA, Goldberg WA: Security of toddler-parent attachment: relation to children's sociopersonality functioning during kindergarten, in Attachment in the Preschool Years: Theory, Research, and Intervention. Edited by Greenberg MT, Cicchetti D, Cummings EM. Chicago, IL, University of Chicago Press, 1990, pp 221–245

Egeland B, Farber EA: Infant-mother attachment: factors related to its development and changes over time. Child Dev 55:753–771, 1984

Egeland B, Kreutzer T: A longitudinal study of the effects of maternal stress and protective factors on the development of high risk children, in Life-Span Developmental Psychology: Perspectives on Stress and Coping. Edited by Green AL, Cummings EM, Karraker KH. Hillsdale, NJ, Lawrence Erlbaum, 1991, pp 61–84

Ekman P, Friesen W, Ellsworth P: Emotions in the Human Face. Elmsford, NY, Pergamon, 1972

Emde RN, Buchsbaum HK: "Didn't you hear my mommy?": autonomy with connectedness in moral self-emergence, in The Self in Transition: Infancy to Childhood. Edited by Cicchetti D, Beeghly M. Chicago, IL, University of Chicago Press, 1990, pp 35–60

Emde RN, Gaensbauer TJ, Harmon RJ: Emotional Expression in Infancy: A Biobehavioral Study. Psychological Issues Monograph No 37. New York, International Universities Press, 1976

Emde RN, Johnson WF, Easterbrooks MA: The dos and don'ts of early moral development: psychoanalytic tradition and current research, in The Emergence of Morality. Edited by Kagan J, Lamb S. Chicago, IL, University of Chicago Press, 1988, pp 245–277

Erikson EH: Studies in interpretation of play, I: clinical observation of child disruption in young children. Genet Psychol Monogr 22:557–671, 1940

Escalona S: The Roots of Individuality. Chicago, IL, Aldine, 1968

Falk D: Primate Diversity. New York, WW Norton, 2000

Fein GG: A transformational analysis of pretending. Dev Psychol 11:291–296, 1975

Fein GG, Apfel N: Some preliminary observations on knowing and pretending, in Symbolic Functioning in Childhood. Edited by Smith N, Franklin M. Hillsdale, NJ, Lawrence Erlbaum Associates, 1979

Feinman S, Lewis M: Social referencing and second order effects in 10-month-old infants. Child Dev 54:878–887, 1983

Feldman R, Greenbaum CW, Yirmiya N: Mother-infant affect synchrony as an antecedent of the emergence of self-control. Dev Psychol 35:223–231, 1999

Fenson L, Ramsay D: Decentration and integration of play in the second year of life. Child Dev 51:171–178, 1980

Fenson L, Kagan J, Kearsely RB, et al: The developmental progression of manipulative play in the first two years. Child Dev 47:232–235, 1976

Field T: Gaze behavior of normal and high-risk infants during early interactions. J Am Acad Child Psychiatry 20:308–317, 1981

Fivush R: Gender and emotion in mother-child conversations about the past. Journal of Narrative and Life History 1:325–341, 1991

Flavell JH, Green FL, Flavell ER: Development of knowledge about the appearance-reality distinction. Monogr Soc Res Child Dev 51:i–v, 1986

Fogel A: Affect dynamics in early infancy: affective tolerance, in Emotion and Early Interaction. Edited by Field T, Fogel A. Hillsdale, NJ, Lawrence Erlbaum, 1982, pp 25–26

Fonagy P, Target M: Attachment and reflective function: their role in self-organization. Dev Psychopathol 9:679–700, 1997

Fonagy P, Gergely G, Jurist E, et al: Affect Regulation, Mentalization, and the Development of the Self. New York, Other Press, 2002

Freud A: Normality and Pathology in Childhood: Assessments of Development. New York, International Universities Press, 1965

Freud S: The interpretation of dreams (1900), in Standard Edition of the Complete Psychological Works of Sigmund Freud, Vols 4 and 5. Translated and edited by Strachey J. London, Hogarth Press, 1953

Gilligan C: In a Different Voice: Psychological Theory and Women's Development. Cambridge, MA, Harvard University Press, 1982

Goldberg S: Social competence in infancy: a model of parent-infant interaction. Merrill Palmer Q 23:163–177, 1977

Goldberg WA, Easterbrooks MA: Toddler development in the family: impact of the father involvement and parenting characteristics. Dev Psychol 55:740–752, 1984

Gouin-Decarie T: Intelligence and Affectivity in Early Childhood: An Experimental Study of Jean Piaget's Object Concept and Object Relations. New York, International Universities Press, 1965

Greenspan SI: Intelligence and Adaptation: An Integration of Psychoanalytic and Piagetian Developmental Psychology. Psychological Issues Monograph No 47–48. New York, International Universities Press, 1979

Greenspan SI: Psychopathology and Adaptation in Infancy and Early Childhood: Principles of Clinical Diagnosis and Preventive Intervention. Clinical Infant Reports No 1. New York, International Universities Press, 1981

Greenspan SI: The development of the ego: insights from clinical work with infants young children. J Am Psychoanal Assoc 36 (suppl):3–55, 1988

Greenspan SI: The development of the ego: biological and environmental specificity and the psychopathological developmental process. J Am Psychoanal Assoc 37:605–638, 1989a

Greenspan SI: The Development of the Ego: Implications for Personality Theory, Psychopathology, and the Psychotherapeutic Process. New York, International Universities Press, 1989b

Greenspan SI: Infancy and Early Childhood: The Practice of Clinical Assessment and Intervention With Emotional and Developmental Challenges. Madison, CT, International Universities Press, 1992

Greenspan SI: Playground Politics: Understanding the Emotional Life of Your School-Age Child. Reading, MA, Addison-Wesley, 1993

Greenspan SI: Developmentally Based Psychotherapy. Madison, CT, International Universities Press, 1997a

Greenspan SI: The Growth of the Mind and the Endangered Origins of Intelligence. Reading, MA, Addison-Wesley Longman, 1997b

Greenspan SI, Porges SW: Psychopathology in infancy and early childhood: clinical perspectives on the organization of sensory and affective-thematic experience. Child Dev 55:49–70, 1984

Greenspan SI, Shanker S: The First Idea: How Symbols, Language, and Intelligence Evolve, From Primates to Humans. Reading, MA, Perseus Books, 2004

Greenspan SI, Wieder S: The Child With Special Needs: Encouraging Intellectual and Emotional Growth. Reading, MA, Perseus Books, 1998

Greenspan SI, Wieder S, Lieberman A, et al: Infants in Multirisk Families: Case Studies in Preventive Intervention. New York, International Universities Press, 1987

Grossmann K, Grossmann KE, Spangler G, et al: Maternal sensitivity and newborns' orientation responses as related to quality of attachment in Northern Germany. Monogr Soc Res Child Dev 50:233–256, 1985

Harlow HF: Motivation as a factor in the acquisition of new responses, in Current Theory and Research in Motivation: A Symposium. Lincoln, University of Nebraska Press, 1953, pp 24–29

Harris PL: Children and Emotion. New York, Basil Blackwell, 1989

Harris PL, Kavanaugh R: Young children's understanding of pretense. Monogr Soc Res Child Dev 58(1, Serial No 231), 1993

Harris PL, Brown E, Marriott C, et al: Monsters, ghosts, and witches: testing the limits of the fantasy-reality distinction in young children. British Journal of Developmental Psychology 9:105–123, 1991

Harter S, Whitesell N: Developmental changes in children's emotion concepts, in Children's Understanding of Emotion. Edited by Saarni C, Harris PL. New York, Cambridge University Press, 1989

Hendrick I: Facts and Theories of Psychoanalysis, 2nd Edition. New York, Knopf, 1939

Hunt JM: Intrinsic motivation and its role in psychological development, in Nebraska Symposium on Motivation, Vol 13. Lincoln, University of Nebraska Press, 1965, pp 189–282

Inhelder B, Lezine I, Sinclair H, et al: Le debut de la function symbolique, in Handbook of Child Psychology, 4th Edition, Vol 4. Edited by Hetherington EM, Mussen PH. New York, Wiley, 1972, pp 187–243

Interdisciplinary Council on Developmental and Learning Disorders Clinical Practice Guidelines Workgroup, SIGC: Interdisciplinary Council on Developmental and Learning Disorders' Clinical practice guidelines: redefining the standards of care for infants, children, and families with special needs. Bethesda, MD, Interdisciplinary Council on Developmental and Learning Disorders, 2000

Izard CE: The Face of Emotion. New York, Meredith & Appleton-Century-Crofts, 1971

Kagan J: The Second Year: The Emergence of Self-Awareness. Cambridge, MA, Harvard University Press, 1981

Kaye K: The Mental and Social Life of Babies: How Parents Create Persons. Chicago, IL, University of Chicago Press, 1982

Kaye K, Fogel A: The temporal structure of face-to-face communication between mothers and infants. Dev Psychol 16:454–464, 1980

Kernberg OF: Borderline Conditions and Pathological Narcissism. New York, Jason Aronson, 1975

Kimmert MD, Campos J, Sorce FJ, et al: Social Referencing: Emotional Expressions as Behavior Regulators, in Emotion: Theory, Research, and Experience, Vol 2: Emotions in Early Development. Edited by Plutchik R, Kellerman H. Orlando, FL, Academic Press, 1983, pp 57–86

Kleinman A: Social Origins of Distress and Disease. New Haven, CT, Yale University Press, 1986

Kohut H: The Analysis of Self: A Systematic Approach to the Psychoanalytic Treatment of Narcissistic Personality Disorders. New York, International Universities Press, 1971

Kraus R, Glucksberg S: The development of communication: competence as a function of age. Child Dev 40:255–266, 1969

Lachman FM, Beebe B: The contribution of self- and mutual regulation to therapeutic action: a case illustration, in The Neurobiological and Developmental Basis for Psychotherapeutic Intervention. Edited by Moskowitz M, Monk C, Kaye C, et al. Northvale, NJ, Jason Aronson, 1997, pp 94–121

La Greca A: Helping Children Cope With Disasters and Terrorism. Washington, DC, American Psychological Association, 2002

Lester BM, Hoffman J, Brazelton TB: The rhythmic structure of mother-infant interaction in term and preterm infants. Child Dev 56:15–27, 1985

Lewis M, Feiring M: Infant, maternal and mother-infant interaction behavior and subsequent attachment. Child Dev 60:831–837, 1987

Lowe M: Trends in the development of representational play in infants from one to three years: an observational study. J Child Psychol Psychiatry 16:33–47, 1975

Lyons-Ruth K, Zeanah C: The family context of infant mental health, I: affective development in the primary caregiving relationship, in Handbook of Infant Mental Health. Edited by Zeanah C. New York, Guilford, 1993, pp 14–37

Mahler MS, Pine F, Bergman A: The Psychological Birth of the Human Infant: Symbiosis and Individuation. New York, Basic Books, 1975

Main M, Kaplan N, Cassidy J: Security in infancy, childhood and adulthood: a move to the level of representation. Monogr Soc Res Child Dev 50:66–104, 1985

Markus H, Kitayama S: Culture and the self: implications for cognition, emotion, and motivation. Psychol Review 98:224–253, 1990

Marvin R, Stewart RB: A family systems framework for the study of attachment, in Attachment in the Preschool Years: Theory, Research, and Intervention. Edited by Greenberg MT, Cicchetti D, Cummings EM. Chicago, IL, University of Chicago Press, 1991, pp 51–87

Maslin-Cole C, Spieker SJ: Attachment as a basis of independent motivation: a view from risk and nonrisk samples, in Attachment in the Preschool Years: Theory, Research, and Intervention. Edited by Greenberg MT, Cicchetti D, Cummings EM. Chicago, IL, University of Chicago Press, 1990, pp 245–272

Matas L, Arend R, Sroufe L: Continuity of adaptation in the second year: the relationship between quality of attachment and later competence. Child Dev 49:547–556, 1978

McCune-Nicholich L: Beyond sensorimotor intelligence: measurement of symbolic sensitivity through analysis of pretend play. Merrill Palmer Q 23:89–99, 1977

Meltzoff A: The roots of social and cognitive development: models of man's original nature, in Social Perception in Infants. Edited by Field TM, Fox NA. Norwood, NJ, Ablex Publishing, 1985, pp 1–30

Meltzoff A: Foundations for developing a concept of self: the role of imitation in relating self to other and the value of social mirroring, social modeling, and self practice in infancy, in The Self in Transition: Infancy to Childhood. Edited by Cicchetti D, Beeghly M. Chicago, IL, Chicago University Press, 1990, pp 139–164

Meltzoff A, Moore K: Imitation of facial and manual gestures by human neonates. Science 198:75–78, 1977

Miyake K, Chen S, Campos J: Infant temperament, mother's mode of interaction, and attachment in Japan: an interim report. Monogr Soc Res Child Dev 50:276–297, 1985

Nelson K: Structure and strategy in learning to talk. Monogr Soc Res Child Dev 38(1–2, Serial No 149), 1973

Nelson K: Event Knowledge: Structure and Function in Development. Hillsdale, NJ, Lawrence Erlbaum, 1986

Nelson K, Gruendel JM: Generalized even representations: basic building blocks of cognitive development, in Advances in Developmental Psychology, Vol 1. Edited by Brown AL, Lamb ME. Hillsdale, NJ, Lawrence Erlbaum, 1981

Osofsky JD, Eberhart-Wright A: Affective exchanges between high risk mothers and infants. Int J Psychoanal 69:221–231, 1988

Papousek H: The common in the uncommon child, in The Uncommon Child. Edited by Lewis M, Rosenblum L. New York, Plenum, 1981, pp 317–328

Papousek H, Papousek M: Early ontogeny of human social interaction: it's biological roots and social dimensions, in Human Ethology: Claims and Limits of a New Discipline. Edited by Foppa K, Lepenies W, Ploog D. New York, Cambridge University Press, 1979, pp 456–489

Pastor D: The quality of mother-infant attachment and its relationship to toddlers' initial sociability with peers. Dev Psychol 23:326–335, 1981

Pederson DR, Moran G, Sitko C, et al: Maternal sensitivity and the security of infant-mother attachment: a Q-sort study. Child Dev 61:1974–1983, 1990

Peller L: Libidinal phases, ego development, and play. Psychoanal Study Child 9:178–198, 1954

Piaget J: The stages of intellectual development of the child, in Childhood Psychopathology. Edited by Harrison S, McDermott J. New York, International Universities Press, 1962, pp 157–166

Pipp-Siegel S, Pressman L: Developing a sense of self and others. Zero to Three 17:17–24, 1996

Pipp S, Fischer KW, Jennings S: Acquisition of self-and-mother knowledge in infancy. Dev Psychol 47:86–96, 1987

Polan HJ, Hofer MA: Psychobiological origins of infant attachment and separation responses, in Handbook of Attachment: Theory, Research, and Clinical Application. Edited by Cassidy J, Shaver PR. New York, Guilford, 1999, pp 162–180

Radke-Yarrow M, Zahn-Waxler C, Chapman M: Children's prosocial dispositions and behavior, in Handbook of Child Psychology, 4th Edition, Vol 4. Edited by Hetherington EM, Mussen PH. New York, Wiley, 1983, pp 469–545

Reiss D: The represented and practicing family: contrasting visions of family continuity, in Relationship Disturbances in Early Childhood. Edited by Sameroff AJ, Emde RN. New York, Basic Books, 1989, pp 191–220

Rheingold H: The social and socializing infant, in Handbook of Socialization Theory and Research. Edited by Goslin D. Chicago, IL, Rand McNally, 1969, pp 779–790

Rothbart MK, Derryberry D: Development of individual differences in temperament, in Advances in Developmental Psychology, Vol 1. Edited by Lamb ME, Brown AL. Hillsdale, NJ, Lawrence Erlbaum, 1981, pp 37–86

Rubin KH, Fein GG, Vandenberg B: Play, in Handbook of Child Psychology, 4th Edition, Vol 4. Edited by Hetherington EM, Mussen PH. New York, Wiley, 1983, pp 136–148

Sander L: Issues in early mother-child interaction. J Am Acad Child Adolesc Psychiatry 1:141–166, 1962

Scaife M, Bruner JS: The capacity for joint visual attention in the infant. Nature 253:265–266, 1975

Schank RC, Abelson RP: Scripts, Plans, Goals, and Understanding. Hillsdale, NJ, Lawrence Erlbaum, 1977

Schweder R, Mahapatra M, Miller J: Cultural and moral development, in The Emergence of Morality in Young Children. Edited by Kagan J, Lamb S. Chicago, IL, University of Chicago Press, 1987, pp 1–90

Sinclair H: The transition from sensorimotor to symbolic activity. Interchange 1:119–126, 1970

Singer DG, Singer JL: The House of Make-Believe: Children's Play and Developing Imagination. Cambridge, MA, Harvard University Press, 1990

Small M: Our Babies, Ourselves: How Biology and Culture Shape the Way We Parent. New York, Anchor Books, 1998

Smetana J: Preschool children's conceptions of transgressions: effects of varying moral and conventional domain-related attributes. Dev Psychol 21:18–29, 1985

Spelke ES, Owsley C: Intermodal exploration and knowledge in infancy. Infant Behavior and Development 2:13–27, 1979

Spitz RA: Hospitalism: an inquiry into the genesis of psychiatric conditions in early childhood. Psychoanal Study Child 1:53–74, 1945

Spitz RA: The First Year of Life: A Psychoanalytic Study of Normal and Deviant Development of Object Relations. New York, International Universities Press, 1965

Sroufe LA: Socioemotional development, in Handbook of Infant Development. Edited by Osofsky J. New York, Wiley, 1979, pp 462–516

Sroufe LA: Infant-caregiver attachment and patterns of adaptation in preschool: the roots of maladaptation and competence, in Minnesota Symposium in Child Psychology. Edited by Perlmutter M. Hillsdale, NJ, Lawrence Erlbaum, 1983, pp 41–83

Sroufe LA: Emotional Development: The Organization of Emotional Life in the Early Years. New York, Cambridge University Press, 1996

Sroufe LA, Waters E: Attachment as an organizational construct. Child Dev 48:1184–1199, 1977

Sroufe LA, Fox NA, Pancake V: Attachment and dependency in developmental perspective. Child Dev 54:1615–1627, 1983

Sroufe LA, Egeland B, Carlson E: One social world: the integrated development of parent-child and peer relationships, in Relationships as Developmental Context: The 29th Minnesota Symposium on Child Psychology. Edited by Collins WA, Laursen B. Hillsdale, NJ, Lawrence Erlbaum, 1999, pp 44–52

Stern D: The goal and structure of mother-infant play. J Am Acad Child Psychiatry 13:402–421, 1974a

Stern D: Mother and infant at play: the dyadic interaction involving facial, vocal, and gaze behaviors, in The Effect of The Infant on Its Caregiver. Edited by Lewis M, Rosenblum L. New York, Wiley, 1974b, pp 187–214

Stern D: The first relationship: mother and infant. Cambridge, MA, Harvard University Press, 1977

Stern D: The early development of schemas of self, of other, and of various experiences of "self with other," in Reflections on Self Psychology. Edited by Lichtenberg J, Kaplan S. Hillsdale, NJ, Analytic Press, 1983, pp 49–84

Stern D: The Interpersonal World of the Infant: A View From Psychoanalysis and Developmental Psychology. New York, Basic Books, 1985

Stewart RB, Marvin R: Sibling relations: the role of conceptual perspective-taking in the ontogeny of sibling caregiving. Child Dev 55:1322–1332, 1984

Talberg G, Couto RJ, O'Donnell ML, et al: Early affect development: empirical research. Int J Psychoanal 69 (part 2): 239–259, 1988

Tennes K, Emde RN, Kisley A, et al: The stimulus barrier in early infancy: an exploration of some formulations of John Benjamin, in Psychoanalysis and Contemporary Science, Vol 1. Edited by Hold R, Peterfreund E. New York, Macmillan, 1972, pp 206–234

Thomas A, Chess S: Genesis and evolution of behavioral disorders: from infancy to early adult life. Am J Psychiatry 141: 1–9, 1984

Trevarthen C: Communication and cooperation in early infancy: a description of primary intersubjectivity, in Before Speech: The Beginning of Interpersonal Communication. Edited by Bullowa MM. Cambridge, England, Cambridge University Press, 1979, pp 321–347

Tronick E: The primacy of social skills in infancy, in Exceptional Infant, Vol 4. Edited by Sawin DB, Hawkins RC, Walker LO, et al. New York, Brunner/Mazel, 1980, pp 144–158

Tronick EZ: Emotions and emotional communication in infants. Am Psychol 44:112–119, 1989

Tronick EZ, Gianino AF Jr: The transmission of maternal disturbance to the infant. New Dir Child Dev 34:5–11, 1986

Ullmann E, Hilweg W: Childhood and Trauma: Separation, Abuse, War. Aldershot, England, Ashgate, 1999

Waelder R: The psychoanalytic theory of play. Psychoanal Q 2:208–224, 1933

Waters E, Wippman J, Sroufe LA: Attachment, positive affect, and competence in the peer group: two studies in construct validation. Child Dev 50:821–829, 1979

Watson J: Behaviorism. New York, People's Institute, 1925

Werner H, Kaplan B: Symbol Formation. New York, Wiley, 1963

White RW: Ego and Reality in Psychoanalytic Theory (Psychol Issues Monogr Vol 11, No 3). New York, International Universities Press, 1963

Winnicott DW: Ego distortion in terms of true and false self, in The Maturational Processes and the Facilitating Environment. New York, International Universities Press, 1960, pp 140–152

Wolf D: Being of several minds, in The Self in Transition. Edited by Cicchetti D, Beeghly M. Chicago, IL, University of Chicago Press, 1990, pp 183–213

Wolf D, Rygh J, Altshuler J: Agency and experience: actions and states in play narratives, in Symbolic Play. Edited by Bretherton I. Orlando, FL, Academic Press, 1984, pp 195–217

Wooley JD, Wellman HM: Young children's understanding of realities, nonrealities, and appearances. Child Dev 61:946–964, 1990

Zahn-Waxler C, Radke-Yarrow M: The development of altruism: alternative research strategies, in The Development of Prosocial Behavior. Edited by Eisenberg M. New York, Academic Press, 1982, pp 109–137

Zahn-Waxler C, Robinson JD, Emde RN: The development of empathy in twins. Dev Psychol 28:1038–1047, 1992

23

Conceptual Research

ANNA URSULA DREHER, Dr.PHIL.

TRANSLATION BY
EVA RISTL

ONE OF THE MAXIMS of Western science was formulated by Descartes, who postulated that ideas should be "clare et distincte," and in fact, scientists are constantly occupied with a task that Peirce (1878), in a classical essay, accurately described as "How to make our ideas clear." Now, after the linguistic turn, we no longer want to make *ideas* "clare et distincte." Today, we are content if the *language*, and especially the concepts we use to convey our ideas and to communicate about the phenomena of interest to us, do not provoke too many misunderstandings, contradictions, and irritations.

In psychoanalysis, it is mostly, but not only, the clinical phenomena that we seek to grasp theoretically. We speak with our patients and reflect about them. However, we do not merely speak *with* our patients; we also speak *about* them—and our interactions with them—and we publish case studies. Language thus has a double function: as ordinary language in the talking cure, and as scientific language when we discuss case studies, introduce our ideas and theories at conferences, or present research findings. In all these contexts, we normally use concepts such as transference and countertransference, trauma and memory, consciousness and unconscious processes, affects and motives, attach-

ment, and many more. In these clinical, as well as scientific, contexts, there is the recurring set of questions: Do these concepts have the same meaning for all of us? Do we, when we use a particular concept, refer to the same phenomena? Do we mean the same thing when we say the same thing?

The complaints about the semantic inexactitude of psychoanalytic concepts—and sometimes about their contradictory or inconsistent use and occasionally about an "anything goes" or even idiosyncratic use—are legend. Yet, arbitrary use overextends concepts, reduces their explanatory and discriminatory power, and, last but not least, makes them less precise, in the same way as an orthodox holding on to traditional uses may freeze a science. The question arises, therefore, whether there can be a reasonable and systematic way to grasp, structure, discuss, and evaluate the differing uses, as well as the differing underlying theoretical understandings of analytic concepts.

Working Definition

Psychoanalytic conceptual research is a possible way to clarify concepts. As a working definition, I offer the fol-

We gratefully acknowledge the Research Advisory Board of the International Psychoanalytical Association for funding of the writing of this chapter and of the translation.

lowing: *conceptual research* is concerned with the systematic and methodical investigation of the explicit and implicit meanings of psychoanalytic concepts and conceptual fields in their clinical and extraclinical use. The subject of scientific investigation is not limited to, for example, clinical *phenomena* such as transference patterns; it can equally encompass changes *in the use of the concept* of transference. To prevent a misunderstanding from the start: conceptual research does not intend to investigate just concepts; rather, it has the aim to clarify the rules of a reasonable concept *use* that meets clinical and scientific requirements.

For this purpose it is useful, first, to reconstruct the important points of change in the history of the concepts and conceptual fields under study. It is equally indispensable, however, to investigate the current use of these concepts—and keep in mind the pressure for change brought about by empirical, particularly clinical, findings and theoretical developments both inside and outside psychoanalysis. The aim of such conceptual studies is not to write a history, but to describe and evaluate a concept in all its relevant meaning aspects. This will help us not only to learn from old mistakes and thus avoid their repetition but also to preserve whatever reasonable elements there are in a concept. Even though it may not be possible to standardize the use of our concepts, it is nonetheless important to find a clarifying communication about commonalities and, in particular, differences—an indispensable precondition for a constructive dialogue within our different analytic schools and cultures as well as with other sciences. One point in advance: *There is no such thing as conceptual research as a unified and standardized procedure*, just as empirical research per se or the experiment as such do not exist. Conceptual research is rather to be understood as a *research program* (Lakatos and Musgrave 1970): if there is research interest, individually planned and structured projects for the clarification of a concept may be initiated.

Some of Freud's Thoughts on the Development of Concepts

Conceptual research thus defines itself by its *subject*, the use of concepts, and its *aim*, the clarification of concepts, the problematical nature and necessity of which were pointed out by Freud (1923/1955):

> Psychoanalysis is not, like philosophies, a system starting out from a few sharply defined basic concepts, seeking to grasp the whole universe with the help of these and, once it is completed, having no room for fresh dis-

coveries or better understanding. On the contrary, it keeps close to the facts in its field of study, seeks to solve the immediate problems of observation, gropes its way forward by the help of experience, is always incomplete and always ready to correct or modify its theories. There is no incongruity (any more than in the case of physics or chemistry) if its most general concepts lack clarity and if its postulates are provisional; it leaves their more precise definition to the results of future work. (pp. 253–254)

In some way, Freud outlined the frame for a *systematic* conceptual reflection, too, when he described psychoanalysis as a science built on the interpretation of the empirical (*Deutung der Empirie*). He said that such a science would

> not envy speculation its privilege of having a smooth, logically unassailable foundation, but will gladly content itself with nebulous, scarcely imaginable basic concepts, which it hopes to apprehend more clearly in the course of its development, or which it is even prepared to replace by others. For these ideas are not the foundations of science, upon which everything rests: that foundation is observation alone. They are not the bottom, but the top of the whole structure, and they can be replaced and discarded without damaging it. (Freud 1914/1957, p. 77)

This characterizes well the field of tension in which our concepts must be seen: on the one hand, concepts need to have clear and consistent—maybe even formal—definitions; on the other hand, concepts should meet clinical requirements.

> [It is only] after more thorough investigation of the field of observation [that] the time may have come to confine them in definitions. The advance of knowledge, however, does not tolerate any rigidity even in definitions. Physics furnishes an excellent illustration of the way in which even "basic concepts" that have been established in the form of definitions are constantly being altered in their content. (Freud 1915/1957, p. 117)

Integration of the "New"

Of course, these problems have not essentially changed since Freud: for our basic concepts, this "constant alteration in content"—an oscillation between preservation and change—still applies. In each science that is still vital, the problem of continually integrating the "new" arises, whereby the new is always confronted with a canon of established concepts. In fact, the new is encountered in psychoanalysis every day in widely ranging forms—in clinical work, in classifying diagnostics, and in research—and raises numerous issues, such as the following:

- Given that the handling of new material that a patient brings to treatment is a determining moment in everyday clinical activity, how should we integrate the new perceptions and experiences into the previous ideas about mode and pattern of transference in the case at hand?
- What happens to our established diagnostic categories when, as has variously occurred in the past decades, specific forms of auto-aggressive behavior, self-mutilation, or eating disorders come increasingly into the focus of clinical as well as theoretical interest? Do we use familiar concepts such as hysteria, or do we develop new diagnostic concepts for this set of symptoms, and if we do, what is the relationship of the new to the old concepts?
- What are the consequences of the "new" knowledge presented by our research for the meaning of concepts? We have seen such an issue raised for some time in infant research, in which some of our developmental concepts—especially the phase theory, based on drive development—are being critically questioned by theories and findings from attachment research. This issue also arises when new findings from imaging procedures change our analytic ideas about how memory functions and how, for instance, psychic traumata are dealt with (see Kandel and Squire 2000; Markowitsch 1999). Traumatic experience changes not only psychic processes—in a certain sense the software (the mind)—but also structures of the brain (the hardware, so to speak) and, thus, the entire course of information processing, especially the possibility to recall memories of the traumatic experience. These findings may even have consequences for clinical work with traumatized people.

Concepts do change; they "live" just like scientific language games in general. Sometimes it is possible to integrate the "new" into our familiar system of concepts, sometimes it may make sense to modify the established use, and sometimes it may be necessary to give up old concepts and introduce new ones. Such change is more clearly seen as we gain greater historical distance from the concept in question. Thus, today—in the light of recent research findings from developmental psychology regarding the different competencies of the infant—we would no longer speak of a "phase of infantile autism," a concept that Mahler still suggested in the 1970s (Mahler et al. 1975). But, of course, there are also recent examples: The empirical findings of Kantrowitz (1997), for instance—the investigations of the patient's impact on the analyst and on the patient-analyst match—have shown that the metaphor of the blank screen for the role and function of the analyst must be abandoned. These examples are intended to illustrate the possible fates of concepts in empirical sciences.

Change and Clarification of Concepts

Thomas Kuhn (1962) has shown that theory change processes in living and evolving sciences are not just linear, cumulative, and continuous but often occur in leaps during moments of crisis and that scientific progress is not necessarily achieved from a steady accumulation of new findings. A modified perspective on the familiar can also be provoked by new methods or by a shift in individually preferred scientific worldviews and mentalities: movements toward cognitive sciences, evolutionary biology, and, currently, the neurosciences ("decade of the brain") are prominent examples in the life sciences. One can see, for instance, how a concept like "declarative and procedural memory systems" flows into our psychoanalytic language games about memory, recall, and the unconscious; in the meantime, analysts also speak of priming effects and episodic memory. Non-negligible parameters in theory development and change also include struggles for institutional power and prestige, for research money, or for securing the "air sovereignty" in discourse for one's own concepts and metaphors—ranging from attempts to dogmatically delineate one's own doctrine to formations of sects. Playing an equal role are factors such as the noncritical taking over of new language games often proposed by idealized authorities. All these factors, also discussed by theorists in the sociology of knowledge, are difficult to grasp but nevertheless influential.

Mechanisms similar to those that are known from the history of sciences regarding theory change as a whole also apply to change in concepts. Sandler (1983) presumed that changes do not show in the same way at all places of our theoretical edifice—and thus not in all concepts simultaneously—but that there are always concepts that are subject to particular tensions and criticism, to a particular pressure to change, and that therefore are of particular interest for conceptual research. Sandler outlined thoughts on the change of psychoanalytic concepts, structurally similar to those of Kuhn on the dynamic change of theories. From his experiences with the London Hampstead Index Project (Bolland and Sandler 1965; Sandler 1987), Sandler proposed to pay special attention to two phenomena: 1) the elasticity of the meaning-space of a concept and 2) the implicit conceptualization by the analyst at work.

An analytic concept can be presented best in an elastic, multidimensional connotative meaning-space, where the number as well as the weighting of dimensions or aspects of meaning may change over time. "Elasticity" of concepts means that concepts can, in a way, react to changes and absorb, endure, and integrate them. Such a view is, of course, different from the conviction that psychoanalytic concepts have an unchanging denotative meaning that can be presented in a formalized form. The way analysts "play" with concepts in an elastic *meaning-space*, in a context-dependent (actually a case-dependent) manner, is, as we know, also a central aspect of the clinician's creative work. Elastic concepts take up the strain of theoretical change, absorbing it, while more organized newer theories or part-theories can develop. But elasticity does not mean elasticity at any price, for it is not so that "anything goes." Achieving an adequate degree of elasticity means walking a fine line between a fixed or even dogmatic definition and a quasi-private concept use. No concept should be overextended or become as arbitrary in its meaning, as has happened lately, for example, to the analytic trauma concept. Blum (2003) describes the situation sharply when he considers the trauma concept as situated between two unsatisfactory poles:

> The concept of psychic trauma has been both unduly compressed and stressed beyond the confines of consensual definition. Trauma may be so narrowly defined that the ego is considered to be totally overwhelmed, with no possibility of adequately registering the trauma or responding to it. At the other extreme, trauma may be loosely identified with any noxious experience or developmental interference. (p. 416)

With the "implicit conceptualizations" by experienced clinicians, Sandler attempted to descriptively grasp a particular process: the usefulness of a concept like transference must show its validity in clinical practice, where each analyst is continually trying to put relevant phenomena into words, thus subsuming them under concepts. The explicit, codified meaning of these concepts often turns out to be unsatisfactory for one's work with an actual patient. As an experienced clinician, one may therefore be tempted to adapt a concept to one's needs, gradually developing a kind of subjective meaning-space, from case to case and from case reflection to case reflection. This subjective meaning-space overlaps with the established one; the one socially shared with the reference group but, nevertheless, possibly showing interesting divergences.

These processes are implicit to the extent that they are, often for a long time, not precisely put into words, let alone published. It is not unusual for scientists to reflect on these adaptation processes of concepts and to *systematically* attempt to make the boundary between "explicit" and "implicit" more permeable. For instance, a working party of the European Psychoanalytic Federation (whose members are Werner Bohleber, Jorge Canestri, Paul Denis, Peter Fonagy) is currently trying to grasp the implicit conceptualizations of analysts. On the basis of extensively documented clinical material (verbal remarks, nonverbal

and emotional reactions, interpretations, perceptions, ideas and reflections of the analyst), the working party is attempting to identify, in addition to the public theories, the analyst's implicit theories in order to construct a grid for mapping private (implicit) theories in clinical practice. Similar research work to clarify analysts' concept use by eliciting the implicit conceptualizations can be found in work by Sandler and colleagues (1987) concerning the use of the concept "psychic trauma."

An Example: The Meaning-Space of "Transference"

What is to be understood by this meaning-space can be briefly illustrated with the concept of transference, surely one of our most important clinical concepts, with a long, complex history (see Sandler et al. 1992). The concept lends itself well to demonstrate a problem that presents itself similarly with many of our concepts, namely, the *reference problem*: What are we referring to in the world when we speak of transference? According to Freud: to a burnt-in cliché—that is, to an unconscious, ontogenetically acquired relationship pattern that is being actualized in the here and now of the analytic encounter. Is this pattern observable? This question is not easy to answer, because for psychoanalysis transference is primarily not an observable behavior, nor is it simply a manifest narrative or just a repetitive pattern of affect. Rather, transference is a theoretical concept under which an analyst subsumes a number of clinical perceptions and experiences. There is, therefore, no behavior that as such *is* transference. There are only very different phenomena that in the clinical situation can be *seen* and interpreted *as* indicators of transference, and these are essentially unconscious patterns.

If one were to subject the concept of transference to a systematic meaning analysis, the following dimensions or aspects of meaning based on clinical phenomena would result (see also Dreher 1999):

- *Repetition*—addressed by Freud in his idea of new editions of indelible impressions of a stereotype template originating early in a patient's life history
- *Change over time*—concerned with the question of if and how transference patterns change over a lifetime and how new editions are elaborated through "deferred action" *(Nachträglichkeit)*
- *Form of appearance*—dealing with the problem of whether transference phenomena are expressed in narrative or enacted form and, especially, by what pattern of affects they are accompanied

- *Meaning of unconscious elements in narratives as well as in enactments*
- *Relevance of interactive processes*—looking at the meaning and role of the transference, as well as the interplay of transference, countertransference, and the analytic situation
- *Psychic functionality*—asking how the "here and now" is connected with the "there and then"

This list is certainly not exhaustive, although it includes the most important aspects of the meaning-space of "transference." Only the consideration of all aspects—that is, a holistic view of the concept—makes it useful for our work in the clinical situation. It is this very complexity and richness of the concept that have made it so powerful and effective in the history of psychoanalysis—a complexity that is sometimes lost when the concept is applied in research contexts.

There have been, for instance, a number of attempts to grasp transference phenomena by measuring it. One of these procedures, the Core Conflictual Relationship Theme (CCRT) method of Luborsky (Luborsky and Crits-Christoph 1990), aims to "understand transference" by enabling external raters to extract, on the basis of transcribed manifest narratives, the core relationship conflicts of a person. The method proceeds in a very differentiated and systematic way and is suitable for distilling manifest relationship conflicts from narratives. Equally, no one would argue that such conflicts are irrelevant to transference. The procedure can, however, capture only one of many clinically relevant aspects of transference. Neither the unconscious moments, nor the enacted transference reactions, nor the intertwining with countertransference, nor the questions about psychic functionality can be adequately grasped with this method. Not infrequently, a *pars pro toto* mistake shows up when analytic concepts are operationalized in empiristic research technologies: one manages to grasp one, certainly important, aspect among many, but one fails to do justice to the complexity of analytic concepts. There is often the danger of "oversimplification" (A. Green, quoted in Sandler et al. 2000)—or, as I would put it, the danger of an empiristic flattening of analytic concepts in the research process.

Specific Features of Psychoanalytic Concepts

Psychoanalytic concepts have a number of particular qualities that make it difficult to grasp the corresponding phenomena by way of observation or measurement. First, these concepts are interwoven with the place where many analytic concepts have their historical origin: the central place where they must prove their worth—the analytic situation. In the latter place, analysts gain a special kind of experience with other people and with themselves, and some even consider this kind of experience unique. Two subjects, patient and analyst, meet each other, and it does not satisfy a psychoanalytic consideration merely to objectively register the behavior of the two actors; the analytic consideration is above all concerned with the attention to and the understanding of two dynamically intertwined inner worlds, including their conscious and unconscious determinants. Two biographical pasts meet each other—pasts we think of not simply as stored in and recallable from episodic memory systems, but also as, for instance, represented in the past and present unconscious (see Tulving 2002 for a discussion of episodic memory).

A particular role therein is played by the tension between psychic reality and external reality, two realities that are not just simply in a representational relationship that could be constructed by objective methods. Analysts attempt to put the totality of these experiences in the analytic situation into scientific language, to make them communicable, replicable, and subject to criticism via the concepts used. The meaning of these clinical concepts refers particularly to the *subjectivity* of the analytic experience, including the controlled emotional participation of the analyst in the analytic process, as well as his or her attention to, for instance, his or her own bodily reactions—a subjectivity not easily accessible from an objectivizing, third-person perspective.

Another specific feature of analytic concepts is that their complexity is increased by the fact that their meanings are embedded into the theoretical presuppositions of the analytic *Weltbild*—namely, the ideas about structure and function of the human psyche. This feature can cause problems at times when the concepts are used in contexts other than clinical ones. Our ideas about conscious and dynamically unconscious processes, our thoughts about how object relations are sedimented, and our analytic convictions about the effects of drives and affects, about fantasies and cognitions, and about experience and behavior are certainly not shared by everyone. There are, indeed, still fundamental differences between the analytic model of the mind and, for example, empiristic, cognitivistic, and neuroscientific models.

Beyond all that, the person of the analyst is also relevant for the use of concepts from a rather different perspective: concepts are in a special way tied to the analytic identity of practicing and researching analysts. Analytic concepts are part of our everyday, usually unquestioned, toolbox, the inventory of terms that are taken for granted to describe reality. It requires some effort to take a distanced or even critical attitude toward one's own concept use. Perhaps it is this very matter-of-course quality of one's concepts that is a source of resistance against any other conceptual understanding, particularly since in many cases analysts create their identity through analytic socialization and by using the language of their analytic reference group or research cohort. Not infrequently, the rules of the narcissism of the small difference apply here: the closer the conceptual understanding of two discussants, the more pronounced their criticism and delineation must become. Such mechanisms are obstacles for any communication about concepts and about proposals for their change.

Further Sources of Variety in Concept Use

Of course all this explains only to a certain extent the great variety in the use of our concepts. Some further factors can be identified:

1. The long history of analytic schools, in the wake of which traditions of partly hermetically closed language games came into existence, which in most cases were linked to prominent names such as Freud, Jung, Klein, Bion, Winnicott, Kohut, and Lacan
2. The history of the worldwide spread of psychoanalysis, with its differentiated regional cultures (Here it is not sufficient to distinguish an Anglo-Saxon North American, Continental European, or South American psychoanalysis; the differences can be traced to the individual societies and subgroups. From a conceptual research viewpoint, it would be a useful endeavor to work out an up-to-date taxonomy of the regional analytic dialects.)
3. The different convictions as to which epistemological status psychoanalysis has or should strive for in the canon of sciences (The range of opinions goes from a strictly empirically oriented, natural science–based understanding to a hermeneutic one, with an orientation at the single clinical case, to opinions attributing to psychoanalysis a status of complete independence and uniqueness—each with a specific view about function and meaning of concepts.)
4. The changed understanding of concepts that may be brought about by the desired closeness of psychoanalysis to one of the currently prominent sciences (biology, cognitive science, or, the latest trend, neuroscience) if a transfer of knowledge or an approximation to their respective language games is wished

5. The consequences of embedding psychoanalysis into the different medical, and thus economic, systems of various countries (One should name here the often criticized so-called medicocentrism [Parin and Parin-Matthèy 1986]—namely, the subsuming of psychoanalytic thinking and psychoanalytic concepts under a strictly medical view of nosology, diagnostics, and therapy. One may mention, in this context, answers to important questions such as, What is normal? To what degree can mental disturbances be understood as an illness? and What are the possible aims of an analytic cure? [Dreher 2002; Sandler and Dreher 1996].)

Whatever other factors may have generated the variety in use of analytic concepts, this situation is judged differently: some complain about the Babel of languages, while others do not. Some recognize a creative evolutionary potential here, whereas others see a danger for the unity of psychoanalysis, and there are good reasons, by all means, for both points of view. Yet, what remains the indispensable basis and impetus for concept development has been known since Freud: "observation alone"—that is, the observations in the clinical situation and the constant attempts to conceptualize them adequately. Between these two spheres—the phenomena and the language used to describe them—lies the "practical-theoretical gap" that Green describes: "No theory will ever be able to cover all of the field of psychoanalytic practice, and no psychoanalytic practice will fit totally and exactly within the limits of the field of any existent theory" (Green 2003, p. 29). The question is, however, Does this gap have to remain invariably wide, a *mysterious* gap forever? Put another way: Don't the constant attempts to differentiate concepts and make them more precise express the continuous effort to grasp the phenomena ever better with language and, if the practical-theoretical gap cannot be closed completely, at least to minimize the gap to the fullest extent possible? So what would a *systematic* as well as *methodical* approach look like that would be useful in reducing the long-standing conceptual confusion?

History and Practice of Conceptual Research in Psychoanalysis: Some Examples

If we were to list everything that might be helpful for the clarification of a concept, we might find the following thematic areas, each with corresponding questions:

- The investigation of the historical context of a concept's origin (Which problems was the concept intended to solve when it came into being?)

- The history of a concept's use viewed against changes of psychoanalytic theory (Were there changes, and if so, which were the main changes in the understanding of the concept?)
- The current use of a concept in clinical and extraclinical practice (Which are the most important variants of current usage, and to which extent are they compatible?)
- A critical discussion and, possibly, formulation of a suggestion for a different use of the concept (Which well-founded suggestions could be made for a better use?)

To integrate these aspects and to do justice to each of them, we must of course use different research methods. A systematic literature analysis, for instance, also committed to philological standards, would help in reconstructing the development of a concept by allowing us to map out the crucial points of its change in analytic history since Freud (as demonstrated by Sandler et al. 1992 regarding concepts relevant to the therapeutic process; see also Sandler et al. 1997). In addition, such studies can contribute to a *preliminary* clarification of the concept or help identify and work out any residual ambiguities. Furthermore, systematic conceptual research comprises procedures that allow us to generate evidence of the explicit as well as implicit use of a concept *in clinical practice* (e.g., by way of expert interviews). Here one has to consider one particular aspect that turns this kind of research into a *psychoanalytic* one: while it is true that a simple inventory of the present use of a concept could be put together by applying behaviorist or philological methods, it is not sufficient when we want to include aspects of a concept's current use in clinical work, especially those aspects that have not yet been made explicit.

As a historical prototype of such conceptual research, we can see the work of the already mentioned Hampstead Index Project, in which a research team of analysts attempted to systematically categorize, on the basis of small units of observation from analytic treatments, these observations under analytic concepts, in close discussion with the analysts treating the respective patient. At times, these categorizations turned out to be not so simple, causing quite controversial discussions about how the analysts themselves understood the material of their cases and which concepts would best grasp the respective units. This lack of agreement in turn provoked attempts at clarification through discourse about the concepts themselves.

With similar interests in the use of analytic concepts, a group of researchers at the Sigmund Freud Institute in Frankfurt, Germany, instigated a project in the 1980s that investigated the concept of psychic trauma (Sandler et al. 1987, 1991). At the time, the concept had been chosen because it played a central role in the formulation of post-

traumatic stress disorder, which the Vietnam veterans' associations had fought for; in the debates of the false memory phenomenon in the context of sexual abuse; and in attempts to understand experiences from the treatment of Holocaust victims, linked to the questions of if and how it is possible that traumatizations could be transferred from one generation to another. In all these considerations and discussions, the use of the concept had undergone a considerable extension.

Along with questions concerning contents, the main purpose of the Frankfurt pilot study was, however, to develop an inventory of methods for conceptual research. (A discussion of the research procedures and results of this project and also of the Hampstead Index itself can be found in Dreher 2000.) Among other methods (e.g., the already mentioned literature analysis), this inventory comprised semistructured interviews *by* experienced psychoanalytic clinicians, members of the research project (in the role of conceptual researchers), *of* experienced psychoanalytic clinicians (in the role of "experimental subjects"). The latter were asked to present three case studies in which "trauma" had played a central role and to discuss them with the interviewers. The data gathered were then analyzed and evaluated in group discussions by the researchers of the project. Eliciting implicit aspects of the concept's use from the explicit statements of the trauma experts was a central task. Of course, the results reflect the state of the discussion 20 years ago—and thus are predominantly of historical value only. Today, as the trauma concept is much more a focus of wider interest, not only of psychoanalytic interest, an update is warranted, especially against the background of neuroscientific findings on how trauma is dealt with.

Of course, there are many more current "hot spots" in the analytic theoretical edifice, such as the concept *unconscious*, for example, which is being increasingly used by memory researchers. In which sense do they use this term? In psychoanalysis the meaning of *unconscious* is essentially based on Freud's considerations and has been clinically confirmed over decades. In memory psychology, on the other hand, the meaning of "unconscious" is based on manifold *experimental* results and is closely related to the concepts of implicit memory and implicit knowledge or also to that *anoetic* quality of memory systems, a term that Tulving (2002) used to describe those memory contents not accessible to consciousness. Psychoanalysis, which in the past was certainly not unjustly called the "science of the unconscious," has evidently lost its monopoly on the concept *unconscious*, and it would be of great current interest to clarify the conceptual field surrounding this concept and to contour the specific psychoanalytic connotation of "*dynamic* unconscious."

Many studies in psychoanalysis have focused on concepts, and it is useful to consider them definitely as expressions of a "research program" with a common methodological justification. A retrospective review reveals *precursors* of such *systematic* conceptual investigations already in Freud's work, when he practiced the integration of empirical investigation and conceptual differentiation that we can see in, for example, the concepts of *sexual* or *unconscious* (see particularly Lecture 20 in Freud 1916–1917/1957). Indeed, conceptual studies have a long tradition, and I would just like to mention a few briefly: MacIntyre's (1958) work advises against the use of "the Unconscious" as a noun because of the danger of an ontological misunderstanding, suggesting instead an adjectival use as in "unconscious processes." Pulver (1970) warned against an inflationary use of the term *narcissism*, and certainly there are the prominent dictionaries of psychoanalysis that are the result of careful investigation by groups of researchers. These encyclopedias are useful tools in orientating oneself better among the variety of concept meanings. In the analytic tradition, Laplanche and Pontalis (1973), then also Moore and Fine (1990), have been reliable companions; the more recent volume by de Mijolla (2002) will perhaps play this role in the future. What becomes evident in such a chronological sequence, however, is that even excellent dictionaries of basic analytic terms, though competent aggregations of the knowledge and understanding of their decade, need to be updated from time to time. The *modified* understanding of a central concept such as *narcissism*, for instance—an understanding initiated by Kohut's work and not yet included by Laplanche and Pontalis but systematically integrated by Moore and Fine—may serve as an illustration.

In the history of psychoanalysis, attempts to clarify concepts in discourse are, especially in the English-speaking world, nothing new. One must only think of *concept study groups* at individual analytic institutes that see their work as just that: the *study* of concepts. The work of the members of these study groups contributes to the clarification of their own use of concepts but does not necessarily lead to publications. An excellent example is the renowned Ernst Kris Study Group of the New York Psychoanalytic Institute. (Its work is documented in the monograph series of the Kris Study Group; see, e.g., Fine et al. 1971; Abend et al. 1986.)

The explicit intention to discuss concepts controversially as well as to seek consensus or record dissent can be found especially in *panel discussions* on a concept. Such panels have a typical pattern, with speech, reply, and conclusion from all arguments, and can definitely be seen in the tradition of the Socratic dialogues. A closer look at this predominantly American tradition shows how imaginative and clarifying such investigations can be, and they could surely be characterized as a *variant* of conceptual research (see Blacker 1981; Escoll 1983; Rothstein 1983).

Panel discussions typically follow a specific procedure:

1. Historical retrospective on the concept's use, with reference to current inconsistencies or contradictions
2. Presentations of concept usage by proponents of the different theoretical orientations, based especially on how they use the concepts in their own clinical practice
3. Plenary discussion on the different concept usages
4. A summary and synthesis, by the chairperson, of the arguments
5. A published report by the panel reporter (making the discussion accessible to a scientific public), as in the long-standing tradition of such reports in the *Journal of the American Psychoanalytic Association*

The aim of these panels is to clarify concepts by simultaneously including clinical experience und theoretical convictions. Panels and the concept study groups are established and generally accepted *models* for activities that, so to speak, meet the minimum requirements for conceptual *research*.

An Intermediate Remark: Conceptual Reflection— Conceptual Research

The idea that an autonomous conceptual research could yield gains, for both clinical work and scientific endeavors, has become accepted in contemporary psychoanalysis. The Hampstead and, later, the Frankfurt project groups initially used the term *conceptual research* only as a loose working title; in the meantime, the *label* has established itself. Who is doing conceptual research? Every clinician who uses a concept to describe his or her case? Every empirical researcher who tries, as part of a study, to transfer aspects of a concept into measuring procedures for the purpose of operationalization? Anyone who thinks about a concept anywhere in any way, or who criticizes how others use a concept? Of course, *psychoanalytic conceptual research* is not a protected term. However, I suggest making a distinction between conceptual research and conceptual reflection—one that can be seen as complementary to the above-mentioned working definition:

- Reserve the term conceptual *research* for activities that are exploring the use of concepts, including their function in conceptual fields, in a systematic way and applying adequate—empirical as well as hermeneutic—methods.

- Distinguish between *reflection* on concepts and conceptual *research*. Conceptual reflection is a necessary, but not a sufficient, condition for conceptual research. Whoever *reflects* on concepts (actually a routine activity for every clinician and researcher) is certainly doing something important and useful, yet this activity does not automatically qualify as *research*.

Some Essentials of the Research Process

Beyond the ever-important reflection in conceptual research, there is first a need for *appropriate* empirical data. Such data alone can reflect a concept's actual use and show how a concept is used in practice and how its users illustrate and legitimize its use. In arriving at a comprehensive picture of both issues, factual use and justification of that use, it is not enough to select suitable methods; it is, in particular, also important to choose representative samples, either historical authors, experts, or clinical practitioners.

The actual questions under study may of course vary considerably with regard to the desired historical longitudinal perspective, as well as the current cross section that is of interest. The inventory of possible methods is very broad, ranging from different forms of literature analysis, to various interview techniques (from nonstructured to structured interviews), to questionnaires, expert ratings, group discussions, and the like. As far as the logical consistency of conceptual fields is concerned, simulation models may indeed be useful. Especially when we are dealing with expert knowledge, the circle of specialists does not have to be limited to psychoanalysts. Thus, in any consideration of the canon of conceptual research methods, exactly the same caveats apply that are pertinent to any other kind of research. Methods are, above all, means to an end, and the all-important question is whether they contribute to reaching the aim: suggestions for an improved concept use for the scientific community.

That structuring reflection and discussion in a research team belong to the procedure of a research process is well understood; however, it is not so obvious that this *discourse* is being *systematically applied* and considered as *essential*. Without such attempts to communicate about the rules of concept use and to look for social consensus—in addition to the historical and empirical inventory of methods—the aim of conceptual research would hardly be attainable. In the course of such a research process, a concept is repeatedly put on the test-bench of reflection, discussion, and criticism by the members of the research team: on the basis of their previous knowledge and the systematically ac-

quired knowledge base, the research team must consider and integrate the clinical understanding extracted from the data collection, as well as the aggregated expert knowledge. The structure of this procedure, oriented equally by hermeneutic as well as empirical principles, is designed to gradually elaborate the meaning-space of a concept. Such working through, with the aim of continually approaching a better concept use, is at its best that "progressive spiral" described within the context of the Hampstead Index Project (Sandler 1987; see also Leuzinger-Bohleber et al. 2003 for a discussion of these research questions).

In its claim, conceptual research goes beyond the limits of school traditions and is often interdisciplinary, too; the bond to our *common ground* should not, however, be lost. Therefore, the integration of clinical knowledge is indispensable. Making sure that this essential meaning of our concepts remains preserved and no reduction occurs thus becomes a gripping tightrope walk between preservation and change.

Some Methodological Problems

Having described how conceptual research works, I now turn to some issues regarding the scientific status of such research.

Especially researchers from empiristic traditions hold the view that only observable—or, even better, measurable—phenomena can be the subject of research. Furthermore, the methods applied should be oriented toward the ideal of the experiment in the natural sciences. The aim of such studies is to formalize theories and models with as much explanatory and predictive power as possible. For many it is above all the choice of the *right method* that will determine whether something is seen as *scientific*.

Conceptual research defines itself not primarily by its methods, but by its subject, the use of concepts, and by its aim, their clarification. Conceptual research is in its procedure *empirical*, when factually describing concept use, as well as *historico-reconstructive*, when tracing a concept's development, and *evaluative*, when involving critical discussion of the collected data and the elaboration of proposals for clinically and scientifically adequate use. In serving these different functions, it is self-evident that conceptual research has to use different methods from various research traditions.

Conceptual research, like empirical research, can recur to qualitative as well as quantitative methods. Nevertheless, because of the subject of interest, it is understood that conceptual research works intensively with language use and meaning-spaces; in addition to the data collection used in describing the concept use, an essential aspect is the analysis and interpretation of verbal data (e.g., from expert interviews or group discussions) and, thus, the application of *hermeneutic methods*, well known and familiar to us analysts. This central attention to language, both as a subject of research and as a data source, can be disturbing only when words are considered as opaque and numbers are always considered to be exact. Where conceptual research and empirical research do indeed differ is in their research *interest*, not necessarily in the class of methods applied, and not at all in their intention to improve analytic knowledge.

Occasionally, when we find analytic research activities divided, for instance, into empirical, clinical, and conceptual research, we may be left with the impression that these traditions stand rather unconnectedly side by side, or are even in competition. Such a view would be reductionist. Only constructive cooperation and mutual acknowledgement will do justice to our complex area of research; only then is the analytic essence in the best Freudian sense, the close relationship between the empirical and the concept, preserved in both contexts, clinic and research. The necessity of *interdependent cooperation* among analytic research traditions is not seen in the same way by all. Target and Fonagy (2003) write, for example: "We do not see a 'developmental line' between conceptual (hypothesis-generating) and empirical (hypothesis-testing) research but, rather, a complementarity" (p. 166).

What becomes visible here, besides the reduction of conceptual research to a merely *complementary* partner of empirical research, is a second misunderstanding: conceptual research is supposed to be hypothesis-generating, while empirical research is supposed to be hypothesis-testing. Behind this differentiation stands the useful separation of two aspects of *each* research process: a creative aspect, the context of discovery, and an affirmative aspect, the context of justification. However, as conceptual research is not concerned with explanation and prediction, but with description, reconstruction, and evaluation, it is not interested in the generating and testing of hypotheses in the same way as empiricism. Most empirical researchers would, by the way, definitely see a developmental line between hypothesis-generation and hypothesis-testing, as it is precisely from this constructive connection of both aspects of each research process that the empirical research technologies result.

In the context of such technologies, one important step concerns the relation between concepts and the phenomena to be investigated. This step is usually called "operationalization" and requires the researcher to determine what in a concept should be precisely observed and measured and which methodic procedures should be used to grasp the aspects of the concept. From the perspective of conceptual research, such detailed definition presents an advantage, compared with some diffuse or idiosyncratic concept use, for it makes its rules traceable. However, just as a concept can be understood differently, it can also be operationalized very differently. The concept of transference is a good example of how various researchers, each with their own technologies, try to grasp transference phenomena on the basis of different operationalizations. These various operationalizations and the conceptual understandings on which they are based can be—as a kind of concept use—compared and evaluated.

It is clear that psychoanalytic concepts present some difficulties within this step of operationalization, since the analysis of the meaning of our concepts requires that we take into account our basic concepts, that is, our *model of the mind*. Thus, for instance, from an analytic perspective, many psychic processes are seen to be dynamically unconscious and, although not directly observable, ascertainable as the result of a process of interpretation and inference. Such a problem—namely, the dependence of the meaning of concepts on preassumptions about the functioning of the psyche—is not that of psychoanalysis alone. The convictions of many cognitive scientists and some neuroscientists are based on the *preassumption*, again not shared by all, that the human mind functions like a computer and that it may actually even be one. Of course, the computer metaphor is considered more "modern" than the system of our fundamental convictions derived from Freud's metapsychological ideas; but that this image of man is generally better, or clinically more adequate, than an analytic one may well be contested.

What makes the handling of our concepts more difficult in the research context is certainly that they change over the course of time. Conceptual research is characterized by its particular interest for these concept *changes*. But—besides the progress in clinical experience and scientific research already mentioned—what actually are the historical and social reasons for concept changes? It should be clear by now that for conceptual investigations, the relationship between language and world, between a concept and the pertaining empirical phenomena, is not simply a two-digit relation, but, according to old semiotic tradition, a triangular one. The person of the concept user comes into play, and thus the dependence of the concept's meaning on historically grown, socially shared language games embedded in different cultures and human life forms. If one adequately considers this matrix, one can become sensitized to the contingent use of concepts. In examining such, in the largest sense, cultural dependencies, conceptual studies can also take the perspective of cultural theory (*Kulturtheorie*), for the changing trends in the research landscape—not only subjects, methods, and aims but also power and organizational structures and the conceptual understanding linked with all these—cannot be principally withdrawn from reflection: What exactly were the reasons two decades ago for the shift in analytic research interests toward empiricism? How do treatment aims change as a function of socioeconomic changes in the health systems? What are the reasons for the current trend toward concepts? All these questions might be addressed in the context of conceptual research in order to further our understanding of conceptual changes.

Conclusion

If we consider conceptual research as a research *program*, we can then undertake a series of different activities examining various areas with different questions. What may also differ are the criteria for concept use that are strived for. Whereas one researcher may mainly be concerned with the logical consistency of conceptual fields, another may be concerned with an intersubjective consensual and reliable grasping of phenomena by standardized instruments. Nevertheless, the decisive point is always the usefulness of our concepts in the clinical situation. In that respect *psychoanalytic* conceptual research is always integrative, in the sense that it takes the different research results on a concept's use into account—focusing on the question whether a concept meets clinical *and* scientific requirements equally well.

Systematic reflections on a concept and its use do not automatically lead to a better understanding among different disciplines; they also do not bring a unified psychoanalysis back. But they can help to make the knowledge about commonalities and differences more precise, and this in turn could facilitate debate. Differing convictions on the meaning of a concept should be not only acknowledged but also examined, as otherwise multiple uses or arbitrary eclecticism may increase. Conceptual research can, by making its own suggestions, stimulate discussions, or at best moderate the discourse, but it cannot lead it alone. A reasonable concept use can in effect be achieved only through good arguments and consensus. Just as the empirical and the conceptual are in a dialectic relationship with each other, so psychoanalytic research activities that have either empirical phenomena or a concept as their subject are dependent on one another. Conceptual research without recourse to the findings from empirical research can be a glass bead game; empirical research without adequate conceptual understanding can be without clinical relevance. Cooperation is conceivable, when it is based on an *acknowl-edgement* of the different methodologies, and not on claims of exclusiveness, as researchers and clinicians strive for a common aim: a theory on a solid empirical basis formulated with good concepts.

References

Abend SM, Porder MS, Willick MS: Borderline Patients: Psychoanalytic Perspectives—The Kris Study Group of the New York Psychoanalytic Institute Monograph No 7. Madison, CT, International Universities Press, 1986

Blacker KH (Reporter): Panel—Insight: clinical conceptualizations. J Am Psychoanal Assoc 29:659–671, 1981

Blum HP: Psychic trauma and traumatic object loss. J Am Psychoanal Assoc 51:415–432, 2003

Bolland J, Sandler J: The Hampstead Psychoanalytic Index: A Study of the Psychoanalytic Case Material of a 2-Year-Old Child. New York, International Universities Press, 1965

de Mijolla A: Dictionnaire International de la Psychanalyse. Paris, Calmann-Levy, 2002

Dreher AU: Was sollte man bedenken, wenn man Übertragung messen will. Zeitschrift für psychoanalytische Theorie und Praxis 14:260–283, 1999

Dreher AU: Foundations for Conceptual Research in Psychoanalysis. Madison, CT, International Universities Press, 2000

Dreher AU: What are the aims of psychoanalysts? in Outcomes in Psychoanalytic Treatment. Edited by Leuzinger-Bohleber M, Target M. London, Whurr, 2002, pp 17–29

Escoll PJ (Reporter): Panel—The changing vistas of transference: the effect of developmental concepts on the understanding of transference. J Am Psychoanal Assoc 31:699–711, 1983

Fine BD, Joseph ED, Waldhorn HF: Recollection and Reconstruction—Reconstruction in Psychoanalysis. The Ernst Kris Study Group of the New York Psychoanalytic Institute Monograph 4. New York, International Universities Press, 1971

Freud S: On narcissism: an introduction (1914), in Standard Edition of the Complete Psychological Works of Sigmund Freud, Vol 14. Translated and edited by Strachey J. London, Hogarth Press, 1957, pp 67–102

Freud S: Instincts and their vicissitudes (1915), in Standard Edition of the Complete Psychological Works of Sigmund Freud, Vol 14. Translated and edited by Strachey J. London, Hogarth Press, 1957, pp 111–116

Freud S: Introductory lectures on psychoanalysis (1916–1917), in Standard Edition of the Complete Psychological Works of Sigmund Freud, Vols 15–16. Translated and edited by Strachey J. London, Hogarth Press, 1957, pp 303–319

Freud S: Two encyclopaedia articles (1923), in Standard Edition of the Complete Psychological Works of Sigmund Freud, Vol 18. Translated and edited by Strachey J. London, Hogarth Press, 1955, pp 235–259

Green A: The pluralism of sciences and psychoanalytic thinking, in Pluralism and Unity? Methods of Research in Psychoanalysis. Edited by Leuzinger-Bohleber M, Dreher AU, Canestri J. London, International Psychoanalytical Association, 2003, pp 26–44

Kandel ER, Squire LR: Neuroscience: breaking down scientific barriers to the study of brain and mind. Science 290:1113–1120, 2000

Kantrowitz JL: The Patient's Impact on the Analyst. Hillsdale, NJ, Analytic Press, 1997

Kuhn TS: The Structure of Scientific Revolutions. Chicago, IL, University of Chicago Press, 1962

Lakatos I, Musgrave A (eds): Criticism and the Growth of Knowledge. Cambridge, England, Cambridge University Press, 1970

Laplanche J, Pontalis J-B: The Language of Psycho-Analysis. London, Karnac Books, 1973

Leuzinger-Bohleber M, Dreher AU, Canestri J (eds): Pluralism and Unity? Methods of Research in Psychoanalysis. London, International Psychoanalytical Association, 2003

Luborsky L, Crits-Christoph P (eds): Understanding Transference: The Core Conflictual Relationship Theme Method. New York, Basic Books, 1990

MacIntyre AC: The Unconscious: A Conceptual Analysis. London, Routledge & Kegan Paul, 1958

Mahler MS, Pine F, Bergman A: The Psychological Birth of the Human Infant: Symbiosis and Individuation. New York, Basic Books, 1975

Markowitsch HJ: Stress-related memory disorders, in Cognitive Neuroscience of Memory. Edited by Nilson LG, Markowitsch HJ. Göttingen, Germany, Hogrefe, 1999, pp 193–211

Moore BE, Fine BD (eds): Psychoanalytic Terms and Concepts. New Haven, CT, American Psychoanalytic Association/Yale University Press, 1990

Parin P, Parin-Matthèy G: Medicozentrismus, in Subjekt im Widerspruch, Aufsätze 1978–1985. Frankfurt am Main, Germany, Syndikat, 1986, pp 61–80

Peirce CS: How to make our ideas clear. Popular Science Monthly 12:286–302, 1878

Pulver SE: Narcissism: the term and the concept. J Am Psychoanal Assoc 18:319–341, 1970

Rothstein A (Reporter): Panel—Interpretation: toward a contemporary understanding of the term. J Am Psychoanal Assoc 31:237–245, 1983

Sandler J: Reflections on some relations between psychoanalytic concepts and psychoanalytic practice. Int J Pyschoanal 64:35–45, 1983

Sandler J (ed): From Safety to Superego: Selected Papers of Joseph Sandler. London, Karnac Books, 1987

Sandler J, Dreher AU: What Do Psychoanalysts Want? The Problem of Aims in Psychoanalytic Therapy. London, Routledge, 1996

Sandler J, Dreher AU, Drews S, et al: Psychisches Trauma: Ein Konzept im Theorie-Praxis-Zusammenhang. Materialien aus dem Sigmund-Freud-Institut, Frankfurt am Main 5, 1987

Sandler J, Dreher AU, Drews S: An approach to conceptual research in psychoanalysis illustrated by the consideration of psychic trauma. Int Rev Psychoanal 18:133–141, 1991

Sandler J, Dare C, Holder A: The Patient and the Analyst: The Basis of the Psychoanalytic Process, 2nd Edition. London, Karnac Books, 1992

Sandler J, Dare C, Holder A, et al: Freud's Models of the Mind: An Introduction. London, Karnac Books, 1997

Sandler J, Sandler A-M, Davies R: Clinical and Observational Psychoanalytic Research: Roots of a Controversy. London, Karnac Books, 2000

Target M, Fonagy P: Attachment theory and long-term psychoanalytic outcome: are insecure attachment narratives less accurate? in Pluralism and Unity? Methods of Research in Psychoanalysis. Edited by Leuzinger-Bohleber M, Dreher AU, Canestri J. London, International Psychoanalytical Association, 2003, pp 149–167

Tulving E: Episodic memory: from mind to brain. Annu Rev Psychol 53:1–25, 2002

PART V

History of Psychoanalysis

SECTION EDITOR: ROBERT MICHELS, M.D.

24

Psychoanalysis: The Early Years

DARIA COLOMBO, M.D.

SANDER M. ABEND

THE EARLY DEVELOPMENT OF psychoanalysis rests primarily on the thought and work of Sigmund Freud. His detailed and unprecedented clinical observations about psychological life and the theories generated from these observations form the central core of psychoanalysis. Freud once described himself as "one of those who have 'disturbed the sleep of the world'" (Freud 1914/1957, p. 21). (The phrase was borrowed from Hebbel's play *Gyges und sein Ring* [V, i].) Freud predicted astutely that his ideas were unlikely to be evaluated by his contemporaries with objectivity and tolerance. His insistence on the importance of childhood sexuality in psychological development and in contributing to adult neurotic syndromes proved to be indeed disturbing and largely unacceptable to most of his scientific and lay contemporaries.

If Freud's focus on childhood sexuality was perhaps his most controversial contribution, it can be argued that his emphasis on the importance of unconscious mental processes was equally difficult for his contemporaries to accept. While the notion of the unconscious mind had surfaced in the work of the Romantic poets, as well as in that of philosophers such as Schopenhauer and Nietzsche, Freud developed the first systematic, thorough, and explicit picture of how the unconscious dimension of the mind exerts its influence on the full spectrum of mental life and behav-

ior. His theory of the mind, first set forth in his 1899 *Interpretation of Dreams* and continuously modified in his later work, contained links to ideas that had been circulating in philosophy, medicine, and literature. Freud's genius lay in his ability to glean brilliantly from his intellectual environment and integrate this knowledge with his clinical observations to arrive at startling and revolutionary conclusions.

The considerable controversy stimulated by Freud's ideas almost immediately led to the proposal of competing views of the nature and etiology of emotional illness and of the principles of clinical practice. Freud's theories have been modified, clarified, and contested by generations of followers, so that the term *classical psychoanalysis* has come to mean what some believe to have been the core of technique and theory set forth by Freud.

To understand Freud's singular contribution, and to appreciate what psychoanalysis in his time came to include and exclude, it is necessary to recognize both the extent to which Freud's work reflected the evolution of his own thinking and the context in which these changes occurred. Freud gathered around him a group of students and disciples who, both in their allegiance and in their dissent, helped to determine the setting in which psychoanalysis—as science, technique, and movement—developed. Freud's theories indeed proved to be disturbing to the sleep of the world; the sleep he was disturbing was that of his own historical period, of which he was as much a product as any of his objectors and followers.

Our review of the early history of psychoanalysis, and of the milieu in which Freud developed his revolutionary theories about human behavior, will focus on the intellectual background from which Freud emerged, on the core features of his discoveries, and on the effect on his developing theory of the revisions, splits, and controversies that ensued during his lifetime.

Early History

Sigmund Freud was born on May 6, 1856, in Freiberg, a small town in Moravia, then a part of the Austro-Hungarian Empire. His father was an impoverished Jewish wool merchant, and Sigmund was the first child of his third marriage to the much younger Amalia Nathansohn. Freud had two half brothers from his father's earlier marriages, the elder half brother being older than Freud's mother. At the age of 4, Freud moved with his family to Leopoldstadt, the traditional Jewish district in Vienna, in the wake of growing financial difficulties. While the family continued to live in very straitened circumstances, Freud, cherished as the talented and brilliant eldest son, was favored with his own room, even as six younger siblings arrived. He was an outstanding student, driven by ambition and enraptured in particular by the natural sciences, although his broad education in the arts would serve him well and later inform his scientific writing with culture and richness.

Freud entered university in 1873, during a time when anti-Semitism was rampant—Jews were being scape-goated for the stock market crash of that same year—and Freud dated his self-awareness as a Jew to this period. Peter Gay has written about the particular tension, during those years, between anti-Semitism and a new openness in which Jewish males were entering the professions at an increasingly high rate and beginning to dream of success in a—if only briefly—more liberal society (Gay 1998, p. 27). Freud chose to study medicine at the university but took a somewhat circuitous route, entering early, at age 17, and finishing late, at age 25, largely as a result of his wide-ranging intellectual curiosity and interest in research (see Gay 1998, p. 28). He studied with Ludwig Feuerbach and with Franz Brentano, influenced by the former's Hegelian approach and by the latter's philosophy of intentionality. Freud actively engaged with the scientific and philosophic ideas of his time: he came of age in an era shaped both by the Helmholz school of physiology, which searched for the physical and chemical basis of natural

phenomena, and by Romanticism, with its emphasis on subjectivity. Eventually, "in a synthesis of these two trends in his education, Freud took subjectivity itself as the object of scientific investigation" (Auchincloss and Glick 1996, p. 3).

After a preparatory education in medicine and physiology, Freud worked as a researcher in the laboratory of the physiologist Ernest Brucke, studying the invertebrate nervous system and imbibing the positivistic, empirical approach that he would later make the foundation of his psychological work. His training was in neuropathology, and his early work on the smallest building blocks of neurological function could be considered the first steps in building a comprehensive theory of mental life.

While Freud's early monographs on this subject began to earn him a small reputation, practical considerations, most prominently the need to earn enough to marry and support a family, led to his taking up clinical neurological practice. Freud had little training in academic psychiatry, which at the time was not interested in the study of the subjective experience of patients. Instead, by entering clinical practice Freud joined a general medical culture in which listening to the patient was indeed central, and it has been argued that Freud's development could not have occurred within the framework of the era's academic psychiatry. It was Freud's decision to open a neurological practice that placed him in frequent contact with a type of patient commonly seen in such settings at that time, the hysteric.

Shift to Psychological Investigations and the Problem of Hysteria

Freud joined the General Hospital in Vienna, working briefly in various departments, including internal medicine, psychiatry (with the brain anatomist Theodor Meynert), and neurology. He narrowly missed making his name for his observation on the anesthetic properties of cocaine. He applied for and obtained the rank of *Privat Dozent* in 1885 and became the recipient of a travel grant.

Interested in disorders of the nervous system, he decided to travel to Paris, to study at the Salpêtrière with the celebrated neurologist Charcot. Freud initially worked on a microscopic study of children's brains and gathered data later used for publications on infantile cerebral paralysis and aphasia. Most significant for Freud was Charcot's understanding of mental illness, in particular his use of hypnosis in the treatment of hysteria. Hysteria was a widespread malady of the time, either believed to be caused by organic brain disturbances in its mostly female sufferers or condemned as a malingerer's ruse; treatment in the former cases involved a variety of ineffective physical manipulations. Charcot, however,

> diagnosed hysteria as a genuine ailment...he had recognized that it afflicts men....Even more daring Charcot had rescued hypnosis from mountebanks and charlatans for the serious purposes of mental healing. Freud was amazed and impressed to see Charcot inducing and curing hysterical paralyses by means of direct hypnotic suggestion. (Gay 1998, p. 49)

Freud also witnessed the strong emotional attachment developed by the hypnotized patients, an observation that he would much later elaborate and conceptualize as transference (see section "Theoretical Revisions and the Beginning of a Movement" later in this chapter). Furthermore, he admired Charcot's devotion to acute observation; Freud's own emphasis on clinical observation would later serve him well and lend him the confidence to overturn received wisdom.

Freud returned to Vienna enthusiastic about Charcot's work and interested in the application of hypnosis to his clinical practice. At the time, susceptibility to hypnosis was thought of as either an artificially induced nervous disorder in already disturbed minds or as purely a product of suggestion, to which anybody could be susceptible. Charcot believed the former, but Freud also traveled in 1889 to Nancy to study with Hippolyte Bernheim, who subscribed to the latter view. Freud also probably came into contact in France with the work of Pierre Janet, who had been experimenting with cathartic treatment. Freud later wrote that as a result of these various studies, he had "received the profoundest impression of the possibility that there could be powerful mental processes which nevertheless remained hidden from the consciousness of men" (Freud 1925/1959, p. 17).

During this period, Freud was employing in his practice the then-current technique of attempting to remove hysterical symptoms using hypnotic suggestion. He noted in 1925, however, that he had also considered hypnosis a tool for inquiring into the origin of patient's symptoms, thus combining from the beginning both the clinical and scientific aspects of his work. But Freud had difficulty hypnotizing many patients and soon became disappointed by the limitations of the technique. He searched for an alternative therapy, and the next step in this search was to be found in his work with Josef Breuer; the results of their collaboration were presented in writings considered to be the immediate antecedent of psychoanalysis.

Freud was in the process of shifting his primary focus from neuroanatomy to detailed observations of mental functioning. In his first book, *On Aphasia: A Critical Study*, published in 1891, he had considered psychological contributions to these disorders (Freud 1891/1953). Freud had dedicated this work to Breuer, an older, established physician who was one of his mentors and a close friend during a time in which Freud was struggling in relative isolation to establish his practice and academic reputation. It was in *Studies in Hysteria* (Breuer and Freud 1893–1895/1955), published a few years later in 1895, and coauthored with Breuer, that a new approach to treating hysterical patients was described. Already in 1893, the two men had written "A Preliminary Communication," in which they proposed the fruitful hypothesis that "hysterics suffer mainly from reminiscences" (Breuer and Freud 1893/1955, p. 7).

The case of Anna O., treated between 1880 and 1881, was Breuer's, who confided its remarkable course to his protégé. Salient features of the case included the link of neurotic symptoms to traumatic memories, and the idea, coined by the patient herself, of the "talking cure"—that is, of a cathartic effect consequent to the retelling of neurosis-inducing memories. Breuer apparently had been reluctant to publish the case himself, however, because of what had turned out to be the sexual origin of the neurotic symptoms. Freud "was the explorer who had had the courage of Breuer's discoveries; in pushing them as far as they would go, with all their erotic undertones, he had inevitably alienated the munificent mentor who had presided over his early career" (Gay 1998, p. 67).

Freud found that the memories at the source of his patients' neurotic symptoms were invariably revealed to be sexual in nature. He wrote, "I was not prepared for this conclusion and my expectations played no part in it, for I had begun my investigation of neurotics quite unsuspectingly" (Freud 1925/1959, p. 24). Despite general skepticism, Freud became convinced that the symptoms of neurasthenia, as well as of hysteria, were caused by sexual disturbances, setting aside the previously held view that such illnesses were a consequence of unspecified weaknesses in the nervous system. He rejected Janet's idea that a splitting of consciousness occurred in hysteria. He also held that the patient's verbal productions had meaning and that psychic as well as physical life followed the principle of determinism. Having arrived at the central concept of psychic determinism, Freud was committed to studying the productions of the mind as causally linked to earlier events, rather than dismissing them as meaningless epiphenomena (Auchincloss and Glick 1996, p. 4).

Freud's First Model of the Mind

In his practice, Freud gradually abandoned hypnosis for the cathartic method. Of the case of Elisabeth Von R., whom he treated in 1892 (the case was published in 1895), in what he called "the first full-length analysis of a hysteria undertaken by me" (Breuer and Freud 1893–1895/1955, p. 139), Freud wrote, "I arrived at a procedure which I later developed into a regular method and employed deliberately. This procedure was one of clearing away the pathogenic psychical material layer by layer, and we liked to compare it with the technique of excavating a buried city" (p. 139.) Many important principles of psychoanalysis appeared in fledgling form in this early case, as Freud not only presented his clinical information but, even more importantly—and a key reason for the richness of his writings—described the process by which his thinking developed. Freud would "carefully note the points at which some train of thought remained obscure or some link in the causal chain seemed to be missing" (p. 139). As Freud listened, he noted the substitution of "physical feelings as a symbol of her mental ones" (p. 144). At one point Freud tried and failed (to the patient's "triumphant" pleasure) to hypnotize her, and shifted to "the pressure technique" instead. "In view of the difficulty he had in hypnotizing his own patients and remembering that Bernheim was able, in the state of post-hypnotic amnesia, to have the subject recall what had happened under hypnosis, Freud told his patients to close their eyes and concentrate" (Ellenberger 1970, p. 518). Pressing his hands on the patient's head, he "instruct(ed) the patient to report to me faithfully whatever appeared before her inner eye or passed through her memory at the moment of the pressure" (Breuer and Freud 1893–1895/1955, p. 145). This was the introduction of free association.

Freud noted that at times the pressure technique would yield extensive material, while at others it appeared to fail. Freud's careful clinical scrutiny, combined with a stubborn confidence, led to fascinating results; he "resolved… to adopt the hypothesis that the procedure never failed" (Breuer and Freud 1893–1895/1955, p. 153) and found indeed that material had been present but had been held back. He writes, "In the course of this difficult work I began to attach a deeper significance to the resistance offered by the patient in the reproduction of her memories and to make a careful collection of the occasions in which it was particularly marked" (p. 154). This is the first use of the term *resistance*, which was to become an important feature of his evolving theory of clinical psychoanalysis.

The Freud in this early case was an uneasy blend of a confident scientist using empirical observations to develop a new theory and an isolated and occasionally defensive figure. He noted at one point of his investigations, "These, incidentally, were not the kind of questions that physicians were in the habit of raising." In his discussion, he wrote,

it still strikes me myself as strange that the case histories I write should read like short stories and that, as one might say, they lack the serious stamp of science….The fact is that local diagnosis and electrical reactions lead nowhere in the study of hysteria, whereas a detailed description of mental processes such as we are accustomed to find in the works of imaginative writers enables me, with the use of a few psychological formulas, to obtain at least some kind of insight into the course of that affection. (Breuer and Freud 1893–1895/1955, pp. 160–161)

At this point, this insight consisted of several critical principles: the importance of close clinical listening; the belief that behavior was meaningful rather than accidental; and the premise that infantile sexuality was the core of unconscious meaning that needed to be uncovered. Freud had received a couch as a gift from a patient in 1890, and he retained from hypnosis the practice of having his patients recline on a sofa while he sat behind them, out of their field of vision.

While his clinical practice afforded him more financial security, he continued to be scientifically isolated, mainly attached to Wilhelm Fliess, a Berlin ear and nose specialist who was his confidant at that time. Freud struggled ambitiously to outline his aims in his posthumously published "Project for a Scientific Psychology," in which he envisioned the biological/neurological substratum for the psychological phenomena he was delineating. His theories were in a process of flux. The concept of defense (*Abwehr*) appeared in 1894. In 1895, he began to refer to his work as "psychoanalysis." By 1896, he was setting forth a theory of neuroses, distinguishing between "actual neuroses," caused by current disturbances in sexual functioning, and "psychoneuroses." The latter, divided between hysteria and obsessions, were thought by Freud to be caused by sexual abuse in childhood, a theory he described in a poorly received 1896 lecture to the Society for Psychiatry and Neurology entitled "The Etiology of Hysteria."

By the fall of 1897, in a letter to Fliess dated September 21, Freud, while still identifying sexuality as the origin of hysteria and while never denying the occurrence of childhood sexual abuse, abandoned the seduction theory as a universal etiological factor. (Freud corresponded with Wilhelm Fliess between 1887 and 1904, in a series of letters in which Freud described the evolution of his ideas. Through his self-analysis, Freud had gradually come to recognize his own intense childhood love for his mother and his corresponding jealousy of his father, a situation he termed "the Oedipus complex," after Sophocles' Oedipus Rex. "This was to be a decisive turning point in psychoanalysis: Freud found that in the unconscious it is impossible to distinguish fantasies from memories, and from that time on he was not so much concerned with the reconstruction of events from the past through the uncovering of suppressed memories, as with the exploration of fantasies" (Ellenberger 1970, p. 488).

This shift, critical for psychoanalysis, has become in recent times a nodal point of controversy, as Freud was attacked by J.M.Masson in 1984 (Masson 1985) as denying the importance of childhood sexual trauma. While this argument hinged on an inaccurate understanding of what Freud's revision of the seduction theory actually entailed, it needs to be understood as the continuation of an ongoing, more significant theoretical divide between the importance of unconscious fantasy and that of "real" trauma, a split that emerged early in the psychoanalytic movement and that had some significant consequences. But it is inarguable that the rejection of the seduction theory was critical for the development of Freud's thinking. Cooper (1985) noted that "[t]he subsequent abandonment of the seduction hypothesis, which I believe was an essential step for the development of psychoanalysis rather than social theory, led to a focus on fantasy and on the sources of fantasy in instinct or drive" (pp. 9–10).

Freud's realization that the childhood sexual seductions described by his patients were largely fantasies, combined with his intense interest in what these fantasies revealed about the complexity and intensity of childhood sexuality, offered a new way to understand what had long been familiar to medical and legal authorities—that is, the complex array of perverse sexual activities enacted by disturbed adults. It also helped to clarify anthropological observations, very well known at the time, about the range of sexual practices encountered in other cultures. But when Freud addressed commonplace events such as such as slips, forgetting names, and childhood memories in *The Psychopathology of Everyday Life* (Freud 1901/1960), he was advancing a claim for the applicability of his discoveries to normal as well as pathological psychology. This work followed *The Interpretation of Dreams* (Freud 1900/1953), first published in 1899, in which Freud used the universal phenomena of dreams to demonstrate the fruitfulness of investigating infantile sexuality through exploring adult fantasy, rather than by direct developmental observation (which would be a later shift made by his daughter Anna Freud). He set forth a technique with which this investigation could be carried out, presented his first model of the mind, and promulgated the concept of an inherent sexual energy, later to be named "libido," thus claiming a biological basis for his new psychological theory.

In *The Interpretation of Dreams*, Freud made the oft-quoted comment that "[t]he interpretation of dreams is the royal road to the knowledge of the unconscious in mental life" (1900/1953, p. 608). Freud attempted to construct a diagram of the mental apparatus with which he could explain the formation of dreams in terms of perception, mem-

ory, symbol formation, and the fate of images. This effort can be viewed as a transitional conceptual bridge between his neurophysiological foundations and his increasing tendency to deal with purely psychological data. Since dreams were universal, Freud, using sample dreams from his own life, as well as those of patients, claimed to elucidate normal as well as abnormal mental life, even as he was introducing a technique, dream interpretation, that could be utilized in the treatment of neuroses. He described dreams as wish fulfillments and identified the method of free association as the key to their interpretation. He described how meanings in dreams are obfuscated by mental operations such as the principles of condensation, displacement, "consideration for representation," and secondary revision. He distinguished between the manifest and latent content of the dream and introduced the censor, a precursor of the superego. Dreams that appeared to be unpleasant merely confirmed his theory of wish fulfillment; the wishes were disguised because of conflict they engendered in the dreamer. Infantile wishes often appeared, disguised, in dreams, and their uncovering was for Freud the key part of the interpretation. The oedipal myth that he had first discussed in letters to Fliess here appeared in a section on typical dreams, to help explain why aggressive dreams about parents or siblings were also wish fulfillments.

In *The Interpretation of Dreams* Freud also proposed a hypothetical model of the mind based on his study of dreams, and made an imaginative leap by claiming that this model served as well to explain the mental operations that underlay the formation of neurotic symptoms. Freud introduced the topographic model of the mind in which mental contents were distributed among three systems, the Unconscious, the Conscious, and the Pre-Conscious. While this model seemed to be describing different loci or areas of the mind, Freud never intended that these divisions should be thought of in a concrete, anatomical fashion.

He employed the term *systems* because he meant to convey that each of the three dimensions of mental life was organized in a distinctive way. The system Unconscious contains wishes from infancy and operates via primary process, a primitive way of thinking based entirely on the pleasure principle. This system is separated by repression from the other systems. The system Conscious, on the other hand, functions according to familiar reason and logic and interfaces with the external world. The system Pre-Conscious refers to mental contents not at the moment in conscious awareness but possibly accessible. Secondary process thinking, in which the reality principle dominates, is characteristic of both the systems Conscious and Pre-Conscious.

In the topographical model, the main emphasis was placed on the censorship barrier between conscious and unconscious material. This emphasis was in accordance with Freud's views on the pivotal role of repression in neurosogenesis and with the then-prevalent focus in psychoanalytic treatment on the lifting of repression and the identification of the unconscious instinctual wishes against which the repressions were arrayed. At this stage, Freud also postulated that the energy attached to repressed sexual wishes, later defined as "libido" in 1905, somehow became converted, as a consequence of repression, into a toxic product, anxiety. Successful psychoanalytic treatment was thus supposed to relieve anxiety.

In *Three Essays on the Theory of Sexuality*, published in 1905, Freud (1905/1953) made the point, as he had in his work on dreams, that neurotic patients merely demonstrated excesses or distortions of normal human psychology. "For Freud…a neurosis is not some outlandish and exotic disease, but rather the all-too-common consequence of incomplete development, which is to say, of unmastered childhood conflicts" (Gay 1998, p. 146). Freud introduced the forerunner of libido—described in economic terms revealing Fechner's influence, as well as in evolutionary terms revealing Darwin's—as he outlined his theories about the infantile origins of biologically rooted sexual drives. He also discussed the reasons for the amnesia of this early period and for the psychological tasks necessary in latency and adolescence for the establishment of normal adult genital sexuality. It is important to recognize that in writing about sexuality, Freud was not unique: Ellenberger points out that "Freud's *Three Essays* appeared in the midst of a flood of contemporary literature on sexology and were favorably received" (Ellenberger 1970, p. 508).

A detailed analysis of what Freud described in these essays is contained elsewhere in this volume (see Chapter 6, "Gender and Sexuality"). For the purpose of understanding the early history of psychoanalysis, several points need to be emphasized. First is the biological underpinnings of Freud's thinking: "Implicit in the concept of psychic determinism is a system of motivation. Freud's motivational system is based on the pleasure-unpleasure principle.…the origins of behavior lie, at least in part, in the biological nature of the organism itself.…the organism is driven" (Cooper 1985, pp. 8–9). This biological basis included the primacy and universality of the sexual instinct, with which Jung most prominently would later disagree. Later hermeneutic critiques of the field would turn away from this biological foundation for different reasons.

The second point that needs to be emphasized is the inherent conceptualization of *conflict* in Freud's model, in which childish fantasy combined with immature cognitive development inevitably led to fears and fantasies about the nature of sexual activity and the dangers believed to be associated with it. Later theoretical revisions would make this conflict and the ego's handling of it more central than the mere identification of the underlying conflict-laden wishes.

The last point to be made is, as previously mentioned, the premise that childhood development can be studied through the prism of adult fantasy rather than simply by direct observation of children. In addition, it is within the context of this discussion that Freud first introduced his ideas about female sexuality, the centrality of penis envy, and the fear of castration, all of which would later occasion significant controversy. (Freud believed that children of both sexes mistakenly believe that every individual either has a penis or has somehow been damaged by losing it. An unconscious belief in the reality of castration, or in the fear of its occurrence, persists long after children learn anatomical differences, and such fantasies may persist in adulthood and cause significant distress. Perhaps of all the propositions Freud offered about sexuality, this has become the most controversial, and the most frequently challenged element of his entire theoretical edifice.) Indeed, each of these issues was a fault line that would soon lead to schisms and dissent; at this point, however, with a model of the mind and an instinct theory based on libido, Freud had a theoretical foundation rooted in a biological, deterministic conception of humankind, along with a clinical armamentarium consisting of free association, interpretation, and the analysis of transference and resistance.

This last principle was at this time the key focus of analytic technique, with the analysis of resistance linked to the idea that unconscious meaning related to infantile sexuality needed to be uncovered. Early psychoanalysis at this point was thus defined by a search for a core meaning—the "excavating (of) a buried city" in Freud's words (Breuer and Freud 1893–1895/1955, p. 139)—rather than by a core methodology; the subsequent shift to the latter approach would eventually enable very different thinkers to claim to be psychoanalytic. The ground for this potentially divisive plurality was established as Freud gradually began to have a wider audience, and it is in this less isolated setting that psychoanalysis further developed.

Theoretical Revisions and the Beginning of a Movement

In 1902, Freud finally obtained a promotion to Professor Extraordinarius at the University of Vienna. He had been a *Privat Dozent* for 17 years, an unusually long time to be fixed at this rank, and was likely hindered by a combination of anti-Semitism and the unpopular nature of his views. Edoardo Weiss, the first Italian psychoanalyst, wrote of

Freud, "While his studies of the central nervous system had been well received by his colleagues, his psychoanalytical writings reduced his scientific reputation sharply. ...In this situation a feeling of personal loyalty towards Freud developed in the small group of his adherents—not all of them physicians" (Weiss 1970, p. 4). Freud had indeed begun to find a sympathetic audience, and in the year of his appointment as professor, his Wednesday meetings, soon known as the Wednesday Psychological Society, began. Initiated at the suggestion of physician Wilhelm Stekel, this small group, consisting along with Stekel and Freud of Alfred Adler, Hugo Heller, Max Graf, and Paul Federn, initially met informally in Freud's study and formed the nucleus of what became in 1908 the Vienna Psychoanalytic Society. Otto Rank, introduced by Adler, became the group's secretary in 1906. Members or frequent visitors eventually included Sandor Ferenczi from Budapest, the Viennese Victor Tausk, Karl Abraham and Max Eitingon from Berlin, C.G. Jung and Ludwig Binswanger from Switzerland, Ernest Jones from England, Edoardo Weiss from Italy and A.A. Brill from America.

As Freud continued to develop his model of the mind, he did so in the context of what was becoming a burgeoning movement, with increasing tension between the tasks necessary to sustain the field's survival and expansion and those concerned with the developments and refinements of psychoanalytic theory. As Cooper (1985) noted,

> Freud's protectiveness of his ideas and his belief that the development of psychoanalysis would best be served by founding a movement rather than a forum for open scientific discussion of competing ideas, while probably essential for the rapid triumph of psychoanalysis within western culture, also contributed to the sectarianism of early psychoanalytic thought and the tendency for each new system to attempt completion and closure. (p. 12)

Jung and Binswanger, after visiting Freud in 1907, founded a psychoanalytic society in Zurich in 1908. The First International Congress of Psychoanalysis met in Salzburg in 1908, and in 1909 the first psychoanalytic journal, *Jahrbuch für Psychoanalytische und Psychopathologische Forschungen*, was founded. Freud was also invited to lecture at Clark University, in Massachusetts, traveling with Ferenczi and Jung to America. In 1910 the International Psychoanalytical Association was founded, at the Second International Congress of Psychoanalysis. "But the very fact that psychoanalysis was proclaimed a 'movement' (and not just a new branch of science) inevitably provoked opposition in psychiatric circles, and crises within the initial group, and an antipsychoanalytic feeling rapidly arose in psychiatric circles" (Ellenberger 1970, pp. 455–456). Edoardo Weiss (1970), in his memories of Freud, wrote,

"Freud himself knew that the concepts of psychoanalysis would be developed and revised. At the same time, he felt quite understandably very protective of the great field of his scientific investigation and theory he had christened psychoanalysis, and he resented any distortion or misinterpretations of his concepts" (p. 5).

While Freud took care to distance himself from some of his followers' work, the first truly significant break was with Alfred Adler, who developed what he called "individual psychology" with a decreased emphasis on the unconscious. Adler believed that the drive for superiority or mastery and the inferiority complexes that could result were more important than the unconscious dynamics that Freud put forth. Adler left the Vienna Psychoanalytic Society with some adherents in 1911, forming a dissident group.

The next significant break, in 1913, was with Jung, who was at the time president of the International Psychoanalytic Association and publisher of its journal. Trained in Switzerland under Eugen Bleuler, Jung early became acquainted with Freud's work and was his passionate advocate. Freud singled him out among his followers as his heir, but the two men increasingly disagreed on the importance of libido theory. Jung began to term his own theory "analytical psychology" as he extended the concept of libido to encompass general, nonsexual forces, and rejected what he saw as Freud's mechanistic view. Another important break was with Otto Rank, who proposed a theory of neurosogenesis based on the birth trauma and discounted the importance of childhood sexual wishes and fantasies. Brenner has noted of these various theoretical dissents that there was a striking "uniformity with which all the otherwise diverse formulations reject the idea of the importance to mental functioning and development of conflicts over sexual and aggressive wishes originating at ages three to six" (Brenner 2000, p. 608).

Freud, in his 1914 *On the History of the Psychoanalytic Movement*, clarified the central tenets of psychoanalysis and declared that "I consider myself justified in maintaining that even to-day no one can know better than I do what psycho-analysis is, how it differs from other ways of investigating the life of the mind, and precisely what should be called psycho-analysis and what would better be described by some other name" (Freud 1914/1957, p. 7). He described the secession of Adler and Jung and "reportedly wrote this essay in order to save psychoanalysis from dilution. . . . He made an organizational decision to enforce his theoretical position about the centrality of the unconscious. From then on, followers would defend his doctrine not only against Jung and Adler's deviance but against all those who would water it down" (Kurzweil 1998, p. 89).

With the departure of Jung and Adler, Freud relied increasingly on Abraham, Ferenczi, and Jones. Ernest Jones, who had met Freud at the First International Congress in 1908, was analyzed by Ferenzci. In 1913 Jones formed the London Psycho-Analytical Society, and later, demonstrating his loyalty to Freud, dissolved the London society because of Jungian dissent, immediately reconstituting it as the British Psycho-Analytical Society in 1919. He became the key advocate for Freud in Britain and North America and was a powerful polemicist and disseminator. He did have his disagreements with Freud, most notably about his theories on female sexuality. He also played a critical role in later attempting to mediate between Anna Freud and Melanie Klein (see Chapter 26, "Psychoanalysis in Great Britain and Continental Europe," in this volume). Freud also supported Abraham's prominence in the movement and was influenced by his papers on the development of libido.

For even as schisms appeared within his group of followers, Freud was himself revising many key aspects of his theory in work he did beginning in the second half of the 1910s and through the 1920s:

> So during the period when Adler increasingly was basing his theory on observations of personality and Jung was stressing archetypal influences—both culturally and more or less "consciously" determined—Freud became ever more involved in elaborations of the unconscious sources of both personality and culture. (Kurzweil 1998, p. 73)

In Freud's 1915 *Papers on Metapsychology*, a series of essays, he approached the superstructure of psychoanalysis with an attempt to describe mental life from the dynamic, economic, and topographical points of view and revised his understanding of various clinical conditions (Freud 1915/1957). In his 1920 *Beyond the Pleasure Principle*, Freud (1920/1955) proposed a new, dual classification of the instincts, adding to Eros (the libidinal instincts) a place for aggression in the form of the controversial and never fully accepted concept of the death instinct. With these modifications, Freud soon found his topographical model inadequate. Introduced in *The Interpretation of Dreams* (1900/1953), this old model

> was challenged by the observation that defenses against unconscious wishes are themselves unconscious and cannot be brought to consciousness by undoing repression. In addition, the analysis of melancholia and obsessional symptoms led to the observation that moral imperatives and self-punitive tendencies can also operate unconsciously. (Auchincloss and Glick 1996, p. 15)

Dropping the idea of a self-preservative drive, Freud hypothesized instead that there must be two biologically derived primary driving psychic forces, libido and aggres-

sion. Wishes expressing either or both of these drives could lead to intrapsychic conflict. To better elucidate this conflict, Freud abandoned the topographical model in favor of a new tripartite schema, which has come to be called the *structural theory*. In *The Ego and the Id* (1923/1961), Freud introduced a new conceptual language in which the mental apparatus was divided into "Id," "Ego," and "Superego," providing Freud with an improved framework with which to describe mental conflicts and their clinical manifestations. The id contained instinctual drives, both libidinal and aggressive; the ego represented the executive functions of the mind and represented the mind's connection with external reality; and the superego encompassed moral prohibitions and ideals. In this new explanatory system, there was a critical shift; now certain aspects of ego and superego functioning were also recognized as located in the unconscious stratum, along with the contents of the id. This recognition allowed Freud to develop a more sophisticated picture of intrapsychic conflict and thus provided a better way to account for the clinical data.

The dual-instinct theory gave clinical weight to both aggression and sexuality. Freud also gradually revised his theory of anxiety as his growing clinical experience led him to reconsider his earlier formulations. In his earlier theories, "Freud held that anxiety appears as a consequence of accumulated, undischarged libidinal cathexes, a situation brought about by the repression of the instinctual drive derivatives" (Arlow and Brenner 1964, p. 59). His new theory of mental conflict held that whenever wishes from the id threaten to emerge in thought or action, anxiety is generated. The anxiety acts as a signal, causing the ego to mobilize repression, along with a broad spectrum of other defenses, in order to block or disguise the anxiety-provoking wish. The invention of the structural model, along with revised theories about anxiety, led to "an emphasis on the centrality of the ego's executive role, both in providing the signal of anxiety and in constructing the defenses which organize the characterologic and symptomatic constructions of ongoing individual life" (Cooper 1985, p. 10).

Freud was modifying and refining not only his theory but also his technique during these years, and disagreements about such central principles as the nature, role, and purpose of transference led to other schisms. Transference had replaced resistance as the focus of the analyst's interpretive work. The term *transference* encompassed the wishes, perceptions, and attitudes that are formed by children in relation to parents and other significant figures, that persist unconsciously in adult life, and that are inevitably transferred onto the analyst. The phenomenon of transference provided the analyst with an emotionally rich stage on which the analysand could be helped to understand the nature of the important unconscious formative influences of childhood, still active in the present. The analysis of the transference took a central position in the technique of treatment. Freud disagreed with one of his closest followers, Ferenczi, who believed in gratifying some aspects of the transference relationship and in utilizing more supportive techniques. As Ellenberger (1970) noted, "In 1919 Freud warned analysts against taking false routes. He disavowed Ferenczi's innovation and precept of the active role of the analyst, and also rose up against the idea of the analyst giving emotional gratification to the patient; the analysis should be conducted in an atmosphere of abstinence" (p. 520). Freud firmly believed that to do otherwise would make the analysis of the transference more difficult, or even impossible.

The codification of clinical practice and of the rules followed by psychoanalysis' growing number of practitioners was of concern to Freud, and as the field gained new adherents, the importance of clarifying it both as theory and as organization became increasingly important. In spite of a difficult beginning, Berlin soon became the center of a flourishing psychoanalytic community, with Karl Abraham, who had left the Burghölzli in Zurich for Berlin, at its center. Karen Horney, Helene Deutsch, and Melanie Klein trained there, all analyzed by Abraham, who had developed some ideas about the female libido that these three analysands would each, in different ways, challenge and modify. Sandor Rado and Franz Alexander arrived in 1921. Some of the basic precepts of analytic training, including the training analyses, the supervision, and the seminars, had been established in Berlin by 1930.

The Later Years and the Major Foci of Dissent

The publication in 1926 of *Inhibitions, Symptoms and Anxiety* (1926/1959) "marked a new phase in the transformation of Freud's theories, from metapsychology to ego psychology" (Ellenberger 1970, p. 517). It was as the significance of Freud's theoretical evolution became absorbed that therapeutic emphasis gradually shifted from the earlier focus on the lifting of repression and the recovery of pathogenic memories to the analysis of ego functions. Anna Freud, presumably with her father's cooperation, published in 1936 the seminal work *The Ego and the Mechanisms of Defense*, in which the nature of the revised technique was clearly summarized (A. Freud 1936/1967). Attention was paid to recognizing, and addressing in interpretations, the various ways in which the patients' egos were defending against forbidden wishes, instead of concentrating on interpreting the nature of those wishes directly, as had been

prevalent in earlier practice. This clinical approach became known as *ego analysis* and the theoretical approach as *ego psychology*. The shift from id analysis toward ego analysis was strongly assisted by Anna Freud and Heinz Hartmann. "While historically the major ego concepts developed as an outgrowth of drive-conflict psychology and remain intimately tied to it via conceptions of defense against drive, Hartmann's…work introduced a significant emphasis on adaptation to the average expectable environment as well" (Pine 1988, p. 572). The followers of Abraham and Eitingon followed this theoretical shift to a focus on defense, while followers of Ferenzci were drawn to Melanie Klein's work (Kurzweil 1998, p. 256).

Several factors contributed to theoretical shifts during the last years of Freud's life, including changes in the intellectual and cultural climate, and new data from growing clinical experience. During the 1930s, the rise of Fascism in Europe led much of its analytic community to emigrate, since many analysts were Jewish, and most were, by nature and inclination, intellectuals, liberals, and free thinkers. This social cataclysm promoted the growth of psychoanalytic interest in Great Britain and in North and South America. The inclusion of many talented individuals and the effect of their dispersal from the first centers in Vienna, Berlin, and Budapest, together with the normal progressive accumulation of clinical experience, fostered the emergence of new trends and clinical developments. The earlier psychoanalytic view had emphasized the genetic viewpoint, which focuses on the intrapsychic experience of the world, rather than the maturation of drives as influenced by the environment. With Anna Freud devoting attention to a developmental framework and Melanie Klein focused on the unfolding of childrens' innate predispositions, conflict arose surrounding what psychoanalysis could say about, and gain from, the earliest years of life and about whether a focus on preoedipal events was either scientifically possible or useful. Later, with the rise of linguistics, there was conflict about whether psychoanalysis is a hermeneutic discipline, "a purely psychological and linguistic effort at understanding meanings, or whether it is a scientific causal discipline with biological roots" (Cooper 1985, p.16). Freud's weakness in describing female sexuality led to a variety of feminist critiques of the field. In some ways, this critique aligned with the controversy over Freud's abandonment of the seduction theory, in which the demotion of real trauma in favor of fantasy was felt to be a denial of sexual abuse; but more than this, it was clear that Freud's work had significant limitations with respect to the understanding of female sexual development.

Consideration of these later trends and critiques is complicated by the difficult task of tracing the influences on Freud of his contemporaries and identifying the residues of ideas introduced by earlier dissenters. Ellenberger has noted that "it is practically impossible to discern the part that disciples play in the shaping of the master's ideas. Not only do disciples bring new advances, but their particular interests, their questions, and the challenge brought by their contradiction of the master's opinions all stand beyond the reach of any complete appreciation" (Ellenberger 1970, p. 544). To this day, there is conflict about the legacy of the dissenters. Some thinkers, especially those who espouse some form of later theory, argue that key disciples and dissenters were introducing vital ideas that Freud himself was unable to accept, ideas which later found their way back, in some fashion, into psychoanalysis. (For example, it has been argued that the exiled Adler's influence was felt in Freud's eventual introduction of aggression into his own theoretical framework with a dual instinct theory [Ellenberger 1970, p. 513]. Cooper has argued that a similar thing happened with Rank and Jung. Rank's "theory of the birth trauma emphasized issues of loss and merging as the original sources of anxiety. ...Freud...eventually revised his own theory of anxiety to take into account the very issues which Rank had raised" [Cooper 1985, p. 10]. Cooper has also argued that Jung's disagreement with libido theory and focus on self concept influenced Freud's understanding of narcissism and played a role in the rise of ego psychology.) However, the majority of mainstream psychoanalysts have seen Freud's theoretical shifts quite differently, as revisions powered by his growing clinical sophistication, and evidence of Freud's own flexibility, creativity, and commitment to what his clinical data gradually taught him. This view sees Freud as reasonably rejecting followers whose beliefs endangered key aspects of psychoanalysis. In a way, definition of the boundaries of the field became increasingly important as a major shift in focus from content (of memories of infantile sexuality) to methodology (analysis of the transference and of ego defenses) occurred, with disagreement among historians and analysts about the relative significance of each. This shift later allowed very diverse thinkers to use psychoanalytic methodology to reach very different conclusions about psychopathology while considering themselves true heirs of Freud.

Conclusion

In spite of the many divisions that, as we have noted, made their appearance early on in the development of psychoanalysis, the main body of work and thought in the field remained centered on Freud and his ideas until the onset of the Second World War. Its central tenets, as conceptualized by Freud, continue to be accepted by various schools of thought, which Cooper (1985) defined as follows:

> The paradigm that Freud constructed, in grossly oversimplified form, consisted of a claim of psychic determinism; a method of investigation—free association; a descriptive-explanatory proposition that behavior is influence or determined by powerful feelings and ideas occurring out of awareness—the dynamic unconscious; and a treatment method based on the recognition of the central role of transference. (p. 6).

Freud came to study neurosis from the vantage point of an established medical practitioner and physiological researcher. He thought in biological terms and he attempted to explain his clinical observations in the light of the then-current understanding of neurophysiology. While he abandoned his 1895 "Project for a Scientific Psychology" and gradually directed his efforts to constructing explanatory models in purely psychological terms, Sulloway (1979), in an extensive critical review, insists that Freud remained a biologist at heart and asserts that his followers overstated the degree of Freud's shift to a psychological focus in order to amplify his reputation for originality. A contemporary reader can easily detect the fundamentally physiological conceptual framework that Freud adapted and incorporated into his psychological theorizing, just as one can see that his confident reliance on his capacity for accurate scientific observation reflects the prevailing positivist assumptions of his time. Freud was convinced that psychological events grow from a biological substrate, and he was also certain that science would some day be in a position to integrate physical and psychological phenomena into a coherent theoretical edifice. This integration, and the question of whether it is necessary, continue to be a prominent feature of the psychoanalytic schools that have developed since his time.

References

Auchincloss EL, Glick R: The psychoanalytic model of the mind, in Psychiatry. New York, Lippincott-Raven, 1996, pp 1–29

Arlow J, Brenner C: The structural model, in Psychoanalytic Concepts and Structural Theory. New York, International Universities Press, 1964, pp 57–85

Brenner C: Observations on some aspects of current psychoanalytic theories. Psychoanal Q 69:597–632, 2000

Breuer J, Freud S: On the psychical mechanism of hysterical phenomena: preliminary communication (1893), in Standard Edition of the Complete Psychological Works of Sigmund Freud, Vol 2. Translated and edited by Strachey J. London, Hogarth Press, 1955, pp 3–17

Breuer J, Freud S: Studies on hysteria (1893–1895), in Standard Edition of the Complete Psychological Works of Sigmund Freud, Vol 2. Translated and edited by Strachey J. London, Hogarth Press, 1955, pp 1–319

Cooper AM: A historical review of psychoanalytic paradigms, in Models of the Mind: Their Relationships to Clinical Work. Edited by Rothstein A. New York, International Universities Press, 1985, pp 5–20

Ellenberger HF: The Discovery of the Unconscious: The History and Evolution of Dynamic Psychiatry. New York, Basic Books, 1970

Freud A: The Ego and the Mechanisms of Defense (1936), in The Writings of Anna Freud, Vol 2. New York, International Universities Press, 1967, pp 1–176

Freud S: On Aphasia: A Critical Study (1891). New York, International Universities Press, 1953

Freud S: The interpretation of dreams (1900), in Standard Edition of the Complete Psychological Works of Sigmund Freud, Vols 4 and 5. Translated and edited by Strachey J. London, Hogarth Press, 1953, pp 1–715

Freud S: The psychopathology of everyday life (1901), in Standard Edition of the Complete Psychological Works of Sigmund Freud, Vol 6. Translated and edited by Strachey J. London, Hogarth Press, 1960, pp 1–310

Freud S: Three essays on the theory of sexuality, I: the sexual aberrations (1905), in Standard Edition of the Complete Psychological Works of Sigmund Freud, Vol 7. Translated and edited by Strachey J. London, Hogarth Press, 1953, pp 135–172

Freud S: On the history of the psychoanalytic movement (1914), in Standard Edition of the Complete Psychological Works of Sigmund Freud, Vol 14. Translated and edited by Strachey J. London, Hogarth Press, 1957, pp 7–66

Freud S: Papers on metapsychology (1915), in Standard Edition of the Complete Psychological Works of Sigmund Freud, Vol 14. Translated and edited by Strachey J. London, Hogarth Press, 1957, pp 105–260

Freud S: Beyond the pleasure principle (1920), in Standard Edition of the Complete Psychological Works of Sigmund Freud, Vol 18. Translated and edited by Strachey J. London, Hogarth Press, 1955, pp 1–64

Freud S: The ego and the id (1923), in Standard Edition of the Complete Psychological Works of Sigmund Freud, Vol 19. Translated and edited by Strachey J. London, Hogarth Press, 1961, pp 12–66

Freud S: An autobiographical study (1925), in Standard Edition of the Complete Psychological Works of Sigmund Freud, Vol 20. Translated and edited by Strachey J. London, Hogarth Press, 1959, pp 7–70

Freud S: Inhibitions, symptoms and anxiety (1926), in Standard Edition of the Complete Psychological Works of Sigmund Freud, Vol 20. Translated and edited by Strachey J. London, Hogarth Press, 1959, pp 75–175

Gay P: Freud: A Life for Our Times. New York, WW Norton, 1998

Kurzweil E: The Freudians: A Comparative Perspective. New Brunswick, NJ, Transaction Publishers, 1998

Masson JM (ed): The Complete Letters of Sigmund Freud to Wilhelm Fliess: 1887–1904. Cambridge, MA, The Belknap Press of Harvard University Press, 1985, pp 264–266

Pine F: The four psychologies of psychoanalysis and their place in clinical work. J Am Psychoanal Assoc 36:571–596, 1988

Sulloway FJ: Freud, Biologist of the Mind. New York, Basic Books, 1979

Weiss E: Sigmund Freud as a Consultant: Recollections of a Pioneer in Psychoanalysis. New York, Intercontinental Medical Book Corporation, 1970

25

Psychoanalysis in North America From 1895 to the Present

SANFORD GIFFORD, M.D.

The Beginnings of Analysis in America, 1895–1909

Some psychoanalytic texts were available in the United States as early as 1895, when Freud gave his famous "Introductory Lectures" at Clark University, at least for readers of German. Our initial receptiveness to analysis was partly based on a misunderstanding, as if Freud's theories were merely another contribution to the popular psychotherapies of suggestion that were flourishing at the turn of the century. This period, called the "Age of Reform" (Hofstadter 1955), was one of ebullience, when the United States was highly receptive to new ideas from abroad in politics and the arts and sciences. New concepts of a dynamic unconscious were already popular here, derived from hypnosis and the suggestive therapies of Charcot, Bernheim, and Janet, which were also the sources of Freud's early theories (Breuer and Freud 1893–1895).

William James and Havelock Ellis had reviewed Freud's book in 1894 and 1899, respectively, and Adolf Meyer had discussed Freud's theories of sexuality in 1906. William James (1902) had welcomed all varieties of what he called "the mind-cure movement," including reports of hypnotic treatment, fugue states, multiple personality, and faith-healing. But his outlook was briskly pragmatic, and he hailed the treatment of neurosis by suggestion, in contrast to nineteenth-century concepts of mental illness as hereditary and untreatable. He extolled its "practical fruits" as congenial to the optimistic American temperament and "perhaps our only decidedly original contribution to the systematic philosophy of life" (James 1902, p. 96)

Among the early readers of Freud, Dr. Robert Edes (1895) discussed Freud's theory of hysteria in "The New England Invalid." Edes was an internist, one of many physicians practicing "medical psychotherapy" (Gifford 1978) for the common neuroses, applying hypnosis and the "waking suggestion" of Charcot and Bernheim, or the "moral re-education" of Dubois and Déjerine. Some general physicians established small sanitaria for the treatment of neuroses: Edes as director of Dr. Adams's Nervine Asylum in Boston; George Gehring in Bethel, Maine; and Austen Riggs in Stockbridge, Massachusetts (Kubie 1960).

Others who practiced the psychotherapies of suggestion were the clinical psychologists, such as William James; Josiah Royce, the philosopher; Hugo Münsterberg; Boris Sidis; and G. Stanley Hall. Neurologists such as Morton Prince, E.W. Taylor, and James Jackson Putnam in Boston, and Smith Ely Jelliffe in New York, treated patients with neuroses in their offices. This office-based approach to treatment was in contrast to the treatment provided by most psychiatrists of that era, who typically were custodians of chronic psychotic patients in state hospitals. There were exceptions among psychiatrists, such as Adolf Meyer and William A. White, who believed that psychoses could be treated. Some mental hospitals—such as Manhattan State Hospital in New York; the Phipps Clinic at Johns Hopkins; St. Elizabeths Hospital in Washington, D.C., and the Boston Psychopathic Hospital, McLean Hospital, and Worcester State Hospital in the Boston area—had a strong interest in psychotherapy.

Among these enthusiasts for psychotherapy, the first Americans to identify themselves as "Freudians" were J.J. Putnam and A.A. Brill. Each was drawn to analytic theories by different routes, and by coincidence both were guided to Freud by Ernest Jones. Jones, a Welshman exiled to Canada from 1908 to 1913, traveled widely in the United States as an indefatigable proselytizer for Freud's ideas. He returned to England in 1913. As a "temporary American," Jones could be called our very first analyst, but Freud (1921) hailed Putnam as "the first American to interest himself in psychoanalysis." Putnam's (1906) report on the treatment of hysteria "according to Freud's method of psychoanalysis" was the first analytic paper in English, although Putnam's approach was still close to Freud's earlier "cathartic method."

Jones visited Boston in early 1909, where he met Putnam at Morton Prince's house, at one of their regular meetings to discuss the new psychotherapies of suggestion. This encounter increased Putnam's confidence in analytic methods, and both Putnam and Jones attended a meeting of the American Therapeutic Society (Jones 1909). This society was organized by Morton Prince, who gave an ebullient opening address on the psychotherapies of suggestion. Putnam spoke enthusiastically about Freud's new contributions and the importance of childhood fears in adult neuroses. Jones gave a fuller account of Freud's current theories, firmly differentiating "psychoanalysis" from all other forms of psychotherapy. In contrasting the authoritarian role of the hypnotist and the nonjudgmental analyst, Jones showed how analytic free association was "in almost every respect the reverse of treatment by suggestion" (Jones 1909, p. 101).

This meeting of the American Therapeutic Society marked a high point in the psychotherapy movement, as well as the first public presentation of Freudian theories in America. But its importance for psychoanalysis was overshadowed by the Clark University Lectures, which took place later that year, in September 1909. G. Stanley Hall, a pupil of William James and chief of psychology at Clark, had invited Freud, Sandor Ferenczi, and Carl Jung to celebrate the twentieth anniversary of Clark University. Jones, who had joined Freud's party in New York, and A.A. Brill were also present. The five lectures that Freud gave, to an academic and general audience, were the closest Freud would come to a "popularization" of analysis (Rosenzweig 1909/1992). Freud's meeting with Putnam, who invited the Europeans to his Adirondack camp, initiated Putnam's intimate correspondence with Freud and Jones, which lasted until his death in 1918 (Hale 1971b).

Ernest Jones had met A.A. Brill the year before, in Zurich, where both were independently studying analysis with Carl Jung, and together they paid a visit to Freud in the summer of 1908. Brill had obtained Freud's permission to translate his papers and books into English. After the Worcester meetings, Jones made himself Freud's roving emissary in North America, speaking about analysis at medical meetings of all kinds. He persuaded Putnam, somewhat reluctantly, to found the American Psychoanalytic Association in 1911 as a national organization. After his meeting with Freud in 1908, Brill returned to Manhattan State Hospital as a self-proclaimed analyst and founded the New York Psychoanalytic Society in 1911, a few months before the founding of the American Psychoanalytic Association.

Freud's abiding distaste for America and his mistrust of Americans can be dated from his American trip, when he attributed his prejudice, half whimsically, to the ill effects of our cooking on his digestion. But his real fears were based on the propensity of Americans for popularization and the dilution of analysis with the base metal of psychotherapy (Gay 1988).

The Early Decades, 1909–1925

The three centers of analytic interest, New York City, Boston, and Baltimore, Maryland–Washington, D.C., were each dominated by a single strong personality, and each had its local peculiarities. The American Psychoanalytic Association was intended for analysts from other parts of the country, and its annual meetings took place just after meetings of the American Psychopathological Association, which represented the psychotherapy movement. Many of the eight founding members of the American Psychoanalytic Association belonged to both associations, and there were occasional motions to merge the two, but Adolf Meyer prevailed in maintaining an independent association for analysis. The International Psychoanalytic Association (IPA) had been founded only a year before, at Freud's suggestion, after the Second Psychoanalytic Congress in Nuremberg, Germany, in 1910. At that time, both the American Psychoanalytic Association and the

IPA included many nonphysicians as members: for example, G. Stanley Hall was president of the American Psychoanalytic Association in 1917–1918 (D'Amore 1978).

The history of analysis in Boston begins with Putnam and his hysteria paper of 1906. Age 62 when he first met Jones at Prince's house, in 1909, Putnam retired in 1912 as the first professor of psychiatry at Harvard Medical School. In 1914, Putnam founded the first Boston Psychoanalytic Society, a small group that met every Friday afternoon in his house until his death in 1918. Its membership, which varied, included Isador Coriat, Putnam's successor, who had first studied with Adolf Meyer at Worcester State Hospital in 1902. Coriat, who had been active in the psychotherapy movement and had joined the Rev. Elwood Worcester's Emmanuel Movement (Gifford 1996) in 1906, became an analyst in 1911–1912 (Sicherman 1978). He remained the only Freudian analyst in Boston during the "Dark Ages" after Putnam's death, and he reestablished the Boston Psychoanalytic Society in 1924–1928. Another early member was L.E. Emerson ("Red-Necktie Emerson"), a clinical psychologist and pupil of Josiah Royce, whom Putnam had appointed to the staff of Massachusetts General Hospital.

Putnam, like Jones, had been active in promoting psychoanalysis by speaking at neurological and psychiatric meetings. He wrote more than 20 papers on psychoanalysis (Putnam 1921/1951) and conducted a vigorous correspondence with Freud and Jones (Hale 1971b). He also strove, unsuccessfully, to interest them in his neo-Hegelian philosophy of ethics.

Putnam was a shy, idealistic man of intense convictions, who was totally lacking in personal ambition. Coriat, his direct successor, was also reserved and scholarly, without the qualities of a charismatic leader. The history of analysis might have been different had Putnam succeeded in appointing Jones to the faculty at Harvard Medical School or had Jones obtained an academic appointment at Johns Hopkins Medical School, where he was rejected by Adolf Meyer (Leys 1981).

Baltimore and Washington were dominated by Adolf Meyer at Johns Hopkins Medical School and William Allanson White at St. Elizabeths Hospital, a federal institution. Meyer, a German-speaking Swiss who had been familiar with Freud's writings from the turn of the century, was a founding member of the American Psychoanalytic Association in 1909. Like his countrymen Bleuler and Jung, Meyer was interested in psychoses and in finding more dynamic ways of treating patients with these disorders. Meyer had been at Worcester State and at Manhattan State in New York from 1902 to 1911. His appointment to head the new Phipps Clinic at Hopkins made him an influential figure in American psychiatry. Though a founding

member of the American Psychoanalytic Association, he continued to have reservations about analytic theory, and his chief interest was in his own dynamic theories, which he referred to as "psychobiology." According to students in the 1930s, Meyer discouraged his residents from analytic training.

The analytic leader in Washington, William A. White, was a New Yorker whose interest in psychiatry and analysis began at Binghamton State Hospital in 1896. There he met Boris Sidis, a protégé of William James and a typical advocate of suggestive psychotherapy but also knowledgeable about analysis. White also met Smith Ely Jelliffe at Binghamton, who also became a lifelong friend. They spent their summer vacations together at Jelliffe's lodge on Lake George, where they literally "analyzed" each other over the years (D'Amore 1976). White became superintendent of St. Elizabeths in 1903 and wrote many papers on psychoanalysis; his book *Mental Mechanisms* (1911) is thought to be "the first...about analysis by an American" (Burnham 1967). His textbook, *Outlines of Psychiatry* (1909), contained a section on analysis that was republished many times and read by generations of medical students. He emphasized the importance of being nonjudgmental as a psychoanalyst, as well as allowing sufficient time ("several months, of at least two or three *séances* each week," recalling the link between analysis and hypnosis).

White was a co-editor with Jelliffe of the *Journal of Nervous and Mental Disease*, which published a monograph series with the first English translations of work by Freud and other European analysts. White and Jelliffe also founded the *Psychoanalytic Review* in 1914, the first analytic journal in English. Through a misunderstanding (D'Amore 1976), Freud refused to contribute to the first issue, and a paper by Jung was published instead.

In 1914 White founded the Washington Psychoanalytic Society, most of whose members were on the staff of St. Elizabeths Hospital. He appointed E.J. Kempf as a full-time research psychiatrist, to apply psychoanalytic methods to work with hospitalized psychotic patients. Kempf was a pioneer in the treatment of schizophrenia and the first to observe primate behavior in order to validate psychoanalytic hypotheses (Kempf and Burnham 1974). The Washington Psychoanalytic Society met once a month, and its membership included several other innovative analysts. Lucile Dooley and Mary O'Malley were the first women analysts, and Trigant Burrow was an early enthusiast of psychoanalytic group psychotherapy. G. Lane Taneyhill introduced the use of the couch, which most American analysts had ignored in those early decades (Noble et al. 1969). After 1918, the society ceased to meet, for obscure reasons attributed to military service. White, who had been president of the American Psychoanalytic

Association in 1915–1916, served in that capacity once again in 1927–1928.

The most important analytic center was New York City, beginning at Manhattan State Hospital on Ward's Island, which Clarence Oberndorf (1953) called, in 1909, "the largest program of training in psychoanalytic psychiatry in the world" (p. 113). Attributing this analytic enthusiasm to Adolf Meyer, Oberndorf (1953) claimed that "[t]hough psychoanalysis was cradled in Boston, it was raised and grew up in New York" (p. 112). The institutional setting of Manhattan State Hospital resembled the Burghölzli in Zurich more than the office practices of Boston's neurologists, but the New York analysts soon set up full-time analytic practices in the city. Brill's suite at 97 Central Park West was in the area where many future analysts settled. By 1913 Oberndorf had established an outpatient psychiatric clinic at Mt. Sinai Hospital, with inpatient consultations. "Thus psychoanalysis began…as an integral part of medical practice, differing radically in this respect from Vienna," Oberndorf (1953, p. 127) concluded. He was already asserting what distinguished American from European analysis: that we "never regarded psychoanalysis as a distinct discipline, but as essentially a branch of psychiatry and medicine."

The early analytic scene flourished in New York, under the energetic, gregarious leadership of A.A. Brill (1911–1947). Brill was an immigrant from an Orthodox Jewish family in Austrian Galicia who felt stifled by his rigid, domineering father (Hale 1971a). He came to New York alone at 16 and settled on the Lower East Side. He supported himself by giving chess and mandolin lessons and worked his way through Columbia Medical School. His warmhearted, optimistic personality attracted followers; he founded the New York Psychoanalytic Society in 1911 with fewer than a dozen members, but the membership rose to 27 the following year. The members met once a month to hear one another's presentations, and their lively discussions lasted long after midnight. Meetings were held in members' apartments, at restaurants like the Café Boulevard, or at the Medical Alliance at 200 East Tenth Street. From the sketchy minutes, administrative matters were simple: motions were for raising the dues from $3 to $4 or for expelling a member with more than three successive absences.

The issue of lay analysis preoccupied the New York Psychoanalytic Society from its first meetings, which had voted to restrict membership to "physicians actively engaged in psychoanalytic work." This criterion was in contrast to the policies of the American Psychoanalytic Association, which had no such restrictions, and the Boston Psychoanalytic Society, which had accepted psychologists like L.E. Emerson. The New York Psychoanalytic Society discussed periodic proposals to "investigate" therapists who had misrepresented themselves as analysts. In 1919, for example, four such therapists were reported to the New York County Medical Society for "practicing medicine without a license." The strong antipathy to lay analysis in the New York Psychoanalytic Society was usually attributed to Brill, who justified that stance by referring to a New York State licensing regulation. According to Daniels (personal communication, 1974), Brill's objections to lay analysis weakened after every European visit to Freud, and reappeared on returning to New York, where nonmedical applicants were rejected who had been analyzed in Europe. Other colleagues of Brill's contrasted his official opposition to lay analysis with his personal respect for certain nonmedical child therapists, often the wives of analysts (Lorand, personal communication, 1975). Some of these therapists treated the children of Brill's colleagues, and Brill advised them to bill their patients for "lessons" rather than therapy.

A compromise was proposed to the New York Psychoanalytic Society (Minutes of Society Meeting 29 Nov. 1921; see Brill 1911–1947), in which the restrictions against membership for nonphysicians were reaffirmed but a special nonvoting category of "Associate Member" was established for "physicians or other professional persons in related fields." Brill claimed that the original constitution of the American Psychoanalytic Association, now lost, denied membership to women (D'Amore 1978); the earliest women members of the American Psychoanalytic Association, Lucile Dooley and Marion Kenworthy, were both admitted in 1926. Brill's claim is puzzling because the New York Psychoanalytic Society, during Brill's tenure, had never had any restrictions against women. Beatrice Hinkle had been elected in 1911, Mary Isham soon after, and Marion Kenworthy in 1919.

Although analysis continued to grow in the 1920s, the appeal of analysis was characterized by a certain superficiality (Burnham 1967; Hale 1971a, 1971b), with wide acceptance but a lack of depth. Burnham (1967) emphasized the inveterate eclecticism and popularization of analysis in the United States, resulting in a psychoanalysis that was "accepted empirically and neglected theoretically, loved and distorted" (p. 213). American analysts tended to ignore Freud's theoretical revisions, his disputes with European colleagues, and the defections of Alfred Adler, Jung, and Otto Rank. As in proselytizing for the earlier psychotherapy movement, American analysts—Brill, Putnam, and Coriat, among others—wrote many popular books for the general reader, although European analysts wrote primarily for their colleagues in scientific journals. Hale (1971a) interpreted the American prejudice against nonmedical therapists as a quest for scientific respectability at a time when American medical education was in a chaotic state, with its diploma mills and inadequate teaching standards, cited by the Flexner Report of 1910, in contrast to the traditional universities and curricula of Europe.

Analytic Training Abroad and the First Institutes, 1925–1938

Until the mid-1920s, there was no real concern with analytic training as such. Membership in the New York Psychoanalytic Society and the American Psychoanalytic Society was open to anyone with a "sincere interest" in analysis and some familiarity with its literature. The first generation of American analysts, such as Putnam, Brill, and Coriat, were entirely self-taught, "becoming analysts" by reading Freud and treating patients accordingly. Although Freud had mentioned the desirability of a personal analysis in 1910 (Freud 1910/1957), Nunberg was the first to propose a didactic or "training" analysis as a requirement in 1918, at the first postwar International Psychoanalytic Congress in Budapest (Freud 1918/1961).

With the founding of the new Berlin Psychoanalytic Institute (1920–1930) in 1920, the standard three-part program was soon established: a personal analysis with a recognized "training analyst," theoretical and clinical seminars, and the analysis of patients under supervision. The success of the Berlin Psychoanalytic Institute was reported on at the Bad Homburg Congress of 1925, and an International Commission on Training was established, with representatives from Vienna, Berlin, Budapest, London, New York, and the American Psychoanalytic Association. Oberndorf was the New York representative, and a committee of the American Psychoanalytic Association was appointed to establish standards for analytic training.

The pattern of European travel for advanced studies had been an American custom for generations, with artists, writers, and scientists following well-worn paths to Paris or Rome. From the late nineteenth century on, German and Austrian universities had a special attraction for physicians, and the University of Vienna had created a minor industry educating Americans in various medical specialties. Hence, Vienna or Berlin was the destination of would-be analysts, for Adolf Stern, H. W. Frink, and Oberndorf in the 1920s, and for Muriel Gardiner, M. Ralph Kaufman, and many others, until the *Anschluss* in March 1938. The Viennese analyst Paul Schilder was popular with Americans for his 3-month summer format. Some European analysts, such as Ferenczi, Paul Federn, and Rank, came to the United States to lecture, and they analyzed a few Americans.

With the need for "institutes" for analytic training, modeled on the Berlin Psychoanalytic Institute, there was a demand for recognized training analysts, preferably well-known Europeans. The New York Psychoanalytic Society was the first American society to become an institute, in 1931, by inviting Sandor Rado from the Berlin Institute. Boston followed (Gifford 1978) by inviting Franz Alexander, who had already spent the academic year 1930–1931 at the University of Chicago. During his year in Boston (1931–1932), Alexander held a part-time research post at the Judge Baker Guidance Center, appointed by William Healy, his chief as well as his analysand. Alexander conducted six or eight "training analyses" before returning to Chicago to found the Chicago Psychoanalytic Institute.

The Boston Psychoanalytic Society then invited Hanns Sachs, a member of Freud's early circle in Vienna and the first "training analyst" at the Berlin Institute in 1920. Sachs' emigration to Boston had been arranged by Irmarita Putnam, an analysand of Freud's, with Freud's explicit approval. Sachs was not a physician, however, and he refused to obey the new "committee rule" that candidates must be approved by the Education Committee. This created some conflict with Ives Hendrick and the reformers, but Sachs continued to teach seminars and reanalyzed many members.

The last Boston Psychoanalytic Society had been reestablished in 1928 by Isador Coriat, Putnam's successor from the first society of 1914–1918. Coriat had presided over a psychoanalytic society from 1924 to 1928, in which he was the only "Freudian" among three to four analysands of Jung; three to four analysands of Rank, who had broken with Freud in 1924; and some analysands of Paul Schilder. These four groups "got along much better together than Freudians got on with Freudians, as soon as there was more than one lone Freudian in the Society!" (Hendrick 1958, p. 16). In 1930 the Boston Society was reorganized, with Martin Peck, a Rankian who was later reanalyzed by both Alexander and Sachs, as president. The final reformation that created an institute was carried out by four young analysts who had just completed their training in Europe: Ives Hendrick and Leolia Dalrymple from the Berlin Institute, and M. Ralph Kaufman and John Murray from Vienna. After 3 years of fierce conflicts, a new constitution was created, and most of the Rankians and Schilderians were "regularized" by having second analyses with Alexander or Sachs. The Boston Psychoanalytic Society and Institute was accepted by the American Psychoanalytic Association in 1933.

Among its conflicts over nonmedical training, the New York Psychoanalytic Society objected to nonphysicians who had obtained full analytic training abroad being recognized as analysts in the United States. After fierce debate, this led to the threat of a separation between the American Psychoanalytic Association and the IPA, which was narrowly averted by Ernest Jones and Anna Freud. A compromise was arranged at the 1929 IPA Congress in Oxford, England, where it was stipulated that the analytic training of American candidates in Europe required permission from the candidate's local analytic society.

There was continuing bitterness among returning American psychologists, teachers, and social workers such as Marie Briehl and Rosetta Hurwitz, who had been denied membership in the New York Institute after completing their analyses and special training in child analysis in Vienna. At the same time, New York and other institutes were admitting nonmedical European analysts, such as Erik Erikson and Berta Bornstein, through an unwritten "grandfather clause." The conservative New York Psychoanalytic Society retained its provision for nonphysicians to join as associate members, after 3 years training "in accordance with the requirements of the International Training Commission."

The third psychoanalytic training center was the Washington-Baltimore Psychoanalytic Society, reestablished in 1930 and recognized as a constituent society of the American Psychoanalytic Association in 1932, after the Washington Psychoanalytic Society, originally formed in 1914, was revived in 1925 as the Washington-Baltimore Psychoanalytic Society. There was also a second group, the Washington Psychoanalytic Association, founded in 1924, with William A. White as president. This second group was more strenuously opposed to nonmedical members than the Washington-Baltimore Society, but it was also led by Ben Karpman, whose analysis by Stekel was considered unacceptable.

Ernest Hadley of Washington had reorganized the Washington-Baltimore Society, in negotiations with A.A. Brill, then president of the American Psychoanalytic Association, and with Clara Thompson of Baltimore (Noble and Burnham 1969, pp. 21–23). The society's history was complicated because of its close relationship with the Washington School of Psychiatry, created by the William Allanson White Psychiatric Foundation. Originally called the *Psychoanalytic* Foundation, its name was changed to the *Psychiatric* Foundation at White's request. In 1940, when the Washington-Baltimore Institute was reestablished, training was conducted by the Institute "in conjunction with the Washington School of Psychiatry." This meant that seminars were attended both by analytic candidates of the Institute and by students of the Washington School. White died in 1938, but the powerful personality of Harry Stack Sullivan continued to influence the Baltimore-Washington Institute.

Sullivan is a difficult figure to portray because of the extreme reactions he evoked. He was admired by some as a genius and an important influence in American psychiatry, but he was also dismissed as an impostor and an impossible human being. Even his staunchest admirers (Chapman 1976; Perry 1982) acknowledged his severe personality problems. Coming from great rural poverty and a family with psychopathology in upper New York State, he had an emotional breakdown in his second year at Cornell. He dropped out of school, supported himself at menial jobs, and finally graduated from a medical "diploma mill" in Chicago. These educational deficiencies contributed to his prickly, self-aggrandizing behavior and secretive, defensive attitudes. He was shy, socially awkward, and unable to present his ideas in coherent written form. Hence, Sullivan's reputation as a great teacher depended on the contending claims of his followers and his critics.

Sullivan's gifts included an intuitive, highly empathic approach to the treatment of young men with schizophrenia, originally at Sheppard Pratt in Baltimore. He was an admirer of Ferenczi, whoses theories about the "active technique" were alienating him from Freud. In 1930–1931, Sullivan sent Clara Thompson, his former student, to Budapest to be analyzed by Ferenczi, apparently in order to obtain a vicarious analysis with Ferenczi by being analyzed by Thompson. Thompson's analysis of Sullivan was abandoned because she could not overcome her awe of her former teacher (Noble and Burnham 1969, p. 30).

During the 1930s, as the four psychoanalytic societies were reorganizing themselves as institutes, the American Psychoanalytic Association was reorganized in 1932 as a federation instead of a scientific society with individual members. These changes were recognized by the IPA in 1936, at the 14th Congress in Marienbad; the Nazis had already come to power in Germany in 1933. At the IPA Congress of 1938 in Paris, the American Psychoanalytic Association notified the IPA that members of foreign analytic societies would not be recognized in the United States. At a time when German-speaking analysts were fleeing from the Nazis, the American response to the refugee problem seemed unconscionably insensitive. There were other signs of American ambivalence toward refugees. When Walter Langer asked the president of the New York Psychoanalytic Institute for help in obtaining affidavits for Viennese refugee analysts, his pleas were rejected, with the comment "What will we do with all these analysts in New York?" (see Langer and Gifford 1978, p. 42).

To summarize: The period of psychoanalytic institutional reorganization began in 1925, when the International Training Commission was proposed, and ended in 1938, when the commission was abolished. Most German-speaking analysts had fled the continent by this time, and the major American institutes for analytic training had been established. The American Psychoanalytic Association was a centralized national association, meeting twice a year for the exchange of scientific ideas and the regulation of training. Before 1938 the first European analysts were already being invited to this country as "approved training analysts." The tripartite structure of analytic training, with a personal analysis, theoretical and clinical seminars, and the supervised analysis of "control" cases, had been established, on the basis of the approach used at the Berlin Psychoanalytic Institute.

Nevertheless, analysis was still a European specialty, in the same sense that "modern architecture" in the 1920s and 1930s was primarily European, with the work of LeCorbusier or the German Bauhaus. The 10th Annual Report of the Berlin Institute (1920–1930) and the reports of returning American candidates indicate that analysis belonged to the avant-garde. The Berlin Institute seemed a well-organized but easy-going institution, with a lively, spontaneous student body and great freedom from regimentation. Its relaxed atmosphere differed greatly from its image as advocated by Hendrick in Boston, a model more rigid and "German" than the model used at the Berlin Institute itself. When Martin Peck visited Freud in 1939 and boasted about the reorganization, Freud dismissed the American "medical fixation" and recommended "a pinch of Attic salt" (Peck 1940).

Immigration and the Europeanization of American Analysis, 1933–1946

With the arrival of the émigré analysts from Europe, the analytic movement entered a new era, in which European ideas and American institutional forms would undergo a mutual interchange. This evolutionary process was overtaken by historical events, with the Nazi occupation of Europe, but there was a strange delay among American analysts in responding to these violent events. The minutes of the New York Psychoanalytic Society seemed almost untouched by international events, and even in Vienna, during the Dollfuss putsch of 1933–1934, Freud could write to Ernest Jones (April 7, 1933):

> We are passing over to a dictatorship of the Right, which means the suppression of social democracy. This will not be a pretty state of affairs and will not be pleasant for us Jews, but we think that special laws against the Jews are out of the question in Austria because of the clauses in our [international] peace-treaty....Vienna is—despite all

the riots, processions, etc. reported in the newspapers— calm and life is undisturbed. (Jones 1953–1957, Vol. 3, p. 181)

In Germany itself, while Grotjahn (1987) was helping Ernst Simmel, his analyst, escape through his consulting-room window, Grotjahn's wife still believed in 1935 that Hitler would last only another 2 years. Helene Deutsch (personal communication, 1966) often said that no one in Vienna encouraged them to leave in 1935 except Robert Waelder, and the Waelders themselves lingered until the *Anschluss*. Felix Deutsch, on a U.S. lecture trip in 1933, observed that Americans were more aware of the potential danger of Hitler than his fellow Austrians. In 1936, according to Kurt Eissler, Anna Freud still advised younger analysts against leaving Vienna.

Freud and his family emigrated to London in 1938, but most Austrian analysts who reached England were urged to move on to the United States as soon as they obtained permanent U.S. visas. The great variety of individual experiences in escaping Europe have woven a rich, tragic tapestry of a forced exodus, and these patterns of emigration influenced the distribution of European analysts in the United States, through personal sponsorship, academic invitations necessary for "affidavits," and the choice of destination.

There are many good histories of this great intellectual migration (Fleming and Bailyn 1969; Fermi 1968; Hughes 1975; Coser 1984). European analysts were one group among the many refugee artists, scholars, and scientists that transformed American cultural life during the Second World War. The analysts most closely resembled the architects of the Bauhaus and the pioneer nuclear physicists—small but influential groups that represented relatively new specialties, already in demand in this country. European analysts were welcomed by friendly colleagues and former analysands, and in New York and Boston psychoanalytic circles the many senior German and Austrian analysts seemed to outnumber the native Americans. In 1933, for example, all 10 founding members of the Boston Institute were Americans, but a decade later, by which time the membership had almost tripled, over half its members were European. Some European analysts complained about the rigidity of institute rules, the proliferation of committee work, and the prejudice against nonmedical applicants. By 1942, however, when the United States entered the war and immigration ceased, Europeans had become the leaders of American analysis.

The prominence of certain émigré analysts, foremost in research and theoretical innovation, made New York the analytic capital of the world. Hartmann, Kris, and Loewenstein were leaders in ego psychology, and René Spitz, Margaret Mahler, and other gifted child analysts explored new fields in early infant development. In the Washington-Baltimore area, there were influential child-analysts like Jenny Waelder-Hall and Lucie Jessner. Frieda Fromm-Reichmann was the foremost practitioner in the analytic treatment of schizophrenia.

As the scientific life of the analytic institutes was undergoing a process of Europeanization, local American customs and institutions played an important role. One American characteristic, first noted by Oberndorf (1953), was the tendency for analysts to hold academic positions in medical schools and schools of social work, a situation in contrast to Freud's isolation from academic medicine. Boston analysts, for example, according to Levin and Michaels (1961), were surprised to learn that over 90% held institutional posts of some kind. There was also a strong tradition of hospital-based psychiatry.

Another American feature was the number of well-established institutions for the treatment of children, such as the Institute for Juvenile Research in Chicago and the Child Study Center at Yale University. There were many such clinics in Boston, from the venerable Judge Baker Guidance Center, Douglas Thom's Habit Clinic, and the Home for Little Wanderers to the new J.J. Putnam Children's Center, founded by his daughter, Marian Putnam.

A major interchange between American and European trends was a "new" psychiatric specialty, psychosomatic medicine. Its American roots were in the early papers of Smith Ely Jelliffe (Burnham 1983) and in the work of Flanders Dunbar's (1935) group at Columbia. The European roots were in the work of Georg Groddeck and Felix Deutsch (1924); the latter was the first to use the term *psychosomatic* in its current sense. The peak of psychosomatic research occurred in 1950–1960, with the journal *Psychosomatic Medicine*, edited by Flanders Dunbar and Carl Binger, which had been founded in 1939. Franz Alexander soon created a center for psychosomatic research at the Chicago Psychoanalytic Institute. Although Felix Deutsch's work had not been well known in Europe, and Alexander (1931/1936) had had no apparent interest in mind-body problems until he reached this country, both Deutsch and the Chicago Psychoanalytic Institute became widely recognized for psychosomatic research in a way that would have been unlikely in Europe. The "psychosomatic movement" drew analysts to hospital and medical school positions, as reflected in the research at Mt. Sinai, New York, by M.Ralph Kaufman (1965) and Sydney Margolin (1953) in the early 1950s and at Rochester, New York, under John Romano and George Engel.

An important native American institution was The Menninger Clinic (and later Foundation), in Topeka, Kansas, which facilitated the migration of refugee analysts throughout the Midwest and the West Coast. Martin Grot-jahn arrived in 1936, followed by Bernard Kamm, David Rapaport, and other distinguished refugees. As a largely psychoanalytic hospital like Ernst Simmel's Berlin sanitarium, Schloss Tegel, Menninger was also a training center for psychiatric residents, many of whom became analysts. As an "open" hospital for the treatment of neuroses, it also belongs in the American tradition of Stockbridge, founded by Austen Riggs and modeled on Dr. Gehring's "retreat" at Bethel, Maine (Kubie 1960). During the 1950s, under the leadership of Dr. Robert P. Knight, the Menninger staff became almost entirely psychoanalytic.

To sum up this period, from 1938 to 1946 the Europeanization of our four newly reorganized analytic training institutes was accomplished with relatively little conflict, as many Americans trained in Europe welcomed their former teachers. The sole area of conflict was lay analysis, often solved by provisions for "affiliate membership." Besides Hanns Sachs in Boston, other eminent European non-M.D.s included Robert Waelder in Philadelphia, Ernst Kris and Edith Buxbaum in New York, David Rapaport in Topeka, and Siegfried Bernfeld, Anna Maenchen, and Erik Erikson in San Francisco.

As ego psychology came to the fore, it was unfairly criticized as a desexualized version of analysis for the American public, but its origins are found in Freud's late papers and in the work of Anna Freud (1936/1946). Hartmann's first major paper, "Ego Psychology and the Problems of Adaptation" (1939/1958), was presented to the Vienna Society in 1937, foreshadowing many later extensions of ego psychology in its links with cognitive psychology and the social sciences. The basic developmental concepts in ego psychology, emerging from new discoveries in child analysis, were synthesized magnificently in Rapaport's paper "Psychoanalysis as a Developmental Psychology" (1957/1967), on the anniversary of Freud's birth. The concept of analysis as a general psychology of normal development was an extension of ego psychology, beyond analyis as a method of treatment, as in Erikson's concept of the life cycle. Even Kohut's later self psychology, with its renewed emphasis on deficiencies in the early mother-infant relationship, can be recognized as a derivation from the "New York School" of ego psychology.

There was a preanalytic American tradition of interest in childhood, going back to G. Stanley Hall (1904) and even John Fiske (1842–1901), whose theories about the effect of prolonged infantile helplessness later influenced Freud. Among the nonanalytic observers of infants and children, such as Arnold Gesell and his group in the 1920s, there was a developmental concept, and Margaret Fries, a student of the Gesells, became an analyst and an observer of newborn behavior. Spitz's first reports on hospitalism and anaclitic depression, and Erikson's (1943) observations on American Indian children, contributed to the acceptance of ego psychology during the war years.

"The Years That Were Fat": Postwar Expansion and Institutional Splits, 1946–1968

Military Psychiatry and the Spread of Analysis

A new element affected the analytic movement after the end of the Second World War: the return from military service of young physicians eager to become analysts. The war had created an increased demand for psychiatrists in order to treat the many unexpected psychiatric casualties among the troops. Medical schools and internships were accelerated, doctors were drafted, and programs in military psychiatry were established.

Military doctors of all kinds who had served as psychiatrists soon became interested in psychiatry and analysis. Among future analysts were those who had treated acute traumatic neuroses on the battlefield, such as Martin Berezin at Guadalcanal, and those eminent analysts who became consultants with high military rank, such as M. Ralph Kaufman, John Murray, and William Menninger. Psychiatrists returned from overseas to teach military psychiatry, full of enthusiasm for quasi-analytic methods of psychotherapy. Roy Grinker and John Spiegel in North Africa had treated soldiers with acute combat reactions close to the frontlines, with methods derived from Breuer and Freud's early "cathartic" treatment of hysteria. Utilizing hypnosis and intravenous barbiturates, Grinker and Spiegel (1945) attempted to "abreact" repressed traumatic experiences and return these young men to their combat units. Their dramatic results were published in a small handbook that was widely distributed throughout the armed forces. Many returning medical officers, fascinated by these experiences, applied for psychiatric residencies and psychoanalytic training. There was a corresponding postwar increase in grants for psychiatric training and research from federal entities such as the Army Stress Committee and the National Institute of Mental Health (NIMH). Veterans Administration (VA) facilities were enlarged to treat returning servicemen, and training grants increased the number of psychiatrists. The Menninger Foundation in Topeka, for example, staffed a 2,300-bed Army and VA hospital that was training 100 psychiatric residents a year, all with a strong psychoanalytic orientation (Friedman 1990).

As this expansive trend reached the medical schools in the 1950s and 1960s, a quarter of some graduating classes planned to become psychiatrists. The chairmen of psychiatric departments in teaching hospitals were increasingly chosen from among psychoanalysts, and many psychiatric residents came to regard analytic training as the inevitable next step in an academic career. After 1946, when the American Psychoanalytic Association allowed more than one institute in a city, new institutes and study groups proliferated, with a pattern of westward migration. From Chicago to Topeka to the West Coast, new training centers followed the "geographic rule," which called for each study group or provisional institute to be sponsored by a parent institute. This led to unusual travels for candidates in outlying areas, who commuted long distances for seminars and supervision. Five new institutes were established during the 1940s, 9 by 1950, 20 in 1966, and 38 in 2003.

Controversies and Institutional Splitting

The first major split had already occurred in 1941, when Karen Horney and her four allies walked out of a regular business meeting of the New York Psychoanalytic Institute. Marianne Eckhardt (1978), Horney's daughter, in an eye-witness account, and Quinn (1987), in a more detailed study, have described the complex issues and the distress experienced by the Institute candidates.

Dissension had occurred among European analysts, but it had involved conflicts with Freud himself. When Jung, Adler, and Rank made their painful departures from analysis, there were theoretical differences, but they also seemed to be enacting oedipal struggles. American institutional splits were among peers—fraternal conflicts between rival factions—perhaps reflecting the native predilection of Americans for social and political clubs, as a "nation of joiners."

Horney's defection from the New York Psychoanalytic Institute was preceded by long-standing dissatisfaction with its dogmatism and rigidity, but her emphasis on social factors played a minor role in the split. The immediate cause of the split was Horney's being deprived of her status as training analyst because her teaching was "disturbing to the students." Horney formed the Association for the Advancement of Psychoanalysis, with its corresponding training facility, called the American Institute of Psychoanalysis. Formerly a prominent teacher in the Berlin Psychoanalytic Institute, Horney had first emigrated to Chicago but had a falling-out with her old Berlin colleague Franz Alexander. In New York her closest followers were Clara Thompson, Bernard Robbins, and William Silverberg. Harry Stack Sullivan joined the group, and although he had moved back to Washington, D.C. in 1939, he believed that a New York branch was important, but it was called the "Washington School."

Horney and Sullivan shared an interest in social and cultural issues, along with Erich Fromm, a prominent member of the Frankfurt School, and the American linguist Edward Sapir. All taught at the Washington School, along with several anthropologists who were sympathetic to analysis, such as Ralph Linton and Ruth Benedict. Horney wrote several popular books that criticized Freud's underestimation of social factors in psychic conflict. Sullivan was editor of *Psychiatry*, the "yellow journal" that welcomed both analysts and social scientists, published by the William A. White Foundation.

Sullivan and Horney seemed an ill-assorted pair, but the new Washington School in New York flourished under their leadership. Classrooms for their seminars were provided by New York Medical College and by the New School for Social Research, which had always been hospitable to unorthodox émigrés. A second split took place in 1943, when 12 members resigned, including Clara Thompson, Sullivan, and Erich Fromm. Again the dispute concerned withdrawal of training privileges, this time from Fromm, ostensibly because he was not a physician, although he had been an accepted member for years. A third split occurred later the same year, over affiliation with New York Medical College, which was opposed by Horney and supported by her early allies William Silverberg, Arnold Robbins, and Judd Marmor. They resigned and created a new analytic training center, reorganized in 1947 as the Society of Medical Psychoanalysts.

The Horney split eventually led to the departure of her Association for the Advancement of Psychoanalysis from the American Psychoanalytic Association. Meanwhile, another split occurred when the Columbia group, led by John A. P. Millet, George Daniels, and Carl Binger, created the Columbia University Psychoanalytic Clinic. They were followed by Abram Kardiner and Sandor Rado. The clinic was recognized in 1945 as an accredited training institute of the American Psychoanalytic Association—the first analytic institute associated with a medical school. This pattern was emulated by the New York University Medical School at King's County Hospital, at Chapel Hill, North Carolina, and at Western Reserve in Cleveland.

Another analytic organization established outside the American Psychoanalytic Association was the Academy of Psychoanalysis, founded in 1956 by Millet, Silverberg, Rado, Franz Alexander, Clara Thompson, and Marmor. Many members from the Washington School joined, but the Academy served a different purpose, as a national scientific society, with no teaching or training function. Any intention of creating a rival organization to the American Psychoanalytic Association was disclaimed, and membership was open to nonmedical analysts and scientists in related fields.

Another divisive issue during the mid-1950s was the protracted controversy over certification in analysis, a quite different issue from recent debates over certification. A proposal was made to the American Psychoanalytic Association that the American Psychiatric Association (APA) create a specialty board in psychoanalysis. By defining analysis as a subspecialty of clinical psychiatry, this proposal was a drastic move toward the "medicalization" of American analysis, as Oberndorf had first advocated. But fierce opposition was evoked from many analysts who adhered to Freud's view that analysis was an independent profession, not "a mere house-maid to psychiatry." The proposal was vigorously supported by enemies of lay analysis, such as Ives Hendrick and Bertram Lewin, who defended native American "medical orthodoxy," and it was opposed by most European analysts. The specialty-board proposal was eventually defeated by the membership of the American Psychoanalytic Association, and its heated debates in local institutes are long forgotten.

Besides the complex divisions within the New York analytic community, there were splits in other institutes during the postwar period. The venerable Philadelphia Psychoanalytic Society, founded in 1937 and approved by the American Psychoanalytic Association in 1939, soon developed undercurrents of dissent (Oral History Workshop #40 1994). The issues concerned analytic orthodoxy, and one of the founding members, Dr. Sidney Biddle, began to circulate "little tracts," instructing his colleagues in the correct teaching and behavior of psychoanalysts. Examples given by Leo Madow suggest an extreme version of "psychoanalytic neutrality," stressing the avoidance of extra-analytic contacts between analyst and patient. The *casus belli* was an encounter between Biddle and LeRoy Maeder on the rooftop of their office building, where Biddle challenged Maeder to resign if he disagreed with Biddle's principles. Maeder returned the challenge, and Biddle announced he and his allies would form their own institute.

From this seemingly trivial disagreement, the Philadelphia Association for Psychoanalysis was organized in 1949 and accepted by the American Psychoanalytic Association in 1950. The original Philadelphia Psychoanalytic Society continued as before, but the effect on both institutes was far from trivial. Analysts who were candidates at the time of the split described their painful choices and sense of betrayal, although most of them followed their own analysts. Many analysands compared their experiences to those of the "children of divorce," kept in the dark while their parents decided their fate, and their hurt feelings and the increasing isolation between the two organizations persisted for decades. Finally, beginning in 1980, there were tentative efforts at a rapprochement (Oral History Workshop #55 2002), which led to the historic reunification of the two institutes. This was the first reconciliation of a split; the process was long, tortuous, and in some ways as painful as the original split.

Another split occurred, in 1950, between the original Los Angeles Psychoanalytic Society of 1946 (LAPSI) and the new Southern California Psychoanalytic Society. The issue seemed to be lay analysis, because there were many prominent refugee analysts in Los Angeles who either were nonphysicians or lacked qualifications for California licensure, such as Ernst Simmel and Otto Fenichel, both of whom were leaders in the original society. Fenichel's premature death occurred in 1946, during a grueling internship he had undertaken to become "qualified." The seceding group was opposed to lay analysis and sympathetic to Franz Alexander, who was about to move to Los Angeles from Chicago. Initially called the Southern California Society for Psychoanalytic Medicine, it became the Southern California Psychoanalytic Society in 1964. Gradually its original medical orientation was reversed, and the society became sympathetic toward nonphysicians, admitting the child analyst Marie Briehl and graduating its first non-M.D. for full training, Peter Loewenberg.

Accounts of the Los Angeles split (Greenson et al. 1975) reported a peaceful coexistence of the two institutes in Los Angeles and a partial resolution of the lay-analysis conflict at the San Francisco Psychoanalytic Institute, where Siegfried Bernfeld, a non-M.D., was a major training-analyst. This bland 1975 account of the two Los Angeles institutes gave no hint of the fierce internal conflicts that were taking place within LAPSI, the original institute. There were internecine rivalries between the American leaders Ralph Greenson and Leo Rangell and a rapidly growing interest in the theories of Melanie Klein, Fairbairn, and the British object relations school. Wilfred Bion was invited to settle in Los Angeles, and there was an influx of British Kleinians, to lecture and proselytize, that threatened to take over the Institute. A site visit from the American Psychoanalytic Association in 1973 seemed to exacerbate the conflict, and only a major threat of disaccreditation, by a special committee led by Joan Fleming, produced a compromise. By 1976 the threat had been dropped by the American Psychoanalytic Association, a split was obviated, and the Kleinian factions became less threatening. More details about these complicated events are provided in the chapter "Fear and Loathing in LA" in Douglas Kirsner's (2000) *Unfree Associations: Inside Psychoanalytic Institutes.*

The Boston split occurred much later (Oral History Workshop #57 2003), in 1974, and showed some unusual features, in that a small group seceded to found a new institute while remaining members of the Boston Psychoanalytic Society. In the late 1960s, dissatisfaction appeared among

the candidates, who were protesting the impersonality of analytic training, and among analysts who had not been appointed training-analysts. A 2-year experiment with a deanship had proved unsuccessful, and in this case the *casus belli* was the action of the Education Committee in terminating the deanship without consulting the Society. This provoked fierce protests, as high-handed and undemocratic, and a series of turbulent meetings of the entire membership followed, with discussions about how to create a better balance between the Society, which had few functions, and the Institute, the seat of all power.

The controversies seemed to be between conservatives and reformers until May 1974, when M. Robert Gardner and four colleagues announced the formation of a separate institute, the Psychoanalytic Institute of New England, usually called PINE. Although its aims were ill-defined, PINE strongly emphasized the importance of remaining a small, congenial group, dedicated to intellectual discussion, unburdened by committee meetings and administrative red tape. The underlying issues, however, concerned the appointment of new training analysts and the exclusive power of the Education Committee. Critics of PINE feared that "the flood gates would open" and large numbers of unqualified training-analysts would be approved by the new institute. After many more months of bruising disputes and mutual hostility, PINE was accepted by the American Psychoanalytic Association as an independent institute, while its members continued to belong to the Boston Psychoanalytic Society. All PINE members shared the Boston Psychoanalytic Society and Institute library and some child-analysis programs. In time, the worst fears of its critics proved groundless: many years elapsed before one new training analyst was appointed by PINE. It remained the small, intimate society that its founders originally envisioned, fulfilling its original aims, although the requirements of the American Psychoanalytic Association involved its limited membership in committee work.

Among these institutional splits, some common features can be identified. Participants in all the splits reported the same lingering distress, pain, and hurt feelings in proportion to their original disagreements. The sense of injustice and betrayal and of mutual hatred among colleagues and close friends lasted for decades, long after the original cause had grown dim. The persistence of these painful feelings has proved an obstacle to recalling our history, leaving a void that has attracted at least one diligent cultural historian. Douglas Kirsner (2000), a professor of philosophy from Melbourne, Australia, has written the only book on psychoanalytic institutional splits, based on interviews with several hundred participants, many of whom are no longer living. He has chosen the histories of four institutes, New York, Boston, Chicago, and Los Angeles, and described them in great detail. His chronicles confirm the American pattern of fratricidal strife among siblings, in contrast to the generational conflicts more common in European splits.

Psychoanalysis in Canada

The history of psychoanalysis in Canada has many unusual features, beginning with Ernest Jones's Canadian sojourn (1908–1913), when he was very active in American psychoanalysis but left no institutional traces in Canada. The later developments of analysis in Canada (Oral History Workshop #28 1989) were complicated by Canada's being very close to the United States, where many early members went for training, with some never to return. Later, the bilingual issue in Montreal became a problem, resulting in the formation of three branches of the Canadian Psychoanalytic Society and Institute: a Toronto branch, the Quebec English-speaking branch in Montreal, and the Société Psychanalytique Canadienne de Montréal. This process was complete in 1968–1969, and by 1988 there were 95 graduates of the French program, when the total membership of the Canadian Psychoanalytic Society and Institute was 325. At that time, Montreal, a city of 6 million, was bilingual, with 1 million native English speakers. According to its members, the three branches met together in perfect harmony, and the only disputes occurred between the Society and the Institute.

In the early years, no distinction was made between French- and English-speaking analysts, and their meetings were presumably conducted in English. The first group met in 1944, at the Allan Memorial Hospital in Montreal, whose director, Ewen Cameron, was strongly opposed to analysis. Their leaders were Miguel Prados, a refugee from the Spanish Civil War, and Father Noel Mailloux, a Dominican friar who was a professor of psychology at the University of Montreal. The other early analysts were also cosmopolitan: André Chentrier, a French non-M.D., and George Zavitzianos, a Greek trained in Paris and the only M.D. The first residents, who called themselves The Four Sad Apples, met in secret, inspired by Prados and Father Mailloux, who urged them to get their training abroad and return.

Many of them left and returned, later joined by W. Clifford M. Scott, a Canadian who had studied at Harvard and Johns Hopkins and completed his training in London. Efforts to form a study group affiliated with the American Psychoanalytic Association were rebuffed in 1952 by Ives Hendrick, because the Canadians accepted lay members for training and were suspected of Kleinian sympathies. The study group organizers turned to the IPA and were accepted in 1957. Among others who returned from training abroad were Henry Kravitz, Bruce Ruddick, and Alastair MacLeod. Alan Parkin, trained in London, was the founder of the Tor-

onto Branch. Many who did not return, such as M. Ralph Kaufman, Douglas Noble, Dorothy Macnaughton, and Cecil Mushatt, were assimilated into their American institutes.

Postwar Expansion in Retrospect

This condensed survey of institutional splits may seem unconscionably long, out of proportion to their lasting effects, but the time and energy consumed by these conflicts was also unconscionable. Many talented analysts, appalled by the personal distress involved, withdrew from professional activities within their local institutes, practiced in isolation, or turned to other fields, rejecting analysis altogether. But, in spite of the impression of endless strife, the outstanding feature of such conflict, in fact, was a confident, optimistic outlook and an unquestioning belief in the continuing expansion of analysis. Analysts foresaw an unlimited horizon, gaining new members, creating new institutes, and finding new applications for analysis.

The three major characteristics of American psychoanalysis were still present: 1) general agreement about Freud's basic theories, in spite of the minor dissents of Horney and Sullivan; 2) continued expansion of certain analytic specialties—child analysis, psychosomatic medicine, and general hospital psychiatry—that flourished In the United States more vigorously than they had in Europe; and 3) widespread interchange between psychoanalysis and other fields, from the social sciences and literature to sleep physiology and animal behavior.

A mutual interest between American anthropology and analysis began with Alfred Kroeber in the 1920s. Kroeber, an eminent California anthropologist who took a sabbatical year in New York in order to undertake an analysis, became the first analyst in San Francisco (Theodora Kroeber 1970). Kroeber assisted Erik Erikson (1943) in studying American Indian children, and Sydney Margolin carried out anthropological fieldwork with the Utes. Mutual interests created a collaboration between Abraham Kardiner and Ralph Linton (Kardiner 1939). Other prominent anthropologists, such as Margaret Mead, Ruth Benedict, and Clyde and Florence Kluckhohn, were sympathetic to analysis. A leading sociologist, Talcott Parsons, undertook analytic training and became an affiliate member of the Boston Psychoanalytic Society.

As we have seen, analysts were leaders in the psychosomatic movement and in the closely related field of general hospital psychiatry, which was an American innovation. The first inpatient psychiatry department in a general hospital was established in 1936 at Massachusetts General Hospital by Stanley Cobb (White 1984), an early member of the Boston Psychoanalytic Society. He invited

Felix Deutsch, Erik Erikson, and other émigré analysts to lecture and teach at Massachusetts General. Similar psychiatry units in general hospitals arose elsewhere, with Flanders Dunbar and George Daniels at Columbia, M. Ralph Kaufman (1965) and Sydney Margolin (1953) at Mt. Sinai in New York, and Roy Grinker at Michael Reese in Chicago. Franz Alexander created a major center for psychosomatic research at the Chicago Psychoanalytic Institute. Another influential training center for psychosomatic research was established by John Romano and George Engel at Rochester Medical School in upper New York State. Romano, who became Chief of Psychiatry, had been analyzed as a Freud Fellow in Boston, but he was not allowed to complete his training in Rochester. George Engel, an analyst and a professor of psychiatry engaged in psychosomatic research, wrote an influential textbook for medical students.

American child psychiatry had been influenced by Anna Freud's seminars in the mid-1920s, Melanie Klein's play technique, and Spitz's direct infant observations. But as we have seen, there were preexisting American institutions, such as the Judge Baker Guidance Center in Boston and the Institute for Juvenile Research in Chicago. In the vast expansion of developmental research during the 1950s, the American format of "team research" evolved, with close collaboration among analysts, clinical psychologists, and social workers. 1950 was declared "The Year of the Child," and a series of multidisciplinary research meetings, published by the Josiah Macy Foundation, were eagerly read by all analysts. New research centers proliferated, with Ernst and Marianne Kris at the Yale Child Study Center, John Benjamin and René Spitz in Denver, Ruth and Gardner Murphy at The Menninger Clinic, and Sibylle Escalona at Einstein Medical College.

Two other American specialties, the psychotherapy of psychoses and group psychotherapy, emerged. The analytic treatment of schizophrenia, which Freud had declared was impossible, began in the early years with William A. White and Edward Kempf at St. Elizabeths and continued with Harry Stack Sullivan at Sheppard Pratt. Its most important institution was Chestnut Lodge, in Rockville, Maryland, where Frieda Fromm-Reichmann and her followers maintained the tradition for decades.

Group therapy was also an American contribution to analysis, from its unlikely beginnings in 1906, in a collaboration among a Boston internist, an Episcopal minister trained in clinical psychology, and a psychiatrist, Isador Coriat, later Boston's second analyst (Gifford 1996). Dr. Joseph Pratt treated tuberculosis by the "class method" (Worcester et al. 1908), which became a group method of treating outpatient neuroses. Influential group therapists like S.R. Slavson (1947) proposed analytic forms of group

therapy, and Paul Schilder, Fritz Redl, and Elvin Semrad became enthusiastic practitioners. Semrad (1973/1978) treated psychiatric casualties during the Second World War by group methods, and Martin Grotjahn (1987) considered analytic group therapy superior to traditional psychoanalysis for certain patients.

In concluding the era of postwar expansion of psychoanalysis, one important feature of the American medical scene was the increasing support of both private and federal funds for both psychiatry and psychoanalysis. The Commonwealth Fund had supported analytic training in Europe for young psychiatrists in the 1920s and 1930s, and the new psychiatric unit of Stanley Cobb at Mass General was funded by the Rockefeller Foundation. But the postwar years brought large-scale government support to all kinds of psychiatric research and training programs in university hospitals. The NIMH instituted a broad program of support for research that was increasingly sympathetic to psychoanalysis. Some leaders at NIMH, such as Robert A. Cohen, William Pollen and Lyman Wynne, were analysts.

The Lean Years, 1968 to the Present

The fat years of continuous expansion lasted almost two decades, from the end of the war to the late 1960s. Exactly when the high tide began to ebb is hard to date and was at first scarcely perceptible. Millet (1966) noted a leveling off in the expected number of new applicants for analytic training, but the American Psychoanalytic Association continued to show steady growth: there were 20 approved institutes and 26 affiliate societies in 1966–1967, and 26 institutes, 31 societies, and 4 approved study groups 10 years later. Knight's presidential address of 1953 had predicted 2,000 members 20 years later, and in 1974–1975 there were 2,758 members.

By the mid-1970s candidates began to feel a scarcity of suitable control patients, and this trend has steadily progressed. As the delays in completing analytic training increased, new applicants were well aware of the time required. Although they realized they could never expect full analytic practices, as their forebears had had, candidates continued to apply for training. Some institutes responded by limiting their entering classes, but most maintained their customary admission criteria.

Under these conditions, recent candidates have shown greater variety, with more unusual backgrounds and more theoretical and research interests. The proportion of women and nonmedical candidates has increased, and there are fewer careerist applicants, for whom analytic training was the next step in academic advancement, now that analysis no longer promises a lucrative practice or academic prestige. For some candidates, analytic training seems the best method of learning psychotherapy, which is no longer taught in many psychiatric residencies. The result may be a smaller, livelier student body and a more stimulating intellectual atmosphere.

In the past 20 years, American psychoanalysis, in terms of practice and training methods, has changed less than the context in which clinical psychiatry, psychiatric research, and even medicine itself are practiced has changed. The decline in popularity has chiefly affected analysis in the number of patients for treatment, while the demand for training has remained relatively high, and popular interest in the history of analysis has increased, judging from the large output of publications. The major institutional changes have been the end of the ancient lay-analysis controversy and the loss of funds for analytic training and research.

The End of the Lay-Analysis Controversy

Despite the traditional American opposition to lay analysts, there have always been constitutional provisions for admitting gifted nonphysicians. At first, these individuals were accepted for theoretical seminars only, to graduate as affiliate members, with an agreement not to practice analysis. Then came special exemptions, such as the grandfather clause that enabled eminent European lay analysts to become training analysts. Other exemptions were instituted through a system of waivers, or petitions to the American Psychoanalytic Association, requesting full clinical training because of research needs, often sought by child therapists or academics engaged in developmental research. Many of these individuals later practiced analysis and became training analysts and prominent teachers. The waiver system succeeded in circumventing the old rules against lay analysis, but the numbers were small: 110 non-M.D.'s out of 2,726 members of the American Psychoanalytic Association, for example, in 1974–1975. Besides the cumbersome and disingenuous nature of the waiver procedure, there was an unfair demand that non-M.D. applicants submit evidence of exceptional scholarship or creativity, when no such requirement was made of the ordinary medical applicant. The discrepancy in incomes between M.D. psychiatrists and Ph.D. academicians also made full training more difficult for nonphysicians. But the unwieldy system functioned as long as its unfair features were not called into question.

In the early 1970s attitudes toward nonmedical analysis seemed to be changing. The so-called Chicago Plan, proposed by the late George Pollock, would have accepted applicants from any background and eventually granted a Ph.D. in Psychoanalysis. The Chicago Plan proposal was defeated at the 1975 annual American Psychoanalytic Association meetings, but discussions in local societies revealed an unexpected groundswell of approval for nonmedical applicants. A proposal by Robert Wallerstein of Mt. Zion Hospital, San Francisco, was more successful in creating a graduate school program for nonphysicians with a doctorate in mental health. The Mt. Zion program lasted 13 years, and many of its graduates later became analysts.

Although these events seemed to foreshadow a change in attitude, there were powerful factions within the American Psychoanalytic Association that opposed any compromise with lay analysis. A succession of American Psychoanalytic Association committees reported on the shifting attitudes, but the final recommendation by the Board of Professional Standards was always for further delay, usually by appointing another committee. In December 1984 an ad hoc committee chaired by Herbert Gaskill of Denver finally reversed this pattern, and the acceptance of the Gaskill Proposal, at the May meetings in 1985, marked a dramatic breakthrough (Shane 1985). An astonishing majority in the American Psychoanalytic Association favored full clinical training for nonphysicians, and the *intent* of the Gaskill Proposal was approved by 68% of the membership. The Gaskill Report still bore the marks of its prolonged and difficult labor, in its attempts to placate the enemies of lay analysis. The report claimed that the proposal would preserve the "essentially medical nature of our organization" and that the number of nonmedical applicants was expected to be small, without disturbing the existing ratio of medical to nonmedical candidates. While the Gaskill Proposal was hailed as "the fruition of a long history of attempts…to deal with the significant issue of lay analysis," the existing system of waivers was not changed. No change in by-laws was required, "thereby retaining the… Association's essential attachment to both medicine and psychiatry" (Shane 1985, p. 10). The need for a constitutional amendment, requiring a two-thirds majority, was also avoided.

These comments about the Gaskill Proposal from the American Psychoanalytic Association newsletter (Shane 1985) clearly reflect ambivalence about change. In fact, 3 months earlier, change was suddenly thrust upon the association by intervening events. In an antitrust suit filed in March 1985 by four psychologists, charges were brought against the New York Psychoanalytic Institute, the Columbia University Center for Psychoanalytic Training, the American Psychoanalytic Association, and the IPA. The suit was based on antidiscrimination and antitrust statutes, accusing the four analytic organizations of operating "in restraint of trade" by not admitting psychologists on the same basis as physicians. The Gaskill Committee, whose proposal was approved in May 1985, insisted that they had not been influenced by the threat of legal action. But, as Samuel Johnson said, "To be hanged in a fortnight... concentrates the mind wonderfully."

The IPA, sued as a codefendant, was outraged at being accused of discriminating against nonmedical applicants, when they had always disagreed with this exclusionary policy of the American Psychoanalytic Association. European and South American analytic societies had always included many nonphysicians, and now, because the American Psychoanalytic Association belonged to the IPA, members of the latter were being asked to contribute their dues to legal expenses incurred by the American Psychoanalytic Association!

At this time, Robert Wallerstein (quoted in Shane 1988) recalled a forgotten episode in early IPA history. In 1938, at the last European IPA Congress in Paris before the war, the American delegation had presented a singularly ill-timed proposal to abolish the International Training Commission of the IPA. The proposal was a parochial American response to the political events of 1938, when the Nazis had put an end to analysis in Germany and Austria. At that time, American analysts made up only 16% of the IPA membership, but by the end of the war and with the great migration of European analysts to the United States, this ratio was reversed and two-thirds of IPA members were living in this country (Knight 1953).

In 1938 the American Psychoanalytic Association was demanding of the IPA exclusive control over all analytic training within the United States, including émigrés with previous membership in the IPA. The Europeans rejected this proposal and postponed discussion to the 1940 IPA Congress, but the war supervened and the next IPA meeting did not occur until 1949. By then, with American analysts in the majority, "everyone acted as if it [the demand for exclusive control] had been approved," according to Wallerstein. "Nobody questioned it and in fact it was written into the IPA bylaws as if it had actually been formally voted."

As for the suit against the IPA in March 1985, the incensed British Society proposed that the American Psychoanalytic Association either extricate the IPA from the suit or agree to pay all its legal expenses. This demand was to be presented at the 1987 IPA Congress in Montreal, and by the skillful diplomacy of Wallerstein, then president of the IPA, a peaceful settlement was reached. The American Psychoanalytic Association accepted IPA training and membership outside the American Psychoanalytic Association and agreed to pay 60% of the IPA's legal expenses.

In 1989, the antitrust suit against the American Psychoanalytic Association and the IPA was settled out of court, and in May 1990, the president of the American Psychoanalytic Association, George Allison, appointed another committee, chaired by Homer Curtis. A constitutional amendment was drafted to accept nonmedical applicants for full clinical training *without a waiver!* They were required to have the highest professional degree in their field, and the waiver system was still retained for nondoctoral applicants. Finally, in July 1991, the Curtis committee's amendment was approved by over 80% of the American Psychoanalytic Association, 17 years after its first attempts to increase eligibility for non-M.D. training.

Recent Changes in American Psychoanalysis

One important change in psychoanalysis in the United States, beginning in 1968 with cuts in federal grants, was the shrinking support for psychoanalytic research and training and for psychodynamic research. At first, this development affected medical school professors and chiefs in teaching hospitals, who had substantial research and training programs supported by the NIMH. Sixty percent of psychiatric research projects were supported by NIMH in 1970, but only 24% in 1991. During the Vietnam War years, analysis was disparaged as elitist and authoritarian, ironically at the same time its student critics were subjecting themselves to authoritarian gurus and antiscientific health faddists. But these young critics correctly saw analysis as part of the medical establishment, no longer the revolutionary movement that had appealed to earlier generations of analysts.

In clinical psychiatry, there was an increasing emphasis on psychopharmacology and a return to nineteenth-century theories of hereditary mental illness. Although the decline in psychoanalysis is often attributed to increasing availability of antipsychotic drugs, this argument is unconvincing because patients with major psychoses are rarely seen in analytic practice. The increased interest in organic psychiatry, however, diminished the dynamic viewpoint that had once made psychiatry attractive to the medical students who later became analysts. The medical profession itself was also changing, with rapid technological advances in treatment and diagnostic procedures. The university hospital became an expensive, high-speed machine, geared to treating patients efficiently and discharging them as quickly as possible, reducing the time for house officers to spend with their patients.

Psychiatric hospitals and psychiatric inpatient services developed the same accelerated schedules and rapid discharges, pressed by insurance companies that increasingly refused to pay for lengthy hospitalizations. With admissions averaging 7–10 days (the "revolving door policy"), the leisurely pace of the psychoanalytically oriented hospitals began to suffer. McLean Hospital, a Harvard teaching hospital, has reduced its services and sold off some of its stately grounds. Chestnut Lodge in Rockville, Maryland, with its long tradition of psychotherapy for patients with psychoses, was compelled to close its doors, in spite of heroic efforts to save it. The greatest loss is the demise of The Menninger Foundation, with its inspiring early history and its superb library and list of publications. These are now dispersed, the books to Baylor University and the archives to the State Archives of Kansas. Finally, the Massachusetts Mental Health Center, the former Boston Psychopathic Hospital of 1912, has just evacuated its last 17 patients and will be demolished.

All physicians, not just psychiatrists, are becoming mired in administrative red tape, including that generated by malpractice insurance, "managed care," CME (continuing medical education) credits to keep one's license, and "recredentialling" to keep one's hospital appointment. Medical red tape has left house officers less time for listening to their patients and has allowed analysts less time for leisurely teaching rounds. Even psychologically astute medical interns, recognizing a patient's emotional needs, are obliged to refer them to psychiatrists, along with nurses and social workers, who have more time to listen.

Besides these unfavorable changes in the medical context, other changes within analysis have affected analysis in a positive way. As restrictions against nonphysicians were lifted, increased numbers of psychologists and social workers produced a greater diversity in our membership. Different points of view augment the trend, already noted, of attracting more original, innovative candidates. Many nonmedical therapists had meanwhile been developing their own training institutions outside the American Psychoanalytic Association, as in membership in the Institute for Psychoanalytic Training and Research (IPTAR), for example, or through Division 39 of the American Psychological Association, which established its own training centers. The Massachusetts Institute for Psychoanalysis (MIP), for example, is a Division 39 institute in Boston that has dispensed with the training-and-supervising-analyst system, but their students' personal analyses and supervision are conducted by BPSI or PINE analysts. As medicine becomes less attractive to potential analysts, future American analytic institutes may resemble the institutes of Europe and South America, with a third or more of their membership made up of nonmedical candidates.

Changes in analytic theory since the ascendancy of ego psychology have been relatively modest, compared with the exhilarating years after the Second World War. There has been an increased diversity and pluralism, with an interest in old and new theories, including those of Melanie Klein and the writings of Wilfrid Bion and Jacques Lacan. A renewed interest in the early mother-infant relationship became one of the sources of Kohut's self psychology, which has some claim to have superseded the conflict- and drive-theories of Freud, though Kohut himself insists that self psychology remains within the mainstream of psychoanalysis. There has been an intense interest in the borderline character, as in the writings of Otto Kernberg, incorporating elements derived from Melanie Klein, Donald Winnicott, John Bowlby, and the British object relations school. An important new direction in analysis is its rapprochement with neuroanatomists, like Mark Solms (2002), who has found validation for Freudian theory in functions of the brain.

While American analysis has remained relatively conservative, compared with the halcyon 1950s, Freud's (1914/1917) disparaging remarks about American analysis come to mind. He deplored America's craving for popularization and attributed this to our native "absence of any deep-rooted scientific tradition." He predicted that "precisely for this reason the ancient centers of culture, where the greatest resistance has been displayed, must be the scene of the decisive struggle over psychoanalysis" (p. 32). Today, when analysis is flourishing in Germany and Scandinavia, and in the newly liberated countries of Central Europe, Freud's early predictions may become relevant again.

Conclusion

As psychoanalysis has passed the 100th anniversary of Freud's *The Interpretation of Dreams* (1900/1953), its development in the United States seems to have come full circle, from modest beginnings, through an enormously expansive postwar phase, to its present diminished role. The decline began with a decrease in new patients, both for treatment and for training. But the psychoanalytic establishment, with its national association and its many component institutes, remains intact, and its scientific activities may even have increased. The number of new applicants for training remains close to previous levels, and many new institutes and study groups have been established in all parts of the country. Once nonmedical candidates were accepted for full training, both within and outside the American Psychoanalytic Association, they contributed increasing numbers to the movement.

A major cause of the reduced number of analytic patients is the greatly increased cost of analysis, without support by health insurance or government stipends, as well as the greater availability and versatility of psychoanalytic psychotherapy (Wallerstein 1986). Economic factors have always exerted an important influence on the development of analysis—favorable in the early years and recently unfavorable. In 1920–1930, postwar depression and inflation in Europe gave American students in Germany and

Austria an inexpensive means of getting analyzed and enjoying "the best years of our lives." Some were supported by fellowships for study abroad, such as that funded by the Commonwealth Fund. After the Second World War, the GI Bill provided government funds for the analytic training of many veterans. In 1948 analytic training was interpreted as professional education rather than treatment, and federal government support for psychiatric residencies came in the form of tax-free stipends rather than salary. The current popularity of analysis in Germany and Scandinavia may be sustained, in fact, because analysis is supported by national health insurance. In the United States at present, there seem to be three types of analysands: candidates-in-training, the very rich, and those individuals poor enough to qualify for institute analyses.

An earlier hypothesis about the waning popularity of psychoanalysis in the United States (Gifford 1978) suggested that the post–Second World War expansion of analysis in this country was the anomaly, not the lean years that followed 1968. In terms of Thomas Kuhn's paradigm of scientific revolutions, the postwar period of growth could be interpreted as a "phase of scientific discovery," with an abundance of new ideas, and the period of decline as a return to the preexisting phase of "normal scientific activity." Thus, the decline in psychoanalytic innovation after 1968 could be seen as a normal phenomenon, the ebb tide after new discoveries, as in other scientific fields with a peak year of theoretical innovation and a later return to baseline levels.

Following this paradigm, Freud might have welcomed a psychoanalytic movement more modest in size, less fixated on its "medical identity," and more open to nonmedical members. A closer interchange between analysis and the humanities and social sciences would have been congenial to Freud, who valued the applications of analysis to other fields as much, or even more, than its therapeutic uses. The current participation of analytic institutes in cultural events, with public discussions of plays, movies, and art exhibits, recalls the cultural "outreach" of the Berlin Institute, with its seminars on the arts and literature and even insect societies.

The waning influence of analysis in psychiatry and medicine has paralleled the ebbing of the European migration, with the deaths of its great leaders and innovators. Although the development of analysis in the United States involved a mutual interchange of European and native elements, it was an unequal interchange, in which nearly all theoretical discoveries came from Europe or from the émigré analysts in the United States. The American contribution included some important native institutions such as child guidance

centers, but our chief characteristic was a boundless energy for organizational activity. This drive to organize was present in the pre–analytic psychotherapy movement, with its incessant lecturing, proselytizing, and writing of popular handbooks. Later the same energy went into creating psychoanalytic societies and institutes and in colonizing a vast westward migration. Many American analysts devoted inordinate amounts of time and energy to administrative and educational activities. They created committees and wrote constitutions, and defended their by-laws with Robert's Rules of Order in local institutes and within the committees of the American Psychoanalytic Institute and the IPA. The best-known native American analysts of the 1950s and 1960s were educators like Bertram Lewin and Robert P. Knight, while theoretical innovations came from Europeans like Hartmann, Rapaport, and Erikson. And these great European figures have not been replaced.

To conclude with a broad generalization, American analysts may be compared to the ancient Roman engineers, pouring their energies into building the mighty edifice of the American Psychoanalytic Association but remaining dependent on European refugees for theoretical innovation. Thus, the Roman genius for engineering, organization, and empire building was dependent on the Greeks as the chief sources of their art, literature, and philosophy. Yet American analysis, in its more modest, postexpansionist phase, may remain an independent profession, smaller in scale, more varied in membership, and closer to Freud's ideals of 1926. In the language of our Bauhaus colleagues, *less may be more.*

References[1]

Alexander F: The Medical Value of Psychoanalysis, 2nd Edition, Revised (1931). New York, WW Norton, 1936

Berlin Psychoanalytic Institute: Zehn Jahre Berliner Psychoanalytisches Institut. Vienna, Austria, International Psychoanalytic Press, 1930

Breuer J, Freud S: Studies on hysteria (1893–1895), in Standard Edition of the Complete Psychological Works of Sigmund Freud, Vol 2. Translated and edited by Strachey J. London, Hogarth Press, 1955, pp 1–319

Brill AA: Minutes of the New York Psychoanalytic Society. AA Brill Papers. Washington, DC, Library of Congress, 1911–1947

Burnham JC: Psychoanalysis and American Medicine: 1894–1918. Psychological Issues Monograph 20. New York, International Universities Press, 1967

---

[1] I have drawn on many personal communications, not referenced in the text, chiefly with Edward and Grete Bibring, Felix and Helene Deutsch, Sandor Lorand, and Martin Grotjahn.

Burnham JC: Jelliffe: American Psychoanalyst and Physician. Chicago, IL, University of Chicago Press, 1983

Chapman AH: Harry Stack Sullivan: The Man and His Work. New York, Putnam, 1976

Coser LA: Refugee Scholars in America. New Haven, CT, Yale University Press, 1984

D'Amore ART: William Alanson White: pioneer psychoanalyst, in William Alanson White: The Washington Years, 1903–1937. Edited by D'Amore ART. Washington, DC, U.S. Government Printing Office, 1976, pp 69–94

D'Amore ART: Historical reflections on the organizational history of psychoanalysis in America, in American Psychoanalysis: Origins and Development. Edited by Quen JM, Carlson ET. New York, Brunner/Mazel, 1978, pp 127–140

Deutsch F: Zur Bildung des Konversionssymptoms. Internazionale Zeitschrift für Psychoanalyse 10:380–392, 1924

Dunbar HF: Emotions and Bodily Changes: A Survey of Literature on Psychosomatic Relationships, 1910–1933. New York, Columbia University Press, 1935

Eckhardt MH: Organizational schisms in American psychoanalysis, in American Psychoanalysis: Origins and Development. Edited by Quen JM, Carlson ET. New York, Brunner/Mazel, 1978, pp 141–161

Edes RT: The New England invalid. Boston Medical and Surgical Journal 133:53–57, 77–81, 101–107, 1895

Erikson E: Observations on the Yurok: childhood and world image. University of California Publications in American Archaeology and Ethnology 35:257–301, 1943

Fermi L: Illustrious Immigrants: The Intellectual Migration From Europe, 1930–41. Chicago, IL, University of Chicago Press, 1968

Fleming D, Bailyn B: The Intellectual Migration: Europe and America, 1930–1960. Cambridge, MA, Harvard University Press, 1969

Freud A: The Ego and the Mechanisms of Defense (1936). New York, International Universities Press, 1946

Freud S: The interpretation of dreams (1900), in Standard Edition of the Complete Psychological Works of Sigmund Freud, Vols 4 and 5. Translated and edited by Strachey J. London, Hogarth Press, 1953, pp 1–715

Freud S: Five lectures on psycho-analysis (1910), in Standard Edition of the Complete Psychological Works of Sigmund Freud, Vol 11. Translated and edited by Strachey J. London, Hogarth Press, 1957, pp 9–55

Freud S: The History of the Psychoanalytic Movement (1914). Translated by Brill AA. New York, Nervous & Mental Disease Publishing Co, 1917

Freud S: Introductory lectures on psychoanalysis (1916–1917), in Standard Edition of the Complete Psychological Works of Sigmund Freud, Vols 15 and 16. Translated and edited by Strachey J. London, Hogarth Press, 1957, pp 9–55

Freud S: Lines of advance in psycho-analytic studies (1918), in Standard Edition of the Complete Psychological Works of Sigmund Freud, Vol 17. Translated and edited by Strachey J. London, Hogarth Press, 1961, pp 159–168

Freud S: The question of lay analysis (1926), in Standard Edition of the Complete Psychological Works of Sigmund Freud, Vol 20. Translated and edited by Strachey J. London, Hogarth Press, 1959, pp 183–258

Freud S: Preface, in JJ Putnam: Addresses on Psycho-analysis (1921). London, Hogarth Press, 1951

Friedman LJ: Menninger: The Family and the Clinic. New York, Knopf, 1990

Gay P: Freud: A Life for Our Times. New York, WW Norton, 1998

Gifford S: Psychoanalysis in Boston: innocence and experience. Introduction to the panel discussion, April 14, 1973, in Psychoanalysis, Psychotherapy, and the Boston Medical Scene, 1894–1944. Edited by Gifford GE Jr. New York, Science History Publications, 1978, pp 106–118

Gifford S: The Emmanuel Movement: Boston 1904–1929. Cambridge, MA, Harvard University Press, 1996

Greenson R, Gabe S, Windholz E: Presentations at the Oral History Workshop #3, Los Angeles, May 1975

Grinker RR, Spiegel JP: Men Under Stress. Philadelphia, PA, Blakiston, 1945

Grotjahn M: My Favorite Patient: Memoirs of a Psychoanalyst. New York, Verlag Peter Lang, 1987

Hale NG Jr: Freud and the Americans: The Beginnings of Psychoanalysis in the United States, 1876–1917. New York, Oxford University Press, 1971a

Hale NG Jr: James Jackson Putnam and Psychoanalysis. Cambridge, MA, Harvard University Press, 1971b

Hall GS: Adolescence, Vols 1 & 2. New York, Appleton, 1904

Hartmann H: Ego Psychology and the Problem of Adaptation (1939). Translated by Rapaport D. New York, International Universities Press, 1958

Hendrick I: The Birth of an Institute: 25th Anniversary, the Boston Psychoanalytic Institute, November 30, 1958. Freeport, ME, Bond-Wheelwright, 1958

Hofstadter R: The Age of Reform: From Bryan to FDR. New York, Random House, 1955

Hughes HS: The Sea Change: The Migration of Social Thought, 1930–1965. New York, Harper & Row, 1975

James W: The Varieties of Religious Experience. New York, Random House (Modern Library), 1902

Jones E: Psychoanalysis in psychotherapy, in Psychotherapeutics. Edited by Gerrish FH. Boston, MA, Badger, 1909, pp 93–105

Jones E: The Life and Work of Sigmund Freud, Vols 1–3. New York, Basic Books, 1953–1957

Kardiner A, Linton R: The Individual and His Society. New York, Columbia Unversity Press, 1939

Kaufman MR: The Psychiatric Unit in a General Hospital. New York, International Universities Press, 1965

Kempf DC, Burnham JC: Selected Papers of E.J. Kempf, 3rd Edition. Bloomington, Indiana University Press, 1974

Kirsner D: Unfree Associations: Inside Psychoanalytic Institutes. London, Process Press, 2000

Knight R: The present status of organized psychoanalysis in the United States. J Am Psychoanal Assoc 1:197–221, 1953

Kroeber T: Alfred Kroeber: A Personal Configuration. Berkeley, University of California Press, 1970

Kubie LS: The Riggs Story: The Development of the Austen Riggs Center for the Study and Treatment of the Neuroses. New York, Hoeber, 1960

Langer WC, Gifford S: An American analyst in Vienna during the Anschluss 1936–38. J Hist Behav Sci 14:37–54, 1978

Levin S, Michaels JJ: The participation of psychoanalysis in the medical institutions of Boston. Int J Pyschoanal 42:271–277, 1961

Leys R: Meyer's dealings with Jones: a chapter in the history of the American response to psychoanalysis. J Hist Behav Sci 17:445–465, 1981

Margolin SG: Genetic and dynamic psychophysiological determinants of psychophysiological processes, in The Psychosomatic Concept in Psychoanalysis. Edited by Deutsch F. New York, International Universities Press, 1953, pp 3–36

Millet JAP: Psychoanalysis in the United States, in Psychoanalytic Pioneers. Edited by Alexander F, Eisenstein S, Grotjahn M. New York, Basic Books, 1966, pp 546–596

Noble D, Burnham DL: History of the Washington Psychoanalytic Society and the Washington Psychoanalytic Institute. Mimeographed monograph for private distribution, 1969

Oberndorf CP: A History of Psychoanalysis in America. New York, Harper & Row, 1953

Oral History Workshop #28 (American Psychoanalytic Association): History of the Canadian Psychoanalytic Society, Roger Dufresne, chair, Montreal, Canada, May 5, 1989

Oral History Workshop #40 (American Psychoanalytic Association): Psychoanalysis in Philadelphia, 1937–94, Selma Kramer, chair, Philadelphia, PA, May 19, 1994

Oral History Workshop #55 (American Psychoanalytic Association): Reunification of the Philadelphia Psychoanalytic Society, Ira Brenner, chair, Philadelphia, PA, May 16, 2002

Oral History Workshop #57 (American Psychoanalytic Association): Psychoanalysis in Boston, Nellie Thompson, chair, Boston, MA, June 19, 2003

Peck MW: A brief visit with Freud. Psychoanal Q 9:205–206, 1940

Perry HS: Psychiatrist of America: The Life of Harry Stack Sullivan. Cambridge, MA, Harvard University Press, 1982

Putnam JJ: Recent Experience in the Study and Treatment of Hysteria at the Massachusetts General Hospital, with Remarks on Freud's Method of Treatment by "Psychoanalysis." J Abnorm Psychol 1:26–41, 1906

Putnam JJ: Addresses on Psychoanalysis (1921). London, Hogarth Press, 1951

Quinn S: A Mind of Her Own: The Life of Karen Horney. New York, Summit Books, 1987

Rapaport D: Psychoanalysis as a developmental psychology, revision of an address given 21 September 1957, at Clark University, Worcester, in memory of Freud's Clark Lectures (1957), in Collected Papers of David Rapaport. Edited by Gill GM. New York, Basic Books, 1967, pp 820–852

Rosenzweig S: Freud, Jung, and Hall the King-Maker: The Historic Expedition to America (1909). St Louis, MO, Rana House Press, 1992

Semrad E: Group discussion, April 14, 1973, in Psychoanalysis, Psychotherapy, and the Boston Medical Scene, 1894–1944. Edited by Gifford GE Jr. New York, Science History Publications, 1978, pp

Shane E: Proposal on nonmedical training approved. American Psychoanalytic Association Newsletter 16:10–11, 1985

Shane E: Interview with Robert S. Wallerstein. American Psychoanalytic Association Newsletter 22:1–18, 1988

Sicherman B: Isador H. Coriat: the making of an American psychoanalyst, in Psychoanalysis, Psychotherapy, and the Boston Medical Scene, 1894–1944. Edited by Gifford GE Jr. New York, Science History Publications, 1978, pp 163–180

Slavson SR (ed): The Fields of Group Therapy. New York, International Universities Press, 1947

Solms M: The Brain and the Inner World: An Introduction to the Neuroscience of Subjective Experience. New York, Other Press, 2002

Wallerstein RS: Forty-Two Lives in Treatment: A Study of Psychoanalysis and Psychotherapy. New York, Guilford, 1986

White BV: Stanley Cobb: A Builder of the Modern Neurosciences. Boston, MA, Countway Library of Medicine, 1984

White WA: Outlines of Psychiatry. Washington, DC, Nervous & Mental Disease Publishing Co, 1909

Worcester E, McComb S, Coriat IH: Religion and Medicine: The Moral Control of Nervous Disorders. New York, Moffat, Yard, 1908

26

Psychoanalysis in Great Britain and Continental Europe

DAVID TUCKETT, M.A., M.Sc., F.INST.PSYCHOANAL.

THE HISTORY OF EUROPEAN psychoanalysis could be written in many ways. The early pioneers, all of whom were European, were based in five psychoanalytic societies in Vienna, Budapest, Berlin, Zurich, and London. Today there are 28 psychoanalytic societies functioning in 19 languages inside a wide variety of national sovereign states, each with its own traditions and mental health services. With such diversity I have chosen to concentrate mainly on ideas.

On the basis of the pioneering developments, the growth of psychoanalytic thinking in Europe should have been (and one day may again be), to a significant extent, a German enterprise. (About one-quarter of analysts in Europe are now working in Germany, mostly within a state-insurance–financed structure.) However, Hitler and the Nazis saw to it that the language and culture in which the founder of psychoanalysis worked were not to be the language and culture in which it matured over the next 65 or so years. Instead, in Europe, psychoanalytic thinking has been developing mainly in a dialogue between specific French and English approaches. The French approach is described in another chapter (see Chapter 27, "Psychoanalysis in the French Community"), so my focus here is on the English. (A drawback of this split is that it has not been possible to discuss the interaction between the French and English traditions, and particularly the work of authors like Joyce McDougall, André Green, and Jean Michel Quinodoz.) Specifically I am going to introduce a set of European-based ideas and debates about mental life and psychoanalytic treatment (the object relations development) and describe both its distinctive approach to the understanding of mental life and its contribution to what I think of as the beginning of a specific evidence-based method for considering the validity and usefulness of new ideas in psychoanalysis.

In fact, the development of a discipline founded on an engaged and critical peer culture, in which new ideas can be taken up, developed, or discarded on the basis of usefulness and validity, has been particularly difficult for psychoanalysis. Worldwide the discipline has "suffered enormously from a refusal to tolerate differences" (Cooper 2003, p. 112), and in the United States, as elsewhere, for many

I would like to acknowledge the invaluable comments by Elizabeth Spillius, Jorge Canestri, and the editors of this volume on earlier drafts of this chapter.

decades new thinking was subjected less to balanced consideration and rather more to "an intellectual reign of terror" (Cooper 2003, p. 112) or to a politics of exclusion and subsequently a politics of plurality (Richards 2003).

Pluralism is present in Europe as in the United Sates and elsewhere. It represents a step forward, but it also has many serious consequences for psychoanalysts as an intellectual community and for psychoanalytic institutions, and especially their training schemes. Questions around competence and truth have become complicated by political exigency, so that it has become very difficult to agree in a practical or operational way on the differentiations that are required to deal with such urgent questions as how a psychoanalyst should and should not practice and what constitutes basic competence (Tuckett 2000, 2003, in press).

I wish to caution the reader at the start that one difficulty with tracing the development of psychoanalysis in one region, even if the discussion is limited to tracing key ideas, is that what one psychoanalyst considers a significant development may not be viewed as such by others. I take the view that what is most interesting are those developments that have the potential to contribute to a modern evidence-based psychoanalytic discipline while at the same time holding true to the revolutionary insights into the human mind offered by Freud.

The Contributions of Ernest Jones

In the shadow of the Holocaust and bearing in mind the importance of the quest for an evidential discipline, Ernest Jones (1879–1958) is a central figure with which to begin. He helped to rescue many Jewish colleagues from central Europe who went on to make their mark in the United States, but he was also the prime facilitator of the development of psychoanalysis in English and in Britain.

A Welshman of extraordinary energy and ability, Jones journeyed to Vienna to learn from Freud and to Budapest for analysis with Ferenczi before returning to start the British Psychoanalytic Society (not to mention, later, the Canadian and the American Psychoanalytic Societies). As he made clear on several occasions, Jones (1940, 1948) is to be credited with a determination that the succession crisis that developed after the death of the charismatic founder, Freud, should be managed by trying to treat the new discipline not as the personal property of a family but as a set of ideas that had to prove its worth in the light of practice and experience. Jones also saw to it that Freud's work was translated into English in an orderly and scholarly way; he effectively founded the *International Journal of Psycho-Analy-*

sis (which he soon established as open to all and the primary means for international psychoanalytic communication), and, most crucially, he encouraged Melanie Klein to come from Berlin to England to develop her work, and supported her after she made the move. (See Winnicott 1958 for a brief account of Jones's achievements, and Gillespie 1992 and Aguayo 2000 for some details of the circumstances surrounding the invitation to Klein.) This last action was important because it ensured that Klein worked within the supportive framework not only of the British empirical tradition but also of its nonconformist tradition of tolerance and rigorous examination of argument—an action that has proved pivotal to the development of psychoanalysis.

Tipped off by James and Alix Strachey, Jones quickly perceived Klein's genius while she was working in Berlin. By inviting her to come to London in 1926, he created the conjunction of that genius with the propitious circumstances provided by the culture of argument and learning from experience within the British Psychoanalytic Society, which he himself both represented and had helped to establish. He placed Klein among the other formidable radical and independent thinkers assembling around him in the period leading to the outbreak of the Second World War: notably, James Strachey, Karin and Adrian Stephen, Susan Isaacs, Joan Riviere, Roger Money Kyrle, Sylvia Payne, Majorie Brierley, Ella Sharpe, John Rickman, Ronald Fairbairn, John Bowlby, and Donald Winnicott.

I stress the importance of Jones's invitation to Klein and the consequent fertile interaction between a genius and the cultural and intellectual environment in which she worked in Great Britain because I believe the developments were mutually reinforcing and crucial. Some evidence for this view can be derived by tracing how Klein's work had very different receptions and led to different consequences, at least for many years, in North and South America.

The Kleinian Development

Klein's central contribution was based on a new method added to Freud's invention of the "analytic hour" (Schwartz 1999), which she used to gain experience of the emotional preoccupations and developing thoughts of small children and the unconscious mental life of adults. Her work in this area started with her play technique for children (Klein 1932), in which she uncompromisingly took the play as representative of unconscious phantasies. She then extended Freud's idea of transference (Klein 1952), eventually coming to uncompromisingly view everything that happened between analyst and patient in terms of what was happening in the adult's inner world and the total situations transferred from the past into the present as well as the emotional defenses and object relations. Klein used the knowledge she thought she had developed from her observations to address and generalize about complex configurations of affect and cognition in the ordinary mental life of child and adult patients, focusing on the pivotal role in normal and pathological development of disturbing impulses and affects. Central to her contribution are her insights into the role of either benign or vicious circles of impulse, anxiety, and defense, and the potential for the saturation of thinking by emotion.

Klein and the Kleinian development have had a central impact on the theory and practice of psychoanalysis in Europe along three main lines: 1) the nature of psychic reality and psychic conflict; 2) the process which psychoanalysis works; and 3) the primary role given to clinical evidence *from the psychoanalytical consulting room* as the evidential data for testing ideas. In this section, I describe both the basis of Klein's thinking and the development of her ideas by the "post-Kleinians"—from Bion, Rosenfeld, and Segal to those of the current generation.

Psychic Reality and Psychic Conflict

Freud had himself shown the world that the child's mind contained in its depths much besides the innocence and freshness that traditionally had so enriched descriptions of infancy. He described mental life as suffused with phantasy based on autoerotic activity and early anal and oral sexuality, as well as all kinds of genital sexual ideas. In that inner world, he considered the dark fears of possibilities that the most gruesome fairy tale had not dared to explore; cruel impulses in which hate and murder rage freely and irrational phantasies mock at reality in their extravagance.

Klein took things further. On the basis of her own psychoanalytic treatment experience with Ferenczi in Budapest and then Abraham in Berlin, and with the opportunity provided by direct work with small children—becoming so to speak more Freudian than Freud—she painted a vision of human infancy dominated by anxieties induced by phantasies of love and hate and by the responses to those anxieties. (It is interesting to note that Jones did not doubt Klein's observational theatre in which the emphasis was at first more on hate than on love just as he had been convinced about Freud's. "I am reminded here of a patient who in a moment of sudden illumination exclaimed[,] 'I knew that Freud's theories were true, but I did not know they were *so* true,'" wrote Jones [1948, p. 11], when considering the plausibility, as he saw it, of Klein's ideas.) Moreover, unlike many other analysts at this time, Klein saw

how sadism, which might otherwise be thought as just destructive, could be a vital component of developing psychic life, enhancing the capacity for symbolization and growth (see her account of the case involving a child, Dick [Klein 1930]).

For those influenced by her, Klein changed in a qualitative rather than quantitative sense the kind of psychic reality with which psychoanalytic theory and practice tried to grapple: a reality dominated by the ubiquity of unconscious phantasy. She emphasized the potentially positive and negative roles of sadistic urges and phantasies in the human psyche. For Klein, human psychic reality is a constant and never very successful effort to manage overwhelming and disturbing affects arising from the conflicts between love and hate as they are experienced in the mind in human relationships.

For Klein, ordinary psychic reality in the adult, as in the child, is deepened and constructed through (what we now conceive of as) the constant interweaving of two omnipresent cognitive and affective mental states (the paranoid-schizoid and the depressive positions) and the ongoing and never-ending dynamic relations between them.

In the *paranoid-schizoid position* (in which we can find ourselves at any time in life), mental experience tends to be dominated by manic omnipotent fantasies and persecution and then dealt with by splitting, projection, introjection, denial, and idealization: the fear of dreaded and expelled "bad" feelings being forced into one self by the other oscillating with a fear of "good" feelings being stolen from one self by the other. The paranoid-schizoid position is most easily described developmentally, although I want to stress that its importance is its continued presence and potential dominance of mental life throughout life. The infant's experience of the paranoid-schizoid position and the phantasies used to understand it is based on his or her frequently changing and rather absolute experience of frustration and satisfaction based on his or her bodily experience. In danger of sudden eruptions of feeling wholly overwhelmed by impulse, anxiety, and confusion, the infant has to find ways to feel safe. To gain protection in even the best of environmental circumstances (with more difficult circumstances simply making this infinitely worse), the child tries to rid himself or herself of frustrating experience; by transforming the mental picture of the other to avoid anxiety, the child creates a new anxiety of being persecuted.

Every child (and then adult) has gradually to face the emotions of being limited, of being mortal, and of being reliant on others for what he or she wants and needs. Painful awareness of feelings of guilt, envy, rivalry, loss, and humiliating frustration go with this giving up of omnipotence and the recognition of our actual qualities and position in the world. Thus, the paranoid-schizoid position is modified in normal infancy by the experience of childhood and the developing capacities to perceive and differentiate that go with development. In particular, the infant's experience of other people in his or her life becomes less partial (all good and wonderful, all bad and persecuting) and more balanced and stable (good and bad, frustrating and satisfying). Otherness or difference can be tolerated and dependency on others can be more accepted so that manic omnipotence and the inability to tolerate disadvantage or difference can be reduced. As the experience of people as less partial stabilizes, they become more potentially "whole," but only if the pain of realizing the reality of loss of omnipotence and of ambivalence is tolerated: the very person whom one loves and depends on for love is also the very person who frustrates. If the conflict of ambivalence, and the painful experiences of envy, jealousy, guilt, and shame, which accompany it, can be tolerated, the opportunity arises for the integration of affect and phantasies into a more rounded, less persecuted, and more realistic personality. A more concerned relation to the self and those around can emerge. It is this configuration of affects and defenses that characterizes the *depressive position*, and Kleinian depictions of psychic reality in the depressive position thus focus on the difficulties of tolerating the mental pain that comes from the realization of what has been split, introjected, projected, idealized, and denigrated and the psychic work that is necessary to sustain it.

The struggle to move from the paranoid-schizoid position to the depressive position tends to exist for the rest of life. Splitting is maintained and even intensified if the painful feelings of realization or confusion are too great so that a reparative or mourning process cannot be begun or tolerated. Similarly a regressive movement back from the depressive position to the paranoid-schizoid position may be initiated whenever something emotionally new (different) and confusing occurs. The paranoid-schizoid position is, so to speak, the potential template for all experience of new and especially frustrating perception. With the template as a basis, new experience can be hated as an intrusive attack on the self and potentially obliterated or gradually recognized as different and accepted in a move back toward the depressive position—the mental state that allows difference and, potentially, integration (see Britton 2003).

In presenting these ideas about the psychic reality described by Klein, I have followed the modern tendency, based on the very significant developments introduced by Bion, to stress how Klein uses the word "position" rather than "phase" to emphasize that throughout childhood, and indeed also in later life, there may be fluctuation between the two organizations. Positions, as Klein implicitly conceived of them, are to be distinguished from developmental stages, which one passes through and leaves behind. It was later colleagues, and especially Bion, who made this distinction even more explicit. He conceived the positions as "states of mind" regardless of the chronological age at which they are experienced. This emphasis has laid the foundation for many analysts to look for moment-to-moment shifts in a session from integration and depressive anxiety toward fragmentation and sometimes persecution and vice versa, rather than looking only for major shifts of character and orientation (for more detailed discussion, see Spillius 1994).

Klein's description of psychic reality and of the configurations of affect and defense she termed the paranoid-schizoid and the depressive positions offered the opportunity to view psychoanalysis as a discipline concerned with mental states. But these conceptions also caused a shift in how we think about the nature of the psychic conflict on which the psychoanalyst will focus. Freud's kernel Oedipus complex—the conflictual tragedy of love and rivalrous hatred whose working-through Freud considered the lynchpin of human psychic development (see, e.g., Blass 2001)—becomes linked with struggles to move from the paranoid-schizoid to the depressive position. Working through the guilt and anxiety of the Oedipus complex goes along with working through the depressive position (see, e.g., Britton 1989). This Kleinian emphasis on the conflict between loving and hating (particularly harboring primitive hatred born from the envy of the other's capacity) has shaped the way, within the Freudian development, that many analysts conceive of mental conflict. It is seen along a somewhat different line from that emphasized in either the Francophone tradition (in which the emphasis is more on the conflicts of genital sexuality) or the North American tradition (in which the emphasis is more on the conflicts between the ego and the instincts).

In terms of ideas about mental structure (i.e., a way to try to explain regularities in psychic functioning), the Freudian notion of a structured conflict between id, ego, and superego—developed in the United States mainly in the direction of understanding the predicament of the ego—has developed within Kleinian-influenced formulations of mental life into a complex theory about the outcome of the individual's struggles with destructive feelings and the way they can influence the capacity for thought. The potential to develop symbolic mental functioning (thinking, learning) depends on the capacity to work through the conflicts of the depressive position and the Oedipus complex. Thinking can become blocked or hypertrophied if the affects from facing the conflict (i.e., envy, guilt, loss) are experienced as too overwhelmingly unpleasant, while the affects that can be achieved by evasion of conflict (mainly triumph) are too pleasurable to give up; when this happens, there is the eroticization (hating and loving) of thought itself, so that the mind does not function properly. Segal's "Notes on Symbol Formation" (1957) and Bion's "A Theory of Thinking" (1962), in which he introduced the Kantian distinction between the thinker and the thought and which has often not been well appreciated in North America, are seminal. (This last comment is based on a peer-review exercise carried out in 1999 when I was editor of the *International Journal of Psychoanalysis*. Whereas European and Latin American members of the editorial boards rated this paper as one of the finest in the literature, many distinguished North American colleagues were doubtful it should have been published.)

Bion (1962) suggested there are two necessary bases for conception: realization and frustration. He explored the term *thought* restrictively by wondering how what he called a "pre-conception" becomes affectively correlated with its experience to become a conception. Broadly, what is at stake is the much discussed problem of meaningful human existence with agency: how is it that one can experience (all of) one's thoughts (and later one's actions) not as alien but as one's own? For Bion, the template for thought is the situation of an infant whose expectation of being satisfied by the mother's breast is frustrated. In that situation the preconception "frustration" can be mated (in other words symbolically associated and affectively linked) with the realization of no breast available for satisfaction. This mating, he argued, is experienced as a no-breast, or as an "absent" breast inside.

The next and crucial step depends on the infant's capacity to bear frustration: in particular, how the infant manages the affective experience and so makes the decision to evade frustration or to modify it. If the capacity for toleration of frustration is sufficient, the "no-breast" inside becomes a thought, and on the basis of this process, an apparatus for "thinking" it develops. This initiates the state described by Freud (1911/1958) in his consideration of the same issue in "Two Principles of Mental Functioning," in which he argued that mental development toward recognition of the reality principle is synchronous with the development of an ability to think and so to bridge the gulf of frustration between the moment when a want is felt and the moment when action appropriate to satisfying the want might culminate in its satisfaction. A capacity for tolerating frustration thus enables the psyche to develop thought as a means by which the frustration that is tolerated is itself made more tolerable.

If, however, the capacity for toleration of frustration is inadequate, the bad internal "no-breast," which a personality capable of maturity ultimately recognizes as a thought, confronts the psyche with the need to decide between evading frustration and modifying it. Incapacity for tolerating frustration tips the scale in the direction of evasion of frustration. The result is a significant departure from the events that Freud describes as characteristic of thought adjusted to the reality principle. What should be a thought, a product of the juxtaposition of preconception and negative realization, becomes felt as a very bad object inducing unpleasure, indistinguishable from a thing-in-itself and fit only for evacuation. Consequently, the development of an apparatus for thinking is disturbed, and instead a hypertrophic development of the apparatus of projective identification takes place. That is, urges, affects, and anxieties are responded to by consistent and repetitive patterns of expulsion through projective identification aimed at producing an experience of conflict-free (and particularly guilt- and anxiety free) states of mind, often at the cost both of mental development and of any real personal relations. As Bion put it, thoughts become treated as if they were indistinguishable from bad internal objects. What we call the mind is then felt to be an apparatus not for thinking thoughts, but for ridding the psyche of accumulations of bad internal objects. Loosely, and on the the basis of the instinctual pleasure to be derived from the experience of evacuation, we can say that the very functioning of the mind is perverted.

Along similar lines, Herbert Rosenfeld (1971, 1987), for example, developed an understanding of what he termed the narcissistic omnipotent character structure: people in the patient's inner world can only be related to as (phantasy) containers (not persons with their own feelings, thoughts, sensibilities and motivations) into which (in phantasy), feeling all powerful, the patient projects those parts of himself or herself that are felt to be undesirable or that cause pain and anxiety. Similarly, Betty Joseph (1987) set out to demonstrate how in the consulting room, projective identification is used perversely in a structured (i.e., regular) way excitedly to maintain the patient's narcissistic omnipotent balance and to prevent the pain required from therapeutic change. In other words, to avoid experiencing the emotional reality of his or her relationship with the analyst, the patient avoids the experience of dependency, anxiety about loss, awareness of envy, guilt, and so forth. John Steiner (1993) developed his idea of the Psychic Retreat—a structured organization of perception and experience to which the patient can withdraw and where he imagines he is protected from the dangers of an open attack on his objects. In this way the patient's hatred is bound in a complex organization in which it is experienced as aimed at him, with a resulting sense of hurt and wrong forming the focus of a continual justified grievance. The patient is then able to avoid the anxieties of the paranoid-schizoid position (e.g., a fear of retaliation) and the pain of the depressive position (e.g., recognition of destructive impulses) by with-drawing into a highly defended state of righteousness.

The Clinical Task

Klein's radical contributions and the developments just mentioned also opened the way for analysts to define and work with the clinical situation in terms of her notion of "the total situation" of the transference developed particularly by Betty Joseph (1985) in her work on enactment and in her development of a "close process" technique (and also by Racker [1957] in South America). (Klein [1952] wrote: "It is my experience that in unravelling the details of the transference it is essential to think in terms of total situations transferred from the past into the present as well as emotion defences and object relations." She went on to describe how for many years transference had been understood in terms of direct references to the analyst, and how only later had it been realized that, for example, such things as reports about everyday life gave a clue to the unconscious anxieties stirred up in the transference situation.) The argument is that the

> patient communicates his psychic world to the analyst by experiencing it and reliving it in the transference. The analyst communicates to the patient his understanding of this relationship—that is, he interprets the relationship itself....The transference is an emotional relationship of the patient with the analyst which is experienced in the present, in what is generally called "the here-and-now" of the analytic situation. It is the expression of the patient's past in its multiple transformations. (Riesenberg-Malcolm 1986, p. 433)

The formulation allows that by interpreting the patient's relationship to the analyst, "the analyst is interpreting simultaneously past and present" (Riesenberg-Malcolm 1986, p. 433). If one accepts this formulation, the implication is that the genesis and resolution of the patient's unconscious conflicts derived from the past can be reached and achieved by interpreting the patient's relationship to the analyst—particularly the use of the analyst and the analyst's ideas and the affects they stimulate. Taken profoundly, it is a logical development of the Freudian notion of the transference, although not perhaps of the way Freud actually practiced. I would differentiate it from the Francophone tradition, in which the ubiquity of the transference is accepted as the engine driving the process but not interpreted directly unless exceptionally. I would also differentiate it from the more conversational traditions that make a distinction between transference and nontransference or address interpretations to the patient within the notion of the need to establish a "treatment alliance" or an opportunity for growth.

Clinical Evidence

The Kleinian development, I have suggested, introduced and took seriously the idea that detailed study of the happenings in the analyst's consulting room provides the primary data of psychoanalysis. This line of development greatly popularized, along with the work of other British colleagues, discussions of psychoanalytic thinking based on line-by-line accounts of the session. In making these contributions (and bearing in mind that in other centers the tradition of detailed clinical presentation did not develop), it made what can now be seen as a significant epistemological contribution.

There is no doubt that the situation in which Klein found herself in London in 1926 was already influenced by the British empirical tradition (Rayner 1991). Nonetheless, Klein's capacity to conceptualize and bring alive clinical material and her emphasis on this material were formative. The distinguished psychoanalytic historian Pearl King (1983) has written,

> In my own opinion, one of Melanie Klein's most important contributions to the British Society, and perhaps to psychoanalysis, and which she may not altogether have been aware of, was that, following Jones, she pioneered the right of psychoanalysts to develop their own understanding of their patients' material, based on the heritage that Freud had bequeathed them. (p. 257)

Thus, although it will seem to some a strange claim, in my view one significant element in the Kleinian development in Europe was its role in helping psychoanalytic epistemology by demonstrating the productivity of moving the discipline further toward a creative dialogue between theory and evidence. While others responded to Freud's death by becoming concerned with the legitimacy of the Freudian heritage, psychoanalysts influenced by Klein worked, as Ernest Jones hoped would be possible, in a tradition in which they were obliged to view their work and their ideas about it in terms of the evidence they could find in the sessions with their patients. They stressed and taught the value of close examination of the details of the clinical encounter and developed the practice of working together in groups, presenting detailed sessions to one another, and critically considering them (see Joseph 1985, p. 448, for an example).

I have mentioned that my claim about the Kleinian contribution to psychoanalytic epistemology may seem strange. Those who are critical of some aspects of the Kleinian development are apt to single out for criticism Klein's and her followers' "certainty" (see, e.g., Bollas 1993)—not exactly a scientific attitude. Moreover, at the time of the great controversies, the general criticism of Klein from the United States and from the Anna Freud camp was that her ideas were implausible and impossibly unscientific—inconsistent with Freud's principles or what was felt to be known about infant and child development (for an example of such criticism, see Brenner 1968). I maintain, however, that whatever truth there may or may not be in such accusations, it is clear that the *practice* of the Klein group—in regard to both the use of clinical discussion and the subsequent "post-Kleinian" development in which ideas have been doubted, revised, and modified, emerging with more capacity to illuminate—speaks for itself. It is the practice of detailed clinical discussion. I have argued at greater length that, in contrast to what happened elsewhere, this has been a major cause of the Kleinian tradition's capacity to develop and grow (Tuckett 2000, pp. 242–245).

I do not, of course, mean to imply that evidence in psychoanalysis is a simple matter. It is not entirely clear what a psychoanalytic clinical fact is, and all the difficulties that exist in determining what a case report can and cannot show are obvious (see Tuckett 1994, 1995; Michels 2000a, 2000b; Widlocher 1994). My contention is only that the presentation of psychoanalytic clinical material by analysts to analysts creates a minimum condition for commensurable arguments from and about the data to take place, a condition that does not exist otherwise (Tuckett 1993, 2000; see also Bernardi 2002). It is this potentiality that has been greatly facilitated by the Kleinian tradition.

Interaction With the Kleinian Development

I have mentioned how, as a result of Ernest Jones's actions, the Kleinian development was nurtured in the particular facilitating conditions of the British Psychoanalytic Society. The fecundity that followed Klein's arrival and continued to develop as ideas were submitted to clinical exemplification and utility led to the major elaborations of psychoanalytic understanding I have outlined, as in the case of the work of Bion, Rosenfeld, Segal, and Joseph, and the subsequent generations of "post-Kleinians." These contributions have taken place in a society that found a way to tolerate difference, which allowed groups and individuals to get on with their research.

When Klein first arrived in 1926, there was initially a tranquil period when her ideas fitted quite easily into what was happening and were eagerly picked up. Disagreements exploded only when a number of factors—some of them very personal, illustrating how ideas in psychoanalysis are often inextricably entangled with personalities—came together. Freud died in 1939, and Jones began to give up his leadership role; this meant that two separate succession cri-

ses were created. They were then intensified by the arrival in London of Anna Freud and a Viennese group—highly traumatized by forced exile and the quite rapid death of Freud, and anxious about the kind of psychoanalysis they encountered. All these factors came together when Klein's own daughter and her daughter's analyst, Glover, thought by some the most likely successor to Jones, were very critical of her: both the small Klein group and the Viennese group seemed to fear for their survival, so that in the middle of wartime these disagreements flared into a theoretical and political dispute in London now known as the Controversial Discussions. (This period is described in a quite remarkable fashion by King and Steiner [1991] and in a number of related biographies and articles [e.g., Grosskurth 1986]; see also Scarfone 2002.) After some years compromise was achieved, so that for about 20 years there was a kind of truce: obvious differences were tolerated under one roof amid largely separate developments and little mutual recognition. However, colleagues had to work with one another to provide training, and they presented to one another in scientific meetings that set up a potential creative interaction—every thinker had, if only in his or her imagination, to relate to and to anticipate the comments of the others.

As time went by, some important Kleinian thinkers (e.g., Heimann) became independent of Klein, and alongside the Klein development and very much engaged with it, other independently minded figures such as Fairbairn, Balint, Winnicott, Bowlby, and Rycroft, as well as more traditionally trained figures such as Sandler, emerged and developed ideas, derived in part by using the Kleinian thinking and in part by modifying it. After Klein's death new generations developed and began to influence the Kleinians themselves, so that compared with analysts from other countries, most British analysts discovered they had a lot in common, despite their differences. In this way, along with the Francophone tradition described in Chapter 27 ("Psychoanalysis in the French Community") of this volume, this broadly Kleinian British development (which became known in North America and elsewhere, but not in Britain, as the object relations school) has gradually established itself in Europe (and increasingly worldwide) as one of the two main schools in psychoanalysis. Many of the same engagements then occurred in many European societies—where those for or against the Kleinian development emerged.

In the space remaining to me, I will try to put some detail on the process I have just outlined by selecting a few of the most important efforts to use and modify the Kleinian work and debate with it in Britain as well as still more briefly turning my attention to the engagement with it in the rest of Europe.

Donald Winnicott

Donald Winnicott—along with Melanie Klein and Wilfred Bion—is one of the most well known British psychoanalysts and one whose reputation is still growing. Like Klein's, Winnicott's experience was based in his work with children—although in this instance as a pioneering pediatrician who had an extraordinary gift for communication. A distinguished collaborator reported that within a few minutes of a child's entering Winnicott's consulting room with any number of others present, both the child and Winnicott were oblivious to the presence of anyone else.

A good example of his acceptance by and communication with children is what happened when he was about to visit a Danish family for the second time after an interval of a few years. The children remembered his playing with them very well and were delighted at the prospect of again meeting an Englishman who could speak Danish. When their father said that Dr Winnicott could not speak a word of their difficult language his children simply did not believe him. (Tizard 1971, p. 226)

In his lifetime, and indeed in the way it is used today, Winnicott's work takes place in a dialogue with the work of Melanie Klein, with whom he seems to have had a profound but always rather disappointed relationship: she was less interested in his ideas than he in hers. He went to her for supervision of his work for 10 years, from 1935 to 1945, and went to a second analysis with one of her closest adherents, Joan Riviere. (Previously he had spent 10 years with James Strachey.) He was also asked by Klein to analyze one of her children. But despite frequent efforts to try to persuade her to modify her theories—with whose basic tenets he was in full agreement—he seems to have felt he could not get her to take him seriously:

Secondly, I feel that…there is something from your end, namely a need to have everything that is new restated in your own terms….What I was wanting on Friday undoubtedly was that there should be some move from your direction towards the gesture that I make in this paper. It is a creative gesture and I cannot make any relationship through this gesture except if someone comes to meet it. I think that I was wanting something which I have no right to expect from your group, and it is really of the nature of a therapeutic act, something which I could not get in either of my two long analyses, although I got so much else. There is no doubt that my criticism of Mrs. Riviere was not only a straightforward criticism based on objective observation but also it was coloured by the fact that it was just exactly here that her analysis failed with me. (Rodman 1987, p. 34, letter 25)

All that no doubt was very complicated with personal and analytic relationships. I mention it now not to try to understand or comment on something that is unlikely ever to be properly understood, but to provide evidence for my view of the context for Winnicott's own thinking—that he was in a continuous engagement with Klein's and her followers' ideas and was continually trying to persuade them to modify their ideas. His preoccupation can be discerned in his papers, but it is in the surviving letters to Klein and her colleagues (as well as to others) that it comes out most clearly. On November 17, 1952, for instance, Winnicott wrote to Klein:

I personally think that it is very important that your work should be restated by people discovering in their own way and presenting what they discover in their own language. It is only in this way that the language will be kept alive. If you make the stipulation that in future only your language shall be used for the statement of other people's discoveries then the language becomes a dead language, as it has already become in the Society. You would be surprised at the sighs and groans that accompany every restatement of the internal object cliches by what I am going to call Kleinians. Your own statements are of course in quite a different category as the work is your own personal work and everyone is pleased that you have your own way of stating it. (Rodman 1987, pp. 33–34)

Winnicott's own central psychoanalytic contributions were often directed at understanding a particular existential problem and its roots in infancy: how is it that human emotional relationships do or do not become endowed with meaning rather than alienation? His answer focused around his notion of the role of illusion and disillusion in mental life (Winnicott 1945, 1953), his ideas about "the use of an object" (Winnicott 1969), and in particular his belief that hatred was a normal phenomena whose eventual fate in the role of the psyche depends on the way it is responded to in the family environment (Winnicott 1958, 1960, 1963).

The main question Winnicott was asking was in fact similar to the one asked contemporaneously by Bion in his theory of thinking already discussed. However, whereas Bion was concerned with how we have realistic "thoughts" endowed with meaning and emotion, Winnicott was interested in the mental experience or representation of the first object. He assumed that "if all goes well," an infant must come to realize that other people "really" are persons like himself or herself with intentions and feelings; however, he took as problematic the process of how we move into a potential world of human relationship, where people are treated with concern, rather than a world of thing-relationships, where people are treated for what they offer to be consumed and so forth. Here Winnicott's differentiation from the Kleinian thinking of the time was not with the actual problem of how to manage conflicting desire and the potentially catastrophic anxieties love and hate can unleash, but with his conviction that what must be stressed is the role of the facilitating environment in making this problem bearable (Winnicott 1960). He considered the role of "holding" by the "good enough" mother and stressed that it is she who must help the child to bear the reality of human life, and especially the disappointments to which it gives rise that generate hatred and despair. For Winnicott, a "good enough" environment does not demand false adaptation from the infant or make false adaptations to the infant. It does not, for instance, pretend that nothing is going on or that it is inconsequential when everyone is manifestly terrified by a life-threatening illness or stirred up by the infant's own sadism.

An important part of Winnicott's thinking concerns the role he attributed to illusion. It is easy to misunderstand, as it is daringly and confusingly original—actually turning the common meaning of the term on its head. He took the Freud-Klein view that early life was dominated by omnipotence and omniscience—what the baby thinks is so, is indeed so—but he famously introduced the idea of the transitional object as a stage along the way of creating a marriage between inner and outer experience through which omnipotence can be given up. The transitional object (Winnicott 1953)—for example, a child's cuddly toy—functions simultaneously in the small child's mind "as" and "as not" what the child believes in "illusion" it is. For Winnicott, only if "illusion" is respected and not challenged too soon, so that disillusionment is made somewhat tolerable, will the child achieve the capacity to treat reality as emotionally real. (The implication will not be missed—those who do not achieve this will not experience life as real; they will be existentially alienated. Winnicott used the term "False Self" for this situation.)

It will be apparent that in this modification of the Kleinian "depressive position" theory, "illusion" is neither some intersubjective assessment nor a state of deception or delusion about how things "are." Rather, it is a state of psychic reality and refers to a potential personal inner sense of connectedness or meaningful relationship, based on the experience of an identity between what to an observer might be considered subject and object. One might say now that Winnicott was introducing what is currently discussed as *mentalization*—that is, the processes through which we become aware of our mind (with its desires and anxieties) through the awareness of the other's mind, and aware of the other's perception of our mind. (*Mentalization* is the term used by Fonagy and Target in a series of papers with the title "Playing and Reality," deliberately borrowed from Winnicott [Fonagy 1995; Fonagy and Target 1996, 2000; Target and Fonagy 1996; see also Chapter 8, "Psychoanalytic Developmental Theory," in this volume].)

For Winnicott, as for all those influenced by the Kleinian development, unconscious psychic reality is privileged over what might be called "intersubjective reality." This point is brought out in a letter to Money-Kyrle written in 1952, in which Winnicott made an extraordinary statement:

> I think we must take it for granted that emotionally there is no contribution from the individual to the environment or from the environment to the individual. The individual only communicates with a self-created world and the people in the environment only communicate with the individual in so far as they can create him or her. Nevertheless in health there is the illusion of contact and it is this which provides the high spots of human life..." (Rodman 1987, p. 43)

This radical statement seems to mean 1) that meaningful emotional relationships depend on the way we represent each other mentally—and that this is an active process of each creating the other out of our own potential to do so; and 2) that what Winnicott calls the high spots in "healthy" adult life occur when there is more or less an identity between the inner experience of two people—something which could not occur if the meaning of the word "illusion" in his letter to Money Kyrle had its more common meaning of "delusion" and, therefore, was applicable to one person's experience but not the other's.

Winnicott's efforts to debate with and modify the Kleinian development can be summed up in his own words from another of his letters:

> "The good mother" and "the bad mother" of the Kleinian jargon are internal objects and are nothing to do with real women. The best a real woman can do with an infant is to be sensitively good enough at the beginning so that illusion is made possible to the infant at the start that this good-enough mother is "the good breast." Similarly in analysis the analyst must always be failing; but if one is to get the full blast of the disillusionment or the hate one must first of all make contact by active and sensitive adaptation so as to become good enough, otherwise nothing happens. (Rodman 1987, p. 38)

A later passage in the letter he wrote to Melanie Klein that I have already quoted highlights another of Winnicott's attempts to modify the Kleinian view, this one directed at technique.

> The worst example, perhaps, was C's paper in which he simply bandied about a lot of that which has now come to be known as Kleinian stuff without giving any impression of having an appreciation of the processes personal to the patient. One felt that if he were growing a daffodil he would think that he was making the daffodil out of a bulb instead of enabling the bulb to develop into a daffodil by good enough nurture. (Rodman 1987, p. 38)

He believed that some Kleinian-influenced analysts were overenthusiastically developing a belief in the value of their interpretations and cautioned (as did Balint 1968) against the possible effect that doing so could repeat previous trauma and also project the image of an omnipotent and all-knowing analyst.

Such criticism may or may not have been justified at that time, but certainly a technical line focusing on the role of the analyst in providing the conditions for nurture in a less obviously obtrusive way was subsequently developed by other British analysts subscribing to Winnicott's thinking, notably Heimann (1989), Milner (1987), Stewart (1992), Casement (1985), and Bollas (1987). These colleagues have developed their own ideas in their own way, but they have focused particularly on the historical absence of a facilitating environment in the patient's past and the complex requirements demanded of the analyst to provide it in the analysis in a way the patient can use to grow.

Meanwhile, in dialogue with this response to their work and from their own reflections on one another's work, the Kleinians themselves, while still focusing most intensively on the internal effects of environmental difficulty, have in recent years been very preoccupied with the risks of creating impasse in the therapeutic situation (O'Shaughnessy 1992; Rosenfeld 1987). They have also increasingly stressed the importance of the environmental situation (historically and as conceived in the analyst's consulting room) as a factor mediating how far the conflicts of mental life can be tolerated and worked through (see, e.g., Brenman 1985; Spillius 1993).

Joseph Sandler and the Quiet Revolution

I have singled out Winnicott's contribution both for its inherent interest and for its role in a debate with Klein's work aimed at trying to modify the Kleinian development in various directions. A second key figure, Joseph Sandler, probably the leading English-speaking theoretician in Europe, created a somewhat different revolution in European psychoanalysis.

Trained in the traditional context of Anna Freud's Hampstead Clinic, Sandler brought some of the core insights from the British Kleinian development into contact with the Viennese and North American traditions (loosely to be designated as ego psychology). He also influenced the Kleinians, prompting them to address certain theoretical difficulties within their own development. Indeed, to the extent that contemporary psychoanalysis has a core common ground focusing on object relations and the conceptualization and understanding of the clinical situation, where similarities and differences can be recognized more precisely, discussed, and evaluated, it is in no small measure the

result of several pathbreaking papers Sandler and various collaborators contributed (see, e.g., Sandler and Rosenblatt 1962; Sandler and Joffe 1969; Sandler and Sandler 1978).

The 1962 paper (among others) was part of Sandler's lifelong preoccupation with developing what might be called a clinical theory. It is significant not just for its content but for the way it opened an avenue for a closer relationship between theory and clinical practice and between theory and research. In the paper, Sandler described his and his colleagues' experience in trying, through the clinical-theoretical discussion project known as the Hampstead Index Project, to recognize their theoretical concepts (such as the superego and other ideas as developed by Anna Freud) in material drawn from ongoing clinical sessions. Sandler (and Rosenblatt) reported that difficulties in rigorously defining clinical events in terms of theoretical concepts led him and his colleagues to begin to reformulate theory so that it could be spelled out and used in clinical practice. In a series of papers with different collaborators, this is what he did over the next 15 years.

One shift that took place was from the "object cathexis" theory toward an object relationship theory:

> It was certainly appropriate, for some considerable time during the development of psychoanalytic theory, to regard an object relationship as the 'cathexis of an object' with libidinal or aggressive energy. This is a way of saying, within the energic frame of reference, that an object relationship is the state of loving, or of both loving and hating, some other person or an aspect of that person. But it is increasingly clear that conceiving of an object relationship as the energic investment of an object is inadequate and simplistic....We know, for example, that object relationships are two-sided, that they equally involve activity on the part of the other person (for example, the caretaking mother)... (Sandler and Sandler 1978, p. 285)

Another shift was toward the notion that the individual is constantly acting to reduce conscious or unconscious representational discrepancy in order to attain or maintain a basic feeling-state of well-being (Joffe and Sandler 1968, p. 453). In addition, Sandler identified how routinely individuals aim at a special form of gratification through their interaction with their environment and with their own selves—actualizing their unconscious fantasies, as he came to term term the process, and so making a link with Joseph's concept of enactment and with the complex field of projective identification to which we will return.

Sandler's achievement was a more serviceable theory, more easily connected to clinical experience. In addition, his reformulation of clinical theory made it a great deal easier to join a variety of different strands of psychoanalytic theory to one another (and especially the British object relations theory to ego psychology). Sandler and Joffe

(1969) conceived feelings as psychic regulators, and then Sandler and Sandler (1978) developed this idea into the whole realm of object relations:

> In the development of object relationships…the part played by affective experience is central. An experience only has or retains meaning for the child if it is linked with feeling. The assumption is made that ultimately all meaning is developmentally and functionally related to states of feeling, and that an experience which does not have some relation to a feeling-state has no psychological significance for the individual at all. (p. 292)

In the same paper, they then placed understanding how the patient regulated affect though the maintenance of specific unconscious role relationships at the heart of the clinical task.

British Object Relations and Its Reception in Continental Europe

British object relations theories and practices, whether in the form of the Kleinian development or in the forms developed by Sandler and by Winnicott and those that followed, have exerted a considerable influence in all the European countries. For various reasons—for instance, the effect of the Nazi period in Germany; the relatively small size of many of the societies—and despite the contribution of a number of gifted thinkers, none of the language cultures except the British and French have really developed their own distinctive body of psychoanalytic thinking. Instead, in those areas where English rather than French is widely spoken—namely, in Germany, the Netherlands, Italy, Scandinavia, parts of Spain and Eastern Europe—colleagues have tried to create an amalgam of available ideas, and in that context British ideas have tended to be quite widely used, along with traditional Freudian ideas and ideas from self psychology and relational psychoanalysis from North America. The way these ideas have been incorporated has varied from place to place, but a major factor in the attractiveness of British object relations theories, at least superficially, has been their perceived clinical relevance. At the same time, the process of transmission from the culture in which the ideas were born into the culture in which they are used has not always been easy.

I will illustrate this proposition by taking advantage of recent attempts to compare the way the concept of projective identification has come to be understood and used in different cultural contexts. Klein (1946/1975) herself introduced the concept without actually naming it:

…the attacks on the mother's breast develop into attacks of a similar nature on her body, which comes to be felt as it were as an extension of the breast, even before the mother is conceived of as a complete person. The fantasied onslaughts on the mother follow two main lines: one is the predominantly oral impulse to suck dry, bite up, scoop out and rob the mother's body of its good contents. (I shall discuss the bearing of these impulses on the development of object-relations in connection with introjection.) The other line of attack derives from the anal and urethral impulses and implies expelling dangerous substances (excrements) out of the self and into the mother. Together with these harmful excrements, expelled in hatred, split-off parts of the ego are also projected on to the mother [Klein herself added a most interesting footnote at this stage, which has often been overlooked. "The description of such primitive processes suffers from a great handicap, for these phantasies arise at a time when the infant has not yet begun to think in words. In this context, for instance, I am using the expression 'to project into another person' because this seems to me the only way of conveying the unconscious process I am trying to describe."] or, as I would rather call it, into the mother. These excrements and bad parts of the self are meant not only to injure but also to control and to take possession of the object. In so far as the mother comes to contain the bad parts of the self, she is not felt to be a separate individual but is felt to be the bad self….Much of the hatred against parts of the self is now directed towards the mother. This leads *to a particular form of identification which establishes the prototype of an aggressive object-relation.* (Klein 1946/1975, pp. 7–8; emphasis added)

It was only in 1952 that she revised this paper for publication and added a further sentence "I suggest for these processes the term 'projective identification.'" Klein also stressed that not only "bad" but also "good" parts of the ego are expelled and projected into external objects, who become identified with the projected good parts of the self. She regarded this identification as essential for the infant's ability to develop good object relations (Klein 1946/1975, p. 9).

Later Kleinian analysts such as Bion (1957), Rosenfeld (1987), and Joseph (1983) extended the concept to a range of situations met with clinically in which the patient seemed to behave concretely toward the analyst as though the analyst was precisely endowed with the patient's projections, which, if recognized and described by the analyst ("contained" in Bion's language) could help make clear to the analyst (or, in other words, to communicate) the underlying problems.

Opening a Europe-wide discussion 2 years ago, Elizabeth Spillius noted the quite surprising amount of interest that projective identification aroused and also how it had evoked annoyance and disapproval (Spillius 2002). She stressed how this ambivalence was there at the start, in

Melanie Klein's own mind. Although it was Klein's own concept, she was never very pleased with the idea.

It is clear from the description above that Klein thought of projective identification as a person's unconscious phantasy and that her interest was in how the phantasy affected the way the subject saw the object (the way the patient saw the analyst). She did not think the analyst should be affected by the phantasy. Thus, she did not agree with Paula Heimann's closely related idea in which Heimann extended the idea of countertransference to include all aspects of the analyst's emotional response to the patient and which Heimann maintained could be a useful source of information about the patient (Heimann 1950). In fact, Hanna Segal told Elizabeth Spillius that in the case of both concepts, Klein thought that the analyst might start to blame the patient for the analyst's own deficiencies. I also recall Heimann telling me of her concern that her idea of the countertransference could be used the same way—if mixed up with the idea of projective identification, which she did not like!

Doubts notwithstanding, for a time Klein's colleagues and many others both used the idea of projective identification and in effect accepted Heimann's ideas about countertransference, simply because both did often seem to allow the analyst to make sense of very difficult clinical situations, especially in work with rather disturbed patients. The adoption of both ideas probably did lead to confusion for a number of years. As Feldman (1994, 1997) and Spillius (2002) have pointed out, it was really Sandler who helped to get matters clarified by adding an important caveat, which might well have appealed to Klein and is now quite widely accepted: he pointed out that a patient does not literally "put" parts of himself or herself into the mind of the other, because projective identification is an unconscious phantasy, but the patient may unconsciously use various evocative and potentially observable behaviors to produce an emotional effect on the analyst; in other words the patient may seek to actualize the phantasy in the relationship with the analyst (Sandler 1976, 1993; Tuckett 1983, 1997). The value of this conceptualization is that it cues the analyst to examine the evidence and sensitizes him or her to observe what is being "done" and to consider why.

Discussing the way the projective identification concept has been received in Germany, Italy, Spain, and the French-speaking world, Canestri (2002), Hinz (2002), and Quinodoz (2002) draw attention to the different ways it has been influenced by the indigenous culture. In all these countries, as in most places in Europe, there are analysts directly influenced by the Kleinian development who essentially work along the same lines as their British colleagues. This collaboration deepens the ideas—assisting in the development of their genesis and their rigorous application.

The development of the projective identification concept began with pioneers like Loch in Germany and Fornari in Italy. There was then an extensive exchange with British visitors. For instance, in the 1980s, Herbert Rosenfeld and other Kleinian analysts began to make regular visits to Germany, where the Kleinian ideas were particularly welcomed in the context of a society seeking to overcome a period of violent destructiveness and cruelty and where there were a large number of guilty secrets that inevitably affected work in the consulting room (see, e.g., Hinze 1986; Schoenhals 1994).

However, outside the groups of workers collaborating closely with British analysts, there is a much larger group in these countries who use the concept within a general theoretical framework of ideas that includes segments of various theories: Freudian-Kleinian when there is a tradition binding them to the French analysis of the past or the present, and Kleinian-Bionian-Winnicottian when they are close in approach to adherents of British psychoanalysis (Canestri 2002). North American self psychology and object relational developments have also added to the mix in recent years, especially in Italy. Canestri suggests that this kind of eclecticism represents the majority group in Italy and Spain and that in these cases there is need for reflection about the coherence of the resulting theory. Arguments about what is now meant by "unconscious," how important external reality is, or how far the person of the analyst is crucial in the psychoanalytic cure are indicators of very fundamental difficulties (see, e.g., Chianese 2003; Sechaud 2003, 2004).

Returning to projective identification: Hinz and Quinodoz make similar points to those of Canestri when considering German- and French-speaking cultures. Their reflections signal the extent to which current European psychoanalysis is pluralistic, but they also highlight the inconsistency in results that sometimes results, so that the relation between theory and clinical work is not always conducive to developing rigor. It is out of an awareness of such difficulties that the European psychoanalytic societies have launched, through the European psychoanalytic federation, a 10-year scientific initiative aimed at researching and clarifying how people work, how candidates are trained to work, and how they evaluate each other (Tuckett, in press).

Public Health and the Development of Research

In Britain and Italy psychoanalysis is an entirely private affair: although some psychoanalysts work within the state healthcare system, they do not practice psychoanalysis there. Thus, patients wishing to avail themselves of psychoanalytic treatment must pay for it themselves. Elsewhere in Europe there is a degree of financial support for psychoanalytic treatment, which is more or less integrated in public health provision. Little has yet been written on the consequences of such differences, but recent pressure on health service budgets, which has been a feature worldwide, has in a number of countries forced an interest in research.

Colleagues in Scandanavia (e.g., Sandell et al. 2000) and Germany (Kächele and Thomä 1993; Leuzinger and Target 2002) have begun studies attempting to evaluate the effect of psychoanalytic treatment, and a group of research workers, working in close collaboration with colleagues from North America, around Joseph Sandler and Peter Fonagy, has gradually begun to be established. As yet, much of this work has been conducted outside or alongside psychoanalytic institutes, but it may be the beginning of a new development that can be linked with the developments of psychoanalytic theory and practice discussed in this chapter. In Europe, as in North America, it remains to be seen over the next 10 years whether psychoanalysis will develop into a more evidence-based discipline or whether it will be unable to do so.

References

Aguayo J: Patronage in the dispute over child analysis between Melanie Klein and Anna Freud: 1927–1932. Int J Psychoanal 81:733–752, 2000

Balint M: The Basic Fault. London, Tavistock, 1968

Bernardi R: The need for true controversies in psychoanalysis: the debates on Melanie Klein and Jacques Lacan in the Río de la Plata. Int J Psychoanal 83:851–873, 2002

Bion WR: Differentiation of the psychotic from the nonpsychotic personalities. Int J Psychoanal 38:266–275, 1957

Bion WR: A theory of thinking. Int J Psychoanal 43:306–310, 1962

Blass R: The teaching of the Oedipus complex: on making Freud meaningful to university students by unveiling his essential ideas on the human condition. Int J Psychoanal 82:1105–1121, 2001

Bollas C: The Shadow of the Object: Psychoanalysis of the Unthought Known. New York, Columbia University Press, 1987

Bollas C: Book review of The Freud-Klein Controversies, 1941–1945. J Am Psychoanal Assoc 41:807–815, 1993

Brenman E: Cruelty and narrowmindedness. Int J Psychoanal 66:273–281, 1985

Brenner C: Psychoanalysis and science. J Am Psychoanal Assoc 16:675–696, 1968

Britton R: The missing link: parental sexuality in the oedipus complex, in The Oedipus Complex Today: Clinical Implications. Edited by Steiner J. London, Karnac Books, 1989, pp 83–102

Britton R: Sex, Death, and the Superego: Experiences in Psychoanalysis. London, Karnac Books, 2003

Canestri J: Projective identification: the fate of the concept in Italy and Spain. Psychoanalysis in Europe 56:130–139, 2002

Casement P: On Learning From the Patient. London, Tavistock, 1985

Chianese D: The person of the analyst in the psychoanalytic cure: the intra-psychic, inter-psychic paradox in different psychoanalytic traditions. Psychoanalysis in Europe 57:24–31, 2003

Cooper A: Commentary. J Am Psychoanal Assoc 52 (suppl):108–114, 2003

Feldman M: Projective identification in phantasy and enactment. Psychoanalytic Inquiry 14:423–440, 1994

Feldman M: Projective identification: the analyst's involvement. Int J Psychoanal 78:227–241, 1997

Fonagy P: Playing with reality: the development of psychic reality and its malfunction in borderline personalities. Int J Psychoanal 76:39–44, 1995

Fonagy P, Target M: Playing with reality, I: theory of mind and the normal development of psychic reality. Int J Psychoanal 77:217–233, 1996

Fonagy P, Target M: Playing with reality, III: the persistence of dual psychic reality in borderline patients. Int J Psychoanal 81:853–873, 2000

Freud S: Formulations on the two principles of mental functioning (1911), in Standard Edition of the Complete Psychological Works of Sigmund Freud, Vol 12. Translated and edited by Strachey J. London, Hogarth Press, 1958, pp 218–226

Gillespie W: The Freud–Klein controversies, 1941–45. Int J Psychoanal 73:161–164, 1992

Grosskurth P: Melanie Klein: Her World and Her Work. New York, Knopf, 1986

Heimann P: On countertransference. Int J Psychoanal 31:81–84, 1950

Heimann P: About Children and Children-No-Longer: Collected Papers of Paula Heimann, 1942–80. Edited by Tonnesmann M. London, Tavistock/Routledge, 1989

Hinz H: Projective Identification: the fate of the concept in Germany. Psychoanalysis in Europe 56:118–129, 2002

Hinze E: The Influence of Historical Events on Psychoanalysis: A Case History. Int J Psychoanal 67:459–466, 1986

Jones E: Sigmund Freud: 1856–1939. Int J Psychoanal 21:2–26, 1940

Jones E: Introduction, in Melanie Klein: Contributions to Psycho-Analysis. London, Hogarth Press, 1948, pp 9–12

Joseph B: On understanding and not understanding: some technical issues. Int J Psychoanal 64:291–298, 1983

Joseph B: Transference: the total situation. Int J Psychoanal 66:447–454, 1985

Joseph B: Projective identification: some clinical aspects, in Projection, Identification, and Projective Identification. Edited by Sandler J. Madison, CT, International Universities Press, 1987, pp 65–76

Kächele H, Thomä H: Psychoanalytic process research: methods and achievements. J Am Psychoanal Assoc 41 (suppl): 109–129, 1993

King P: The life and work of Melanie Klein in the British Psycho-Analytical Society. Int J Psychoanal 64:251–260, 1983

King P, Steiner R (eds): The Freud-Klein Controversies: 1941–1945. London, Tavistock/Routledge, 1991

Klein M: The importance of symbol formation in the development of the ego. Int J Psychoanal 11:24–39, 1930

Klein M: The Psycho-Analysis of Children. New York, Grove Press, 1932

Klein M: Notes on some schizoid mechanisms (1946), in Envy and Gratitude and Other Works: 1946–1963. London, Hogarth Press, 1975, pp 1–24

Klein M: The origins of transference. Int J Psychoanal 33:433–438, 1952

Leuzinger BM, Target M (eds): Outcomes of Psychoanalytic Treatment. London, Whurr, 2002

Michels R: The case history. J Am Psychoanal Assoc 48:355–375, 2000a

Michels R: Commentary. J Am Psychoanal Assoc 48:417–420, 2000b

Milner M: The Suppressed Madness of Sane Men: Forty-Four Years of Exploring Psychoanalysis. The New Library of Psychoanalysis No 3. London, Tavistock/Institute of Psycho-Analysis, 1987

O'Shaughnessy E: Enclaves and excursions. Int J Psychoanal 73:603–611, 1992

Quinodoz JM: Projective identification: what do French-speaking psychoanalysts think? Psychoanalysis in Europe 56:139–147, 2002

Racker H: The meanings and uses of countertransference. Psychoanal Q 26:303–357, 1957

Rayner E: The Independent Mind in British Psychoanalysis. Northvale, NJ, Jason Aronson, 1991

Riesenberg-Malcolm Ruth: Interpretation: the past in the present. Int Rev Psychoanal 13:433–443, 1986

Richards A: A plea for a measure of humility. J Am Psychoanal Assoc 52(suppl):73–89, 2003

Rodman FR (ed): The Spontaneous Gesture: Selected Letters of D.W. Winnicott. Cambridge, MA, Harvard University Press, 1987

Rosenfeld H: A clinical approach to the psychoanalytic theory of the life and death instincts: an investigation into the aggressive aspects of narcissism. Int J Psychoanal 52:169–178, 1971

Rosenfeld H: Impasse and Interpretation: Therapeutic and Antitherapeutic Factors in the Psychoanalytic Treatment of Psychotic, Borderline and Neurotic Patients. London, Tavistock/The Institute of Psycho-Analysis, 1987

Sandell R, Blomberg J, Lazar A, et al: Varieties of long-term outcome among patients in psychoanalysis and long-term psychotherapy. Int J Psychoanal 81:921–942, 2000

Sandler J: Countertransference and role responsiveness. Int Rev Psychoanal 3:43–48, 1976

Sandler J: On Communication from patient to analyst: not everything is projective identification. Int J Psychoanal 74:1097–1107, 1993

Sandler J, Joffe WG: Towards a basic psychoanalytic model. Int J Psychoanal 50:79–90, 1969

Sandler J, Rosenblatt B: The concept of the representational world. Psychoanal Study Child 17:128–148, 1962

Sandler J, Sandler A-M: On the development of object relationships and affects. Int J Psychoanal 59:285–296, 1978

Scarfone D: Controversial discussions: the issue of differences in method. Int J Psychoanal 83:453–456, 2002

Schoenhals H: Kleinian supervision in Germany: a clinical example. Psychoanalytic Inquiry 14:451–461, 1994

Schwartz J: Cassandra's Daughter: A History of Psychoanalysis in Europe and America. London, Allen Lane/Penguin, 1999

Sechaud E: The person of the analyst in the psychoanalytic cure: the intrapsychic-interpsychic paradox in different psychoanalytic traditions: an introduction to the topic. Psychoanalysis in Europe 57:22–24, 2003

Sechaud E: Which unconscious? And for which psychoanalysis? Psychoanalysis in Europe 58:20–23, 2004

Segal H: Notes on symbol formation. Int J Psychoanal 38:391–397, 1957

Spillius EB: Varieties of envious experience. Int J Psychoanal 74:1199–1212, 1993

Spillius EB: Developments in Kleinian thought: overview and personal view. Psychoanalytic Inquiry 14:324–364, 1994

Spillius EB: A brief introduction to the concept of projective identification. Psychoanalysis in Europe 56:115–118, 2002

Steiner J: Psychic Retreats: Pathological Organizations in Psychotic, Neurotic, and Borderline Patients. London, Routledge, 1993

Stewart: Psychic Experience and Problems of Technique. London, Tavistock/Routledge, 1992

Tizard J: Donald W. Winnicott. Int J Psychoanal 52:226–227, 1971

Target M, Fonagy P: Playing with reality, II: the development of psychic reality from a theoretical perspective. Int J Psychoanal 77:459–479, 1996

Tuckett D: Words and the psychoanalytical interaction. Int Rev Psychoanal 10:407–413, 1983

Tuckett D: Some thoughts on the presentation and discussion of the clinical material of psychoanalysis. Int J Psychoanal 74:1175–1189, 1993

Tuckett D: The conceptualisation and communication of clinical facts in psychoanalysis: foreword. Int J Psychoanal 75:865–870, 1994

Tuckett D: The conceptualisation and communication of clinical facts in psychoanalysis: afterword. Int J Psychoanal 76:653–662, 1995

Tuckett D: Mutual enactment in the psychoanalytic situation, in The Perverse Transference and Other Matters: Essays in Honor of R. Horacio Etchegoyen. Edited by Ahumada J, Olagaray O, Richards AK, et al. New York, Jason Aronson, 1997, pp 203–216

Tuckett D: Theoretical pluralism and the construction of psychoanalytic knowledge, in Changing Ideas in a Changing World: The Revolution in Psychoanalysis: Esays in Honour of Arnold M. Cooper. Edited by Sandler J, Michels R, Fonagy P. London, Karnac, 2000, pp 235–246

Tuckett D: A ten-year scientific initiative. Psychoanalysis in Europe 57:22–24, 2003

Tuckett D: Does anything go? Towards a framework for the more transparent assessment of psychoanalytic competence. Int J Psychoanal (in press)

Widlocher D: A Case is not a fact. Int J Psychoanal 75:1233–1244, 1994

Winnicott DW: Primitive emotional development. Int J Psychoanal 26:137–143, 1945

Winnicott DW: Transitional objects and transitional phenomena: a study of the first not-me possession. Int J Psychoanal 34:89–97, 1953

Winnicott DW: Ernest Jones. Int J Psychoanal 39:298–304, 1958

Winnicott DW: The theory of the parent-infant relationship. Int J Psychoanal 41:585–595, 1960

Winnicott DW: Dependence in infant care, in child care, and in the psycho-analytic setting. Int J Psychoanal 44:339–344, 1963

Winnicott DW: The use of an object. Int J Psychoanal 50:711–716, 1969

27

Psychoanalysis in the French Community

DOMINIQUE SCARFONE, M.D.

FROM A NORTH AMERICAN vantage point, understanding the development of psychoanalysis in the French-speaking world is a complex endeavor. From the outset, psychoanalysis in France took a very different path than it did in the United States. As Sherry Turkle (1978) observed, whereas psychoanalysis was perhaps too easily accepted in the United States, resistance was at work in France at the beginning, even though it was there that Freud had made important steps toward his crucial early discoveries. The reverse would eventually be true: whereas psychoanalysis became less fashionable in the United States after its glorious era in the 1940s and 1950s, a psychoanalytic explosion would affect France in the 1960s and 1970s. The reasons for these trends are many, and here the psychoanalyst would need some help from both a historian and a sociologist, for certainly not everything is related to issues internal to psychoanalysis. Cultural, historical, and sociopolitical differences are at work here as in any other domain.

The "French Freud"

Every now and then in Francophone psychoanalytic circles, someone will take some pride in reminding the audience that the word "psychoanalysis" made its very first appearance as a French word. Freud indeed used the term for the first time in a paper about heredity and the etiology of hysteria, written directly in French and published in the *Revue*

Neurologique. Freud's previous brief stay in Paris and Nancy in the 1880s, when he became acquainted with the work of Charcot and Bernheim, whose books he translated into German, is a well-known episode. Looking back at the history of psychoanalysis in France, the idea of a "French Freud" is a major thread among the numerous events that have marked its course, a course rich with enthusiasm and quarrels, intellectual universalism and parochial politics, claims of fidelity to Freud and outright heretical creativeness.

The other word, however, that would aptly describe the beginnings of the otherwise passionate and fascinating relationship between France and Freud would be "ambivalence." For one thing, the enthusiasm shown by the Surrealist leader André Breton toward psychoanalysis was met by Freud's cold skepticism. On the other hand, a number of medical practitioners led by René Laforgue became acquainted with Freud's ideas thanks to the presence of Eugénie Sokolnicka. A Polish-born analyst trained in Vienna, Sokolnicka had links with the Paris literary milieu and was able to penetrate the Paris medical establishment with the help of well-known literary figures. Thus, a small group of physicians started using psychoanalysis with their patients, although in a very idiosyncratic way, but they soon resolved to give the theory a "Latin accent" aimed at alleviating its supposedly Germanic overtones (Roudinesco 1990). These developments took place in the aftermath of the First World War, when anything "Teutonic" was less than palatable in victorious France.

One emblematic figure of psychoanalysis in France—Marie Bonaparte, princess of Greece—showed no ambivalence whatsoever and played a most important historical role on the psychoanalytic world scene as well. After her analysis with Freud, she became a close friend of his and helped the founder of psychoanalysis in numerous ways, including aiding his escape from Nazi Austria and salvaging—against Freud's own advice—the letters to Fliess and the precious manuscripts they contained, among which was the "Project for a Scientific Psychology." In France, Bonaparte was a major catalyst for the implantation of the psychoanalytic organization in 1926 and the founding, in 1927, of the *Revue Française de Psychanalyse*, organ of the newly created Société Psychanalytique de Paris (SPP).

The second major figure of this initial period was another Polish analyst whose name is more readily associated with American psychoanalysis: Rudolph Loewenstein. Loewenstein was trained in Berlin and had moved to Paris in 1925, where he analyzed and supervised many of the early adepts. He supervised Marie Bonaparte prior to becoming her lover. During the 1930s he analyzed a number of people who were later to play a prominent role on the Paris scene: among them Daniel Lagache, Sacha Nacht, and a young neuropsychiatrist by the name of Jacques Lacan. Considering Loewenstein's importance in the United States—where he emigrated in 1942 after having been decorated as a French soldier—it might be said that, despite major differences, French and American psychoanalytic histories have more in common than usually thought. (Heinz Hartmann and René Spitz also briefly resided in Paris before crossing the Atlantic.)

Toward the French Analytic Galaxy

In France, the Second World War put psychoanalysis to sleep, so to speak, for about 6 years. The postwar era therefore marked a new beginning for French psychoanalysts, as well as the opening of a long and rather violent struggle between competing views of what psychoanalysis is and what it takes to become a psychoanalyst. The story is the usual intricate tangle of principled debate and personal rivalry, but one can assert with some confidence that the fiercest battles always concerned what in France is called, not analytic "training," but the "transmission" of psychoanalysis and the "making" *(formation)* of analysts.

In the early 1950s the SPP included 20–30 members and a rapidly growing number of candidates. The creation of a training institute was therefore on the agenda. Two opposing views emerged on that occasion. One group thought of psychoanalysis as a medical profession, while the other

upheld the independence of psychoanalysis from medicine and supported the training of "lay" analysts. The first trend was represented by Sacha Nacht. Deemed authoritarian and "conservative," Nacht faced opposition from a group under the leadership of Daniel Lagache. Marie Bonaparte, herself not a physician, first supported Lagache's group and used in its favor her influence within the International Psychoanalytic Association (IPA). But, for reasons difficult to grasp—possibly very personal ones (Turkle 1978)—in a reversal she supported Nacht. Conflicts then flared up to the point where Lagache and others left the SPP in 1953 and created the Société Française de Psychanalyse (SFP). Jacques Lacan, then president of the SPP, soon joined the dissidents in the SFP.

Lacan had by then begun his *Séminaire* and issued his now famous call for a "return to Freud"; he was also analyzing and supervising about half of the SPP candidates, something about which Loewenstein, from afar, expressed worries to Marie Bonaparte (Roudinesco 1997). The split that led to the creation of the SFP, however, soon prompted the IPA to inquire into Lacan's analytic technique. This inaugurated a long series of episodes with Lacan at center stage. From that point onward, from whatever angle one looked at psychoanalysis in France, Lacan would emerge at every turn, haunting every schism that punctuated psychoanalytic history up until the 1980s.

Lacan, for Better or for Worse

The importance of Lacan, both as a political figure and a *maître à penser* in French psychoanalysis, can too easily be misconceived as the result of mere personal idiosyncrasy. Obviously, Lacan's personality and style played a major role in his destiny, and there is no question that he was a master puppeteer who encouraged the cult that eventually surrounded him. Seducing people who attended his *Séminaire* into starting analysis with him, endlessly entertaining his listeners' curiosity (e.g., by interminably deferring to yet another session of the *Séminaire* the answer to some obscure set of theoretical problems), impressing the audience with seemingly infinite, though sometimes sham, erudition—these were among his numerous effective strategies for widening the circle of his influence (see Roudinesco 1990, 1997; Turkle 1978). Lacan was nevertheless a genuine thinker and, in that sense, a typical representative of the French way of dealing with psychoanalysis. French psychoanalysis, thereby, did take a distinct "hexagonal" flavor, just as psychoanalysis in the United States had espoused many traits of American culture. But whereas pragmatism and utilitarianism marked psychoanalysis across the

Atlantic, the imprint given by French analysts was of a different kind, especially in the case of Lacan.

Lacan was a brilliant neuropsychiatrist who had wide intellectual and cultural interests and was closely related to prominent Parisian intellectual, literary, and artistic figures. Painters such as Picasso and Dali, philosophers and historians such as Sartre and Koyré, and writers such as Bataille and Queneau were among his close acquaintances. He had written his medical dissertation around a case of paranoia (Lacan 1932/1975). He was very interested in this psychic structure, which would eventually provide him with the original paradigm for the construction of his own theory—hence his interest in Freud's structural model and in narcissism and aggressive drives for the understanding of paranoia (Julien 1994).

Lacan made his first appearance on the international scene in 1936 at the IPA Congress in Marienbad, where he first presented his theory of the "mirror stage" after a clinical description by the great psychologist Henri Wallon. The mirror stage is, according to Lacan, a phase in the constitution of the human being occurring when the child is between 6 and 18 months old; still helpless and uncoordinated in his movements, the child anticipates in imagination the unity of—and mastery over—his or her unified body image that is the matrix and prototype of the ego, achieved through identification with the image of the other (Laplanche and Pontalis 1974). Interrupted by Jones after only 10 minutes, Lacan left the congress infuriated and humiliated. After the war, however, he rewrote his paper and presented it again at the Zurich Congress of 1949. The mirror stage is one of the best known Lacanian concepts (Lacan 2001), but only the first of a series of new ideas in the theoretical armature of Lacanism.

It must be stressed that however controversial a personality he may have been, Lacan asked important and difficult questions regarding the status of psychoanalysis. For instance, how can a discipline such as this, which requires freedom of thought and the refusal of every form of certainty (the latter resulting mainly from the defensive productions of the ego), possibly flourish within a rigid structure such as is found in psychoanalytic institutions? How can knowledge that is transmitted mainly through the personal experience of analysis, with its unavoidable transferential biases, sustain a pretense to scientific status? Ultimately, what is a psychoanalyst, and how do we recognize one?

For better or for worse, Lacan directed his efforts at trying to bring theoretical and practical answers to those questions. *Theoretically*, he embarked on a rereading of Freud, which resulted in a reformulation of psychoanalytic theory along more contemporary lines. By the same token, Lacan took hold of the epithet "Freudian" to the point where today, in France at least, it actually means "Lacanian." The

new theory was intended to take a form whose transmission would not necessarily require a personal experience of the couch. University teaching was therefore vested with the mission of formalizing psychoanalytic knowledge, much in the manner of a mathematical science. This inaugurated the era of "mathemes" and topology—Lacan's effort at formulating the workings of the mind in a mathematical guise—which came after Saussure's linguistics and Lévi-Strauss's structural anthropology had ceased serving as "pilot sciences" in Lacan's conceptualization. *Organizationally*, the structure and the practices of Lacan's École Française de Psychanalyse (École Freudienne de Paris, or EFP) were intended to provide a setting where becoming an analyst would supposedly be free from the bureaucratic, ego-centered slants imputed on the traditional forms of training. The new structures were designed to face the problems of institutionalized analysis up front. Reality, however, revealed a different face. In spite of the apparently radical departure from bureaucracy, the new structures allowed Lacan to sit on every committee or council endowed with executive power. Petty or passionate "sibling" rivalries, quarrels, slander, and splits were the expectable results. With the advantage of hindsight, one can either feel sorry that the debate around such vital questions was obscured by the maneuvers of a man in constant need of admiration and power (Reisinger 1991) or wonder whether even asking the kind of questions Lacan raised necessarily calls into question the institutional structures of psychoanalysis. The choice is far from being obvious.

Non-Lacanian France in the Early 1960s

Back in 1953, when leaving the SPP, Lagache and his followers (including Françoise Dolto, Juliette Favez-Boutonier, and Jacques Lacan)—inadvertently and on strictly administrative grounds—excluded themselves from the IPA, hence losing their status as training analysts. When, for the sake of reintegrating the IPA, the newly created SFP was assessed by a visiting committee, Lacan's technique came under closer scrutiny. The assessor's attention was called to his "variable length" analytic sessions—with the variation tending toward ever *shorter* sessions. Confronted by the demands of the IPA accreditation committee, Lacan, who strongly wished to remain within the IPA, *officially* renounced his controversial technique, but everyone knew his practice had not really changed (Roudinesco 1990). In 1961 the IPA was finally ready to give the SFP official status as a component society provided Lacan and Dolto were denied their capacity as training analysts. Two more years of discussion would lead to nothing, and a 10-year long negotiation resulted in a new split. Lacan and a number of his followers left the SFP to create, in 1964, the École Française de Psychanalyse (EFP) (the acronym was shortly to signify École Freudienne de Paris), while the others stayed with Lagache and founded the Association Psychanalytique de France (APF), which was integrated in the IPA in 1965.

The founding members of the APF, many of whom had been Lacan's analysands and his earliest and brightest "pupils" (as he used to call them), had chosen to stay in the IPA out of their feeling that Lacan's "return to Freud" was really a one-way ticket to Lacan himself (Laplanche and Pontalis 1985). They were shortly to become prominent figures of French psychoanalysis, making major contributions to the discipline. Didier Anzieu, Wladimir Granoff, Jean Laplanche, Jean-Bertrand Pontalis, Daniel Widlöcher—these were just a few of the young exponents of this new organization.

The group had also an important hold on the publishing of psychoanalytic works: within the Presses Universitaires de France, Lagache was already in charge of the "Bibliothèque de Psychanalyse" (Psychoanalytic Library), today directed by Laplanche, while Pontalis initiated another major psychoanalytic series, "Connaissance de l'inconscient" (Knowledge of the Unconscious), within the most important French publishing house, Gallimard. The often cited *Vocabulaire de la Psychanalyse* (published in English as *The Language of Psycho-Analysis*) (Laplanche and Pontalis 1974) was undertaken at about the same period and involved a thorough reading of the complete works of Freud, Klein, and others.

The two authors of the *Vocabulaire* also undertook the translation of many of Freud's papers. Their society—the APF—is still today considered a highly select group, its membership kept to a minimum through a very demanding training program. Candidates are required to undergo two *consecutive* supervisions, each lasting for the whole length of the supervised treatment. Therefore, training is very long and candidates usually become members well after having displayed their creative talents elsewhere. When finally obtaining membership, they are usually well-established professionals with a notable academic or clinical career behind them. This elitist image of the APF gives it a rather distinct status among the French psychoanalytic groups.

Thus, in 1964 the French psychoanalytic community consisted of three groups, two of them within the IPA: the Société Psychanalytique de Paris (SPP), which had kept growing and developing, and the smaller Association Psychanalytique de France (APF). Lacan's École Freudienne de Paris (EFP) was the third group.

Although deemed the more "traditional" society and identified negatively as the anti-Lacanian group, the SPP flourished and made numerous original contributions to both theory and practice. For one thing, it kept holding the annual Congress of French-Speaking Psychoanalysts, which gathered analysts mainly from France, Belgium, Switzerland, and French Canada but also from Italy, Spain, Portugal, Greece, and Britain. The format of this Congress is worth mentioning in that instead of the usual series of papers and panels on various matters it is centered around the thorough discussion of one or two main topics. These are presented in the elaborate form of one or two major "reports" whose authors were appointed years in advance. The reports are therefore expected to be genuine contributions to psychoanalysis. The Congress's home is Paris, but every other year it meets in a different European city, with Montreal the only non-European exception. It gives the SPP a wide audience and makes for a lively exchange of ideas with analysts from other countries, languages, and cultures. The *Revue Française de Psychanalyse*, which has published steadily since 1927 (except for the war period), is today the oldest French psychoanalytic journal, displaying a strong vitality and openness to authors of various psychoanalytic creeds.

The SPP also contributed remarkable theoretical advances in many aspects of psychoanalysis. One noticeable example is the theoretical and practical intervention in the field of psychosomatics. Around the mid-fifties, a group of SPP analysts, including Pierre Marty, Michel de M'uzan, Christian David, and Michel Fain, initiated research on the mental functioning of patients with treatment-resistant somatic diseases, and proposed a new conception of psychosomatics that differed from the then prevailing theories of Franz Alexander. Their theory did not rest on disease-specific dynamics but rather highlighted a common mental ingredient that they found to predispose to physical rather than neurotic ailments: poor mentalization. Marty and de M'Uzan (1963) thus described in many somatic patients what they called "*la pensée opératoire*," a state of the thinking process that lacks the usual metaphoric dimension. These patients also harbor poor and scanty dreaming, a penchant for concreteness, and poor differentiation of affects, a condition resembling what a few years later—and independently—the American team of Sifneos and Nemiah would describe as "alexithymia." Marty, de M'Uzan, and others later created the Institute of Psychosomatics (IPSO), where specific forms of treatment, such as psychoanalytic relaxation therapy, were developed for patients who could not benefit from the classical analytic setting. Research and treatment are still carried out at the IPSO, which publishes its own journal, the *Revue Française de Psychosomatique*.

Many SPP analysts have been actively involved in the development of community-oriented psychoanalytic services, such as in the Paris 13th Arrondissement. There, psychoanalytic psychotherapies and psychoanalytic psychodrama are currently offered to patients who are unsuitable for the classic analytic treatment or who cannot afford private therapy. Classical analysis, on the other hand, has been and is still provided for free or at low fee within the SPP Consultation Center. Recently, the SPP was officially acknowledged by the French State as an organization of "public interest." Other experiences directed toward the less affluent communities include the involvement of psychoanalysts in community psychiatry and the treatment of psychotic patients in special settings, as theorized by Philippe Paumelle or in the work of P.-C. Racamier, *"Le psychanalyste sans divan"* ("The couchless analyst") (Racamier 1970). Many other analysts, too numerous to mention here, are involved in special programs for the treatment of psychotic children or mother-infant dyads in various settings such as the "medico-psychological centers." René Diatkine and Serge Lebovici were among the pioneers in this field.

During the last decade, the SPP was able to make its presence felt even more strongly in Paris and other major French cities. In the early 1990s, the SPP started a series of large meetings open to the general public, where vital issues regarding psychoanalysis are widely discussed. Until recently, the SPP had been considered the most conservative in regard to the training of analysts and the progression of its members toward the status of training analyst. Its membership grew steadily nonetheless, with major differences from the Lacanian societies and splinter groups. Despite institutional limitations and problems of its own, the SPP has never been dominated by a charismatic leader; for all the unavoidable rivalries, debate and reforms did not result in new schisms, and the SPP never imposed on its members a single psychoanalytic doctrine. This has certainly played in favor of its survival and present-day vitality.

Amid the conflicts and rivalries between Lacanian and non-Lacanian societies and groups, a number of people felt the need to bypass the institutional and theoretical barriers to a dialogue among analysts, regardless of their affiliation. Such an approach was made possible thanks to the creation of *Confrontations*, promoted by the Canadian-born René Major and the Lebanese-born Dominique Geahchan, both members of the SPP. *Confrontations* was an open discussion forum that soon attracted many participants from every group. A great number of them were Lacanians who were fleeing the mysteries of "mathemes" and other disappointments with Lacan and his son-in-law, Jacques-Alain Miller (Roudinesco 1990). The weekly meetings gave birth to more important symposia and even to an eponymous journal. It was in the wake of these encounters that the philosopher Jacques Derrida gained in influence over a number of French psychoanalysts. *Confrontations*, however, perhaps due to its very nature, was not destined to become a lasting institution. It disappeared in 1983. In recent years, René Major, who in the meantime had left the SPP, tried to revive the same spirit on a much larger scale by inviting analysts from all over the world to meet for the "General Estates of Psychoanalysis" in Paris, in the year 2000.

On the Lacanian Front: A Succession of Schisms

After the second split that led to its creation, the influence and size of the École Freudienne de Paris expanded very rapidly in response both to Lacan's growing notoriety among the intelligentsia and to the new modes of training that were introduced within the the new organization. These changes, however, would lead to yet another schism in 1969, this time within the Lacanian group itself. Ever since its founding, and despite an officially democratic structure, the EFP was governed in a rather autocratic manner by Lacan. While senior members resented the situation and tried to resist Lacan's penchant for absolutism, the growing mass of younger members who had been attracted by Lacan's personal charisma—and therefore by his very specific brand of psychoanalytic theory *and* politics—were less inclined to express dissent. For the most experienced analysts in the group, the rapid growth of the EFP brought to the fore the problem of how to establish a valid training process and, as a corollary, how to make sure that the ability to conduct analysis and the ability to think for oneself (vs. allegiance to a leader) was the deciding factor in admitting new members.

On October 9, 1967, Lacan came up with a "proposal" that was supposed to revolutionize the training process and, in particular, accession to the status of the most prized variety of analyst: the "School Analyst." This title was awarded to a member who, after successfully going through a special procedure called *"la passe,"* would be considered a kind of master analyst. But whereas *la passe* was a quite complex procedure, joining the EFP at its entry-level of "Practicing Analyst" (PA) was quite easy. Based on Lacan's aphorism that "for the conduct of treatment the analyst needs no other authorization but from oneself," the only requirement was for the future PA to *inform* the school that he or she had started a psychoanalytic practice! Although the EFP offered these rank-and-file practitioners no official acknowledgement, it did not escape the critics that, for the public at large, anyone bearing the title of "practicing analyst member of the École Freudienne" enjoyed a de facto professional status (Turkle 1978). To some, this strategy was Lacan's way of ensuring a rapid expansion of his group and of his personal area of influence. Obviously, however, the rapid growth at the grass-roots level counterbalanced the highly selective procedure for accessing the elite subgroup within the school, a procedure that always included the personal presence of…Jacques Lacan. Thus, the Master's influence was assured at both ends of the process.

In 1967 the conditions for adopting the "proposal" were not yet ripe. Fearing opposition from the "old guard," Lacan did not immediately ask for a vote. France's general insurrection of the following year, however, was to provide him with the ideological background and atmosphere needed to put forward his "proposal" again. In a move deemed not unlike Mao Zedong's strategy for gaining control of the Communist Party and absolute power over China, Lacan stirred a revolt at the grass-roots level and induced the younger generation to attack the so-called conservatives (Roudinesco 1990; Turkle 1978). Those in the "old guard," however, did not give Lacan the time to put them aside. Early in 1969, as the vote on the proposal was about to be held, Piera Aulagnier, François Perrier, Jean-Paul Valabrega and a few others left the EFP to create a new psychoanalytic group, the Organisation Psychanalytique de Langue Française (OPLF), usually referred to as the "Fourth Group" (Le Quatrième Groupe) (see below).

After experimenting with "la passe" for a number of years, Lacan eventually called it a failure. Shortly before his death in 1981, he was facing new opposition, so he dissolved the EFP and founded yet another organization. The story is here again very complex and even confusing. Suffice it to say that, much as in a monarchy, power was passed on to Lacan's son-in-law, Jacques-Alain Miller, who still today reigns uncontested over the École de la Cause Freudienne (School of the Freudian Cause) and the World Psychoanalytic Association, while personally editing the transcriptions of Lacan's *Séminaire*.

The Making of an Analyst

Thus, the transmission of the psychoanalytic flame was at the core of the struggles in psychoanalytic groups from the time that psychoanalysis began occupying a visible place in French culture both as a therapy and as an intellectual discipline. One of the cultural and intellectual capitals of the world, Paris hosted in the 1960s the leading fig-

ures in many intellectual fields: philosophy (Sartre, Merleau-Ponty, Ricoeur, Foucault, and, later, Derrida), anthropology (Lévi-Strauss, Dumézil), semiotics (Barthes), linguistics (Jakobson, Benveniste), "new wave" cinema (Godard, Truffaut), theatre and literature (Beckett), and many others. Paris was also the home of radical left-wing politics that were to culminate in the 1968 libertarian upheaval. All this made for an effervescent milieu, where ambitious characters such as Lacan struggled to play a prominent role among the intellectual masters. Psychoanalysis, in this context, quickly became fashionable. It combined its own intellectual appeal with a sociopolitical discourse as it became intertwined, especially for the Lacanians, with the teaching of prominent figures such as Louis Althusser, a Marxist philosopher at the École Normale Supérieure, the major French intellectual nursery (see, e.g., Althusser 1999).

One consequence of Lacan's machinations has been to elicit in his ex-companions a profound reflection on how to avoid falling in to similar impasses concerning the training of analysts and institutional life. The three French non-Lacanian analytic organizations share in this respect a number of basic principles, such as the strictly confidential nature of the candidate's personal analysis (there is no "reporting analyst" of any kind). But there are also major differences. As already mentioned, the Société Psychanalytique de Paris may be regarded as the most traditional, while the Association Psychanalytique de France, for all its elitist reputation, extends its principle of non-intrusion in personal analysis so far as to accept candidates analyzed outside of its ranks.

Supervision of control cases also involves important differences. The SPP, for instance, now has a long experience in group supervision for one of the control cases, the principles and modalities of its training program being otherwise similar to those of the average IPA society. At the APF, the supervisor is not called upon to evaluate the supervisee. Rather, supervisor and supervisee are each separately asked to present a report on their work to other members of the training committee for the sake of validating the case. The work of supervision is therefore kept as close as possible to the original analytic experience of the supervisee and is intended as a way of assisting the candidate in dealing, among other things, with his or her countertransference. Candidates then feel more free to report personal difficulties with their control cases. The training institute directs its efforts at maintaining the "extraterritorial" status of personal analysis—that of the candidate *and* that of the candidate's patients—considering that whenever a "goal-representation" is attached to it, the psychoanalytic process is endangered. For a training analyst, the goal of "producing" a new analyst is, in that respect, no less detrimental than it is for a child analyst to try satisfying the parent's request of "producing" an obedient child: in both cases the analytic attitude is biased, with talking and listening being inhibited (Laplanche 1993).

The OPLF also subjected these problems of training to extensive reflection. Wishing to avoid the repetition of what befell them under Lacan's rule, the founders of this organization carefully tried to design mechanisms by which a psychoanalytic group could perpetuate itself—and grow—on psychoanalytic rather than ideological grounds. In their view, it was fundamentally a matter of taking seriously the hypothesis of the unconscious—of grasping how transference residues can create personal allegiances within psychoanalytic groups, especially toward charismatic figures. The new training philosophy therefore aimed at emphasizing the most important feature in the analyst—or, for that matter, in every individual: the ability to think for oneself. A very detailed policy was elaborated and made public in the first issue of the journal *Topique*. Thus, candidates are considered "participants" in the OPLF on the sole premise of being engaged in a genuine training process, whether within the Fourth Group or in another psychoanalytic organization, and provided they can demonstrate sufficient prior clinical experience in psychopathology as well as a solid general background in the sciences and the "humanities." On this basis, candidate-participants bear no specific title and cannot claim affiliation to the Fourth Group. A candidate can choose his or her analyst from among any psychoanalytical group; personal analysis is never discussed during the training process.

A basic principle in the Fourth Group is of considering training (*formation*) as a continuous process, regardless of accession to membership. Becoming a member gives one the right to vote at administrative meetings, to accept new members, and to take part in teaching and in supervision, here called "fourth analysis" (*analyse quatrième*). In this form of supervision, it is not so much a matter of "overseeing" the candidate-participant's work as of fostering the analytic dialogue that may bring to the fore the eventual countertransferential impasses in the candidate's analytic listening and intervention. It is called "fourth analysis" because it takes into account the four analytic processes involved in the supervisory encounter: that of the patient, that of the candidate, that of the candidate's analyst, and that of the member conducting the supervision. Supervising analysts are not involved in the evaluation process of the candidates they supervise. This restriction is motivated by the wish to favor a genuine cooperation in the supervisee rather than eliciting a submissive attitude toward the supervisor. Every participant is encouraged to get more than the two required supervisions, one or more of them with analysts from other societies.

Becoming a member of the Fourth Group requires going through a procedure of "qualification" (*habilitation*), in which the candidate is expected to demonstrate full maturity as an analyst. To engage in the procedure, the future member must have undergone at least two supervisions and a series of "inter-analytic sessions." These are meetings convened between the candidate and a number of colleagues of his or her choice in which they explore and discuss problems encountered in their practices. It is also a way of counterbalancing the one-to-one relationship of individual supervision.

A participant who feels ready to become a member convenes a meeting with a small group of members of his or her choice, excluding his or her analyst and supervisors. After a number of encounters, this committee eventually recommends the candidate for election at the annual general meeting of the Fourth Group. Thus, in the making of an analyst, the Fourth Group's efforts are directed at countering the bureaucratic attitude, avoiding sectarian trends, emphasizing theoretical heterogeneity, encouraging variety in supervision, and concentrating on problems related to the psychoanalytic process in everyone involved.

The Société Psychanalytique de Montréal (SPM), the French branch of the Canadian Psychoanalytic Society, has developed a model that borrows from the various non-Lacanian French groups (Lussier 1991). While selection of candidates and assessment of their progress in the training are carried out along lines similar to those of the SPP, the SPM's statutes of 1967 guarantee the extra-territoriality of personal analysis. In other words, candidates can choose their personal analyst from a list of "habilitated analysts" that is much larger than the list of training analysts. Ordinary members may ask to be put on the list of "habilitated analysts" 5 years after their election as members provided they have been practicing analysis at least half-time. This aspect of the training is very specific to the SPM and not found elsewhere within the Canadian Psychoanalytic Society. On the one hand, it addresses the SPM's wish to avoid the concentration of power and influence in the hands of a few training analysts within the society, and on the other hand, it makes for a freer analytic process for the candidates, as their personal analysis is not "guided" in any way, not even at the very delicate stage of choosing one's analyst. For example, since no request for training is seriously considered unless the applicant has already been engaged in a personal analysis for at least 2 years, it cannot be expected that every future candidate will have chosen a training analyst for personal analysis. In other branches of the Canadian Psychoanalytic Society, where only training analysts are entitled to analyze candidates, this sometimes entails a compulsory change of analyst—something unthinkable under the SPM's strict observance of the extra-territoriality of personal analysis. It goes without saying that there is no reporting on the personal analysis of candidates.

Once admitted, every candidate must undergo supervision of at least three cases and complete the equivalent of 4 years in supervision. The specific role of training analysts at the Institut Psychanalytique de Montréal (IPM) is to select new trainees, do supervision, and assess the candidates' progress in the training program. Training analysts are elected in that capacity by all members attending the annual business meeting. A majority of two-thirds is required, and the election must be confirmed by a vote among the membership of the larger Canadian Institute, which generally endorses the democratic decision of the local branches.

Training at the SPM is highly individualized rather than organized into "classes." Candidates enter the program throughout the year and may join the weekly basic teaching seminar at any point of its 4-year cycle. In this basic seminar, 3 of the 4 years are devoted to the study of the most important Freudian papers and their functions in contemporary literature; a fourth year is dedicated to the study of major contemporary authors, but this is the only explicitly mandatory aspect of the training. In fact, in addition to this basic seminar and the three supervisions, every candidate is expected to be part of a number of (two or three) study groups of his or her choice from among the 30-odd such ongoing work teams in this society of about 100 members. It is left to the candidate's personal initiative to get admitted to the existing groups and to take an active part in their clinical and/or theoretical work.

During the past decade, the SPM witnessed a rather slow growth of its training institute, the Institut Psychanalytique de Montréal. There are few active members in the IPM, and there is no rush among the SPM membership to belong to the Institute. Among the reasons for this is the feeling that approval by two-thirds of the voting members is hard to obtain and that failure in this regard may be very hurtful. This is probably but one aspect of a more complex situation. In 2003, the Society and the Institute decided to start a review process of their mutual relationship, in which all the important issues will be brought under discussion by the whole membership.

Psychoanalytic Thought in the French Sphere

It is a commonplace yet always astonishing experience for a French-speaking author to be deemed a "Lacanian" of some sort by his or her American colleagues. Although most are somewhat appalled by the idea (with the obvious exception of those upholding their Lacanian identity), this stereotyped view of French psychoanalysis is not entirely gratuitous. We already saw how inescapable a figure Lacan was in the French landscape. Whether one adores or curses him, one always has to take him into account. And the fact is that many of the major original contributions to psychoanalysis in France are either inspired by Lacan or reactions against him.

One of the first of Lacan's analysands to take a clear stand against his teachings was Didier Anzieu. During the Rome congress of 1953, when Lacan read his now-famous paper "Speech and Language in Psychoanalysis" (Lacan 1981) before an already divided audience, Anzieu, who had just terminated his analysis with Lacan, vehemently criticized his linguistic turn (Roudinesco 1990). A founding member of the APF, Anzieu (1989) had embarked on a path of his own in theoretical and clinical research around various issues such as the psychoanalytical use of the Rorschach test and psychoanalytical psychodrama, the creative process in literature and the arts, group analysis, the concept of the ego as a "Skin-Ego" (1989), and the theory of "psychic envelopes" (1990). One of his best known contributions is the masterly book *Freud's Self-Analysis* (Anzieu 1987). Ironically, it was discovered of late that Lacan's case "Aimée," the subject of his psychiatric dissertation in the 1930s, was none other than Anzieu's mother, and that neither Lacan nor Anzieu was aware of this during their work together.

Another of Lacan's early "pupils" who would soon criticize and separate from the master was Jean Laplanche. In 1959, at the historical conference on the unconscious held in Bonneval under the auspices of the major figure of French psychiatry Henri Ey, Jean Laplanche and Serge Leclaire were more or less representing the "Lacanian current." Yet in their presentation, Lacan's theory of the unconscious "structured as a language" was frontally opposed by Laplanche. Laplanche would later renounce Lacan during the 1964 split and become a founding member of the APF. With the encouragement of Daniel Lagache, he had embarked with Jean-Bertrand Pontalis on a vast project: producing the *Vocabulaire de la Psychanalyse*, published in 1967 (English translation: *The Language of Psycho-Analysis*) (Laplanche and Pontalis 1974). This major opus is not merely a psychoanalytic dictionary; it is rather a thoroughly researched exploration of psychoanalytic concepts, examined in both their synchronic and their diachronic dimensions. Translated into many languages, it remains one of the most often cited books of psychoanalysis, in which one is assured to find a reliable account of the fundamental bricks of the Freudian edifice.

After this major endeavor, Laplanche continued to study the foundations of psychoanalysis by looking closely into Freud's thinking and elaborating a number of major concepts that the work on the *Vocabulaire* had helped unearth. One major example is the concept of *étayage* (Freud's *anlehnung*; Strachey's *anaclisis*), at center stage in his very influential book *Life and Death in Psychoanalysis* (Laplanche 1976). For Laplanche, the concept played a role in delimiting the specific domain of psychoanalysis, that of repressed sexuality, by contrast with the domain of self-preservation, the former emerging as if "leaning on" *(anlehnung)* the satisfaction of the vital needs of self-preservation. But Laplanche soon found this concept wanting. In a radical criticism of Freud's "biologism," he noted that the theory of inherited primal fantasies (which he and Pontalis had also helped unearth from Freud's writings) was untenable and that the mechanism of *anlehnung* fell short of explaining the formation of unconscious infantile sexual fantasies.

This brought Laplanche to propose a reformulation of Freud's seduction theory as a truly *general* theory of the origins of the repressed unconscious, rather than a mere etiological hypothesis about neurotic symptoms. This reformulation was carried out in a series of five books *(Problématiques)* that eventually culminated in *New Foundations for Psychoanalysis* (Laplanche 1989). The theory accounts for the "normal" development of the unconscious in human beings, while also providing the tools for understanding the nature and mechanism of psychic trauma (i.e., when sexual messages are not emitted unconsciously but rather violently "intromitted") (Laplanche 1999). Although revisiting Freud's writings, Laplanche's theory of seduction is not a work of "Freudology." The starting points for Laplanche's theory are the analytic setting and the specific phenomena therein; it carries in its wake a theory of transference and of the psychoanalytic process in general (Laplanche 1999).

While still actively pursuing his research, Laplanche is also the scientific director of the French translation of Freud's complete psychoanalytic works, with about half of the work published to this day. Laplanche marked the French psychoanalytic scene in still other ways: he succeeded Lagache in psychoanalytic teaching at the Sorbonne and created the first Ph.D. program in theoretical psychoanalysis. This was a very controversial move, as it was interpreted as the training of analysts outside of psychoanalytic institutes. Laplanche, however, made a clear distinction between training in psychoanalytic *research* within the university and the *transmission* of psychoanalysis within the training programs of analytic institutes. A journal, *Psychanalyse à l'Université*, founded and directed by Laplanche, was also published until the mid 1990s; its publication ceased amid the general crisis of psychoanalytic publishing in France.

The other major journal that ceased its publication in the mid 1990s faced no major economic or editorial crisis.

The founder and director of *Nouvelle Revue de Psychanalyse (New Journal of Psychoanalysis)*, J.-B. Pontalis, the well known co-author of the *Vocabulaire*, had managed to establish his journal as the most serious, original, and generally revered psychoanalytic publication in France. Edited and distributed by the major publishing house, Gallimard, the journal was Pontalis's way of exerting a decisive influence on the psychoanalytic world while at the same time denying any pretense at leaving a personal psychoanalytic *oeuvre*. In this respect, Pontalis's path was very different from that of his close colleague Laplanche.

Analyzed by Lacan and an early member of his *Séminaire*, Pontalis was at the forefront of Paris intellectual life, closely acquainted with Maurice Merleau-Ponty and Jean-Paul Sartre, with whom he collaborated on the editorial board of *Les Temps Modernes*, then a rather important journal. A founding member of the APF, he left Sartre and his journal after disagreements had emerged around Sartre's well-known ambivalence toward psychoanalysis.

A few years after the publication of the *Vocabulaire*, Pontalis wished to do for psychoanalysis what the *Nouvelle Revue Française*—Gallimard's prestigious literary journal—was doing for the world of literature. Hence, the biannual *Nouvelle Revue de Psychanalyse*, a thematic journal whose policy was to never treat a topic unless it could be dealt with from a newer point of view. The 50 issues of the journal produced over its 25-year existence are generally considered major reference works. It was the journal's policy to host papers not only by analysts but also by writers, historians, philosophers, sociologists, and artists. This multidisciplinary work was so appreciated that Gallimard is now publishing a paperback edition of selected issues. In 1995, despite an enviable readership, Pontalis decided to put an end to the journal. He explained in a personal communication that he felt the time had come to make room for other, younger analysts who had editorial projects of their own. Moreover, he did not wish to have to designate an "heir" to head the journal that bore his very personal stamp, a gesture consistent with his vow to leave no distinctive "Pontalisian" concept to psychoanalysis. In recent years, Pontalis has devoted himself to writing about psychoanalysis in a freer literary form, making little use of psychoanalytic jargon and reaching a wider public with fine pieces of meditation such as *Love of Beginnings* (1993), *Windows/Fenêtres* (2003), and other works not yet available in English. Two new journals have emerged that, in a way, are inspired by the *Nouvelle Revue de Psychanalyse* and were both created by members of the APF: *Penser/Rêver (Thinking/Dreaming)*, founded and directed by Michel Gribinski, and *Libres Cahiers Pour la Psychanalyse (Free Notebooks for Psychoanalysis)* founded and directed by Jean-Claude Rolland and Catherine Chabert.

A member of the Société Psychanalytique de Paris, André Green attended Lacan's *Séminaire* for a number of years and always acknowledged Lacan's influence on his work (along with that of Bion and Winnicott). He nevertheless found Lacan's theory wanting in many areas, most of all in its contempt for the affective component of mental life. At the 1969 Congress of French-Speaking Analysts, Green presented a major "report" on the subject, later published in book form with the telling title *Le Discours Vivant* (literally, "Living Discourse") (Green 1999a). The book played a prominent role both in positioning Green as a major contributor to psychoanalytic theory and in giving the SPP a newer, theoretically more assertive stance toward the then expanding influence of Lacan. Instead of the usually defensive attitude toward Lacanism, there emerged for the first time from the ranks of the SPP an elaborate piece of theory directly confronting Lacan's ideas. Green thereby made his mark both as a theoretician and as a clinician, with his theory always linked with practice, mainly his experience with narcissistic and borderline mental functioning. A living encyclopedia, Green touched on almost every aspect of psychoanalysis and the surrounding disciplines, but his most famous contributions dwell on the issues of narcissism (Green 2001), the psychoanalytic setting and process, the work of "the negative" in psychoanalysis (e.g., negative hallucination, denial and negation; Green 1999b), representation, and language and time. His paper "The Dead Mother," however, is probably the one that provided the most suggestive metaphor regarding his clinical work with narcissistic pathologies (Kohon 1999).

From the ranks of the post-Lacanian OPLF–Fourth Group emerged another major opus: the work of Piera Aulagnier, whose seminal book *The Violence of Interpretation* has only recently been translated into English (Aulagnier 2001). After having left Lacan around the issue of training and having founded the Fourth Group and the journal *Topique*, Aulagnier undertook the task of formulating a metapsychology of psychosis. While Lacan's influence is noticeable in Aulagnier's writings, one is struck by her true originality and her clear and precise writing around very difficult issues, such as when she presents the relationship of the psychotic mind to thinking. Two more books and a series of brilliant articles, mostly devoted to the understanding of psychotic thinking, were published prior to her death from cancer in 1990.

Conclusion

A host of other creative authors in French psychoanalysis would deserve to be presented here were it not for space limitations. They demonstrate that for all the quarrels and the splits in the French psychoanalytic movement, something managed to thrive, evolve, and differentiate into a wide array of experiments with Freud's legacy, both in theory and in practice. French-language psychoanalysis is alive and well, extending far beyond its best-known authors. Directly or indirectly influenced by Lacan, but not reducible to the Lacanian idiom, it is at once very classic in its constant reference to Freud and very innovative in its unrelenting intellectual quest for conceptual rigor and clarity, elegance of style, and a genuine dialogue with other disciplines.

References

Althusser L: Writings on Psychoanalysis: Freud and Lacan. New York, Columbia University Press, 1999

Anzieu D: Freud's Self-Analysis. New York, International Universities Press, 1987

Anzieu D: The Skin Ego. Translated by Turner C. New Haven, CT, Yale University Press, 1989

Anzieu D: Psychic Envelopes. Translated by Briggs D. London, Karnac Books, 1990

Aulagnier P: The Violence of Interpretation: From Pictogram to Statement. Translated by Sheridan A. London, Routledge, 2001

Green A: The Fabric of Affect in the Psychoanalytic Discourse (New Library of Psychoanalysis). London, Routledge, 1999a

Green A: The Work of the Negative. Translated by Weller A. London, Free Association Books, 1999b

Green A: Life Narcissism, Death Narcissism. London, Free Association Books, 2001

Julien PH: Jacques Lacan's Return to Freud: The Real, the Symbolic, and the Imaginary. New York, New York University Press, 1994

Kohon G (ed): The Dead Mother: The Work of André Green. London, Routledge, 1999

Lacan J: De la Psychose Paranoïaque Dans ses Rapports Avec la Personnalité (1932). Paris, Le Seuil, 1975

Lacan J: Speech and Language in Psychoanalysis. Baltimore, MD, Johns Hopkins University Press, 1981

Lacan J: Ecrits: A Selection. London, Routledge, 2001

Laplanche J: Life and Death in Psychoanalysis. Translated by Mehlman J. Baltimore, MD, Johns Hopkins University Press, 1976

Laplanche J: Preface, in Fantasme Originaire, Fantasme des Origines, Origines du Fantasme. Paris, Hachette, 1985, pp 7–10

Laplanche J: New Foundations for Psychoanalysis. Translated by Macey D. Oxford, England, Basil Blackwell, 1989

Laplanche J: Une analyse sur commande. Trans Revue de Psychanalyse 3:75–84, 1993

Laplanche J: Essays on Otherness. Edited by Fletcher J. London, Routledge, 1999

Laplanche J, Pontalis J-B: The Language of Psycho-Analysis. Translated by Nicholson-Smith D. New York, WW Norton, 1974

Lussier A: Our training ideology. Paper presented at the Training Analysts' Pre-Congress of the 37th International Psychoanalytic Association Congress, Buenos Aires, July 1991

Marty P, de M'Uzan M: La pensée opératoire. Revue Française de Psychanalyse 27(suppl):345–356, 1963

Pontalis J-B: Love of Beginnings. London, Free Association Books, 1993

Pontalis J-B: Windows/Fenêtres. Lincoln, NE, Bison Books, 2003

Racamier P-C: Le Psychanalyste Sans Divan: La Psychanalyste et les Institutions de Soins Psychiatriques. Paris, Payot, 1970

Reisinger M: Lacan l'insondable. Paris, Les empêcheurs de penser en rond, 1991

Roudinesco E: Jacques Lacan and Co: A History of Psychoanalysis in France, 1925–1985. Chicago, IL, University of Chicago Press, 1990

Roudinesco E: Jacques Lacan: Outline of a Life, History of a System of Thought. New York, Columbia University Press, 1997

Turkle S: Psychoanalytic Politics: Freud's French Revolution. New York, Basic Books, 1978

28

Psychoanalysis in Latin America

CLÁUDIO LAKS EIZIRIK
MÓNICA SIEDMANN DE ARMESTO

IN THIS CHAPTER, we discuss aspects of the development of psychoanalysis in Latin America—primarily in Argentina, where the analytic movement began, and Brazil, where it has grown most rapidly in recent years. We make reference to the situation in other countries as well. Currently, there are around 3,000 analysts affiliated with the International Psychoanalytical Association (IPA) in Latin America, as well non-IPA analysts, mainly Lacanian, about whom there are no reliable figures. The main IPA analytic institutions in Latin America are FEPAL (Latin American Psychoanalytical Federation) and its 26 affiliated societies: 11 in Brazil, 6 in Argentina, and others in Uruguay, Mexico, Chile, Colombia, Peru, and Venezuela. We highlight here the main historical events of the development of psychoanalysis in each country, as well as relevant facts in more recent years.

It is a true challenge to write about the history of a movement as passionate as that of the development of psychoanalysis in Latin America. This task involves not only delving into written accounts and rediscovering the facts that gave rise to legends (and connecting them in perhaps new ways), but also, to a great extent, remembering and working-through all that has shaped us as analysts by means of transference and identifications. To summarize a long history, we are compelled to make sometimes difficult choices about

what to focus on, even though we must acknowledge that many important events and names will be left out.

Psychoanalysis in Argentina

Development of the Discipline

Many years elapsed between the first time Freud and his method were named at an International Medicine Conference held in Buenos Aires in 1910 and the foundation of the Argentine Psychoanalytic Association in 1942. During those years, many philosophers, scientists, and intellectuals became familiar with Freud's work. Some of them exchanged letters with Freud himself, and one even sent an invitation to Freud for him to settle in Argentina. At the beginning of the twentieth century, many people became interested in the workings of the mind because there was a need to find an alternative to positivist materialism as a way of understanding human suffering. Already in the 1930s, there was an active interest in psychoanalysis, as shown by Celes Cárcamo's departure for France, where he went to be trained as a psychoanalyst, after having attempted to apply the method, self-taught, at the Hospital de Clínicas (University Hospital).

Growth and Institutionalization: The Argentine Psychoanalytic Association

Previous historical accounts have stated that there were no psychoanalysts in Buenos Aires until 1938. However, many pioneers were already meeting to study Freud's works and applying this newly acquired knowledge in treating patients at different hospitals. This was the case of Arnaldo Rascovsky, at Hospital de Niños (Pediatric Hospital), as well as Enrique Pichon Rivière and Arminda Aberastury at Hospicio de las Mercedes (the former Psychiatric Hospital). They lacked, however, personal analysis. This situation changed with Angel Garma's arrival from Spain and Celes Cárcamo's return from France in 1938. Both had been trained in Europe as psychoanalysts. Garma had been trained in Berlin and was a member of the German Psychoanalytic Society, and Cárcamo had finished his training at the French Psychoanalytic Society. Shortly thereafter, Marie Glas de Langer, who had been trained in Vienna, joined the group. The first candidates underwent analysis with them and in turn became members of the founding group.

In the group of interested and enthusiastic people starting analysis, different styles of training began to be transmitted according to the experience of the pioneers such as Garma, Cárcamo, and Glas de Langer gained from their respective institutes (German, French, and Viennese). This diversity in styles influenced the origin of one of the main traits of Argentine psychoanalytic thought: its pluralism and open-mindedness, which became the source not only of original creations but also of the potential of articulating different schools and authors. The situation radically changed in just 4 years. The Argentine Psychoanalytic Association was founded in 1942, and Ernest Jones was asked to recognize it as a study group of the IPA.

The Institute of Psychoanalysis was immediately organized, following Eitingon's model of training that prevailed in Berlin and that had been adopted by the English School. Based on the tripartite training still currently in force, it had certain characteristics: the simultaneity of candidates' personal training analysis (referred to as "didactic"); the supervision of clinical cases; and seminars and writings on specific topics. Moreover, to be accepted as members, those who had completed their training had to submit a paper and be approved by two-thirds of the members present at an assembly. Initially, the training course usually took 3 years, but it was gradually extended to 4 years. Two supervisions, each of which lasted 2 years, had to be carried out during these 4 years. The curriculum was determined by the Training Committee of the Institute according to a plan that included a thorough study of Freud's works in their metapsychological, clinical, and technical aspects, as well as study of English School authors, an introduction to child and adolescent psychoanalysis, psychopathology, and group supervision of clinical cases. This plan of study was in force until 1975, when a major review and reform took place, as will be described later in this section.

In 1943, the journal *Revista de Psicoanálisis (Journal of Psychoanalysis)* was first published. It immediately had 185 subscribers and became a significant means of disseminating Freudian thoughts, as well as the ideas of other authors.

The initial years of psychoanalysis in Argentina were characterized by hard work and enthusiasm devoted to creation, institutionalization, and recognition of psychoanalytic work that became known beyond Argentina, since many Latin Americans came to Buenos Aires to be trained and, in turn, founded new societies in their own countries.

Argentine Psychoanalytic Association members usually held activities that helped to connect their society to Buenos Aires University, to other scientific societies, and to several hospitals. Both Garma and Rascovsky delivered lectures and gave classes at the Main Hall (Aula Magna) of the School of Medicine of Buenos Aires University. Their lectures are still remembered because of the large number of interested students who attended them. In addition, many of these students underwent analysis and later became outstanding analysts. The first time that Argentine Psychoanalytic Association members participated in a congress was at a neurology and psychiatry congress held in Buenos Aires.

This connection with hospitals and the university fluctuated depending on the country's political situation. There were times of expansion and others of contraction, especially during military dictatorships. It is worth highlighting, however, that the relationships with hospitals and universities were not carried out by the psychoanalytic institutions as such, but by their members, who either individually or in groups introduced psychoanalysis into psychopathology or psychiatry departments or to the chairs and deans at universities.

In 1949, at the Zurich International Psychoanalytic Congress, the first one held after the Second World War, the Argentine Psychoanalytic Association was recognized as a component society of the IPA. It becomes evident, on reviewing the reports from those years, that there was intensive scientific activity in the psychoanalytic world, both in Latin America and internationally. This burst of activity was the real source from which COPAL (Cousejo de las Organizaciones Psicoanaliticos de America Latina; today's FEPAL) originated. Exchanges with Brazilian, Chilean, Uruguayan, and North American colleagues were relevant, and trips to deliver lectures and courses in other countries furthered development of the field.

The years following 1949 saw the appearance of many papers dealing with a psychoanalytic approach to general medicine, psychosomatic disturbances, psychoses, mother-hood, and femininity. At the same time, Arminda Aberastury and Elizabeth Garma started developing their own line of thought on clinical practice with children and adolescents, thus giving rise to an important growth in clinical practice, which later crystallized into an original style of training in this area. The Child and Adolescent Department of the Argentine Psychoanalytic Association, established in 1974, was the first one to be organized in Latin America.

In the 1950s these pioneers held close relationships with the French and English psychoanalytic communities. Trips to Europe to submit reports on clinical cases and for supervision were quite frequent. There were exchanges with Melanie Klein, Paula Heimann, Herbert Rosenfeld, Donald Winnicott, Serge Lebovici, and Henry Ey, among others. Additionally, Hanna Segal, Ida Macalpine from London, and Paul Hoch from New York went to Argentina to present their ideas. With Arminda Aberastury's translation of Melanie Klein's "The Psychoanalysis of Children" in 1948, Klein's scientific influence became increasingly significant.

Ten years after being founded, the Argentine Psychoanalytic Association was able to open its own building thanks to contributions from members, candidates, and friends. Internal symposia started taking place with the participation of other Latin American colleagues. New generations of psychoanalysts were incorporated into the original group. In 1954, some of them founded the Argentine Association of Group Psychology and Psychotherapy, which a year later held the first Latin American congress dealing with this subject. Furthermore, also in 1955, Willy and Madeleine Baranger settled in Montevideo, Uruguay, to train a small group of analysts who were beginning to work and study there.

Psychoanalysis had had an excellent reception in Buenos Aires. Its thought and discourse became increasingly articulated with those of science and culture. The local population, comprising a large number of immigrants and their descendants, had socially permeable characteristics and a good intellectual level and was greedy for new developments in scientific knowledge, forming the appropriate ground for the growth of psychoanalysis. The bridge for Freud's theory was the already acquired knowledge of psychosomatic issues and the interest that this new discipline had raised. However, as usually happens, the evolution of the field did not go smoothly. The medical and psychiatric worlds were strongly resistant to psychoanalysis, and psychoanalysts were regarded with suspicion by some traditional social groups and accused of being pansexual or in favor of divorce.

The Argentine Psychoanalytic Association, as an institution, continued developing inwardly and outwardly. It started teaching psychoanalysis in several other cities and towns (e.g., Mar del Plata, Mendoza, Córdoba, Tucumán) and deepening its bonds with other Latin American colleagues through successive conferences that resulted in the organization of COPAL in 1960. Regarding the relationship with the international psychoanalytic community, an Argentine psychoanalyst, León Grinberg, was the first Latin American IPA vice-president. The Argentine Psychoanalytic Association also received many visitors who left deep imprints on the local scientific thought, such as Elizabeth Zetzsel, Wilfred Bion, Avelino González, Nathan Ackerman, Luis Guimaraes Dalheim, Peter van der Leeuw, Salomón Resnik, Leo Rangell, Viola Bernard, Bryce Boyer, Walderedo de Oliveira, Donald Meltzer, Adam Limentani, Frances Gitelson, Arthur Mirsky, and Eli Marcovitz. The creation of the Racker Center for Research and Psychoanalytic Assistance represented a further step in the outreach toward the community at large. The center was devoted to patients with modest economic resources who would not otherwise have had access to psychoanalytic treatment.

In the years following these developments, several psychoanalytically oriented institutions were founded. Among them, we may mention the Argentine School of Psychotherapy for Graduates, created by Argentine Psychoanalytic Association members, which has been transmitting psychoanalysis for 40 years; and the Child and Adolescent Psychiatry and Psychology Association, organized by Argentine Psychoanalytic Association members along with professors of the School of Psychology of Buenos Aires University. Another institution founded during this time was the Center for Research in Psychosomatic Medicine, which paved the way for other institutions devoted to this subject.

The Argentine Psychoanalytic Association also developed internally, as its membership grew dramatically despite the fact that at that time admittance was restricted to medical doctors. In 1983, with the return of democracy, a mental health law was passed, and psychologists were allowed to practice as independent psychotherapists, thus being able to enter official training at the Argentine Psychoanalytic Association.

New Challenges

Notwithstanding the growth indicating the consolidation and flourishing of psychoanalysis in Argentina, this process did not lack some dark aspects. Different ways of regarding the institution itself and its workings as a society, as well as differing views on training, led to difficulties in finding harmonious solutions. By the end of the 1960s, times of intense questioning, tinted by political ideologies, arose. An outcome of this questioning was the withdrawal from the Argentine Psychoanalytic Association of two groups of members and candidates (about 30 members and 20 candidates, respectively), the "Plataforma" and "Documento" (Langer et al. 1982). This departure did not put an end to internal controversies. On the contrary, two distinct ways of thinking about the transmission of psychoanalysis resulted.

At the same time, new generations of analysts demanded an increasingly active participation in the decisions concerning the Argentine Psychoanalytic Association. There was discontent among associate members, who up to then had voice but no vote. Scientific pluralism was restricted, and access to training analyst status for full members, who in fact fulfilled training functions, had become very difficult. In almost 30 years of institutional existence, only 20 psychoanalysts had had access to training analyst status, and this number included the Association founders. Those who wanted to start their training analysis (which had to be performed with a training analyst), a requirement to allow later access to the Institute, had to wait for several years. Meanwhile, a peculiar phenomenon took place: those interested in becoming analysts, who were quite numerous, underwent analysis for several years with an associate or full member and, then once admitted, started their training analysis with another analyst. During the years of the so-called therapeutic analysis, which also implied four to five weekly sessions, the would-be candidate had to study and be supervised privately, or had to take another complete training course at any of the various institutions that taught psychoanalysis or psychoanalytic psychotherapies outside the Argentine Psychoanalytic Association, but with Association members as analysts, supervisors, and/ or teachers. Thus, when those who applied for admission into the Argentine Psychoanalytic Association were ultimately accepted, they already had considerable psychoanalytical experience. This took place all throughout the 1960s and into the early 1970s. We could retrospectively think today, at 30 years' distance from the passions those events stirred, that every aspect of this critical situation would inevitably give rise to important movements and deep controversies.

Finally, in 1974, there was the possibility of choosing between two different programs, each with its own authorities. As an alternative to the traditional path, described above, the Barangers—Willy and Madeleine—and Jorge Mom proposed a plan, previously worked out with many colleagues, to restructure the Argentine Psychoanalytic Association at every level. In this program, professors were allowed to choose the subjects they would rather teach, and candidates could choose their own curriculum, to the extent that they fulfilled certain conditions governing the 24 mandatory seminars. The requirements concerning training analysis and supervisions did not change. Regarding social regulations, there were some modifications: associate members would be able to both vote and participate in the organization of the different administrative departments. Full members could ask to become training members, which no longer represented a category but a function. However, to become a full member, it was necessary to fulfill certain conditions within a finite period of time.

Such was the program ultimately adopted, but not without consequences. This decisive step meant the beginning of what came to be a traumatic event for many analysts: the splitting of a group of colleagues (64 members, both associate and full members, and 70 candidates), who founded the Buenos Aires Psychoanalytic Association, acknowledged by the IPA as a provisional society at the Jerusalem Congress in 1977 (with the official support of the Argentine Psychoanalytic Association) and recognized as a component society at the New York Congress in 1979.

These were difficult times, during which mutual accusations were cast; moreover, in some people's minds there had been a split between "good" and "bad" analysts—"pure" as opposed to "extremely flexible" analysts. This division involved, in fact, an unprecedented event both in the Argentine psychoanalytic environment and in the international community.

After several years, both societies came closer again, as indicated by the intense joint activity carried out—along with the Mendoza Psychoanalytic Society and the Córdoba Study Group—when the First Argentine Congress was organized in 1988. Argentine congresses continue to be held, rotating venues among Buenos Aires, Córdoba, Mendoza, and Rosario, which are the cities where the IPA component societies are located.

From the 1960s onward, important psychoanalytic centers started developing in some of the provinces, supported by members of Argentine Psychoanalytic Association and, after the split in the 1970s, by those of the Buenos Aires Psychoanalytic Association. The Mendoza Psychoanalytic Society was acknowledged as a provisional society in 1981 and as a component society in 1983. In 1991, the Córdoba Study Group was accepted as a provisional society, and it became a component society a few years later. In Rosario, a town with a long-standing psychoanalytic tradition, a study group that had been organized there was recognized as a provisional society at the Nice Congress in 2001.

The developments recounted above are the landmarks on the road of psychoanalytic development that culminated in the creation of societies. But, in fact, there are throughout the country groups of mental health professionals studying and undergoing psychoanalysis, applying its ideas to their hospital and private practice. Many of them go to Buenos Aires regularly. The Argentine Psychoanalytic Association has for many years had a department for the interior, which organizes courses and sends teachers and supervisors to regions as distant as Río Gallegos in the south or Salta in the north of the country.

In 1991, almost 50 years after the foundation of the first psychoanalytic society in Argentina, a meeting resulting in the fruitful collaboration and exchange among all recognized societies took place in Buenos Aires: the First Latin American IPA International Congress. The congress was a great success because of both the number of participants enrolled (3,300) and the scientific contributions of the presenters. Moreover, at this congress, and for the first time, all the members of the international psychoanalytic community would choose the first Latin American IPA president for the 1993–1997 period. Both the Argentine Psychoanalytic Association and Buenos Aires Psychoanalytic Association presented their candidates, and Dr. Horacio Etchegoyen, from the Buenos Aires Psychoanalytic Association, was elected.

Contemporary Perspectives

What is the state of affairs concerning Argentine psychoanalysis in the last few years? There are currently six Argentine societies, with the newest association, the Argentine Society of Psychoanalysis, having been created just a few years ago. The newest society comprises a group of members and candidates who decided to separate from the Argentine Psychoanalytic Association, founding a new study group. It was acknowledged as a provisional society in 2001, and this decision was supported by the other Argentine societies.

The six IPA societies together comprise 1,223 members and numerous candidates. There are, in addition, many schools and institutions outside the IPA that maintain different theoretical orientations. Some of them are pluralistic, and some adhere to just one theoretical frame of reference. Lacan's ideas have had a strong impact on the profession, mostly outside the IPA component societies, and these groups have created their own associations. There is, however, a remarkable growth of the French School, both Lacanian and post-Lacanian, in the "traditional" societies. Notwithstanding, training continues being pluralistic, with the prevailing and alternating influence of the British and French schools of thought at different times, depending on various factors.

In the last years, the direct connection between psychoanalytic institutions and universities has increased as psychoanalytic societies search for official recognition. One may officially qualify as a psychiatrist or psycholo-

gist, but not as a psychoanalyst. This search for recognition is partly related to the fact that more recent generations perform their clinical practice mostly in relation to the new public health systems. Consequently, master's degree programs in some psychoanalytic specialties/specializations have been organized in cooperation with certain universities.

We conclude this review of the development of psychoanalysis in Argentina with Fidias Cesio's (2000) assessment of the current status of psychoanalysis in Argentina: "The Argentine psychoanalytic movement maintains the drive that the pioneers endowed it with, and which has turned our country into one of the most active psychoanalytic centers in the world." This growth is likely to continue, despite the economic and political difficulties that Argentina is currently going through. The country's psychoanalytic institutions will be able to support the depth and thoroughness already achieved, in the same atmosphere of freedom and openness that characterized that of those who initiated the psychoanalytic enterprise (Argentine Psychoanalytic Association 1982, 2002; Cesio 2000; Langer et al. 1982; Wender et al. 1995).

Argentine Psychoanalytic Thought

All the institutional and training activity described in the previous section has given rise to what many call "the Argentine School": works, research, and publications that cover a broad spectrum of interests and developments.

As we have previously mentioned, at the very beginning the most meaningful traits of Argentine psychoanalytic thought were its pluralism and openness. Issues of grand disparity were tackled: the psychosomatic phenomena (Angel Garma), the psychoses (Pichon-Riviere), sexuality (M. Langer, A. Raskovsky), dreams (A. Garma), different psychopathological syndromes, child psychoanalysis, the psychoanalytical theory of technique, psychoanalysis applied to mythology and the works of literature, among others. Distinct schools of thought (Kleinian, Viennese, North American, German) were present, while, simultaneously, less-known works by Freud were being translated and published.

Nevertheless, with the passing of time, this scientific pluralism, which was certainly not eclectic, started to fade away somehow, when the contributions of the English School, predominantly represented by Melanie Klein and Wilfred Bion, were adopted as the mainstream thought. After 1968, the work of French authors and the contributions of Winnicott were introduced. Both lines of thought influenced Argentine scientific production. There then occurred a considerable increase in the works devoted to metapsychology, as well as a deepening in the study of the different aspects of the psychoanalytical process. Concepts such as transference and countertransference, the communication and semiotic in psychoanalytic therapy, analytic field theory, lethargy and diverse perspectives of the understanding of the oedipal tragedy, bond theory and its application in group therapies—all are examples of the deepening of psychoanalytic inquiry at that time. Numerous authors produced major developments, and it is impossible to mention them all. Yet, it is relevant to point out the participation of analysts such as Mauricio Abadi, Enrique Racker, David Liberman, Jose Blecher, Willy and Madeleine Baranger, Jorge Mom, Jaime Szpilka, Fidias Cesio, Isidoro Berenstein, Janine Puget, and Horacio Etchegoyen for having left an imprint on the analysts who followed them. The journals of the Argentine Psychoanalytic Association and the Buenos Aires Psychoanalytic Association, as well as the countless books produced, are a clear proof of their creativity.

From the 1980s onward, the influence of Serge Leclaire, Jacques Lacan, Guy Rosolato, Pierre Marti, Janine Chasseguet-Smirgel. Piera Aulagnier, and Andre Green, among others, became more evident, along with a relative decrease of the British School influence. On the other hand, North American authors such as Otto Kernberg, Heinz Kohut, Margaret Mahler, and Peter Blos also left a considerable mark. At present, Argentine analytic thought (regarding adults and children) has returned to a more pluralist stage—so much so that reading and discussing works with different theoretical approaches has become feasible. Discussing issues on the basis of distinct viewpoints—Kleinians, Winnicottians, Kohutians, Lacanians—may be an enriching challenge but no easy task. Fortunately, Freud continues to be a core reference.

The most recent developments have focused on the clinic and theory of ideals, the ego ideal, the work on the negative, the transgenerational, the not-representable, narcissism, the metapsychological understanding of psychoses, and the pathologies of impulsiveness. They cast a different light with which to see the previous concepts.

Psychoanalysis in Brazil

The experience of immigration structured the formation of a Brazilian national character. Brazil, a country of 8,547,403 km^2 and a current population of 174,632,935 inhabitants, has remarkable ethnic and cultural diversity and, at the same time, serious socioeconomic differences. Initially inhabited by several Indian tribes, Brazil was colonized by the Portuguese from 1500 onward, and in the following centuries these first European settlers admixed

with the Indians, the Africans (brought as slaves during the sixteenth century), and the Spanish to constitute the main foundations of this new ethnic group. (The presence of the Dutch and French in the northeastern part of the country was an additional influence.) During the nineteenth and twentieth centuries, new waves of immigration occurred, bringing Germans, Italians, Japanese, Arabs, Russians, and Poles, especially to the southern and southeastern regions. Thus, immigration is a cultural phenomenon that has been fully integrated in the country's history, helping create a multiracial society whose various ethnic expressions, despite sporadic tension accompanied by violence and a certain still existing level of prejudice, now present a predominantly tolerant association.

As with Brazilian society at large, the implementation of psychoanalysis in Brazil presented a certain synergy that can be observed among its different constitutive elements. The history of the Brazilian psychoanalytic movement can be divided into three periods. The first began in 1919 with the publication of the first translations of Freud: short-lived groups interested in psychoanalysis were established, with the presence of outstanding psychiatrists and intellectuals from São Paulo, Rio de Janeiro, and Porto Alegre. The second period began in 1937 with the arrival of the German psychoanalyst Adelheid Lucy Koch in São Paulo to officially begin training psychoanalysts according to the standards established by the IPA. During this period, a dedicated group of pioneers, facing great difficulties, endeavored to structure a training system and build solid institutions, furthering the presence of psychoanalysis in the culture. The third period, beginning in the early 1950s and continuing today, with the successive recognition of the São Paulo Society (1951), the Psychoanalytic Society of Rio de Janeiro (1955), the Brazilian Society of Psychoanalysis of Rio de Janeiro (1959), and the Psychoanalytic Society of Porto Alegre (1963), has been characterized by the full institutionalization and development of a psychoanalytic practice that is accompanied by production of theory, publications, congresses, and an intense interfacing with culture, as well as by the inevitable vicissitudes of institutional scientific life.

Currently, Brazil has 1,038 psychoanalysts affiliated with the IPA and, in addition to the already mentioned centers, analytic societies or study groups in Recife, Brasilia, Pelotas, Ribeirão Preto, and Campo Grande, as well as nuclei in several other cities. The Brazilian Psychoanalytic Association (ABP) was founded in 1967, having as its first president Mario Martins. The ABP is a federation of all Brazilian societies and study groups and organizes a Brazilian Congress every 2 years, which is generally open to nonmembers as well.

Development of Psychoanalysis in São Paulo

The main name in the beginning of psychoanalysis in São Paulo is that of psychiatrist and intellectual Durval Marcondes (1899–1981), who took the first initiative to organize a psychoanalytic movement in that city, beginning in 1924, when he graduated from medical school and took out a subscription to the *International Journal of Psycho-Analysis*; in 1926 he began corresponding with Freud, who encouraged him in successive letters.

Initially there were two attempts to bring over European analysts who had trained along the IPA lines, to implement a local training system. The first was in 1932, when René Spitz was invited; however, because of the difficulty in exchanging letters due to the revolution that was taking place in São Paulo at the time, Spitz decided to go to the United States instead. The next attempt was by request of Abraham Brill, then IPA president, who suggested that a certain number of competent and very able Jewish physicians who were being persecuted in Germany should come to Brazil. Durval Marcondes tried to interest two important political leaders (the owner of the main São Paulo newspaper and the State Governor) who were making an effort to create a model university, the University of São Paulo. Although both did show an interest in the possibility of establishing a psychoanalytic discipline, the project did not go any further, because it was opposed by the Chief Professor of Psychiatry, who was against psychoanalysis.

A third opportunity arose in 1936, during the Marienbad Congress. Ernest Jones, then IPA president, heard that Dr. Adelheid Koch intended to emigrate from Germany because of the persecution against Jews, and was trying to get to Palestine, the United States, or Argentina. Jones remembered the requests by Durval Marcondes and suggested that Koch could move to Brazil. With Jones's and Fenichel's authorization to work as a training analyst, Koch and her family arrived in Brazil on November 15, 1936, on her 40th birthday.

Adelheid Lucy Koch (1896–1980) had graduated from the Medical School of the University of Berlin in 1924 and entered the Psychoanalysis Institute in 1929. She did her training analysis with Otto Fenichel and supervisions under Salomé Kempner and Tereza Benedek. She became a member of the German Society in 1935 with the paper "Aspects of Resistance in a Narcissistic Neurosis" (Sagawa 1994).

After a few months to settle in, Dr. Koch went to see Durval Marcondes in July 1937 and immediately began her pioneering work of analyzing future analysts, teaching seminars, and doing supervisions. For this purpose, a room at Dr. Durval Marcondes' office was used. She began with three physicians, one of them Marcondes himself, and a female sociologist. The inclusion of a sociologist made a lasting mark on the initial nucleus of São Paulo in that it accepted from the beginning nonphysicians as candidates. In the following years, Koch accepted new candidates, and her work, together with the work of those who finished their analyses and took up training functions, promoted the creation of the Psychoanalytic Group of São Paulo in 1944; it was officially recognized as a component society of the IPA in 1951.

The constitution of the Psychoanalytic Group of São Paulo was based on the synergy between Marcondes and Koch. Marcondes was the cultured, aristocratic psychiatrist from São Paulo, closely connected to art, a former teacher of literature who spoke and wrote very well, a friend of intellectuals, physicians and politicians, and a participant in the Modern Art Week in 1922. Adelheid Koch was the immigrant psychoanalyst who had trouble with the language and with the new, unknown culture and had to perform many different tasks, maintaining an analytic attitude amid such challenging circumstances, including a threat of being denounced for charlatanism for practicing psychoanalysis, which was considered an irregular and unacceptable method by some physicians.

In this association, aspects of the Brazilian cultural structure were reproduced against the background of the transformations that were occurring in a society that was changing rapidly and becoming more modern, in which the arrival of psychoanalysis was one of the effects of the cultural and scientific project that had been moving the economically and politically rising classes. Even facing conservative barriers in the traditional academic and psychiatric worlds under the influence of the predominant positivism, psychoanalysis managed to become part of the Brazilian modernization project. The facts reported here took place during the period between the two World Wars and immediately afterward, which marked the transition of Brazil from a predominantly agrarian-export economy to a modern economy with industry and integrated communications. The meeting between the two cultures, the traditional São Paulo one of Durval Marcondes and the immigrant European one of Adelheid Koch, shaped the character of a psychoanalytic movement in continuous development, within the guidelines established by its pioneers; it was not merely by chance that São Paulo became the location where the first psychoanalyst of Latin America settled and taught.

In the following decades, until the present day, the Psychoanalytic Society of São Paulo grew in terms of number of members and candidates, in its role as a center of excellence in clinical practice, and in chances for analytic training. In spite of going through a number of internal tensions throughout the years, the society managed to keep its unity within such a big city. A generous policy of investments in scientific activities, an emphasis on publications, and the inauguration of new and modern facilities constituted a trend in the last decade. The Psychoanalytic Society is responsible for publishing three journals: *Revista Brasileira de Psicanálise* (*Brazilian Journal of Psychoanalysis*), on behalf of the Brazilian Association; *IDE*, the society's journal; and the *Jornal de Psicanálise*, produced by the society's Institute of Psychoanalysis and dedicated to training matters. An active policy of a permanent scientific program, and strong ties with the cultural and university environment (with joint events and exhibits on psychoanalysis and art, literature, and the movies), keep the membership high and keep the Psychoanalytic Society in the position of one of the leading institutions in the cultural and scientific life of São Paulo (Lobo 1994; Luz 1976; Nosek 1996; Sagawa 1994, 2001; Sister and Taffarel 1996; Vollmer 1995).

The Immigrant Analysts and Psychoanalysis in Rio de Janeiro

As in São Paulo, the first decades of the twentieth century witnessed incipient expressions of interest in psychoanalysis in Rio de Janeiro, in the form of lectures and work performed by physicians and psychiatrists to disseminate Freudian ideas. Beginning in 1944, a group of young psychiatrists attempted to bring an IPA-trained psychoanalyst to Rio de Janeiro to begin analytic training. They invited Garma and Raskovsky to give lectures in Rio de Janeiro and counted on the help of both of them to invite Georg Gerö and, then, Daniel Lagache, who did not accept the invitation. Since the attempt was fruitless, the idea of establishing a psychoanalytic nucleus in Rio was put off, and in 1946 Alcyon Bahia, Danilo Perestrello, Marialzira Perestrello, and Walderedo Oliveira traveled to Buenos Aires for analytic training. There they met Mário and Zaira Martins, who would become the pioneers in psychoanalysis in Porto Alegre.

Another group of psychiatrists who had remained in Rio contacted Ernest Jones, then president of the IPA, and once again requested that an analyst be suggested. Jones named Dr. Mark Burke, a member of the British Society, who had been James Strachey's patient. Burke arrived in Rio on February 2, 1948. A man with a great musical culture, and a violinist with a rare talent for languages, he would soon speak Portuguese correctly. Already in February he began to analyze several candidates. Thus, the Brazilian Institute of Psychoanalysis was started, and, wishing to increase its training activities, the Institute requested another name from Jones, which led to the arrival of the German analyst Dr. Werner Kemper at the end of 1948. He immediately began to analyze another group of physicians. Both Dr. Burke and Dr. Kemper started to teach seminars in 1949, and in Kemper's group, initially, Dr. Luiz Dahlheim (who later would become an important analyst) acted as interpreter and intermediary between the students and the teacher.

Their cooperation lasted only a short time, since, in April 1951, the Board of Directors of the Institute found out that Kemper had transformed his wife, Katrin, a graphologist, into a training analyst and sent her analytic training candidates. Since he would not agree to interrupt his wife's work, Kemper was dismissed from the Institute.

After this incident, there were now three groups in Rio: Burke's, Kemper's, and the Argentines (i.e., the four who had trained in Buenos Aires). The group that remained around Kemper would later become the current Sociedade Psicanalítica do Rio de Janeiro (Rio de Janeiro Psychoanalytic Society). The group that had begun training with Burke, after several difficulties caused by his return to Europe in 1953, joined by those who returned from Argentina and with the support of the São Paulo Society, formed the Sociedade Brasileira de Psicanálise do Rio de Janeiro (Brazilian Society of Psychoanalysis of Rio de Janeiro).

The information available on Mark Burke (1900–1975) is scarce and concerns mainly two points: his perfected and efficient technical capacity on the one hand, and his difficulty in adapting to a new environment on the other. Used to the silence in London, it appears to have been hard for him to stand the noisier atmosphere in Rio, especially when it interfered with his analytic work. At the end of 1953, Burke returned to London, interrupting the training of his group. They were obliged to find another way of finishing it.

As for Werner Kemper (1899–1975), there is sufficient but contradictory information, about which we will only mention what appears most relevant. Kemper trained at the Berlin Society and was the patient of Carl Müller-Braunschweig; he was supervised by, among others, Fenichel. Kemper was the son of a Protestant pastor and was described as a gentleman, friendly, sensible, and full of romantic idealism. During this turbulent period, and in the postwar era, there was a well-known opposition between Schultz-Henke, who developed a "neo-analytic" viewpoint (an amalgam of the theories of Adler, Jung, and Freud), and Müller-Braunschweig, who proposed to return to classical psychoanalysis as taught by Freud. Kemper had cordial relations with both, and after the war ended he tried, unsuccessfully, to smooth out their differences.

Among the information available, it should be mentioned that Kemper had worked with patients, had taught seminars, and had been a chief of the Polyclinic at the

Göring Institute in Berlin. There are reports that having been the analyst of Erna Göring, the wife of the Institute Director (who was a relative of Hitler's powerful minister), helped reduce the Nazi persecution of Polyclinic members. He was also the analyst of Reitmeister, the director of the outpatient department of the Polyclinic, who was arrested and executed by the Gestapo for his supposed connection to the Rote Kapelle (Red Orchestra) resistance group. Kemper said that he had unsuccessfully tried to obtain information through his patient Erna to save Reitmeister, and later replaced him as Institute director. There is information that his intervention enabled Edith Jacobson, who was in the resistance, to be released from prison and to get to the United States via Prague.

After the war ended, Kemper held an important position in attempts to reorganize German psychoanalysis, but at the same time he was facing personal and professional difficulties, not knowing what he would be able to do from then on. From a political standpoint he was in an uncomfortable position with the occupying forces: he appears to have been considered pro-American by the Russians because he participated in an international society run according to bourgeois models, and considered a communist by the Americans because he had worked at an institute with a strong social content and had socialist ideas. Jones suggested that Kemper went to Brazil for several possible reasons: he was compensating the effort of German analysts in having tried to keep up some psychoanalysis during the Nazi period, he was counterbalancing the presence of an English analyst with a German one in Rio, and, by living as a pioneer in a tropical world, he was trying to find idealism within himself again, at a time when he felt worn out and desolated because of the difficulties he had undergone and his lack of prospects in Germany.

In the episode that led to his dismissal from the Brazilian Institute of Psychoanalysis, Kemper showed an authoritarian attitude: he did not accept the arguments presented by his peers; he insisted instead on encouraging and protecting the work performed by his wife, who did not have any training and used her own methods, very different from the usually accepted ones. (For example, she had social contact with patients.) All the same, Kemper continued to work—he even went to prison for a few hours for supposedly practicing medicine illegally—and finished training several new analysts, as well as participating in structuring the first acknowledged Society of Rio de Janeiro. He returned to Germany in 1967 (Almeida Prado 1978; Fúchtner 2000; Perestrello 1987; M. Perestrello, personal communication, 2002; Victer 1991, 1996).

The early days of the institutionalization of psychoanalysis in Rio de Janeiro had the intense, dedicated participation of a growing number of young candidates who, on the one hand, learned from the pioneers despite the latter's limitations and, on the other, developed a great capacity to face complex situations and crises in associative life. Several members and candidates were very active at the university, both in the medical and psychology schools, as well as in the cultural life of the city.

In later years, during the 1970s, a crisis emerged when a candidate of the Rio de Janeiro Psychoanalytic Society Institute, Amilcar Lobo, was charged with taking part in torture in his capacity as an army doctor. His training analyst, Leão Cabernite, said he was not aware of these facts and attributed the charges to an anti-analytic movement. A long and painful ethical and institutional crisis developed in the next years, mainly after the end of the military dictatorship, and this was a consuming and challenging process throughout the 1990s, involving not only local institutions but also the IPA. After long and painful discussions, there was an acknowledgement of several mistakes and wrongdoings. The group of Society members that kept the subject under permanent questioning, the Grupo Pró-Ética (Pro-Ethics Group), constituted a new IPA institution in the city, the Psychoanalytical Association of the State of Rio de Janeiro—Rio IV.

The current state of psychoanalysis linked to the IPA in that city shows the presence of four solid institutions, all of them training new analysts according to technical and ethical standards, and in full dialogue with the culture. In addition to the already mentioned societies, there is the Rio III Psychoanalytic Group (constituted by former members of the Brazilian Society of Rio de Janeiro). There are two analytic journals, which publish papers from members of the societies, as well as relevant contributions that deal with the interface with the scientific and intellectual milieu: *Trieb*, published by the Brazilian Society of Rio, and *Psicanalítica*, published by the Rio Society.

The international conference "Identifying Marks of Psychoanalysis in Latin America," sponsored by the *International Journal of Psychoanalysis*, was held in Rio de Janeiro in 2004. The IPA's 44th International Psychoanalytical Congress will be held for the first time in Brazil in 2005, in Rio, where the first Brazilian (and second Latin American) elected to preside over the IPA, Cláudio Eizirik, from Porto Alegre, will take office.

Psychoanalysis in Porto Alegre

The third main psychoanalytic center in Brazil is Porto Alegre, capital of the southernmost state of the country. Psychoanalytic ideas appeared there in the 1920s and developed in the following decades, through lectures and translations of Freud's books made by psychiatrists and professors of the medical school.

After his analytic training in Buenos Aires, where he was analyzed by Angel Garma, Mario Alvarez Martins went back to Porto Alegre in 1947, with his wife, Zaira Martins, a child analyst, beginning the analytic movement in that state. Mainly stimulated by their Argentinean colleagues, Mario Martins, Cyro Martins, José Lemmertz (both of the latter also trained in Buenos Aires), and Celestino Prunes (who trained in Rio, with Kemper) structured the Porto Alegre Psychoanalytic Society (SPPA), which was recognized by the IPA in 1963. Since its origin, the SPPA has been closely connected with psychiatry, Federal University of Rio Grande do Sul, and the cultural milieu. Many of its members and candidates were and still are members of departments of psychiatry in the main medical schools of the city. At the same time, one of the pioneers, Cyro Martins, one of the best known writers of the state, was very active in the diffusion of psychoanalysis in the cultural milieu. The SSPA, in its development, shows a blend of the activities and personal trends of Mario and Cyro Martins (who were not relatives): the former turned inward, developing a continuous, persistent, and patient work of training candidates, teaching and facing internal tensions; the latter performed his analytic function but, through his many books and lectures, also opened new channels and stimulated young people to join in and become interested in psychoanalysis.

These two trends must be stressed: the internal work aiming at a training with high standards, and the close links with psychiatry and a strong influence in the intellectual area. Possibly connected with the first trend, only in the late 1980s were psychologists accepted for training, which eventually corrected a distortion that had produced criticisms and the search for other training institutions. In the ensuing decades, members of the SPPA were also very active in developing group analytic psychotherapy, a trend that decreased in the 1990s. At the same time, members of the Society were extremely active in the development of psychoanalytic psychotherapy, and today analysts and candidates are teaching it at universities. Since 1993 the SPPA has had its own quarterly journal, *Revista de Psicanálise da SPPA*. The FEPAL Congress of 2000 was held in the nearby city of Gramado, organized by members of the SPPA.

A new study group was established in Porto Alegre in 1992, becoming a component organization of the IPA in 2001, as Sociedade Brasileira de Psicanálise de Porto Alegre. Its founding members were former members of the SPPA and colleagues who had recently trained in Argentina and were back in Porto Alegre. In spite of inevitable initial tensions, the main current trend is toward a collaborative effort for the sake of developing psychoanalysis. There is room for both institutions in the city, as well as for other training centers.

Overview of Contemporary Psychoanalysis in Brazil

As previously mentioned, there are currently psychoanalytic societies recognized by the IPA in Recife, Brasília, and Pelotas, and study groups in Ribeirão Preto, Campo Grande, and Rio de Janeiro, as well as nuclei in several other cities, each under the sponsorship of one of the official societies.

In terms of analytic ideas, Freud is the most important author, as is borne out by the objective evaluation of papers and their references in the main Brazilian journals. Melanie Klein was very influential in São Paulo, Porto Alegre, and Rio de Janeiro—an influence that decreased in the last decade. Bion is one of the most studied authors, mainly in São Paulo (where his work shaped the analytic thinking of its membership), as well as in Porto Alegre. In Recife, French psychoanalysis is a strong influence, following the training of the city's pioneer, José Lins de Almeida, and other colleagues in Paris.

In recent years, there has been a growing tendency to study authors from different traditions, such as the British post-Kleinians (Segal, Betty Joseph, Steiner), contemporary Freudians (Sandler, Fonagy), and independents (Winnicott). The French tradition is also increasingly known, mainly through the work of Lacan, Green, Laplanche, Chasseguet-Smirgel, and MacDougall. In spite of a relatively lower interest in ego and self psychology, some American authors, such as Kernberg and Wallerstein, are influential. Since the beginning of the analytic movement in Brazil, as shown previously, there were close ties with Argentina and the work of its authors, mainly Racker, Liberman, and the Barangers. Currently, influential authors from Argentina are Horácio Etchegoyen, Norberto Marucco, and Isidoro Berenstein.

Brazilian psychoanalysis, as well as Brazilian culture, presents a blend of traditions and a specific local development. Is there a Brazilian psychoanalytic thinking? This question was the subject of several debates in the past few years, and the current scenario shows that several Brazilian analysts are producing a growing mix of theoretical and clinical contributions to the field—among them Fábio Herrmann, with his theory of the analytic fields; Renato Mezan, with his studies on the cultural impact of psychoanalysis; and Elias Rocha Barros, with his contributions to analytic technique.

In all analytic institutions there is a very active scientific life and a growing interface with the surrounding culture. More recently, the influence of psychoanalysis in medicine and psychiatry decreased, but there are several active university centers, where research and doctoral studies in psychoanalysis attract many students. The delay, in some societies, to allow psychologists to train as analysts was an unfortunate policy that led many talented colleagues to look for their training elsewhere.

The main challenges currently faced by psychoanalysis in Brazil are: to keep its relevance as an effective treatment; to maintain high standards of training, in spite of economic difficulties; to find a proper way of regulating it as a profession; to expand its presence in the university and the culture; and to make Brazilian theoretical and clinical production better known abroad (Eizirik 2002).

Psychoanalysis in Other Latin American Countries

We are going to present a very brief account of the development of psychoanalysis in other countries of the region, with the caveat that each of these histories, because of its richness and importance, deserves more attention than is permitted within the scope of a textbook chapter.

Mexico

In Mexico, a group of psychiatrists began to meet in the 1940s (in Mexico City) to study Freud's works and then founded the Sigmund Freud Study Group. Later, they trained in Buenos Aires at the Argentine Psychoanalytic Association, at Columbia University, in Paris, and at The Menninger Clinic. When they returned to Mexico, they were joined by others to constitute the Mexican Study Group of Psychoanalytic Studies, under the sponsorship of the Argentine Psychoanalytic Association. In 1957, the IPA recognized the Mexican Psychoanalytic Association (APM) as a component organization (J. Vives and T. Lartigue, personal communication, 2004).

In its early days, the APM accepted only psychiatrists as candidates (with the exception of the biologist Luis Feder and the chemist Estela Remus), a situation that led many psychologists to create their own training institution. Later, the APM opened access to doctors in psychology and professionals with training in analytic psychotherapy. In the 1980s, the APM created a graduate center for training in analytic psychotherapy; today it has a doctoral program in psychotherapy and two master of science programs (one on analytic psychotherapy and the other on child and adolescent psychotherapy). Although in the first days members of the APM were very active in several universities, this presence decreased in the following decades, but it was again stronger in the past decade. The first Mexican congress was held in Cuernavaca, in 1961, and since then it has been held each year in a different city

of the country. The journal of APM, *Cuadernos de Psicoanálisis*, has been published twice a year since 1965. There is now a program of education at a distance, linking the APM with several groups in development in different cities of Mexico.

Another society—the Monterrey Psychoanalytic Society (ARPAC)—was formed in Monterrey by psychiatrists trained at APM and was recognized by the IPA in 1993. It is a young and very active society, with strong university and community links, offering a graduate program in psychoanalysis. The ARPAC hosted the FEPAL congress of 1996 (Vives and Lartigue 2004).

Venezuela

The analytic movement in Venezuela began formally in 1965, when the first study group was constituted, with five members: Drs. Hernán Quijada (trained in Paris), Jaime Araújo and Antonio Garcia (both trained in Santiago de Chile), Guillermo Teruel (trained in London), and Manuel Kizer (trained in Buenos Aires). In 1971, with the inclusion of other colleagues, the Venezuelan Psychoanalytic Association (ASOVEP) was recognized by the IPA. Training of candidates began in 1969, and an intensive program of visits by distinguished analysts from the three IPA regions was developed. In 1975 a crisis emerged in the association that can be attributed to analytic intolerance among colleagues. This crisis led to an intervention by the IPA and required the help of members of the Colombian Society, who gave seminars and supervisions. There was a reconciliation in 1977.

A new crisis began in 1989, caused by disagreements concerning criteria of selection, promotion of members and candidates, and administration of the institute and the association. A group of members decided to create the Study Group of Caracas, which was recognized by the IPA as a component society in 1993, as the Psychoanalytic Society of Caracas.

Nowadays, both the Venezuelan Psychoanalytic Association and the Psychoanalytic Society of Caracas develop their training programs, and the main theoretical influences are Freud, Klein, the post-Freudians, the post-Kleinians, and members of the French and the American schools. There are also two other active training institutions: the Caracas School of the Freudian Field (where Lacan gave his last seminar, in 1980), with a Lacanian orientation, and the Jungian School of Psychoanalysis. All groups have strong ties with universities, hospitals, and graduate programs. Sometimes there are joint activities among them. Despite difficult social and economic conditions in Venezuela in the last few years, which affected the possibilities of access to analytic treatment and training, there is an acceptable amount of clinical work and candidates in training, as well as scientific programs in all institutions (R. Lander, personal communication, 2004).

Uruguay

The origins of psychoanalysis in Uruguay lie in the 1940s, while its development can be divided into two periods: the first runs from 1943 to 1961 and can be called the prehistory of the Uruguayan Psychoanalytic Association (APU), and the second extends to the present day. In the first period, Dr. Valentín Pérez Pastorini, a psychiatrist and professor at the medical school, had analysis with Angel Garma in Buenos Aires and influenced many young colleagues to study Freudian ideas. After his death, two of his patients, Drs. Rodolfo Agorio and Gilberto Koolhaas, took the lead, and a growing number of people interested in psychoanalysis tended to congregate around them. Several attempts were made to invite a training analyst, a condition demanded by the IPA for accepting the beginning of official activities in Uruguay. Hanna Segal spent a month in Montevideo in 1952, working with the group and considering the possibility of emigration, but she eventually abandoned the idea. Finally, in 1954, Willy and Madeleine Baranger left Argentina, settled in Uruguay, and began their training activities. The act of foundation was signed in 1955 by 11 analysts. In 1957 the IPA, on the recommendation of the Argentine Psychoanalytic Institute, recognized the Uruguayan Study Group, and in 1961 the IPA recognized the Uruguayan Psychoanalytic Association as a component organization (Garbarino et al. 1995).

In the following decades, the APU grew, both in numbers of members and candidates and in the quality of its training and continuous theoretical and clinical contributions to the analytic literature. The system of training was restructured and became more flexible in the 1970s; the initial Kleinian influence decreased as Lacan and other French authors were progressively included, leading to the current pluralistic atmosphere. The APU faced the loss of members who emigrated during the military dictatorship, and in recent years Uruguay has faced difficult economic and social problems that have affected both training and analytic practice. In spite of this, APU keeps a continuous scientific program, maintains close links with the cultural milieu, and ensures regular publication of its journal, *Revista Uruguaya de Psicoanálisis* (which first appeared in 1956). A FEPAL congress was held in Montevideo in 2002. A major recent achievement was the recognition by the Uruguayan government of analytic training in the APU as a master's degree. As for the quality of its members' work, it can be illustrated by a study on controversies in psychoanalysis (Bernardi 2002). Taking as example the debates held in Buenos Aires and Montevideo during the 1970s, when the dominant Kleinian ideas came into contact with Lacanian thought, Bernardi, after a careful examination of different examples of argumentative discourses, showed that the major difficulties encountered did not hinge on characteristics pertaining to psychoanalytic theories (i.e., the lack of commensurability between them), but on the defensive strategies aimed at keeping each theory's premises safe from the opposing party's arguments.

Chile

One of the first analysts with a complete training to arrive in Latin America, Allende Navarro (who had trained in Switzerland), was a pioneer of psychoanalysis in Chile; he began to analyze colleagues who would later become analysts. In 1934, Ignácio Matte Blanco returned to Santiago, after concluding his training at the British Society. The group of analysts that formed around these pioneers founded the Center of Psychoanalytic Studies, in 1946. In 1949, the IPA officially recognized the Chilean Psychoanalytic Association. Matte Blanco was a central figure in the development of psychoanalysis in Chile. He was a full professor in the Department of Psychiatry at the University of Chile Medical School, and master of a body of knowledge that integrated, at a high level, his abilities as an analyst, a psychiatrist, and a university professor. The greater part of the struggle to overcome the difficulties created by environmental influences fell on his shoulders; he was a stimulating leader of several generations of Chilean analysts, at the same time pursuing the objective of integrating psychoanalysis with psychiatry. In 1966, Matte Blanco left Chile and moved to Rome, to take up permanent residence in Italy and to continue to develop his theoretical contributions to psychoanalysis.

The Chilean Psychoanalytic Association continued to grow, and several of its members moved in the 1960s to other countries: Otto Kernberg went to the United States, where he would become one of the leading international analytic authors and the president of the IPA (from 1995 to 1999); Paulina Kernberg, a leading author in child analysis, also went to the United States; Ruth Riesemberg went to England, where she is a respected member of the Kleinian group; Hernán Davanzo took an important part in the development of psychoanalysis in Ribeirão Preto, Brazil; and Ramón Ganzarain went to The Menninger Clinic in Topeka (Arrué 1995; Cesio 2000).

In spite of tensions at various levels, including internal ones and opposition in the University setting, as well as the military dictatorship, psychoanalysis developed in the last decades, and the Chilean Association is now a solid and growing institution, with its own journal and a good number of candidates. Many of its members have important positions at the university and a regular program of interface with the culture. The IPA Congress was held in Santiago in 1999.

Peru

Peru was the first country in the Spanish-speaking world in which psychoanalysis was introduced. This happened, in 1915, through the correspondence between Freud and Honorio Delgado, enabling the latter to be the first representative of psychoanalysis in Latin America (Engelbrecht and Rey de Castro 1995). Delgado was a psychiatrist and the leading figure of the period between 1915 and the mid-1930s. Despite initial interest in psychoanalysis and several articles published in newspapers about it, Delgado eventually turned away from the field. In the 1930s, psychoanalysis attracted greater attention again, through the influence of the psychiatrist Carlos Alberto Seguin, who had undergone analysis in New York and, in spite of not concluding a full training program, had the main achievement of introducing a counter-model to traditional psychiatry as then represented by Delgado. The four founding members of the Peruvian Study Group and also some other of its future members were psychiatrists of the Seguin school before they turned to psychoanalysis.

In the late 1960s, the history of psychoanalysis in Peru entered its institutionalization phase. Saul Peña, Carlos Crisanto, and Max Hernández, all of whom had been trained in London, have worked in Lima since 1969, 1972, and 1974, respectively. Together with members of the second generation they founded the Peruvian Psychoanalytic Society, recognized by the IPA as a component society in 1987. From then on, contributions by Peruvian authors appeared at international congresses and national psychiatric and psychotherapeutic meetings, and in publications. At the same time, a growing dialogue between psychoanalysis and the human sciences developed. Conferences were systematically organized by the Peruvian Society in order to discuss several interdisciplinary matters, among them Peruvian myths.

A group of analysts has been collaborating for years with an anthropologist and a historian in the Seminário Interdisciplinario de Estudios Andinos (SIDEA), investigating and interpreting ancient Peruvian myths and traditions. The studies of Max Hernandez on the psychobiography of the Inca Garcilaso de la Vega were published and presented in several international events. Two major international conferences were organized by SIDEA, "At the Threshold of the Millennium" (1999) and "At the End of the Battle" (2001), with an enormous participation of analysts and members of the cultural and scientific communities. There is an ongoing training program at the society, the already mentioned interface with the culture, and

a presence in the analytic international community of several members of the Peruvian Psychoanalytic Society (Engelbrecht and Rey de Castro 1995; Lemlij 2002).

Colombia

In Colombia, Freud's works were read by a select group of intellectuals soon after their appearance. Only after they were translated into Spanish by Luis Lopez-Ballesteros during the years 1922 and 1934 and published nearly simultaneously with the originals in German did they become more known in Colombia. One of the Colombian intellectuals influenced by Freud's ideas was the medical student José Francisco Socarrás, who would play a leading role in the future development of psychoanalysis in his country. In 1929 he introduced the teaching of analytic ideas in the School of Psychology; in 1930 he wrote his thesis on the fundamental principles of psychoanalysis. He then went to Paris, where he trained and returned to Bogotá in 1950. Arturo Lizarazo did his training in Chile; he went back to Colombia in 1948 and became the first to start the practice of psychoanalysis in that country (Villarrel 1995).

The two pioneers worked together and faced great resistance, even being attacked by some of the most well-known psychiatrists and by some priests as well. They were among the founding members of the Colombian Study Group, which was accepted as such by the IPA in 1957. Carlos Plata Mujica returned from his training in Buenos Aires in 1958 and has been a leading figure in Colombian psychoanalysis ever since. In 1961, the Colombian Psychoanalytic Society was recognized by the IPA as a component organization. In 1962, 10 analysts left the Colombian Society and founded the Colombian Psychoanalytic Association. In spite of the tensions, resignations, and splits, which led to the formation of two other analytic groups linked to the IPA in Colombia, there is a continuous growth and presence of Colombian analysts in the international scene.

Conclusion

What cruel, obscure instinct pushes us through time and through places that are defended? This question, posed by the Brazilian poet Carlos Drummond de Andrade (1963), apparently is not difficult for a psychoanalyst to answer. Even so, there are several possibilities, and within them we perform our daily clinical work. The great difficulties we encounter in giving some sense to a life "stepping on books and letters during pathetic trips through lost kingdoms" may, however, be faced using the psychoanalytic method that we work hard to apply. When we wish to cast a retrospective gaze on complex social situations, however, without having the instruments of history available as a specific branch of knowledge, these difficulties appear impossible to overcome. And yet, just as we are fascinated by the joint trips we take with each of our patients, with whom we "walk a long distance," the search for some meaning for our situation as psychoanalysts belonging to an institution within its historical perspective ultimately becomes a task not to be refused. In this way, we can understand our origins, how we became what we are, and the reasons why our institutions followed their particular course over time.

The fragmentary, incomplete data carved out by our subjectivity from among the mass of information available may throw no more than a pallid light on the conditions in which some analysts became characters in the progressive implementation of psychoanalysis in Latin America.

Among its many leading figures, major contributions to psychoanalytic thinking were made by Angel Garma (in his studies of dream phenomena, psychosomatic conditions, and analytic process), Heinrich Racker (on countertransference, in its meanings, uses, and presentations, and as an instrument for understanding the patient's mind), David Liberman (on the analytic dialogue and complementarity in the styles of analyst-patient communication), Ignácio Matte Blanco (on his studies of the different logic of conscious and unconscious phenomena, with the latter operating in terms of propositive functions), and Willy and Madeleine Baranger (on the dynamic analytic field that is established in each analysis, with its specific bipersonal unconscious fantasy).

One important feature in all accounts is the relation of the psychoanalytic movement in each country with its surrounding culture and the way they influenced each other. Maybe the experience of immigration described in this chapter, and the blend of social and economic difficulties with an impetus for growing and developing new fields, could help to explain the specific features of this region.

In briefly reviewing aspects of a history that mixes grandeur and misery, and achievements and failures, and in describing what existed prior to the introduction of psychoanalysis and how the field developed, we hope to have shared with our readers the experience of trying to understand something of the feelings and thoughts of those pioneers who launched the multiple foundations of the flourishing Latin American psychoanalytic movement of today.

References

Almeida Prado MP: Subsídos à história da Sociedade Brasileira de Psicanálise do Rio de Janeiro. Revista Brasileira de Psicanálise 12:139–147, 1978

Andrade CD: Antologia Poética. Rio de Janeiro, Brazil, Editora do Autor, 1963

Argentine Psychoanalytic Association: La Historia del Psicoanálisis en la Argentina. Buenos Aires, Argentine Psychoanalytic Association, 1982

Argentine Psychoanalytic Association, Publications Committee: 60 Años de Psicoanálisis en Argentina. Buenos Aires, Grupo Editorial Lumen, 2002

Arrué O: Chile, in Psychoanalysis International: A Guide to Psychoanalysis Throughout the World, Vol 2: America, Asia, Australia, Further European Countries. Edited by Kutter P. Stuttgart, Germany, Frommann-Holzboog, 1995, pp 74–93

Bernardi R: The need for true controversies in psychoanalysis. Int J Psychoanal 83:851–873, 2002

Cesio F: La Gesta Psicoanalítica en América Latina. Buenos Ares, Editorial La Peste, 2000

Eizirik CL: Emigration of European analysts to Brazil. Presentation at the Plenary Session the Ninth International Meeting of the International Association for the History of Psychoanalysis, Barcelona, Spain, July 25, 2002

Engelbrecht H, Rey de Castro A: Peru, Psychoanalysis International: A Guide to Psychoanalysis Throughout the World, Vol 2: America, Asia, Australia, further European countries. Edited by Kutter P. Stuttgart-Bad Cannstatt, Germany, Frommann-Holzboog, 1995, pp 160–173

Füchtner H: O caso Werner Kemper. Pulsional Revista de Psicanálise 138:49–89, 2000

Garbarino MF, Maggide Macedo I, Newe JC: Uruguay, in Psychoanalysis International: A Guide to Psychoanalysis Throughout the World, Vol 2: America, Asia, Australia, further European countries. Edited by Kutter P. Stuttgart-Bad Cannstatt, Germany, Frommann-Holzboog, 1995, pp 174–185

Langer M, del Palacio J, Guinsberg E: Memoria, Historia y Diálogo Psicoanalítico. Mexico City, Folios Ediciones, 1982

Lemlij M: At the end of the battle, in Psychoanalysis International: A Guide to Psychoanalysis Throughout the World, Vol 2: America, Asia, Australia, further European countries. Edited by Kutter P. Stuttgart-Bad Cannstatt, Germany, Frommann-Holzboog, 1995, pp 51–53

Lobo R: As mudanças e históricas a chegada da psicanálise ao Brasil, in Álbum de Família: Imagens, Fontes, e Idéias da Psicanálise em São Paulo. Edited by Nosek L, Montagna P, et al. São Paulo, Brazil, Casa do Psicólogo, 1994, pp 49–55

Luz CL: A psicanálise em São Paulo—Jubileu de Prata: homenagem a Durval Marcondes e Adelheid Koch. Revista Brasileira de Psicanálise 10:507–509, 1976

Nosek L: São Paulo Psychoanalytic Society, in The Actual Crisis of Psychoanalysis: Challenges and Perspectives. Report of the IPA House of Delegates Committee, 1996, pp 28–30

Perestrello M: Históire da Sociedade Brasileira de Psianálise do Rio de Janeiro: Suas Origens e Fundaçao. Rio de Janeiro, Ed. Imago, 1987

Sagawa RY: A história da sociedade Brasileira de psicanálise de São Paulo, in Álbum de Família: Imagens, Fontes, e Idéias da Psicanálise em São Paulo. Edited by Nosek L, Montagna P, et al. São Paulo, Brazil, Casa do Psicólogo, 1994, pp 15–28

Sagawa RY: A Construção Local da Psicanálise. Marília, Brazil, Editora Interior/Psicanálise, 2001

Sister BM, Taffarel M: Isaias Melsohn: a Psicanálise e a Vida— Setenta Anos de Histórias Paulistanas e a Formação de um Pensamento Renovador na Psicanálise. São Paulo, Brazil, Ed. Escuta, 1996

Victer R: Elementos para uma compreensão da pré-história da SPRJ. Revista de Psicanálise do Rio de Janeiro 1:77–83, 1991

Victer R: Na busca das correntes históricas da SPRJ. Boletim Científico da Sociedade Psicanalítica do Rio de Janeiro 17: 125–133, 1996

Villarreal I, Colombia, Psychoanalysis International: A Guide to Psychoanalysis Throughout the World, Vol 2: America, Asia, Australia, Further European Countries. Edited by Kutter P. Stuttgart-Bad Cannstatt, Germany, Frommann-Holzboog, 1995, pp 103–115

Vollmer FG: Brazil, in Psychoanalysis International: A Guide to Psychoanalysis Throughout the World, Vol 2: America, Asia, Australia, further European countries. Edited by Kutter P. Stuttgart-Bad Cannstatt, Germany, Frommann-Holzboog, 1995, pp 40–54

Wender L, Torres D, Vidal I: Argentina, in Psychoanalysis International: A Guide to Psychoanalysis Throughout the World, Vol 2: America, Asia, Australia, further European countries. Edited by Kutter P. Stuttgart-Bad Cannstatt, Germany, Fromman-Holzboog, 1995, pp 1–26

PART VI

Psychoanalysis and Related Disciplines

SECTION EDITOR: MORRIS EAGLE, M.D.

29

Freud and His Uses of Interdisciplinary Sources

JOHN KERR

IN CONSIDERING THE INTRIGUING possibilities of interdisciplinary studies in relation to psychoanalysis, one does well to pause at the outset to take in some cautionary considerations derived from the history of the field. What one discovers thereby is that psychoanalysis, though putatively anchored in the privacy of the clinical setting, has long drawn its interpretive hypotheses from a diverse variety of sister disciplines. In a manner of speaking, psychoanalysis is, and has always been, an interdisciplinary field (see Esman 1998; Kitcher 1992). That said, it has also been the case that for most of its history, psychoanalysis has not properly observed this fact about itself, assuming to the contrary that its findings were entirely of its own creation and, indeed, that they rather trumped the findings of other fields. With both of these beliefs having held back progress for many decades, it is the purpose of this brief introduction to draw attention to them so that they may be all the more readily discarded in favor of a more open, more informed, and more profitable outlook as analysts envision collaboration with scholars from other disciplines.

Freud and the Beginnings of Applied Analysis

Interdisciplinary studies in psychoanalysis have a surprisingly long history. Though it is not usually noted, the fact is that the first official publication of the fledgling psychoanalytic movement was not a journal but a monograph series under Freud's editorship, *Papers in Applied Psychology*, devoted to what has come to be called "applied analysis." The first four titles give some idea of the scope, not to say ambitiousness, of the series: Freud's own *Delusions and Dreams in Jensen's* Gradiva, Franz Riklin's *Wish Fulfillment and Symbolism in Fairy Tales*, Karl Abraham's *Dreams and Myth*, and Otto Rank's *Myth of the Birth of the Hero*. Thus did two psychiatrists and a university student join a neurologist in crafting psychoanalytic reinterpretations of various mythic and literary motifs.

However, these early efforts, like those that followed in Freud's monograph series, were not truly interdisciplinary in a modern sense. Most analysts who dip into these early volumes will be struck by how jejune the analytic interpretations now seem—an understandable failing, given how young the whole field was. A more penetrating reading of the monographs reveals something else, moreover (something that drew harsh criticism at the time), namely, that although their authors are essentially amateurs vis-à-vis the intellectual territory they are exploring, the studies announce their conclusions with great fervor and conviction. It is as though the authors are in possession of a great truth, before which all other truths are secondary and inconsequential.

The source of this attitude is easy to trace; it stems directly from Freud himself. A single historical anecdote will do here. On November 30, 1911, Freud took it upon himself to write to Carl Jung, then president of the International Psychoanalytic Association, to voice his displeasure over a presentation the night before at the Vienna Psychoanalytic Society. The presentation had been made by one of Jung's protégées, Sabina Spielrein, so it was not inappropriate for Freud to complain to the mentor:

> What troubles me most is that Fraulein Spielrein wants to subordinate the psychological material to biological considerations; this dependency is no more acceptable than a dependency on philosophy, physiology, or brain anatomy. ψ-A *fara da se*. (quoted in McGuire 1974, pp. 468–469)

The ψ-A (the Greek Psi-Alpha) was, of course, shorthand for Psychoanalysis. The Italian phrase *fara da se* means "goes by itself." Psychoanalysis goes by itself.

The nature of Freud's assertion was not lost on Jung, nor would it have been lost on any of Freud's colleagues at the time. From the very first published mentions (Freud 1896c/1962, p. 151; 1896b/1962, pp. 162, 164; 1896a/1962, pp. 193, 220–22) of the exact term "psychoanalysis," Freud had consistently taken the stance that his method of therapy simultaneously constituted a method of investigation, and that this method of investigation had its own rules and procedures and was capable of generating its own robust and original findings. It had, perhaps, been a source of embarrassment that the first occasion for these announcements was the promulgation of the ill-fated "seduction theory," as it is now called. That potentially instructive misstep aside, Freud had continued to make the same claim in succeeding works. Thus, the theory presented in 1905 in *Three Essays on the Theory of Sexuality*, to take the most pertinent example, was said to be the fruit of "the ever-increasing number of psycho-analyses of hysterical and other neurotic patients which I have carried out during the last 10 years" (1905/1953, p. 163). In subsequent editions, Freud simply increased the number of years as appropriate until the number reached "25" in the fourth edition (Freud 1905/1953, p. 163, n. 2), after which he let it stand.

Logicians and methodologists, and others as well, have been less than kind in recent decades to Freud's claims about the sturdiness of his procedure as a research method, though, in truth, they have added little to what his critics had to say back at the outset. We may leave it, with Rubovits-Seitz (1998), that there are times when an interpretation of unconscious motivations may be warranted in the clinical setting, though our reasoning will necessarily be based on "post-positivist" evidentiary standards. Meanwhile, historians of science have been even less kind to Freud's various claims for originality. In fact, as is now clear beyond the pos-

sibility of further disputation, virtually all of Freud's psychoanalytic "discoveries" were available to him from other sources. Put in other words, Freud himself did not do psychoanalysis as a way of discovering things. At best, he tried out hypotheses he had gleaned extraclinically to see how they would fly in the consulting room, this while otherwise welding them into a distinctive overarching synthesis.

Yet, the nature of Freud's claims was quite otherwise. And the "climate of opinion," to use Auden's famous phrase, that grew up around him, both within psychoanalysis and without, was shaped by the claims far more than by the actuality. It is important to be clear about this as we approach the general topic of how psychoanalysts may collaborate with scholars and practitioners in other disciplines, because the claims have been a source of great mischief for most of the preceding century.

Development of Applied Analysis: Pitfalls and Potential

To the extent that psychoanalysts were under the impression that their interpretive rubrics had been empirically demonstrated by the practice of clinical psychoanalysis, they felt free to make very bold assertions as to the fundamental nature of human nature, including, most pointedly, the human unconscious. Possession of such a grand warrant did not foster modesty vis-à-vis other disciplines.

A few examples may suffice here. Bruno Bettelheim enjoyed a splendid career as a psychiatrist-educator with psychoanalytic credentials (now known to be suspect; see Pollak 1997). In the field of applied analysis, he had few equals, that is, if we are to judge by book sales to the general public. His all-time bestseller, *Freud and Man's Soul* (1982), is no more than a nicely turned rhetorical attack on Strachey's translation. It is indeed pertinent to know that behind what Strachey sometimes translates as "mental apparatus" is the German word *seele*, which is much better rendered as "psyche" or "soul." Also worth reminding ourselves is that Freud wrote with the vividness of ordinary speech when he theorized about relations of the "I" and the "it." "Ego" and "id" are pseudo-technical terms. But it is *not* fair to go on from such observations to assert, as Bettelheim does, that Freud is above all a great humanist and intuitive philosopher of the soul, and not the scientist-psychologist of Strachey's translation. Freud certainly thought of himself as a scientist—when it came time to collect his award, he was disappointed that the Goethe Prize for Literature, which he won, was not the Nobel Prize for Medicine, which he did not. And Freud's prose is embedded in the rhetoric of science, pace Bettelheim. There is no other way to read it, in any language.

Why would Bettelheim bother with such a claim, and why would it go largely undisputed by his colleagues? In part, Bettelheim is simply uninformed as to the revolution in modern historical studies of the origins of psychoanalysis. But, in another sense, he is even more simply an heir to a tradition that grew up in the wake of the discovery, and publication, of the famous "Project for a Scientific Psychology." The disconcerting aspect of the Project at the time of its publication was that it was clearly a neurological document, pure and simple, and yet it was equally clearly the basis for the famous Chapter 7 of *The Interpretation of Dreams*. (Should we take time out here to remind ourselves that in German the title of this book is *Traumdeutung*, which in the German language invoked and resonated with *Sterndeutung*, the word for "astrology"? Perhaps, but this doesn't save the intellectual origins of the seventh chapter.) To counteract the possibility that people would get the correct impression that in fact the famous Chapter 7 was recooked neurological speculation, albeit of a very high order for the time, a new legend was promptly promulgated that after writing the Project, or at the turn of the century at the latest, Freud turned away from neurology as a way of anchoring his theory and turned instead toward something identified vaguely as "pure psychology." This left hanging what "pure psychology" might be worth, as Holt (1989) later asked pointedly, but it otherwise kept the claims intact at a time when the field was not ready for a thoroughgoing look at its own history. Just how tenacious this legend was can be judged by the fact that 9 years after Henri Ellenberger's massive *Discovery of the Unconscious* (1970) appeared, and a new look at the history of the field had inescapably begun, a thoroughly estimable and historically informed survey of Freud's early theorizing by Kenneth Levin (1979) appeared that nonetheless saw fit to repeat the turn-to-pure-psychology thesis gratuitously in its epilogue. Unfortunately for Levin, his book appeared more or less simultaneously with Frank Sulloway's *Freud, Biologist of the Mind* (1979), which pointedly demolished the "pure psychology" legend once and for all. Not neurology but evolutionary biology, including some manifestly fallacious doctrines then current, guided the further evolution of Freud's theorizing after 1900.

Freud as biologist manqué being no more acceptable to analytic practitioners than Freud as neurologist manqué, Bettelheim found a new rhetorical niche for the hero: he could be a great humanist with a bad translator. Other Bettelheim works are more specific in their theses and thus open to more specific rejoinder. Here let me single out *The Uses of Enchantment*, which postulates, among other things, that fairy tales such as the frog prince are emblematic of a specifically feminine fear of masculine sexuality. As it happens, the identical argument had been made as long ago as 1908 in German by Franz Riklin in his monograph *Wish Fulfillment and Symbolism in Fairy Tales*, which had appeared as the second number of Freud's monograph series *Papers on Applied Psychology*. Anyone who checks will see that for methodological warrant, Riklin relied on the assertion that the meaning of the fairy tale was clear "to the initiated" (see Kerr 1993), which warrant is as good as any Bettelheim can claim. But more to the point, Bettelheim is simply off-base with his gender specification. For every frog prince there is also a frog princess, or at least some other fairy tale in which the animal-hero is specifically an animal-heroine, as folklorist Barbara Fass Leavy (1994) has pointed out.

This fact, to be sure, is something only known to folklorists; moreover, among folklorists it is only the beginning of wisdom. For there are indeed gender differences to be observed in stories of this kind in the folk literature, as Leavy (personal communication, July 1903) further notes, but they are more subtle—and analytically interesting. For example, though the female human figure in such stories scarcely ever has difficulty bringing herself to kiss the frog, given the promissory note that this will all work out in princely fashion, in a majority of the gender-reversed stories the male human figure simply cannot bring himself to go through with it (usually he fails on the third and crucial try), with the result that the frog-princess remains enchanted. Then, too, frog-princes ordinarily do very well after their transformation, readily adapting themselves to the world of men, whereas the adventures and difficulties of the frog princess are typically only just beginning after her transformation. And so forth.

It would seem that Bettelheim's fault in the aforementioned works lies in straying beyond the boundaries of his own disciplinary expertise, such as it may have been. But what then to make of a work such as Peter Gay's (1998) biography of Freud, which in important places sees fit to rely on the judgments of psychoanalysts while neglecting the judgments of many of Gay's fellow historians? Gay is, or was, Sterling Professor of History at Yale. Nothing wrong with those credentials. Yet the book is open to serious objection on historical grounds. At bottom, Gay is guilty of accepting at face value the heroic significance of Freud's self-analysis and, having thus committed himself to a "Great Man" approach to his topic, of neglecting all the ways in which contemporary developments were in fact shaping the origins and further development of the field—and for this he has been scored by a diverse array of historians and clinicians (Breger 2000; Kerr 2003; McGrath 1992; Swales 1988). Gay's Freud, like Bettelheim's, went by himself.

While we are on the subject of Gay (1975), we should take in his assertions about Mondrian , which can serve as our final example of the pitfalls of applied analysis, namely, that the artist avoided figurative painting out of anxiety in the face of the sensual world. This characterization is reminiscent of, though a good deal less tendentious than, Phyllis Greenacre's earlier contention that the artist was motivated more specifically by primal scene anxiety. The pair of contentions has been examined by the psychoanalyst and psychiatrist Aron Esman (1994), who points out several salient facts neglected by Gay, Greenacre, and other psychoanalytic commentators. For most of his early career, Mondrian did in fact paint figuratively—and, after 1915, under the influence of the Fauvists, with pure colors, if you want to know. Moreover, when he wasn't painting landscapes, which in the Dutch tradition did not typically include human figures, he "earned his living in part by executing glorious, meticulous, but richly sensuous watercolors of chrysanthemums and amaryllis flowers" (Esman 1994, p. 335). As for his alleged aversion to the human body, it is worth noting that apart from his art, he had a passion for the Charleston and developed into a fan of Fred Astaire. All of which still leaves hanging how to approach his much more famous, and indeed defining, later canvasses, such as Victory Boogie Woogie, with their dazzling arrays of geometric forms rendered in pure color. But the secret of those canvasses, for those who would like to go still further into the puzzle, would seem to lie as much in a mystical sensuality—Mondrian used to joke as a young man that he worried that some green would rub off on his coat during his walks in nature—finally availing himself of a mature technique, rather than in any late-blooming defensive obsessionality.

The last example of applied analysis is a hopeful one, in that Esman is a psychoanalyst and a psychiatrist whose interest in art and art history represents an avocation rather than a profession. In fact, there is no reason why psychoanalysts cannot make contributions to other disciplines, as Esman has, provided they inform themselves and proceed with methodological caution and interpretive modesty. And it would be easy to cite works that meet this standard. Milton Viederman's (1986) brief essay on Magritte, for example, announces quite a daunting set of analytic theses in its very first paragraph, only to follow with a whole panoply of methodological cautions and caveats in its second. And it distinctly adds to the credibility of the endeavor that Viederman (1986, pp. 970–971) sees fit to quote a letter from the painter to a friend commenting on his meeting with two psychoanalysts and their interpretations of his work: "Just between ourselves, it's terrifying to see what one is exposed to in making an innocent picture." In the same vein, Viederman goes on to introduce the reader not only to Magritte's famous reticence about his past but also to his distinctive approach to painting, an approach that the painter expressly denied had anything to do with symbolism. A challenging and self-consciously diffident puzzle,

Magritte. Viederman judiciously does not try to solve the puzzle so much as to introduce us to him.

Limitations of Psychoanalytic Data for Interdisciplinary Inquiry

There are, as both contemporary and nineteenth-century psychologists have demonstrated, such things as unconscious processes. An interpreter accustomed to this truth, and accustomed to sifting through the data with this truth in mind, would seem to be operating with an advantage, not a handicap. To be sure, when one moves beyond the clinical encounter, there is necessarily a dearth of certain kinds of information, such as are normally to be extracted from shifts in associations, transference-countertransference fits, and the like, as observed via the analyst's preexisting interpretive armamentarium (see Rubovits-Seitz 1998). Applied analysis simply will never have the same kind of information base, with all *its* limitations, that regular analysis has.

Too often, however—this failing is especially evident in the sister discipline of "psychohistory"—the problem is further compounded when a belief in the efficacy of unconscious processes is coupled with a less-than-sure grasp of the available data, so that an unconscious motivation is invoked precisely where there is a gap in the historical record. Sheer folly. Because we do not know why this or that historical figure took the fateful step he or she did on a particularly fateful day does not let us leap straightaway to some theory about castration anxiety, primal scene anxiety, or, to pick a more contemporary motif, empathic failure on the part of an important selfobject, to relieve our sense of intellectual uncertainty. Any of these motives may have, in fact, been in play. But to demonstrate their relevance one actually needs more data, not less. One needs to be able to say that all the obvious conscious motives would seem not to have applied. This requires a thorough understanding of our subject's character, of his or her typical responses in such situations, and of his or her circumstances at that moment. Only when we can add up all these and see that we are still short of the mark should we begin casting about for unconscious motives.

It would help tremendously if the subject of our inquiry left behind a diary in which he or she confessed being at a loss to know why a certain course of action suddenly seemed like the "right" thing to do. Likewise, it would help if those closest to the person wrote in their diaries that the king or queen seemed quite out of sorts that morning. But we would just be beginning. We would still want to know something about our subject's childhood, about any dreams and slips that he or she had recently, about whatever hopes and fears had lately been stirred up, and about whatever else we might be able to get our hands on in the historical record. Now in all of this, it would be additionally helpful if we were personally familiar with some kings and queens, so as to know how kings and queens tend to act, and failing that, if we had read widely about kings and queens. It would also be helpful if we had some knowledge, however gained, of the typical conflicts and anxieties that come with being a sovereign, perhaps with a special look at how they might play out a little differently depending on gender. And so forth. A psychoanalyst might well do this better than a nonanalyst, but it is a tall order in any case, and most especially so if one is otherwise maintaining a full caseload.

Unless we have the kind of data that we require—to repeat, this will be somewhat different than the data we are accustomed to dealing with—we can do no better than make suggestions and draw analogies. We are reduced to theme-hunting. This is why an apostate like Frederick Crews can step away from his earlier study of Hawthorne (Crews 1966) with no more than a shrug: Maybe those thematic echoes weren't oedipal after all.

Theme-hunting and the search for analogies are lately prominent in a very different direction: in recent attempts to weld psychoanalytic ideas together with the latest findings of neurology and nonlinear system dynamics, or chaos theory. Too often the attempts stand, or fall, on the strength of very loose analogies. Both these intellectual domains have obvious relevance to the human condition, and owing to the availability of illuminating texts written for the nonspecialist reader, advances in these fields are beginning to be noticed by the analytic community. Yet, what is called for is circumspection: It will be a long time still before knowledge in either field reaches the kind of specificity that would be truly helpful to the analyst, or before an analytic hypothesis can be operationalized and tested by outsiders. In the meantime, we might be content to think of the new knowledge as usefully limiting rather than liberating. That is, we might check to see if any of our favorite notions now stand controverted, as, for example, Schachter (2002) has done in the case of genetic constructions of the transference vis-à-vis the limits of predictability within chaos theory.

Potential of Psychoanalysis for Interdisciplinary Studies: Example of Attachment Theory

Well, then, does psychoanalysis have nothing to offer to other academic disciplines? Even a cursory look around

the campus would persuade us that this is not so. The entire field of biography has been transformed in the past hundred years, owing in part to the advent of the psychoanalytic perspective on personal history. This is not to say that biographers are writing psychohistories; but they are writing biography in a different way than they did a century ago, and in some important ways what they now consider important, and worth interpreting, represents the legacy of the psychoanalytic tradition. Literary criticism isn't the same as it was 20 or 30 years ago, either, thanks in part to the Lacanians and their descendants, though whether this is a benign development or not is open to debate. Developmental psychology has also undergone a transformation, albeit a more recent one, courtesy of John Bowlby's theory of attachment. And that theory, let us remind ourselves, was seen by its originator *as a psychoanalytic theory*, specifically as an object relations theory. Ethology is also different than it was, thanks to the same theory—and the same theorist.

Bowlby's example deserves to be discussed in some detail, since in many ways it constitutes a model. It is not accidental that his ideas have gained currency in other disciplines. From the first, he made it a point not only to inform himself as to what was going on in other disciplines but to keep in personal contact with leading nonanalytic figures. During the years 1953–1956, for example, he was a member of the Psychobiology of the Child Study Group organized by Ronald Hargreaves of the World Health Organization; other participants included Erik Erikson, Julian Huxley, Jean Piaget and Barbel Inhelder, Konrad Lorenz, Margaret Mead, and Ludwig von Bertalanffy. Bowlby also enjoyed a close friendship with the Cambridge ethologist Robert Hinde, who in turn introduced him to the American psychologist Harry Harlow. The result was that Bowlby was uniquely situated to keep abreast of important new developments as they happened—and to influence them in his turn. Thus, Hinde, who had previously been studying songbirds, switched to studying mother-infant pairs in rhesus monkeys, while his good friend Bowlby started wondering about the possibilities of cross-species validation of the hypotheses he was about to put forward about the nature of the child's tie to the mother in humans.

Meanwhile, in America, for quite different reasons, Harry Harlow had also turned to virtually the same topic area. As Morris Eagle (personal communication, July 2003) recounts, Harlow's theoretical predicament was almost isomorphic with Bowlby's. American psychology was then still under the sway of the behaviorist theories of Clark Hall, who argued that both cognitive motives, like the need for exploration, and what we would now call attachment motives derived from so-called primary drives, such as hunger and sex. That is to say, in Hullian terms, an animal explores because in this way it sometimes finds food and is thus positively reinforced; similarly, an infant stays in close proximity to its mother for the same reason. The parallel with classical psychoanalytic theory of that era was quite close, as Eagle points out. Moreover, as Eagle further points out, just as some analytic thinkers such as Ives Hendricks and Robert White were beginning to question the primacy of basic drives vis-à-vis cognitive motives, Harlow had already done studies showing the same thing vis-à-vis Hullian drive psychology: In Harlow's experiments, the animals exhibited various motives, such as curiosity and the search for novelty, in ways that could not be simply reduced to their association with the satisfaction of so-called primary drives (e.g., hunger). But it was when he turned to the mother-infant bond and produced his famous experiment with the wire mother and the terry cloth mother that Harlow finally demolished the Hullian synthesis once and for all. It was the rarest of things for academic psychology—a truly decisive experiment. John Bowlby heard about it—and saw the film—before the results were officially published. It persuaded Bowlby that there was indeed a cross-species basis for the kinds of mechanisms that he was about to postulate in his own paper "The Nature of the Child's Tie to the Mother" (Bowlby 1957). Put another way, Harlow's finding encouraged Bowlby to take the same theoretical step, vis-à-vis classical psychoanalytic instinct theory, that Harlow was about to instigate decisively in American psychology.

Yet, the story does not stop there. As Steven Suomi (personal communication, August 2003) recounts, Bowlby returned the favor by encouraging Harlow to turn to the study of psychopathology. Indeed, legend has it that Bowlby's influence was decisive on a crucial methodological point. Harlow began trying to induce psychopathology through the use of rejecting surrogate mothers in the raising of his rhesus monkeys, but he was not getting very far. He complained as much to Bowlby during one of the latter's visits. Bowlby is said to have responded with great surprise, for as far as he could tell, Harlow's laboratory was full of the craziest rhesus monkeys he had ever seen. Indeed it was; only the monkeys who had developed the severe psychopathology were not the rejected ones but the severely deprived ones who had been used in the original crucial experiments. (Another version of the story has it that it was Robert Hinde, not Bowlby, who made the comment, though for the record, Suomi recounts that he heard the Bowlby version directly from Harlow himself.) Thus began a whole new, seminal line of primate research, one with obvious application to the human condition and, not incidentally, to psychoanalytic theory (for a fuller account, see Blum 2002). Indeed, most analysts would be as-

tonished, and I think inspired, if they were to acquaint themselves more intimately with what is currently going on in primatology under the direction of Suomi and others.

Bowlby was clearly unusual in the determination and effectiveness with which he pursued interdisciplinary collaboration. He was also unusual, at least in his era, for his theoretical eclecticism. Many of his colleagues read "The Nature of the Child's Tie to the Mother" and concluded that he had left the fold. Happily, this kind of intellectual conformity no longer obtains within psychoanalysis—and is no longer the obstacle to effective collaboration across disciplines that it once was. Indeed, we are obliged to note here that psychoanalysis is no longer a single thing. Rather, as Victoria Hamilton (1996) demonstrated in her elegantly conceived survey, psychoanalysis today is actually composed of a number of disparate communities, each with its own interpretive assumptions and, perhaps not surprisingly, its own workaday bibliography. Auden's phrase needs updating—today there are at least four or five distinct climates of opinion. Nor have analysts themselves failed to notice the new state of affairs, with the leading journals now regularly running papers that seek to identify a "common ground."

Interdisciplinary Sources of Psychoanalytic Theory

But it is not just its new pluralism that we need to focus on in considering the relation of psychoanalysis to other disciplines. Rather, we need to go back to Freud's original claim and take another look. The facts of the matter were always quite otherwise from what Freud claimed. One does not have to go far in any particular direction to find the interdisciplinary nature of psychoanalysis leaping forth from the historical record (again, see Esman 1998). Earlier, we touched on the embarrassment that the Project once seemed to pose for analysts. Few analysts, however, are familiar with Peter Amacher's (1962) subsequent reconnaissance into the past and what he found: namely, that Freud's was scarcely the only "project" out there. A number of leading neurological and biological theorists of the day made their own intriguing, if premature, attempts to deduce the laws of psychology from what was then known about the central nervous system. To be sure, Amacher appended to his researches a thesis to the effect that Freud now stood revealed as psychophysical reductionist, and thus for humanists a rather low type. This earned him a well-turned critique from the historian of science Paul Cranefield (1966), who pointed out most astutely that the figures Amacher was alluding to, such as Sigmund Exner or Ernst Brücke, were anything but the intellectual hard hats of Amacher's account. They were, in fact, highly cultivated men with interests in such things as music, art, and literature, areas in which they also wrote treatises! They were, to coin an awkward term, *interdisciplinarians.* So, too, was Freud.

Or one can look into the minutes of the Vienna Psychoanalytic Society. Consider those for the evening of November 29, 1911, which occasion was the impetus for Freud's letter to Jung quoted at the outset maintaining that psychoanalysis "goes by itself." Included in the discussion were Wagner's Flying Dutchman, Freud's paper on rescue fantasies, Eugen Bleuler's theory of instincts coming in matched pairs, the Greek myth of Glaukos, Elie Mechnikov's theory of a death instinct, Nietzsche's notion of the superman, Gustav Fechner's psychophysics, and, most surprisingly, issues of textual exegesis centered around the Book of Genesis. Freud may have complained about eclecticism the next day to Jung, but it was Freud himself who brought up the exegetical issues attending the Book of Genesis.

Or, as the foregoing example suggests, one can look at Freud's own sources. An intelligent survey of the influences, cited and uncited, on Freud's thinking would take a separate volume (see Kitcher 1992). But for some idea, the reader need go no further than his or her bookshelf and the index to the Standard Edition. Freud's work includes an incredibly rich variety of references.

Or consider, to take one final example, the theory of the Oedipus complex, which was for decades the very emblem of analytic orthodoxy. Did it emerge wholesale from the consulting room, the fruit of the unprejudiced examination of the facts, to use one of Freud's phrases? Scarcely. To begin with, we should note that the Oedipus in question in the complex is Sophocles' Oedipus, and not the Oedipus of the more extensive mythological record. Next, we should observe with Peter Rudnytsky (1987) that this Oedipus was terribly important at the end of the nineteenth century specifically because his dilemma had become emblematic of the human condition as it was contemplated by nineteenth-century idealist German philosophy. That is to say, German idealist philosophers saw man as tragically torn between the natural, from which he springs, and the spiritual, to which he must aspire, and in turn they saw Sophocles' drama, which they regularly cited, as dramatizing man's tragic duty to seek the truth of his origins, no matter where it took him. Further, we should take in Peter Swales's (1996) demonstration that the first clinical mention of Sophocles' hero comes in connection with a patient who is scarcely oedipal in the ordinary sense, his mother having died when he was all of 22 months old; rather he is oedipal in the specific sense that his earliest childhood is surrounded in mystery. The patient's name is Oscar Fell-

ner, though analytic readers will know him as "Herr E." of the Freud-Fliess correspondence. Fellner's mother died giving birth to Fellner's younger sister, as Swales has discovered, leaving Fellner with multiple mysteries to solve about his origins. And this aspect of the Oedipus story continued to be important; it was regularly conjoined in Freud's writings for a number of years with a theme taken from psychiatric pedagogy, namely, the unfortunate consequences of keeping children ignorant of the mystery of where babies come from. Then, too, we should note with John Forrester (1980) that the idea that the Oedipus complex was fundamentally triangular in nature and that it was the central complex in neurotic psychopathology was actually quite late in coming, only being fully put forward in 1910–1911. Moreover, as Forrester has moved, and I have seconded strongly (Kerr 1993), in making the Oedipus complex central and all other complexes derivative, Freud was borrowing his procedure from mythological studies. Meanwhile, the notion of a "complex" had come from experimental psychology, the term having originally been coined by Theodore Ziehen of Berlin and then the concept experimentally refined by Carl Jung and his associates in Zurich. And the final theory became finally enshrined only when it could be anchored in evolutionary biology as a universal psychic inheritance from prehistory in a ceremony that required that Freud first brush himself up on the length and breadth of the anthropology of his day. Quite an interdisciplinary fellow, this Oedipus.

Conclusion

Psychoanalysis never went by itself. But that was scarcely a weakness. Recognizing the true state of affairs, however, does leave an important question hanging. If psychoanalysis is, and always has been, an interdisciplinary endeavor, does it have anything uniquely its own to offer? If there is a "common ground" to be found in today's pluralistic world of different analytic schools, does it comprise something that scholars and researchers from other fields would do well to pay attention to?

Here we might take our cue from the history of the field. The reader may have already guessed from what was said earlier, or heard elsewhere, that the early critics and opponents of psychoanalysis were not the intellectual Luddites, riddled with their own complexes and barely concealing their anti-Semitism, that Ernest Jones would have had the field believe (see Decker 1977). In fact, the early critics, who were always respectful of Freud personally, were for the most part either objecting to facets of psychoanalysis, such as the exclusive focus on sexuality, that are no longer part of the "common ground" or else raising methodological issues that are now accepted as valid by psychoanalysts themselves. Still, there is a feature of their criticism, such as it survives in the historical record, that deserves mention. The fact is that many of them evinced a feeling, despite themselves, that they might be missing something—that there might be something to this psychoanalysis, some kind of secret knowledge, that they were losing out on.

Exactly so. Here we might take a page from pediatric psychiatry. If one wants an accurate history of a complaint, it is best to ask the parents. But if one wants to know how much suffering was entailed—there is research on this (see Leventhal and Conroy 1991)—one should ask the child. The same applies for the relation of psychoanalysis as a field to other disciplines. Psychologists might be able to demonstrate the potency of unconscious processes, but only in laboratory setups. Poets and writers might be able to capture the flavor of unconscious themes and issues, but only in make-believe. Ethologists might be willing to concede, as Konrad Lorenz did, that trauma and conflict between motivational systems can be real shapers of behavior, and that individual differences and the impact of personal history can be seen in most mammal species, but they cannot tell us for sure how such things might turn out for better or worse in an individual human lifetime. And so forth.

One can and should get one's hypotheses about what matters from anywhere and everywhere. But, to know how things really are for real individuals in the real world, how much suffering is entailed, and how much of many other things besides, it is necessary to put our questions to individuals and to wait, really wait, to get their answer. The sustained effort to get to know people one-on-one in an atmosphere of appreciation and respect will always generate a particular kind of knowledge. To be sure, practitioners in other fields, from anthropology to oral history to serious journalism, also sometimes obtain intensive intimate knowledge of their respondents. Yet only the analytic situation allows the subject to explore and to play beyond what he or she already knows—and thus beyond what he or she is otherwise willing to tell a truly interested other. To that extent, analysts can obtain a kind of understanding that cannot be duplicated anywhere else. Practitioners of this craft should never have to apologize. Or pretend that their field goes by itself.

References

Amacher P: Freud's Neurological Education and Its Influence on Psychoanalytic Theory (Psychological Issues Monograph Series, No 16). New York, International Universities Press, 1962

Bettelheim B: Freud and Man's Soul. New York, Knopf, 1982

Blum D: Love at Goon Park: Harry Harlow and the Nature of the Science of Affection. London, Penguin, 2002

Bowlby J: The nature of the child's tie to the mother. Psychoanal Study Child 30:230–240, 1957

Breger L: Freud: Darkness in the Midst of Vision. New York, Wiley, 2000

Cranefield P: Freud and the "School of Helmholtz." Gesnerus 23:35–39, 1966

Crews F: The Sins of the Fathers: Hawthorne's Psychological Themes. New York, Oxford University Press, 1966

Decker H: Freud in Germany: revolution and reaction in science, 1893–1907 (Psychological Issues Monograph Series, No 41). New York, International Universities Press, 1977

Ellenberger HF: The Discovery of the Unconscious: The History and Evolution of Dynamic Psychiatry. New York, Basic Books, 1970

Esman A: Piet Mondrian: the fusion of art and life. Psychoanalysis and Contemporary Thought 17:325–344, 1994

Esman AA: What is "applied" in "applied" psychoanalysis? Int J Psychoanal 79:741–756, 1998

Forrester J: Language and the Origins of Psychoanalysis. New York, Columbia University Press, 1980

Freud S: The aetiology of hysteria (1896a), in Standard Edition of the Complete Psychological Works of Sigmund Freud, Vol 3. Translated and edited by Strachey J. London, Hogarth Press, 1962, pp 191–221

Freud S: Further remarks on the neuro-psychoses of defence (1896b), in Standard Edition of the Complete Psychological Works of Sigmund Freud, Vol 3. Translated and edited by Strachey J. London, Hogarth Press, 1962, pp 157–185

Freud S: Heredity and the aetiology of the neuroses (1896c), in Standard Edition of the Complete Psychological Works of Sigmund Freud, Vol 3. Translated and edited by Strachey J. London, Hogarth Press, 1962, pp 143–156

Freud S: Three essays on the theory of sexuality, I: the sexual aberrations (1905), in Standard Edition of the Complete Psychological Works of Sigmund Freud, Vol 7. Translated and edited by Strachey J. London, Hogarth Press, 1953, pp 135–172

Gay P: Art and Act. New York, Harper & Row, 1975

Gay P: Freud: A Life for Our Times. New York, WW Norton, 1998

Hamilton V: The Analyst's Preconscious. Hillsdale, NJ, Analytic Press, 1996

Holt R: Freud Reappraised: A Fresh Look at Psychoanalytic Theory. New York, Guilford, 1989

Kerr J: A Most Dangerous Method: The Story of Jung, Freud, and Sabina Spielrein. New York, Knopf, 1993

Kerr J: Review essay: Is Freud dead? Questions and answers for the practicing analyst. Psychoanalytic Dialogues 13:141–161, 2003

Kitcher P: Freud's Dream: A Complete Interdisciplinary Science of Mind. Cambridge, MA, MIT Press, 1992

Leavy B: In Search of the Swan Maiden: A Narrative on Folklore and Gender. New York, New York University Press, 1994

Leventhal B, Conroy L: The parent interview, in Textbook of Child and Adolescent Psychiatry. Edited by Wiener JM. Washington, DC, American Psychiatric Press, 1991, pp 78–83

Levin K: Freud's Early Psychology of the Neuroses: A Historical Perspective. Pittsburgh, PA, University of Pittsburgh Press, 1979

McGrath W: Freud and the force of history, in Freud and the History of Psychoanalysis. Edited by Gelfand T, Kerr J. Hillsdale, NJ, The Analytic Press, 1992, pp 79–97

McGuire W (ed): The Freud/Jung Letters. Princeton, NJ, Princeton University Press, 1974

Pollack R: The Creation of Dr. B.: A Biography of Bruno Bettelheim. New York, Simon & Schuster, 1997

Rubovits-Seitz P: Depth Psychological Understanding: The Methodological Grounding of Clinical Interpretation. Hillsdale, NJ, Analytic Press, 1998

Rudnytsky P: Freud and Oedipus. New York, Columbia University Press, 1987

Schachter J: Transference: Shiboleth or Albatross? Hillsdale, NJ, Analytic Press, 2002

Sulloway FJ: Freud, Biologist of the Mind. New York, Basic Books, 1979

Swales P: Protecting Freud's image from Sigmund: review of Peter Gay's Freud: A Life for Our Times. Los Angeles Times, Book Reviews, May 8, 1988, p. 1

Swales P: Freud, his ur-patient, and their romance of Oedipus: the role of "Herr E." in the conception of psychoanalysis. Presentation before the Institute for the History of Psychiatry, Weill Cornell Medical Center, New York, December 4, 1996

Viederman M: Rene Magritte: coping with loss—reality and illusion. J Am Psychoanal Assoc 35:967–998, 1986

30

Psychology

JOEL WEINBERGER, PH.D.

KENNETH N. LEVY, PH.D.

Psychoanalysis is not a particular branch of medicine. I do not see how anyone can refuse to see this. Psychoanalysis is part of psychology—not even a medical psychology in the old sense of the term...but simply of psychology. (Freud 1927, pp. 392–393)

IN THIS CHAPTER, we examine the relationship between psychoanalysis and psychology, focusing on the interface between academic psychology and psychoanalysis. This relationship is a complicated one and can be characterized mainly as a tale of two psychologies: academic psychology (including research-oriented clinical psychology) and psychoanalytic psychotherapy (applied clinical psychology). We examine the historical development of the relationship between these disciplines as well as their contemporary relationship. To accomplish this task in a comprehensive fashion is a huge endeavor, well beyond the scope of a single chapter. We therefore focus on two specific areas to illustrate our points: unconscious processes and interpersonal relationships (attachment). These two themes were chosen because the intrapsychic and the interpersonal are central to the psychoanalytic enterprise and because there are a great deal of data on each. We conclude the chapter with recommendations for the future of the relationship between the two disciplines.

Academic Psychology and Psychoanalysis

Academic psychology and psychoanalysis have a long and ambivalent relationship (Hornstein 1992). The pioneers of academic psychology were at odds with one another from the moment they first heard of Freud's work. This dissension can be illustrated through their reactions to his appearance at Clark University in 1909 (which many of them attended). Edward Bradford Titchener thought little of Freud's work. He did not even consider psychoanalysis to be psychology because of its emphasis on unconscious processes and its applied focus. Titchener insisted that psychology be a science of consciousness and that it be "pure" (i.e., have no applied focus) (Hornstein 1992). William James, in contrast, although not an unabashed admirer of Freud's psychoanalysis, had a generally positive reaction. He was even reported to have declared to Freud that "the future of psychology belongs to your work" (1920). (James is often portrayed as disparaging the entire notion of unconscious processes and therefore of being opposed to Freud's views. This characterization is, however, a misunderstanding of his work; see Weinberger 2000.)

The founder of behaviorism, John Watson, was extremely ambivalent about psychoanalysis. On the one hand, he saw it as unscientific and even closely akin to superstition (Watson 1919); on the other hand, he seemed compelled to try to account for the phenomena identified by Freud in behavioristic terms, thereby acknowledging their reality. B.F. Skinner seemed similarly ambivalent. Skinner (1953) discounted the possibility of any mental entities or organizations such as id, ego, and superego but acknowledged the veracity of Freud's observations qua observations. He told one of us (J.W.) that Freud was the only "mentalistic" theorist he cited favorably because of his brilliant observations of behavior, but that he believed Freud's mentalistic explanations were bogus (B.F. Skinner, personal communication, May 1988).

Views such as those of Watson and of Skinner led to efforts to reformulate psychoanalysis in behaviorist terms. This often took the form of "translating" psychoanalytic concepts into behaviorist terminology. The best-known and most comprehensive example of such an effort at "translation" was probably the work of Dollard and Miller (1950). (This tradition of translating Freud into the current language of academic psychology was revived more recently by Erdelyi [1985] in a wonderful book that tried to translate Freud 's work into more modern cognitive terms.)

Psychoanalytic thinking enjoyed a heyday in academic psychology in the 1950s through a program of research termed the "New Look" (Dixon 1971, 1981). This work employed subliminal presentation of stimuli in an effort to demonstrate unconscious phenomena termed "perceptual defense," "perceptual vigilance," and "subception." *Perceptual defense* referred to difficulty in recognizing threatening stimuli (high recognition threshold), whereas *perceptual vigilance* referred to unusual ease in recognizing such stimuli (low recognition threshold). *Subception* involved physiological reactions to threatening stimuli while denying phenomenal awareness of them. These phenomena seemed to corroborate psychoanalytic thinking. First, unconscious events were apparently being demonstrated, and second, they seemed to be of a psychoanalytic nature. For example, hysterics, who according to psychoanalytic theory employ defenses, demonstrated perceptual defense (Dixon 1981), whereas paranoids, who are said to always be on the lookout for danger, demonstrate perceptual vigilance (Dixon 1981).

The New Look came to a screeching halt in about 1960 as its studies came to be intensively criticized and the psychoanalytic understanding of their results was rejected (Eriksen 1959; Goldiamond 1958). Later reviews of the literature indicated that these criticisms were oversold (Dixon 1981) or that those who made these criticisms bought into the soon-to-be-replaced behaviorist paradigm (Erdelyi 1974; Weinberger, in press). Nonetheless, with a few exceptions (two of which are reviewed below), psychology saw the New Look as a dead end. This ushered in a period of extreme hostility on the part of academic psychology toward psychoanalysis. Consider the following quote from a still prominent psychologist:

> The latter [psychoanalytically oriented clinicians] employ symptom-underlying disease models in which the "disease" is a function of conscious or (more often) unconscious inner agents akin to the supernatural forces that once provided the explanatory concepts of physics, biology, and (more recently) medicine. General medicine has progressed from the demonology that dominated it during the dark ages. As scientific knowledge has increased, magical explanations have been replaced by scientific ones. In contrast, theories of psychopathology, in which demons reappear in the guise of "psychodynamic forces," still reflect the mystical thinking that once predominated in science. (Bandura and Walters 1963, pp. 30–31)

Nor has this hostility abated with time. More recently, Greenwald (1992) pronounced that unconscious phenomena "are limited to relatively minor cognitive feats.... it appears to be intellectually much simpler than the sophisticated agency portrayed in psychoanalytic theory" (p. 766). He concluded that "it will be time, at last, to abandon psychoanalytic theory" (p. 775).

Psychotherapy and Psychoanalysis

As Shakow and Rapaport (1964) pointed out 40 years ago, parts of clinical psychology have achieved much integration with psychoanalysis. However, a gap still exists within applied clinical psychology because of the somewhat unique path that clinical psychologists have followed toward professionalism and the (until recently) exclusionary training practices of the American Psychoanalytic Association. Because of these historical factors, the relationship between psychoanalysis and psychology is a strange one.

Although psychoanalysis relies on empirical evidence to support many of its basic tenets, particularly in this era of evidence-based medicine, thereby demonstrating its connection to academic psychology's pro-research tenets

(Sackett et al. 1996), psychoanalysts often accept the need to do so only reluctantly, thereby showing their estrangement from research-based academic psychology. The few active collaborations that take place are usually focused on specific findings consistent with a particular author's preconceived ideas. Some analysts have asserted the separateness of psychoanalysis from disciplines like psychology and see little need for empirical support or minimize the relevance of psychological research.

Nonpsychoanalytic clinicians and theorists have practiced their own form of exclusion. Beginning with attacks on psychoanalytically oriented psychotherapy by Eysenck (1952), who claimed that they lacked scientific credibility, this kind of thinking still reverberates today in the form of so-called empirically supported treatments (all of which are short-term and virtually none of which are psychodynamic). Proponents of this view suggest that clinical training be restricted to so-called empirically supported treatments, which would effectively exclude psychoanalytic treatment from graduate schools and clinical internships. Insurance reimbursement has also been affected by this view.

In fact, with regard to the treatment of borderline personality disorder (BPD), a disorder common in psychoanalytic practice (Doidge et al. 1994; Friedman et al. 1998) and for which psychoanalytic therapy is most promising and most likely to be uniquely effective (Shakow and Rapaport 1964), many managed care companies (e.g., Massachusetts Behavioral Health Partnership, which manages Massachusetts' Medicaid mental health dollars) have defined special benefits for a cognitive-behavioral therapy called Dialectical Behavior Therapy (DBT; Linehan 1993), and certain companies will only reimburse DBT treatment of BPD. In addition, departments of mental health in several states (e.g., Illinois, Connecticut, Massachusetts, New Hampshire, North Carolina, and Maine) have now enthusiastically endorsed DBT as the treatment of choice for clients with BPD. These states have provided funding and coordination for training in DBT.

Thus, psychoanalysts often critique clinical researchers for their lack of clinical richness and relevance, whereas clinical researchers often argue that psychoanalytic treatment is completely without proven effectiveness. Although it is true that psychological research often fails to capture the richness and complexity of human experience, as some psychoanalysts assert, it is untrue that psychoanalysis is not in need of empirical support. As Spence (1994) and others (Fonagy 2000; Masling and Cohen 1987) point out, not all the evidence needed to support psychoanalytic ideas comes from the consultation room. Fonagy (2000), a psychoanalyst and psychologist, eloquently noted that clinical data offer fertile ground for theory building, but not for distinguishing good theories

from either bad or better ones. Fonagy argued further that "the proliferation of clinical theories currently in use, is the best evidence that clinical data are more suitable for generating hypotheses than for evaluating them" (p. 228). It is true that psychoanalysis needs more empirical investigations as some clinical researchers assert. It is not true, however, that psychoanalytic theories are totally devoid of such support, as those working in the Eysenck tradition contend. In fact, one could argue that much of the movement in psychoanalysis has been stoked by empirical findings from developmental attachment research, psychotherapy research, and social and cognitive psychology in areas such as implicit processes. Some of this work has been conducted by psychoanalytically oriented researchers (e.g., attachment), but a significant portion of this research was conducted by nonpsychoanalytic psychologists (e.g., the study of social cognition).

Despite the difficulties and conflicts outlined above, there has been much that scientific/academic psychology and psychoanalysis have provided to each other. It would be impossible to review all of these contributions in one chapter. We therefore offer brief reviews of two areas—unconscious processes and interpersonal relationships (attachment)—to illustrate the cross-fertilization between academic psychology and psychoanalysis. We chose these two areas because, as stated earlier, they are exemplars of intrapsychic and interpersonal functioning. In our review, we focus on relatively recent research. The reader interested in studying a wider corpus is referred to a compendium edited by Barron and colleagues (1992). Especially rewarding is a series edited by Bornstein and Masling (2002a, 2002b) devoted to psychoanalytically oriented research.

Unconscious Processes

Central to psychoanalytic thinking is the concept that much, if not most, human mental functioning can be attributed to unconscious processing. Freud (1926/1959) went so far as to say that psychoanalysis might be characterized as the study of unconscious processes. Subsequent psychoanalytic theorists have retained this emphasis (cf. Westen 1998). Until relatively recently, academic psychology disagreed, abjuring the very existence, and therefore the study of, unconscious processes (Weinberger, in press). Over the past 25 years, this stance has changed, and academic psychology's study of unconscious processes has burgeoned. Psychologists now routinely study such topics as implicit memory, implicit learning, and automaticity. There is also some empirical research on unconscious processes more directly tied to psychoanalytic thinking, including what has been termed "subliminal psychodynamic activation" and a research program that integrates psychoanalysis with subliminal stimulation and measurement of brain waves spearheaded by Howard Shevrin (Shevrin et al. 1996).

Implicit Memory

Implicit memory is inferred when a person does something indicating that he or she was affected by a prior experience but has no conscious recollection of that experience (Schacter 1987). The memory of the experience is implicit in the person's behavior, hence the term. Academic psychologists tend to study this phenomenon through testing brain-damaged individuals evidencing the amnesic syndrome, much as Poetzl (1917) studied unconscious recall through investigating brain-damaged war-wounded soldiers back in the time of Freud. It can also be investigated in brain-intact individuals through subliminal priming. *Subliminal priming* involves presenting a stimulus too quickly or faintly to be consciously noticed (subliminally). The stimulation nonetheless can affect subsequent judgments, evaluations, and behaviors; it therefore "primes" these reactions (cf. Weinberger, in press).

Implicit memory can be implicated in both fears and preferences. Moreover, it begins much earlier in life than does explicit (conscious) memory. It is at virtually full strength from early childhood (by age 4) and perhaps before language acquisition (Naito and Komatsu 1993; Schacter 1996), whereas explicit memory develops throughout childhood and into adolescence (Kail 1990; Naito and Komatsu 1993). Although it weakens with age, implicit memory does not deteriorate to nearly the same degree as does explicit memory and is powerful even into old age. The effects of implicit memory are also long-lasting. Simple and affectively neutral experiences like word-stem completions and skills learning show evidence of retention for weeks and even months without the need for intervening practice or reminders. (Implicit learning can be analogized to learning to ride a bicycle, in that you never forget.)

No one has systematically investigated implicit memory for emotionally meaningful and charged experiences. It is fair to expect that, if anything, such experiences would be even more strongly retained than would affectively colorless events. Implicit memory may therefore underlie some of the lasting effects of unreported childhood experiences. Defenses would not be implicated in such instances; it is merely the way the mind operates. Experiences would be coded implicitly before explicit memory is well developed. The person would continue to respond to them and to similar events in a way that suggested some memory of them but would legitimately have no recollec-

tion of them. Phobias, fears, preferences, and fetishes might be produced in this way.

A clinical vignette, almost a century old, may illustrate this point. In 1911, the great French neurologist Edouard Claparede (1995) hid a pin between his fingers and pricked an amnesic patient (who had Korsakoff's syndrome) when he took her hand. She became upset but quickly forgot the incident. Later, she was fearful of taking Claparede's hand but could not say why. An example more familiar to psychologists and one that illustrates the differential development of implicit and explicit memory is that of "Little Albert." John Watson, the founder of behaviorism, succeeded in causing a preverbal child (Little Albert) to become phobic of white furry objects (and not so incidentally of Watson himself) by banging a loud gong whenever poor Albert reached for a white rat presented to him. It would not be surprising if Little Albert retained his fears but could not consciously explain them. This is exactly what Watson expected, and he used this case to poke fun at psychoanalysis. Albert would have an implicit memory of being terrified, but his explicit memory was not sufficiently developed for him to be able to consciously recollect Watson's abuse of him.

Implicit Learning

Implicit learning involves registering relationships among experiences without any awareness of having done so (Reber 1993). Reber (1993) created artificial grammars to investigate implicit learning. He presented people with strings of letters connected by arbitrary rules. After viewing several such sets of letter strings, his participants were presented with another series of letter strings and asked to determine which of them were consistent with the first series. People were capable of making such determinations even though they had no awareness of the rules governing the associations between the letters. In fact, their performance at this task worsened when they were told that such rules existed and that they should try to determine what they were.

Of more obvious relevance to psychoanalysis were studies conducted by Lewicki and his colleagues, who demonstrated that implicit learning applied to meaningful social stimuli (Lewicki 1986). For example, Lewicki presented participants with a series of behavioral descriptions of people that *implied* but never explicitly referred to certain personality traits. No participant was able to verbalize these connections. Nonetheless, they affected subsequent ratings of the traits of people they knew. Lewicki further showed that people learned these covariations even when they made no logical sense. For example, he presented threatening words auditorily in combination with photos of people sporting something innocuous like a hat. Participants judged subsequently presented hat-wearing people as threatening. The conclusion to draw from these studies is that the unconscious is very good at forming connections but very poor at critically evaluating them. It picks up covariations in the environment regardless of whether they are sensibly or coincidentally related. In other words, unconscious processes are powerful but are uncritical and do not reality-test. A real-world example of such processes is what has come to be called *implicit prejudice* (Fiske 1998). For example, Caucasians seem to have come to associate African American faces and names with negativity, even when this does not reflect their actual experiences or conscious beliefs (Greenwald et al. 1998). They are quicker to push a button labeled as negative when presented with a black face or a stereotypical African American name than they are a button labeled as positive.

Like implicit memory, implicit learning capabilities are apparent very early in life. Lewicki found that preschool children could easily pick up complex and simultaneous covariations of color, object, and spatial location of experimenter. These abilities are equivalent to those of an adult and are beyond an adult's (let alone a child's) ability to consciously recognize. Implicit learning is also quick and robust. Hill and Lewicki (1997) showed that once a connection between two events has been unconsciously made, people would behave as though that relationship continues to exist long after the two events no longer co-occur. One trial can be enough to pick up a covariation and begin this process. This learning can then bias the processing of subsequent experiences such that the covariations learned are maintained even in the face of subsequent disconfirming experiences.

Implicit learning, like implicit memory, is normative. It is not the result of conflict, defense, or even affective arousal, although all of these may be expected to affect what is attended to and therefore learned unconsciously. Implicit learning simply picks up whatever covaries in the environment, whether it makes sense or not. The fruits of this learning will persist, even if the environment changes. That is, people will continue to act as if something is so even when it is not. And people are unable to report on any of it because it is unconscious. Implicit learning can explain some of the unrealistic and maladaptive connections people seem to evince but have no awareness of and may even deny.

Automaticity

Automaticity is a sophisticated model of habit formation originally investigated by Schneider and Shiffrin (1977; Shiffrin and Schneider 1977). Notions of automaticity practically dominate social psychological writings on uncon-

scious processes. In simple language, automatic processing involves the activation of well-learned behaviors. Once such behaviors have been activated, they proceed mechanically, almost reflexively. There is no need to attend to or monitor them. In fact, once begun, these behaviors are almost impossible to control or stop. They have virtually no flexibility, and in this way resemble an obsessive thought, a compulsion, or a ritual. Changing an automatic process is extremely difficult. Attempts to do so feel unpleasant and even frightening, like trying to resist a compulsion.

Virtually anything can become automatic; all that is required is sufficient practice. Many of our everyday behaviors are automatic (e.g., driving a car, tying our shoelaces). Automaticity makes functioning more efficient and easy until one tries to change. Imagine trying to drive on the left side of the road in England if you are used to driving on the right side in the United States (or vice versa). Even though failure to do so could be life-threatening, it is very difficult to make the change. It is also very unpleasant to try. Automatic processes need not come from conscious practice. They can develop through implicit learning that occurs repeatedly. The result is automatic but the origin of the behavior is unconscious. The person may not even realize that he or she engages in that behavior, but it is just as automatic and hard to change as more mundane automaticity.

Maladaptive behaviors seen in psychotherapy may fall into the category of automated implicit learning. Such behaviors can include enactments and ways of relating as well as manners of speech and carriage. They would be very hard to change simply because they have become automatic, and patients would resist such change. This could help to explain some of the pain and resistance associated with the working-through process. The patient knows what he or she has to do but finds it difficult, frustrating, and unpleasant to do it. It takes a very long time and constant repetition to make such changes permanent.

More Directly Psychoanalytic Research Into the Unconscious

Two research programs employ subliminal priming to investigate specifically psychoanalytic propositions concerning unconscious processes. One approach was conceived by Lloyd Silverman (1976) and is termed *subliminal psychodynamic activation*. The other is a combination of psychodynamic, cognitive, and neurophysiological methods that was spearheaded by Howard Shevrin (Shevrin et al. 1996).

Subliminal Psychodynamic Activation

Subliminal psychodynamic activation involves presenting a person with a subliminal stimulus that is designed to capture an important psychoanalytic proposition. The person's subsequent responses are assessed to see if he or she is affected by the stimulus in a way that psychoanalytic theory would predict. Most recent work has involved the stimulus MOMMY AND I ARE ONE, or MIO, which was designed to foster a fantasy of merger (Silverman et al. 1982). Studies have demonstrated that this subliminal stimulus was able to improve mood (Weinberger et al. 1998) and, more impressively, led to better outcomes when it preceded psychotherapeutic and educational interventions (Silverman and Weinberger 1985). Several meta-analyses (a statistical way to combine the results of many studies in order to determine whether an effect is genuine and reliable) revealed that the MIO effects were genuine and reliable (Hardaway 1990; Weinberger and Hardaway 1990). They also revealed that the MIO message was more effective than alternative positive messages, even when the latter included references to mother. Another meta-analysis (Bornstein 1990) revealed that the effects were stronger when the stimulation was subliminal (out of awareness) than when it was supraliminal (in awareness). More recent research (Sohlberg et al. 1998) indicates that the message is effective only when the recipient has a relatively positive internal representation of mother. This work shows that the psychoanalytic unconscious can be investigated experimentally using the tools of academic psychology. In such studies, the results support certain psychoanalytic conceptions of unconscious processes.

Activation of Event-Related Potential by Stimuli

The Shevrin group's work, which is more individualized and clinical than is subliminal psychodynamic activation, is comprehensively detailed in a volume by Shevrin and colleagues (1996). Through extensive testing and clinical interviewing, the research team chooses words that seem to best capture a person's conscious conflicts, as well as words that seem to best capture a person's unconscious conflicts. Pleasant and unpleasant words are also chosen for control purposes. These words are then presented both subliminally and supraliminally to the person. Brain responses in the form of event-related potentials (ERPs) are recorded to determine the effects of these stimuli. Findings generally indicate that the unconscious conflict words most easily activated ERPs when presented subliminally, whereas the conscious conflict words produced the most easily discriminable ERP patterns when presented supraliminally. Ordinary pleasant and unpleasant words evinced no particular pattern of ERP response. The results support the psychoanalytic concept of unconscious conflict as well as the analyst's ability to identify important features of it. As Shevrin and colleagues (1996) put it: "The subjective clin-

ical judgments of the psychoanalyst concerning the nature of unconscious conflict in each subject are supported by the objective measurement of unconscious processes and their correlated brain responses" (p. 134).

Interpersonal Relationships (Attachment)

Attachment Theory

Not all contributions relevant to psychoanalysis and psychology have come from the side of non–psychoanalytically oriented researchers. Psychoanalysis has also inspired research that has had a major impact on psychology's view of human functioning. John Bowlby's attachment theory is a major case in point.

Although Bowlby was a psychoanalyst, he clashed with his supervisor Melanie Klein over the issue of whether to involve the mother in the psychoanalytic treatment of a child. This difference in focus was the beginning of Bowlby's eventual estrangement from the psychoanalytic community. In contrast to object relations theorists, such as Winnicott, who retained much of Freud's emphasis on sexual and aggressive drives and fantasies, Bowlby, in his attachment theory, focused on the affective bond in close interpersonal relationships. Bowlby believed that Klein and other psychoanalysts overestimated the role of infantile fantasy, neglecting the role of actual experiences. Additionally, in contrast to most psychoanalysts of the time, Bowlby was also empirically minded. Rather than draw inferences about childhood from the free associations, dreams, transferences, and other mental productions of adults primarily seen in psychoanalytic treatment, Bowlby wanted to study and work directly with children. His focus was on the observable behavior of infants and their interactions with their caregivers, especially their mothers, and he encouraged prospective studies of the effects of early attachment relationships on personality development. In this sense he was again different from many of his object relations colleagues, who focused instead on adults' mental representations of self and others in close relationships, often revealed during psychoanalysis and psychotherapy, although these colleagues also believed that these representations were the result of early relationships with parents. Nevertheless, although Bowlby was critical of certain aspects of classic psychoanalytic formulations, he always considered himself a psychoanalyst, and his work clearly falls within the framework of psychoanalysis because he retained and extended many of Freud's clinical and developmental insights.

Attachment theory and research provide a powerful and valuable heuristic framework for conducting psychoanalytic research, testing psychoanalytic hypotheses, and enriching the perspective of psychoanalytic clinicians and investigators. They also help us to understand normative development and the operation of interpersonal functioning. Although Bowlby was a psychiatrist and psychoanalyst, much of the work in attachment theory has been carried out by clinical and developmental psychologists. The landmark research by Ainsworth and colleagues (1978) on the relationship of maternal sensitivity to attachment patterns, and the subsequent research by Sroufe, Hamilton, and Waters (Hamilton 2000; Waters et al. 2000; Weinfield et al. 2000) on the continuity of infant attachment into adolescence and young adulthood, have provided strong empirical evidence for two basic psychoanalytic tenets: 1) early childhood relationships are important in shaping adult relationships, and 2) meaning systems are important in understanding an individual's unique life and living perspective and resulting behavior. Additionally, the seminal work of Mary Main and her colleagues in developing the Adult Attachment Interview (AAI) and relating mothers' and fathers' attachment representations to their children's attachment patterns, as well as Fonagy and Target's creative research on reflective function, provides fertile ground for the future growth of psychoanalysis and its scientific evolution.

Basing their approach on Bowlby's attachment theory, Ainsworth and colleagues conducted a seminal study to observe the effects of childrearing behaviors employed by mothers on the development of attachment patterns in their offspring. They developed a measurement technique called the Strange Situation (Ainsworth et al. 1978). The Strange Situation involves a series of standard episodes staged in a playroom during which the infant, the caregiver, and a "stranger" interact in a comfortable setting and the behaviors of the infant are observed. First, the baby has the chance to explore toys while the mother is present. Then a stranger enters, converses with the mother, and invites the baby to play. Next, the mother leaves the baby with the stranger for a few minutes and then reenters the room to reunite with the baby. After this reunion, the mother leaves the baby a second time, this time all alone, followed by the stranger's return, and finally the mother's return for a second reunion. Ainsworth was able to categorize infants into three distinct groups on the basis of their reunion behavior with their mothers after this brief separation. From their observations of infants and caregivers, Ainsworth and colleagues (1978) identified three distinct patterns or styles of infant-mother attachment: secure (63% of the dyads tested), avoidant (21%), and anxious-ambivalent (16%). Later, a fourth category, disorganized/disoriented, was added (Main and Solomon 1990).

All four categories of infants are *attached* to their mothers, yet there are significant individual differences in the quality of these attachment relationships, and these differences can be reliably measured. The *avoidant* dyad is characterized by quiet distance in the mother's presence, often acting unaware of the mother's departure and avoiding the mother upon reunion. The *anxious-ambivalent* dyad (sometimes called *anxious-resistant*) is characterized by much emotional protest and anger on the part of the infant, who becomes extremely distressed on the mothers' departure, and often continues crying long after his or her mother's return. These reunions are also characterized by the infant's seeking attention, yet being unable to experience the mother's ministrations as soothing and comforting. The *disorganized/disoriented* dyad is characterized by disorganized or disoriented behaviors in the parent's presence, suggesting a temporary collapse of behavioral strategy. For example, the infant may freeze with a trancelike expression and hands in the air or may approach the parent but then fall prone and huddled on the floor. The *secure* dyad is characterized by the confident use of the mother as a "secure base" to explore the playroom with considerable ease and comfort in the mother's presence. Although a secure infant may experience distress on the mother's departure, on her return, the secure baby approaches her for comfort and is soothed more readily. The secure baby seeks proximity and interaction with the mother and then resumes his or her exploration of the environment. The Ainsworth (1978) study has been replicated and extended by many subsequent investigators (see, e.g., van IJzendoorn and Bakermans-Kranenburg 1996 for a review) and replicated with samples of children from other nations (van IJzendoorn 1995).

In addition, consistent with Bowlby's theory, the attachment patterns identified by Ainsworth are closely associated with differences in caregiver warmth and responsiveness (Ainsworth et al. 1978; see Main 1995 for a review). Ainsworth and colleagues (1978), and Grossmann and colleagues (1985) in a German sample (see also Grossmann and Grossmann 1991), found that maternal sensitivity during infancy strongly predicted the security of infants' attachments to their mothers. For example, Ainsworth and colleagues (1978) observed child-mother interactions at home and found that children's behaviors in the Strange Situation were related to mothers' general responsiveness. Mothers of children who displayed secure behaviors in the laboratory setting were found to be most responsive to infant signals at home. Mothers of anxious-ambivalent children were found to respond to their children inconsistently, belatedly, or inappropriately, so that the children could never be certain of their mother's availability. Mothers of avoidant children disliked physical contact with their babies and were selectively unresponsive to their infants' distress signals. Ainsworth and colleagues (1978) drew the conclusion that a child's expectations about mother's responsiveness were influenced not only by actual physical separation from the mother but also by the child's everyday relationship with her. Other studies have also provided strong support for the link between maternal sensitivity and attachment security. For example, mothers of securely attached infants, in contrast to mothers of insecurely attached infants, tend to hold their babies more carefully, tenderly, and for longer periods of time during early infancy (Main et al. 1985). Additionally, mothers of securely attached infants respond more frequently to crying, show more affection when holding the baby, and are more likely to acknowledge the baby with a smile or conversation when entering the baby's room compared with mothers of babies who are later independently deemed insecurely attached.

Several longitudinal studies have investigated the influence of these infant attachment styles on subsequent functioning and adaptive potential (Hamilton 2000; Waters et al. 2000). In terms of stability, Hamilton (2000) found a 75% correspondence for secure-insecure attachment status between infancy and late adolescence, with the strongest stability in the preoccupied group. Waters and colleagues (2000) followed 50 individuals for 20 years, finding 64% stability in attachment classification. There was greater than 70% stability for individuals with no major negative life events, and less than 50% stability for those who, for example, lost a parent or endured parental divorce. Thus, longitudinal research, although preliminary, indicates that attachment patterns remain relatively stable over time, even into early adulthood (age 20). When attachment styles do change, they appear to change in ways that are predictable and consistent with attachment theory (Fraley and Spieker 2003; Lewis 2000).

Employing Ainsworth's typology of attachment patterns, Main and colleagues (1985) developed the Adult Attachment Interview to assess aspects of adults' internal working models of attachment with regard to their parents. The AAI is a semistructured interview designed to elicit thoughts, feelings, and memories about early attachment experiences, and to assess the individual's state of mind with regard to early attachment relationships (C. George, N. Kaplan, M. Main, "The Berkeley Adult Attachment Interview," unpublished manuscript, Department of Psychology, University of California, Berkeley, 1985). Main and her co-workers found that parents' narrative reports of interactions with their own parents could predict their children's attachment security classification in a laboratory procedure with about 80% accuracy and thus demonstrated a link between symbolic processes of adults and attachment behavior of their infants. These laboratory associations extended to observations in the home. Similar levels of association also have been found in 21 of 24 studies that have assessed both mother and child attachment patterns (van IJzendoorn and Bakermans-Kranenburg 1996).

Over the last several years, Peter Fonagy and colleagues (1998) have been developing a complex and subtle scale to assess individuals' ability to comprehend feelings, beliefs, intentions, conflicts, and other psychological states in their accounts of current attachment experiences. This capacity, termed *reflective function* (RF) by Fonagy, refers to awareness of mental process in the self and in the other—that is, the ability to take account of one's own and others' mental states in understanding why people behave in specific ways. Briefly, the Reflective Function Scale is a clinical scale that ranges from −1 (negative RF, in which interviews are overly concrete, totally barren of mentalization, or grossly distorting of the mental states of others) to 9 (exceptional RF, in which interviews show unusually complex, elaborate, or original reasoning about mental states). The midpoint of the scale is 5 (or ordinary RF, in which interviews indicate fairly coherent, if somewhat one-dimensional or simplistic, reasoning about mental states).

RF can be reliably coded and has been found to be independent of social class, socioeconomic status, ethnic background, education, or verbal intelligence (Fonagy et al. 1991, 1996; Levy 2003). Fonagy and colleagues (1991) found that parental RF mediated the relationship between parental attachment organization and the child's attachment security assessed in Ainsworth's Strange Situation. When both father and mother were rated as having ordinary or high RF, they were three to four times more likely to have secure children than were parents whose RF was rated as low. Fonagy and colleagues (1996) found that BPD patients were rated significantly lower on RF than other psychiatric patients. In addition, in abused psychiatric patients, high RF was a protective factor against the diagnosis of borderline personality disorder.

Attachment and Psychopathology

A number of studies have linked insecure attachment and disorganized attachment status to a range of clinical disorders and conditions, including emotional distress and substance abuse (Riggs and Jacobvitz 2002), BPD (e.g., Fonagy et al. 1996), psychiatric hospitalization (e.g., Allen et al. 1996), and suicidal ideation (e.g., Adam et al. 1996). Attachment constructs have increasingly been used to understand the etiology, treatment, and prognosis of borderline pathology (e.g., Fonagy et al. 1995). For example, clinical researchers and theorists have understood fundamental aspects of borderline conditions, such as unstable, intense interpersonal relationships, feelings of emptiness, bursts of rage, chronic fears of abandonment, and intolerance for aloneness, as stemming from insecure attachment organization (e.g., Gunderson 1996; Levy and Blatt 1999). These theorists have noted that attachment constructs provide a comprehensive model for assessing the representational world of borderline patients.

Attachment and Psychotherapy Outcome

The clinical applications of attachment theory have recently begun to be explored through theory development (Blatt and Levy 2003; Diamond et al. 1999; Eagle 2003; Holmes 1996, 1996; Slade 1999) and empirical methods (Dozier et al. 1994; Fonagy et al. 1996). This research has suggested that patient attachment patterns are both a prognostic indicator of outcome and a vehicle for understanding aspects of the psychotherapeutic process.

Psychotherapy Outcome as a Function of Attachment Status

In the discussion that follows, we should keep in mind that different terms are used in the child and adult attachment literatures to describe conceptually similar patterns. In the infant research, the term *avoidant* is used to describe infants who avoid approaching the caregiver upon her return during the Strange Situation procedure, whereas in the research based on the Adult Attachment Interview, the terms *dismissing* and *dismissively attached* are used. These terms describe individuals who dismiss or devalue attachment relationships. The anxious-ambivalent pattern outlined in infant research is referred to as *preoccupied* in the adult literature. This category is characterized by anxiety about relationships and intense longing. Some self-report measures of attachment have also distinguished between two types of avoidant attachment in adults, dismissing and fearful. *Fearful* avoidant individuals strongly desire close relationships but avoid them out of fear of rejection or disappointment. Lastly, the disorganized/disoriented pattern described in infant literature is referred to as *unresolved/disorganized* in adult literature.

Fonagy and colleagues (1996) found that whereas securely attached patients functioned better than other patients both at admission and on discharge, dismissively attached patients had the greatest amount of relative therapeutic improvement in long-term, intensive, psychoanalytic therapy. Meyer and colleagues (2001), in contrast, found that "securely attached" outpatients had significantly greater improvement in psychosocial functioning over 6 months of treatment than did patients with other attach-

ment patterns. Meyer et al. found that a secure attachment style, in contrast to insecure attachments, was associated with fewer symptoms prior to treatment and with greater therapeutic improvement. Likewise, Mosheim and colleagues (2000) found that securely attached inpatients—patients rated as comfortable and confident in past and present relationships—tended to benefit more than other patients from 7 weeks of inpatient treatment. Cryanowski and colleagues (2002), in a naturalistic study of 162 men and women treated for major depression with interpersonal psychotherapy, found no attachment pattern differences in the recovery rate. They did, however, find that fearful avoidance was related to a longer time to recovery. In contrast, Kilmann and colleagues (1999), using a three-session attachment-focused group for insecurely attached women, found that fearful avoidance predicted the greatest treatment gains. Thus, securely attached patients appear to benefit more than other patients from brief treatment.

Among insecurely attached patients—the dismissively attached—more severely impaired patients appear to do better in long-term intensive treatment (Fonagy et al. 1996; see also Blatt 1992; Blatt and Ford 1994). Meyer and Pilkonis (2002) speculate that patients with "dismissing attachment may require more concentrated interventions, helping them overcome their characteristic detachment. Once they do connect emotionally with a therapist, however, improvement might be all the more dramatic."

Psychotherapy Process as a Function of Attachment Status

With regard to the impact of attachment on psychotherapy process, Hardy and colleagues (1998) examined responses to patient attachment patterns and found that therapists tended to adopt more affective and relationship-oriented interventions in response to clients with preoccupied interpersonal styles and more cognitive interventions with patients characterized by dismissing styles. Hardy and colleagues (1999) studied 16 patients in psychodynamic interpersonal therapy. Consistent with predictions, they found that "therapists responded to preoccupied styles with reflection and to dismissing styles with interpretation" (Hardy et al. 1999, p. 51). Eames and Roth (2000) found that a self-report assessment of attachment patterns of 30 adult outpatients correlated with the quality of their therapeutic alliance and with ruptures in the alliance. Securely attached patients tended to form an effective alliance, whereas fearful avoidant patients tended to rate their alliance as weaker. Interestingly, some evidence also suggested that preoccupied and dismissive attachment styles were both associated with more positive alliance ratings, but for different reasons:

Patients who yearn for intimacy and fear abandonment might strive with particular persistence to establish a close alliance, given their concerns about a possible rejection. In contrast, patients with dismissive styles might defensively deny problems in the alliance or establish only a superficial relationship while remaining reluctant to connect and self-disclose on a more genuine, personal level. (Eames and Roth 2000)

Consistent with this interpretation, preoccupied attachment was associated with more ruptures, and dismissing attachment was associated with fewer ruptures.

Dozier (1990) found that dismissing patients are often resistant to treatment, have difficulty asking for help, and retreat from help when it is offered. Dismissing individuals often become more distressed and confused when confronted with emotional issues in therapy (Dozier et al. 2001). This observation led Dozier and colleagues to study, using the AAI, patterns of relationship between patient and therapist attachment styles. Patients in treatment with therapists who were dissimilar to them on the preoccupied to dismissing dimension of attachment on the AAI had better therapeutic outcomes and stronger therapeutic alliances than their counterparts (Dozier et al. 1994; Tyrell et al. 1999). Clinicians classified as secure/autonomous on the AAI tended to challenge the patient's interpersonal style, whereas clinicians classified as insecure on the AAI were more likely to complement the patient's interpersonal style (Dozier et al. 1994; Tyrell et al. 1999). Patients had the best outcome if treated by securely attached clinicians (defined on the AAI) or by clinicians at the opposite side of the secure/autonomous continuum from the patient (based on AAI classification) (e.g., patient rated preoccupied on AAI and therapist rated at the dismissing end of the autonomous category) (Dozier et al. 1994).

In a second study, Tyrell and colleagues (1999) conducted adult interviews with 54 severely disturbed patients and 21 of their case managers. Patients were usually classified as insecurely attached, whereas most case managers were classified as securely attached. Interactions were found between the attachment styles of patients and case managers on measures of the quality of the alliance, life satisfaction, and psychosocial functioning. Those interactions involved a preoccupied versus dismissive attachment style, indicating that complementary combinations regarding case managers and patients' attachment styles worked best. Preoccupied patients fared best when they worked with dismissing case managers, and dismissing patients fared best with preoccupied managers.

Finally, Rubino and colleagues (2000) had 77 therapists-in-training review video vignettes of simulated ruptures in the therapeutic alliance and then asked them how they would respond when interacting with actual patients. Generally, therapists with anxious-attachment styles tended to respond with less empathy, especially to patients with secure and dismissive attachment. Rubino and colleagues (2000) have speculated that "more anxious therapists may interpret ruptures as an indication of their patients' intentions to leave therapy, and their own sensitivity towards abandonment might diminish their ability to be empathetic" (p. 416).

Consistent with prior research on client-clinician match (e.g., Beutler et al. 1991), the dissimilarities between patients and therapists interpersonal style appear to be advantageous, indicating that patients benefit from interventions that counteract their problematic style of relating to others. Overly emotional patients may require emotion-containing interventions, whereas emotionally detached patients may need interventions that facilitate their affective expression and connection (cf. Hardy et al. 1999; Stiles et al. 1998). Different interpersonal or attachment styles of patients pull for different types of interventions from the therapist (Hardy et al. 1998, 1999). Although preoccupied patients pull for emotional-experiential interventions, they appear to benefit from a more cognitive-behavioral strategy that helps them modulate overwhelming feelings. Likewise, avoidant patients pull for rational-cognitive interventions but appear to benefit from strategies that facilitate emotional engagement (Hardy et al. 1999). Therapists need to recognize how a patient's attachment style influences their response to the patient and their ability to establish a therapeutic alliance.

Attachment Status as a Psychotherapy Outcome Measure

Three studies have employed attachment constructs as a psychotherapy outcome measure. Levy and colleagues (Levy 2003; Levy and Clarkin 2002; Levy et al. 2002) used the AAI to assess change in attachment status and reflective function in 45 patients over the course of a long-term, randomized clinical trial or in patients diagnosed with BPD. Levy et al. found that all but two patients were initially rated as insecure, with the majority having a primary AAI classification of "unresolved" for trauma and/or loss. The majority of patients showed a change in attachment status after 1 year of treatment—some patients shifted from "unresolved" and "insecure" to "secure," others to "cannot classify" or to a mixed attachment. In addition, they found a significant increase in patients' reflective function.

Fonagy and colleagues (1995) reported on changes in attachment status on the AAI amomg 35 nonpsychotic inpatients following 1 year of intensive psychodynamic psychotherapy. Although all 35 inpatients were classified as having insecure attachment during their initial Adult Attachment Interview, 14 (40%) of them showed a shift to a secure classification on discharge. Travis and colleagues (2001) examined change in attachment patterns over the course of time-limited dynamic psychotherapy in 84 clients and found that a significant number of clients changed from an insecure to a secure attachment pattern. Also, significant relationships were also found among changes in attachment, Global Assesment of Functioning scores, and symptom levels.

In summary, the attachment literature suggests that attachment patterns of both patients and therapists influence the process and outcome of psychotherapy. The attachment organization of the patient is expressed in his or her response to the therapist, and these in turn influence the therapist's response to the patient. In addition, the study of attachment organization and the underlying cognitive-affective interpersonal representations of self and other, and evaluation of their change in the therapeutic process, could facilitate further understanding of the mechanisms of therapeutic change (see, e.g., Blatt et al. 1996).

Conclusion and Recommendations

Notwithstanding an often-conflicted relationship between psychology and psychoanalysis and the many obstacles to integration, significant pockets within academic psychology have evolved to contribute both directly and indirectly to psychoanalysis. We have briefly reviewed two areas: unconscious processes and interpersonal relationships (attachment). In addition, as we have seen, psychoanalysis has also contributed much to the richness of psychology. Nevertheless, the relationship between psychoanalysis and psychology is in serious need of repair. Medical psychoanalysis either ignored or was indifferent to academic psychology for many decades. Although there has been a sea change in recent years, with increased interest in the implications of cognitive psychology and neuroscience for psychoanalysis (Westen and Gabbard 2002a, 2002b), and as a result more clinically relevant diagnostic (Westen and Shedler 1999) and psychotherapy research (Clarkin and Levy 2003; Fonagy et al. 1996; Milrod et al. 2000), the neglect has taken a toll on the presence of psychoanalytic viewpoints in academic psychology.

In the 1960s and 70s many psychology departments included psychoanalytically oriented faculty members. A review of the editorial board of the journal *Psychoanalytic Psychology* in the mid-1980s revealed that more than two-thirds of the members were faculty in academic psychology departments and many others held positions in medical schools. Today, less than a handful of the editorial board

members have an academic position. Bornstein and Masling (2002a) note that increasingly fewer psychology departments have psychodynamic clinical faculty members and ever fewer programs list themselves as psychodynamic. Of related interest, in 2001 the American Psychoanalytic Association sponsored a symposium on the relationship between psychoanalysis and academic psychology. Many distinguished psychoanalyst-psychologists participated. When asked about the future of academic psychology, one distinguished participant suggested it might be too late to save psychoanalysis within academic psychology. Another prominent psychologist, an institute director, suggested it might be time for psychoanalysts to abandon psychology departments in favor of humanities departments. Although we appreciate the important perspectives our colleagues from the humanities bring to psychoanalysis, we also believe that psychology brings an important perspective to psychoanalysis and contributes immeasurably to its richness.

In light of the contributions of psychology to psychoanalysis, we believe it is important for psychoanalytic institutes not only to tolerate, accept, and embrace psychological research but to encourage training in cutting-edge research designs and methods. In addition, psychoanalysis has to be more open to findings from scientific disciplines such as psychology. Given the current state of psychoanalytic psychology in academic psychology, we believe it is important to increase the number of psychoanalytically oriented faculty in psychology departments, which can now (with only a few exceptions) be counted on two hands. These faculty will need to become highly sophisticated in basic research methods and constructs, and this may require highly sophisticated nonclinical training. Seed money from psychoanalytic associations will need to be available so that pilot data for larger federally funded grants can be obtained. These psychoanalytic funding sources need to expand the kinds of questions they fund so that instead of individual studies, the infrastructure for research programs can be developed. In addition, we recommend that institutes develop more flexible training programs so that those with both clinical and research-oriented career goals can obtain analytic training. The steps outlined will allow for more direct mentoring of psychology students into both psychoanalytic research and clinical training, and will greatly enrich psychoanalysis.

We end with a quote from Noble laureate Eric Kandel (1998) that we think is relevant:

> The future of psychoanalysis, if it is to have a future, is in the context of an empirical psychology, abetted by imaging techniques, neuro-anatomical methods, and human genetics. Embedded in the sciences of human cognition, the ideas of psychoanalysis can be tested, and it is here that these ideas can have their greatest impact. (p. 468)

References

Adam KS, Sheldon-Keller AE, West M: Attachment organization and history of suicidal behavior in clinical adolescents. J Consult Clin Psychol 6:264–272, 1996

Ainsworth MDS, Blehar ME, Wall S, et al: Patterns of Attachment: A Psychological Study of the Strange Situation. Hillsdale, NJ, Lawrence Erlbaum, 1978

Allen JP, Hauser ST, Borman-Spurrell E: Attachment theory as a framework for understanding sequelae of severe adolescent psychopathology: an 11-year follow-up study. J Consult Clin Psychol 64:254–263, 1996

Bandura A, Walters RH: Social Learning and Personality Development. New York, Holt, Rinehart, & Winston, 1963

Barron JW, Eagle MN, Wolitzky DL (eds): Interface of Psychoanalysis and Psychology. Washington, DC, American Psychological Association Press, 1992

Beutler LE, Engle D, Mohr D, et al: Predictors of differential response to cognitive, experiential, and self-directed psychotherapeutic procedures. J Consult Clin Psychol 59:333–340, 1991

Blatt SJ: The differential effect of psychotherapy and psychoanalysis on anaclitic and introjective patients: The Menninger Psychotherapy Research Project revisited. J Am Psychoanal Assoc 40:691–724, 1992

Blatt SJ, Ford RQ: Therapeutic Change: An Object Relations Perspective. New York, Plenum, 1994

Blatt SJ, Levy K: Attachment theory, psychoanalysis, personality development, and psychopathology. Special issue: attachment research and psychoanalysis, III: further reflections on theory and clinical experience. Psychoanalytic Inquiry 23:102–150, 2003

Blatt SJ, Stayner DA, Auerbach JS, et al: Change in object and self-representations in long-term, intensive, inpatient treatment of seriously disturbed adolescents and young adults. Psychiatry 59:82–107, 1996

Bornstein RF: Critical importance of stimulus unawareness for the production of subliminal psychodynamic activation effects: a meta-analytic review. J Clin Psychology 46:201–210, 1990

Bornstein RF, Masling JM (eds): Empirical Perspectives on the Psychoanalytic Unconscious: Empirical Studies in Psychoanalytic Theories, Vol 10. Washington, DC, American Psychological Association, 2002a

Bornstein RF, Masling JM (eds): The Psychodynamics of Gender and Gender Role: Empirical Studies in Psychoanalytic Theories, Vol 10. Washington, DC, American Psychological Association, 2002b

Claparade E: Recognition and selfhood. Conscious Cogn 4:371–378, 1995

Clarkin JF, Levy KN: A psychodynamic treatment for severe personality disorders: issues in treatment development. Psychoanalytic Inquiry 23:248–267, 2003

Cyranowski JM, Bookwala J, Feske U, et al: Adult attachment profiles, interpersonal difficulties, and response to interpersonal psychotherapy in women with recurrent major depression. J Soc Clin Psychol 21:191–217, 2002

Diamond D, Clarkin JF, Levine H, et al: Attachment theory and borderline personality disorder. Psychoanalytic Inquiry 19:831–884, 1999

Dixon NF: Subliminal Perception: The Nature of a Controversy. London, McGraw-Hill, 1971

Dixon NF: Preconscious Processing. New York, Wiley, 1981

Doidge N, Simon B, Gillies LA, et al: Characteristics of psychoanalytic patients under a nationalized health plan: DSM-III-R diagnoses, previous treatment, and childhood trauma. Am J Psychiatry 151:586–590, 1994

Dollard J, Miller NE: Personality and Psychotherapy: An Analysis in Terms of Learning, Thinking, and Culture. New York, McGraw-Hill, 1950

Dozier M: Attachment organization and treatment use for adults with serious psychopathological disorders. Dev Psychopathol 2:47–60, 1990

Dozier M, Cue KL, Barnett L: Clinicians as caregivers: role of attachment organization in treatment. J Consult Clin Psychol 62:793–800, 1994

Dozier M, Lomax L, Tyrrell CL, et al: The challenge of treatment for clients with dismissing states of mind. Attach Hum Dev 3:62–76, 2001

Eagle M: Clinical implications of attachment theory. Special issue: attachment research and psychoanalysis, III: further reflections on theory and clinical experience. Psychoanalytic Inquiry 23:27–53, 2003

Eames V, Roth A: Patient attachment orientation and the early working alliance: a study of patient and therapist reports of alliance quality and ruptures. Psychotherapy Res 10: 421–434, 2000

Erdelyi MH: A new look at the new look: perceptual defense and vigilance. Psychol Rev 81:1–25, 1974

Erdelyi MH: Psychoanalysis: Freud. New York, WH Freeman, 1985

Eriksen CW: Unconscious processes, in Nebraska Symposium on Motivation, 1958. Edited by Jones MR. Lincoln, University of Nebraska Press, 1959

Eysenck HJ: The effects of psychotherapy: an evaluation. J Consult Psychol 16:319–324, 1952

Fiske ST: Stereotyping, prejudice and discrimination, in Handbook of Social Psychology, 4th Edition, Vol 2. Edited by Gilbert DT, Fiske ST. New York, McGraw-Hill, 1998, pp 357–411

Fonagy P: On the relationship of experimental psychology and psychoanalysis. Comment on "Experimental psychology and psychoanalysis: what we can learn from a century of misunderstanding." Neuro-Psychoanalysis 2:222–232, 2000

Fonagy P, Steele M, Steele H, et al: The capacity for understanding mental states: the reflective self in parent and child and its significance for security of attachment. Infant Ment Health J 12:201–218, 1991

Fonagy P, Steele M, Steele H, et al: Attachment, the reflective self and borderline states: the predictive specificity of the Adult Attachment Interview and pathological emotional development, in Attachment Theory: Social, Developmental, and Clinical Perspectives. Edited by Goldberg S, Muir R, Kerr J. Hillsdale, NJ, Analytic Press, 1995, pp 233–279

Fonagy P, Leigh T, Steele M, et al: The relation of attachment status, psychiatric classification and response to psychotherapy. J Consult Clin Psychol 64:22–31, 1996

Fonagy P, Steele M, Steele H, et al: Reflective-Functioning Manual: Version 5.0. For Application to the Adult Attachment Interviews. Unpublished manuscript, University College London, 1998

Fraley RC, Spieker SJ: Are infant attachment patterns continuously or categorically distributed? A taxometric analysis of strange situation behavior. Dev Psychol 39:387–404, 2003

Freud S: Inhibitions, symptoms and anxiety (1926), in Standard Edition of the Complete Psychological Works of Sigmund Freud, Vol 20. Translated and edited by Strachey J. London, Hogarth Press, 1959, pp 75–175

Freud S: Concluding remarks on the question of lay analysis. Int J Psychoanal 8:392–401, 1927

Friedman RC, Bucci W, Christian C, et al: Private psychotherapy patients of psychiatrist psychoanalysts. Am J Psychiatry 155:1772–1774, 1998

Goldiamond I: Indicators of perception, I: subliminal perception, subception, unconscious perception: an analysis in terms of psychophysical indicator methodology. Psychol Bull 55:373–411, 1958

Greenwald AG: New Look 3: unconscious cognition reclaimed. Am Psychol 47:766–779, 1992

Greenwald AG, McGhee DE, Schwartz JLK: Measuring individual differences in implicit cognition: the Implicit Association Test. J Pers Soc Psychol 74:1464–1480, 1998

Grossmann KE, Grossmann K: Attachment quality as an organizer of emotional behavioral responses in a longitudinal perspective, in Attachment Across the Life Cycle. Edited by Parkes CM, Steveson-Hinde J, Marris P. London, Tavistock/Routledge, 1991, pp 93–114

Grossmann K, Grossmann KE, Spangler G, et al: Maternal sensitivity and newborns' orientation responses as related to quality of attachment in Northern Germany. Monogr Soc Res Child Dev 50(1–2):233–256, 1985

Gunderson JG: Borderline patients' intolerance of aloneness: insecure attachments and therapist availability. Am J Psychiatry 153:752, 1996

Hamilton C: Continuity and discontinuity of attachment from infancy through adolescence. Child Dev 71:690–694, 2000

Hardaway R: Subliminal symbiotic fantasies: facts and artifacts. Psychol Bull 107:177–195, 1990

Hardy GE, Stiles WB, Barkham M, et al: Therapist responsiveness to client interpersonal styles during time-limited treatments for depression. J Consult Clin Psychol 66:304–312, 1998

Hardy GE, Aldridge J, Davidson C, et al: Therapist responsiveness to client attachment styles and issues observed in client-identified significant events in psychodynamic-interpersonal psychotherapy. Psychotherapy Research 9:36–53, 1999

Holmes J: "Something there is that doesn't love a wall": John Bowlby, attachment theory, and psychoanalysis, in Attachment Theory: Social, Developmental, and Clinical Perspectives. Edited by Goldberg SM. Hillsdale, NJ, Analytic Press, 1995, pp 19–43

Holmes J: Attachment, Intimacy, and Autonomy. Using Attachment Theory in Adult Psychotherapy. Northvale, NJ, Jason Aronson, 1996

Hornstein GA: The return of the repressed: psychology's problematic relations with psychoanalysis, 1909–1960. Am Psychol 47:254–263, 1992

James W: The Letters of William James, Vol 2. Boston, MA, Atlantic Monthly Press, 1920

Kail R: The Development of Memory in Children, 3rd Edition. New York, WH Freeman/Times Books/Henry Holt, 1990

Kandel ER: A new intellectual framework for psychiatry. Am J Psychiatry 155:457–469, 1998

Kilmann PR, Laughlin JE, Carranza LV, et al: Effects of an attachment-focused group preventive intervention on insecure women. Group Dynamics: Theory, Research, and Practice 3(2):138–147, 1999

Levy KN: Change in attachment organization in treated patients diagnosed with borderline personality disorder. Invited presentation, Rapaport-Klein Study Group, Austen Riggs Center, Stockbridge, Massachusetts, June 2003

Levy KN, Blatt SJ: Psychoanalysis and attachment theory: developmental levels of attachment. Psychoanalytic Inquiry 19:541–575, 1999

Levy KN, Clarkin JF: Change in social cognition and behavior in borderline personality disorder: a preliminary report. Invited presentation, NIMH, New Directions in Personality Disorder, Minneapolis, Minnesota, May 2002

Levy KN, Clarkin JF, Diamond D: Change in attachment representations in patients with borderline personality disorder during the course of long-term psychotherapy treatment. Paper presented at the Society for Psychotherapy Research, Santa Barbara, CA, June 2002

Lewicki P: Nonconscious Social Information Processing. San Diego, CA, Academic Press, 1986

Lewis M, Feiring C, Rosenthal S: Attachment over time. Child Dev 71:707–720, 2000

Linehan MM: Cognitive-Behavioral Treatment of Borderline Personality Disorder. New York, Guilford, 1993

Main M: Attachment: overview, with implications for clinical work, in Attachment Theory: Social, Developmental, and Clinical Perspectives. Edited by Goldberg S, Muir R, Kerr J. Hillsdale, NJ, Analytic Press, 1995, pp 233–279

Main M, Solomon J: Procedures for identifying infants as disorganized/disoriented during the Ainsworth Strange Situation, in Attachment in the Preschool Years: Theory, Research, Intervention. Edited by Greenberg M, Cicchetti D, Cummings E. Chicago, IL, University of Chicago Press, 1990, pp 95–124

Main M, Kaplan N, Cassidy J: Security in infancy, childhood and adulthood: a move to the level of representation. Monogr Soc Res Child Dev 50:66–104, 1985

Masling J, Cohen IS: Psychotherapy, clinical evidence, and the self-fulfilling prophecy. Psychoanalytic Psychology 4:65–79, 1987

Meyer B, Pilkonis PA: Attachment style, in Psychotherapy Relationships That Work. Edited by Norcross JC. New York, Oxford University Press, 2002

Meyer B, Pilkonis PA, Proietti JM, et al: Attachment styles and personality disorders as predictors of symptom course. J Personal Disord 15:371–389, 2001

Milrod B, Busch F, Leon AC, et al: Open trial of psychodynamic psychotherapy for panic disorder: a pilot study. Am J Psychiatry 157:1878–1880, 2000

Mosheim R, Zachhuber U, Scharf L, et al: Quality of attachment and interpersonal problems as possible predictors of inpatient-therapy outcome (in German). Psychotherapeut 45:223–229, 2000

Naito M, Komatsu S: Processes involved in childhood development of implicit memory, in Implicit Memory: New Directions in Cognition, Development, and Neuropsychology. Edited by Graf P, Masson MEJ. Hillsdale, NJ, Lawrence Erlbaum, 1993, pp 231–264

Poetzl O: The relationship between experimentally induced dream images and indirect vision. Psychological Issues 3 (no 7):41–120, 1960

Reber AS: Implicit Learning and Tacit Knowledge: An Essay on the Cognitive Unconscious. New York, Oxford University Press, 1993

Riggs SA, Jacobvitz D: Expectant parents' representations of early attachment relationships: associations with mental health and family history. J Consult Clin Psychol 70:195–204, 2002

Rubino G, Barke C, Roth T, et al: Therapist empathy and depth of interpretation in response to potential alliance ruptures: the role of therapist and patient attachment styles. Psychotherapy Research 10:408–420, 2000

Sackett DL, Rosenberg WM, Gray JA, et al: Evidence based medicine: what it is and what it isn't. BMJ 312:71–72, 1996

Schacter D: Implicit memory: history and current status. J Exp Psychol 13:501–518, 1987

Schacter DL: Searching for Memory. New York, Basic Books, 1996

Schneider W, Shiffrin RM: Controlled and automatic human information processing, I: detection, search, and attention. Psychol Rev 84:1–66, 1977

Shakow D, Rapaport D: The influence of Freud on American psychology. Psychological Issues 4 (no 13), 1964

Shevrin H, Bond JA, Brakel LAW, et al: Conscious and Unconscious Processes: Psychodynamic, Cognitive, and Neurophysiological Convergences. New York, Guilford, 1996

Shiffrin RM, Schneider W: Controlled and automatic human information processing, II: perceptual learning, automatic attending and a general theory. Psychol Rev 84:127–190, 1977

Silverman LH: Psychoanalytic theory: "the reports of my death are greatly exaggerated." Am Psychol 31:621–637, 1976

Silverman LH, Weinberger J: Mommy and I Are One: implications for psychotherapy. Am Psychol 40:1296–1308, 1985

Silverman LH, Lachman FM, Milich RH: The Search for Oneness. New York, International Universities Press, 1982

Skinner BF: Science and Human Behavior. New York, Free Press, 1953

Slade A: Representation, symbolization, and affect regulation in the concomitant treatment of a mother and child: attachment theory and child psychotherapy. Psychoanal Inquiry 19:797–830, 1999

Sohlberg S, Billinghurst A, Nylen S: Moderation of mood change after subliminal symbiotic stimulation: four experiments contributing to the further demystification of Silverman's "Mommy and I are one" findings. J Res Pers 32:33–54, 1998

Spence DP: The special nature of psychoanalytic facts. Int J Psychoanal 75:915–925, 1994

Stiles WB, Honos-Webb L, Surko M: Responsiveness in psychotherapy. Clinical Psychology: Science and Practice 5:439–458, 1998

Travis LA, Binder JL, Bliwise NG, et al: Changes in clients' attachment styles over the course of time-limited dynamic psychotherapy. Psychotherapy: Theory, Research, Practice, Training 38:149–159, 2001

Tyrell CL, Dozier M, Teague GB, et al: Effective treatment relationships for persons with serious psychiatric disorders: the importance of attachment states of mind. J Consult Clin Psychol 67:725–733, 1999

van IJzendoorn MH: Adult attachment representations, parental responsiveness, and infant attachment: a meta-analysis on the predictive validity of the AAI. Psychol Bull 117:387–403, 1995

van IJzendoorn MH, Bakermans-Kranenburg MJ: Attachment representations in mothers, fathers, adolescents, and clinical groups: a meta-analytic search for normative data. J Consult Clin Psychol 64:8–21, 1996

Waters E, Merrick S, Treboux D, et al: Attachment security in infancy and early adulthood: a twenty-year longitudinal study. Child Dev 71:684–689, 2000

Watson JB: Psychology From the Standpoint of a Behaviorist. Philadelphia, PA, Lippincott, 1919

Weinberger J: William James and the unconscious: redressing a century-old misunderstanding. Psychol Sci 11:439–445, 2000

Weinberger J: The Rediscovery of the Unconscious. New York, Guilford (in press)

Weinberger J, Hardaway R: Separating science from myth in subliminal psychodynamic activation. Clin Psychol Rev 10:727–756, 1990

Weinberger J, Kelner S, McClelland DC: The effects of subliminal symbiotic stimulation on free-response and self-report mood. J Nerv Ment Dis 185:599–605, 1998

Weinfield N, Sroufe A, Egeland B: Attachment from infancy to early adulthood in a high-risk sample: continuity, discontinuity, and their correlates. Child Dev 71:695–702, 2000

Westen D: The scientific legacy of Sigmund Freud: toward a psychodynamically informed psychological science. Psychol Bull 124:333–371, 1998

Westen D, Gabbard GO: Developments in cognitive neuroscience, I: conflict, compromise, and connectionism. J Am Psychoanal Assoc 50:53–98, 2002a

Westen D, Gabbard GO: Developments in cognitive neuroscience, II: implications for theories of transference. J Am Psychoanal Assoc 50:99–134, 2002b

Westen D, Shedler J: Revising and assessing Axis II, Part I: developing a clinically and empirically valid assessment method. Am J Psychiatry 156:258–272, 1999

31

Anthropology

ROBERT A. PAUL, PH.D.

WE NOW HAVE BEHIND us a century that witnessed the emergence, efflorescence, and—it must be admitted—(partial) decline of the fields of both psychoanalysis and (cultural) anthropology. From this perspective, we can take stock of what, if anything, was accomplished in the efforts to forge a link between them.

Relationship Between Psychoanalysis and Anthropology

Parallels

The fields of psychoanalysis and anthropology were both invented by secularized Western European Jews who were close contemporaries: Freud was born in 1856; both Durkheim and Boas, the main founders of the modern academic discipline of anthropology, were born in 1858. Each field represented a challenge to the existing self-knowledge of western civilization: psychoanalysis by revealing unconscious thought "beneath" it, and anthropology by taking a respectful and relativistic empirical approach to other ways of life "outside" it.

Both disciplines take seriously, and try to make sensible, ideas and practices that might seem bizarre or whimsical from the ordinary, rational point of view of the modern Western observer. Both rely for the most part not on the hypothetic-deductive or experimental research method, but on the prolonged immersion of the investigator in the rich and complex details of a particular case. Both also rely

on the subjectivity and interpretive and empathic capacities of the observer. Both disciplines, in principle, straddle and draw on the biological as well as the cultural disciplines, though this dichotomy remains a tension that sometimes veers toward the one and sometimes toward the other pole in both fields.

Both psychoanalysis and anthropology provide opportunities for the typical Western observer to achieve a creative alienation from ordinary habits of thought so as to achieve greater self-awareness. And both disciplines, while having once enjoyed a period of great influence on the intellectual world at large, have now to some degree been relegated to places closer to the corners and margins of informed scholarly and public opinion, for better or for worse.

Differences

Despite the parallels described above, the relationship between the two fields has never been an easy or even a very friendly one, and there are as many forces separating them as those that might seem to unite them. While both ethnographic field work and psychoanalytic clinical work afford to the person who undertakes them unparalleled access to empirical knowledge in depth of the ways of thinking and feeling of other people, there are crucial differences in the way this knowledge is collected and the kind of knowledge that results.

The most obvious difference is that one discipline is a research endeavor, the other a treatment. The people being studied by the ethnographer do not want to change and have not asked to be observed. They put up with the investigation of their lives with varying degrees of willingness, and often with monetary or other inducements. On the other hand, the ethnographer does not require them to delve into matters they would prefer to keep hidden (though they may well volunteer these in the course of conversation). The people observed by the analyst, by contrast, have come voluntarily—indeed, they pay handsomely for the privilege—for the purpose of being treated and, they hope, made better in some way by the process they undergo. In return, they are asked to abandon the usual restraints on discourse and to explore the very matters about which they have the most shame, guilt, and dread. The idiomatic discourse of psychoanalysis, arising as it does from the diagnosis and treatment of disorders, almost inevitably implies that there is something wrong with the object of observation, but this discourse, when applied to ethnography, is bound to rub many people the wrong way by apparently pathologizing the objects of study.

Add to these differences the following—that psychoanalysis is a procedure that can only be conducted with a tiny minority of educated western subjects, and could not logistically or otherwise be carried out in the field under almost any imaginable conditions; that the conduct of psychoanalysis requires of the practitioner a thorough knowledge of the cultural milieu in which both he or she and the analysand live, whereas the ethnographer, by design, attempts to acquire such knowledge from an initial position of ignorance; that the rules of confidentiality and the ethical considerations that should prevail in all our dealings with others normally do not allow the truthful publication of the most interesting and potentially valuable aspects of a psychoanalytic treatment, so that psychoanalysis is in the odd position of having access to vast amount of fabulous data, none of which can be shared with anyone or put to further use—and one can see that the orientation of the psychoanalyst and the ethnographer are, as the great psychoanalytic anthropologist George Devereux (1978) proposed, complementary endeavors that cannot be conducted simultaneously, and even may be, to some extent, mutually exclusive and contradictory.

Devereux's dictum is applicable not just at the intellectual level but also at a highly pragmatic one: not only is it difficult, and in some cases impossible, to receive full professional training as both an anthropologist and a psychoanalyst, but the requirements and commitments of a career carrying out the clinical practice of multiyear, 4- or 5-day-a-week analyses effectively preclude the possibility of also pursuing the long-term residence in another community necessary for good ethnographic research.

Freud's Early Interdisciplinary Foray

In spite of these difficulties, a number of researchers and thinkers over the years have been drawn to the subject matter and intellectual projects of both disciplines. These individuals have sought in various ways to combine the two disciplines, integrate them, incorporate one into the other, or otherwise cross the real boundaries that do separate them. In the 90 years since Freud's fateful foray into anthropology with his book *Totem and Taboo* (1913/1958), a field of "psychoanalytic anthropology" has emerged and flourished and has made a number of contributions to knowledge worth surveying.

Totem and Taboo is based on the premise that customs, practices, and beliefs can be subjected to the same sort of analysis that had already shown such success in making sense of such phenomena as dreams, jokes, everyday slips of the tongue, and, most importantly, the symptoms of the disorders known as the "transference neuroses," as well as the unconscious fantasies that underlie and animate them. This premise reflects the further belief that the history of human civilization follows a unilineal developmental trajectory analogous to the one that characterizes the life span of an individual person. By this analogy, the rituals and beliefs of contemporary society reflect memories of events that occurred during the infancy and childhood of civilization, while the primitive peoples of today give us a glimpse into what life was like during the primordial stages of the evolution of culture. These views represent extensions of the then-current anthropological assumption that human civilization had indeed passed through a series of stages on its ascent to modern civilization, and that contemporary non-Western peoples represented stages now surpassed by the West.

The text to which Freud submits his interpretive theories is *Totemism and Exogamy* by Sir James G. Frazer, a four-volume comparative work that had appeared in 1910 when Sir James's prestige as the great anthropologist of the age was at its peak. Frazer examined the evidence for a link between "totemism"—the supposed original religion of the primordial stage of human life featuring a special set of attitudes toward animals—and "exogamy"—the practice whereby members of clans, named after particular animals and holding that animal sacred, are not allowed to marry clan-mates, but must exchange wives with members of other clans with other animal names.

Convinced that the original form of human life had been the polygynous family (such as that which characterizes gorillas), as Darwin had maintained, Freud hypothesized an event that was supposed to explain how the family, in a precultural state of nature, was transformed into the first level of human culture, that of totemism and exogamy. This well-known theory has it that after the sons of the primal father of the family, or "horde" (as Darwin had called it), rebelled against the involuntary celibacy enforced by the jealous senior male, who maintained a monopoly on sexual relations with the women of the group, and killed and cannibalized him, they were seized with remorse. In retrospective guilt, they imposed on themselves the worship of the now-deified father imagined in animal form, along with the prohibitions on killing the paternal animal and on committing "incest"—that is, sex with women of the same horde (thus renouncing the sexual objects for whom they had committed the crime). Exogamy is just the flip side of the prohibition on incest—one must marry outside instead of within the group if one's group mates are forbidden—while "totemism" is the set of beliefs and customs surrounding the memory of the murder of the primal father (symbolized as the totem animal) and the fear of retribution that followed it.

The Challenge of Cultural Anthropology

Freud's theory of the primal crime was accepted by his early disciples, and it continued to inspire work based on similar premises by a number of analysts, such as Theodor Reik, Otto Rank, and Géza Róheim (about whom more in a moment). But in the field of anthropology (and I will here limit myself mainly to the field of cultural anthropology as it developed in America), the intellectual and professional revolution inspired by Franz Boas at the turn of the twentieth century summarily rejected Frazer and all he stood for: the "armchair" comparative method, the premise that civilization had undergone a single evolutionary or unilineal developmental process, and the consequent belief that contemporary primitives were survivors of an earlier historical epoch. Instead, basing their ideas on the principles of cultural relativism and a belief that there are vastly many human stories, not just one, modern anthropologists were to be first and foremost fieldworkers who immersed themselves as participant observers in the lives and lived worlds of other peoples. These peoples were to be understood in their own terms and through their own eyes, with no assumptions about their place in any hierarchy, evolutionary or otherwise. Works such as Freud's, even without the controversial story of the primal crime and the privileging of the Oedipus complex as the foundation of civilization, now seemed to belong to an antiquated genre from which contemporary anthropologists wished to distance themselves. The reception of *Totem*

and Taboo in anthropology thus ranged from bemused indifference to outright rejection. (In my book *Moses and Civilization*, however, I have rescued Freud's "primal crime" theory, unconvincing as it may be if taken as an explanatory theory, from the dustbin of history and have shown in detail how it accurately analyses the core myth of Judeo-Christian civilization [Paul 1996].)

Malinowski

Ironically, given his characterization in received wisdom as an opponent of psychoanalytic thinking, Bronislaw Malinowski, the great Polish/British anthropologist and ethnographic fieldworker par excellence, was one of the anthropologists most receptive to Freud's ideas, and to the idea of the Oedipus complex, recognizing, as his diaries (1967) make clear, its applicability to himself. His attempt (Malinowski 1927) to delineate a "matrilineal complex" characteristic of the Trobriand Islanders of the Southwest Pacific whom he studied was intended as a "friendly amendment" to psychoanalytic theory, preserving the notion of a core nuclear family complex but replacing Freud's unilineal approach to a supposed world civilization with a viewpoint informed by the new cultural relativism and respect for the diversity of societies. In amending Freud's theory, Malinowski showed that in cultures where descent is reckoned through the maternal line, the leading incestuous fantasies revolve around the sister, not the mother, while the struggles over authority refer to the mother's brother, not the father, as the one who wields power over the young man's fate.

For better or worse, psychoanalysis in the early 1920s was in no mood to have its core tenets challenged in any way, and far from accepting Malinowski's ideas, Ernest Jones (1925) rejected them out of hand. What might have been an alliance based on a synthesis that accepted oedipal dynamics while recognizing the variations in outcome and resolution of them was not to be, at least not just then. But Malinowski's claims did act as a challenge to Géza Róheim, another of Freud's faithful inner circle, who was partially goaded into undertaking fieldwork himself with the explicit intention of refuting Malinowski's ideas about the supposed Trobriand matrilineal complex.

Róheim

Róheim, a Hungarian geographer, folklorist, and anthropologist trained in Berlin, underwent analysis with his countryman Ferenczi and became a fervent adherent of psychoanalysis, and especially of Freud's theory of the primal horde, which he used to organize vast amounts of ethnographic material (gathered and published by others) about the culture of the aboriginal peoples of Australia. He accepted Freud's equation of the thought of neurotic individuals and that of primitive peoples, though he was quick to clarify that this did not imply that primitive people were neurotic: it was their cultural forms, not they themselves, that displayed themes and modes of symbolization typical of the fantasies of Western neurotic individuals. Thus, just as Freud in *Totem and Taboo* compared to Frazer's concept of contagious magic the "contagion" in the thought of obsessional neurotic individuals, Róheim (1992) argued, for example, that a clinical case report on a patient with a phobia about how things were handed to him for fear he would not grow paralleled the widespread belief in folklore that babies must not be handed through windows or over the threshold because they would not grow. He traced this to oedipal dynamics thus: "the house in this case represents a woman, the window represents the vagina, and passing through or lifting over represents coitus. For we know from analysis that a fear that something will not grow is a castration-fear" (p. 13).

This is the sort of apparently formulaic overconfidence in the handling of "symbols" that has won such psychoanalytic interpretations a bad name in many circles. Yet when approached with a sympathic and analytically informed attitude, Róheim's excursions in the vast forest of symbols, customs, and rituals available to him in the ethnographic record of his day should be read today for the many nuggets of insight they contain. He was the first to chart this territory, and in effect he invented the field of psychoanalytic anthropology.

In 1929, with financial backing from Marie Bonaparte and Freud's blessing, Róheim and his wife undertook ethnographic fieldwork in several locales, most importantly the central Australian desert and also the Normanby Islands, close by to the Trobriands and, like them, having peoples with cultures characterized by a matrilineal descent system. Even anthropologists who are not in sympathy with Róheim's psychoanalytic approach continue to regard the quality of his ethnographic work as excellent.

It was no great surprise that he argued, contra Malinowski, that the Normanby Islanders had a regular Oedipus complex despite their matrilineal kinship system. But more importantly, after his fieldwork, Róheim relied less on the primal horde scenario as a key to the decoding of cultural symbolism, and in place of Freud's phylogenetic theory, he developed an ontological theory of cultural difference that was to have wide ramifications (Róheim 1974).

According to this theory, childhood traumas that typically occur in a particular cultural setting lead to a distinctive characterological outcome among adults of that culture, one reflected in institutions that represent projections of childhood fantasies induced by the shared typical trauma.

So, for example, Róheim argued that the hypermasculinity found among the peoples of Central Australia, and reflected in their elaborate men's cults and high valuation of war, can be traced to childhood sleeping arrangements. It is common for mothers to lie on top of their infants during sleep, and this, Róheim reasons, would produce an unusually strong fear among men as they matured of being dominated and rendered passive by women, to which they would then react with unusually strong assertions of male pride and preeminence. By contrast, Róheim identified the key ontological factor among the Normanby Islanders as the custom whereby fathers threateningly take their sons' genitals in their mouths, producing a high level of castration anxiety that leads to the defensive occlusion of paternity and the corresponding elaboration of the idea of *matriliny*, a system of kinship reckoning in which fathers play a minor role.

Kardiner

This formulation of the impact of the childrearing situation on adult character and on cultural and social institutions was systematized by Abram Kardiner (1939; Kardiner et al. 1945), a psychiatrist who had been analyzed by Freud but who took a growing interest in the influence of culture on personality. He developed a model of Basic Personality Structure in the course of his teaching at the New York Psychoanalytic Institute and at Columbia University. Whereas Róheim was trained in both psychoanalysis and anthropology, and had carried out both clinical analyses and ethnographic fieldwork, Kardiner, as a psychiatrist, solved the problem of how to merge psychoanalytic and anthropological perspectives by collaborating with anthropologists, working with them in seminars to arrive at a psychodynamic understanding, for which he provided the expertise, of the data they brought back from the field. Kardiner's model proposed that a society is characterized by certain "primary" institutions, such as the kinship system, itself determined by the system of economic production that prevails. An effect of these primary institutions is a particular form of childrearing situation, such as whether children need to be immobilized by swaddling or a cradleboard to free women for horticultural or agricultural work or at what age weaning can or must take place, given the labor demands on the mother, the availability or lack of alternative caregivers from an extended family, and so on.

The typical childrearing situation, in turn, as Róheim had proposed, leads by way of certain repetitive "traumas" or chronic stressors to a characteristic Basic Personality Structure, in which certain fantasies and dynamic issues are more salient than others because of the experiences the child has in the typical infantile situation. The culture then exhibits a set of "secondary institutions" in the realm of expressive culture, such as art, folklore, myth, religion, and ritual, that reflect in symbolic form the leading concerns and dynamics of the Basic Personality Structure of the group in question.

So, to take an example from Kardiner's collaboration with the anthropologist Ralph Linton (Kardiner 1945), a key primary institution of the Marquesas Islanders of Polynesia is *polyandry*, whereby many men consort with a single powerful woman. Holding sexual attractiveness to multiple partners to be the highest value in this system, women wean infants early so as not to spoil their figures, and also practice the (counter-oedipal) female infanticide that, in turn, perpetuates the surplus of men that produces the need for polyandry. The result is that childhood for Marquesans is orally frustrating and threatening, while oedipal rivalry between boys and fathers is muted because of the relative lack of status of males and the fact of multiple male caregivers, no single one of whom emerges as a powerful rival. The Basic Personality Structure that develops in these conditions is, according to this analysis, focused on greed and frustrated oral strivings, dominated by threatening women, and lacking a father-based superego (which in turn produces the sort of men suited to the unprotesting subordination necessary in the polyandrous household arrangement). It follows as no great surprise, then, that Marquesan secondary institutions, according to Linton and Kardiner, include folklore motifs of cannibal women who eat their children, together with a shifting and diffuse pantheon of gods who can be asked serially for divine favors but who lack any great power to discipline, punish, or reward the worshiper.

Whiting

A major further refinement of the ontogenetic model was developed by the anthropologist John Whiting and his coworkers (Whiting and Child 1953). Whiting was very concerned to frame anthropological propositions as testable hypotheses that would hold up to the canons of contemporary social science research. His ingenious solution to the question of how to do this was to use the comparative data on hundreds of different cultures that he and others had helped compile and catalog in the database known as the Human Relations Area Files (HRAF). This monumental project had attempted to systematize all known ethnographic data by organizing it according to headings such as "kinship system," "supernatural beings," "age at weaning," and so on. Whiting saw that one could use this resource to perform natural experiments to test the causal claims implicit in Róheim's ontogenetic model and Kardiner's Basic Personality Structure theory by seeing whether the

institutions and traits thought to be related held up as correlated in a random sample of cultures from the HRAF. In this way, it was hoped, impressionistic interpretations such as those of Róheim or Kardiner could be either empirically supported or not through objective and quantified tests.

Thus, for example, to test the Kardiner/Linton analysis of the Marquesan material, one could code for two variables, "age at weaning" and "belief in orally threatening female supernaturals," and see how much they were or were not correlated in a random sample of societies from the HRAF catalog. In a well-known real example, Whiting and his co-authors (1958) found a strong correlation between lengthy exclusive mother-child sleeping arrangements (such as those Róheim had observed in Australia) and substantial postpartum sex taboos (often associated with men's cults or other forms of strong separation of the sexes). They then supported the hypothesis that this sleeping arrangement exacerbated the Oedipus complex, leading in turn to secondary institutions (Whiting called them "projective systems") necessary to respond to and resolve these conflicts, such as harsh male initiation rites. Later, Burton and Whiting (1961) revisited the issue and were able to show that cross-sex identity among boys resulting from prolonged exclusive attachment to the mother was a better predictor of strong correlations than was oedipal conflict (though a contemporary observer might not see these as necessarily opposed).

Culture and Personality School

Whereas for a variety of reasons—his Freudian orthodoxy in a culturally relativist time, his ungainly writing style, and his relatively brief presence in the United States—Róheim remained a marginal figure in anthropology, Kardiner's influence spread through the anthropologists with whom he collaborated and out into the world of anthropology in general. Kardiner influenced anthropology to such an extent that his model focusing on the childrearing situation became the standard model for the then-dominant Culture and Personality school of anthropology. Many of the leading figures of this school, such as Ruth Benedict, Margaret Mead, and Gregory Bateson, were not particularly sympathetic to psychoanalysis as such but accepted the fundamental importance of childrearing practices and associated unconscious dynamics or patterns for understanding culture.

The 1940s and 1950s represent the high-water mark of the dominance in American cultural anthropology of the Culture and Personality school, which, whether strictly speaking psychoanalytic or not, accepted the causal importance of childhood and unconscious determinants in behavior and in cultural and social phenomena. Many ethnographies of the time routinely included information on childrearing practices and attempted some sort of synthesis of individual and collective data. Life histories of members of different cultures became prominent as an ethnographic genre, often with either implicit or explicit psychodynamic formulations about character and its relation to culture. The prestige of psychoanalysis was then at its highest in American intellectual life, and the same social class of intelligentsia that was drawn to anthropology for its implied critique of contemporary conformist society was also drawn to psychoanalysis, which still to some degree enjoyed the status of a radical and avant-garde movement. Great anthropologists of the stature of Clyde Kluckhohn (1944), Weston LaBarre (1954), and Anthony F.C. Wallace (1969) incorporated psychoanalytic thought into their work as a matter of course, and clinically trained psychoanalysts such as George Devereux (1951), L. Bryce Boyer (1979), and Erik Erikson (1943) wrote influentially about various Native American societies on the basis of their own ethnographic experience.

Culture and personality theory even became part of the war effort, as distinguished anthropologists were recruited to analyze the cultures of our enemies and allies. Ruth Benedict's great study of Japanese culture *The Chrysanthemum and the Sword* (1946), written from afar during wartime without benefit of actual ethnographic fieldwork, may stand as the prototypical and best representative of this category of works, one that sought to define for each culture a "national character" and placed great importance on childrearing customs. Surely the most notorious and perhaps fateful effort along these lines was *The Great Russians: A Psychological Study* (1950) by Geoffrey Gorer and John Rickman. Rickman, a British psychiatrist and analyst, contributed some very elegant literary sketches, describing his experiences as a doctor with the Friends' War Victims Relief Unit in Russia during the years 1916–1918. But the section by Gorer on Russian national character attempted to draw far-reaching conclusions about Russian character and culture from the widespread practice among the peasantry of "swaddling" infants for most of the first year of life—wrapping them so tightly they were unable to move any but facial muscles, and letting them out only to be nursed and bathed.

Gorer reasoned that while they are swaddled, Russian infants could not explore the world physically to establish the boundary between "me" and "not me." He further supposed that the inability to move and express discomfort would lead to a furious rage that would form a dramatic contrast with the indulgence in movement and sensual pleasure that would characterize those times when the swaddling was removed. At the same time, the restraints

(rationalized by adults as necessary to prevent the otherwise unruly baby from tearing himself apart) would represent security and so would be seen as vital despite the restrictions they imposed. Drawing on Kleinian theory, Gorer assumed that this childhood experience would lead to depression and generalized guilt, combined with a tendency to periodically give way to sensuous indulgence, drinking, and even violence alternating with remorse—a character portrait he was able without much difficulty to find amply illustrated in the pages of Dostoevsky and other writers.

Read with distance and charity today, the "swaddling hypothesis" not only seems fairly reasonable and at least partly accurate but also almost indistinguishable, except for the jargon, from popular and widely accepted contemporary theories derived from the work of Pierre Bourdieu (1977) on what he called the *habitus* (just another word for "character") expressed in a habitual unconscious physical posture and bearing, resulting from the socialization of behavior that leads to typical cultural behaviors. Nonetheless, Gorer's idea became a flashpoint for a reaction against national character studies in general. It was remarkably easy to caricature or ridicule as a reduction of vast sociopolitical forces to "diaperology," as one critic put it. According to critics, national character studies were reductionistic and no different from stereotyping, and erroneously reified "cultures" as coherent units that could be compared and counted, as in Whiting's method, when in fact there is as much personality variation within a culture as between cultures. By the mid-1960s Culture and Personality as a major trend in anthropology was on the decline, and by the 1970s the very term *culture and personality* was gone altogether, replaced by the less provocative and more inclusive *psychological anthropology*, which included not only psychodynamic but also cognitive, social psychological, and other theoretical approaches.

Contemporary Developments

At the same time, challenges and rivals to psychoanalysis, both as a psychological theory of personality and as a therapy, began a steady increase. The 1960s and 1970s saw the emergence of a much more politically engaged stance for many scholars and intellectuals, including anthropologists, in the wake of the antiwar and civil rights movements, and for whatever reasons psychoanalysis began to seem to many to be part of the problem and not part of the solution. The feminist and gay rights movements in particular often portrayed Freud himself and his thought as retrograde, oppressive, and "essentialist" (though of course, many of the most influential feminist thinkers have either been analysts, such as Juliet Mitchell, Julia Kristeva, Nancy Chodorow, and Jessica Benjamin, or others who were at least strongly influenced by or critically engaged with psychoanalysis). In this climate, psychoanalysis ceased to be taken for granted as part of the theoretical armamentarium of the average expectable intellectual, including anthropologists, and was relegated to the sidelines in much of academic psychology as well as psychiatry.

Human Universals and Cultural Variation

Notwithstanding these developments, even as cultural anthropology in its growing postmodernist phase moved away from seeing itself as a positive science and grew distrustful of explanatory theories in general (preferring a more pragmatic, situated, and highly localized critique of inequality), psychoanalysis continued to attract the interest of a small number of anthropologists who were uncomfortable with the loss of cultural anthropology's mission as the empirical and comparative study of humankind, rather than as the ethnographic description of particular historical moments in particular places. Exemplary of such thinkers is Melford E. Spiro, who was originally trained as an anthropologist in the heyday of Culture and Personality but later underwent clinical psychoanalytic training as well. Spiro's analyses of his fieldwork on the Micronesian island of Ifaluk, on an Israeli kibbutz, and in Burma just before the coup that isolated that country (now renamed Myanmar) always included a strong psychodynamic point of view, but he did not challenge the Boasian doctine of cultural relativism until he reexamined Malinowski's *Sex and Repression* (1927), an experience that led to his publication of *Oedipus in the Trobriands* (1982).

In that work, after a careful reading of Malinowski's ethnography, Spiro concluded that the Trobrianders do have an Oedipus complex, indeed a very strong one, and went on to contend that "the only appropriate response to the question, 'Is the Oedipus complex universal' is 'How could it possibly not be?'" (1982, p. 162). The fact that it is universal does not, however, imply for Spiro that it is therefore cross-culturally uniform, which, as the Trobrianders demonstrate, it manifestly is not. This coexistence of universal with cultural variation is possible, Spiro explained, because the Oedipus complex has "three important dimensions— structure, intensity, and outcome" (p. 163), and "although the structure of the Oedipus complex, while variable in principle, seems to be universal in fact, this is not the case in regard to its other two attributes—its intensity and outcome—in which cross-cultural variability is...an ethnographic fact" (p. 164).

Spiro's analysis, whereby cultural variation coexists with human universals, suggests an analogy with Chomskyan linguistics, according to which existing languages, which are certainly very different from one another, are nonetheless different "surface" manifestations of a universal "deep structure." Thus, cultural variation and difference does not imply complete cultural relativity or the notion of the human mind as a "blank slate" filled with ideas from the environment; rather, it allows for a core of something like human nature, itself often incomplete and unmanifest, on which cultural variation is elaborated depending on geographic, historic, ecological, political, and other conditions in the external world. I myself (Paul 1982) used an analogy with Chomsky's "generative grammar" and a modified version of Lévi-Strauss's structural analysis (also implicit in Spiro's interpretation of the Trobriand Oedipus complex) in my attempt to find order and relative unity in a wide array of Tibetan cultural symbolism, taking as my starting point the simultaneous necessity for both conflict and continuity in the process of the succession of generations. I showed how a few specifiable logical dilemmas arising from this situation gave rise to a vast array of symbolic expressions in Tibetan culture, each very different on the surface but similar in representing transformations of the same underlying dynamics.

Evolutionary Psychology

The retreat from radical cultural determinism among some psychoanalytic anthropologists and the positing of some specifiable core universal and possibly innate human characteristics that are amenable to greater or lesser degrees of culturally induced variation, elaboration, and transformation have been paralleled by another theoretical development that has had a major impact on anthropology as well as on many other fields: the development, since the 1970s, of a new evolutionary perspective, appearing first as "sociobiology" and more recently as "evolutionary psychology." The latter owes more than a little to the British psychoanalyst John Bowlby (1969, 1973, 1980), who, like John Whiting, frustrated with the lack of empirical observations and testable hypotheses in psychoanalysis, used evolutionary theory in his formulation of "attachment theory." In this formulation, Bowlby put his Winnicottian psychoanalytic perspective on the preoedipal mother-infant bond into operational form suitable for both field observation and laboratory experiments. In doing so, Bowlby originated the concept of the "environment of evolutionary adaptedness" (EEA), by which he meant the period of a million years or more during which the protohuman ancestors of *Homo sapiens* evolved the biological range of capacities of modern humankind. This period, usually understood to correspond roughly with the Pleistocene, was characterized by human societies in relatively small bands who, without much sophisticated technology, lived by scavenging, hunting, and foraging for wild fruits and vegetables.

According to the theory, it was in this period that elements of "human nature" were evolved as adaptations to that particular lifestyle. The infant relied absolutely on the care and protection of his or her mother for a prolonged period in that environment, leading to a hard-wired capacity for strong early mother-infant attachment that was accompanied by anxiety and depression when this bond was threatened or lost.

The concept of the EEA could of course be generalized more widely, and it led to the view that many behavioral traits observed in modern societies, including many that appear dysfunctional, may have been adaptive when they were evolved but are no longer so under the conditions of modern life in complex technological society. Thus, to take a classic example, a taste for sweets is adaptive in an environment in which ripe fruits grow naturally but are relatively scarce. In a society that produces vast quantities of artificially sweetened products, however, the same craving leads to such symptoms of poor nutrition as obesity, tooth decay, and so on. The premise of evolutionary psychology is that the human mind, far from being either a blank slate or a general information processing device, consists of a large number of specific "modules" (of which Chomsky's universal language acquisition device [LAD] would be the type case) that evolved during the EEA to adapt to living conditions that prevailed at that time, and that these underlie and can explain contemporary behaviors. The latter, in turn, can be tested in the laboratory or in experiments to see if they conform to predictions made on the basis of evolutionary theory.

In a way, this new evolutionary paradigm resuscitates the idea that, as we saw, prevailed in Freud's time to the effect that there was indeed a primordial condition of humankind, and that elements of it have endured in the form of innate capacities and tendencies in the human unconscious even as society, culture, and technology have evolved at a breakneck pace to outdate them. Randolph Nesse and A. Lloyd (1992) have, in this spirit, argued that the classical psychoanalytic defense mechanisms, which are today apparent most usually as symptoms of disorder or pathology, originally evolved as adaptations in the EEA that served inclusive fitness–enhancing functions. By this logic, for example, the mental alertness for potential "contagion" that seemed to Freud (1913/1958) to underlie both obsessive-compulsive anxieties and Frazerian sympathetic magic would, in the EEA, have served an adaptive function by leading to the avoidance of things that really are

"contagious," such as sick or dead people, human waste products, and so forth.

Despite what might appear to be real convergences, psychoanalysis and evolutionary psychology have largely either ignored each other or, in the case of evolutionary psychology, viewed the other as an intellectual fossil rather than as a potential source of insights and hypotheses. This lack of interchange has occurred even though many of the discoveries of evolutionary psychology not only are compatible with but often actually replicate psychoanalytic ideas without attribution. Nevertheless, despite this mutual distrust, some contemporary psychoanalytic anthropologists have attempted to reconcile psychoanalytic and current evolutionary thinking. John Ingham, who had earlier written an ethnography of Mexican folk Catholicism informed by a sophisticated psychoanalytic perspective (Ingham 1986), sought to integrate psychoanalytic, evolutionary, as well as many other contemporary perspectives in his book *Psychological Anthropology Reconsidered* (Ingham 1996). This book might be seen as a contemporary example in the same synthesizing genre as Weston LaBarre's 1954 classic *The Human Animal*. Likewise, *Reinterpreting Freud From a Modern Psychoanalytic Anthropological Perspective*, by Dan Forsyth (2002), is an ambitious integration of psychoanalytic, evolutionary, and sociocultural perspectives on fantasy and, in particular, on what David Spain (1992) has called "oedipality" in *Homo sapiens*. Taken together with Spiro's *Oedipus in the Trobriands* (1982) and the fascinating comparative study of oedipal tales around the world, *Oedipus Ubiquitous*, by Allen Johnson and Douglass Price-Williams (1996), Forsyth's book ought to put to rest any controversy over the question of whether the Oedipus complex exists and is universal. It does and it is, though it is universal as a generative structure subject to locally varying manifestations and transformations in different cultural and social settings.

Life History Determinants and Complex Emotional Factors

At the other end of the spectrum from those intrigued by hard-wired evolutionary commonalities in humans as a basis for psychoanalytic theorizing are those who take the great strength of psychoanalysis to be not its generalizing formulations but rather its close attention to the details of particular lives in the context of the particularities of different cultural settings, with an emphasis on life history determinants and complex emotional concomitants of unique individual actions and choices. Nancy Chodorow's *The Power of Feelings* (1999) is a recent exposition of this position, and so to some degree is Gananath Obeyesekere's *The Work of Culture: Symbolic Transformation in Psychoanalysis and*

Anthropology (1990). Some fine exemplars in this genre would include Vincent Crapanzano's study of a marginalized Moroccan in *Tuhami* (1980), Obeyesekere's study of Sri Lankan women who wear long matted locks and the life history events that have led to their choices in *Medusa's Hair* (1981), and Jean Briggs's detailed study of a few months in the life of an Inuit 3-year-old as she is socialized into her elders' psychosocial world in *Inuit Morality Play* (1998). Waud Kracke's (1981, 1992) exquisitely insightful writings explore the subtle transferential and countertransferential dimensions of the relations between the anthropologist and his friends (and informants) among the Parintintin people of Paraguay.

Gender

The question of gender has dominated much social thought in recent decades, and though psychoanalytic theories about this topic have been far from unchallenged, even within psychoanalysis, psychoanalytic anthropologists have continued to bring to bear on this subject both studies of gender relations in particular societies and attempts at cross-cultural comparisons that may shed light on the nature of human gender more broadly. Spiro's *Gender Ideology and Psychological Reality* (1997), for example, explores the psychodynamics that render belief in the superiority of males and the dangerousness of women among Burmans plausible and motivational, despite their being manifestly false, while David Gilmore, in his comparative study *Manhood in the Making* (1990), finds commonalities in similar beliefs about masculinity in a wide selection of different societies. While such ideologies are in fact more the rule than the exception, they are particularly pronounced and have been studied with great psychoanalytic sophistication in regions such as the Mediterranean world (Brandes 1980; Gilmore 1986; Saunders 1981) and Papua New Guinea (Herdt 1981, 1989; Gillison 1993; Tuzin 1980).

The uncanny similarity of symbolic detail between men's cults in native South America and in Papua New Guinea, two regions with no historic connection to each other, has always seemed to suggest to those open to its implications a degree of commonality in human symbolic and fantasy life that could not be reduced to or encompassed by a purely culturally constructionist point of view. (While a Jungian approach might seem entailed, few anthropologists have been much influenced by Jung.) For example, in both areas, men's cults play on long hollow "flutes" and swing bullroarers (noisemaking instruments fashioned by tying an object to the end of a string and swirling it around) to reproduce the voice of the ancestors, and prohibit women from uncovering these secrets under pain of violent punishment, including gang rape or death. A clas-

sic article by the leading contemporary psychoanalytic student of comparative folklore, Alan Dundes (1976), represents a modern classic of the genre pioneered by Róheim of the psychoanalytic interpretation of ritual symbolism. Dundes traced the symbolism of the bullroarer to male anxieties and concerns about homosexuality and anality.

In their contribution to a recent volume they edited examining the parallels between the two regions, Thomas Gregor and Donald Tuzin (2001) addressed the issues in psychoanalytic terms in a way that may be taken to exemplify the current state of the art in psychoanalytic anthropology. Following Robert Murphy's (1959) question about why, if the Oedipus complex is indeed universal, we aren't all swinging bullroarers, Gregor and Tuzin followed Murphy in supposing that the elaboration of secret men's cults and the ritual symbolism that characterizes them is particularly likely to occur in societies where the social division into same-sex groups is not mitigated by other cross-cutting social ties. In horticultural societies such as those that flourish under the ecological conditions that prevail in the tropical forests of Amazonia and Melanesia, women typically are the garden workers while men hunt and engage in warfare. Each activity is off-limits to the other, but the defensive assumption of male superiority and the threat of women's pollution force the men to be much more secretive and phobic about what they are up to.

Gregor and Tuzin reasoned further that in such societies, while young girls are able early on in their lives to join the older women in gardening activities, boys in middle childhood cannot engage in either hunting or war effectively, and so are excluded from the world of the older men just as their sex excludes them from the world of women. This results in the creation of a relatively isolated and unmonitored subsociety of boys whose fantasy life reflects the concerns and understandings of sexuality, authority, secrecy, taboo, and anality developmentally associated with this age group. These concerns and fantasies then become the dominant ideas of the men's cult these boys go on to form as they enter adulthood.

Here one can see the continuing influence of the Kardiner-Whiting model: the ecology demands a certain economic adaptation—tropical horticulture combined with hunting and war—which in turn leads to a particular social institution—the strong gendered division of labor—at the level of primary institutions. This social institution, in turn, produces as a consequence a particular childrearing situation, in which middle childhood boys are excluded from productive activity and from either adult male or female groups, and so form gangs who indulge in the sorts of fantasies such gangs of boys indulge in everywhere, only much more so. Finally, the childrearing situation having produced a certain set of typical fantasies regnant in the

Basic Personality Structure (of the men), these fantasies inform the ritual symbolism of the secondary institutions, the men's cults and their emphasis on taboo, secrecy, symbols of dominance and hierarchy, ritual purity and pollution, and their policy of "no girls allowed."

Significantly, when Tuzin (1997) returned after a long absence to his field site among the Ilahita Arapesh of Papua New Guinea, he found that the men's cult had quite suddenly collapsed as missionary-inspired Christianity spread in the region. Far from improving matters, however, this collapse led to increases in conflict, especially between men and women, suggesting that cultural forms do indeed act, as Spiro (1965) suggested, as "culturally constituted defense mechanisms" that, far from beings themselves symptoms of neurosis, actually serve to prevent the development of individual neurosis.

Conclusion

As this brief survey has, I hope, demonstrated, the field of psychoanalytic anthropology, despite its distance from any mainstream and the relatively small numbers of its practitioners, has made some highly intriguing and subtle contributions to our understanding of the dynamics of human social and cultural life. The formulations arrived at are as powerful and multifaceted as they are enduring and persuasive. It now remains to be seen what a new century will produce to build on this foundation.

References

Benedict R: The Chrysanthemum and the Sword: Patterns of Japanese Culture. Boston, MA, Houghton Mifflin, 1946

Bourdieu P: Outline of a Theory of Practice. Translated by Nice R. New York, Cambridge University Press, 1977

Bowlby J: Attachment and Loss, Vol 1: Attachment. New York, Basic Books, 1969

Bowlby J: Attachment and Loss, Vol 2: Separation: Anxiety and Anger. New York, Basic Books, 1973

Bowlby J: Attachment and Loss, Vol 3: Loss: Sadness and Depression. New York, Basic Books, 1980

Boyer LB: Childhood and Folklore: A Psychoanalytic Study of Apache Personality. New York, Library of Psychological Anthropology, 1979

Brandes S: Metaphors of Masculinity: Sex and Status in Andalusian Folklore. Philadelphia, University of Pennsylvania Press, 1980

Briggs JL: Inuit Morality Play: Emotional Education of a Three-Year-Old. New Haven, CT, Yale University Press, 1998

Burton RV, Whiting JWM: The absent father and cross-sex identity. Merrill-Palmer Q Behav Dev 7:85–95, 1961

Chodorow NJ: The Power of Feelings: Personal Meaning in Psychoanalysis, Gender and Culture. New Haven, CT, Yale University Press, 1999

Crapanzano V: Tuhami: Portrait of a Moroccan. Chicago, IL, University of Chicago Press, 1980

Devereux G: Reality and Dream: Psychotherapy of a Plains Indian. New York, International Universities Press, 1951

Devereux G: Ethnopsychoanalysis: Psychoanalysis and Anthropology as Complementary Frames of Reference. Berkeley, University of California Press, 1978

Dundes A: A psychoanalytic study of the bullroarer. Man 11:220–238, 1976

Erikson E: Observations on the Yurok: childhood and world image. University of California Publications in American Archaeology and Ethnology 35:257–301, 1943

Forsyth DW: Reinterpreting Freud From a Modern Psychoanalytic Anthropological Perspective. Lewiston, NY, Edwin Mellen Press, 2002

Frazer JG: Totemism and Exogamy: A Treatise on Certain Early Forms of Superstition and Society, Vols 1–4. London, Macmillan, 1910

Freud S: Totem and taboo (1913), in Standard Edition of the Complete Psychological Works of Sigmund Freud, Vol 13. Translated and edited by Strachey J. London, Hogarth Press, 1958, pp 1–161

Gillison G: Between Culture and Fantasy: A New Guinea Highlands Mythology. Chicago, IL, University of Chicago Press, 1993

Gilmore DS: Mother-son intimacy and the dual view of women in Andalusia: analysis through oral poetry. Ethos 14:227–251, 1986

Gilmore DS: Manhood in the Making: Cultural Concepts of Masculinity. New Haven, CT, London, Yale University Press, 1990

Gorer G, Rickman J: The People of Great Russia: A Psychological Study. New York, Chanticleer Press, 1950

Gregor TA, Tuzin DF: The anguish of gender: men's cults and moral contradiction in Amazonia and Melanesia, in Gender in Amazonia and Melanesia: An Exploration of the Comparative Method. Edited by Gregor T, Tuzin D. Berkeley, University of California Press, 2001, pp 309–336

Herdt GH: Guardians of the Flutes: Idioms of Masculinity. New York, McGraw Hill, 1981

Herdt GH: Father presence and ritual homosexuality: paternal deprivation and masculine development in Melanesia reconsidered. Ethos 17:326–370, 1989

Ingham JM: Mary, Michael, and Lucifer: Folk Catholicism in Central Mexico. Austin, University of Texas Press, 1986

Ingham JM: Psychological Anthropology Reconsidered. New York, Cambridge University Press, 1996

Johnson AW, Price-Williams D: Oedipus Ubiquitous: The Family Complex in World Folk Literature. Stanford, CA, Stanford University Press, 1996

Jones E: Mother-right and the sexual ignorance of savages. Int J Psychoanal 6:109–130, 1925

Kardiner A: The Individual and His Society: The Psychodynamics of Primitive Social Organization. New York, Columbia University Press, 1939

Kardiner A, Linton R, Du Bois CA, et al: The Psychological Frontiers of Society. New York, Columbia University Press, 1945

Kluckhohn C: Navajo Witchcraft. Boston, MA, Beacon Press, 1944

Kracke WH: Kagwahiv mourning: dreams of a bereaved father. Ethos 9:258–275, 1981

Kracke WH: Myths in dreams, thought in images: an Amazonian contribution to the psychoanalytic theory of primary process, in Dreaming: Anthropological and Psychological Interpretations. Edited by Tedlock B. Santa Fe, NM, School of American Research Press, 1992, pp 31–54

LaBarre W: The Human Animal. Chicago, IL, University of Chicago Press, 1954

Malinowski B: Sex and Repression in Savage Society. New York, Harcourt, Brace, 1927

Malinowski B: A Diary in the Strict Sense of the Term. Translated by Gutermann N. New York, Harcourt, Brace World, 1967

Murphy R: Social structure and sex antagonism. Southwestern Journal of Anthropology 15:89–98, 1959

Nesse RM, Lloyd A: The evolution of psychodynamic mechanisms, in The Adapted Mind: Evolutionary Psychology and the Generation of Culture. Edited by Barkow J, Cosmides L, Tooby J. New York, Oxford University Press, 1992, pp 601–626

Obeyesekere G: Medusa's Hair: An Essay on Personal Symbols and Religious Experience. Chicago, IL, University of Chicago Press, 1981

Obeyesekere G: The Work of Culture: Symbolic Transformation in Psychoanalysis and Anthropology. Chicago, IL, University of Chicago Press, 1990

Paul RA: The Tibetan Symbolic World: Psychoanalytic Explorations. Chicago, IL, University of Chicago Press, 1982

Paul RA: Moses and Civilization: The Meaning Behind Freud's Myth. New Haven, CT, Yale University Press, 1996

Róheim G: The Riddle of the Sphinx, or Human Origins (1934). Translated by Money-Kyrle R. New York, Harper & Row, 1974

Róheim G: The Significance of stepping over (1922), in Fire in the Dragon and Other Psychoanalytic Essays on Folklore. Edited by Dundes A. Princeton, NJ, Princeton University Press, 1992, pp 11–17

Saunders G: Men and women in southern Europe: a review of some aspects of cultural complexity. Journal of Psychoanalytic Anthropology 4:435–66, 1981

Spain DH: Oedipus rex or edifice wrecked? Some comments on the universality of oedipality and on the cultural limitations of Freud's thought, in Psychoanalytic Theory After Freud: Essays Marking the 50th Anniversary of Freud's Death. Edited by Spain D. New York, Psyche Press, 1992, pp 198–224

Spiro ME: Religious systems as culturally constituted defense mechanisms, in Context and Meaning in Cultural Anthropology. Edited by Spiro M. New York, Free Press, 1965, pp 100–113

Spiro ME: Oedipus in the Trobriands. Chicago, IL, University of Chicago Press, 1982

Spiro ME: Gender Ideology and Psychological Reality: An Essay on Cultural Reproduction. New Haven, CT, Yale University Press, 1997

Tuzin DF: The Voice of the Tambaran: Truth and Illusion in Ilahita Arapesh Religion. Berkeley, University of California Press, 1980

Tuzin DF: The Cassowary's Revenge: The Life and Death of Masculinity in a New Guinea Society. Chicago, IL, University of Chicago Press, 1997

Wallace AFC: The Death and Rebirth of the Seneca. New York, Knopf, 1969

Whiting JWM, Child I: Child Training and Personality: A Cross Cultural Study. New Haven, CT, Yale University Press, 1953

Whiting JWM, Kluckhohn R, Anthony A: The function of male initiation ceremonies at puberty, in Readings in Social Psychology. Edited by Maccoby E, Newcomb T, Hartley E. New York, Holt, Rinehart, Winston, 1958, pp 359–370

32

Literature

EMANUEL BERMAN, Ph.D.

Freudian Approaches to Literature: "Applied Analysis"

Freud as Sensitive Listener and Conquistador

On May 31, 1897, Sigmund Freud wrote to his friend Wilhelm Fliess about Goethe's personal sources of inspiration: "So Shakespeare was right in juxtaposing fiction and madness (fine frenzy)" (quoted in Masson 1985, p. 251). We could think of that moment as a starting point of the stormy love affair between psychoanlysts and literature. To better understand the upheavals of this affair, we need to pinpoint some contradictory sides in Freud's character, clearly expressed in his attitude toward literature and art (Berman 1997b, 2003). We could speak of a tale of two Freuds.

One Freud is the *sensitive listener.* His curiosity, open-mindedness, patience, and empathic capacity enable him to discern subtle nuances and emotional currents both in the life stories of his patients and in novels, poems, and dramas that he avidly reads. This sensitivity was of great help in Freud's self-analysis. Not getting much inspiration from contemporary or past psychiatrists and psychologists, Freud mobilized writers and artists to be his guides. The most striking example again appears in a letter to Fliess, on October 15, 1897:

> I have found, in my own case too, being in love with my mother and jealous of my father, and I now consider it a universal event in early childhood....If this is so, we can

understand the gripping power of *Oedipus Rex*.... Everyone in the audience was once a budding Oedipus.... Fleetingly the thought passed through my head that the same thing might be at the bottom of *Hamlet* as well. (Masson 1985, p. 272)

Oedipus and Hamlet are invited to Freud's couch, to lie side by side with him. "Analyzing" them is an expression not of condescending superiority, but rather of a sense of identification and shared destiny. Numerous literary and theatrical figures—the protagonists of Jensen's *Gradiva* (Freud 1907/1959), Richard III, Lady Macbeth, Ibsen's Rebecca Gamvik (Freud 1916/1957)—are Freud's fantasized siblings in his self-analytic search for insight and relief from his conflicts, anxieties, and depressions.

Freud's excitement with literature is lifelong; we can find in his writings references to all of Shakespeare's plays, as well as to dozens of other writers of his own and earlier generations. Grinstein (1968), in his thorough exploration of Freud's dreams, demonstrated time after time the depth of the influence of books Freud read and how their emotional impact can be discerned in aspects of his dreams, going far beyond his own conscious associations to these books.

The second Freud is the *conquistador,* the youthful admirer of Hannibal who strives to build an empire of his own. This is the Freud who, in his discussion of psychoanalytic studies of literature and art, writes:

> It was only to be expected from the beginning that, whatever the regions into which psycho-analysis might penetrate, it would inevitably experience the same strug-

gles with those already in possession of the field. These attempted invasions, however, have not yet stirred up the attention…which awaits them in the future. (Freud 1914/1957, p. 37)

Of course, there was one Freud, not two. These two sides are interrelated and complementary (Ylander 2001). The courage and stamina of Freud the *conquistador* may have been helpful in allowing him to develop a different mode of listening, utterly different from the professional methods of his milieu (Berman 2002), and they were crucial in gaining broad attention for the subtle insights made by Freud the listener.

Freud's interests in literature were rich and varied. He was intrigued by the relation of art to fantasy (an issue developed in "Creative Writers and Daydreaming" [Freud 1908/1959]), by the impact of the author's life on his or her works of fiction (as studied in "Dostoyevsky and Parricide" [Freud 1928/1957]), and specifically by the relation of writers to their protagonists. He was also concerned with the impact of fiction and drama on the emotions of the readers or the spectators; while comparing, in the October 15, 1897 letter, the effectiveness of Sophocles' dramas with the ineffectiveness of later "dramas of fate," Freud raised the question of audience response as a path to understanding the unique characteristics of particular works. Audience response was further studied by Freud in his work on jokes (Freud 1905/1960), which can give us, alongside clinical studies of transference, a model for exploring the rhetorical-interactional dimension of literature (see Skura 1981, particularly pp. 178–185). And in "The Theme of the Three Caskets" (Freud 1913/1958), Freud explored literary themes with the hope of understanding the deeper layers of human reality. Freud became attentive to his own warning: "But we must stop here, or we may really forget that Hanold and Gradiva are only creatures of their author's mind" (Freud 1907/1959, p. 93).

Of course, our present understanding of the interrelatedness of transference and interpretation, to which I will return, gives us an added perspective on Freud's remarks about Oedipus. We may notice that his reading of *Oedipus Rex* is highly selective. He focuses on the impulses of Oedipus, while bypassing the murderous impulses of Laius (see Ross 1982, who speaks in this context of "the Laius complex"). This bias can be easily related to the shift of responsibility for neurosis from the parent (in the "seduction theory") to the child (in the Oedipus complex model), and to Freud's emphasis on the distorting transference of the patient while disregarding the analyst's actual personality and countertransference, and its impact on the analysand's experience. Such personal biases are unavoidable, of course; taking them into account may reduce our tendency to treat interpretations as discoveries of definitive truth.

The moments when the need to invade and possess became dominant for Freud may have eventually colored the troublesome aspects of "applied analysis," a term which came to be equated in the literary and scholarly milieu with patronizing omniscient tendencies—with reductionistic readings that disregard the rich specific traditions of literature and other arts and treat writers ("pathography") and figures alike as disturbed and ignorant patients awaiting our helpful interpretation. These interpretations, moreover, gradually became too predictable. What was initially a fresh and exciting discovery often turned—a few generations later—into a stale formula.

Elaboration and Critique of Freud's Approach

The interpretations of literature of Freud's early followers often expressed both sides of Freud's position regarding applied psychoanalysis. Otto Rank, for example, was outstanding in the early analytic circle in his systematic scholarship in literature and in cultural history. In *The Double* he introduced numerous examples of the double in literature: works of Heinz Ewers, E.T.A. Hoffmann, Oscar Wilde, Edgar Allan Poe, Fyodor Dostoyevsky, and many others. He studied the biographies of some of these authors, describing them as "decidedly pathological personalities who, in more than one direction, went beyond even that limit of neurotic conduct otherwise allowed to the artist" (Rank 1914, p. 35). He also discussed anthropological theories regarding the double in numerous cultures and concluded with a rich theoretical explication connecting this theme with issues of narcissism.

Ernest Jones's (1949) book *Hamlet and Oedipus* is a thorough exploration of Freud's oedipal interpretation, first mentioned in the 1897 letter to Fliess and spelled out in *The Interpretation of Dreams* (Freud 1900/1953, pp. 264–266). Jones represents the classical tradition at its best, thanks to his thorough knowledge and use of all studies of Shakespeare available at the time; this background enabled him to go, in many points, beyond Freud's intuitive impression. Still, the basic conception is identical, and it has invited many critical and polemical evaluations throughout the years. Questions have been raised regarding the artificiality of reducing Hamlet's matricidal impulse to a theory-derived patricidal core (Wertham, in Faber 1970), or the risk that a narrow emphasis on Hamlet's personal pathology may blind us to his insights into the surrounding social pathology (Friedman and Jones 1963). Jacobson (1989) questions the basic assumptions of Jones regarding the hidden a priori "meaning" of works of literature and their direct relation to the unconscious mind of the author:

By contrast, the author argues that works like *Hamlet* actually subvert the distinctions we ordinarily make between conscious and unconscious intention, between manifest and latent content, even between language and the material world. It is suggested that *Hamlet* itself is peculiarly concerned with the problems and dangers arising from the attempts by Shakespeare's characters to interpret each other's acts and words. Every such interpretation is shown to be ultimately an act of self-revelation. This, the argument concludes, is true not only for the characters in the play, but for each of its readers. (p. 271)

Jacobson presents a more mutual image of literature and analysis: We may turn to the play to better understand our dilemmas as interpreters; Shakespeare may interpret us. The centrality of mutual interpretations (and misinterpretations) within drama has also been studied by Simon (1985), who shows how often such interpretations are central in a play's plot (e.g., in *King Lear*).

Felman (1982) pinpointed a risky paternalistic assumption in "applied analysis": "While literature is considered as a body of *language—to be interpreted*—psychoanalysis is considered as a body of *knowledge*, whose competence is called upon *to interpret*" (p. 5). Spitz (1985) showed how pathography

assumes that creative activity does not represent for the artist a real 'working through' of basic conflict.…This view severely limits the pathographer's capacity to deal with aspects of creating that are relatively conflict-free and prejudices him in favor of the Romantic notion of the artist as deeply troubled, as limited in some way. (p. 51)

The bridge that "applied analysis" erects between art and psychoanalysis may be too narrow, allowing traffic in one direction only: teaching rather than learning. Preoccupied with content, "applied analysis" often reduces attention to the unique structural characteristics of each art, an attention that requires the analyst to become a student in a new field.

Reaction to Psychoanalytic Literary Analysis

As Freud predicted, the psychoanalytic colonialist invasion was met with fierce animosity by local liberation movements with xenophobic views, wishing to expel psychoanalysts (along with Marxists, historians, philosophers and other "intruders") from the homeland of literature. This led at times to shallow, defensive, anti-analytic readings, narrowly focusing on manifest content while avoiding what was beneath the surface, and outlawing the study of the personal context in which the work was created. Both sides were impoverished by the confrontation.

A good example of such impoverishing polarization is the stormy debate about Carroll's *Alice in Wonderland* in the 1930s, when psychoanalyst Paul Schilder (1937/1938) described Carroll as "a particularly destructive writer…[who might] increase destructive attitudes in children…without the help of an adult, the child may remain bewildered, and, alone, may not find his way back to a world in which it can appreciate love relations, space and time and words" (p. 166). Schilder's apparent fantasy of rescuing children from the book's impact aroused many attempts to rescue literature from analysts; critic Joseph Wood Krutch (1937) said: "I have never heard of a child who confessed to being dangerously terrified by 'Alice' or of an adult who attributed his downfall to a trauma received from the book in infancy" (p. 125).

Schilder, in his alarmist tone, disregarded potential constructive developmental uses of Carroll's bizarre world, a point raised by later analytic scholars, starting with Grotjahn (1947, p. 41): "repression and sublimation are achieved easier and with healthier results when the communication with the creative unconscious is kept alive, free and open." At the same time, Krutch—through defensive naivete, and clinging to the surface—denied the potential sources of anxiety in *Alice* and their dynamic significance. Only by transcending that controversy, noticing subjective elements on both sides, and overcoming their blind spots, can we seriously study the complex emotional currents of *Alice in Wonderland.*

Actually, both Schilder and Krutch appear to have been defending against the regressive potential of the book. Krutch did so by denying this regressive potential and clinging to a forced naive view overlooking any anxiety. Schilder did so by projecting and externalizing (e.g., only a disturbed author could imagine such crazy scenes, they are very far from "our" sane world), as well as by seeking mastery through the role of the rescuer. Indeed, both interpretations have a strong transferential quality in their struggle to protect the innocent from danger, whether the potential victim is the child (Schilder) or literature (Krutch). At the same time, we could attempt to study the characteristics of *Alice* through the collective/cumulative response of many different and divergent critics (whether they are professional scholars or naive students—in both cases the range of experiences is similar; see Berman 1993, pp. 3–4, 12–13). What do we learn about the book's ambivalence regarding its protagonist, about its subtle game of touching and not touching, of frightening and pacifying, of uncovering horrors and covering them up whimsically, of being cynical and innocent?

Changing Relationship Between Psychoanalysis and Literature

While several authors (e.g., Baudry 1984) have convincingly emphasized the basic methodological weakness of "applied analysis"—namely, the lack of an analysand who can react to the analyst's interpretation, dispute it, or correct it—Esman (1998) reminds us that "'applied' analysis is a public performance....its interpretations/constructions are...subject to review/reconsideration/correction/rejection by the community of scholars" (p. 745). Moreover, many commonalities can be shown between the blind spots of applied analysis and the pitfalls endangering clinical analytic technique if that technique is based on a "one person psychology" only: an authoritative stance that may at times turn authoritarian, belief in impartial objectivity, a search for veridical reconstructions, insufficient attention to the analyst's subjectivity and the impact of countertransference on interpretation, and images of patients (and artists) as primarily irrational and prone to projective distortions.

In the clinical context, the sharp conceptual separation of transference (explored mostly in patients) and interpretation (attributed solely to analysts) may have blocked the study of the inherent inseparability of transferential currents and interpretive endeavors. These two may intermingle both within the analysand (whose transference may include attempts to figure out the analyst's subjectivity, as Aron [1996] and others have pointed out) and within the analyst (whose interpretive efforts are colored by unique life experiences and transferential reactions to the analysand, unearthing his or her own subjectivity as well). Of course, the unique roles of analyst and analysand are not interchangeable, and their mutual impact must be understood in the context of profound asymmetry; the complex combination of deep mutuality and of disciplined asymmetry contributes to the capacity of the analytic encounter to be illuminating and transforming for both participants.

The same dynamic forces that cast aside for some decades Ferenczi's quest for greater mutuality in the clinical encounter (see Berman 1999, 2004) also blocked for decades any chance for a truly mutual—and therefore neither omniscient nor domineering—illuminating and mutually transforming interdisciplinary encounter between art and psychoanalysis.

Developments in Psychoanalysis

To understand the gradual change in the encounter between literature and psychoanalysis, we must follow some developments within psychoanalysis during the last century.

Decline of Reductionism

One development has been continuous: Reductionism has necessarily decreased with the expansion of psychoanalytic understanding to more aspects of emotional life. As more explanatory models have become available (oedipal and pre-oedipal, drive-related and pertaining to separation-individuation, focusing on conflict or on developmental arrest, rooted in object relations or in self integration, etc.), the need to reduce clinical or literary phenomena to one hypothetical source has decreased, and more respect can be guaranteed to the uniqueness of each person or work of literature.

This trend can be traced to Freud's (1900/1953, p. 283) notion of overdetermination and to Waelder's (1936) concept of multiple function. The latter is already a part of ego psychology, an outgrowth of its increasing emphasis on the multiplicity of human needs mediated by the regulating functions of the ego. This new emphasis added complexity to the psychoanalytic theory of motivation. At the same time, the emphasis on regulation may have moderated some of the more subversive, revolutionary elements of Freud's thought (Wright 1984).

Ego Psychology

Ego psychology (as developed by, e.g., Anna Freud, Heinz Hartmann, Ernst Kris, Erik Erikson) has also contributed to the erosion of Freud's initial dichotomy between manifest and latent (in the dream and in other aspects of personality), resulting in the abandonment of the view of observable phenomena as merely a shell that needs to be cracked and thrown away. Erikson's (1954) reanalysis of Freud's "dream specimen," the dream of Irma's injection, is a good example. Erikson conducts what is actually a careful literary analysis of the dream's text, in which he derives much insight from the narrative qualities of the manifest dream, and then relates it to more latent aspects that can be deciphered only with the help of Freud's own associations and additional knowledge about his life at the time.

The attention to the visible, and the interest of ego psychology in individual differences based on defensive structure, paved the way to a psychoanalytic consideration of issues of style and artistic devices, issues that were out of place in Freud's own content-focused thinking. Questions of sentimentality and dryness, sarcasm and involvement, laconic and expansive treatment of experiences—all are crucial in determining the atmosphere and emotional impact of works of literature. The possibilities of exploring the dynamic (and defensive) significance of form materialize in Holland's (1968) classical work *The Dynamics of Literary Response*. Kris's (1952) concept of "regression in the service of the ego" freed psychoanalysis from a simplistic equation of regression and pathology. (The lack of such a concept was felt, for example, in Schilder's alarmist view of *Alice in Wonderland*.)

Object Relations

A central contribution of object relations models in psychoanalysis is the deepening of our understanding of self-other ("self-object") relations—an issue crucial to the understanding of author-figure, author-story, reader-figure, and reader-story relations, and, in a less direct but no less meaningful way, author-reader relations. It allows us to conceptualize the source of each figure in the author's representational world—self representations and object representations—and to follow its subtle subsequent transformations. Of course, only thorough and rich information regarding the process in which a book or story was created makes it possible to conduct such a study.

All object relations models cast doubt on any simplistic dichotomous division between object and subject, self and other. Margaret Mahler, in studying "the psychological birth of the human infant," taught us how much the separate, individuated existence of one's personality is not given, but is rather a developmental challenge—how much obstacles in the separation-individuation process may sabotage or distort the achievement of this goal. In completely different terms, Melanie Klein emphasized the fluidity of the experiential boundary between self and other—its vulnerability to constant processes of introjection and projection that may lead us to "locate" our contents in the other or "locate" within us experiences of the other. The development of the idea of projective identification (by Bion, Ogden, and others) as not merely an inner fantasy but an actual interpersonal process may make it particularly valuable in understanding the emotional undercurrents of writing and reading. A similar goal is achieved in Heinz Kohut's self psychology through the concept of the *selfobject*, which could be understood as an aspect of the other (parent, initially) that becomes a building block of the self. Both Klein's and Kohut's thinking has been applied to literature (e.g., Layton and Schapiro 1986; Segal 1994; Wolf 1980).

The most profound erosion of the object-subject dichotomy is inherent in the work of D. W. Winnicott, who gave a central role to transitional objects (mostly in childhood) and transitional phenomena (throughout life) that create an intermediate space between self and other and between reality and fantasy: "The place where cultural experience is located is in the potential space between the individual and the environment (originally the object). The same can be said of playing. Cultural experience begins with creative learning first manifested in play" (Winnicott 1971, p. 118). Winnicott's thinking has indeed inspired many applications to literature, although not all questions regarding such an application have been fully resolved (Skura 1981, pp. 185–190).

It is not surprising that object relations models led to a reformulation of the dynamics of the analytic situation and eroded the distinction between interpretation and transference and between objectivity and subjectivity. There is now a strong trend toward conceptualizing the analytic process "primarily as an encounter between two people, rather than as a setting whose purpose is the examination of the intrapsychic process of one of them" (Abrams and Shengold 1978, p. 402). The more modest and self-critical contemporary approach to interpretation is expressed in Winnicott's comment regarding the need for interpretations: "If I make none the patient gets the impression that I understand everything. In other words, I retain some outside quality by not being quite on the mark—or even by being wrong" (Winnicott 1962/1965, p. 167).

Lacan

Another radical challenge to traditional interpretation is Jacques Lacan's view "that the lack of meaning—the discontinuity in conscious understanding—can and should be interpreted as such, without necessarily being transformed into meaning" (Felman 1987). Lacan's (1956/1972) "Seminar on 'The Purloined Letter'" has become one of the most quoted and debated psychoanalytic studies of literature. In contrast to the earlier interpretation of Marie Bonaparte (1933/1949, pp. 483–85), which subjects Poe's story to an examination based on the clinical understanding of psychopathology, Lacan mobilizes literature for an examination of psychoanalysis (through the equation of detective Dupin with the psychoanalyst) based on linguistic and literary understanding. This primacy of linguistic-literary notions may explain Lacan's popularity in academic literary circles, where at times psychoanalysis becomes equated with Lacan's work (a mistaken equation, even in France). Lacan's view that the unconscious is structured as a language, and thus his emphasis on words and verbal nuances in his clinical practice, turned literary scholars into the pioneers of Lacan's thought.

A prominent literary spokesperson for Lacan's work is Shoshana Felman. Her original approach comes into full fruition in "Turning the Screw of Interpretation" (Felman 1982), a study of Henry James's *The Turn of the Screw*. Felman combines a discussion of the story itself with a study of the stormy debate aroused by Edmund Wilson's "Freudian" interpretation of it, published in 1934. The ghosts haunting the governess, the story's protagonist, do not really exist, suggests Wilson: "they are but figments of the governess' sick imagination, mere hallucinations and projections symptomatic of the frustrations of her repressed sexual desires" (Felman 1982, p. 97). This interpretation aroused a barrage of indignant refutations. Felman takes no sides in the confrontation between the two views of the ghosts, "psychoanalytic" and "metaphysical," believing "that the reality of the debate is in fact more significant for the impact of the text than the reality of the ghosts" (p. 98). She shows how central motives of the story (a danger that must be averted, violent aggression inflicted by an injurious alien force, attack and defense, the enemy's defeat) are all repeated in the polemic against Wilson. The story itself can be seen as raising unanswered questions (in its rhetoric, thematic content, narrative structure), but Wilson's attempt to reply to the text's questions is too literal, and "the literal is 'vulgar' because it stops the movement constitutive of meaning" (p. 107). Felman suggests an alternative:

> ...not so much to capture the mystery's solution, but to follow, rather, the significant path of its flight; not so much to solve or answer the enigmatic question of the text, but to investigate its structure; not so much to name and make explicit the ambiguity of the text, but to understand the necessity and the rhetorical functioning of the textual ambiguity. The question underlying such a reading is thus not "what does the story mean?" but rather "how does the story mean?" (Felman 1982, p. 119)

In the process of fulfilling these goals, Felman demonstrates the correspondence between the governess's demand for confession, which leads to her killing the child entrusted to her, and Wilson's attempt to force the text to "a confession," to extort its secret: "To 'grasp' the child, therefore, as both the governess and Wilson do, to press him to the point of suffocating him, of killing or of stifling the silence within him, is to do nothing other than to submit, once more, the silent speech of the unconscious to the very gesture of repression" (Felman 1982, p. 193).

Reevaluation of Countertransference

Skepticism regarding omniscient interpretation goes hand-in-hand with the growing realization that countertransference is omnipresent and unavoidable—that the analyst's emotional life is no less influential than the analysand's. Starting with the pioneering work of Winnicott, Paula Heimann, and Margaret Little, the question of overcoming countertransference gave way to the question of understanding it and attempting to draw on it. Heinrich Racker (1968/1982) noted:

> The first distortion of truth in "the myth of the analytic situation" is that analysis is an interaction between a sick person and a healthy one. The truth is that it is an interaction between two personalities, in both of which the ego is under pressure from the id, the superego and the external world; each personality has its internal and external dependencies, anxieties, and pathological defenses; each is also a child with his internal parents; and each of

these whole personalities—that of the analysand and that of the analyst—responds to every event in the analytic situation...The analyst's objectivity consists mainly in a certain attitude towards his own subjectivity and countertransference. (p. 132)

This view of analyst and analysand as undergoing parallel experiences naturally leads to an important question: If the analyst's interpretive task is colored by (counter)transference, doesn't the analysand's transference to the analyst involve potentially valid interpretive observations? Merton Gill (1982), in his work on transference, goes in this direction and objects to defining transference in terms of distortion. Gill casts doubt on analysts' pretense to be able to judge what is the truth about themselves in order to define what distortion is. He believes transference inevitably combines accurate observations and projections—perceptions of the present and influences of the past. Rather than dismiss the analysand's responses as unrealistic, the analyst accepts their potential realistic dimension, while trying to elucidate their personal meaning in the analysand's life.

Contemporary Perspectives

The present phase of psychoanalysis, with its greater modesty, its distancing from pretenses of being an objective natural science, and its better awareness of our subjectivity and limitations, may supply a more suitable ground for true interdisciplinary bridges—bridges built for two-way traffic, not planned for invasion armies—with other areas in the social sciences and the humanities, as well as with literature and all other arts (Simon 1993).

New Ways of Reading Literature

The study of literature has undergone changes in parallel with the evolution of psychoanalytic thought. In literary studies, the positivistic strictures of New Criticism gave way to greater interest in the subjectivity of the reader as a co-creator of the text (Reader Response Criticism) and to critical deconstructions of the absolute significance formerly attributed to texts (Berman 1993). The renewed legitimacy of biographical research as relevant to the understanding of the personal sources of literature (without the reductionistic, pretensious, and condescending judgments of older "pathography") may pave the way to a fruitful collaboration of analysts and literary scholars in developing an intersubjective model of writing and reading. This implies patiently exploring the full cycle in which a text is created out of the inner world of an artist, colored by the author's self and object representations (which may be creatively transformed into figures with the aid of splits, condensations, and displacements); by the writer's wishes, anxieties, and conflicts; and, in collaborative art such as theater and film, by those of other collaborators as well—actors, musicians, designers, and others. Subsequently, the work acquires numerous additional shades and meanings as it reverberates with the subjective world of each individual reader (or viewer); it is transformed by the unique transitional space created, and at times, when truly effective, it transforms the reader's subjectivity in the process.

The experience of the reader, whether a layman or a professional, is conceived in this perspective as combining an attempt to uncover and spell out the work's meanings, with unavoidably personal identifications and emotional reactions—positive, negative and ambivalent. It therefore necessarily combines transference (to the work of literature as a source of insight and growth), countertransference (the fantasy of author and figures as patients—maybe sick patients—to be analyzed), and interpretation (the striving to understand more deeply). The different transferential currents—transference and countertransference to literature in the sense described here (Felman 1982, pp. 7–8)—cannot be sharply separated, and both levels influence the interpretive effort. This awareness is consistent with the view that no work of literature has a "real" meaning; rather, it acquires a unique meaning for each reader, which is neither a discovery of existing "deep content," nor a "mere projection," but rather a new significance emerging in the transitional space opened up by the fresh encounter (Berman 1997a). This may be said to be an intersubjective exchange between the inner worlds of writer and reader mediated by literature itself.

Of course, our skepticism regarding absolute pronouncements of a work's meaning does not free us from striving to reach thoughtful judgments regarding the relative cogency, consistency, and contribution of various transferentially informed interpretations. One may say, "It's the delicacy of balance, the admissibility of all relevancies and the artful capacity to weigh and prioritize, that leads to interpretations that in turn contribute to ongoing discussions, whether in the clinical situation or in public discussions of aesthetics" (Berman 2003, p. 122).

Psychoanalysis and Literature: A Mutual Endeavor

Changing theoretical trends in psychoanalysis also change our relationship with various aspects of Freud's work. When we become disenchanted with Freud the empire-builder, when we rely less on his grand metapsychology or on his authoritative technique, we are driven back to Freud

the listener. I have in mind in particular Freud's legacy in listening to the individual's inner voice, which is one of his unique contributions. Identification of psychopathology, in comparison, was well developed in psychiatry before Freud; when Freud turned toward pathography, he stepped out of his own unique domain.

To enrich our listening, and to use Freud's unique model creatively, we need to mobilize once more Freud's most reliable allies. Literature and art can become springboards to improving our skills in listening to the other, as well as our self-analytic skills. Artists can do more than become our imaginary patients; they can also serve as imaginary analysts and supervisors. A poem, a story, a film, and our associations and affective reactions to them—all can serve us just as Freud's dreams and associations served him during his pioneering self-analysis. Self-analysis and analytic work on a text, film (Berman 1997a, 1998a, 1998b), or painting can become intertwined and mutually reinforcing, deepening each other. The more creative and unconventional the art, the more art can become "our analyst" rather than "our disturbed patient."

Another aspect of greater interdisciplinary mutuality is our willingness to subject psychoanalytic texts to a literary examination. Well-known examples are Marcus's (1974) study of Freud's Dora case as a work of literature, putting it in the context of novels written around the turn of the century; Mahony's (1982, 1986, for example) thorough studies of Freud's literary style, both in case studies and in theoretical works; Cixous's (1976) reading of Freud's "The Uncanny"; influential readings of Freud by Derrida (1980/1987); and, on another level, the work of psychoanalysts such as Schafer (1980) and Spence (1987), who emphasize narrative and metaphoric elements in psychoanalytic theory as a whole.

As I have already noted, a much closer attention to the analyst's countertransference (in its broadest sense) has been a crucial factor in the progress of clinical psychoanalysis, from Ferenczi onward. This attention has gradually become a part of an intersubjective understanding of the analytic dyad, an understanding that surpasses the early one-sided definitions of countertransference as merely a counterreaction, definitions that had denied defensively the unavoidable mutuality of influence in the comprehensive transference/countertransference cycle ("transference is the expression of the patient's relations with the fantasied and real countertransference of the analyst" [Racker 1968/1982, p. 131]).

Many aspects of the psychoanalytic process, with all its richness and complexity, could be used in studying literature psychoanalytically (Skura 1981). A much greater attention to the role of the analyst's transferences (including the nuances, described earlier, of experiencing the work of art as "patient" or as "analyst/supervisor") may be a crucial condition for progressing toward an intersubjective and interdisciplinary psychoanalytic study of literature, in which psychoanalysts contribute to a deeper understanding of the complex cycle created between author, work of literature, and readers, including the psychoanalyst or the literary scholar as better educated (but still unavoidably subjective) readers.

A fascinating example of fruitfully recasting the role of the psychoanalyst—from an expert striving to objectively discover "true meaning" from behind well-defended and secure closed doors, to an expert whose major expertise resides in a self-analytic attention to his or her own subjectivity in experiencing and interpreting the story—can be found in Eifermann's (1987/1993) study of the personal-biographical determinants of an earlier interpretation she wrote of "Little Red Riding Hood." Through her self-analysis, Eifermann realized that, for example, her focus on the mother's unprotective attitude, and on the girl's overobedient and denying reaction, was related to her own relationship with her mother in childhood, as expressed in two episodes associated in her mind with "Little Red Riding Hood." While Holland (1975) demonstrated how personal-biographical-characterological variables colored the ways a number of students experienced/interpreted Faulkner's "A Rose for Emily" through their individual "identity themes," Eifermann makes it clear that the analyst's professional interpretation can be subjected to the same kind of scrutiny.

The centrality of transferential currents can be demonstrated in opposing interpretations of Kafka's story "The Metamorphosis" (Berman 2003). One is a psychoanalytic interpretation published by a prominent Israeli novelist, Yehoshua (1985). Yehoshua highlights the incestuous wishes of Gregor Samsa directed toward his sister. He analyzes Gregor's metamorphosis into an insect, the central theme of the story, as an anal regression defending against these wishes. Yehoshua continues a line of psychoanalytic interpretations focusing on Gregor's sexual drives and related guilt, although most earlier commentators emphasize not Gregor's desire for his sister but rather oedipal dynamics and punishment by a castrating father: "the motivation of Kafka's conflict ridden psyche and his works… [is] the anxiety resulting from repressed sexual desires… [and] guilt feelings for the murderous intent against the father" (White 1967, p. 194).

An opposite interpretation of Kafka's story is made by Kohut, who speaks of Gregor as "the child whose presence in the world has not been blessed by the empathic welcome of self-objects" (Kohut 1977, p. 287). This line of thought is more fully elaborated by Schaefer (1988), who describes the family as traumatically rejecting Gregor, arousing in him experiences of "depersonalization, estrangement and derealization" (p. 322). A similar viewpoint appears in a stage interpretation of the British director Steven Berkoff, in two productions of a dramatized version of Kafka's story, in England and in Israel, also in the 1980s. (Theater, unlike literature, is an art in which the author's work reaches its audience already mediated by the director's and the actors' transferential interpretations; see Berman 1991.) Berkoff portrays Gregor as an innocent, helpless victim of his disturbed and destructive family, in a way bringing to mind R.D. Laing's view of the identified patient as echoing disguised family pathology.

While both Yehoshua and Schaefer emphasize Gregor's yearnings toward his sister, Yehoshua sees the yearnings as blatantly incestuous; whereas Schaefer believes the sister "becomes for him the mother of early childhood, the feeding, nurturing, mirroring, and confirming preoedipal mother" and contends "there is nothing in the story to suggest that she is the erotically desirable, oedipal mother" (Schaefer 1988, p. 324).

Identifications are prominent in all versions. Schaefer and Berkoff identify with Gregor and are enraged with his selfish, uncaring family. Yehoshua is contemptuous of Gregor and identifies with the suffering of the family, which has to live with its unbearable regressed member. An integrative meta-analysis of the contrasting interpretations of Kafka's story may offer us an additional perspective: "The Metamorphosis" as a story that arouses intense anxiety that the search for "who is to blame" may alleviate, as well as a conflict between opposing identifications (Could it be me? Or is it a remote other, utterly different from me?) The reader's identifications fluctuate (Gans 1998). It is very difficult to remain "outside." We are drawn inward and become—in fantasy—horrified Gregor; we may even become enraged and defiant in a way that he, in his submissiveness, cannot afford to be (Schaefer's or Berkoff's attack on the family). Or, as a defense against such a fearful identification, we become the family members who ostracize monstrous Gregor (Yehoshua's judgmental diagnostic attitude, in which "he is in an anal regression" can be seen as a sublimated version of "he is a disgusting cockroach") and eventually want to kill him.

I believe this example clearly demonstrates the ubiquity of subjective reactions—transferential in the broad sense of the word—in the critical exploration of literture, including its psychoanalytic exploration.

Conclusion

Psychoanalytic explorations of literature will remain heterogeneous. They can benefit from both positive and negative transferences, and our emotions cannot be legislated. But it is worthwhile to pay attention to the general climate of this field. Transference is also *counter*-countertransference, both in the clinical setting and in the interdisciplinary encounter. If we often come with the agenda of showing writers their pathology, from the point of view of our presumed maturity and health, we are likely to arouse defensiveness, antagonism, resistance, and a negative distrustful transference among authors and literary scholars alike. If we more often come with a curious openness to the unique contribution of the other, a more trusting transference may develop, with a better potential for richer joint listening and mutually fruitful contact.

Writers and psychoanalysts meet at times as patients and therapists; but even this real encounter can be conceptualized in various ways. We could focus on the analyst wisely helping the writer with personal difficulty; but we could also notice the analyst's fascination with the writer's creativity and his or her capacity to learn from the patient's insights. Simon (1988), in his study of Bion and Beckett as "imaginary twins," demonstrates the mutual impact these two individuals had upon each other's work for years after their therapeutic encounter in 1934–1935.

The potential for becoming partners in a true interdisciplinary dialogue about literature will increase—I conclude—when we diminish the pretense of objective knowledge and authoritative understanding of "true deep meaning." We may gain more respect and interest if we mobilize a powerful tool we possess, a major component of our analytic legacy from Freud onward: a capacity to listen to subjective and intersubjective nuance, both in ourselves and in the other (be it an actual other, as an author or a critic, or a fictional other, as a figure). This capacity—which is itself related to the artistic-creative side of psychoanalysis as a profession—could help in highlighting the transitional space created among the writer, the work of literature, and readers, thus enhancing our sensitivity to the multiple meanings and complex emotional influences of literature.

References

Abrams S, Shengold L: Some reflections on the topic of the 30th congress: affects and the psychoanalytic situation. Int J Psychoanal 59:395–407, 1978

Aron L: A Meeting of Minds: Mutuality in Psychoanalysis. Hillsdale, NJ, Analytic Press, 1996

Baudry F: An essay on method in applied psychoanalysis. Psychoanal Q 60:69–85, 1984

Berman E: Psychoanalysis and theater: imaginary twins? Assaph: Studies in Theater 7:1–19, 1991

Berman E (ed): Essential Papers on Literature and Psychoanalysis. New York, New York University Press, 1993

Berman E: Hitchcock's Vertigo: the collapse of a rescue fantasy. Int J Psychoanal 78:975–996, 1997a

Berman E: Something there is which doesn't love a wall (on Robert Frost). Psychoanalytic Dialogues 7:641–650, 1997b

Berman E: The film viewer: from dreamer to dream interpreter. Psychoanalytic Inquiry 18:193–206, 1998a

Berman E: Arthur Penn's Night Moves: a film that interprets us. Int J Psychoanal 79:175–178, 1998b

Berman E: Sandor Ferenczi today: reviving the broken dialectic. Am J Psychoanal 59:303–313, 1999

Berman E: The Long Journey: Introduction to S. Freud, Psychoanalytic Treatment (1890–1938) [in Hebrew]. Tel Aviv, Israel, Am Oved, 2002

Berman E: Reader and story, viewer and film: on transference and interpretation. Int J Psychoanal 84:119–129, 2003

Berman E: Impossible Training: A Relational View of Psychoanalytic Education. Hillsdale, NJ, Analytic Press, 2004

Bonaparte M: The Life and Works of Edgar Allan Poe: A Psycho-Analytic Interpretation (1933). London, Imago, 1949

Cixous H: Fiction and its phantoms: a reading of Freud's Das Unheimliche. New Literary History 3:525–548, 1976

Derrida J: The Postcard: From Socrates to Freud and Beyond (1980). Chicago, IL, University of Chicago Press, 1987

Eifermann R: Interactions between textual analysis and related self-analysis (1987), in Essential Papers on Literature and Psychoanalysis. Edited by Berman E. New York, New York University Press, 1993, pp 439–455

Erikson EH: The dream specimen of psychoanalysis. J Am Psychoanal Assoc 2:5–56, 1954

Esman AA: What is "applied" in "applied" psychoanalysis? Int J Psychoanal 79:741–756, 1998

Faber MD: The Design Within: Psychoanalytic Approaches to Shakespeare. New York, Science House, 1970

Felman S (ed): Literature and Psychoanalysis. The Question of Reading: Otherwise. Baltimore, MD, Johns Hopkins University Press, 1982

Felman S: Jacques Lacan and the Adventure of Insight. Cambridge, MA, Harvard University Press, 1987

Freud S: The interpretation of dreams (1900), in Standard Edition of the Complete Psychological Works of Sigmund Freud, Vols 4 and 5. Translated and edited by Strachey J. London, Hogarth Press, 1953, pp 1–715

Freud S: Jokes and their relation to the unconscious (1905), in Standard Edition of the Complete Psychological Works of Sigmund Freud, Vol 8. Translated and edited by Strachey J. London, Hogarth Press, 1960, pp 9–238

Freud S: Delusions and dreams in Jensen's "Gradiva" (1907), in Standard Edition of the Complete Psychological Works of Sigmund Freud, Vol 9. Translated and edited by Strachey J. London, Hogarth Press, 1959, pp 7–95

Freud S: Creative writers and daydreaming (1908), in Standard Edition of the Complete Psychological Works of Sigmund Freud, Vol 9. Translated and edited by Strachey J. London, Hogarth Press, 1959

Freud S: The theme of the three caskets (1913), in Standard Edition of the Complete Psychological Works of Sigmund Freud, Vol 12. Translated and edited by Strachey J. London, Hogarth Press, 1958, pp 291–301

Freud S: On the history of the psychoanalytic movement (1914), in Standard Edition of the Complete Psychological Works of Sigmund Freud, Vol 14. Translated and edited by Strachey J. London, Hogarth Press, 1957, pp 7–66

Freud S: Some character types met with in psychoanalytic work, I: the exceptions (1916), in Standard Edition of the Complete Psychological Works of Sigmund Freud, Vol 14. Translated and edited by Strachey J. London, Hogarth Press, 1957, pp 309–315

Freud S: Dostoyevski and parricide (1928), in The Standard Edition of the Complete Psychological works of Sigmund Freud, Vol 21. Translated and edited by Strachey J. London, Hogarth Press, 1957, pp 177–194

Friedman N, Jones RM: On the mutuality of the Oedipus complex: notes on the Hamlet case. American Imago 20:107–131, 1963

Gans JS: Narrative lessons for the therapist: Kafka's The Metamorphosis. Am J Psychother 52:352–364, 1998

Gill MM: Analysis of Transference. New York, International Universities Press, 1982

Grinstein A: On Sigmund Freud's Dreams. Detroit, MI, Wayne State University Press, 1968

Grotjahn M: About the symbolization in Alice's adventures in Wonderland. American Imago 4:32–41, 1947

Holland NN: The Dynamics of Literary Response. New York, Oxford University Press, 1968

Holland NN: Five Readers Reading. New Haven, CT, Yale University Press, 1975

Jacobson D: Hamlet's other selves. Int Rev Psychoanal 16:265–272, 1989

Jones E: Hamlet and Oedipus. New York, WW Norton, 1949

Kohut H: The Restoration of the Self. New York, International Universities Press, 1977

Kris E: Psychoanalytic Explorations in Art. New York, International Universities Press, 1952

Krutch J: Psychoanalyzing Alice. The Nation 144:124–130, 1937

Lacan J: Seminar on "The Purloined Letter" (1956). Yale French Studies 48:30–72, 1972

Layton L, Schapiro BA (eds): Narcissism and the Text: Studies in Literature and the Psychology of the Self. New York, New York University Press, 1986

Mahony P: Freud as a Writer. New York, International Universities Press, 1982

Mahony P: Freud and the Rat Man. New York, International Universities Press, 1986

Marcus S: Freud and Dora: story, history, case history. Partisan Review 41:12–23, 89–108, 1974

Masson JM (ed): The Complete Letters of Sigmund Freud to Wilhelm Fliess, 1887–1904. Cambridge, MA, Harvard University Press, 1985

Racker H: Transference and Countertransference (1968). London, Maresfield, 1982

Rank O: The Double: A Psychoanalytic Study (1914), Chapel Hill, University of North Carolina, 1971

Ross JM: Oedipus revisited: Laius and the Laius complex. Psychoanal Study Child 37:169–200, 1982

Schaefer M: Kafka's The Metamorphosis: a contemporary psychoanalytic reading. Annual of Psychoanalysis 16:319–339, 1988

Schafer R: Narration in the psychoanalytic dialogue. Critical Inquiry 7:29–53, 1980

Schilder P: Psychoanalytic remarks on Alice in Wonderland and Lewis Carroll (1937). J Nerv Ment Dis 87:159–168, 1938

Segal H: Salman Rushdie and the sea of stories: a not-so-simple fable about creativity. Int J Psychol 75:611–618, 1994

Simon B: The imaginary twins: the case of Beckett and Bion. Int Rev Psychoanal 15:331–352, 1988

Simon B: Criteria for evaluating interdisciplinary papers for the Journal of the American Psychoanalytic Association. J Am Psychoanal Assoc 41:1199–1204, 1993

Simon B: "With cunning delays and evermounting excitement": or, what thickens the plot in psychoanalysis and tragedy? in Psychoanalysis: The Vital Issues, Vol 2. Edited by Gedo J, Pollock G. New York, International Universities Press, 1985

Skura MA: The Literary Use of the Psychoanalytic Process. New Haven, CT, Yale University Press, 1981

Spence DP: The Freudian Metaphor. New York, WW Norton, 1987

Spitz EH: Art and Psyche: A Study in Psychoanalysis and Aesthetics. New Haven, CT, Yale University Press, 1985

Waelder R: The principle of multiple function: observations on overdetermination. Psychoanal Q 5:45–62, 1936

White J: Psyche and tuberculosis: the libido organization of Franz Kafka. Psychoanalytic Study of Society 4:185–251, 1967

Winnicott DW: The aims of psycho-analytical treatment (1962), in The Maturational Processes and the Facilitating Environment. London, Hogarth, 1965, pp 166–170

Winnicott DW: Playing and Reality. London, Tavistock, 1971

Wolf ES: Psychoanalytic psychology of the self and literature. New Literary History 12:41–60, 1980

Wright E: Psychoanalytic Criticism: Theory in Practice. London, Methuen, 1984

Yehoshua AB: An attempt to describe the insect [in Hebrew]. Moznaim 58:7–8, 1985

Ylander F: Discussion of E. Berman's paper, "Reader and writer, viewer and film: transference, countertransference, and interpretation." Presentation at the International Psychoanalytic Congress, Nice, July 2001

33

The Arts

ELLEN HANDLER SPITZ, Ph.D.

ALMOST FROM ITS ORIGINS, psychoanalysis has been applied outside the clinical sphere to works of art and used as a mode of understanding in at least three major areas of concern to those who are involved with the arts: 1) the nature of creative work in the arts and the life histories of artists, 2) the interpretation of works of art, and 3) the nature of aesthetic encounters with works of art. Importantly, unlike clinical psychoanalysts, writers who apply psychoanalytic ideas to the arts do not undertake their projects in response to a presenting complaint, nor have they any therapeutic goal. When the writer interprets art of the past, there is rarely any interpersonal context for evolving transferences. Thus, in the absence of live interpersonal exchanges, interpretations in the realm of the arts normally lack the intersubjective validation fundamental to clinical practice.

Yet, even when the object of inquiry is not a live human being but an *objet d'art*, a literary work, or a musical composition or performance, there continues to be dialogue, for works of art *do* answer back when they are attended to, and the finest of them are endowed with transhistorical powers to co-create and to transform—even if transiently—their viewers and audiences. Therefore, works of art are best seen as relational rather than as fixed. Nonetheless, the applied psychoanalyst differs from the practicing analyst in his or her motives, methods, and goals—all of which are quintessentially nontherapeutic.

Over the years, boundary issues have occasionally interfered with a positive reception on the part of art critics, artists, art historians, philosophers, and scholars in other disciplines toward psychoanalysts who have wandered into the aesthetic domain and toward nonanalysts who have attempted to import psychoanalytic theories into the realm of the arts. These boundary issues concern not only territorialism in its most basic form—that is, protective defense of what is perceived to be one's own rightful space and resentment at the invasion—but also failures on the part of psychoanalytically informed authors to specify the limits of their projects. For reasons such as these, outsiders to psychoanalysis have sometimes considered analytic forays into their territory as presumptuous and unilluminating. Correspondingly, practicing psychoanalysts have occasionally deemed superficial and hyperintellectual the efforts of nonclinical academic authors who draw on psychoanalytic theory mechanically without an experience-near grasp of its richly nuanced emotional implications and unconscious resonances. The danger always looms: superficiality and premature closure.

Sometimes, in my teaching, I have adopted the shortcut strategy of showing examples of psychoanalysis embarrassingly used; I present illustrations of psychoanalysis treated formulaically and of art objects reductively beheld. Here is an example: Describing "Sunrise in the Catskills," a nineteenth-century American Romantic landscape painting by Thomas Cole, an art historian writes:

> The narcissistic assertion of the foreground promontory in its extension into the middleground peak is muted into a more clearly oedipal rivalry between foreground and middleground planes…
>
> The narcissism of the earlier painting…has been replaced by an erotic object attachment, an attempt at both identification and rivalry along oedipal lines…

Despite the maternal promises of the distant meadow-lands, the deepest affective moments within Cole's sublime works remain centered around the male-male conflict of the central space. (Wolf 1982, pp. 185, 194, 201)

The males in question seem to be trees, since there are no human figures depicted. Thus, trees, rivers, flat lands, hills, and peaks all become conflated simplistically with human gender and generational conflict. The notion of narcissism seems egregiously misconstrued. In short, theory is mapped on to a painted image, and, predictably and absurdly, it is found to be a mismatch. Reading such phrases, we can see how jargon stupefies, and how someone who knows too little about the ideas he is using, no matter how perceptive a critic, can easily slip into making a travesty not only of those ideas but of the objects of his inquiry.

However, when psychoanalytic theory as an approach to the arts is more solidly grounded, when it is combined sensitively with other approaches rather than taken as sovereign, and when it is conjoined with qualitatively fine experiences in the arts themselves, the interdisciplinary marriage bears fruit, and the unique value of psychoanalytic ideas in the realm of the aesthetic is made manifest. One stellar example of such excellence is Leo Steinberg's (1984) tour-de-force *The Sexuality of Christ in Renaissance Art and in Modern Oblivion*, in which, without resorting to any jargon whatsoever, Steinberg exploits his deep understanding of psychoanalytic thought to unmask sweeping cultural repressions that have persisted, unnoticed, or denied, and uninterpreted, for centuries.

More contemporarily, Margaret Iverson's forthcoming *Art Beyond the Pleasure Principle* (in press) offers a brilliant, moving, carefully researched discourse on Maya Lin's minimalist, conceptualist, incredibly moving Vietnam War memorial design in Washington, D.C. Iverson makes use of the psychoanalytic notion of the "fetish" to explicate the ways in which a public monument can serve both to disavow traumatic knowledge and, at the same time, to induce memories of trauma by standing simultaneously for and against loss. Drawing on the work of Julia Kristeva (1987/1992), Iverson invokes the image of a scar that heals yet maintains afterward the path of the gash. She quotes psychoanalyst Octave Mannoni's (1969) formulation of fetishism—"I know, but all the same..."—to develop her depiction of Maya Lin's work in the context of the fraught political and ideological battles that stormed around it, mirroring the already deep rifts that had splintered American culture in the wake of this wasteful war. Citing Freud's (1910a/1957) fantasy about the imaginary Londoner who might pause in sorrow before a monument to Queen Eleanor of Aquitaine rather than attend to his present love, Iverson asks whether the purpose (or fate) of such a monument is actually to foster what she calls "the necessary art

of forgetting." Telling her reader the precise moment at which tears filled her own eyes when she walked along the wall for the first time, she reveals how Maya Lin's monument negotiates passages between private grief (the highly polished black granite reflecting each mourner's face as he or she passes by) and public mourning. With the help of psychoanalysis, she demonstrates how Maya Lin's stark design acts like a "lightning rod" for emotions that continue to swirl around the Vietnam War—principally, anger and outrage. Such feelings and attitudes, she persuasively argues, are, by virtue of the monument's design, "displaced onto issues of aesthetics—modernism as against tradition, abstraction as against figurative art." Iverson's interpretive work, in short, stands as an exemplary instance of the application of psychoanalysis to the arts—thoughtful, heartfelt, original, and inspiring.

A Three-Part Paradigm

Following the paradigm mapped out by Spitz (1985), we divide our field of inquiry into three areas previously identified (artistic creativity, the interpretation of works, and the nature and genesis of audience response). Each of these topics correlates with a specific chapter in the development of psychoanalytic theory per se and also with a chapter in the history of criticism in the arts. Freud (1922/1955) said that the best way to understand psychoanalysis is to study its origins and history. Following his counsel, we may take the evolution of psychoanalysis in its relation to the arts as falling into a three-stage sequence beginning with the *Studies on Hysteria* (Breuer and Freud 1893–1895/1955) and *The Interpretation of Dreams* (1900/1953), in which Freud reports his discovery of the dynamic unconscious; develops his notions of repression (mental conflict), repetition, and transference; and maps out a topographic model of the mind. In this first stage, Freud views artistic form as a pleasurable disguise, however complex and elaborate, for content originally derived from forbidden wishes of an erotic and/or an aggressive nature.

With the development of ego psychology (stage two) by Anna Freud (1936/1966), Heinz Hartmann (1939), Ernst Kris (1952), and others, the viewpoint of psychoanalysis toward the arts shifts. Now, rather than taking the buried and disguised wishful content of art as our primary focus, it is the elaboration of artistic form that comes into the limelight. Our new question in this stage has to do with how form arises, and for some authors, form is thought of as representing, at least in part, the relatively autonomous functioning of the ego. Here, in other words, a position is taken that at least some aspects of artistic form develop more or less independently of the drives and of instinctual energy.

Finally, with the advent of object relations theory (stage three), as exemplified by the writings of Margaret Mahler and such British-based authors as Melanie Klein and her followers, especially including D. W. Winnicott, Hanna Segal, and Marion Milner, aesthetic experience is traced back to a young child's first relationship with her mother, to the stages of "symbiosis" and separation-individuation (Mahler 1968, 1972), to play, and to transitional objects and phenomena (Winnicott 1953, 1966)—things and sounds that evoke the qualities of that formative relationship. In this model, a work of art is seen as representing an "intermediate area of experience" (Winnicott 1953) between the self and the outside world. Artistic form and content fuse; any attempt to separate them is considered tantamount to depriving the work of its status as art.

Can these three approaches be integrated, or are they fundamentally incompatible? While psychoanalytic theorists who have attempted to integrate them in the past (e.g., Kernberg 1976) have not altogether managed it, still a measure of unification among the various modes of psychoanalytic interpretation is clearly feasible. In the case of the artist's relation to his or her work, a classical Freudian approach seems highly pertinent in that it traces—via inquiries into the artist's life—the nature of the intrapsychic conflicts that infiltrate, and sometimes motivate, but ever appear masked in many works of art. Here too, however, ego function (as it relates to means, media, method, and style) and object relations theory have their niches as well. In the case of the interpretation of works, ego psychology and object relations theory seem even more relevant in that they are concerned with unconscious fantasy that involves both id and ego; this matters because when we interpret psychoanalytically, we search surface and depth and all the clever ways in which these categories resist and defy their reification. Object relations theory also has much to contribute, from a developmental perspective, to the subject of aesthetic response. Thus, the three approaches do not in fact represent ultimately separable categories but, rather, mutually interdependent interpretive modes.

As an artist, one must continually step back from one's work in progress to appraise it critically and to revise it; as a critic, one's perceptual acuity, inventiveness, general and specialized knowledge, and unconscious fantasy determine to a high degree the quality of one's aesthetic encounters and judgments. As an audience member, one seeks to re-create in imagination, and resonate in fantasy, with many aspects of the works one perceives. Hence, although to separate these contingent categories serves the needs of academic discourse, what actually occurs during creation, criticism, and aesthetic encounters is a set of experiences whose psychic differences consist in emphasis rather than in kind and in which each mode is implicit in the others.

A parallel interdependence may be observed among various aspects of psychoanalytic theory. Thus, early drive theory involved a recognition—as yet unformulated—of an agency in conflict with the drives, later to be developed into ego psychology. And in ego psychology, there is an implicit awareness of and concern with id analysis—with drives and their derivatives, the wishes out of which unconscious fantasies are made and against which specific defenses are mobilized. Moreover, the full analysis of each drive includes a concern with its objects as well as with its aim, impetus, and source (see, in this regard, the work of Pine 1990). Thus, object relations theory is inextricably tied to the earlier paradigms from which it sprang. We would do well, therefore, to regard the analysis of drives, ego psychology, and object relations theory not as separate approaches but as parts of a whole with varying stresses or accents. Similarly, art criticism shifts among expressive, objective, and phenomenological modes, all of which exist on a continuum. The approaches of romantic, formalist, response-theory, as well as ideologically driven and contextual, criticism in the arts and literature are mutually interdependent (see Abrams 1953). Furthermore, because of its absorption into our intellectual and cultural milieus, twentieth-first-century psychoanalysis now plays (although not always openly), in concert with them, a unique and salient role.

Contribution of Freud

Freud's love of and interest in art are well documented by his sizable art and antiquities collection ("I have sacrificed a great deal for my collection of Greek, Roman and Egyptian antiquities," he wrote in 1931, "and actually have read more archaeology than psychology" [letter to Stephan Zweig, September 7, 1931]), as well as by his several papers and books devoted to the subject and the numerous incidental references to art and literature scattered throughout his oeuvre. Although his perspectives on the arts evolved to some extent during his lifetime, his tastes remained stable, and he never attempted to systematize his cultural theories as he did his clinical findings. His general approach—which set the stage for what comes later in the psychoanalytic writings of others in this domain after his death—can, however, be characterized.

Freud's major concern, with few exceptions, is with the relation between an artist's inner life and his artistic product. He sees the cultural object as expressive of, as redolent of, as the result of, internal themes and conflicts. "Art," he states,

> brings about a reconciliation between two principles
> [pleasure and reality]. An artist is originally a man who

turns away from reality because he cannot come to terms with the renunciation of instinctual satisfaction which it [reality] at first demands, and who allows his erotic and ambitious wishes full play in the life of phantasy. He finds the way back to reality, however, from this world of phantasy by making use of special gifts to mould his phantasies into truths of a new kind which are valued by men as precious reflections of reality. (Freud 1911/1955, p. 244)

Through art, in other words, Freud goes on to say, one actually *becomes* the king or hero or the chosen beloved of one's dreams but without expending all the energy necessary and without being blessed with the luck necessary to achieve such goals in the "real" world of living beings. The artist's success, he avers, is predicated on the fact that others share his dissatisfaction with this obligation, that is, to replace the pleasure principle with the reality principle. Art offers ersatz gratification; it confers temporary but highly satisfactory wish fulfillments and ones sanctioned, moreover, by the surrounding culture.

This formulation makes, of course, perfect sense when we apply it to contemporary popular arts, including, if we wish, widely prevalent commercial art, the art of advertising, say, and movies, television shows, hard rock and rap and country and world music, as well as thrillers, mysteries, romantic novels, and even video games (if we are willing to take them too as a species of popular art). And we must not omit the current phenomenon of *Harry Potter*. The explanation works less well, however, for some of the fine art of our day, which, whether gallery- or electronically based, is sometimes so focused on ideological and political themes that it eschews and even mocks aesthetic gratification as an artistic goal, offering scant pleasure to its beholders. A case in point is the prominent international Documenta exhibition held every 5 years in Kassel, Germany, or, closer to home, the Whitney Biennial in New York City.

Freud also emphasizes communication. Interestingly, in this, he concurs with his older contemporary, Leo Tolstoy (1898/1995). The value of aesthetic experience, for both thinkers, stems from a process of identification. Here, however, we must be cautious. Freud does *not* say that the specific latent content of an artist's work must resonate with, be mirrored in, or even be revealed to its viewer. The object of identification that counts, as he sees it, is far more subtle. It is nothing more or less than the quintessential process of circumventing renunciation: what delights an audience and constitutes the very essence of aesthetic experience is, for Freud, the successful outwitting of the censor by making possible the gratification of wishes in fantasy. This is what gives us our deepest pleasures in art. Thus, while instinctual matter lies at the core of all art, it is its elaboration into form by the "special gifts" of the artist that brings about a convergence of reality and

pleasure and provides the grounds for identification and communication.

Speculatively but persuasively, Freud (1908/1959) traces a path from children's imaginative play through daydreaming and fantasy to the work of artists. In various writings (e.g., 1900/1953, 1905, 1907, 1910a/1957), he underscores the continuity of art with other modes of mental functioning, such as jokes and dreams. The artist exists on a continuum with others who are not, at least principally, artists: "Might we not say that every child at play behaves like a creative writer, in that he creates a world of his own, or, rather, re-arranges the things of his world in a new way which pleases him?" (Freud 1908/1959, p. 143). Thus, Freud conjures the image of a child/artist rearranging objects in unique configurations that please him, and in doing so he paves the way for D. W. Winnicott and other more recent writers, who have elaborated this derivation of artistic activity from childhood play. Freud's image also prefigures subsequent theories concerning the experiences of audiences for works of art. When art seems new and compelling, it challenges us implicitly to reorient ourselves. It charges us to reconceive phenomena in novel reorderings that disrupt our previously unexamined assumptions and tastes. It confronts us with truths heretofore unacknowledged and with fresh possibilities for the fusion of our inner and outer realities. It puts us, in other words, into the place of a child who is experimenting. It forces us to create our own world—or at least some aspects of it—anew.

It is important, then, to resist those who would attack Freud for taking art merely as a way of circumventing prohibition by permitting instinctual gratification in an indirect way, for, as we can see, Freud was well aware and profoundly respectful of the potential of art (as content transformed) to bring us in touch with deep inner truths. Freud was not, furthermore, oblivious to his own rather cursory treatment of artistic form. He apologizes for it in the opening paragraph of his "The Moses of Michelangelo":

> I may say at once that I am no connoisseur in art, but simply a layman…the subject matter of works of art has a stronger attraction for me than their formal and technical qualities, though to the artist their value lies first and foremost in these latter. I am unable rightly to appreciate many of the methods used and the effects obtained in art. (Freud 1914/1958, p. 214)

Nonetheless, he speculates on the nature of artistic form by asking us to consider why it is that when ordinary persons tell us their daydreams, we often feel bored or repelled, whereas when the daydreams of artists are transformed into poetry or drama, sculpture, music, or painting, we awaken from our lethargy and experience intense delight. He analogizes the pleasure of artistic form to sexual foreplay in that it gives pleasure of its own while simultaneously readying us for the even greater pleasure we get from the full liberation of sexual tension. He goes on to propose that the artist's work provides a kind of model for us, "enabling us thenceforward to enjoy our own dreams without self reproach or shame" (Freud 1908/1959, p. 153). Thus, Freud hints that form and content work hand in hand and that art, at its strongest, may function to liberate audiences by empowering them to dare to enter into more intimate contact with their own internal worlds, unlocking boundaries that formerly seemed fixed. This notion, which attempts to explain how it is that art can have (as we know it does) such dramatic effects on us, whether via music or dance or theater or literature or visual art, constitutes Freud's most telling contribution to the philosophy of art and to aesthetics. It is, furthermore, a contribution highly pertinent to much of the art of our own time, which, whether or not it eshews ideology, takes risks, shocks into awareness, and opens (both technically and conceptually) onto new horizons that are hallmarks of this new century.

Today's art brings us sensations of human selves that fluctuate and metamorphose not only geographically (through exile and displacement) but also physically. For physical metamorphoses, one thinks of art-related surgeries, as in the disturbing work of the French performance artist Orlan, who has since 1990 undergone a series of plastic surgeries in order to transform her body into new forms modeled on Venus, Diana, and Mona Lisa, thus critiquing the enslavement of women to the ideals of beauty. One thinks also of prostheses, hormonally and surgically induced gender changes, and cyborgs. What is amazing is that Freud's own actual tastes in art, while passionate and highly developed, were clearly retrograde. He clung to the plastic arts of Near and Far Eastern antiquity and preferred them to the exuberant avant-garde art of his own era—in fin-de-siècle Vienna—that swished about him with a dazzling brilliance that failed utterly to gain his notice (see Schorske 1980).

Contribution of Ego Psychology

Since Freud's lifetime, other psychoanalytic authors have dealt with the problems of artistic form and content and made their own significant contributions to our understanding. Notable among them is Ernst Kris, who was an art historian in Vienna at the eminent Kunsthistorisches Museum before becoming a psychoanalyst and who emigrated to New York in advance of the Nazi terrors of the Second World War. In "Aesthetic Ambiguity" (1952), Kris tackles the complex relationships that exist between

artistic production and aesthetic response. He asks how these two experiences are linked. Clearly they are: picture once more the artist who, during the process of creation, simultaneously plays the role of her own evolving work's first consumer and critic. Imagine her as a painter standing motionless, brush in hand, contemplating her canvas for long moments in silence. Physically inert, she is hard at work on the painting. She is also communicating with it as its initial beholder. Here we have a condensed image of the problem Kris addresses. "Aesthetic creation," he states, "is aimed at an audience" (1952, p. 254), and he actually defines as aesthetic *only* those self-expressions that communicate. But here again, as with Freud, we must be careful, for Kris does not mean—reductionistically—that the content of a work, separated from its form, communicates. On the contrary, he understands "communication" to involve far more than what he takes to be the "prior intent" of the artist, as he puts it. Rather, communication consists in "the re-creation by the audience" of the artist's work.

Expressing it this way, Kris comes very close to the notions of two American philosophers who were contemporaries of his, John Dewey (1934) and Susanne Langer (1953), who likewise held that works of art are best taken as mutual co-creations. Authentic responses to works of art, moreover, according to these thinkers, inevitably entail contributions of self. What counts as aesthetic experience is a collaborative, interactive adventure. For Kris, as for Dewey and Langer, artists must not be seen as active while audiences remain passive; rather, both parties should be seen as active. In the example given above, the painter who is standing motionless before her canvas must be understood as fully engaged, absorbed, and active, just as she is when actually daubing the canvas with her brush or mixing her colors.

This notion, of course, matches a quintessential psychoanalytic tenet, namely, that the process of a psychoanalytic treatment, the work of therapy, involves a genuine partnership. Furthermore, although both individuals engage, they need not, and indeed cannot, be engaged in precisely the same way. Kris postulates a similarity between the processes of artist and audience, not an identity. By turning away from the artist's "prior intent," inner conflicts, and away from any preexistent condition that must be unearthed, Kris implies that for communication to occur, what is (or was) emotionally charged for a particular artist at the time of her work's creation need not be so for her audience; thus, information about an artist's life and purposes may be simply irrelevant for our aesthetic experience of any particular work she has created. Emphasis shifts, in Kris's model, from the hidden to the manifest. What matters now is what we can actually perceive in the work itself and what has been presented to us by the work—how it resonates with whatever we bring to it in the moments of our interaction with it. An example that springs readily to mind is the work of the Belgian surrealist painter René Magritte (1898–1967), whose images often seem highly charged and whose symbols are ripe with meaning. When we come upon them in reproduction or in a museum, we may be moved to respond to them emotionally; yet, the actual occurrences in Magritte's own life that caused him to create them may have no manifest connection with the particulars of our own lives (see Spitz 1994 for further discussion).

Central to Kris's approach is the role played by ambiguity. He introduces his notion of the "potential of a symbol," which is "the obverse side of its overdetermination" (1952, p. 255). In other words, as psychoanalysis teaches concerning symbols in general, symbols in works of art arise from a condensation of many psychic (and external) factors, some of which are unconscious—in this case, either repressed or otherwise unknown to the artist. A potent symbol, however, is potent not merely because of its genesis but because it wields the power to initiate a parallel process in its audience and to inspire a multiplicity of associations in us. Importantly, these two phenomena—the repressed matter vis-à-vis the artist and the repressed matter vis-à-vis any individual audience member—need not correspond. They cannot in fact be identical. What is crucial for Kris is that symbols judged to possess genuine aesthetic merit be deemed so on the basis of their ability to stimulate primary process thinking in the members of their audience. A valuable work of art puts us in contact with our own unconscious. This idea comes close to that of Freud when he says that the work of art enables us to enjoy our own daydreams without self-reproach. For both Kris and Freud, then, art offers its audiences a safe realm in which boundaries may be crossed with minimal risk. Kris stresses that to function aesthetically the symbol must involve us in a shift from secondary to primary process.

Yet, although this condition is necessary, it is not sufficient. We can easily imagine nonartistic situations (think of heated political arguments) that generate precipitous shifts in psychic level with no accompanying aesthetic pleasure. Kris adds, therefore, the notion of psychic distance, familiar to philosophers as "aesthetic" distance or "disinterest" (see Kant's [1790/1952] *The Critique of Judgment*). Distance matters because when form and latent content move too close together, we find that we do not have art but something else, for example, pornography or propaganda or magic. To elaborate this point, the failure of aesthetic distance may turn a work into a kind of fetish that actually stimulates erotic feelings and real acts (as in pornography) or political passions and acts (as in propaganda). Impor-

tantly, we might add, going beyond both Kant and Kris, the experience of aesthetic distance is historically and culturally (as well as personally) relative. One looks today at nudes by Titian, Velasquez, or Ingres, for example, contemplatively, just as one looks at Goya's "Executions of May Third" or Picasso's "Guernica" despite their manifest subject matter because their carefully crafted aesthetics and their ambiguities invite a many-layered response rather than primitive emotion and acting out.

When, on the other hand, form and latent content grow too remote, we tend to feel bored with the resultant works; they do not attract us. We are unable to participate in them, and thus we simply withdraw, dismissing them as incomprehensible and worthless. The most effective images avoid these twin pitfalls. They are able to effect changes in us in terms of both psychic level and distance. Redolent of ambiguity, they can and should be interpreted from within the context they themselves create. Therefore, the highest value or best chances for the survival of works of art belong to those works that, according to Kris (1952), possess "as high a degree of interpretability [ambiguity] as is compatible with containing within themselves their own sources of integration" (p. 264). I can think of no finer example of this brilliant point than Shakespeare's 154 sonnets, which, despite all the fraught and perhaps never-to-be resolved questions concerning their genesis and intended recipients, continue to be revered for their subtlety, wisdom, and passion. In this poetry, the implied recipients are incorporated in effect by the poet's use of varied but ambiguous modes of address and intimacies of expression such that to envision any given recipient in one way rather than another will serve to alter all attendant meanings, metaphors, associations, and references—not absolutely, but significantly.

Kris actually uses poetry as an example of ways in which form can alert us to the latent ambiguity of art. Meter and rhyme, for example, give us license to depart from our usual method of reading and invite us to attend differently, to shift our focus from a preoccupation with transparent meaning to the individual components—the words themselves—with their interrelationships, sounds, and musicality, and to the images they conjure and to the structure and rhythms of the text. Apropos, Kris refers to a footnote of Freud's that can be applied to the ambiguities not only within poetry but within the plastic and performing arts as well:

> In a line of associations ambiguous words (or, as we may call them, "switch-words") act like points at a junction. If the points are switched across from the position in which they appear to lie in the dream, then we find ourselves upon another set of rails; and along this second track run the thoughts which we are in search of and which still lie concealed behind the dream. (Freud 1905/1953, p. 65)

This notion of "switch-words," when applied to the reading of poetry, lets us see how form can stimulate primary process functioning. One highly condensed symbol thus takes on new meanings depending on shifts in the context into which it is placed. One might think here of art intended originally to be religious, such as a devotional image (an "Ecce Homo," perhaps—an image of Christ crowned with thorns and displaying his wounds), which, when removed from its church wall niche and placed in an art museum thousands of miles away, sheds its spiritual aura, shifts from sacred to secular, and at the same time achieves, by way of compensation, an enhanced aesthetic, historical, and documentary value. Still, however, as psychoanalysis would have us understand, vestiges of the repressed spiritual meanings continue subtly to inhere, inducing in some beholders an element of the uncanny.

Kris's original concept of "regression in the service of the ego" has fallen into relative disuse among most contemporary psychoanalytic thinkers (however, see Knafo 2002), but it retains its heuristic value for students of the arts. It is a particularly useful notion with regard to the problematic link we have been considering between artistic activity and aesthetic and emotional response. Kris's idea involves the intermittent relaxation of the ego functions (such as thought, planning, control, and critical judgment) so as to permit access to the primary process. He sees the artist not as a prisoner of regressive forces within himself but, quite the contrary, as endowed with a strong observing ego and thus able, to some degree, to regulate the interplay and shifts among psychic levels within himself. Aesthetic creation, according to Kris, is largely purposive and controlled.

A small child's experiences with easel painting are relevant here. Kris (1955) describes how at first a child may be thrilled by the bright colors and viscous texture of the tempera medium and be motivated instinctually to smear and mess with it as she moves her paint-laden brush across the paper. Gradually, however, she becomes fascinated by what is actually happening on the paper itself. She looks at the marks she has made and focuses her attention on her growing ability to manipulate her brush. At this point in the process, instinctual energies are left behind, and the ego begins to function semiautonomously. At this point, the child begins to behave as an artist does. In clinical and developmental terms, Kris (1952) suggests that "as maturation proceeds, as the inner world grows, as new pleasures in fantasy and mastery become accessible, the structure of the activity itself influences the process of neutralization" (p. 37). We might cite the relevance here of this formulation to examples drawn from modern art: Josef Albers's exploration of color relationships, Piet Mondrian's concern with graphic structure and design, Jackson Pollock's

performances of the elastic relations between freedom and order through the medium of calligraphic line. It seems reasonable to describe the activity of these artists as involving, in large measure, skill, technique, and problem-solving capacities—in short, functions of the ego.

Another contemporary of Freud who also contributed to this dialogue on the relation between art and ego is Otto Rank. Briefly, Rank (1932) conceives of form as representing a kind of "ego ideal." Artistic form, he holds, embodies the human desire to transcend our given biological and social determinants. Thus, it reveals—in architecture especially perhaps—the attempt of human beings to gain control over aspects of the external environment. At the same time, however, Rank explains recurring elements in aesthetic form by tracing them to biological sources. The spiral, for example, which is a ubiquitous design used frequently to ornament ancient pottery, is derived by him from the human intestines, and similar examples abound. Our sense of rhythm may emanate from infantile somatic sensations, and our emotional responses to music may correlate with an affinity between its tempo and the pulse. Studies show, moreover, that, while we listen to music, our bodies sometimes react by releasing endorphins, a phenomenon that explains why music often serves as an alleviator of pain (Langone 2003). Yet another psychoanalytic author, Phyllis Greenacre (1957/1971), writing about the childhood of artists, underscores Rank's interest in biological *Anlagen* by deriving a predisposition toward later adult aesthetic experience from a heightened and broadly based sensuality in early childhood.

It is important before leaving the field of ego psychology to point out that, within it, a psychoanalytic approach that depends *purely* on the so-called autonomous functions of the ego would suffer from twin shortcomings. One is that it would remove itself from the wellsprings of psychoanalytic thought, which are founded on notions of unconscious conflict and fantasy derived from the vicissitudes of instinctual pleasures as they struggle repetitively, ingeniously, and valiantly against various forms of internal and external resistance. The other is that an exclusive preoccupation with form can be limiting. Formal problems are often diverting, it is true, and their solutions fascinating; not all form carries meaning. For a work of art to be truly great, there must be content in Freud's sense—that is, not merely perception but a reaching down into the depths of the unconscious. Aristotle understood this when he spoke of a catharsis of pity and fear, and perhaps the greatest artists of every age have known it. Although we can (and do) spend many profitable hours dwelling on form and technique in Rembrandt, Goya, or Van Gogh, their works have survived because their content is nontrivial. They have painted the deepest fears and wishes of mankind.

Contribution of Object Relations Theory

Prototypically developmental, the approach of D.W. Winnicott to the arts is best found in his seminal paper on the transitional object (Winnicott 1953). The blanket or soft toy animal is taken by Winnicott to be a precursor of an adult's eventual investment in cultural objects of many kinds, including works of art. Winnicott regards the baby's blanket as transitional in several senses: it is a step along the way to full symbolization; it is transitional in that any question as to whether its soothing properties are inherent within it or are created by the baby himself must remain unasked and labile; and it represents a developmental marker between total dependence on an object and relative independence from it, an independence that accrues from the internalization of an ego-supportive environment. Thus, a child's attachment to a transitional object betokens the fact that he or she is well on the way toward internalization. (I am indebted for this description of the transitional object to a personal communication from Dr. Morris Eagle, October 9, 2003.) Winnicott sees attachments to transitional object as normal, healthy, and, even possibly with modifications, universal in development and claims that the highly personal significance they manifest is a function of whatever reciprocal cuing develops in the mother-child partnership. From this attachment, Winnicott derives an individual's capacity not only to invest in cultural objects and experiences of all kinds but also to forge creative links between inner and outer worlds. Like Freud, he cites—with great respect—children's imaginative play and claims that it forms a bridge between infantile illusion or fantasy—objectified initially in the transitional object—and aesthetic experiences in adulthood, a line of thought pursued also by Greenacre (1971) in her work on the childhood of the artist.

Winnicott stresses that the question we must never ask a child about her teddy bear or blanket is "Did you *make* this object or did you *find* it?" This is because, as with an artist, the child's experience includes both of these modes, and to challenge her might inhibit her further from elaboration of fantasy. Instead of intruding with our rationalism, we must be knowingly complicit in her transformation of the ragged blanket or scruffy toy into a supremely valued object.

Taking this, then, as paradigmatic of our relationships to works of art, we see how a radical separation of form from content destroys any work as art and any experience as aesthetic. This is so because such a severing involves moving outside the experience in such a way that the experience is reduced to something less or other than what

it was. An analogy to the psychoanalytic situation seems apt. The psychoanalyst operates within boundaries given by a developing dialogue that takes place between two individuals, and ideally he or she does not interrupt this privileged space-time to introduce material from outside or to judge the emerging material on grounds imported from elsewhere. The treatment, therefore, seen in this Winnicottian light, resembles a field of play; like a work of art, it comes gradually into being over time during the enactment per se.

A distinctive feature of Winnicott's theory is that whereas Freud concerns himself almost exclusively with intrapsychic processes, Winnicott posits a third area of experience, an "intermediate space," as he terms it, in which inner and outer, fantasy and reality, are commingled. He is alive, furthermore, to the "thing-ness" of the art object. His theory has special resonance for the dramatic and performing arts, in which his so-called intermediate space can actually be seen as the very stage itself and all that transpires thereon. Transitional phenomena, moreover, differ from dreams and daydreams in that they are not purely mental constructs. Transitional objects have palpable representation and existence in the external world. They cannot, therefore—as is true likewise of materials, instruments, and tools used by artists—be easily controlled. As mothers know to their chagrin, blankets are frequently lost. With respect to working artists, Winnicott implicitly reminds us that, whatever conflicts and secret desires he may have, an artist must cope every day in his studio with the recalcitrances of paint or stone, with the vagaries of his computer, with the technicalities of his camera, with the delicate adjustments of his untuned harp, or with, perhaps, the limitations of even the most agile human body moving through space.

As has been noted, there is a clear interdependence among various modes of aesthetic experience. Philosophers interested in understanding and describing this interdependence have sometimes spoken of experiencing an art work from within and from without. Most of us do, in fact, when attending a concert or an opera, or when visiting an art gallery, alternate between full absorption in the art or music and a return to a clear consciousness of self. The "aesthetic distance" between ourselves and any composition varies as we experience it. What does psychoanalysis have to offer by way of explanation of the most privileged of such moments when, in an aesthetic encounter, we find ourselves fully transported "within" a work of art, feel fused with it, and the illusion becomes real? When we dwell momentarily within its aura of magic and power?

Such moments are characterized by a deep rapport of subject and object—a state in which, as psychoanalyst

Christopher Bollas (1978) notes, the subject feels "captured in a reverential moment with an aesthetic object" (p. 394) by a "spell which holds self and other in symmetry and solitude [in which] time crystallizes into space [and we experience] the uncanny pleasure of being *held* by a poem, a composition, a painting" (pp. 385–386, emphasis added). This description returns us to Winnicott, who has described what he calls a "holding environment," which mothers create again and again for their children. A work of art, similarly, may create such states of absorption and embrace for its listeners, beholders, or readers. Or it may push us away, and then open its arms again for another embrace. (For an elaboration of this notion and a phenomenological account of aesthetic experience, see Spitz 2001.) What psychoanalysis offers here, through the work also of Margaret Mahler on separation-individuation, is a developmental model that can help explain the power of such experiences and how they can exert their influence on us long after our childhood years have passed.

Conclusion

The finest interdisciplinary dialogue between psychoanalysis and the arts—because there is no clinical agenda—assiduously avoids the diagnosis of artists. It comprehends the force of Isaac Bashevis Singer's wry comment that "in art, truth that is boring is not true." It seeks, in parallel with its subject, to draw closer to the fount from which imagination springs. It searches for intuitive feelings of rightness and never pretends to final solutions. It trades in high degrees of both candor and suspicion (see Gay 1976). It knows the connections between memory and desire and never privileges reason over unreason or vice versa. It emphasizes the reality of meanings and espouses the truth that, like events, meanings too reverberate throughout history—both personal history and history on a global scale. It teaches the importance of studying these meanings as they circulate, colliding with and superseding one another. It enables us to see how it is that we ourselves, in studying these meanings—through art and through psychoanalysis—take part in altering them.

When psychoanalytic interpretations adhere to works of art and become internalized, the works themselves seem to morph, and our aesthetic experience with them modulates, as well. The finest work of this kind, when all is said and done, not only illuminates and changes its objects but grows itself, proliferates, and inspires and, like the greatest works of art themselves, turns individuals back to their own lives reanimated, expectant, and renewed.

Suggestions for Further Reading and Research

Most published work in psychoanalysis and the arts relies on Freudian psychoanalysis, and among Freud's papers there are several others that deserve special mention in this context. "Family Romances" (Freud 1909/1959) offers richly nuanced suggestions with respect to understanding artists' desires for idealization and devaluation in their imagery; it complicates our notions of symbolism by showing how the present and past mutually revise each other in terms of the imagery we simultaneously remember and invent. "Leonardo da Vinci and a Memory of His Childhood" (Freud 1910b/1957) is arguably Freud's most famous paper on art, and despite its egregious exaggerations and inaccuracies, it continues to enthrall readers and to spawn an entire literature of responses, with more to come. "'Wild' Psycho-Analysis" (Freud 1910c/1957) proves a useful paper insofar as it cautions authors lest they jump too quickly to (erroneous) psychoanalytic conclusions, while "Formulations on the Two Principles of Mental Functioning" (Freud 1911/1955) divides the field into primary and secondary functioning, pleasure and reality, innovation and repetition, all of which have important roles to play vis-à-vis any serious consideration of formal elements in the arts. "Mourning and Melancholia" (Freud 1917[1915]/1957) and "The Uncanny" (Freud 1919/1955) are brilliant works relevant for the oeuvre of specific artists—those who dwell in trauma, tragedy, and mystery, respectively—and "The Note Upon 'The Mystic Writing Pad'" (Freud 1925/1955) offers metaphors for creative mental processes and for the structure of various works, as do "Fetishism" (Freud 1927/1957) and "The Splitting of the Ego in the Process of Defense" (Freud 1940/1955). In short, it is not simply the papers Freud wrote ostensibly about the arts that can prove useful to us now, but the larger corpus of his work, in which—sometimes in unexpected nooks—he offers stunning aperçus and struggles to define concepts that can help us grapple with newly emerging art of our twenty-first century.

References

Abrams MH: The Mirror and the Lamp. New York, Oxford University Press, 1953

Bollas C: The aesthetic moment and the search for transformation. Annual of Psychoanalysis 6:385–394, 1978

Breuer J, Freud S: Studies on hysteria (1893–1895), in Standard Edition of the Complete Psychological Works of Sigmund Freud, Vol 2. Translated and edited by Strachey J. London, Hogarth Press, 1955, pp 1–319

Dewey J: Art as Experience. New York, Paragon Books, 1934

Freud A: The ego and the mechanisms of defense (1936), in The Writings of Anna Freud, Vol 2. New York, International Universities Press, 1966

Freud S: The interpretation of dreams (1900), in Standard Edition of the Complete Psychological Works of Sigmund Freud, Vols 4 and 5. Translated and edited by Strachey J. London, Hogarth Press, 1953, pp 1–715

Freud S: Fragment of a case of hysteria (1905a), in Standard Edition of the Complete Psychological Works of Sigmund Freud, Vol 7. Translated and edited by Strachey J. London, Hogarth Press, 1955, pp 7–122

Freud S: Three essays on the theory of sexuality (1905b), in Standard Edition of the Complete Psychological Works of Sigmund Freud, Vol 7. Translated and edited by Strachey J. London, Hogarth Press, 1953, pp 125–243

Freud S: Delusions and dreams in Jensen's "Gravida" (1907), in Standard Edition of the Complete Psychological Works of Sigmund Freud, Vol 9. Translated and edited by Strachey J. London, Hogarth Press, 1959, pp 3–95

Freud S: Creative writers and daydreaming (1908), in Standard Edition of the Complete Psychological Works of Sigmund Freud, Vol 9. Translated and edited by Strachey J. London, Hogarth Press, 1959, pp 142–153

Freud S: Family romances (1909), in Standard Edition of the Complete Psychological Works of Sigmund Freud, Vol 9. Translated and edited by Strachey J. London, Hogarth Press, 1959, pp 235–244

Freud S: Five lectures on psycho-analysis [The Clark Lectures] (1910a), in Standard Edition of the Complete Psychological Works of Sigmund Freud, Vol 11. Translated and edited by Strachey J. London, Hogarth Press, 1957, pp 9–55

Freud S: Leonardo da Vinci and a memory of his childhood (1910b), in Standard Edition of the Complete Psychological Works of Sigmund Freud, Vol 11. Translated and edited by Strachey J. London, Hogarth Press, 1957, pp 59–137

Freud S: "Wild" psychoanalysis (1910c), in Standard Edition of the Complete Psychological Works of Sigmund Freud, Vol 11. Translated and edited by Strachey J. London, Hogarth Press, 1955, pp 221–227

Freud S: Formulations on the two principles of mental functioning (1911), in Standard Edition of the Complete Psychological Works of Sigmund Freud, Vol 12. Translated and edited by Strachey J. London, Hogarth Press, 1955, pp 215–226

Freud S: The Moses of Michelangelo (1914), in Standard Edition of the Complete Psychological Works of Sigmund Freud, Vol 13. Translated and edited by Strachey J. London, Hogarth Press, 1958, pp 211–238

Freud S: Mourning and melancholia (1917[1915]), in Standard Edition of the Complete Psychological Works of Sigmund Freud, Vol 14. Translated and edited by Strachey J. London, Hogarth Press, 1957, pp 237–260

Freud S: The "uncanny" (1919), in Standard Edition of the Complete Psychological Works of Sigmund Freud, Vol 17. Translated and edited by Strachey J. London, Hogarth Press, 1955, pp 219–256

Freud S: Two encyclopaedia articles: (A) psychoanalysis (1922), in The Standard Edition of the Complete Psychological works of Sigmund Freud, Vol 18. Translated and edited by Strachey J. London, Hogarth Press, 1955, pp 235–254

Freud S: Fetishism (1927), in The Standard Edition of the Complete Psychological works of Sigmund Freud, Vol 21. Translated and edited by Strachey J. London, Hogarth Press, 1957, pp 52–157

Freud S: Splitting of the ego (1940), in Standard Edition of the Complete Psychological Works of Sigmund Freud, Vol 23. Translated and edited by Strachey J. London, Hogarth Press, 1955, pp 275–278

Gay P: Art and Act: On Causes in History: Manet, Gropius, Mondrian. New York, Harper & Row, 1976

Greenacre P: The childhood of the artist, in Emotional Growth (1957), Vol 2. New York, International Universities Press, 1971, pp 479–504

Hartmann H: Ego Psychology and the Problem of Adaptation. New York, International Universities Press, 1939

Iverson M: Art Beyond the Pleasure Principle (in press)

Kant I: The Critique of Judgment (1790). Translated by Meredith JC. Oxford, England, Clarendon Press, 1952

Kernberg O: Object Relations Theory and Clinical Psychoanalysis. New York, Jason Aronson, 1976

Knafo D: Revisiting Ernst Kris' concept of "regression in the service of the ego." Psychoanalytic Psychology 19:24–49, 2002

Kris E: Psychoanalytic Explorations in Art. New York, International Universities Press, 1952

Kristeva J: Black Sun: Depression and Melancholia (1987). Translated by Roudiez LS. New York, Columbia University Press, 1992

Langone J: The sounds of serenity. The New York Times, August 26, 2003, D7

Langer SK: Feeling and Form: A Theory of Art. New York, Charles Scribner's Sons, 1953

Mahler MS: On Human Symbiosis and the Vicissitudes of Individuation. New York, International Universities Press, 1968

Mahler MS: On the first three sub-phases of the separation-individuation process. Int J Psychoanal 53:333–38, 1972

Mannoni O: Clefs pour l'imaginaire. Paris, Seuil, 1969

Milner M: On Not Being Able to Paint. New York, International Universities Press, 1957

Pine F: Drive, Ego, Object, and Self: A Synthesis for Clinical Work. New York, Basic Books, 1990

Rank O: Art and Artist. New York, Knopf, 1932

Schorske CE: Fin-de-Siecle Vienna: Politics and Culture. New York, Knopf, 1980

Spitz EH: Art and Psyche: A Study in Psychoanalysis and Aesthetics. New Haven, CT, Yale University Press, 1985

Spitz EH: Museums of the Mind: Magritte's Labyrinth and Other Essays in the Arts. New Haven, CT, Yale University Press, 1994

Spitz EH: An essay on beauty: two madonnas, the scent of violets, and a family of acrobats. Figurationen: Gender/Literature/Kultur 2:27–34, 2001

Steinberg L: The Sexuality of Christ in Renaissance Art and in Modern Oblivion. Chicago, IL, University of Chicago Press, 1984

Tolstoy L: What Is Art? (1898). Translated by Pevear R, Volokhonsky L. London, Penguin Books, 1995

Winnicott DW: Transitional objects and transitional phenomena. Int J Psychoanal 34:89–97, 1953

Winnicott DW: The location of cultural experience. Int J Psychoanal 48:368–72, 1966

Wolf B: Romantic Re-vision. Chicago, IL, University of Chicago Press, 1982

34

Philosophy

JONATHAN LEAR, Ph.D.

PSYCHOANALYSIS AND PHILOSOPHY share more than an interest in the core concepts of the human condition—freedom, happiness, mental life, desire; they both purport to be strategies for changing one's life. At least, that's the way it was at philosophy's beginning, and it is a promise philosophy held out during the first centuries of its existence. If we are to understand the relation between philosophy and psychoanalysis, we need to learn what happened to that promise.

"Our conversation concerns no ordinary topic," Socrates says, "but the way we should live" (Plato, *Republic* I, 352d). (This is my translation, which I use to bring out the point; but elsewhere in this essay I rely on the translation of G.M.E. Grube and C.D.C. Reeve [1992].) For Socrates, this is the fundamental question for humans: *How should one live?* It is pressing for each person, he thought, because humans are inevitably born into a dilemma. On the one hand, each person's life is *already* an answer to this question, even if the person has not explicitly thought about it as such. Human life is not a mere biological category; it is saturated with norms and values. A person's life reflects his or her sense of *what matters* (given the constraints under which he or she must live). On the other hand, humans are born into a cultural world: they absorb values in childhood with little understanding of what they mean or why they matter. So while they may dedicate their lives to their sense of what matters, their sense of what matters

may never rise above the clichés and prejudices of the environment into which they were born. For Socrates, this is the hallmark of a wasted life. A worthwhile life, for Socrates, is one that somehow takes itself into account and lives according to its own accounting.

Note that Socrates' question is not itself a moral question. It asks, in an open-ended way, What would it be to live well? For Socrates, as for all the ancient Greek philosophers, the key is happiness: What is involved in humans living happy lives? The Greek word for happiness is *eudaimonia*—which literally means "well off when it comes to daimons, demons, or spirits." It is living with good spirits. (Whether the spirits are within or without is left indeterminate.) Less literally, it means living a full, rich, meaningful life. It is sometimes translated as "flourishing." The question then becomes, What is involved in living a full, rich, meaningful life? What is it for us genuinely to flourish? (It might be that living a moral life is an answer, but that has to be shown. It is not presupposed in the question from the start.)

Philosophy, at least in the Socratic tradition, is an activity that will help us be able to answer that question for ourselves. Socratic philosophy was not just a theoretical inquiry; it had a therapeutic aim. We shall soon examine the details of Socratic technique. But, for the moment, notice that if changing one's life is the aim of philosophical activity, then the Socratic question is fundamental not only for each person but for philosophy as well.

I should like to thank Morris Eagle and Gabriel Lear for valuable comments on an earlier draft.

If one's reads through Plato's works, one will see serious forays into metaphysics, science, literary criticism, mythology, psychology, politics and aesthetics—but all of those inquiries are disciplined by an overriding interest in how to live. And though we shall concentrate on Socrates and Plato, as the inventors of philosophy, it is worth noting that the subsequent philosophical schools—of Aristotle, the Stoics, Epicureans, and Skeptics—were all concerned with philosophy as an activity that could change one's life. Even Aristotle's most abstract thinking—metaphysics—was to help humans better understand their place in the world. And understanding *that*, Aristotle thought, was part of a process of coming to recognize that one's life ought to be oriented toward such understanding. For the happiest human life, he argued, was oriented toward contemplation (see *Nicomachean Ethics* X, 6–9). So, provided one did it in the right sort of way, doing philosophy about the highest things was itself a changing of one's life for the better.

Psychoanalysis shares with philosophy the same fundamental question. Though analytic patients may not have thought about it explicitly, they come to analysis with a sense that something is going wrong in their own attempts to live well. They may have no real sense of what is going wrong or with what it would be like to live better. But they have come for treatment, and the treatment is a peculiar form of conversation. It is a conversation about their life and how they are living it; it is a conversation about whatever it is that comes into their minds. We shall look later at some of the peculiarities of this conversation. But, for the moment, consider this broad-scale feature: people come to analysis for help; they want help in figuring out how to live better; and analysis purports to be a conversation that can help them in that project. Were he alive today, Socrates would be interested; for this is the project he took to be fundamental.

The Socratic Method

For Socrates, conversation is the key. While each of us is confronted with the question of how to live, none of us can answer it well on our own. This is one manifestation of our *finite* nature: none of us has God's vantage point; each of us looks out on the world from a limited perspective that was not of our choosing. It is all but impossible to gain a reasonable perspective on our perspective entirely on one's own. We need the conversation of others to test our perspective; indeed, to find out what it is. But what sort of conversation should it be?

In the early dialogues, Socrates used a method of cross-examination, or *elenchus*. (To call these dialogues "early" is by now a figure of speech. Until recently it has been fashionable to think that the dialogues in which Socrates is involved in cross-examination reveal the historical Socrates and that, therefore, Plato wrote those dialogues earlier than other dialogues in which Socratic method is abandoned. These assumptions have undergone serious criticism. It nevertheless remains a useful metaphor for thinking about the structure of certain problems, as will be illustrated in this essay.) Socrates and an interlocutor would start out with one of life's basic values—say, acting courageously. Courage is called a virtue—an *aretē*—but another translation is *excellence*. That is, it is agreed that living courageously would be a fine way to live. But Socrates has this crucial insight: people may agree that living courageously is a fine way to live *and they may nevertheless have no idea what courage is.* As a result, they have no real understanding of what living well is. They are inducted into current fashions, but no one seems to have any idea whether the fashions are more than that. So not only do people not know what, say, courage is; they don't know that they don't know. As a result, people think they have an answer to the question of how to live—live courageously!—and they use that answer to disguise from themselves that they have no idea what they are talking about. The purported answer to the question turns out to be a defense against confronting the question with any seriousness.

The Socratic method is designed to undo this defense. Socrates asks his interlocutor to state what, say, courage is. The interlocutor thinks he knows and offers an account; through a series of questions and answers Socrates elicits a contradiction. Once the interlocutor sees that he is in contradiction, *something* about his life must change. In the best possible circumstances, he would recognize that he didn't really know what courage is, and then he could begin a real inquiry into how it is best to live. Another possibility is that he revises some of his other beliefs in order to hold onto his account of courage. Still another possibility is that he evades the problem by rushing off. But, even then, life cannot be the same; for the contradiction has been brought to his attention, and this, at least, must be an occasion for discomfort.

As a therapeutic technique, the Socratic method does not rest on a sophisticated account of the psyche. It is as though the psyche were a mere container of beliefs and desires. And it seems as though Socrates tacitly assumes that the psyche is home to many truths as well as to falsehoods (see Vlastos 1983, 1991). For if the interlocutor's psyche doesn't contain many truths about courage (as well as important falsehoods), there would be no way to elicit a contradiction. And perhaps the *hopefulness* of Socrates' technique consisted in the confidence that, once the contradiction was elicited, the truths would outweigh the falsehoods.

Note, too, that Socrates assumes that the only impediment to rationality is lack of self-awareness. He takes his therapeutic job to be done when he brings the contradictions to light. Indeed, he famously argues that it is impossible for anyone knowingly to do bad. Roughly speaking, he argues that it is built into the concept of action that when one acts one is aiming at something one takes to be good. Thus, it is only through ignorance that one could aim at something bad. In this way, Socrates passes over as impossible a phenomenon that psychoanalysts treat seriously: that humans may be motivated to live in contradiction. Not only do they act against their own sense of what is best for them—which Socrates argues is impossible—but *that* is why they are doing it. To take a common example, consider cigarette smoking. On the standard model of irrational behavior, there may be people who smoke in spite of the fact that they know it is likely to make them ill in the long run, and they genuinely do not want to get ill. On this model, the pleasures of the moment weigh most heavily with them and cloud their judgment of their long-term goal. This is familiar enough. But now consider a stranger case: a person smokes not primarily for the immediate physical pleasures, but from the *excitement* of knowing he may be throwing away his own life. We cannot legitimately say that such a person is simply throwing away his own life. It is precisely because his life—his long-term health—genuinely matters to him, that risking it is exciting. If his life didn't matter to him, then neither would the risk to it, and there would be no excitement. Precisely because it violates his own best judgment of how to live, he is drawn to it. Thus, merely bringing the contradiction to light may be of no help; indeed, it may even be counterproductive.

The problems with Socratic method are by now well known, but it is worth mentioning the most serious. First, there is no evidence that cross-examination helped the interlocutors. Perhaps it helped Socrates in his own efforts to figure out how to live. And it may have helped generations of readers of Platonic dialogues. But there is an outstanding question of whom, if anyone, did the Socratic method benefit?

Second, although the method revealed the interlocutor as living according to unexamined clichés, the clichés were also the values of the time. Thus, there should be no surprise that the Socratic method provoked anger among some citizens. It would be easy enough to assume that Socrates was challenging the fundamental values of society. The death of Socrates has been much written about, but one way to view it is as a psychotherapeutic catastrophe. Obviously, Western civilization may have benefited from two and a half millennia of pondering the death of Socrates. And we may well suspect that Socrates had precisely that outcome in mind. Perhaps his "patient" was Western civi-

lization itself. But, in the short run at least, a purported mode of therapy is open to criticism if it provokes the patient to act out his murderous wishes—and kill the analyst.

Cooperative Conversation

In the *Republic* Socrates abandons the method of cross examination. Indeed, the failure of that method is put on vivid display in Book I. There Socrates is questioning a narcissist: Thrasymachus is a bold rhetorician who likes to win admiration through making speeches. He complains to Socrates in the following exchange:

> THRASYMACHUS: I'm not satisfied with what you're now saying. I could make a speech about it, but, if I did, I know that you'd accuse me of engaging in oratory. So either allow me to speak, or, if you want to ask questions, go ahead, and I'll say, "All right," and nod yes and no as one does to old wives' tales.
> SOCRATES: Don't do that contrary to your own opinion.
> T: I'll answer so as to please you, since you won't let me make a speech. What else do you want?
> S: Nothing, by god! But if that's what you're going to do, go ahead and do it. I'll ask my questions.
> (*Republic* I, 350d–350e)

Thrasymachus, for his part, abandons one of the basic rules of Socratic conversation, to state only what you believe. If he can't make speeches, then he will sabotage the conversation with false compliance: "Enjoy your banquet of words," he says to Socrates. "Have no fear, I won't oppose you." Socrates, for his part, gives in to his own temptation for talking regardless of the fact that his interlocutor has hunkered down into narcissistic noncompliance. "Come, then, complete my banquet by continuing to answer as you've been doing" (*Republic* I, 352b).

At the beginning of Book II, Glaucon, a bright and honest young man (and a brother of Plato's), politely but firmly tells Socrates that his method has failed. From that moment on, the Socratic method is jettisoned. In its place there is a cooperative conversation between like-minded investigators. From a psychoanalytic point of view, this is a striking transition. For this is the moment when the ideal of therapeutic conversation is abandoned in favor of joint research through thought-experiment and shared logical thought. Obviously, there is still some hope that shared inquiry into truth will be a benefit to the inquirers. The overall aim of the inquiry is to prove that it is better to live a just life, and knowing that will be a benefit to the inquirers, as they structure their lives toward justice, resist temptations to injustice, and so on. But, therapeutically speaking, these are rather limited aims. First, the inquirers are already in pretty good shape; and the more fundamental goal of eliciting contradiction and facing up to psychic conflicts no longer arises. Second, one of the lessons of the *Republic* is that therapy on adult individuals already brought up in a decadent society will be of little use. Rather, one needs a political solution in which children are brought up well from the start. The issue then is not of undoing past psychic harm, but of preventing it from occurring in the first place.

Contributions to Dynamic Psychological Thinking

Ironically, it is precisely in the inquiry recounted above that a serious theory of the psyche is first laid out. Here are a few of the contributions to dynamic psychological thinking that the *Republic* makes.

A Theory of Psychic Formation

The human psyche is itself shaped by the internalization of meanings that are transmitted from the culture to the child via parents, nursemaids, and teachers. These meanings are often taken into the psyche before the child is in a position to grasp their (full) meaning. But they will come to play a significant role in shaping a person's outlook (*Republic* II, 377–378).

A Dynamic Theory of Psychic Structure

The psyche is itself divided into characteristic parts: a desiring, id-like part, which Plato calls appetite (*epithumia*), that strives after food and sex; a narcissistic component, which Plato calls spirit (*thumos*), that strives after recognition and admiration; and reason (*logos*), which strives to understand how things really are. Each part of the psyche is thus a desiring part; the parts differ according to the type of thing they are after (*Republic* IV, 435e–444a).

A Theory of Neurotic Conflict

Neurotic conflict occurs when none of the psychic parts is successful at organizing and disciplining the others (*Republic* IV, 444a; see also Books VIII, IX). So, for example, the narcissistic component might experience a certain sexual temptation as shameful, but id-like desire goes for it anyway. The impasse is intrapsychic conflict in which powerful feelings of temptation struggle against feelings of shame, humiliation, and worthlessness. Socrates tells the story of Leontius, who, when he was walking back to town, saw some corpses outside the walls of the city:

> He had an appetite to look at them but at the same time he was disgusted and turned away. For a time he struggled with himself and covered his face, but, finally, overpowered by the appetite, he pushed his eyes wide open

and rushed towards the corpses, saying, "Look for yourselves, you evil wretches, take your fill of the beautiful sight!" (*Republic* IV, 439e–440a)

A Dynamic Theory of Personality Organization

For instance, we can speak of a narcissistic personality when the narcissistic component in the psyche takes control and imposes some kind of organization over the other parts. In the narcissist, the more id-like desires for sex are disciplined to an overriding desire for admiration. Now it becomes important to have sexual relations with someone who will contribute to one's glory. And reason is deployed as a primarily calculative faculty: figuring out which are the next good moves if one is to achieve celebrity. Thus, we have the formation of what Plato calls *timocratic* man, the lover of honor (*Republic* VIII, 549c–550).

A Dynamic Theory of Typical Pathologies of Personality Organization

For example, the wealthy businessman—the "oligarch"—will have organized his life around acquiring and preserving wealth. Socrates sees such a personality as inevitably conflicted. The attraction of money is that it enables people to buy things to satisfy their desires. But if a coherent personality is to be achieved, the desires have to be held in check. The id-like desires are repressed, thus enabling the person to acquire wealth and save it. Narcissistic desires are subordinated to acquiring wealth: being wealthy is what makes this person proud. Reason is subordinated to calculating how best to acquire more money. This is a personality organization, but it is inherently unstable because although it is organized in the name of desire, the desires are repressed (*Republic* VIII, 553c–554e).

An Object Relations Theory of the Transmission of Pathology

In the social world, the oligarch will typically encourage his neighbors to indulge the very desires he represses. So, think of the head of Visa encouraging his neighbors to overspend on their credit cards. It is only if *they* indulge their desires that he can succeed at his project. Thus, his social world has basically the same structure as his own psyche: his neighbors are the representative of the teeming desires, and he is the figure holding them in check. But inevitably the oligarch's son will take in these messages of excess in the surrounding environment. Thus, there will be dissolution within the family structure. This is brought about against the oligarchical father's express wishes, but it occurs inexorably nevertheless, given the messages he unconsciously transmits (*Republic* VIII, 554b–559e).

An Account of the Limits of Psychological Integration

"Republic" is the translation for *poleteia*, which can also mean *constitution*. The English translation follows earlier Latin translations, entitled *Res Publica*, literally, the public thing. The Latin translators particularly emphasized the political aspects of the text, but I suspect that *Constitution* is a better title. For the book is concerned with the question of constitutionality: What is it to be constituted? What is it to function as a differentiated unity? The inquiry is into the very idea of constitutionality—whether it arises in political entities, in the human psyche, or in the cosmos. Now, in the specific case of the human psyche, there are definite limits to the possibility of integration. A prime reason is the presence "probably in everyone" of a particularly unruly type of desire:

> They are awakened in sleep, when the rest of the soul—the rational, gentle, ruling part—slumbers. Then the beastly and savage part, full of food and drink, casts off sleep and seeks to find a way to gratify itself: You know there is nothing it won't dare to do at such a time, free of all control by shame or reason. *It doesn't shrink from trying to have sex with a mother as it supposes or with anyone else at all*, whether man, god or beast. It will commit any foul murder, and there is no food it refuses to eat. In a word, it omits no act of folly or shamelessness. (*Republic* IX, 571b–571c)

These are desires that basically can only be dealt with by repression. A few exceptional people may be able to get rid of them, but even in them weak ones may remain. For everyone else, they need to be "held in check." This means that there will always be pressure on any form of psychic integration. Note that this account implies the next point.

A Theory of Dreams as Expressions of Unconscious and Illicit Desires

Socrates is also interested in showing how a society's shared sense of reality can be distorted. He argues that the culture's most magnificent artifacts—the myths of the gods, Homer's poems, the tragedies—have hidden messages that have shaped the souls of the citizens in ways they do not understand. As a result, people experience themselves and each other according to preformed images, and nevertheless take themselves to be experiencing things the way they really are. In his famous allegory of the Cave, Socrates is trying to give an account of "the effect of our education or lack of it on our nature" (*Republic* VII, 514a). Unbeknown to ourselves, we are actually prisoners in a cave, looking at shadows projected on a wall and mistaking them for reality. Psychologically speaking, the important point is that the outcome of our education (*or lack of it*) is not primarily a set of beliefs, even

a set of false beliefs, about the world. Rather, it is a worldview: a way of experiencing events and interpreting them so that they all hang together, but in such a way as to keep us imprisoned. And thus Plato gives us the next point.

A Theory of Illusion and the Rudiments of a Theory of Transference

Moreover, there is even an account of a precursor to negative transference. Suppose that someone were able to break out of this illusion. The image is of someone breaking his shackles, ascending out of the cave to see things in the light of the sun, then returning to the cave to help his fellow prisoners. Here is a man with a true understanding of reality but zero therapeutic technique.

> If this man went down into the cave again and sat down in his same seat, wouldn't his eyes—coming suddenly out of the sun like that—be filled with darkness? And before his eyes had recovered—and the adjustment would not be quick—while his vision was still dim, if he had to compete again with the perpetual prisoners in recognizing the shadows, wouldn't he invite ridicule? Wouldn't it be said of him that he'd returned from his upward journey with his eyesight ruined and that it isn't worthwhile even to try to travel upward? And, as for anyone who tried to free them and lead them upward, if they could somehow get their hands on him, wouldn't they kill him? (*Republic* VII, 516e–517a)

To which Glaucon responds: "They certainly would."

Implications of Conversation With Glaucon

There are two important features about this less-than-successful therapeutic encounter. First, the prisoners in the cave have a preformed schema in terms of which they interpret this disruption in their environment. Rather than experience this person as having something new to say, they interpret him in terms of familiar, old categories. Given that unbeknown to themselves they live in a cave, dominated by shadows mistaken for reality, they are necessarily unaware of the bases of their judgments. And, of course, this structure of judgment provides an outlet for ridicule and aggress: it thereby motivates the prisoners to stay precisely where they are. Thus does this unconsciously motivated structure of judgment hold them captive.

Second, Socrates is trying to explain his own murder. On the surface, what could be more puzzling: Socrates, one of the finest men who ever lived, put to death by democratic vote of one of the greatest civilizations of all time. But the Socrates of the *Republic* describes an unconsciously motivated structure of judgments and evaluations in terms of which the outcome is unsurprising. "They'd kill me, wouldn't they?" Socrates asks. *They certainly would,* Glaucon responds.

Crisis in Philosophy: Abandonment of the Therapeutic Ideal

This is the barest outline, but perhaps enough has been said to make it clear that the *Republic* is a book of astonishing psychological sophistication. By way of contrast, consider the simplistic conception of the psyche as a bare container that was the background assumption for the Socratic method. We might reasonably have hoped that as Plato's theory of the psyche increased in sophistication, there would be a corresponding increased sophistication in therapeutic technique. If so, we would have been disappointed.

From a psychoanalytic point of view, we have to face this irony: at precisely the moment when Socrates devises a viable and sophisticated theory of dynamic psychology, he abandons interest in individual psychotherapy. Instead he turns to politics. This is a direct consequence of his psychological theory. The human psyche is fundamentally shaped in childhood by cultural messages, and after that it is rigid and inalterable. Given an ill-formed adult, there is really not much you can say to him that will be of any help. Thus, the Socrates of the *Republic* writes off as a loss the entire adult population of contemporary Athens. He engages instead in a thought-experiment in political utopianism: what would be involved in starting from scratch, in establishing a psychopolitical order in which children were brought up right? This now seems like the only question worth pursuing. And it is pursued with two young men who seem remarkably to have escaped much of the psychological damage that had been inflicted by the culture on their contemporaries. Socrates even suspects they must be divinely inspired to have escaped the corruption. The idea of carrying out an individual therapy on an actual individual in the actual environment now seems hopeless.

From this new Socratic perspective, it seems as if there is now only one type of conversation worth having: namely, a conversation among people who are already in pretty good shape about what a good life would be. Socrates, as we have seen, conducts his conversation with two fine young men, and it seems Plato wrote the *Republic* in order that the conversation might continue over the generations. The book is meant to be read by fine young men and women in the future, and perhaps some day some of them will be in a position to fashion the psychopolitical environment. For, as Socrates says, not until rulers become philosophers or philosophers become rulers will people be happy. They will know how to shape a society in which young people are brought up well, and only then will happiness and harmony become a political and psychological reality.

This, it seems to me, is a crisis moment in philosophy. It is at just this moment that philosophy turns away from a therapeutic ideal toward a conversation among the good. Yet it is at just this moment that a new kind of question becomes possible. As we have seen, Socrates the therapist did not have an account of psychological structure. His conversations were meant to elicit false beliefs, and if the interlocutor could recognize them as such and get rid of them, he could stop living falsely. But once Socrates has a theory of psychological structure, a new question becomes possible: might a conversation change the structure of the psyche? Is there any form of words that might alter psychological constitution? The Socrates of the *Republic* thinks the answer to this is no. And thus at the moment when the development of a sophisticated therapeutic technique becomes possible, Socrates gives up his therapeutic ambitions. He is now concerned with the form and content of words that should be transmitted to children; for words do influence psychic formation. But once psychic structure is in place, there is little or nothing that conversation can do to bring about therapeutic alteration—at least, so thinks Socrates in the *Republic*. Thus, at the moment a crucial question becomes possible, it is basically ignored.

Philosophy and Psychic Change

How might a conversation change the structure of the psyche? This question is not about changing a person's beliefs—this one can do through argument—nor about changing a person's desires—this one can do through moral education, persuasion, and so on. It is, rather, about how basic psychic organization can change. And how could such a change occur merely through conversation? This is the question that philosophy raises—and leaves hanging.

This is not an appropriate place to review the entire history of philosophy. But it seems safe to say that this question is taken up most seriously in the Christian tradition. Since Christianity believes in the reality of sin, the reality of vice, *and* the possibility of redemption for everyone through confession, it has an inherent concern with how this comes about. Of course, the Christian answer is a religious one: through God's grace. And since philosophy, at least since the Enlightenment, has been a predominantly secular inquiry, it has by and large ignored medieval and early modern Christian thought. Ironically, one way to view psychoanalysis is as an attempted secular appropriation of the Christian therapeutic tradition.

It is precisely because modern (secular) philosophy has ignored the question of psychic change through conversation that philosophy and psychoanalysis have seemed, at least on the surface, to be such different types of activity. What, then, are the possible routes philosophy can take, given that it ignores this question? One way to explore the consequences is according to this dilemma: *either* philosophy cuts itself off altogether from the Socratic question of how to live, *or* it continues on with that question but without a concern for dynamic psychological structure. On the first lemma, philosophy becomes an abstract inquiry into the most basic world-structuring concepts: for example, the nature of causation, logic, what it is to be a mental state, meaning, and the conceptual foundations of physics. This would be the pursuit of knowledge for its own sake about the basic structure of mind and world. On the second lemma, philosophy would still purport to give some account of how to live via an inquiry into, say, freedom or happiness. But it would ignore challenges raised by the idea that the human psyche is complex, dynamically structured with significant repressed components. So, for example, approaches to ethics or morality that are influenced either by the British Empiricists or by Kant might assume that an understanding of human psychology is important, but the psychology they would assume would be basically one of beliefs and desires. This is a psychology of *propositional attitudes*: belief *that* something is the case; desire *that* something be acquired; hope or fear *that* something should come to pass; angry *that* something has happened. The philosopher Donald Davidson has convincingly shown that a psychology in which mental states are propositional attitudes will inherently tend to show the person to be rational (Davidson 1984). And while one can show how, in such a psychology, motivated irrationality is nevertheless possible, this remains basically a technical exercise (see Davidson 1980, 1982). When it comes to central philosophical questions—say, the nature of freedom—the significance of the dynamic unconscious is by and large ignored.

Does this matter? Obviously, I think the answer is yes: ignoring the phenomenon of dynamic psychological structure has had serious deleterious consequence for philosophy *and for psychoanalysis*. In the remainder of this chapter, I give a brief sketch of what some of these consequences are, and then, in a more constructive spirit, I indicate how this gap may be overcome through a joint program of philosophical-psychoanalytic inquiry.

Reflection Function and Psychic Functioning

There is a distinguished philosophical tradition—alive in contemporary philosophy but descended at least from Kant—that locates our freedom in self-conscious awareness. How could this be? In *Being and Nothingness*, Sartre (1956, pp. 595–615) argues that once one becomes reflectively aware of a given psychological impulse, a choice is, as it were, forced on one: how is one to act with respect to it? One may ignore it, go along with it, endorse it, acquiesce to it, reject it and so on, but it is no longer possible for the impulse simply to be a given of psychological life. As Harvard philosopher Richard Moran (2001) puts it,

> When I am reflectively aware of some attitude or impulse of mind, I am thereby made aware that its persistence in me (as a "facticity") is not a foregone conclusion stemming from the inertia of psychic life, and in particular that its counting as a reason for me in my current thought and action *is my affair* [emphasis added]. (p. 140; see his general discussion of this problem, pp. 138–151)

It is now in the realm of things I can react to and do something about. Christine Korsgaard, another Harvard philosopher, makes a similar point in her book *The Sources of Normativity:*

> [O]ur capacity to turn our attention on to our own mental activities is also a capacity to distance ourselves from them, and to call them into question. I perceive, and I find myself with a powerful impulse to believe. But I back up and bring that impulse into view and then I have a certain distance. Now the impulse doesn't dominate me and now I have a problem. Shall I believe? Is this perception really a *reason* to believe? (Korsgaard 1996, p. 93; discussed by Moran 2001, p. 142)

And Thomas Nagel, commenting on Korsgaard, gives this gloss:

> [T]he reflective self cannot be a mere bystander because it is not someone else; it is the very person who may have begun with a certain unreflective perception, or desire or intention, but who is now in possession of additional information of a special, self-conscious kind. Whatever the person now concludes, or chooses, or does, even if it is exactly what he was about to do anyway, will either have or lack the endorsement of the reflective view. Given that the person *can* either try to resist or not, and that he is now self-conscious, anything he does will imply endorsement, permission, or disapproval from the reflective standpoint. (Nagel 1996, pp. 200–201)

Roughly speaking, the reason is that in reflection lies responsibility. If I become aware of some psychological datum—say, a tempting impulse, an occurrent thought about another person, a feeling of shame—there will always be a further question of how I should live with respect to it. Should I give into the impulse? Is my judgment of the other person a prejudice? Is there really anything to be ashamed about? We thus bring the impulse into the domain of rational assessment and thereby manifest our freedom with respect to it.

Obviously, it is tempting to use this conception of our rational freedom to illuminate the therapeutic process. Perhaps *this* is what Freud really meant by his claim that in psychoanalysis one "makes the unconscious conscious." And yet, any analyst who has had an person with an obsessional neurosis as a patient will likely have come across someone for whom reflection is a manifestation of their unfreedom. Consider this story of O: to all appearances O is a psychologically minded fellow, indeed, he devotes much time to bringing various impulses to conscious awareness and wondering what to do about them. That is, he devotes *too much* time to it. He is addicted to reflecting on his impulses; there is some weird motivation to keep reflecting. What an "ideal" analysand! He's willing to come in and associate until the cows come home; he'll draw his own connections and even make tentative interpretations. Yet none of it seems to do him much good. He is, as it were, *stuck* in his analytic activity. But he's a sharp student of philosophy: he just completed an essay on the importance for freedom of having one's "second-order" desires in harmony with one's "first-order" impulses (see Frankfurt 1988). Indeed, that is the project on which he takes himself to have embarked. In name at least, his intellectual inquiry and the larger concerns of his life are of a piece. The problem is, he can't ever quite get around to living.

This is a caricature to be sure, but the overall structure is accurate and familiar. O's problem is that his entire faculty of reflective self-consciousness has been taken over by his obsessional personality. On the one hand, he is active in his thinking; on the other hand, he has no choice but to think. Philosophers have tended to assume that if there is going to be a problem for reflective freedom, it is going to be either because our impulses are too strong or our capacity for reflection is too weak or undeveloped. No doubt this is often the situation (see Freud 1909/1955, pp. 166–209), but it need not always be thus. It is possible for some obsessionally neurotic persons to experience their impulses as weak but to experience reflective thought as powerful and not entirely in their control. What are they to do, reflect on that? Obviously, this description covers a wide spectrum of cases. At the extreme, there is compulsive reflection; and the compulsiveness may incline us to conclude that the patient has lost the ability genuinely to reflect. But the more interesting case from a philosophical point of view is less severe. Mr. O is *able* to reflect all right—there is no air of compulsiveness—it's just that reflecting seems somehow to have taken the place of living. Instead of reflecting on his life being of a piece with his living that life, reflecting on his life has become his life. In such a case, thoughtful reflection becomes a form of unfreedom.

Here, then, is an example of a significant philosophical insight—that our rational freedom is somehow manifest in our ability to reflect—that is limited by ignorance of the vicissitudes of dynamic psychological structure. No doubt there is something correct in the idea that in reflection we manifest our freedom; but now we see it's got to be *the right sort* of reflection. But what could that mean? It cannot be about the content or about the steps of the reflection itself. It must rather be about how that reflection is woven into overall psychic functioning. But then how are we to explain the difference between the form of psychic functioning in which reflection is a manifestation of our unfreedom and the form in which it is a manifestation of our freedom? One obvious way would be to give an account of the transition from one condition to the other. Suppose, now, that that transition could itself be achieved through reflective conversation. This would be the situation in which a certain kind of reflective conversation itself facilitated a transformation of overall psychic functioning. This would simultaneously be a movement from unfreedom to freedom. Thus are we brought back to the question that arose with Plato: How might a conversation change the structure of the psyche? This is the question psychoanalysis tries to answer, and we can now see that it is of central philosophical importance.

Conclusion: The Future of Psychoanalytic-Philosophical Investigation

Conversely to the dilemma described in the previous section, psychoanalysis suffers when it is split off from its philosophical roots. Psychoanalysis is essentially a therapeutic activity: it aims at promoting a certain outcome. But if we lack a clear understanding of what this outcome is, we cannot be confident that our activities are aiming at it. But what is psychoanalysis aiming at? Psychic health? Mental freedom? The capacity to love? But what do these concepts mean?

Psychoanalysts have shed valuable light on the goals of psychoanalytic treatment, but we have just begun to think about the deeper meanings. Without a clear conception of the goal of psychoanalysis, and of how to aim at it, we cannot say with confidence whether we are helping people or harming them. We cannot even say with confidence what we are doing. There is astonishing variation within the mental health community both in goal and in method of treatment. Although some of this reflects honest disagreement, too much of it reflects a lack of thinking through what the values of a talking cure could be.

I shall conclude this essay by mentioning a few areas for psychoanalytic-philosophical investigation.

Transference

The phenomenon of transference suggests that there is no straightforward way to initiate and carry on a conversation about how to live. Each interlocutor will typically be assigning peculiar roles to the other that occur within highly structured, yet idiosyncratic worlds of meaning, much of which remains unconscious. Thus, the purported inquiry into how to live will be distorted by other issues about which no one is very clear. To take a caricatured example, the purported conversation could be experienced by one person as the insatiable hectoring of a maternal figure, but by the other as the very activity of conversation that keeps him so busy he never has to face up to what he is like. It is not enough to say that the conversation needs to get clear on what the transferences are. We need an understanding of what this could possibly mean, for clearly, understanding the transferences as we have just done—as an intellectual cognition—is of no help. That too can be more of the intellectualization that keeps any genuine conversation at bay. On the surface, it looks as though there is no place from which genuine conversation can occur. Inside the transference one is assigned a preordained role; outside the transference the conversation is too remote to engage the interlocutor. So, what would it be like to take up the transference in the right sort of way—that is, a way that facilitates genuine conversation about how to live?

Psychic Change Through Conversation

Psychoanalysis brings about changes in *the structure* of a person's psyche—and it does so through conversation. How can any conversation do this? Psychoanalysis does not change this or that desire, or this or that wish or fantasy; it transforms the very way the psyche functions. One typical outcome of a successful analysis is that a person has a less punishing superego. What does this mean? Not just that the voice of the superego becomes less cruel in *what* it says, but that there are important changes in *how* the superego speaks to the ego. There is increased communication—harmonious and reciprocal—between superego and ego, so much so that the distinction between these two psychic faculties starts to blur. Psychologically speaking there is a factual question as to how any conversation could bring this about. Indeed, one is inclined to think that this is the question of the therapeutic action of psychoanalysis. But if so, we need to ask what it is about this psychic change that makes it therapeutic (see Lear 2003a)?

Perhaps naively, we may have thought that the conversation about how to live was valuable because it helped us recognize who we are and what we and the world we inhabit are like. On the basis of that increased understanding,

we could make better life choices. But psychoanalysis shows us that a conversation about how to live might not just reveal what we are like, it might fundamentally alter it. In which case, the conversation isn't just an *inquiry* into how to live; it's a transformation of the conditions of life itself. Thus, it seems that just as one is getting into a position where one could raise the question of how to live in a genuine way, *one has already answered it*. On what grounds can one be confident that one has answered it for the better?

Activity and Passivity in the Mind

Psychoanalysis reveals that the mind is a heterogeneous place. Not only does a person have beliefs and desires, hopes, fears, and resentments, he or she also has wishes and fantasies. These are forms of imaginative activity that operate for the most part unconsciously and according to their own rules. Of course, they often intersect with (and influence) beliefs and desires; they often get expressed in actions. But they are not constrained by the limitations of rationality that apply to the standard model of belief, desire, and action in human life (see Davidson 1980, 1984). Psychoanalysis has been extraordinarily successful in charting the form and efficacy of unconscious fantasies.

But what significance do these fantasies have for human happiness and freedom? Obviously, we know that certain fantasies are painful, inhibiting, crippling. But, philosophically speaking, the question is about the significance of having any kind of fantasy life at all. On the one hand, fantasies are forms of mental activity; on the other, we seem to suffer passively many of their consequences. They bypass our will more or less completely, though we can have some control over them, either through further imaginative activity or through a psychoanalytic conversation. What are we to think about this? Are fantasies part of our heteronomous nature, coming in an important sense "from outside" us, and acting on us? Is true autonomy then impossible, given that we are always subject to fantasies? Or should we just junk the concepts of autonomy and heteronomy as too crude to capture human psychic reality? Or should we *re-think* those concepts to help us conceptualize our shifting relations to our own fantasies? Might we rethink the concepts so that the fantasies we "suffer" can also become an expression of our "autonomous" nature?

The Idiosyncrasy of Meaning

As we saw in the *Republic*, Socrates' interest in therapeutic conversation ground to a halt with his discovery of dynamic psychological structure. There was no longer any point in trying to transform the individual through therapeutic conversation; rather, one should focus on the psychopolitical transformation of society. Psychoanalysis, by contrast, wants to rescue the therapeutic conversation for the individual. Freud insists that therapeutic conversation must be primarily aimed at the individual because unconscious meaning is permeated with idiosyncrasy. In primary process, the mind is making all sorts of loose associations to contingent events. Freud happens to see a botanical monograph in a shop window and dreams about it at night. Many others no doubt passed that shop window without any particular psychic consequences. But for Freud the mere image of the monograph comes to stand for the central struggles of his life. And each of those struggles is itself embedded in a nest of associations that is idiosyncratic through and through. What consequences does this idiosyncrasy of meaning have for human happiness? Can philosophy make sense of the idea that there are layers of meaning that are not public, that are utterly particular to the individual, and that often have great resonances for the meaning of their lives?

Naturalistic Moral Psychology

We want an account of human beings that makes psychological sense of the fact that they are capable of living moral or ethical lives. How does the recognition of a norm—of how one *should* live—actually grab hold of us and influence how we *do* live? We also want an account of the so called "moral emotions" like guilt and shame. These are powerful emotions by which we hold ourselves accountable. How do they work? What is the source of their power? How is it that they can vary in primitiveness and sophistication? How do they fit or disrupt human flourishing?

The idea that moral psychology should be naturalistic expresses the aim that we humans should be depicted as part of nature, whatever that means precisely. Our emotions and intuitions should not be seen as flowing from a mysterious intuition or supernatural source. Rather, we ought to be able to make sense of emotions like shame and guilt arising in animals like us, human animals.

The dilemma, which the philosopher Bernard Williams lays out clearly, is that, on the one hand, the standard empirical approaches—whether cognitive psychology, neurobiology, evolutionary theory, or sociobiology—do not have the conceptual resources from which we can genuinely derive the rich phenomena of cultural and ethical life. The theories tend to be reductionist and thus fail to capture the complexity of human evaluative life. On the other hand, if we turn to the philosophers, we tend to get a moral psychology that is a moral*ized* psychology—that is, one that begs the question by building moral outcomes into the basic structure (Williams 1995b).

Williams suggests that the way to overcome this dilemma is by turning to psychoanalysis:

A non-moralized, or less moralized, psychology uses the categories of meaning, reasons and value, but leaves it open, or even problematical, in what way moral reasons and ethical values fit with other motives and desires, how far they express those other motives, and how far they are in conflict with them. Thucydides and (I believe) the tragedians, among the ancient writers, had such a psychology; *and so, in the modern world, did Freud* [emphasis added]. (Williams 1995a, p. 202)

Williams does not explicitly say why he believes this, but he *shows* why in his own magisterial work on the structure of shame, *Shame and Necessity* (Williams 1993). There he demonstrates how one can only make sense of the complexity and richness of shame if one construes it in terms of intrapsychic object relations. Basically, one needs to posit the gaze of an internalized other. And Williams shows how crucial shifts in the experience and meaning of shame can be understood only via transformations of intrapsychic structure. As the philosopher Richard Wollheim (1984, 1999) has shown, the same is true of guilt and the other emotions of moral self-assessment.

In this way, psychoanalysis can help philosophers take a step beyond Nietzsche. Nietzsche was in many ways masterful in showing how a supposedly moral approach to life can arise out of unconscious emotions of resentment and envy. But how? Nietzsche points to the dynamism, but he doesn't explain it. In significant part, this is because he does not have a theory of intrapsychic structure, nor does he have a theory of internal object relations. Thus, he is not in a position where he can develop a systematic account of the transformations in object relations that facilitate and express psychic change. Psychoanalysis, with its account of intrapsychic transformations, allows us to develop a sophisticated and nonmoralized approach to moral psychology (Lear 2003b).

The Nature of Human Happiness and Freedom

Given that the mind is dynamically organized and much of its functioning is unconscious, what do human happiness and freedom consist of? Really, this is just the Socratic question all over again; only this time it assumes we must ask it via a psychoanalytic engagement with the human spirit.

References

Aristotle: Nicomachean Ethics. Translated by Rowe C. Oxford, England, Oxford University Press, 2002

Davidson D: How is weakness of will possible? in Essays on actions and events. Oxford, England, Clarendon Press, 1980, pp 21–42

Davidson D: Paradoxes of irrationality, in Philosophical Essays on Freud. Edited by Wollheim R, Hopkins J. Cambridge, England, Cambridge University Press, 1982, pp 289–305

Davidson D: Inquiries into Truth and Interpretation. Oxford, England, Clarendon Press, 1984

Frankfurt H: Freedom of the will and the concept of a person, in The Importance of What We Care About. Cambridge, England, Cambridge University Press, 1988, pp 80–103

Freud S: Notes upon a case of obsessional neurosis (1909), in Standard Edition of the Complete Psychological Works of Sigmund Freud, Vol 10. Translated and edited by Strachey J. London, Hogarth Press, 1955, pp 151–318

Grube GME, Reeve CDC (trans and eds): Plato: Republic. Indianapolis, IN, Hackett Publishing Co, 1992

Korsgaard C: The Sources of Normativity. Cambridge, England, Cambridge University Press, 1996

Lear, J: Therapeutic Action: An Earnest Plea for Irony. New York, Other Press, 2003a

Lear J: The idea of a moral psychology: the impact of psychoanalysis on philosophy in Britain. Int J Psychoanal 84:1351–1361, 2003b

Moran R: Authority and Estrangement: An Essay on Self-Knowledge. Princeton, NJ, Princeton University Press, 2001

Nagel T: Comment on Korsgaard, in The Sources of Normativity. Edited by Korsgaard C. Cambridge, England, Cambridge University Press, 1996, pp 200–209

Sartre J-P: Being and Nothingness. New York, Washington Square Press, 1956

Vlastos G: The Socratic elenchus. Oxford Studies in Ancient Philosophy 1:27–58, 1983

Vlastos G: Socrates: Ironist and Moral Philosopher. Cambridge, England, Cambridge University Press, 1991

Williams B: Shame and Necessity. Berkeley, University of California Press, 1993

Williams B: Naturalism and morality, in World, Mind and Ethics. Edited by Altham JEJ, Harrison R. Cambridge, England, Cambridge University Press, 1995a, pp 202–203

Williams B: Nietzsche's minimalist moral psychology, in Making Sense of Humanity and Other Philosophical Papers. Cambridge, England, Cambridge University Press, 1995b, pp 65–76

Wollheim R: The Thread of Life. Cambridge, England, Cambridge University Press, 1984

Wollheim R: On the Emotions. New Haven, CT, Yale University Press, 1999

35

Politics and International Relations

VAMIK D. VOLKAN, M.D.

STARTING WITH SIGMUND FREUD, psychoanalysts have ventured beyond the couch and applied their understanding of individual psychology to collective human behavior in general. However, when they have adapted their knowledge and insight to writings about politics, diplomacy, and related issues, their contributions have not been received with enthusiasm by those outside psychoanalysis. Politicians and diplomats could not find useful guidelines in these psychoanalytic insights that would allow them to develop practical strategies to deal with specific national or international problems.

In this chapter, I first review the difficulties encountered in the collaboration between psychoanalysts and those who practice the arts of politics and diplomacy or who are scholars of political science. Next, I focus on some new psychoanalytic observations on the psychology of large groups, such as ethnic or religious groups, and the relationships of these large groups with their political leaders. Finally, I explore some predictable "rituals" performed by enemy groups—in peace and in war. It is hoped that these findings will prove useful in the development of practical and humane strategies for dealing with massive human phenomena and of closer cooperation between psychoanalysis and political science.

Difficulties in Collaboration

There is a "natural" human resistance to experiencing anxiety or other unpleasant affects. Accordingly, as a whole, people resist exploring hidden aspects of national or international affairs that may induce these affects. Furthermore, increased awareness and exploration of disturbing shared mental processes produces a responsibility for dealing with them. Politicians and diplomats, like the rest of us, usually resist assuming new responsibilities that may complicate existing ones. Thus, they may unconsciously prefer to explain complicated situations through intellectualization, rationalization, displacement, projection, and other mental mechanisms. In political or diplomatic affairs, as in psychoanalysis, it takes time to work through newly gained insights and to take new actions. For this reason, political and diplomatic efforts should be considered processes rather than hit-or-miss activities.

Estonia regained its independence in 1991 after the collapse of the Soviet Union. On the surface, Estonians were elated; however, they also had hidden shared anxieties. In reality, the new republic faced many problems. Among them was the fact that one out of every three persons living in Estonia was a Russian-speaking former Soviet citizen; most of these persons were ethnic Russians. Estonia's population numbered 1.5 million people; ethnic Estonians perceived the 500,000 ethnic Russians as enemies and former oppressors.

For purposes of "national interest," the Estonian government instituted a difficult and often humiliating language examination for Russian speakers living in Estonia in order to avoid granting most of them Estonian citizenship. The explanation of this political decision was highly rationalized. For example, a lack of funds was used as an excuse for not developing a more humane and fair method for the language examinations. This in turn became a sore point in Estonian-Russian relations. The Russian government did not want to "relocate" Russians living in Estonia into Russia; this was not a practical or realistic consideration. But Russians in Russia did not want ethnic Russians in Estonia to be humiliated and subjected to unfair practices like the language examination.

A couple of years after Estonia regained its independence, a team from the University of Virginia's Center for the Study of Mind and Human Interaction (CSMHI), working with the Carter Center in Atlanta, Georgia (under former president Jimmy Carter), began a 5-year project in Estonia to assist in the adjustment to a new political and psychological reality. The interdisciplinary team included psychoanalysts, who brought psychoanalytic insights and tools to the project, and former U.S. diplomats who could help with negotiations between Estonians and Russians. During the first 2 years, high-level Estonian politicians (including the current president, Arnold Rüütel) and scholars, leaders of Russian-speaking communities in Estonia, and diplomats and scholars from Moscow convened in Estonia every 3–4 months for 4 days of unofficial dialogue. The CSMHI/Carter Center team facilitated these meetings.

Slowly, the Estonian participants learned about and faced anxiety-provoking shared sentiments that had been previously hidden: 1) mostly unconsciously, but also consciously, they wished all the Russian-speakers to disappear magically (to die), and 2) since they had lived under foreign domination for nearly a millennium, they felt "independence" was dangerous, because it might invite a new occupation by "others," which could erase Estonians as an ethnic group from the face of the earth. Under the overt elation of being independent lay the shared irrational (psychological) thought that their large-group identity could be lost. When a ferry named "Estonia" sank in the Baltic Sea, instead of grief, most Estonians felt anxiety because the loss of the ferry *actualized* their hidden expectation of their disappearance as a people.

After learning about their covert shared thought processes, with the facilitators' help, Estonian participants faced the accompanying unpleasant affects. During early meetings, some of their faces had literally turned purple with anger and anxiety. After 2 years of dialogue, they could speak about previously unacceptable thoughts and freely express the feelings associated with them. They could now "play" with their unacceptable wishes and also accept the realities associated with the new Estonia. They also could "think" of new political strategies, free from the influence of their shared anxieties.

With the help of the Estonian participants, the new government eventually accepted the facilitator team, which provided them with various methods for language examinations (the CSMHI/Carter team also included a linguist) and restructured the language examinations in a more systematic and humane way. This removed the constant humiliation of the Russian speakers in Estonia to a great extent and opened a door to better collaboration between ethnic Estonians and ethnic Russians living in Estonia. In addition, the language examinations could no longer serve as a focus for displaced expressions of Estonians' irrational thoughts and affects (Apprey 1996; Neu and Volkan 1997; Volkan 1997).

Of course, the Estonia project was most unusual. Given the pervasive influence of *realpolitik* on governments, it is not surprising that psychoanalytic observations are not embraced with open arms by politicians, diplomats, or political scientists. Since Ludwig von Rochau (1853/1972) introduced the concept of *realpolitik*, this idea has evolved, in general, to mean the rational evaluation and realistic assessment of the options available to one's large group and its enemies without considering psychological processes. It gave birth to what become known, especially in the United States, as *rational actor models* of politics and diplomacy.

As the shortcomings of various rational actor models became evident, in the late 1970s and early 1980s some political scientists, and even some government decision-makers and diplomats, began to borrow concepts from cognitive psychology to explain "faulty" decision making. But they did not look to psychoanalysis for insights (Volkan et al. 1998). Exploration of shared, unconscious forces was avoided despite a long history of attempts to introduce psychoanalysis into politics and diplomacy, including the efforts of Harold Laswell (1927, 1930), a pioneer in the study of psychosocial warfare. Other difficulties that complicate collaboration between psychoanalysts and practitioners and scholars of politics and international relations come from psychoanalysis itself. The following points illuminate this assertion.

Factors Limiting Contributions of Psychoanalysis to Politics

Not Having a Psychology of Large Groups in Its Own Right

Politics and diplomacy necessarily deal with the psychology of large groups, the psychology of leader-followers, and the psychology of relationships between enemy groups and their leaders. Freud was interested in these topics, but he also left a legacy that discouraged his followers from pursuing them. In his letter to Albert Einstein, Freud (1933/ 1964) was pessimistic about human nature and the role of psychoanalysis in preventing wars or war-like situations. Although Jacob Arlow (1973) later suggested some optimism in some of Freud's writings on this subject, Freud's pessimism played a role in limiting psychoanalytic contributions to the fields of politics and diplomacy.

There were, of course, exceptions (Fornari 1966/1975; Glower 1947). However, those exceptions followed Freud's lead in another area, and this too blocked the potential influence of psychoanalysis on politics and diplomacy: these writers, like Freud, focused on individuals' unconscious perceptions of what the image of political leaders and the mental representations of a large group symbolically stand for instead of on large-group psychology and leader–follower relations in their own right. Psychoanalysis remained primarily an investigative tool of an individual's internal world and was not used as a tool to examine massive human movements. Freud's (1921/1955) well-known theory on large-group psychology, for example, reflects a theme that mainly focuses on the understanding of the individual: the members of the group sublimate their aggression against the leader in a way that is similar to the process of a son turning his negative feelings toward his oedipal father into loyalty. In turn, the members of a large group idealize the leader, identify with each other, and rally around the leader.

Freud's theory is based on a "male-oriented" psychological process. More importantly, as Robert Waelder (1971) noted, Freud was speaking only of *regressed* groups. Given such shortcomings, in the last decade or so some psychoanalysts who study large groups and their leaders shifted their approach from emphasizing the image of the leader to focusing on the mental representation of the large group itself as seen by the individual. For example, Didier Anzieu (1971, 1984), Janine Chassequet-Smirgel (1985), and Otto Kernberg (1980, 1989) wrote about shared fantasies of members of a large group. They suggested that large groups represent idealized mothers (breast mothers) who repair all narcissistic injuries. But, again, their theories focus on individuals' perceptions. It is assumed that external processes that threaten the group members' image of an idealized mother can initiate political processes and influence international affairs. Nevertheless, an approach that focuses on individuals' perceptions that a large group represents a mother image does not offer *specificity* concerning a political or diplomatic process. Thus, it does not excite practitioners of politics and diplomacy or receive much attention from political scientists. What the psychoanalytic tradition lacks is the study of both large-group psychology in its own right and the specific elements of various mass movements.

Not Exploring Analysts' Own Large-Group Sentiments During Their Training

A future analyst's personal analysis usually does not include a full exploration of the analysand's ethnic, national, or religious affiliations. Unless the psychoanalyst-to-be suffers from malignant prejudice or paranoia, his or her large-group sentiments are not brought up on the couch. The human "need to have enemies and allies" (Volkan 1988) in a large-group context is not discussed. We also know that analysts and analysands often shy away from addressing sensitive large-group issues. Some aspects of a large-group history induce "anxiety" (Loewenberg 1991; Rangell 2004). For example, an analyst who is a survivor of the Holocaust may resist exploring the transgenerational transmission of trauma in an analysand who is a child of other survivors or of Jewish persons affected by the Holocaust. During the last two decades, I have had many opportunities to supervise young German psychoanalysts who resisted bringing their German analysands' Nazi-connected family history to the couch (Volkan et al. 2002). Similarly, when reading Israeli and Arab psychoanalysts' writings on the Middle East conflict, we cannot escape noticing that when it comes to ethnic, national, religious, or even ideological sentiments, psychoanalysts, like politicians, diplomats and just about everyone else, may exhibit prejudices and respond to propaganda and manipulations by political leaders (Varvin and Volkan 2003).

Evaluation of international processes and leader–follower relations correctly takes experience in the international field and the difficult "working through" of the meaning and functions of large-group sentiments. Otherwise, there will be contamination with prejudicial affects that change perceptions. More than 25 years ago, I wrote a book on the conflict between Cypriot Greeks and Cypriot Turks (I belong to the second group); the subtitle of my book was "A Study of *Two* Ethnic Groups in Conflict" [emphasis added] (Volkan 1979). Looking back, I must admit that I had no deep knowledge of the suffering of the Greek side and, indeed, had no wish to know about their experiences and perceptions of events. Freud himself has left us some evidence that when it comes to large-group issues, psychoanalysts have prejudices, and this, I believe, is an obstacle to their suggesting practical solutions for ethnic or religious problems—even though they try to be neutral. In his correspondence with Albert Einstein, Freud (1933/1964) made "racist" remarks about Turks and Mongols. He also jokingly referred to his patients as "negroes" (Tate 1996). These were not necessarily vicious or hateful attacks, and racism in general was prevalent— and to a great degree, accepted—in Europe in the late nineteenth and early twentieth century. Freud may have identified with the aggressor in an attempt to defend against mounting anti-Semitism, but his remarks nevertheless should serve to remind psychoanalysts that our own personal analyses, self-analyses, and extensive study and training in human nature do not free us from investment in certain cultural norms, the attitudes of our own large group, or even racism.

Analysts Not Working in Interdisciplinary Settings

In his or her practice, an analyst is often a lonely figure: he or she alone (though with the analysand's input, of course) assesses the patient's internal conflicts and adaptations and decides what to interpret and how to react. When it comes to the myriad complicated issues in political and international affairs, it is difficult simply to sort out unfolding events, let alone figure out what hidden, shared psychological processes are attached to them. Most psychoanalysts are knowledgeable about how small therapy groups work; others have written about the psychology of organizations composed of hundreds or even thousands of individuals (Abse 1974; Bion 1961; Foulkes 1957; Zaleznik 1984). They then tend to apply these insights to religious, national, or ethnic groups that may include millions of individuals. Large groups, such as ethnic groups, have their own specific psychological processes (Volkan 1988, 1997, 1999a, 1999c, 2004). In their clinical practices, psychoanalysts learn the histories and psychic realities of their individual patients. Often, however, they are not sufficiently familiar with the histories of large groups and the shared mental representations of such histories. They tend to treat large groups as they would treat individuals with psychopathology.

Following Otto Fenichel's (1935) concern about uncritical expansion of psychoanalytic interpretation into areas that are not amenable to direct psychoanalytic observation, German psychoanalyst Alexander Mitscherlich (1971) emphasized the need to work closely with those in other social science disciplines. Such collaborative studies are always exceptions in psychoanalytic work, however. Accordingly, such studies suffer from a lack of historical knowledge and related issues and cannot illuminate specific areas that interest politicians and diplomats. To deal with this problem, when I established CSMHI in 1987 within the Medical School of the University of Virginia, I invited high-level (former) diplomats, political scientists, historians, and others to join the Center as appointed faculty, to work alongside the psychoanalysts, psychiatrists, psychologists, and other mental health professionals.

Thus far, I have focused on the difficulties facing psychoanalysts in their attempts to contribute to the fields of politics and diplomacy. These problems need to be acknowledged. Before proceeding further, I must say that I agree with most psychoanalytic conceptualizations about individuals' perceptions of what images of leaders and large groups signify to them. Like Freud, I am pessimistic about psychoanalytic contributions to "curing" large-group conflicts, taming massive aggression and destruction, and diminishing the derivatives of aggression within human nature. On the other hand, I am optimistic about using psychoanalytic insights and concepts to deal with and modify certain specific and limited political and international situations. For this to happen, psychoanalysts must be willing to work with historians, political scientists, diplomats, and others within an established team. The first thing to do is to work though the competition between the disciplines in order to establish a true team spirit. It is also imperative that people from different disciplines be willing to work together for many years in long-term projects and processes (just as psychoanalysts are involved with their analysands), focusing on specific "conflicts" (see Volkan 1999b).

Background for Concepts of Collaboration in Politics and Diplomacy

In my own life and professional career, I have spent over 25 years in international relations and unofficial diplomacy, which has provided opportunities to suggest certain concepts that have close connections with politics and diplomacy. In evolving these concepts, I had three "laboratories":

1. *Dialogues between high-level officials and scholars of opposing groups.* I took part in unofficial dialogues between high-level officials and scholars of opposing groups (e.g., Arabs and Israelis, Georgians and South Ossetians, Turks and Armenians, and, as already mentioned, Estonians and Russians). During these meetings, representatives of each antagonistic group (besides exhibiting aspects of their individual personalities) became spokespersons for their specific large-group psychological processes.

2. *Visits to traumatized societies.* I visited many traumatized societies with other analysts and mental health professionals as well as colleagues from other disciplines (Northern Cyprus after the 1974 war, Kuwait after the 1990 Iraqi invasion, Croatia after separating from Yugoslavia, post–Enver Hoxha Albania, and refugee camps in Georgia and South Ossetia, for example). In such societies, there is a focus on "we-ness" in which a psychology that separates "us" from "them" is clearly observable. In some locations we conducted hundreds of psychoanalytic interviews. We collected data about individuals' internal worlds, including their fantasies

and dreams and how they intertwined their internal processes with external political, military, economic and legal issues. This taught us a great deal about the psychology of politics and diplomacy.

3. *Meetings with political leaders.* I met a dozen or so political leaders, from President Carter and former Soviet leader Mikhail Gorbachev to PLO Chairman Yasser Arafat and Northern Cyprus President Rauf Denktash. I spent considerable time with some of them, less time with others. During these meetings, I observed how specific leaders had perceived and reacted to specific political and diplomatic situations.

The following section contains new or modified concepts related to politics and diplomacy. Each concept, however, is discussed only briefly (for extensive examination of them, see Volkan 1988, 1997, 1999c, 2004). This list is provided so that the concepts can be evaluated critically. Also, those psychoanalysts who are willing to work in the field of political psychology may find them useful. I have chosen to include items here that are in some way related to a fundamental concept, large-group identity.

Focus on Specific Political and Diplomatic Issues

Large-Group Identity: The Tent Metaphor

We can visualize the classical Freudian theory about large groups and their leaders by imagining people arranged around a large maypole, which represents the group's leader, as if joined in a May Day dance of identification with each other and of idealization and support of the leader. We can build upon this metaphor by imagining a large cloth over the people, a "tent canvas" of large-group identity. Following Erik Erikson's (1956) description of individual identity, we can describe the large-group identity of thousands, or millions, of people—most of whom will never meet one another in their lifetimes—who share a persistent sense of sameness (we-ness) while also sharing some characteristics with people who live under other tents. While people under a large-group tent are divided into subgroups (clans, occupations, religious sects, and so on), they wear the tent canvas as a shared garment. If the tent shakes—especially as a result of threats or attacks from "others"—or the tent's pole becomes unsteady (the leader becomes paranoid or dies), and if there is significant wear-and-tear on the cloth, group identity becomes even more important to the people. It may even become their primary garment (psychologically), eclipsing their usual individual garments (their personal identities).

From a large-group psychological, political, and diplomatic perspective, the psychoanalyst's focus should not be on personal perceptions that the pole represents an oedipal father or that the tent canvas is like a nurturing mother. Rather, analysts should focus on large-group identity—its formation and the group's need to protect it at any cost. People rally around the leader so that the pole keeps the tent canvas erect. The main purpose of the leader becomes the protection of large-group identity; this influences political and diplomatic processes. An examination of the tent canvas and its components, which become exaggerated under stressful conditions and with which group members become preoccupied, offers specific elements on which to focus. This leads to a more fruitful collaboration between psychoanalysts and policy-makers. Psychoanalytic consultations may help develop useful strategies (e.g., third party neutrals could shore up opposing camps' large-group identities during negotiations).

Sharing the tent canvas as a common garment connects multitudes of people and may dominate their individual psychological processes. It is difficult to understand the psychology of suicide bombers unless we see them as "spokespersons" of their large-group identity who are doing what they feel and think is necessary to maintain that identity. In times when the large-group identity is threatened, consideration for individual lives becomes secondary. In our routine lives, we are not necessarily aware of our connections with our large-group processes. We do not wake up each morning feeling intensely American, Polish, or Syrian. Belonging to a large group does not necessarily elicit overwhelming feelings of patriotism, for example, each time we see our nation's flag. Our relationship with our large-group identity, in ordinary times, is like breathing. While we breathe constantly, we do not usually notice it unless our ability to breathe is threatened, such as when we have pneumonia or are caught in a smoke-filled house on fire. When representatives of enemy groups come together, they often react as if they have entered a burning building. Psychoanalytic insights can be used to bring in fresh air so that conflicts and misunderstandings may be resolved, paving the way for successful negotiations.

Chosen Glories and Chosen Traumas

To provide fresh air and to not add fuel to the fire, analysts need to study what types of components/threads are woven into the tent canvasses of the involved parties. Some "threads" tell us how individual and large-group identities are interwoven: we have a great deal of information on how certain early identifications with the adults around us connect our personal identities with our large-group identities. I do not focus here, in this brief chapter, on identification and other concepts that connect individual and group identities (see Volkan 1999a, 1999c for extensive explanations). Instead, I discuss two "threads" that bring specificity to each ethnic, national, or religious tent canvas. Political leaders instinctively know how to focus on these two elements and use them for political propaganda and for political movements. I call them "chosen glories" and "chosen traumas."

Chosen glories are mental representations of a large group's past triumphs and the heroes and martyrs associated with them (Moses 1982; Volkan 1988, 1997, 2004). They are specific phenomena for specific large groups; they induce a heightened sense of "we-ness." During the Gulf War, for instance, Saddam Hussein tried to galvanize his followers by associating himself with Sultan Saladin, who defeated the Christian Crusaders in the twelfth century, thus reviving a past glorious event and its hero. Chosen glories are passed from generation to generation through caretaker-child interactions and through participation in ceremonies that recall the past success. However, they influence large-group identity less pervasively than chosen traumas because the latter bring with them powerful experiences of loss and feelings of humiliation, vengeance, and hatred that are shared.

A *chosen trauma* is the shared mental representation of a negative event in a large group's history in which the group suffered catastrophic loss, humiliation, and helplessness at the hand of another large group. There are countless clinical investigations of members of large groups that have suffered massive trauma from the actions of an enemy group; there are also many investigations of the second and third generations of a group on whose ancestors overwhelming trauma was inflicted. These investigations clearly show how the mental representations of a shared tragedy are transmitted to subsequent generations in varying levels of intensity (see Volkan et al. 2002 for a selected review of the literature on the transmission of Holocaust images).

There is far more to the transmission of massive trauma than children mimicking the behavior of their parents or hearing stories about the event told by the older generations. Rather, it is the end result of mostly unconscious psychological processes through which survivors *deposit* into their progeny's core identities their own injured self-images. Thus, the parent's injured self-image "lives on" in the child. Then the parent (now within the child, so to speak) unconsciously assigns to the child specific tasks of reparation that rightfully belong to the survivor (i.e., to reverse shame and humiliation, turn passivity to activity, tame the sense of aggression, and mourn the losses associated with the trauma). Since all the injured self-images that individual parents in a traumatized group transmit to

their children refer to the same event, a shared image of the tragedy develops, and over generations, it evolves into the group's chosen trauma. By sharing the chosen trauma, succeeding generations are unconsciously knit together. The chosen trauma becomes a specific thread of a specific large group's tent canvas; it is now also highly mythologized.

When enemy representatives come together for negotiations, they inevitably reactivate their chosen traumas (as well as their chosen glories, but to a much lesser degree) in order to deal with the anxiety concerning the threats against their large-group identity. The main unconscious reason to reactivate a chosen trauma is to hold on to the group's identity when it is threatened. For example, during unofficial talks with Estonians, Russians would recall centuries of being attacked and occupied by the Mongols, or the disproportionate losses and sacrifices they suffered to protect the "civilized" world during the Nazi period. The appearance of preoccupation with chosen traumas while negotiating current issues may confuse negotiators and third-party neutrals. Psychoanalytic insights about chosen traumas and why they appear at certain times—to protect large-group identity—can be useful in putting negotiations back on track.

Time Collapse

When political leaders reactivate a large group's chosen trauma through political propaganda, related emotions and perceptions are experienced as if the trauma were a recent occurrence, and they become fused with the emotions and perceptions related to current political, diplomatic and/or military issues. They may even be projected into the future. What is "remembered" from the past is felt in the present and is expected for the future, coming together in a *time collapse*.

The concepts of chosen trauma and time collapse are critical for understanding the tragedies in Bosnia in 1992 and in Kosovo in 1999. The shared mental representation of the Battle of Kosovo in 1389 is the Serbian chosen trauma. Despite the fact that the leaders of both sides—Ottoman Sultan Murat I and Serbian Prince Lazar—were both killed, and despite the fact that Serbia remained autonomous for some 80 years after the battle, the Battle of Kosovo evolved as a major chosen trauma for Serbians (Emmert 1990). Lazar's "ghost" and the images of the battle were resurrected by Slobodan Milošević, Radovan Karazić, and other Serbian leaders to reactivate the 600-year-old "memory" of humiliation and the accompanying desire for revenge. The time collapse that was facilitated through sophisticated propaganda (Gutman 1993) readied the Serbian people emotionally for the atrocities they would eventually commit against Bosnian and Kosovan

Muslims. For example, Lazar's remains were put into a coffin and were taken for a year-long trip throughout Serbia, visiting many villages and towns where speeches and religious ceremonies created an atmosphere as if he had been killed recently. The creation of this particular time collapse happened in front of the world (for details, see Volkan 1997). Psychoanalysts studying the concepts of chosen trauma and time collapse could forecast a malignant outcome.

Large-Group Regression and Rituals

Large groups regress when the large-group identity is threatened and/or damaged. Psychoanalysts have identified certain signs and symptoms of this regression, such as blind rallying around a leader, the loss of individual identity for group members, the development of a new "shared morality" that allows destroying or killing "others" without much guilt feelings, and an increasingly primitive and absolutist belief system held by the group. Those persons perceived to be in conflict with the group are labeled as "them" versus "us," thus creating a sharp division between the group and the enemy. In addition, new findings on signs and symptoms of large-group regression (Volkan 2004) include the reactivation of the group's chosen glories and traumas, the group's experiencing of legal and geographical boundaries as a "second skin," and group concerns about "blood" (identity as a people). More importantly, regressed groups are involved in certain rituals, some of which, if not diagnosed and dealt with constructively (perhaps with the help of outside neutral parties), may lead to malignant developments.

During the regression and during efforts to relieve the regression, a regressed group becomes like a snake shedding its skin. In a sense, the regressed group asks, "Who are we now?" and is intent on getting rid of unacceptable elements "contaminating" its identity. I call this obligatory group process *purification*. Purification may be benign, such as removing foreign words from the group's language, or may be deadly, such as so-called ethnic cleansing. Again, there is a large-group psychology of such activities that can be illuminated by psychoanalysts who are willing to work in the field.

Minor Differences

Particularly when it is regressed, a large group resists being the same as or even similar to an enemy in any way. Antagonist groups may have major differences in religion, language, history and myths. But when enemy representatives meet for negotiations, the most troublesome immediate issues may well be *minor differences*, a concept introduced by Freud (1917/1957). However, he was not aware of how minor differences appearing in large-group interactions can become deadly. Minor differences are perceived as dangerous signals of similarity. Enemies are both real and fantasied (Stein 1990); they are the reservoirs for a large group's bad externalizations and projections. To be the same as or similar to an enemy spoils the stability of externalization and projection. What has been put *out there* could boomerang.

Minor differences can be found practically everywhere: food, clothing, architecture, or any other characteristic. For instance, Thomas Butler (1993) examined the minor differences between the dialects involved in pronunciation of certain words by Serbians and Croatians. Donald Horowitz (1985) writes about minor differences with deadly consequences in the way Sinhalese and Tamils dress in Sri Lanka. Minor differences also complicate situations during political or diplomatic efforts (Volkan 1988, 1997a). During negotiations, when the issue of minor differences becomes a major obstacle, psychoanalytic consultation may help the neutral facilitators develop strategies for the protection of the antagonist groups' identities while dealing with the issue.

Accordion Phenomenon

After some airing of chosen traumas and glories or their derivatives (which may be observed directly and/or indirectly), the opposing groups in diplomatic negotiations often experience a rapprochement. This closeness is then usually followed by a sudden withdrawal from one another, then again by closeness, and so on. This pattern may be repeated many times during negotiations. It can be likened to the playing of an accordion. The psychology of this phenomenon is similar to the psychology of minor differences. I have observed that effective discussion of real-world issues, such as banking adjustments, economic concessions, legal contracts, or disarmament, cannot take place unless "accordion playing" is allowed for a time during the political or diplomatic discussions between the representatives of the opposing large groups. This makes it possible for the pendulum-like swings in sentiment to be slowly replaced by more realistic and stable conceptualizations. Sometimes "neutral" facilitators mistakenly urge the opposing parties to make agreements during a period of premature closeness. Psychoanalysts can advise the groups not to push for agreement too soon and instead to allow time for stabilization of the *psychological borders* of the opposing parties.

Mourning

Politics and diplomacy are always connected with the psychology of mourning, a concept familiar to psychoanalysts. Mourning, in the psychoanalytic sense, accompanies political and diplomatic activities and war and warlike conditions because there will always be *losses* pertaining to prestige, identity, and security, as well as people and property/land. Mourning is an obligatory response to loss or threat of loss. Politicians and diplomats always react to losses and gains, as does everyone. Furthermore, like individuals, large groups mourn. While psychoanalysts know about the individual's mourning processes (Freud 1917 [1915]/1957; Pollock 1989), the evolution of large-group mourning (Volkan 1988) takes a different course and initiates societal or political processes in response to loss. This is a vast area, not detailed here, in which psychoanalytic observations can be greatly beneficial. During the dialogue series between Egyptians and Israelis between 1980 and 1986 that was sponsored by the American Psychiatric Association, one meeting occurred soon after the Israeli withdrawal from the Sinai. During the withdrawal, the Israeli residents of Yamit, a border region containing Israeli settlements, refused to evacuate the area, and the Israeli forces bulldozed Yamit. Egyptians accused Israelis of destructive acts. What was "given back" to the Egyptians was a destroyed region. During the meeting, representatives of the opposing countries were very emotional and could not negotiate issues in a realistic way. The facilitating team was able to note that the destruction of Yamit was associated with the Israelis' mourning process concerning their "losing" Sinai. Even though the Sinai did not belong to them, the Israelis had developed images of Sinai as an area buffering them from the enemy. Reaction to loss was accompanied with the expression of aggression. When Egyptian participants comprehended the idea that Israelis had a right to mourn for "losing" Sinai, the atmosphere of the meeting room changed considerably and unofficial negotiations could be resumed in earnest.

Conclusion

The previous observations are by no means complete; there are many psychoanalytic conceptualizations that are pertinent to politics and diplomacy. The concepts chosen for this chapter illustrate, in a sense, a new way of thinking about psychoanalytic contributions to national and international conflicts. Alongside theoretical writings about what political leaders and ethnic, national, or religious groups represent for the individual, analysts could offer insights concerning practical aspects of politics and diplomacy. In illustrating those often-unseen psychological processes that accompany relations between opposing parties and nations, psychoanalysts also need to be protective of

"reality." To focus on psychology does not minimize the existence of realistic difficulties, but psychology may provide a new perspective from which to view these realities.

In addition to the efforts of some individuals and of academic centers such as the Center for the Study of Mind and Human Interaction to bring psychoanalysis together with politics and diplomacy, both the American Psychoanalytic Association and the International Psychoanalytical Association (IPA) seem to be more aware of the desire for such a rapprochement. Recently, the American Psychoanalytic Association's annual meetings included panels and study groups dealing with these topics. Even before September 11, 2001, the IPA had formed a committee to work with the United Nations. After 9/11, IPA's Working Group on Terror and Terrorism was established. This working group has already published a book (Varvin and Volkan 2003) that can be used as a vehicle for further collaboration between psychoanalysis and the fields of political science and diplomacy.

References

Abse DW: Clinical Notes of Group-Analytic Psychotherapy. Charlottesville, University Press of Virginia, 1974

Anzieu D: L'illusion groupale. Nouvelle Revue de Psychanalyse 4:73–93, 1971

Anzieu D: The Group and the Unconscious. London, Routledge & Kegan Paul, 1984

Apprey M: Heuristic steps for negotiating ethno-national conflicts: vignettes from Estonia. New Literary History 27: 199–212, 1996

Arlow J: Motivations for peace, in Psychological Basis of War. Edited by Winnik HZ, Moses R, Ostow M. Jerusalem, Israel, Jerusalem Academic Press, 1973, pp 193–204

Bion WR: Experiences in Groups. London, Tavistock, 1961

Butler T: Yugoslavia mon amour. Mind and Human Interaction 4:120–128, 1993

Chasseguet-Smirgel J: The Ego Ideal: A Psychoanalytic Essay on the Malady of the Ideal. New York, WW Norton, 1985

Emmert TA: Serbian Golgotha: Kosovo, 1389. New York, Columbia University Press, 1990

Erikson EH: The problem of ego identification. J Am Psychoanal Assoc 4:56–121, 1956

Fenichel O: Über psychoanalyse, Krieg und Frieden. International Arztl Bulletin 2:30–40, 1935

Fornari F: The Psychoanalysis of War (1966). Translated by Pfeifer A. Bloomington, IN, Indiana University Press, 1975

Foulkes SH, Anthony EJ: Group Psychotherapy. London, Penguin, 1957

Freud S: Taboo of virginity (1917), in Standard Edition of the Complete Psychological Works of Sigmund Freud, Vol 11. Translated and edited by Strachey J. London, Hogarth Press, 1957, pp 191–208

Freud S: Mourning and melancholia (1917[1915]), in Standard Edition of the Complete Psychological Works of Sigmund Freud, Vol 14. Translated and edited by Strachey J. London, Hogarth Press, 1957, pp 237–260

Freud S: Group psychology and the analysis of the ego (1921), in Standard Edition of the Complete Psychological Works of Sigmund Freud, Vol 18. Translated and edited by Strachey J. London, Hogarth Press, 1955, pp 65–143

Freud S: Why war (1933)? in Standard Edition of the Complete Psychological Works of Sigmund Freud, Vol 22. Translated and edited by Strachey J. London, Hogarth Press, 1964, pp 199–215

Glower E: War, Sadism, and Pacifism: Further Essays on Group Psychology and War. London, Allen & Unwin, 1947

Gutman RA: A Witness to Genocide: The 1993 Pulitzer Prize-winning Dispatches on the "Ethnic Cleansing" of Bosnia. New York, Maxwell MacMillan International, 1993

Horowitz DL: Ethnic Groups in Conflict. Berkeley, University of California Press, 1985

Kernberg OF: Internal World and External Reality: Object Relations Theory Applied. New York, Jason Aronson, 1980

Kernberg OF: Mass psychology through the analytic lens. Article presented at Through the Looking Glass: Freud's Impact on Contemporary Culture. Philadelphia, PA, September 23, 1989

Lasswell HD: Propaganda Technique in the World War. New York, Knopf, 1927

Lasswell HD: Psychopathology and Politics. Chicago, IL, University of Chicago Press, 1930

Loewenberg P: Uses of anxiety. Partisan Review 3:514–525, 1991

Mitscherlich A: Psychoanalysis and aggression of large groups. Int J Psychoanal 52:161–167, 1971

Moses R: The group-self and the Arab-Israeli Conflict. Int Rev Psychoanal 9:55–65, 1982

Neu J, Volkan VD: Developing a Methodology for Conflict Prevention: The Case of Estonia. Atlanta, GA, The Carter Center, 1999

Pollock GH: The Mourning-Liberation Process, Vols 1 and 2. Madison, CT, International Universities Press, 1989

Rangell L: Affects: in an individual and a nation. Mind and Human Interaction 13:242–257, 2004

Stein HF: The international and group milieu of ethnicity: identifying generic group dynamic issues. Canadian Review Studies in Nationalism 17:107–130, 1990

Tate C: Freud and his "Negro": psychoanalysis as ally and enemy of African Americans. Journal for the Psychoanalysis of Culture and Society 1:53–62, 1996

Varvin S, Volkan VD (eds): Violence or Dialogue? Psychoanalytic Insights on Terror and Terrorism. London, International Psychoanalysis Library, 2003

Volkan VD: Cyprus—War and Adaptation: A Psychoanalytic History of Two Ethnic Groups in Conflict. Charlottesville, University Press of Virginia, 1979

Volkan VD: The Need to Have Enemies and Allies: From Clinical Practice to International Relationships. Northvale, NJ, Jason Aronson, 1988

Volkan VD: Bloodlines: From Ethnic Pride to Ethnic Terrorism. New York, Farrar, Straus, & Giroux, 1997

Volkan VD: Psychoanalysis and diplomacy, part 1: individual and large group identity. Journal of Applied Psychoanalytic Studies 1:29–55, 1999a

Volkan VD: The Tree Model: a comprehensive psychopolitical approach to unofficial diplomacy and the reduction of ethnic tension. Mind and Human Interaction 10:141–206, 1999b

Volkan VD: Das Versagen der Diplomatie: Zur Psychoanalyse Nationaler, Ethnischer und Religiöser Konflikte. Giessen, Germany, Psycho-Social Verlag, 1999c

Volkan VD: Blind Trust: Large Groups and Their Leaders in Times of Crisis and Terror. Charlottesville, VA, Pitchstone Publishing, 2004

Volkan VD, Akhtar S, Dorn RM, et al: Psychodynamics of leaders and decision-making. Mind and Human Interaction 9: 129–181, 1998

Volkan VD, Ast G, Greer W: The Third Reich in the Unconscious: Transgenerational Transmission and Its Consequences. New York, Brunner-Routledge, 2002

von Rochau AL: Grundsätze der Realpolitik (1853). Frankfurt, Germany, Ullstein, 1972

Waelder R: Psychoanalysis and history, in The Psychoanalytic Interpretation of History. Edited by Wolman BB. New York, Basic Books 1971, pp 3–22

Zaleznik A: Charismatic and consensus leaders, in the Irrational Executive. Edited by Kets de Vries MFR. New York, International Universities Press, 1984, pp 112–132

36

Neuroscience

MARK SOLMS, PH.D.

THIS CHAPTER INTRODUCES the reader to one of the most promising developments in psychoanalysis in recent years: neuropsychoanalysis. My aim in this chapter is twofold; first, to describe the history of the relationship between psychoanalysis and neuroscience that led up to the neuropsychoanalytic development, and second, to provide a brief overview of the current status of psychoanalytic theory, viewed through a neuroscientific lens.

Historical Background

Neuropsychoanalysis is, in a sense, as old as psychoanalysis itself. Sigmund Freud, the founder of psychoanalysis, was an active neuroscientific researcher for more than 20 years. Between 1877 and 1900 he published more than 200 neuroscientific titles (including numerous reviews) on a wide range of neuroanatomical, clinical neurological, and psychopharmacological topics (Freud, in press). Not surprisingly, his neuroscientific background was a seminal influence on his psychoanalytic thinking and, therefore, on many foundational psychoanalytic concepts (Solms and Saling 1986). Freud's neuroscientific background is particularly clearly demonstrated by his 1895 "Project for a Scientific Psychology," in which almost all of his basic psychological concepts are formulated in neuroscientific terms (e.g., consciousness and the unconscious, primary and secondary process, ego, drive, repression, mechanism of neurosis, function of dreams).

It is easy to forget that psychoanalysis was always intended to be more than a therapeutic procedure. Today many psychoanalytic institutes serve as little more than technical colleges, the essential purpose of which is to produce practitioners ("dentists of the mind," to borrow Riccardo Steiner's amusing phrase). Accordingly, modern psychoanalysts for the most part have no interest in science; indeed, some are positively antiscientific. They know (and care) very little about developments in mental science beyond the narrow confines of the psychoanalytic curriculum. But for Freud and many other pioneers of psychoanalysis, the first and last aim of the discipline was to understand *how the mind works*. For them, the human mind was a piece of nature, part of the natural world, and the task of psychoanalysis—no less than that of any other natural science—was to discern the construction of this aspect of the world and the laws that govern its functioning. Psychoanalytic therapy was, at bottom, nothing more than an *application* of our accumulated scientific knowledge about the inner workings of the mind. To the extent that our theory was wrong, to that extent our therapeutic capacity was accordingly diminished.

Freud inevitably began his analytic research with *basic assumptions* derived from elsewhere (Freud 1920/1955), most notably from his neuroscientific education. Then he shaped these assumptions in the light of his clinical observations. It is true, therefore, that psychoanalytic knowledge is derived essentially from analytic observation. Nevertheless, it would be highly questionable to claim—if anyone seriously does—that the psychoanalytic method is the *only* way to test Freud's ideas about how the mind works. Indeed, it is questionable whether exclusive reliance on a single method is ever desirable in science. Every method has both strengths and weaknesses. Accordingly, good science relies on multiple methods and seeks *multiple, converging lines of evidence.*

Some psychoanalysts justify their disinterest in neuroscience in particular by reference to a supposed precedent set by Freud (1900/1953), who famously "carefully avoid[ed] the temptation to determine psychical locality in any anatomical fashion" (p. 536). Freud abandoned his "Project" in 1896 and proposed instead that we conceptualize the apparatus of the mind as a *virtual* entity, an *abstraction*—that we picture it as something like "a compound instrument, to the components of which we give the name of 'agencies,' or (for the sake of greater clarity) 'systems'" (p. 536). For Freud the mind was something located not *in* the physical elements of the brain but rather, as it were, *between* them. This "functionalist" approach enabled Freud to draw theoretical inferences about the workings of the mind from his clinical (psychological) observations, without having to constantly translate them into the language of anatomy and physiology. This approach is not, however, antineuroscientific. In fact, it has since been widely adopted by modern scientists (usually without acknowledgement to Freud)—and utilized in mind-brain research—most notably by cognitive psychologists, about whom more will be said below.

What psychoanalysts who cite Freud's precedent seem *not* to realize, moreover, is that for him it was simply a matter of expedience—of what was most practicable *at that time.* Freud always recognized, and acknowledged, that it would be preferable if we *could* translate our psychological models into the language of physical science, and he always looked forward to a day when we would be able to do so:

> The deficiencies in our description would probably vanish if we were already in a position to replace the psychological terms by physiological or chemical ones. . . . Biology is truly a land of unlimited possibilities. We may expect it to give us the most surprising information and we cannot guess what answers it will return in a few dozen years to the questions we have put to it. They may be of a kind which will blow away the whole artificial structure of our hypotheses. (Freud 1920/1955, p. 60)

Indeed, Freud's philosophy of mind was such that he clearly recognized that any model of how the mind works *must* be compatible with both its psychological and its physiological realization (Solms 1997b). There can only be one part of nature called the human mind, and it can only obey one set of laws. The metapsychological models

that Freud developed were abstractions, derived mainly from psychological observation, but, as he clearly pointed out in the passage quoted above, they were also translatable *in principle* into physiological and chemical terms, if only the methods were available.

The psychoanalytic method has served us well as a generator of hypotheses about how the mind *might* work, but—especially with regard to its basic constituents and other universals (e.g., taxonomy of the drives, imperatives of the maturational process)—it has proved less than ideal for *testing* the hypotheses it generates (i.e., for deciding between competing alternatives). The clear advantage of physical descriptions over psychological ones, in this regard, is their very *tangibility.* Tangibility begets testability. Psychological observations of the kind that interest psychoanalysts are such fleeting and fugitive things. If the abstractions derived from them could only be translated into anatomical or physiological terms, they would immediately be translated into something concrete, easily observed, and readily measured—something far more manipulable and therefore more conducive to the levels of confidence aspired to by a natural science. It is not at all surprising that Freud looked forward to the day when it would be possible to do so.

It seems that Freud was more aware of the uncertainty attaching to theoretical inferences derived from psychoanalytic observation than most of his followers were. We all know how difficult it is to know anything *definite* about even an individual case, let alone a whole class of mental phenomena, or the human mental apparatus as a whole. Yet it must be admitted that psychoanalysts often speak about the human mind and its workings as if they really did *know* how it all fits together. In fact all we have—and ever have had—are more or less insecure *hypotheses* about these things. Hypotheses by their nature are provisional: subject to appropriate testing. But self-critical research—even research using the analytic method—has been sorely lacking in psychoanalysis, especially since Freud's death. Accordingly, postwar psychoanalysis has tended mainly to be characterized by regurgitation of existing theory and cogitation over perennial conundrums.

As the mainstream of cognitive science progressed, therefore, these inward-looking tendencies resulted in an increasing isolation of psychoanalysis and a gradual reduction in public confidence in the value and validity of its propositions.

What changed most of all in the rest of mental science was that it took full advantage of technical progress in neuroscience, which had advanced enormously since Freud's day. For Freud (1940[1938]/1964, p. 97) the single biggest hurdle that had to be overcome before the "unsatisfactory" gap between psychoanalytic theory and cerebral anatomy could be bridged was "our complete ignorance of the *dynamic* nature of the mental process." In other words, in Freud's view, once neuroscience had evolved methods that could accommodate the dynamic nature of mental life, the neural correlates of Freud's theoretical fiction—the mental apparatus—could be identified. As a result of advances in neuropsychological methodology (i.e., "dynamic localization"; cf. Solms 2000b), and—above all—in functional imaging technology, neuroscience can now deal with the dynamic nature of mental life and therefore *is* now in a position to provide answers to the sorts of questions that Freud put to it in 1895. Mainstream psychiatry today is, accordingly, no longer dominated by psychoanalysis—instead it draws on models derived from the dynamics of neurotransmission—and mainstream psychology is dominated by models derived from the neural networks of cognitive neuroscience.

The example of cognitive psychology is highly instructive. As stated above, modern cognitive models of the mental apparatus, like our metapsychological models, are functionalist abstractions. They are justified ontologically in almost identical terms to those that Freud (1900/1953) used to justify his novelty of constructing an imaginary mental apparatus composed of virtual "agencies" or "systems" that have no tangible existence in the physical elements of the nervous system (Semenza 2001). Thus, for example, like Freud (1900/1953), cognitive psychologists today infer the existence of virtual structures: *systems* subserving abstract functions like "consciousness," "perception," and "memory." These systems are divided into functional modules (information processing units) such as—in the case of the memory system—"encoding," "consolidation," "storage," and "retrieval," or "short-term" and "long-term," stages. Nobody denies the scientific value of these abstractions, given the theoretical work they have allowed us to perform—even though nobody can actually *see* them. We may rightfully claim the same value for our own metapsychological constructions.

But cognitive psychologists went further. They took the step that Freud so eagerly anticipated: they attempted, increasingly successfully in recent decades, to "translate" their psychological terms and concepts into anatomical and physiological ones (i.e., correlate them with brain functions). Making use of the methodological and technical advances in the neurosciences that psychoanalysts chose to ignore, they systematically identified the neurological structures and functions involved in the dynamic information processing systems they had hitherto conceptualized in purely functional terms. They did so by studying the mental phenomena that operationalized the "systems" that constituted their hypothetical models, using the chemical, physiological, radiological, and other methods

then newly available. For example, the functions of the "memory system" were studied under varying physical conditions—which could, with the new methods, be manipulated and measured by a vast array of in vivo and experimental methods—and the results were compared with predictions based on the existing cognitive theories. This not only revealed the brain correlates of the mental functions in question, and therefore of the underlying theoretical constructs, but also the numerous *shortcomings* of the relevant theory. The theory was accordingly advanced.

There is no reason why the same cannot be done with our psychoanalytic abstractions. This is the essential rationale behind the neuropsychoanalytic movement, which is now in its infancy.

Major Developments in Relation to Neuroscience Since Freud

Interdisciplinary research in psychoanalysis and neuroscience did not begin suddenly one day in mid-1999 (when the journal *Neuro-Psychoanalysis* was first published) or mid-2000 (when the inaugural annual congress of the International Neuro-Psychoanalysis Society was held). The developments that took place between 1896 (when Freud abandoned his "Project") and 1999 can be usefully divided into three overlapping phases or trends. (See www.neuro-psa.org for a complete bibliography of publications at the interface of psychoanalysis and neuroscience from the years 1895 through 1999.)

Contributions From Analyst-Neurologists

The first coherent trend was the combined work of clinicians such as Paul Schilder, Smith Ely Jelliffe, Erwin Stengel, Ed Weinstein, and Mortimer Ostow. These psychoanalysts (like Freud himself and many of his earliest followers) were all neurologists. As such, in their clinical work they could not help but make psychoanalytic observations on the many fascinating mental changes that occur when different parts of the brain are diseased. In Ostow's case, this extended also to psychoanalytic observations on the mental effects of psychotropic drugs. The small number of psychoanalysts who treated epileptic patients in the early years of psychoanalysis (when epilepsy was still considered a "neurosis," that is, a functional disorder of the nervous system) should also be included under this heading. The same applies to those rare colleagues—like Jerome Frank—who subjected the mental sequelae of psychosurgical procedures to analytic scrutiny.

Needless to say, there is much about the mental life of neurological patients that strikes the psychoanalyst as being theoretically important for a proper understanding of the presenting symptoms but that completely passes by the analytically untrained observer. As a result, these analyst-neurologists gained many important new insights into the mechanisms underlying the neurobehavioral disorders they studied. Unfortunately, however, the scientific context within which they worked was not receptive to such insights, with the result that their valuable contributions—which make wonderfully interesting reading today—were more or less ignored by both fields during their lifetimes.

Contributions From Nonanalytic Neuroscientists

The second coherent trend arises from the purely neuroscientific work of nonanalysts. Prior to the advent of *Neuro-Psychoanalysis*, these scientists would never have published their findings in a psychoanalytic journal, and yet their subject matter overlapped considerably with core topics of interest to mainstream psychoanalysis: functions of consciousness, the nature and extent of unconscious mental processing, memory in all its manifestations (including infantile memory, emotional learning, unconscious memory, autobiographical memory, and misremembering), child development in all its complexity (including the perennial nature-nurture issues, which could now finally be laid to rest empirically), sexuality and gender, instinctual mental life, drives and motivation, dreaming, inhibition, self-regulation, the mechanisms of mental illness, and so forth.

In this vast sea of psychoanalytically relevant (but nonanalytic) research, some of the main trends of which are summarized below, neuroscientists addressed directly many profound questions that were the traditional preserve of psychoanalysis—typically without even realizing that their work would interest us. They were marching, as it were, to the beat of a different drum. I am referring, for example, to the work of Joseph LeDoux (on emotional learning), Antonio Damasio (on consciousness), and Jaak Panksepp (on instincts)—about all of whom more below. It is tempting to believe that their progress would have been more rapid, or at least psychologically deeper and richer, if the historical divisions between our disciplines had not prevented them from taking advantage of the theoretical yield of a century of psychoanalytic inquiry into exactly the same questions. Today these colleagues are all actively involved in the neuropsychoanalytic movement (e.g., they speak at our congresses, serve on the editorial board of our journal, and publish in its pages).

Speculative Syntheses

Despite the fact that most psychoanalysts—until the closing years of the twentieth century—remained unaware of, or uninterested in, these increasingly relevant developments, not *all* of them did so. Scattered publications appeared (mainly in the mainstream psychoanalytic literature), drawing attention to theoretical implications for psychoanalysis of one or another new finding regarding the brain. The widespread interest in lateral hemispheric specialization that occurred during the era of "split-brain" research, in particular, led to a flurry of such publications. For example, numerous analytic commentators drew attention from the 1970s onward to apparent similarities between the inferred functions of the right and left cerebral hemispheres and those of the metapsychological systems *Ucs* (Unconscious) and *Pcs-Cs* (Preconscious–Conscious), respectively. Consistent with this, they also drew analogies between structural hemispheric disconnection and functional "repression."

As the obvious relevance for psychoanalysis of new findings in the neurosciences increased by the decade, so did the number of such synthetic, essentially speculative publications—reasoning by analogy, as it were, about what the psychoanalytic equivalent *might be* of various brain mechanisms, and (to a lesser extent) vice versa. In very recent years, the monumental text by Allan Schore (1994), synthesizing just about everything we know about the ventral frontal region of the developing brain with developmental theory in psychoanalysis, stands as an outstanding example of this kind of contribution. Fred Levin's *Mapping the Mind* (1991) is also a well-known representative of this increasingly fashionable genre. The main value of this type of interdisciplinary work is that it draws attention to possible correlations deserving of serious research interest; but it is not, in itself, empirical work.

The Advent of Neuropsychoanalysis

The development of neuropsychoanalysis was the brainchild of Arnold Pfeffer, a New York psychoanalyst who had a deep interest in behavioral neurology and neuropsychiatry in his early career, in the immediate postwar period, before he devoted himself exclusively to psychoanalysis. Pfeffer kept abreast of ongoing developments in neuroscience and became increasingly convinced during the 1980s that the new findings and technology emanating from neuroscience had important implications for the future of his own science, which by then was in something of a crisis, perhaps especially in New York. Pfeffer therefore fatefully decided to invite the neuroscientist James

Schwartz (renowned for his work, with Eric Kandel, on the molecular mechanisms of memory) to convene a series of educational seminars on recent advances in basic neuroscience for an invited group of colleagues at the New York Psychoanalytic Institute. These legendary seminars—which extended over two academic years in 1991–1993—were followed by lively interdisciplinary discussions, which frequently continued for several *hours* after the end of the formal proceedings. A floodgate was opened. The seminars were rapidly broadened, to include not only members of other psychoanalytic societies and institutes in the New York area but also a growing number of interested neuroscientists, and eventually a wide cross-section of other mental health professionals.

By 1993–1994 the educational program had shifted from basic neuroscience to behavioral neuroscience, and accordingly it was convened by a behavioral neurologist, Jason Brown, rather than a bench neuroscientist. By 1994 the group felt ready to tackle the neuroscience-psychoanalysis interface directly, and I was asked to take over the program. Today these meetings (held on the first Saturday of every month) are open to all, and they still form the cornerstone of the larger educational and research program organized under the auspices of the New York Psychoanalytic Institute, in what has become the Arnold Pfeffer Center for Neuro-Psychoanalysis. We have reverted to the format of inviting leading neuroscientists working on topics of psychoanalytic interest to present their findings to an interdisciplinary audience for the purposes of interdisciplinary discussion and debate.

Initially when I took over the seminars, however, I tried to encourage a shift from the trend described above—where psychoanalysts merely reinterpreted the established findings of neuroscientific researchers in analytic terms and speculated on their possible implications. I tried to encourage the psychoanalysts in the audience to involve themselves directly in interdisciplinary *research*. I did this by presenting over a period of 2 years (together with my wife and scientific collaborator, Karen Kaplan-Solms) transcribed sessions of analytic work with patients with focal brain lesions. My intention in doing so was to introduce a method that was capable of making simultaneous psychoanalytic *and* neuroscientific observations on the same clinical material. The method was, in essence, an extension of the classical method of behavioral neurology, namely, *clinico-anatomical correlation*. However, whereas in classical behavioral neurology the researcher gathers and describes the psychological data that constitute the clinical side of the correlation within a *cognitive* or *behavioral* technical and theoretical framework, I suggested that we do so within a *psychoanalytical* framework. That is, instead of subjecting the mental changes that occur with focal brain lesions to cognitive-behavioral analysis (as traditionally occurs)—and then perhaps reinterpreting the findings psychoanalytically—we studied the neurological patients *directly* in a psychoanalytic setting. This enabled us to observe, in the frame within which psychoanalytic constructs are conventionally operationalized (thereby ensuring face validity), how the "functions" of the mind—as we conceptualize them in psychoanalysis—are differentially altered by damage to different neuroanatomical structures. This in turn made it possible for us to identify *empirically*, at least in broad outline, how our "mental apparatus" is represented in (or between) the structures of the brain. This also enabled us to *test* existing speculative syntheses of the kind described above. For example, it was possible to establish in the Arnold Pfeffer seminars that patients with damage to the right and left hemispheres did *not* display the mental changes in an analytic setting predicted by the hypothesis that the affected regions are the functional-anatomical equivalents of the metapsychological systems Ucs and Pcs-Cs, respectively. (This question formed the main topic of the 1996–1997 academic years. It was addressed by way of session-by-session study of eight clinical cases, four with left perisylvian lesions and four with equivalent lesions on the right.)

This method has the additional benefit of throwing new light on the underlying mechanisms of the neurobehavioral disorders in question, thus extending the pioneering work of the early analyst–neurologists described in the previous section. Readers interested in learning more about this method should consult the book by Kaplan-Solms and Solms (2000), which specifically explicates and demonstrates the method and summarizes the early discussions of the Arnold Pfeffer seminars. It is gratifying to be able to report that numerous colleagues around the world, including two formal study groups (one in New York and one in Frankfurt-Cologne), are now using this same method, with a view to confirming, correcting, and extending the work begun at the Pfeffer seminars.

The Arnold Pfeffer Center provided a model for other psychoanalytic institutes, and similar groups soon formed in almost all the major institutes throughout the world. These groups, in turn, formed themselves into the International Neuro-Psychoanalysis Society in 2000 (www. neuro-psa.org). The Society hosts an annual congress on topics of inter-disciplinary interest (2000: emotion; 2001: memory; 2002: sexuality; 2003: the unconscious; 2004: the right hemisphere; 2005: dreaming). These congresses have from the first attracted participants of the highest caliber from both the psychoanalytic and the neuroscientific communities. The Society also publishes the journal *Neuro-Psychoanalysis*, which is now in its fifth volume. The initial format of the journal was to publish target articles on topics of mutual interest to neuroscience and psychoanalysis, together with open peer commentaries by leading representatives of the two disciplines. In this way, via the congress and the journal, the spirit of interdisciplinary communication and collaboration that was initiated in the auditorium of the New York Psychoanalytic Institute broadened out onto an international stage. The editorial structure of the journal comprises two advisory boards, one psychoanalytic and the other neuroscientific. The names on these boards read like a "Who's Who" in both fields, which in itself provides testimony to the enthusiasm that leading authorities in both fields today feel for the important task of integrating these two parallel disciplines.

It is important not to leave the reader with the impression that clinico-anatomical correlation is the *only* valid method in neuropsychoanalytic research. Clinico-anatomical correlation is only the first step. There are many different ways of proceeding from there. For example, a small group of neuropsychological colleagues (and some students in my own labs) are currently subjecting the clinico-anatomical correlations we drew between psychoanalytic concepts and functional brain anatomy (Kaplan-Solms and Solms 2000) to cognitive-neuropsychological scrutiny. That is, they are *experimentally* testing predictions that flow from the *clinical* neuropsychoanalytic correlations, thereby attempting to falsify them. Other colleagues and research groups are using *functional imaging* techniques and *neuropharmacological probes* to test neuropsychoanalytic hypotheses. There are no limits to the methods that can be employed, although I personally would implore researchers to ensure that the hypotheses they test at least derive from correlations in which the psychoanalytic side of the equation was—at least initially—validly (i.e., clinically) operationalized.

What is particularly important about this line of research is that it is getting published in the most prestigious neuroscientific journals, thereby bringing a psychoanalytic point of view into the mainstream of contemporary mental science (e.g., Fotopoulou et al. 2004; Solms 2000a, 2004; Turnbull et al. 2002, 2004). This development would have been unimaginable just a few years ago. But considering what psychoanalysts *should* have to say to neuroscientists studying subject matter that has been their traditional stomping ground for more than 100 years, now that a vehicle of cross-disciplinary communication has been established, perhaps this is not so surprising.

Research Findings

Some authors believe that the psychoanalytic model of the mind may serve as a sort of template to guide the multitude of incredibly detailed neuroscientific research programs currently under way, in order to better discern the emerging theoretical "big picture" (see Solms and Turnbull 2002). This recasts Freud as a sort of Charles Darwin of the mind, in that his seminal model of the mental apparatus may serve the same role for modern behavioral neuroscience that Darwin's evolutionary theories served for modern molecular genetics (Solms 2004). Who would have thought that a Nobel laureate for medicine and physiology at the dawn of the 21st century—namely neuroscientist Eric Kandel (1999)—would describe psychoanalysis as "still the most coherent and intellectually satisfying view of the mind [that we have today]" (p. 505)?

In the following subsections, I review some of the main strands of evidence for this increasingly accepted view and simultaneously summarize some of the main research findings that have accumulated over the past several years at the interface of psychoanalysis and neuroscience. To keep things simple, I have organized my review around *very basic* Freudian concepts; I do not even attempt to tackle the complex theoretical questions that have been the main focus of contemporary psychoanalytic debate. Readers interested in a more sophisticated treatment of the topics reviewed below are referred to Kaplan-Solms and Solms (2000) and Solms and Turnbull (2002). Neuropsychoanalytic integration is still in its infancy—and therefore still occupied mainly with correlation rather than verification. (A psychoanalytic theory cannot be *tested* by neuroscientific methods before its constituent parts have been *described* in neuroscientific terms; any alternative approach runs the risk of testing apples by measuring pears.) The reader of this brief review will, however, observe that the first wave of research in this area has been *gratifyingly consistent with many of our most basic theoretical propositions*.

The Unconscious

When Freud introduced the notion that many, indeed most, of the mental processes that determine our everyday thoughts, feelings, and volitions occur unconsciously, his scientific contemporaries derided the notion as patently impossible, even logically incoherent (Freud 1915/1957). But today one would be hard pressed to find a cognitive neuroscientist who did not consider unconscious mental processing to be a proven fact and an indispensable explanatory concept (Bargh and Chartrand 1999).

How else are we to understand the fact that patients with "split brains" (in which the hemispheres are surgically disconnected) blush and giggle with uncomfortable feelings when pornographic pictures are projected to their isolated right hemispheres, even though they have no self-awareness of the source of these feelings (Galin 1974,

p. 573)? Such patients typically "rationalize" their manifest behaviors and emotions—explaining them away through plausible but invented motives and causes, just as Freud claimed we all do with our everyday unconscious intentions. Gazzaniga (1992) has argued on the basis of split-brain and other evidence that the (reflexively conscious) left hemisphere acts as a sort of "interpreter" of ongoing decisions made unconsciously by the inarticulate right hemisphere, much as Freud's conscious ego was thought to rationalize the inexplicable influences on our ongoing cognition and behavior of the unconscious "repressed." Although these correlations do not validly *localize* the conscious ego in the left hemisphere, they do demonstrate experimentally the reality of the phenomena that Freud conceptualized under the broad *descriptive* heading of "the mental unconscious."

The same fact is demonstrated by patients with damage to some memory-encoding structures of the brain, who are unable consciously to remember events that occurred after their brain damage but nevertheless demonstrate unequivocal evidence that the "forgotten" events influence their subsequent behavior. The most famous example of this type is the case of H.M., whose performance on various neuropsychological tasks has improved significantly over the years that he has been tested, since both his hippocampi were surgically removed (Scoville and Milner 1957)—despite the fact that he denies any conscious recollection of the testing sessions themselves or any sense of familiarity with the neuropsychologists who tested him. Cognitive neuroscientists have made sense of such facts by inferring the existence of multiple memory systems, some of which process information consciously (i.e., manifestly or "explicitly") and others unconsciously (i.e., latently or "implicitly").

Also of considerable interest is the fact that the brain structures that mediate conscious memory are not functional during the first 2 years of life, which provides an elegant neuropsychological explanation of the phenomenon called "infantile amnesia." As Freud surmised, it is not so much that we *forget* our earliest memories as that we *cannot recall them to consciousness;* but this does not by any means preclude them from having significant effects on subsequent behavior.

Repression

The observations described above abundantly confirm the existence of unconscious mental processing. But they do not support Freud's *dynamic* conception of the unconscious. Ramachandran (1994) took this step in accounting for some unexpected observations he made on the phenomenon of *anosognosia*—a symptom caused by damage to the right parietal lobe of the brain, in which the patient is unaware of the devastating effects of this damage, including such gross physical defects as paralysis of the left arm and leg. After artificially stimulating the damaged right hemisphere of one such patient (Mrs. M.)—by means of caloric stimulation, which Bisiach and colleagues (1991) had previously demonstrated was capable of temporarily lifting some symptoms of anosognosia—Ramachandran observed that the patient suddenly became aware that her left arm was paralyzed—indeed, that it had been paralysed continuously since she suffered a stroke several days before. Eight hours after the effects of the caloric stimulation had worn off, the patient not only reverted to the belief that her arm was normal, she also *selectively forgot* the part of the interview in which she had acknowledged that the arm was paralyzed. Ramachandran's conclusion is worth quoting at length:

> Her admission that she had been paralysed for *several days* suggests that even though she had been continuously denying her paralysis, *the information about the paralysis was being continuously laid down* in her brain, i.e., the denial did not prevent memory…we may conclude that *at some deeper level she does indeed have knowledge about the paralysis.…*[However,] when tested eight hours later, she not only reverted to the denial, but also "repressed" the admission of paralysis that she had made during her stimulation. The remarkable theoretical implication of these observations is that memories can indeed be selectively repressed.…Seeing [this patient] convinced me, for the first time, of the reality of the repression phenomena that form the cornerstone of classical psychonalytical theory. (Ramachandran 1994, p. 324; emphasis added)

The fact that we perceive and know things without consciously recognizing them has also been demonstrated in other ways, in various fields of contemporary neuroscience. What is important about Ramachandran's observations (since confirmed by others, including by analytic observation; see Kaplan-Solms and Solms 2000) is the additional fact that we know things unconsciously that we do not *want* to recognize consciously. This fact has also been demonstrated experimentally, very recently, in *normal* subjects (Anderson and Green 2001). As the British neuropsychologist Martin Conway pointed out in a 2001 commentary on this research in *Nature*, if significant repression effects can be artificially generated in neurologically and psychiatrically healthy people in innocuous laboratory conditions, then far greater effects are likely in the maelstrom of real-life emotional trauma (Conway 2001).

Perhaps more pertinent to the real-life context is recent neuroscientific research into the neural basis of *emotional* learning. LeDoux (1996), for example, demonstrated the existence of a pathway connecting perceptual information with the subcortical structures that mediate learned "fear" responses, a pathway that bypasses the hippocampus (and thereby, conscious remembering) entirely. By means of such mechanisms, objectively innocuous stimuli can trigger personally traumatic memories of which the subject is completely unaware, producing apparently irrational behaviors. Freud inferred a closely analogous mechanism for neurotic symptoms from his earliest clinical observations in cases with inexplicable fears and phobias.

Indeed there is even evidence to suggest that the exact conditions that might lead one to have an amnesia (loss of conscious memory) for the events surrounding a traumatic experience might also lead to a particularly powerful unconscious memory that has direct influence on the way the person acts and feels. Because these influences are operating unconsciously, the person would have little understanding of why the actions and feelings occur. (LeDoux 1999, p. 44).

Not surprisingly, LeDoux—writing in *Neuro-Psychoanalysis*—has concluded:

> [A]lthough I have never actually tested aspects of psychoanalytic theory in my research on emotions and the brain, "psychoanalytic-like" concepts (such as the unconscious)…have been key to the way I have interpreted my research findings over the years. (LeDoux 1999, p. 44)

Even the link between repression and neurotic symptoms has recently found direct neuroscientific support. Howard Shevrin's laboratory at the University of Michigan reported an experiment (Shevrin et al. 1996) with persons with social phobia in which the brain activity evoked by visual representation of pathogenic repressed ideas related to the phobia, previously identified by psychoanalysts from recorded interviews, was objectively different from brain activity associated with analogous but unrepressed ideas. The difference was found only when the repressed material was presented unconsciously (subliminally).

The Pleasure Principle

Mainstream cognitive scientists now concede, on the basis of evidence such as that reviewed in the previous subsections, that consciousness is extremely limited. Bargh and Chartrand (1999), in a recent review of the relevant literature, concluded that at least 95% of our motivated actions are unconsciously determined. Libet (1985) went so far as to suggest that conscious volition is almost *entirely* illusory. But Freud went even further. He did not claim merely that large portions of our mental life are unconscious; he claimed also that the unconscious portion of the mind includes a system that operates according to *different functional principles* from the rational, reality-constrained ones governing the functional activities of the executive ego. The fundamental property of this type of unconscious thinking, according to Freud (1915/1957), is that it is *wishful* to a degree that blithely disregards reality constraints such as those contributed by objective perceptions, the arrow of time, and the rules of logic.

These are the sort of unconscious mechanisms that are now being invoked to account for some neurobehavioral disorders, such as "confabulation." Some patients with amnesia, such as that displayed by H.M. in the case discussed earlier—demonstrate additional symptoms, due to the involvement of other brain structures, principally in the anterior forebrain. These patients are *unaware* that they are amnesic (i.e., they are anosognosic for their amnesia) and, perhaps for this reason, they fill the gaps in their memory with fabricated recollections known as *confabulations*. Katerina Foutopoulou recently studied a patient of this type who failed to recall, over 13 consecutive days in my London lab, that he had ever met me before, or even that he had undergone an operation to remove the tumor in his brain that caused his amnesia. As far as he was concerned, there was nothing wrong with him. When asked about the scar on his head, he confabulated wholly implausible explanations: he had undergone dental surgery, or a coronary bypass operation. In reality, years before, he had indeed undergone these procedures—which, in contrast to his brain operation, had had successful outcomes. Similarly, when asked who I was and what he was doing in my lab, he variously confabulated that I was a colleague, a drinking partner (whom he was visiting for a tipple), a client consulting him about his area of professional expertise, a teammate in a sport that he had not participated in since he was at college decades before, or a mechanic repairing one of his numerous sports cars (which, in reality, he did not possess). What struck me clinically was the *wishful* quality of these confabulations, an impression that was confirmed objectively through blind ratings of a consecutive series of 155 confabulations (Fotopoulou et al. 2004). Similar observations have been reported by Conway and Tacchi (1996) and Turnbull and colleagues (in press).

These neuropsychological investigators interpret their findings in strikingly psychoanalytical terms, claiming in essence that the lesions in anterior forebrain structures that produce confabulation not only *damage* cognitive control mechanisms that regulate normal memory search processes but also *release from inhibition* the implicit wishful influences on perception, memory, and judgment that Freud inferred for his dynamic system Ucs (from the study of neurologically normal people). The implicit features of the dynamically unconscious mind that Freud *hypothesized* to account for his observations of neurotic symptoms, dreams, slips, jokes, and the like are directly *observable* in the behavior of patients with damage to these anterior forebrain cognitive control mechanisms.

> A man believes that he has seen a long-deceased friend instead of accepting that he is surrounded by strangers. Another believes that he is living in a comfortable hotel (and on holiday) instead of accepting that he is confined to a hospital (and recuperating from a serious illness). He also believes that it is perpetually visiting time. A woman believes that she goes home at night and enjoys a party, rather than that she is stuck in a hospital bed. The pleasure of the underlying wishes (the pleasure principle) is readily apparent. In all of these cases, the primary process overrides adaptive constraints to a far greater degree than would normally be tolerated by the secondary process (the reality principle). (Solms 2000c, p. 136)

In a recent discussion of this topic in *Neuro-Psychoanalysis*, behavioral neurologist Neill Graff-Radford (2000) concluded, "I find it remarkable that Freud, from the analysis of normal individuals, described some of the features of the mind [now] revealed in the confabulating amnestic syndrome" (p. 150).

The Id

Freud argued that the "primary process" of the mind, just exemplified, is dominated by unconstrained *instinctual* mechanisms—which in turn reveal the fundamentally *biological* nature of human mental life. For Freud, we humans, no less than other living creatures, are *animals* and therefore driven by evolutionarily conserved "drives." To his Victorian contemporaries, the implication that human behavior was at bottom governed by urges that served no higher principle than the enhancement of reproductive fitness was downright scandalous. The moral outrage waned during the subsequent decades of the twentieth century, but Freud's conception of man-as-animal was then sidelined by other forces—not least of them the behaviorist tradition, then dominant in experimental psychology, which reduced all motivation to *learning* mechanisms. Today, following the collapse of behaviorism, the tide has turned, and Freud's view that human beings are indeed driven by a set of hard-wired instinctual mechanisms is finally receiving the scientific attention it deserves. Indeed, as affective neuroscientist Jaak Panksepp's recent masterful review of the field attests (Panksepp 1998), the instinctual mechanisms that govern human motivation are far more primitive than even Freud imagined. We share the "basic emotion command systems" that determine our core values not only with our nearest primate relatives but with *all mammals*. In other words, at the deep level of mental or-

ganization that Freud called "the id," the functional anatomy and chemistry of our brains are not essentially different from that of our favorite barnyard animals and household pets. This is not to say that modern neuroscientists accept Freud's classification of human instinctual life into a simple dichotomy between sexuality and aggression (or destructiveness):

> Affective neuroscience has now provided an empirically based set of neuropsychological conceptualizations by which some of the subcomponents of the id can be more systematically discussed. These kinds of resolved discussions were not possible when the id was simply an amorphous psychic wellspring for everything else that emerged along "developmental lines." By accepting the existence of a variety of affective brain functions, we are in a much better position to describe how the "epigenetic landscapes" of the mind unfold as organisms absorb the lessons of various life experiences through the interplay of nature and nurture. (Panksepp 1999, p. 77)

Simply put, modern neuroscience has identified at least four basic mammalian instinctual mechanisms:

1. *The SEEKING system.* This system is also known as the "reward" (Rolls 1999), "wanting" (Berridge 2003), or "curiosity-interest-expectancy" system (Panksepp 1985), a subcomponent of which is called the PLEASURE-LUST system.
2. *The ANGER-RAGE system.* This system governs "hot" (angry) aggression but not "cold" (predatory) aggression, which is controlled by the SEEKING system, or "male dominance" behavior, which has a more compound organization.
3. *The FEAR-ANXIETY system.* A portion of this system was discussed above in relation to unconscious memory.
4. *The PANIC system.* This system, also known as the "separation-distress" system, is closely linked with more complex social instincts such as those that govern maternal bonding and mother-infant attachment.

Despite the many differences between this classification and Freud's, the all-purpose SEEKING system bears a remarkable similarity to Freud's broadened conception of sexuality (his libidinal drive).

Of special interest is the link between the neurochemistries that mediate these systems and the drugs developed by modern psychopharmacology, which seem to exert their therapeutic influence via these same systems. Interestingly, the perceived antagonism between psychoanalysis and the newer psychopharmacological therapies was not shared by Freud, who enthusiastically anticipated the day when "id energies" would be controlled directly by pharmacological means:

The future may teach us to exercise a direct influence, by means of particular chemical substances, on the amounts of energy and their distribution in the mental apparatus. It may be that there are still undreamt-of possibilities of therapy. But for the moment we have nothing better at our disposal than the technique of psychoanalysis, and for that reason, in spite of its limitations, it should not be despised. (Freud 1940[1938]/1964, p. 182)

Today integrated treatments, combining psychotherapy with psychoactive drugs of various kinds, are widely recognized as best practice for some disorders (Andreasen 1997; Roose et al. 1998).

Also of special interest, alongside these empirical and clinical considerations, are the striking *theoretical* similarities between Freud's conceptualization of the relationship between instinctual drives and affective consciousness and those of modern neuroscientists studying the same relationships. In essence, the contemporary neuroscientific view (e.g., Damasio 1999a; Panksepp 1998) is that consciousness evolved as a fundamentally *affective* property of the nervous system, rooted in primitive drive-regulating structures, with the purpose of enabling the organism to *evaluate* its current physiological state in relation to prevailing environmental conditions. The similarity between this conception and Freud's (1911/1958) is so close that it prompted Antonio Damasio (1999b) to write that "Freud's insights on the nature of affect are consonant with the most advanced contemporary neuroscience views" (p. 38).

The Meaning of Dreams

Current neuroscientific interest in Freudian theory is probably nowhere more apparent than in the field of sleep and dream science. When REM sleep and its near-perfect correlation with dreaming were discovered in the 1950s (Aserinsky and Kleitman 1953, 1955; Dement and Kleitman 1957a, 1957b), and when its cholinergic brainstem mechanism was laid bare in the 1970s (Hobson et al. 1975), Freud's (1900/1953) dream theory appeared to lose all scientific credibility: "The primary motivating force for dreaming is not psychological but physiological since the time of occurrence and duration of [REM] sleep are quite constant, suggesting a preprogrammed, neurally determined genesis" (Hobson and McCarley 1977, p. 1346).

However, more recent research has revealed that dreaming and REM sleep are doubly dissociable states, controlled by quite different—although interactive—brain mechanisms (Solms 1997a, 2000a). Dreaming turns out to be generated by a network of *forebrain* structures centered principally around the instinctual-motivational circuitry discussed earlier (Braun et al. 1997a; Maquet et al. 1996;

Nofzinger et al. 1997; Solms 1997a, 2000a). This line of research has prompted a host of new theories about the dreaming brain (Pace-Scott et al. 2003), some of them strongly reminiscent of Freud's. Most intriguing in this respect is the observation that dreaming stops completely when fibers in the ventromesial frontal lobe are severed; a symptom that coincides with a general reduction in motivated behavior (Solms 1997a). The lesion producing this syndrome is exactly the same as the damage that was deliberately produced in "prefontal leukotomy," a procedure once used to control hallucinations and delusions. This operation was replaced in the 1960s by drugs that dampened activity in the same (dopaminergic) fibers. A currently influential hypothesis (Solms 2002) suggests that this system, the SEEKING system—centrally implicated in hallucinations and delusions (which share many formal features with dreams) and addictions—might be the primary generator of dreams. If this hypothesis is confirmed, then, considering the similarity between Panksepp's SEEKING system and Freud's libidinal drive, the "wish-fulfillment" theory of dreams could yet again set the agenda for mainstream sleep and dream science (Shevrin and Eiser 2000). Either way, few neuroscientists today would still claim—as they once did with impunity—that dreams are "motivationally neutral" (Hobson 1988), and still fewer that they have "no primary ideational, volitional, or emotional content" (Hobson and McCarley 1977, p. 1347).

Conclusion

Whatever "undreamt-of" therapeutic possibilities the future might bring—both psychological and pharmacological—both psychoanalysis as a discipline and patients in general can only benefit from a better understanding of how the mind *really* works. In this respect, much of what Freud hypothesized on the basis of his early clinical observations will be surpassed by subsequent knowledge. Even as we are rediscovering in neurological terms the phenomena that he conceptualized under headings such as "the unconscious," "repression," "the id," and "libido," we are recognizing that his monolithic conceptions cannot possibly do justice to the sheer multiplicity of new mechanisms thereby revealed. But that is not the point. As modern neuroscience begins to tackle the really big questions of human psychology that so preoccupied Freud, even as we fully expect to discover that he was wrong in this respect and that, so we are finding, his first-pass theories still provide us with "the most coherent and intellectually satisfying view" we have of the global structure and functions of the human mind. As suggested in *Newsweek* magazine, "it is not a matter of proving Freud right or wrong, but of finishing the job" (Guterl 2002, p. 51). In this respect at least, there is every reason to be optimistic about the future of psychoanalysis.

References

Anderson M, Green C: Suppressing unwanted memories by executive control. Nature 410:366–369, 2001

Andreasen NC: Linking mind and brain in the study of mental illnesses: a project for a scientific psychopathology. Science 275:1586–1593, 1997

Aserinsky E, Kleitman N: Regularly occurring periods of eye motility, and concomitant phenomena, during sleep. Science 118:273–274, 1953

Aserinsky E, Kleitman N: Two types of ocular motility occurring in sleep. J Appl Physiol 8:1–10, 1955

Bargh J, Chartrand T: The unbearable automaticity of being. Am Psychol 54:462–479, 1999

Berridge KC: Pleasures of the brain. Brain Cogn 52:106–128, 2003

Bisiach E, Rusconi M, Vallar G: Remission of somatoparaphrenic delusion through vestibular stimulation. Neuropsychologia 29:1029–31, 1991

Braun A, Balkin T, Wesenten N, et al: Regional cerebral blood flow throughout the sleep-wake cycle—an (H₂O)-O-15 PET study. Brain 120:1173–1197, 1997

Conway M: Repression revisited. Nature 410:319–20, 2001

Conway M, Tacchi P: Motivated confabulation. Neurocase 2: 325–38, 1996

Damasio A: The Feeling of What Happens: Body and Emotion in the Making of Consciousness. New York, Harcourt Brace, 1999a

Damasio A: Commentary to Panksepp. Neuropsychoanalysis 1: 38–39, 1999b

Dement W, Kleitman N: Cyclic variations in EEG during sleep and their relation to eye movements, body motility, and dreaming. Electroencephalogr Clin Neurophysiol Suppl 9: 673–690, 1957a

Dement W, Kleitman N: The relation of eye movements during sleep to dream activity: an objective method for the study of dreaming. J Exp Psychol 53:543–553, 1957b

Fotopoulou A, Solms M, Turnbull OH: Wishful reality distortions in confabulation: a case report. Neuropsychologia 42: 727–744, 2004

Freud S: The interpretation of dreams (1900), in Standard Edition of the Complete Psychological Works of Sigmund Freud, Vols 4 and 5. Translated and edited by Strachey J. London, Hogarth Press, 1953, pp 1–715

Freud S: Formulations on the two principles of mental functioning (1911), in Standard Edition of the Complete Psychological Works of Sigmund Freud, Vol 12. Translated and edited by Strachey J. London, Hogarth Press, 1958, pp 218–226

Freud S: The unconscious (1915), in Standard Edition of the Complete Psychological Works of Sigmund Freud, Vol 14. Translated and edited by Strachey J. London, Hogarth Press, 1957, pp 166–204

Freud S: Beyond the pleasure principle (1920), in Standard Edition of the Complete Psychological Works of Sigmund Freud, Vol 18. Translated and edited by Strachey J. London, Hogarth Press, 1955, pp 1–64

Freud S: An outline of psycho-analysis (1940[1938]), in Standard Edition of the Complete Psychological Works of Sigmund Freud, Vol 23. Translated and edited by Strachey J. London, Hogarth Press, 1964, pp 139–207

Freud S: The Complete Neuroscientific Works of Sigmund Freud, Vols 1–4. London, Karnac (in press)

Galin D: Implication for psychiatry of left and right cerebral specialization: a neurophysiological context for unconscious processes. Arch Gen Psychiatry 31:572–83, 1974

Gazzaniga MS: Nature's Mind. New York, Basic Books, 1992

Graff-Radford N: A cognitive neuroscience perspective on confabulation. Neuropsychoanalysis 2:148–150, 2000

Guterl F: What Freud got right. Newsweek, Nov 11, 2002, pp 50–51

Hobson JA: The Dreaming Brain. New York, Basic Books, 1988

Hobson JA, McCarley R: The brain as a dream state generator: an activation-synthesis hypothesis of the dream process. Am J Psychiatry 134:1335–1348, 1977

Hobson JA, McCarley R, Wyzinki P: Sleep cycle oscillations: reciprocal discharge by two brainstem neuronal groups. Science 189:55–58, 1975

Kandel E: Biology and the future of psychoanalysis: a new intellectual framework for psychiatry revisited. Am J Psychiatry 156:505–524, 1999

Kaplan-Solms K, Solms S: Clinical Studies in Neuro-Psychoanalysis: Introduction to a Depth Neuropsychology. London, Karnac, 2000

LeDoux J: The Emotional Brain. London, Weidenfeld & Nicholson, 1996

LeDoux J: Psychoanalytic theory: clues from the brain. Neuropsychoanalysis 1:44–49, 1999

Levin F: Mapping the Mind: The Intersection of Psychoanalysis and Neuroscience. Hillsdale, NJ, Analytic Press, 1991

Libet B: Unconscious cerebral initiative and the role of conscious will in voluntary action. Behavioral and Brain Science 89:567–615, 1985

Maquet P, Peters JM, Aerts J, et al: Functional neuroanatomy of human rapid-eye-movement sleep and dreaming. Nature 383:163–166, 1996

Nofzinger EA, Mintun MA, Wiseman MB, et al: Forebrain activation in REM sleep: an FDG PET study. Brain Res 770: 192–201, 1997

Pace-Schott E, Solms M, Blagrove M, et al: Sleep and Dreaming: Scientific Advances and Reconsiderations. New York, Cambridge University Press, 2003

Panksepp J: Mood changes, in Handbook of Clinical Neurology. Edited by Vinken P, Bruyn G, Klawans H. Amsterdam, Elsevier, 1985, pp 271–285

Panksepp J: Affective Neuroscience: The Foundations of Human and Animal Emotions. Oxford, England, Oxford University Press, 1998

Panksepp J: Emotions as viewed by psychoanalysis and neuroscience: an exercise in consilience. Neuropsychoanalysis 1: 15–38, 1999

Ramachandran V: Phantom limbs, neglect syndromes, repressed memories, and Freudian psychology. Int Rev Neurobiol 37: 291–333, 1994

Rolls E: The Brain and Emotion. Oxford, England, Oxford University Press, 1999

Roose S, Johannet M: Medication and psychoanalysis: treatments in conflict. Psychoanalytic Inquiry 18:606–620, 1998

Schore A: Affect Regulation and the Origin of the Self: The Neurobiology of Emotional Development. Hillsdale, NJ, Lawrence Erlbaum, 1994

Scoville W, Milner B: Loss of recent memory after bilateral hippocampal lesions. J Neurol Neurosurg Psychiatry 20: 11–21, 1957

Semenza C: Psychoanalysis and cognitive neuropsychology: theoretical and methodological affinities. Neuropsychoanalysis 3:3–10, 2001

Shevrin H, Eiser A: Continued vitality of the Freudian theory of dreaming. Behavioral and Brain Sciences 23:1004–1006, 2000

Shevrin H, Bond JA, Brakel LAW, et al: Conscious and Unconscious Processes: Psychodynamic, Cognitive, and Neurophysiological Convergences. New York, Guilford, 1996

Solms M: The Neuropsychology of Dreams: A Clinico-Anatomical Study. Mahwah, NJ, Lawrence Erlbaum, 1997a

Solms M: What is consciousness? J Am Psychoanal Assoc 45: 681–778, 1997b

Solms M: Dreaming and REM sleep are controlled by different brain mechanisms. Behav Brain Sci 23:843–850, 2000a

Solms M: Freud, Luria and the clinical method. Psychoanalysis and History 2:76–109, 2000b

Solms M: A psychoanalytic perspective on confabulation. Neuropsychoanalysis 2:133–138, 2000c

Solms M: The neurochemistry of dreaming: cholinergic and dopaminergic hypotheses, in The Neurochemistry of Consciousness: Advances in Consciousness Research series, Stamenov M, series editor. Edited by Perry E, Ashton H, Young A. Amsterdam, John Benjamins Publishing, 2002, pp 123–131

Solms M: Freud returns. Scientific American 290:82–88, 2004

Solms M, Saling M: On psychoanalysis and neuroscience: Freud's attitude to the localizationist tradition. Int J Psychoanalysis 67:397–416, 1986

Solms M, Turnbull O: The Brain and the Inner World: Introduction to the Neuroscience of Subjective Experience. New York, Other Press, 2002

Turnbull OH, Jones K, Reed-Screen J: Implicit awareness of deficit in anosognosia in emotion-based account of denial of deficit. Neuropsychoanalysis 4:69–86, 2002

Turnbull OH, Owen V, Evans CEY: Negative emotions in anosognosia. Cortex 41:67–75, 2004

Turnbull O, Jenkins S, Rowley M: The pleasantness of false beliefs: and emotion-based account of confabulation. Neuropsychoanalysis (in press)

Glossary

RICHARD ZIMMER, M.D., EDITOR

PETER M. BOOKSTEIN, M.D., ASSOCIATE EDITOR

EDWARD KENNY, M.D., ASSOCIATE EDITOR

ANDREAS K. KRAEBBER, M.D., ASSOCIATE EDITOR

Abstinence   The technical principle that the analyst must refrain from gratifying the wishes of the patient. By refraining from providing gratification, the analyst encourages these wishes to be put into words by the patient so that they can be analyzed.

Acting out   The expression in action outside of a psychoanalytic session of feelings and thoughts that were aroused within the session. By substituting an action or behavior for self-reflection or words, a person deprives himself or herself of knowledge of an important part of his or her inner experience.

Adaptation   The individual's capacity to deal with the external environment, either by accommodating to the demands of REALITY or by actively modifying reality in a personally or socially beneficial way.

Affects   In classical PSYCHOANALYSIS, emotions, and particularly their physiological manifestations, that are derivative (i.e., transformed) expressions of libidinal and/or aggressive DRIVES. The EGO, as an executive AGENCY, deals with affects, with special importance given to ANXIETY, which serves as a signal.

Agency   The capacity to recognize contingencies in human interactions and to participate in exchange with others through action. Agency is distinguished from a sense of agency, which develops through repeated acknowledgments of one's agency by others and by repetition of experiences that confirm one's capacities to bring about desired results. The term is also used to refer to any of the three major subdivisions of the mind in Freud's STRUCTURAL THEORY: ID, EGO, and SUPEREGO.

Aggression   The manifest strivings, in thought, action, feeling, or FANTASY, to dominate, prevail over, or be destructive to others. The term also refers to the DRIVE that gives rise to such manifestations.

Alexithymia   Inability to know and to describe one's own feelings. Alexithymia differs from intolerance of feelings and may be seen in patients with disorders on the border between somatic and psychological illness.

Alpha function (Bion)   The process through which the mother receives the primitive affective experiences of the infant, communicated through PROJECTIVE IDENTIFICATION; processes them through her REVERIE; and returns them in a modified form to her infant, thereby serving to both modulate these experiences and imbue them with meaning.

Ambivalence   The state of having simultaneous contradictory feelings toward an OBJECT. Ambivalence is always present but may become a clinical issue if one of the feelings is intolerable and repressed. If this occurs, the threat of the repressed feeling coming to awareness may generate ANXIETY or mobilize DEFENSES that affect functioning.

We gratefully acknowledge the following individuals for providing definitions for this glossary: Aisha Abbasi, M.D.; Ann Appelbaum, M.D.; Maurice Apprey, Ph.D.; Morton Aronson, M.D.; Elizabeth Auchincloss, M.D.; Rosemary Balsam, M.D.; Michael Beldoch, Ph.D.; Anna Burton, M.D.; A. Scott Dowling, M.D.; Wayne Downey, M.D.; Peter Dunn, M.D.; Aaron Esman, M.D.; Henry Evans, M.D.; Stephen Firestein, M.D.; Karen Gilmore, M.D.; Eugene L. Goldberg, M.D.; Lee Grossman, M.D.; Jeffrey K. Halpern, M.D.; Samuel Herschkowitz, M.D.; Wendy Jacobson, M.D.; Benjamin Kilborne, Ph.D.; Lewis Kirshner, M.D.; Anton Kris, M.D.; Kimberlyn Leary, Ph.D.; Eric Marcus, M.D.; Andrew Morrison, M.D.; Peter Neubauer, M.D.; David D. Olds, M.D.; Sharone B. Ornstein, M.D.; Ernst Prelinger, Ph. D.; Ellen Rees, M.D.; Robert Scharf, M.D.; Eleanor Schuker, M.D.; Susan P. Sherkow, M.D.; Robert Tyson, M.D.; Milton Viederman, M.D.; and Arnold Wilson, Ph.D.

Anaclitic object   A person on whom an individual is totally dependent for survival, seen most clearly in the infant's ATTACHMENT to the mother. The loss of the OBJECT precipitates a severe DEPRESSION. This infantile dependency is also present in severely depressed adults.

Anality   SYMPTOMS and CHARACTER traits in the adult that are analogous to the infantile delight in messiness and to the new-found capacity to control SELF and others by retaining or expelling feces. DEFENSES such as REACTION FORMATION and RATIONALIZATION further define the anal character. Associated traits include excessive concern with order, cleanliness, and tidiness, and irrational retention of information, money, or things that are no longer useful.

Anal phase   The phase of psychosexual development in which pleasure arises primarily from the anal zone, specifically from the retention and expulsion of feces. AMBIVALENCE typifies this phase.

Analyzability   A prospective analysand's capacity to undergo psychoanalytic treatment. It takes into account 1) the descriptive and dynamic diagnoses (e.g., symptom NEUROSIS, CHARACTER DISORDER), 2) the patient's capacity for perseverance in difficult tasks, and 3) the patient's ability to relate positively to the analyst in his or her role as helping professional. The analyst's impression should suggest that the analysand can fruitfully employ the method of FREE ASSOCIATION. Only the actual analytic collaboration will demonstrate whether the preliminary assessment of analyzability will be corroborated.

Anhedonia   The condition of being unable to experience pleasure, typically as a manifestation of DEPRESSION or MASOCHISM.

Anonymity   In clinical PSYCHOANALYSIS, the withholding of personal facts about the analyst in order to facilitate the emergence of fantasies about the analyst as a transferential OBJECT. Currently, many analysts feel that selective self-disclosure may be technically useful in certain clinical situations.

Anxiety   An unpleasant AFFECT characterized by physiological manifestations of autonomic discharge and a subjective apprehensiveness. Psychologically, the danger is unconscious and should be contrasted with fear, which is a response to an external and realistic danger.

Applied analysis (applied psychoanalysis)   The use of psychoanalytic INSIGHTS originally developed from the clinical situation in order to understand history, culture, literature, or biography.

Attachment   The biologically based bond between child and caregiver that ensures the safety, survival, and emotional well-being of the child. The quality of the attachment bond—whether it is secure or insecure—appears in clinical observation and empirical research to have powerful implications for the quality of psychic STRUCTURE and the subsequent relationships a person develops.

Attachment theory   A view that postulates an innate need for ATTACHMENT to a caregiver as the primary motivating force in human development. Varying patterns or failures in early attachment are thought to predispose to or be consistent with later developmental pathologies or to particular modes of OBJECT relatedness.

Autistic phase (Mahler)   The state of the first few weeks of extrauterine life marked by an absence of awareness of a mothering agent and by the hallucinatory, omnipotent satisfaction of needs.

Autonomous ego function   An aspect of the EGO that operates with little or no conscious or unconscious conflict (e.g., aspects of perception, recent memory, motility, intelligence, and communication). These functions can of course also be drawn into conflict, and many analysts question whether there is any function of the ego that is totally conflict-free.

Autonomy   The relative independence of the individual, which rests on the development of a reasonably constant sense of what is internal and external, and the psychological presence of important others. Developmental achievements of the first 3 years of life are instrumental in the subsequent acquisition of autonomy, which is a critical maturational issue of adolescence. EGO FUNCTIONS are said to be autonomous when they lose their links to their origins in intrapsychic conflict (see CONFLICT, INTRAPSYCHIC). Some analysts question the concept of AUTONOMOUS EGO FUNCTIONS.

Bipolar self   In SELF PSYCHOLOGY, the two-part STRUCTURE that is the core of an individual's personality and sense of SELF. It consists of the pole of the GRANDIOSE SELF, expressed by ambitions, and the pole of the idealizing parental imago, expressed by ideals and experienced as embodied in the parental OBJECT. In the PSYCHOANALYTIC SITUATION the grandiose self may be activated and forms the basis of the MIRROR TRANSFERENCE. The idealized parental imago may be activated and forms the basis of an IDEALIZING TRANSFERENCE.

Birth trauma   The hypothesized experience of overwhelming anxiety for the newborn as he or she emerges from the womb of the mother. Otto Rank proposed that it was the prototypical experience of ANXIETY and was responded to with REPRESSION. He believed that subsequent developmental crises follow from this traumatic loss of the original experience of union with and likeness to the mother.

Bisexuality   A psychological makeup in which the individual may choose either a man or a woman as a sexual OBJECT. Freud believed that bisexuality was universal in the UNCONSCIOUS. On a conscious level, research has demonstrated that most individuals have a primary preference for either a male or a female sexual object, while only a minority of individuals are bisexual.

Body ego   The sense of one's body in three respects: what the body feels (i.e., external and internal sensory input), what the body does (e.g., internal/external movement), and how the body fits into the external world (its place, position, and extensions).

Body image   The unconscious mental REPRESENTATION of one's own body, which may be anatomically incomplete or inaccurate and which may structure some psychological SYMPTOMS.

Borderline personality organization   A primitive CHARACTER structure represented by a fluid and labile sense of IDENTITY; desperate fear of ISOLATION and aloneness, along with chaotic intimate relationships in which the other is both intensely needed and experienced as toxic and rejecting; and the use of archaic DEFENSES of SPLITTING and PROJECTIVE IDENTIFICATION. This personality often manifests with eruptive anger in chaotic relationships, yet in nonintimate situations these individuals often function well.

Castration anxiety   The fear, occurring in both sexes, that the most sexually pleasurable parts of the genital anatomy (i.e., the penis and clitoris), which are most valued because they symbolize GENDER, may be damaged or lost. This fear is particularly intense in children ages 4–6 but continues unconsciously throughout life in displaced form (e.g., as inordinate ANXIETY in the face of the feared loss of health, youth, beauty, or wealth).

Cathexis   The investment of attention, interest, or mental energy (either libidinal or aggressive), the quantity and quality of which determines the level of engagement between SELF and other. In the TRANSFERENCE, patients withdraw their cathexis (or investment) from past figures and reinvest in the clinician as a new figure.

Character   The aggregate of relatively enduring and stable personality traits in an individual. Examples of these habitual modes of feeling and thinking are obsessionality and HYSTERIA. CHARACTER develops over time and is related to infantile solutions to particular conflict. It is slow to change, even with psychoanalytic INTERVENTION.

Character disorder   A disturbance in the structure of an individual's personality in which there are rigidly held patterns of behavior that get the individual in trouble or lead to the defeat of his or her own aims but that cause him or her no subjective distress.

Co-construction   A process that integrates the experiences of two individuals in a dyad. Each individual constructs the experience of "SELF" and "other"; each one's experience of "self" is affected by the other's experience of him or her as "other." For example, a "co-constructed" NARRATIVE of an analysis is created by the back-and-forth interaction between the narrative of the analyst's experience of self and patient, and the patient's experience of self and analyst, and their wish to have a shared narrative of the shared experience.

Component instincts   Different early forms of the sexual DRIVE directed at specific body areas such as the oral mucosa or genitalia, or associated with specific activities that may be erotically charged. These components frequently occur as complementary pairs, such as SCOPOPHILIA and EXHIBITIONISM or SADISM and MASOCHISM, and gradually combine to form mature sexuality in the course of psychic development.

Compromise formation   The EGO's solution to a problem presented by the competing demands of ID, SUPEREGO, the REPETITION COMPULSION, and external REALITY. Every psychic action has MULTIPLE FUNCTIONS and can be understood as a compromise formation.

Compulsion   A repetitive, ritualized action, the need for which forces its way into consciousness regardless of whether the person wishes to perform the action. Failure to perform this action often generates ANXIETY.

Condensation   A mental process in which a number of disparate thoughts or feelings are simultaneously represented by a single thought, feeling, or image. Condensation is a characteristic of PRIMARY PROCESS thinking and is frequently seen in operation in dreams and SYMPTOMS.

Conflict, intrapsychic   The condition arising from the opposition of competing motives, at least one of which is unconscious. The motives may arise from sexual or aggressive wishes, the wish to satisfy one's moral sense, the wish to conform to the demands of REALITY, and the wish to maintain a positive image of the SELF. Resolution of conflict involves a COMPROMISE FORMATION that takes into account the opposing motives, resulting in a SYMPTOM, a CHARACTER trait, or sublimation.

Conscious   The state of mental awareness of external and internal events—past, present, and future. Within Freud's TOPOGRAPHIC THEORY, the system Conscious could be differentiated from the system UNCONSCIOUS and the system PRECONSCIOUS on the basis of accessibility to reflection. The system Cs receives information from the external world as well as from the body and PSYCHE, and operates on the basis of SECONDARY PROCESS, characterized by logical thought that can be expressed in language.

Construction   See RECONSTRUCTION. Although these terms are used interchangeably, many contemporary analysts prefer *construction*, as it more accurately reflects that the NARRATIVES of the patient's past experiences, either external or INTRAPSYCHIC, that are elaborated in the analytic setting are not necessarily accurate renditions of these experiences, but rather renditions that explain more of the data or explain it in a more satisfying way than previously held renditions.

Container/Contained   Respectively, the recipient of projected affects who modifies these affects by accepting them inside himself or herself and tolerating them, and the projected unacceptable AFFECT. Bion asserted that the container/contained aspect of the mother-infant relationship was an important mechanism of early emotional growth, as well as a paradigm for an aspect of the therapeutic action of PSYCHOANALYSIS.

Conversion   The transformation of unacceptable thoughts or impulses into physical SYMPTOMS, resulting in the clinical picture of a physical ailment caused or exacerbated by psychical rather than physiological forces. The symptom is simultaneously an expression of the unacceptable thought and a DEFENSE against it, rather than a nonspecific physical response to stress or ANXIETY.

Countertransference   Originally, the unconscious reactions of the analyst to the patient derived from earlier situations in the life of the analyst, displaced onto the patient. As such, these feelings were felt to be an impediment to analytic treatment and to require self-scrutiny and self-analysis on the analyst's part to minimize their effects. Gradually, the term has come to include all the analyst's emotional responses to the patient, conscious and unconscious. With this expansion of meaning of the term, there has been wider interest in the countertransference as a source of analytically useful data about the inner life of the patient.

Day residue   The precipitating stimulus for a dream that is an event from waking life in the day before the dream. The event acquires significance from unconscious connection with repressed conflicts and appears in the dream in a displaced and symbolic form.

Death instinct   An INSTINCT postulated by Freud impelling the individual toward death and self-destruction. Its existence has always been a controversial question among psychoanalysts. Clinically, only AGGRESSION and the striving for power have been documented, not the biological DRIVE toward a return to the inanimate by way of self-destruction.

Declarative memory   The type of memory characterized by active, conscious recall of specific facts and events, usually verbal in nature. It is often contrasted with PROCEDURAL MEMORY, which refers to implicit learned behaviors or rules for various functions.

Defense   An unconscious mental operation aimed at avoiding ANXIETY. Examples of defenses are DENIAL, REPRESSION, REACTION FORMATION, SOMATIZATION, and INTELLECTUALIZATION. Failure of such responses may lead to conscious ANXIETY or to SYMPTOM formation.

Deferred action   The control of impulses so that one may think and choose alternative actions rather than act immediately. Alternately, the onset of a SYMPTOM or feeling when a significant time has elapsed after its precipitant.

Denial   A DEFENSE mechanism in which knowledge of an unacceptable thought, feeling, wish, or aspect of external REALITY is repudiated.

Depersonalization   The feeling that one's SELF is strangely unfamiliar or missing or that one is watching oneself behave in accordance with external REALITY but without emotional participation. Depersonalization may be a normal reaction to an acute and overwhelming danger, internal or external, or an abnormal reaction to what seems to be only a minor danger.

Depression   An emotional state (AFFECT, mood, or disorder) usually characterized by feelings of sadness, reduced energy, and self-esteem, and often accompanied by feelings of GUILT and self-reproach, loss of appetite, insomnia, and suicidal impulses. It is frequently precipitated by actual or fantasized experiences of abandonment, loss, or disappointment.

Depressive position (Klein)   The psychic organization that developmentally succeeds the PARANOID-SCHIZOID POSITION. It begins when the infant realizes that his or her loved good OBJECT and hated bad object are actually two aspects of the same object. Feelings of GUILT toward the object for AGGRESSION directed toward it, and desires to make REPARATION to the object (from which ultimately derive a capacity for mature object love and for sublimations), characterize the depressive position.

Derealization   A feeling of estrangement from the external world in which the enviornment is experienced as unreal, strange, and, if familiar, changed in some profound way. Perception and judgment remain intact even though the person experiencing derealization may feel threatened or afraid of the changes that seem to have taken place.

Derivative   The conscious expression, in modified form, of repressed contents of unconscious wishes, fears, and fantasies. Examples of derivatives are dreams, daydreams, SYMPTOMS, play, artistic creations, and TRANSFERENCE fantasies and ENACTMENTS.

Desire   A state of yearning for satisfaction or attainment; a particular feeling stronger than a wish, different from a need, and akin to intense longing. Often the longing in desire is more intense and satisfying than its attainment.

Developmental arrest   An interruption, as a result of TRAUMA, constitution, or both, in the expectable unfolding of psychological development of an individual. This may profoundly affect the quality of the adult personality of the individual.

Differentiation subphase (Mahler)   The subphase of the SEPARATION-INDIVIDUATION process during which the infant begins to show greater interest in the external world beyond the mother, and appears to be psychologically "hatching" from the mother-infant symbiosis. This subphase occurs between the ages of 5 and 10 months.

Disavowal   The unconscious repudiation of awareness of some painful aspect of external REALITY in order to diminish ANXIETY or even more painful AFFECTS.

Displacement   The severing of the connection between a thought or feeling and its OBJECT, and the ATTACHMENT of that thought or feeling to a substitute object. This mechanism is commonly observed in dreams and in the formation of PHOBIAS.

Dissociation   The separating off of two or more mental states within an indivdual so that the individual is unaware of one state while he or she is in the other. Often a result of psychic TRAUMA, it may allow the individual to maintain allegiance to two contradictory truths, while not being conscious of the contradiction. An extreme manifestation of dissociation is multiple personality, in which a person may exhibit several independent personalities, each unaware of the others.

Dream work   The mental process by which the DAY RESIDUE and the dream thoughts are transformed into the manifest dream. The process makes use of archaic modes of thinking, primarily CONDENSATION and DISPLACEMENT. The dream thoughts are transformed into visual images, which are then linked together into a relatively coherent story by means of SECONDARY REVISION (OR ELABORATION).

Drives   The motivating force for all human behavior, according to Freud's drive theory. Each drive consists of a source (somatic), a pressure, an aim (the means to achieve gratification), and an OBJECT, which provides the gratification. The primary drives, according to Freud, are the sexual and aggressive drives.

Dual instinct theory   A theory holding that the struggle between two opposing but complementary instinctual forces is central in the psychic life of the individual. Though currently the term is used mostly to refer to the sexual and aggressive DRIVES, other dual instinct models have been proposed, including those in which the opposing forces are life instinct/DEATH INSTINCT, sexual instinct/self-preservative instinct, and self love/OBJECT love.

Dynamic unconscious   Mental contents that are out of awareness because they have been subject to REPRESSION. It is distinguished from the system UNCONSCIOUS, which comprises the rules and principles that govern unconscious mental processes.

Ego   One of three major subdivisions of the mental apparatus (along with ID and SUPEREGO). Operations of the ego may be conscious or unconscious. The ego serves to mediate between the internal world, the external world, and the superego. It perceives the needs and wishes of the individual and the qualities of the environment and integrates these perceptions so as to achieve (through modification of internally arising needs and action taken on the environment) optimal gratification of internal needs and wishes in such a way as to be acceptable to external world and superego.

Ego apparatus   The psychic STRUCTURE associated with the execution of all of the functions of the EGO (e.g., REALITY TESTING, thought processes, defensive functions).

Ego defect   A failure or weakness of some EGO FUNCTION or functions that would normally be expected in a healthy individual. Ego functions that are often involved are SELF-OBJECT differentiation, defensive functioning, modulation of DRIVES and AFFECTS, and REALITY TESTING. Constitutional factors, psychic TRAUMA, and early maternal deprivation may all play a role in the genesis of an ego defect.

Ego-dystonic   Thoughts, feelings, personality traits, or behaviors that are experienced by the individual as incompatible with the dominant view of the SELF. Compare EGO-SYNTONIC.

Ego functions The specific capacities employed by the individual in the assessment of and mediation between the demands of the ID, the SUPEREGO, and external REALITY. Examples are perception, defensive functioning, impulse control, and REALITY TESTING.

Ego ideal A set of standards that reflects an exemplary view of the SELF. It derives from multiple sources, including idealized images of the parent, qualities perceived as necessary to maintain the love of the parents, and vestiges of infantile fantasies of omnipotence and perfection.

Ego psychology The area of psychoanalytic theory that focuses on the EGO as a STRUCTURE, the operation of its varying functions, and how they serve the aims of the individual's ADAPTATION and negotiation between the demands of internal needs and wishes, constraints of conscience, and exigencies of external REALITY.

Ego-syntonic Thoughts, feelings, personality traits, or behaviors that are experienced by the indvidual as compatible with the dominant view of the SELF. Compare EGO-DYSTONIC.

Empathy The imagining of another's subjective experience through the use of one's own subjective experience. Empathy has been posited by self psychologists as the defining means by which the data of PSYCHOANALYSIS are gathered.

Emotional refueling (Mahler) The experience of the infant, during the PRACTICING SUBPHASE of the SEPARATION-INDIVIDUATION process (10–15 months of age), in which he or she is able to restore the elation and confidence of being physically separate from the mother and of exercising developing cognitive and motor skills through momentarily reconnecting with the mother. During this phase, the mother needs to be available so that the child can turn to her periodically for this "refueling."

Emptiness A painful feeling in which the SELF is experienced as devoid of contents, thoughts, emotions, or inner images of relationships with others. It may be associated with feelings of worthlessness and having nothing to give to others.

Enactment The expression, in action, of TRANSFERENCE impulses or fantasies and their associated memories as a substitute for experiencing, understanding, or remembering them. Some measure of enactment is inevitable in all analyses and, if interpreted by the analyst, may be therapeutically useful.

Envy The emotion associated with the idea that someone else has something that you want. Envy is a form of AGGRESSION, since it embodies a wish not only to have what the other person has but to deprive the person of what is valuable and make them suffer for having possessed it. Envy is often confused with JEALOUSY, which involves three parties and has the aim of winning the exclusive love of the OBJECT over a rival for that love.

Eros A mental energy that binds elements of experience from relationships, gratifications, or DESIRES into larger units or patterns. These coalesce into fantasies tinged with sexual excitement.

Erotogenic masochism As defined by Freud, a propensity to seek physical or mental suffering for the purposes of conscious or unconscious sexual gratification.

Erotogenic zone A body part that serves, when stimulated, as a source of erotic excitation or gratification. Freud postulated a developmental series of such zones: the mouth, the anus, and the phallic/genital organs. Under particular circumstances, however, virtually any organ, mucous membrane, or cutaneous surface might fulfill this function.

Evocative memory The capacity to retrieve a memory by virtue of conscious will, in the absence of an externally perceived cue. It is distinguished from recognition memory, in which the memory is retrieved in response to an external cue.

Exhibitionism Pleasure in attracting attention to oneself. It is a normal part of child development and may be integrated into a well-functioning adult personality. The term also refers to the PARAPHILIA of exposing the genitals to strangers as a means of achieving orgasm.

Expressive psychoanalytic psychotherapy A form of treatment that relies on the basic psychoanalytic concepts of TRANSFERENCE, COUNTERTRANSFERENCE, and unconscious MOTIVATION, even though it may not adhere to some conventions of formal PSYCHOANALYSIS, such as the use of a couch. It seeks to encourage the expression, understanding, and WORKING-THROUGH of thoughts and feelings that may have been previously unavailable to conscious awareness.

Externalization A mental process that results in the individual attributing internal phenomena or his or her own agency in INTERPERSONAL phenomena to the external world.

False self The SELF experience that emerges and organizes in response to another's needs, expectations, and demands (as opposed to the TRUE SELF that emerges and organizes in response to one's own needs, expectations, and demands).

Family romance A FANTASY, common in LATENCY-age children, in which, as a result of disillusionment with their family of origin, children imagine they had parents very different from their own. These fantasy parents are endowed with ideal characteristics that they wish their own parents had, such as royalty, wealth, power, or special kindness.

Fantasy/Phantasy An unconsciously organized INTRAPSYCHIC "story" about oneself and others. Fantasies shape perceptions of the external world and determine the nature of INTERPERSONAL interactions. Freud believed UNCONSCIOUS FANTASIES were originally elaborated consciously in words and images and became unconscious through REPRESSION. The Kleinians added the concept of very early fantasies, elaborated before the attainment of language and experienced primarily on a somatic level, which they believe are part of a developmental continuum with the higher-level fantasies described by Freud. As a convention, the term *phantasy* is used to connote this broader Kleinian definition of fantasy life.

Feminine masochism A term used by Freud to describe one of three forms of MASOCHISM in which men or women identify with certain aspects of the role of the woman that are experienced as submissive: being castrated, being penetrated, or giving birth to a baby. This identification is reflected in masochistic submissive behavior or sexual fantasies.

Femininity See MASCULINITY/FEMININITY.

Fetish/Fetishim A PARAPHILIA (or perversion) in which a body part, inanimate object, or piece of clothing substitutes for the genitals as the aim of the sexual DRIVE.

Fixation The unchanged, unmodulated persistence of earlier patterns of thought or ADAPTATION into advanced levels of maturing development, when their manifestations may be deemed inappropriate. This developmental stasis is often a consequence of early TRAUMA.

Frame The rules and regulations of social interaction that produce necessary boundaries to sustain the PSYCHOANALYTIC SITUATION and permit creative understanding in the

PSYCHOANALYTIC PROCESS. These include arrangements between patient and analyst regarding time and frequency of sessions and payment of the fee. For patients whose disorders include difficulty in negotiating boundaries, the analytic frame becomes an important focus of the treatment.

Free association   The principal method or "FUNDAMENTAL RULE" of psychoanalytic treatment, in which the patient says whatever comes to mind, without conscious editing. Implicit in this rule is the understanding that difficulties in doing so will inevitably be encountered. The analyst attempts to assist the patient, through INTERPRETATION, to create greater freedom of association.

Fundamental rule   In clinical PSYCHOANALYSIS, the injunction to the patient at the onset of treatment to report whatever comes to mind, regardless of its seeming lack of relevance or logic, social inappropriateness, or feelings of SHAME or embarrassment that it might stir.

Gender/Gender identity   Comprising two aspects of the experience of the SELF: core gender identity and gender role identity. *Core gender identity* refers to the individual's anatomical self-image, usually as either male or female, rarely as hermaphrodite. *Gender role identity* is the sense of oneself as being masculine or feminine, in comparison to perceived familial/cultural norms on a continuum.

Genital phase/Genitality   The final phase of psychosexual development as conceived by Freud, and the psychic characteristics of this stage. The genital stage begins at the onset of puberty. The integration of OBJECT love with genital sexuality is a primary developmental attainment of this stage.

Good enough mother   The mother who can take care of, anticipate, and gradually allow frustration in a developmentally appropriate way, allowing the baby's TRUE SELF to emerge.

Grandiose self   In SELF PSYCHOLOGY, a normal STRUCTURE in the path of development of a cohesive sense of SELF. This structure is reactivated in the treatment of patients with narcissistic personality disorder. Its expression includes omnipotence and EXHIBITIONISM. In development, it represents the child's attempt to recover an experience of perfection in infancy, experiencing all perfection as residing in the self and all imperfection as residing in the external world. The grandiose self may develop into mature ambition and healthy and realistic self-esteem. In less optimal circumstances, demands of the unmodified grandiose self may persist and lead to rages when the needs for confirmation are not met by the outside world.

Group psychology   The mental processes in operation when several individuals join together to act in concert with each other. Freud noted in particular the IDEALIZATION of and IDENTIFICATION with the leader of the group leading to reduction of individual SUPEREGO controls.

Guilt   A feeling of remorse, accompanied by expectations of negative consequences, for specific thoughts, feelings, or actions (or lack thereof) that are felt by the individual to be wrong or bad. Guilt is a response to failing to come up to one's own internal standards, whereas SHAME is associated with being seen to be bad in the eyes of others.

Hallucinatory wish fulfillment   An infantile mental mechanism in which a wish is experienced as fulfilled even if it has not been fulfilled in REALITY. This experience is based on memory traces of experiences of satisfaction. In normal psychological development, the infant learns to replace hallucinatory wish fulfillment with actions directed to the outside world, with the aim of evincing actual satisfaction of wishes.

Hermeneutics   The theory, science, and art of interpretation. Psychoanalysis may be regarded as a hermeneutic discipline, and the study of the sources, methods, and validation of psychoanalytic interpretations is an important aspect of contemporary PSYCHOANALYSIS.

Homeostasis   A state of stable psychic equilibrium, in which the different agencies of the mind work together in harmony so as to achieve reasonable satisfaction of the individual's needs and ADAPTATION to external REALITY, without being overwhelmed by AFFECTS or external stimuli.

Horizontal split   In SELF PSYCHOLOGY, a process by which unwanted qualities of the SELF are warded off by placing them outside of consciousness, while the desirable qualities of the self remain conscious. The primary DEFENSE associated with the horizontal split is REPRESSION.

Hypnosis/Hypnotic suggestion   A state of altered consciousness variously described as DISSOCIATION, focused attention, or split AFFECT, accompanied by changes in brain waves, induced by special techniques. Under hypnosis, individuals may be induced to recall previously repressed memories or convinced that they remember events that never occurred. Individuals may be instructed to carry out specific behaviors after the hypnotic trance is ended.

Hypochondriasis   An excessive preoccupation with bodily concerns, often involving imagined serious illness, sometimes bordering on the delusional.

Hysteria   A common diagnosis during the earlier epoch of PSYCHOANALYSIS, encompassing somatic symptoms (e.g., paralyses or blindness in the absence of physical etiology, fugue states, dissociative episodes). The treatment of hysterical patients led Freud to the theory of unconscious conflict as the etiology of NEUROSIS.

Id   In Freud's STRUCTURAL THEORY, the source of the INSTINCTS, manifested in biological urges pressing for satisfaction, as well as repressed infantile wishes. The content of the id is always unconscious.

Idealization   The attribution in FANTASY of ideal or wished-for characteristics in others that do not accurately reflect the REALITY of these people.

Idealizing transference   An attitude in which the therapist is seen in glowing, elevated terms. From a self psychological perspective, this attitude—including the yearning for a good SELFOBJECT—is viewed as an inevitable element in the treatment of narcissistic phenomena. Alternatively, IDEALIZATION is considered to be a DEFENSE against underlying AGGRESSION and hatred, frequently leading to destructive disillusionment.

Identification   An unconscious process in which a person models his or her ways of thinking and acting after those of an important figure in life such as a parent. Influenced by AFFECT, identification is an ongoing process that occurs throughout life, though being especially important in one's early years and in adolescence.

Identity   The enduring experience of the SELF as a unique, coherent, and relatively consistent entity over time.

Identity diffusion The lack of a consistent sense of SELF due to a failure of integration of diverse senses of self. This leads to either the presentation of an assumed IDENTITY to others, the overflow of poorly modulated AGGRESSION, fragmented or shifting self-presentations, or the appearance of being simply rudderless and adrift in the world.

Imaginary Commonly used to denote productions of the mind that are largely fantastical and do not adhere rigidly to perceptions or the constraints of external REALITY. Lacan uses the term to denote a register of mental activity dominated by images; it is opposed to the symbolic register, in which mental activity makes use of SYMBOLS, and thought occurs by the manipulation of these symbols.

Implicit memories/Procedural memories Memories that are not readily available in words or images and are not conscious. Their presence is revealed by behavioral and emotional patterns that are elicited without the subject's awareness. Examples include riding a bicycle, playing a musical instrument, the subtleties of social eye contact, and automatic emotional responses in patterned situations.

Incorporation The FANTASY of taking on the traits of another person by taking them in bodily (e.g., by eating them). The fantasy of incorporation is typical of the ORAL PHASE of development.

Individuation The process through which the developing child distinguishes his or her own individual characteristics and increasingly experiences himself or herself as different from the OBJECT.

Induction phase The initial phase in clinical PSYCHOANALYSIS. It is characterized by unclear and often shifting TRANSFERENCES, unlike the more persistent transferences that are said to characterize the MIDPHASE.

Infantile amnesia The normal, universal inability to remember experiences from the early years of life. It is based on either the inability of the developing brain to deposit these experiences such that they are recoverable in memory, or the REPRESSION by the mind of disturbing early mental contents.

Infantile neurosis According to Freud, a normal developmental phase in children in which the intense conflicts of childhood, particularly those of the OEDIPAL PHASE, with its attendant ANXIETY and GUILT, are brought to some sort of adaptive resolution and repressed. Definitions of the infantile neurosis have varied widely among psychoanalysts, and some believe that it regularly resurfaces in the course of PSYCHOANALYSIS and is thereby resolved.

Infantile sexuality The full range of sexual thoughts, feelings, fantasies, and activities throughout childhood. Freud asserted its importance in the formation of character and SYMPTOMS. More narrowly defined, it comprises the manifestations of psychosexual development prior to LATENCY unfolding in a pattern of sequential, overlapping phases. See PSYCHOSEXUAL PHASES.

Inhibition The withdrawal from a particular activity that would ordinarily be assumed to be well within one's purview in order to avoid the ANXIETY associated with that activity. The withdrawal may be conscious or unconscious.

Insight An understanding of some previously unrecognized truth about one's SELF, one's behavior, or the actions and MOTIVATIONS of others. It may accrue gradually or be experienced as a flash of recognition, and may be associated with feelings of either relief or pain.

Instinct Freud postulated that somatic energic forces, sexual and aggressive, provided the energy that stimulated mental activity. In this view, all mental life could be seen as derivative of sexual or aggressive instinctual forces.

Instinctual aim The REPRESENTATION of the specific action on the OBJECT that will satisfy an instinctual wish, for example, to suck on the breast or to penetrate in genital intercourse.

Instinctual object The REPRESENTATION of a person or thing, either an external "other" or an internal memory of "other," toward which instinctual energy is directed. Freud's concept of INSTINCT reflects an organic state integrating physiological DRIVE and psychological MOTIVATION.

Intellectualization The exaggerated use of intellectual measures such as abstract philosophizing, speculative thought, or pedantic logic as a DEFENSE against ANXIETY or other unwelcome AFFECTS. It is commonly mobilized in adolescence. It may be associated with obsessional or paranoid thinking.

Internalization The unconscious psychological processes by which an individual adopts aspects of the environment. Three separate components—INCORPORATION, INTROJECTION, and IDENTIFICATION—are regularly distinguished, according to developmental features.

Internalized object relation The mental REPRESENTATION of persons in the external world and their interactions with the SELF. These OBJECT RELATIONS are created by specific defensive and adaptational processes that include IDENTIFICATION and INTROJECTION and form a template that organizes our world into a stable way of situating ourselves in relation to others.

Internal object (Klein) The mental REPRESENTATION of the OBJECT and of aspects of its relation with the SELF.

Interpersonal The interactions between individuals that are responsible for psychological change and growth, often contrasted with INTRAPSYCHIC referring to processes occurring in the mind of one individual.

Interpretation A communication by the analyst aimed at expanding the patient's self-knowledge by pointing out connections in the patient's mental life of which he or she was previously unaware. The analyst's interpretations are key factors in the unfolding of the PSYCHOANALYTIC PROCESS.

Intersubjective/Intersubjectivity The aspect of INTERPERSONAL experience that is characterized by the interaction of two individuals with different subjective experiences of themselves, each other, and the events between them, and that is best understood by examining the subjective contributions of each to the interaction. The intersubjective school of PSYCHOANALYSIS places this aspect of the TRANSFERENCE-COUNTERTRANSFERENCE matrix at the center of inquiry in clinical psychoanalysis, implicitly making a demand on the analyst for greater awareness of the impact of his or her own subjective experience on the evolution of the TRANSFERENCE.

Intervention Any of the psychoanalyst's activities in clinical PSYCHOANALYSIS meant to facilitate the unfolding of the analytic process and the patient's self-understanding. Examples are questions, clarifications, INTERPRETATIONS, confrontations, and educative or supportive statements.

Intrapsychic Located within the mind of the individual. An intrapsychic conflict (see CONFLICT, INTRAPSYCHIC) would be one between two contradictory wishes of the individual rather than between the individual and the external world.

Introjection A process of internalizing OBJECT images and their affective relation to images of the SELF. It differs from IDENTIFICATION in that modification of the EGO is a less central aspect of introjection than of identification. Introjections (i.e., introjected object images) form the basis of the primitive SUPEREGO: optimally, these images ultimately coalesce into a structuralized superego, which may then be modified through identifications and other ego processes.

Introspection The attempt to examine and understand one's own inner psychological and emotional experiences and constructions.

Isolation The disconnection of relevant ideas from one another, or of ideas from AFFECTS, in order to avoid ANXIETY or psychic pain.

Jealousy The emotion associated with the idea that someone that you love is in love with someone else. The aim of the jealous person is to win the love of the beloved from the rival. Jealousy differs from ENVY because it involves three parties and because the wish to destroy the rival is secondary to the wish to become the person who is more loved.

Latency A developmental phase extending from age 6–7 years to age 10–11 years, originally identified by Freud as the period between the oedipal phase and puberty that is distinguished by quiescence in regard to libidinal and aggressive DRIVE. During this phase, the child's focus shifts to school and peers, and there is the advent of concrete operational thought and an expanded repertoire of EGO capacities. Most modern analysts agree that the oedipal struggles have not disappeared but are warded off by the newly acquired SUPEREGO and the DEFENSES of EXTERNALIZATION, REACTION FORMATION, and sublimation.

Latent content The unconscious dream thoughts, stimulated by the DAY RESIDUE and the associatively linked infantile, sexual, and aggressive wishes, that underlie the manifest dream and are tranformed into the manifest dream through DREAM WORK.

Libido The souce of psychic energy deriving from the organism's sexual wishes, drawn from all levels of psychosexual development, not just genital sexuality.

Libido theory An early model of mental life postulated by Freud that sought to explain SYMPTOMS such as ANXIETY and NEURASTHENIA as the result of variations in the distribution and discharge of sexual energy.

Manifest content The dream as it is recalled by the dreamer. The manifest content is the product of the DREAM WORK and is to be differentiated from the LATENT CONTENT, which is unconscious.

Masculinity/Femininity Respectively, male and female GENDER role identities that develop after the establishment of core gender identity. These include early identifications and fantasies of oneself as male or female and internal representations of gendered OBJECT RELATIONS. Most individuals consider themselves primarily masculine or feminine, but each individual nevertheless has a wide range of unconscious and preconscious FANTASIES and wishes that derive from multiple identifications.

Masochism Broadly, the seeking of pleasure in pain. Freud described three kinds of masochism—EROTOGENIC MASOCHISM, in which conscious sexual pleasure is derived from pain, suffering, or humiliation; MORAL MASOCHISM, in which defeat or humiliation is unconsciously sought out without any conscious sexual pleasure; and FEMININE MASOCHISM, which is the pleasure derived by women (or by men who are having a FANTASY of being a woman) in submitting and being penetrated. Many modern analysts believe the term falsely lumps together a variety of clinical phenomena with very different meanings that have in common only a seeking of unpleasure.

Melancholia A pathological depressive reaction to loss, characterized by persistent self-hatred and self-reproaches. Freud distinguished melancholia from normal MOURNING, emphasizing in melancholia an inability to come to terms with the AMBIVALENCE toward the lost OBJECT and an unconscious IDENTIFICATION with hated aspects of that OBJECT.

Mentalization The developmental attainment in which the child becomes aware of the existence of the mind and of the sense that other people in the environment are motivated by activities of their minds that are in some ways like, and in some ways different from, those of the child's mind.

Metapsychology The construction of high-level abstract theories that are intended to serve as a basis for understanding more specific clinical phenomena.

Midphase The second of three phases (with INDUCTION phase and TERMINATION phase) of a clinical PSYCHOANALYSIS. Hallmarks of the midphase are the establishment of the TRANSFERENCE NEUROSIS, the patient's understanding of the nature of the work of psychoanalysis (e.g., FREE ASSOCIATION, the analysis of RESISTANCES), and his or her voluntary participation in it. Many analyses do not follow such a clearly defined course.

Mirror transference In SELF PSYCHOLOGY, that aspect of the SELFOBJECT TRANSFERENCE in which the patient experiences the analyst solely or primarily in his function of confirming or validating the patient's GRANDIOSE SELF.

Moral masochism One of the three types of MASOCHISM (with EROTOGENIC MASOCHISM and FEMININE MASOCHISM) desribed by Freud. Moral masochism implies that a person has an unconscious need to be punished, arising from a sense of GUILT, manifesting in self-defeating or self-destructive behavior without conscious sexual excitement.

Motivation The cause of behavior. Analysts disagree on whether DRIVES, AFFECTS, or wished-for relations with objects, or combinations of these, are the primary motivating forces. In a psychoanalytic view, many actions are unconsciously motivated, and probably all actions have multiple psychological sources of motivation.

Mourning The INTRAPSYCHIC process of responding to loss. This process regularly requires an alternation between the wish to reverse the loss and the wish to accept it and regain that portion of oneself bound up with what has been lost. It involves coming to terms with both positive and negative feelings about what has been lost. Mourning is always painful; inability to adequately mourn can lead to a state of pathological grief or DEPRESSION.

Multideterminism The concept that all mental and behavioral events are not random but are caused by the convergence of multiple factors, including the needs of the EGO, SUPEREGO, and ID, COMPULSIONS to repeat, developmental and maturational influences, and the effects of memories, symbolic meanings, and relations with others.

Multiple function, principle of   The concept, first put forward by Waelder, that every psychic action reflects the EGO's attempt to find a compromise solution to the problem presented by the competing demands of ID, SUPEREGO, and external REALITY.

Mutative   A quality of an INTERPRETATION in PSYCHOANALYSIS. A mutative interpretation is one that changes the patient's perspective on himself or herself and his or her relationship with the world. The response of a patient to a mutative INTERPRETATION has an emotional quality, rather than being purely cognitive, and offers the possibility for change in behavior.

Narcissism   An individual's love, regard, and valuation of his or her own SELF. Normal narcissism is represented in adequate self-care, realistic self-confidence, and pride. Heightened narcissism is seen in vanity, insistence on privilege, exaggerated assumptions of superiority over other people, or outright grandiosity. The more intense a person's narcissism, the more aggressively he or she may react to real or imagined insults, and the greater his or her vulnerability to humiliation and SHAME.

Narrative   A recounting of events that provides a sense of history; selecting and bringing together a series of discrete events to form a coherent story with implicit elements of cause and effect. An individual's narratives of his life may play an important part in his view of himself in relation to the world. Narratives are subject to constant revision; in treatment, observing the way in which these narratives are revised provides a window into the mental functioning of the patient. Revision of narratives as a result of INTERPRETATION and INSIGHT can be an important part of the therapeutic action of clinical PSYCHOANALYSIS.

Negation   A spontaneous statement of denial that something has occurred or has meaning. Such denial often indicates that actually the opposite is unconsciously believed. Negation can permit repressed thoughts to enter consciousness without their accompanied feelings or connotations.

Negative hallucination   The nonperception of something that is actually present, involving any of the senses. This experience is the inverse of a hallucination, which is the subjective perception of an external phenomenon not in fact present.

Negative therapeutic reaction   The worsening of SYMPTOMS in response to the therapist's effort to foster INSIGHT. Many different dynamics may underlie such a response, including GUILT over lessened suffering or improved functioning, or ENVY of the analyst's capacity to help.

Neurasthenia   A state of excessive fatigability, lassitude, irritability, lack of concentration, and hypochondria. In Freud's early work, he attributed these SYMPTOMS to physiological consequences of inadequate sexual satisfaction due to masturbation. Both the term and Freud's understanding of it are important in the history of PSYCHOANALYSIS but are not considered clinically relevant in modern psychoanalysis.

Neurosis   A category of symptomatic disturbance arising from intrapsychic conflict (see CONFLICT, INTRAPSYCHIC) that interferes with normal functioning but that does not interfere with REALITY TESTING. Compare with PSYCHOSIS, in which reality testing is impaired.

Neutrality   The position of nonjudgmental listening adopted by a psychoanalyst toward his or her patient, avoiding suggestion, advice, or choosing sides in the patient's intrapsychic conflicts (see CONFLICT, INTRAPSYCHIC). Modern analysts have questioned both the realistic attainability and the clinical value of neutrality as it was originally described by Freud. Today, analysts vary widely as to what they believe constitutes a stance of neutrality.

Neutralized energy   A postulated form of psychic energy that results from a process in which sexual and aggressive elements are fused, providing impetus for the performance of psychic work not dominated by either libidinal or aggressive feelings.

Normality   As commonly used, psychological health or appropriate behavior. Some psychoanalysts have attempted to posit a relatively normal EGO that pursues reasonable pleasures and accomplishments in relationships with others. However, there is no consensus among psychoanalysts as to what constitutes "normality" from a psychoanalytic point of view.

Object   A person who is the focus of one's wishes and needs. The object may be internal (the individual's mental image of the object) or external (the actual person external to the subject), part (a body part, function, or gratifying or frustrating aspect of the object) or whole (an image of the entire object that takes into account its multiple attributes.)

Object constancy   Integration of originally separate, unconscious mental REPRESENTATIONS of "good" and "bad" OBJECTS into more realistic and stable representations combining the "good" and "bad" qualities.

Object relations   Refers both to the actual relationships of subject and OBJECT and to the internal FANTASY of the nature of the object (the "other"), as well as the nature of the relationship of self and object.

Object relations theory   A theory of psychological STRUCTURE and development that postulates that the internalized REPRESENTATIONS of OBJECTS, and the FANTASIES of the relationship of self and object, are determining factors in the development of psychic structure.

Object representation   The individual's mental image of an OBJECT in his or her life. The REPRESENTATION contains aspects of the actual external OBJECT but is also colored by the individual's fantasies about the object.

Obsession   A recurrent thought that intrudes on an individual's mind and cannot be banished from consciousness by an exercise of will. Obsessions are closely related to COMPULSIONS but differ in that obsessions occur within the realm of thought, whereas compulsions impel the individual to action.

Oedipus complex   An aggregate of mental processes that develops from the child's incestuous wishes toward the parent of the opposite sex. There are associated conflictual feelings toward the parent of the same sex as both a rival for the love of the incestuous OBJECT and a loved object himself or herself. This conflict is resolved through an IDENTIFICATION with the same-sex parent. (The "negative" Oedipus complex involves an identification with the parent of the opposite sex in order to receive the love of the parent of the same sex.)

Oral-incorporative mode   A mode of relating to objects that is characterized by the prominence of FANTASIES of eating and swallowing the object and making it part of the individual's own body, thus abolishing individual characteristics of the OBJECT.

Oral-intrusive mode   The earliest of the infantile developmental stages. It provides the prototypes of both love (LIBIDO) and hate (AGGRESSION), manifesting, respectively, through feeding/ taking in and biting/spitting out. The oral-intrusive mode reflects the infant's aggressive insertion of SELF into the body of the mother through demand for constant feeding, or biting. Later expressions of clinging and demandingness may be traced developmentally to oral intrusiveness.

Orality   All the psychic interests, impulses, CHARACTER traits, and DEFENSE mechanisms that stem from the libidinal and aggressive DRIVES associated with the mouth, particularly during the ORAL PHASE of psychosexual development, when these drives and the defenses against them are the dominant organizing forces of mental life. Greed, dependency, demandingness, impatience, curiousity, and sarcasm are character traits associated with orality.

Oral-retentive mode   A mode of relating to OBJECTS that is characterized by the prominence of fantasies of holding on by closing or grasping with the mouth.

Oral phase   The PSYCHOSEXUAL PHASE, consisting of approximately the first 18 months of life, in which sensations of the oral zone and strivings attached to these sensations are dominant in the organization of psychic life.

Overdetermination   The concept that all aspects of psychic life, including SYMPTOMS, FANTASIES, dreams, personality traits, and behaviors, are caused by a number of intersecting psychic factors.

Parameter   A term coined by Eissler to describe deviations from a standard psychoanalytic technique. The term and concept are little used today.

Paranoia   A condition in which the subject holds to irrational beliefs, often circumscribed to one area of life, generally characterized by both grandiosity and persecutory ideas.

Paranoid-schizoid position (Klein)   The earliest psychic organization, characterized by a predominance of AGGRESSION over LIBIDO, and by primitive DEFENSES such as SPLITTING and PROJECTIVE IDENTIFICATION. Through SPLITTING, the mother is perceived alternately as a good (gratifying) or bad (frustrating) OBJECT, and the intense aggression stirred by the bad object is projected, so that it is experienced as persecutory. Remnants of this psychic organization persist throughout life and alternate with the higher level DEPRESSIVE POSITION.

Paraphilia   A form of sexual behavior in which the the aim of the sexual impulse is diverted from coitus and in which organsm is obtained through other means or in which other activities are required for adequate sexual functioning. Examples are FETISHISM, pedophilia, EXHIBITIONISM, sexual MASOCHISM, and SADISM. Replaces *perversion*, which many analysts have moved away from as imprecise and implicitly judgmental.

Parapraxis   Slips of the tongue, errors, bungled actions, and memory lapses that usually surprise the subject. These occurrences, like neurotic SYMPTOMS, are COMPROMISE FORMATIONS between forbidden wishes or ideas and DEFENSES against them.

Part object (Klein)   The individual's experience of the OBJECT as only one aspect of the object rather than the entire object in its full complexity. This aspect may be a particular body part (e.g., the breast) or an experience of the object dominated by one AFFECT (e.g., the good or the bad object) or of a function of the object (e.g., feeding, containing.) The experience of the object as a part object is a hallmark of the PARANOID-SCHIZOID POSITION.

Pathological grandiose self (Kernberg)   The central mental STRUCTURE in narcissistic personality disorder, which consists of a CONDENSATION of elements of the idealized object, the ideal SELF, and the real self. Though it may describe similar phenomena to Kohut's GRANDIOSE SELF, it differs in that, according to Kernberg, it is a result of a pathological line of development rather than the persistence of a normal developmental phase.

Penis envy   ENVY of power and strength in others, unconsciously attributed to the other's possession of a bigger or "better" penis. While originally attributed primarily to girls' envying the larger, more visible penis of boys, penis envy is considered today by many analysts to be a symbol of the social advantages of males in society.

Phallic phase   That period of psychosexual development, beginning at about 2 years of age and culminating in the oedipal phase, during which the sensations from the PHALLUS (penis or clitoris), and the wishes and impulses connected with these sensations, are dominant in the organization of psychic life.

Phallus   Used literally to refer to the mental REPRESENTATION of the genitalia (the penis or clitoris), and figuratively to refer to personality traits such as pride and assertiveness, as well as a type of CHARACTER in which such traits are prominent.

Phantasy   See FANTASY/PHANTASY.

Phobia   A SYMPTOM involving the avoidance of an OBJECT or situation that stimulates ANXIETY. A phobia involves the DISPLACEMENT of a feeling away from its actual object onto one that bears some symbolic connection to it, along with a PROJECTION of a forbidden urge onto the phobic object.

Pleasure principle/Unpleasure principle   The basic regulatory aim of all mental activity, according to Freud, in which the individual seeks to maximize pleasure and to avoid unpleasure. Frustration in achieving immediate gratification leads to recognition of environmental constraints and modifications in the pleasure principle so that immediate pleasure is delayed in the interest of eventual satisfaction and self-preservation. Freud called this developmental achievement the REALITY PRINCIPLE and juxtaposed it with the pleasure principle.

Practicing subphase (Mahler)   The subphase (10–12 to 16–18 months of age) of the SEPARATION-INDIVIDUATION process that is initiated by the infant's maturational capacity to create physical distance from mother, beginning with crawling and peaking with running, and is at its height with the achievement of upright locomotion. The subphase is distinguished by a) elation, as the toddler experiences a "love affair with the world", and excitement about exploration and his or her own growing EGO capacities; and b) the toddler's capacity to reassure himself or herself by returning to mother's physical body if ANXIETY intrudes.

Preconscious   One of the three components (with CONSCIOUS and UNCONSCIOUS) of the mental apparatus in Freud's TOPOGRAPHIC THEORY. The preconscious contains word residues that can connect an unconscious or conscious feeling, thought, or image with a linguistic REPRESENTATION. Elements of the preconscious are not conscious but are easily brought into conscious awareness through focusing attention on them.

Preoedipal The psychic organization, including DRIVES, DEFENSES, and SELF REPRESENTATIONS and OBJECT REPRESENTATIONS, specific to the phases of development before the OEDIPUS COMPLEX. Preoedipal organization is associated with more primitive forms of PSYCHOPATHOLOGY, such as narcissistic or borderline personalities, but the persistence of some preoedipal features of psychic life is ubiquitous, and these features may become prominent in regressive states even in individuals who are primarily organized around oedipal conflicts.

Primary process A primitive form of thought described by Freud, closely linked with the PLEASURE PRINCIPLE. It seeks immediate discharge of impulses through HALLUCINATORY WISH FULFILLMENT and makes use of the mechanisms of DISPLACEMENT and CONDENSATION in its REPRESENTATIONS of satisfactions. Developmentally it gives way to the SECONDARY PROCESS, which is associated with the REALITY PRINCIPLE and obeys higher-level rules of logic. In Freud's original TOPOGRAPHIC THEORY, the primary process was believed to be the form of thinking that governed all the activities of the UNCONSCIOUS. Later, in the structural model, Freud understood that many mechanisms governed by the SECONDARY PROCESS can also occur at an unconscious level.

Primal scene The childhood perception of parental sexual intercourse, whether actually observed, actually overheard, or only imagined, and the meaning the child attaches to it.

Primary gain In reference to a psychological SYMPTOM, refers to the psychic gain derived from its function in the resolution of an intrapsychic conflict (see CONFLICT, INTRAPSYCHIC). It is distinguished from SECONDARY GAIN, which refers to the gain derived from the SYMPTOM's use in the manipulation of the external world.

Primary identification The earliest form of IDENTIFICATION with an OBJECT, which occurs before the infant can distinguish the SELF from the object. This is different from later forms of identification, in which the growing infant or child distinguishes outside influences as external and then takes them in.

Procedural memory A form of memory for motor patterns, habits, and skills. Procedural memory is nonverbal and unconscious. A skill such as skiing or surgery is learned with conscious input, but many of the components of the skill are neither conscious nor verbally expressible. The concept has been applied by some contemporary analysts to understand some aspects of TRANSFERENCE, which can be conceptualized as habitual modes of object relatedness learned as procedures in the first few years of life.

Prohibition A mechanism of the SUPEREGO whereby impulses, wishes, or thoughts are deemed unacceptable and prevented from entering consciousness or from being acted on.

Projection The DEFENSE mechanism in which an individual attributes to another person an unacceptable thought, feeling, or attribute, such as an aggressive or sexual impulse, which is his or her own.

Projective identification The DEFENSE mechanism, originally described by Klein, through which an intolerable aspect of the individual's mental life is projected into another person, accompanied by the FANTASY that this projected element controls the other person from within. In an INTERPERSONAL context, the target of projective identifications may have powerful feelings stirred in him or her, as if he or she is actually taken over by the projected element. Bion added that in addition to functioning as a mechanism of defense, projective identification also functions as a primitive form of communication and can ultimately be a vehicle for emotional growth in the mother-infant interaction.

Psyche The realm of the mind, as distinguished from the realm of the body, or soma.

Psychic determinism The hypothesis that mental events are not random and that behavior can be understood to be determined by unconscious as well as conscious influences.

Psychic reality Reality as it is constructed in the mind of an individual at a particular moment. The components of this "reality" are perceptions, memories, wishes, and fears. It is distinguished from OBJECTIVE or historical REALITY.

Psychoanalysis Psychoanalysis was conceived by Freud as a theory of mind, an investigative method, and a form of treatment for mental disorders. As a method of treatment, it involves multiple sessions per week for several years. Psychoanalysis utilizes FREE ASSOCIATION, observations about unconscious mental functioning, and the examination of TRANSFERENCE and COUNTERTRANSFERENCE as major means by which to understand and therapeutically influence the patient.

Psychoanalytic boundaries A set of conditions that compose the FRAME, including setting, time limit, confidentiality, payment of a fee, avoidance of dual relationships, and abstinence regarding sexual or physical contact. These conditions facilitate the emergence of the TRANSFERENCE while also protecting both the patient and the analyst from potential exploitation.

Psychoanalytic method The technique of classical PSYCHOANALYSIS involving multiple sessions per week with the patient lying on a couch out of view of the analyst and endeavoring to say everything that comes to mind. The analyst uses the patient's associations and the information derived from TRANSFERENCE and COUNTERTRANSFERENCE to enhance the patient's self-understanding.

Psychoanalytic process The experience within a patient who is responding to the PSYCHOANALYTIC METHOD. Analysis of RESISTANCE leads the patient to master unpleasurable feelings, particularly with respect to the analyst; this leads to the emergence of previously unconscious thoughts and feelings with a new set of resistances, which are, in turn, interpreted. At the same time, unfolding feelings within the analyst help him or her to better understand the patient's emotions and DEFENSES and facilitate his or her capacity to interpret.

Psychoanalytic situation The totality of the conditions—practical, psychological, and INTERPERSONAL—that are present when patient and analyst come together for the purposes of psychoanalyzing the patient. It may be seen as having three components: the patient who brings a disposition to use a relationship with an analyst to transform aspects of his or her emotional life; the analyst who listens with the aim of understanding the patient's UNCONSCIOUS; and the setting, including practical arrangements such as time and fee, and agreed-on methods and procedures, such as the injunction to free-associate.

Psychodynamics The organized constellation of unconscious wishes and DEFENSES against those wishes that underlie a piece of human behavior. Implicit in psychoanalytic theory is the idea that all human behaviors and mental events have psychodynamic underpinnings.

Psychopathology Psychological states or STRUCTURES, transitory or enduring, that either cause active psychological pain to the individual, get in the way of the individual's optimal functioning, lead to patterns of action in the external world that repeatedly bring the individual into trouble, or can be seen by the external observer to inevitably lead to harmful consequences.

Psychosexual phases A series of sequential, overlapping stages in the developing infant and child—oral, anal, phallic, and genital—each representing predominant sensual investment in different bodily zones (e.g., sucking, biting, or mouthing in the ORAL PHASE; expelling or retaining feces in the ANAL PHASE; and manipulating the genitals in the PHALLIC PHASE). FIXATION at one of these stages may color adult personality development and CHARACTER type.

Psychosis A category of mental disorders typified by a loss of REALITY TESTING, as opposed to NEUROSIS or CHARACTER pathology, in which REALITY TESTING remains intact. Phenomenologically, psychotic disorders may include delusions, idiosyncratic thinking, hallucinations, abnormal affective states, and bizarre behaviors.

Psychosomatic Physical SYMPTOMS or diseases in whose expression psychological factors play an important role. The sufferer may or may not be aware of this connection. These symptoms and diseases are associated with actual physiological dreangements; they are not IMAGINARY or factitious.

Psychotic process The changes in thinking and experiencing that are associated with PSYCHOSIS. These changes may include PRIMARY PROCESS thinking (e.g., CONDENSATION and DISPLACEMENT), delusions, idiosyncratic thinking, and hallucinations.

Rapprochement subphase (Mahler) The subphase of the SEPARATION-INDIVIDUATION process following the PRACTICING SUBPHASE. It extends from about 16 to 25 months of age. The infant has mastered upright locomotion and now becomes more aware of physical separateness from the mother. The need to share every experience with mother is heightened as the infant's exuberance wanes with the recognition that she is not participating in his or her "delusion of parental omnipotence." During this subphase, the toddler is in a crisis of AMBIVALENCE, seeking to coerce the mother and yet also escape her orbit.

Rationalization A DEFENSE mechanism in which apparently sensible explanations are used to justify something unconsciously considered unacceptable.

Reaction formation A DEFENSE mechanism in which a person convinces himself that he feels exactly the opposite way from how he does feel. The most common form of reaction formation involves substituting exaggerated feelings of love for hate.

Reality PSYCHOANALYSIS has distinguished between "outer" or "objective" reality and "inner" or "psychic" reality. The former consists of consensually validated judgments of the nature of the external world. The latter, subjective, unique, and idiosyncratic to the individual, is determined by unconscious wishes, perceptions, memory traces, and fantasies about early experiences and OBJECT RELATIONS. In life, the two are in constant dialectic interaction; "psychic" reality may distort "external" perceptions and judgments, while too great a focus on "external" reality may constrict the imagination.

Reality principle A basic organizing principle of the mind that developmentally succeeds the pleasure principle in response to both growing cognitive capacities and experiences of frustration. The individual no longer seeks immediate satisfaction of needs and discharge of impulses, but interposes an assessment of the environment and actions directed toward the environment with the aim of effectively maximizing pleasure and minimizing unpleasure within the confines of the external reality of the situation.

Reality testing The process of distinguishing between inner thoughts and feelings and outer perceptions, or between the subjective and objective elements in the judgment of external reality.

Reconstruction In clinical PSYCHOANALYSIS, the process of elucidation and recollection of repressed experiences. Though once considered a central mechanism of the therapeutic effect of analysis, analysts have come to see its role as less important and have increasingly understood that it is PSYCHIC REALITY, rather than objective reality, that is retrieved in reconstruction.

Regression Change in psychological phenomena in a direction that is the reverse of its usual, progressive direction. Freud distinguished three forms of regression:

> **Topographic** Involvement of psychic energy (e.g., from unconscious to perceptual in dreams)
> **Structural** Reversion of portions of the tripartite STRUCTURE of the mind to earlier forms (e.g., regression from mature SUPEREGO function to primitive superego function)
> **Temporal** A reversion to modes of psychological functioning of an earlier time of life.

Regression in the service of the ego Forms of REGRESSION that, though they may be originally instituted for defensive purposes, lead to a return to a more innovative and adaptive mental function and organization.

Reparation (Klein) The idea that the GUILT experienced by the individual for his or her aggressive wishes toward his or her OBJECT may be ameliorated through efforts to repair the fantasied damage done by the aggressive impulses. It is associated with the attainment of the DEPRESSIVE POSITION.

Repetition compulsion A tendency to repeat patterns of behavior or to re-create situations that may be painful or self-destructive.

Repression The expulsion of unacceptable psychic content from consciousness. The psychic content is seemingly forgotten via a motivated unconscious action but is potentially retrievable for conscious consideration.

Resistance An unconsciously mobilized DEFENSE that arises in the course of psychoanalytic treatment. While such defenses may or may not be adaptive in everyday life, in psychoanalytic treatment they constitute an obstruction to the patient's and analyst's joint effort to uncover the patient's unconscious wishes and fantasies. The analysis of these resistances constitutes a major part of a psychoanalytic treatment.

Return of the repressed The reemergence into consciousness or preconsciousness of previously repressed ideas and AFFECTS. This may occur under circumstances of stress, leading to manifest ANXIETY, deregulation of affect, or the emergence or intensification of SYMPTOMS. In the context of psychoanalytic therapy, however, the return of the repressed may signal that the EGO may now be strong enough to resolve previously overwhelming, and therefore repressed, conflicts.

Reverie Used by Bion to refer to the mental state of a mother with her infant. It is a state in which she is filled with what she imagines to be her child's inner life, in the past, the present, and the future. This state, according to Bion, is the mother's tool for receiving and understanding the affective communications from her infant; in so doing, she is able to contain and modify her infant's intense affective life so that he can manage intense emotional states more capably. Some analysts use this model in analytic work as a way of thinking about how the analyst helps the patient deal with affect states that are difficult to manage.

Ritual A sequence of connected behaviors enacted in a specific context. Rituals have meanings that are both conscious and unconscious. A ritual can be either a normal form of expression or a SYMPTOM. When used as a symptom, a ritual is constructed so that it contains a compromise between unacceptable wishes and DEFENSES against those wishes.

Rorschach The "ink blot" test in which, by scoring the subject's responses to a set of 10 ambiguous forms on cards, inferences can be made about mental functioning and diagnosis, including psychological DEFENSES and major conflicts.

Role responsiveness As used by Sandler, refers to a COUNTERTRANSFERENCE response in the analyst in which he or she feels impelled to behave in a way so as to play out a role that the patient unconsciously has assigned to him or her.

Sadism The seeking of pleasure in the act or FANTASY of inflicting pain or humiliation on another. Also refers to a PARAPHILIA (perversion) in which conscious sexual excitement is found in inflicting pain or humiliation.

Schizoid This term has been used in different contexts with various meanings. Bleuler described some nonpsychotic personality types as schizoid because, as with schizophrenia, they showed a divorce between the mind's emotional and intellectual functions. More recently, the term *schizoid character* has come to encompass a broader group of individuals and connotes an individual who is withdrawn, derives a majority of gratification from a vivid FANTASY life, and may be suspicious of others while overestimating himself. Fairbairn, in his clinical descriptions of schizoid dynamics, referred to this broader group. Melanie Klein described schizoid DEFENSES, particular to the PARANOID-SCHIZOID POSITION, which include SPLITTING, PROJECTIVE IDENTIFICATION, and INTROJECTION.

Scopophilia Sexual pleasure derived from looking, often at another person's body or sexual organs. It is linked with its complementary COMPONENT INSTINCT, EXHIBITIONISM, and clinically the two often occur together in the same individual.

Screen memory A memory that is remembered with particular emotional intensity, often containing some prominent visual detail. Though such memories have a very real quality, their details are often inconsistent with the chronology of the memory. The elements of these memories are often SYMBOLS associatively linked to repressed aspects of the historical event to which the memories allude. In this way, they may function in a similar way to dreams.

Secondary gain The gratification from a SYMPTOM that derives from the use of that symptom to manipulate others or to obtain concrete benefit in the external world. It is distinguished from the PRIMARY GAIN of the symptom, which is the solution of intrapsychic conflict (see CONFLICT, INTRAPSYCHIC).

Secondary process A type of thinking characterized by rationality, order, and logic. It arises during development in accordance with the REALITY PRINCIPLE, which aims to replace HALLUCINATORY WISH FULFILLMENT with adaptations to REALITY. It is distinguished from PRIMARY PROCESS, a more primitive mode of mental activity associated with the PLEASURE PRINCIPLE. Ordinarily both processes contribute to mental life, although in different proportions at different times.

Secondary revision (or elaboration) The part of the DREAM WORK that reorganizes and links together the elements of the dream into a relatively coherent NARRATIVE.

Seduction theory Freud's early hypothesis that the TRAUMA of childhood sexual seduction by adults was the cause of hysterical SYMPTOMS. He later abandoned this theory as he came to realize that many of the accounts of seductions were fantasized rather than real, and to understand the importance of repressed fantasies in the genesis of neurosis. He never explicitly took the position that all such memories were fantasies, and certainly modern psychoanalysts recognize lasting psychological damage that can arise from childhood sexual abuse.

Self A psychic STRUCTURE consisting of the individual's subjective sense of "I," an AGENCY of the mind that is a center of initiative in relation to the external world, and the total individual (including both mind and body). Kohut emphasized the sense of continuity over time and cohesiveness in space as an important aspect of the self; in SELF PSYCHOLOGY, *the self* refers both to experience-near subjective aspects of the individual's mental life and to an abstract concept of a mental structure, whose vicissitudes are a central focus of clinical attention.

Self-actualization A course of action that results in the positive potentialities and special abilities of the individual finding expression in the external world, and the pleasurable subjective experience of the individual when he or she is able to successfully pursue such a course of action.

Self-cohesion The subjective experience of the SELF as whole, well-functioning, relatively internally consistent, relatively enduring over time, and not subject to serious disruption as a result of disappointments in the self or others.

Selfobject (Kohut) In SELF PSYCHOLOGY, the individual's experience of another person as functioning as part of the SELF or as necessary to fulfill a need of the self. The selfobject dimension of experience is usually unconscious but can be made conscious. It exists along a continuum from archaic to mature. Common selfobject needs include a person's need for affirmation and IDEALIZATION.

Selfobject transference (Kohut) The aspect of the patient's experience of the analyst in which the analyst functions as part of the patient's self. There are three major types of selfobject TRANSFERENCES:

Mirror transference The patient requires validating or affirming responses from the analyst. See MIRROR TRANSFERENCE.

Idealizing transference The patient requires merger with an admired analyst. See IDEALIZING TRANSFERENCE.

Twinship transference The patient requires merger with the analyst as a person who is similar to himself or herself. See TWINSHIP TRANSFERENCE.

Kohut believed that these transferences represented developmentally necessary experiences in the establishment of a stable and cohesive sense of SELF.

Self psychology (Kohut)   The psychoanalytic theory originated by Heinz Kohut. It places central importance on the sustained, empathic immersion in the patient's subjective experience and the vicissitudes of the SELFOBJECT TRANSFERENCE. In self psychology, Freud's tripartite model of ID, EGO, and SUPEREGO is seen as subordinate to the self-selfobject configurations.

Self representation   The individual's mental image of himself or herself. This REPRESENTATION is made up of experiences of internal stimuli, fantasies about the SELF that are elaborated in relation to OBJECTS, and internalized perceptions of the way in which others experience oneself.

Self-state dreams   In SELF PSYCHOLOGY, dreams in which the MANIFEST CONTENT reflects the current condition of the SELF and the SELFOBJECT TRANSFERENCE rather than the disguised fulfillment of a wish.

Separation anxiety   The child's fear of being physically separated from the mother. It is a fundamental anxiety of early childhood and is likely to accompany each developmental advance. It is common for separation anxiety to persist in some form into later childhood and even adulthood, manifesting as "homesickness" or ANXIETY associated with separation from any important OBJECT.

Separation-individuation (Mahler)   The process of "psychological birth" of the child in the first 3 years of life. Unlike biological birth, separation-individuation is a gradual INTRAPSYCHIC unfolding that begins with the "symbiotic dual unity" of the mother-infant dyad and moves through the following phases: differentiation, practicing, rapprochement, and "moving toward OBJECT CONSTANCY." The crowning achievement is the establishment of optimal "distancing from and INTROJECTION of the lost symbiotic mother."

Sexual identity   This broad term includes the experience of the SELF in four separate categories: biological sex; GENDER (composed of core gender identity and gender role identity); sexual behavior (actual and fantasied, including OBJECT choice and nature of activity); and reproduction (fantasies and behaviors). It is fully established after puberty, finding its expression in FANTASY and DESIRE in physical sexuality.

Shame   An AFFECT linked to a sense of wrongdoing in the presence of others, either in REALITY or in FANTASY.

Signal anxiety   An unconscious affective response to an anticipated danger situation. Signal anxiety mobilizes defensive activity so as to avert the conscious experience of ANXIETY; when unsuccessful, it may lead to panic states or to neurotic SYMPTOM formation.

Somatic compliance   The participation of the body in the expression of unconscious psychic conflict. It implies a readiness of specific organs or body parts to provide a somatic outlet for psychological processes either because of their unconscious meaning or because a constitutional weakness predisposes them to be used in this way.

Somatization   The use of the body to express psychological states.

Splitting   The separating of positive feelings and perceptions, either toward the SELF or toward others, from negative feelings and perceptions so that the self or OBJECT is seen as either "all good" or "all bad." Freud described it as a DEFENSE mechanism; Klein posited that it was a normal developmental stage in the perception of self and other, and only later mobilized as a defense.

Stimulus barrier   The psychological mechanism that protects the individual from excessive and overwhelming stimulation, internal or external.

Stranger anxiety   The reaction of the infant as he inspects the faces of individuals who are not the mother, with confidence of the availability of the mother. This reaction may range from curiosity and wonderment to marked ANXIETY. Its onset is generally at about 8 months of age, when the differentiating infant achieves sufficient INDIVIDUATION to recognize the mother and distinguish her from others.

Structural change   A change in the enduring patterns, or STRUCTURES, of an individual's mental life, resulting in changes in subjective experience and/or behavior. Structural change is an important goal of psychoanalytic treatment. Improved capacities to delay gratification, to regulate AFFECT and self-esteem, to tolerate painful feelings, to develop a more reasonable conscience, and to have more flexible expectations for the SELF and the ability to maintain self-esteem characterize structural change that may occur in a successful psychoanalytic treatment.

Structural theory   The theory, introduced by Freud in 1923, of the tripartite model of the mind consisting of three separate systems, the EGO, ID, and SUPEREGO. With the structural theory, Freud attempted to address problems not explained by his earlier theorizing referred to as his TOPOGRAPHIC THEORY, such as why DEFENSES against unconscious impulses were also unconscious, and the phenomenon of unconscious GUILT.

Structure   A grouping of mental processes that is enduring, changing only slowly over time, and that functions with some degree of AUTONOMY with respect to other mental processes. Freud divided the mental apparatus into three structures: the EGO, ID, and SUPEREGO. Other theorists have used the term to refer to enduring configurations that reflect experience with, and fantasies about, important others during development; this more general use of the term is the more common connotation for contemporary analysts.

Sublimation   A resolution of intrapsychic conflict (see CONFLICT, INTRAPSYCHIC) by changing the sexual or aggressive aim of an urge and finding a substitute gratification. The term differs from other resolutions (INHIBITIONS, SYMPTOMS, CHARACTER traits) in that it implies a constructive or socially admirable outcome that is satisfying and flexible.

Superego   One of three major agencies of the mind (along with ID and EGO) as described in Freud's STRUCTURAL THEORY. It is the seat of the individual's system of ideals and values, moral principles, PROHIBITIONS, and moral injunctions. It observes and evaluates the SELF and may either criticize, reproach, and punish, or praise and reward. It is thus an important modulator of self-esteem.

Supportive psychoanalytic psychotherapy   The form of psychotherapy based on psychoanalytic understanding and principles that seeks to support the patient's EGO by strengthening adaptive DEFENSES, modifying unhealthy defenses, improving REALITY TESTING, and using the therapist as an auxiliary ego or SUPEREGO. In contrast to PSYCHOANALYSIS and EXPRESSIVE PSYCHOANALYTIC THERAPY, supportive psychotherapy involves more direct focus on symptoms and other areas of immediate concern, with a greater tendency to avoid exploration of the TRANSFERENCE and unconscious themes. Also, the technical INTERVENTIONS are characterized by a greater emphasis on advice giving, with a deemphasis on INTERPRETATION.

Suppression The conscious process of "putting out of mind." It is the conscious counterpart of the unconscious process of REPRESSION.

Symbiotic phase (Mahler) The developmental phase, lasting from about 6 weeks to 1 year of age, that is the immediate forerunner of the SEPARATION-INDIVIDUATION PROCESS. In this phase, the infant's behavior suggests that he experiences the mother and himself as a unit, in which the mother is experienced as a need-satisfying extension of himself, and there is little affective differentiation between SELF and OBJECT.

Symbol A thing that is used to stand for, or represent, something other than itself. The UNCONSCIOUS makes use of symbols as a way of simultaneously expressing and concealing unconscious thoughts. The connection between the symbol and its referent is outside of conscious awareness. This process plays an important part in dreams and in the formation of some psychological SYMPTOMS.

Symbolic equation A mental process, described by Segal, that is a forerunner of SYMBOLIZATION proper. In this process, the mind chooses a SYMBOL for an OBJECT but treats it as if it is literally and concretely the object. For example, a patient might experience the analyst's use of the word "attack" as an actual physical assault on him, or be fearful of being seen smoking a cigarette because he would experience himself as actually performing fellatio.

Symbolization The unconscious process by which one OBJECT or concept comes to represent another object or concept. The associative link may be sensory (e.g., visual, auditory), temporal (i.e., relating to time), or concrete (i.e., similar objects such as a friend's brother substituting for one's own brother). Though some SYMBOLS may be universal, symbols always have personal meanings that are unique to the individual.

Symptom An EGO-DYSTONIC manifestation of mental life that is the result of an unconscious attempt to solve an intrapsychic conflict (see CONFLICT, INTRAPSYCHIC). Examples are obsessional thoughts, COMPULSIONS, slips of the tongue, PHOBIAS, hysterical paralysis, INHIBITIONS, and ego-dystonic CHARACTER traits.

Termination phase The concluding period of an analysis, subsequent to the decision that the objectives for which treatment was undertaken have been substantially achieved. From that point onward until the appointed final day, there is enhanced focus on the imminent separation of patient and analyst, leading to reverberations in emotion and FANTASY that revisit the important themes that emerged in the analysis. The prospect of termination may stir symptomatic recurrences that are usually brief.

Therapeutic alliance The sense of constructive collaboration between the patient and the analyst as they work together on the patient's problems. Some research suggests that this element is a predictor of successful treatment. Some differentiate between a TRANSFERENCE, which tends to be irrational, and the therapeutic alliance, which is said to be more real. Others believe that this state is just an aspect of a positive transference.

Topographic theory Freud's early effort to classify mental functioning and contents in terms of their relationship to consciousness. A mental event, such as a wish, idea, or feeling, is termed *unconscious* when it exists outside of conscious awareness and cannot be made conscious via focal attention, and *preconscious* when such attention leads to conscious awareness. The STRUCTURAL THEORY, which divided the mind into ID, EGO, and SUPEREGO, expanded on rather than replaced the topographic theory.

Training analysis The personal analysis that is required of prospective analysts. The training analysis is intended to help prospective analysts become aware of their own psychological processes and to master unconscious conflicts that would otherwise lead to interference with participation in the analytic treatment as an analyst.

Transference In clinical PSYCHOANALYSIS, the patient's emotional experience of and fantasies about the analyst, which, though they may be based in part on actual perceptions of the analyst, recapitulate experiences with and fantasies about important OBJECTS in the patient's childhood.

Transference neurosis In clinical PSYCHOANALYSIS, the analysand's reexperiencing of his or her characteristic psychic conflicts and modes of DEFENSE, finding their expression in fantasies about the analyst. These fantasies recapitulate experiences with and fantasies about important OBJECTS in the patient's childhood.

Transitional object An inanimate OBJECT (e.g., a blanket or teddy bear), existing in REALITY and highly invested with FANTASY, that is used for the purposes of emotional growth. It preserves the illusion of the comforting, soothing mother when the mother is not available, while also promoting AUTONOMY, since the transitional object is under the child's control.

Transitional phenomenon A process, relationship, or activity (as opposed to an inanimate OBJECT) used as a symbolic REPRESENTATION of an important object (usually the mother) for the purposes of counteracting painful feelings in relation to that object, particularly related to the object's absence. These processes incorporate aspects of both FANTASY and REALITY; they constitute the basis of play and creativity.

Transmuting internalization (Kohut) In SELF PSYCHOLOGY, the process of internal STRUCTURE building through the INTERNALIZATION of SELFOBJECT functions originally provided by the OBJECT. Kohut believed this occurred as a result of nontraumatic empathic failures on the part of the selfobject. The internalization of the analyst's (or parent's) mirroring function enables the patient to regulate affective experience and to more effectively manage disappointment and rage.

Trauma An experience in which external events overwhelm the capacity of the EGO to process and manage them, evoking intense feelings of helplessness. The meaning of the event, not its REALITY characteristics, defines it as traumatic.

True self An experience of the SELF that emerges in response to one's own needs and wishes (as opposed to the FALSE SELF experience, which emerges in response to another's needs, expectations, and demands).

Turning against the self A DEFENSE in which an aggressive impulse is redirected from another to the SELF. It is commonly found in masochistic individuals.

Twinship transference In SELF PSYCHOLOGY, that aspect of a patient's TRANSFERENCE in which the patient experiences the analyst as just like himself or herself and wishes for an experience of merger or oneness with the analyst as "twin."

Uncanny The quality of an experience of a mysterious or magical type, not able to be explained scientifically, but for which Freud believed a psychoanalytic explanation was possible. Premonitions and states of dejá vu are common examples.

Unconscious   Refers to mental contents that are beyond the reach of conscious thinking. For Freud, dreams and parapraxes provided evidence of the existence of the unconscious and its impact on mental life. He distinguished between the DYNAMIC UNCONSCIOUS, meaning the sum of all repressed mental contents, and the system Unconscious, which is the seat of the DRIVES, is governed by the PLEASURE PRINCIPLE, and operates according to the logic of PRIMARY PROCESS thinking. In his later writings, the term was used in a primarily descriptive way: most DEFENSES and SUPEREGO conflicts, for example, operate on an unconscious level but are not necessarily part of either the system Unconscious or the dynamic unconscious. In contemporary PSYCHOANALYSIS, nonverbal enactments in the analytic setting are viewed as another manifestation of unconscious themes.

Unconscious fantasy   NARRATIVES about the SELF in relation to others that are either consciously elaborated and then repressed, or elaborated outside of conscious awareness. They represent compromises between DRIVES or wishes and the DEFENSES against them, and are constituted as well by the individual's perception of himself or herself in relation to others. The fantasies form a template for behavior in the real world. When these fantasies are brought to consciousness through analysis, their power as motivators of maladaptive behavior is lessened.

Undoing   A DEFENSE mechanism in which unacceptable unconscious wishes, feelings, and impulses are disguised by substituting behavior that appears to be their opposite.

Vertical split   In SELF PSYCHOLOGY, a process by which conscious but unwanted qualities of SELF are warded off, as by an impenetrable wall, and separated from conscious desirable self elements. The DEFENSES associated with vertical split are DENIAL, DISSOCIATION, and DISAVOWAL.

Whole object (Klein)   The experience of the OBJECT as one object comprising both good and bad characteristics, toward whom both love and hatred may be felt. It is characteristic of the DEPRESSIVE POSITION.

Working alliance   The spoken or unspoken agreement between patient and analyst to work toward understanding and recovery. It is differentiated from the THERAPEUTIC ALLIANCE in that the working alliance implies an understanding of how the work of analysis proceeds, and the patient's voluntary adherence to his or her role as analysand and to the the rules, conventions, and methods of the analysis.

Working-through   A phase of clinical PSYCHOANALYSIS during which the dynamics of conflict are repeatedly revisited in experiences of the present, past, and the TRANSFERENCE. It aims at transforming intellectual understanding into emotional knowledge; unconscious conflicts are resolved or replaced by more adaptive compromises, leading to an increase in adaptive functioning and a decrease in SYMPTOMS.

Name Index

Page numbers in *italics* indicate chapters in this volume.

Abadi, Mauricio, 440
Abend, Sander M., 222–223, 235, *375–384*
Aberastury, Arminda, 436, 437
Ablon, J. S., 323, 329
Abraham, Karl, 46, 247, 381, 383, 453
Abrams, S., 119, 230
Ackerman, Nathan, 437
Ackerman, S. J., 323, 325, 329, 330
Adler, Alfred, 135, 149, 282, 381, 384, 390, 395
Agorio, Rodolfo, 446
Aguayo, J., 408
Ainsworth, Mary, 150, 161, 163, 469–470
Akhtar, Salman, 9, 17, *39–51*
Albee, Edward, 8–9
Albers, Josef, 507
Alexander, Franz, 222, 302, 383, 391, 394, 395, 396, 397, 399, 426
Allison, George, 400
Althusser, Louis, 428
Alvarez, A., 207
Amacher, Peter, 458–459
Anthony, A., 483
Anzieu, Didier, 108, 426, 430, 527
Aquinas, Thomas, 287
Arafat, Yasser, 529
Araújo, Jaime, 445
Aristotle, 287, 514
Arlow, Jacob, 24, 124, 232, 236, 285, 527
Aron, Lewis, 101, 109, 206, 210, 211, 494
Atwood, G., 123, 182
Auden, W. H., 458
Augustine, 287
Aulagnier, Piera, 428, 432, 440

Bachrach, H. M., 307, 308
Bahia, Alcyon, 442
Bakermans-Kranenburg, M., 165
Balint, Michael, 135, 136, 195, 204, 207, 208, 413
Bandura, A., 464
Baranger, Madeleine, 437, 438, 440, 444, 446, 448

Baranger, Willy, 437, 438, 440, 444, 446, 448
Barber, J., 321, 325
Bargh, J., 542
Barke, C., 472
Barkham, M., 471
Barnett, L., 472
Barron, J. W., 465
Bassin, D., 101, 102, 107
Bateson, Gregory, 483
Beebe, B., 339
Behrends, R., 219
Benedek, Tereza, 123, 441
Benedict, Ruth, 396, 398, 483, 484
Benjamin, Jessica, 18, 45, 94, 99, 101, 109, 138, 211, 399, 485
Berenstein, Isidoro, 440, 444
Beres, D., 124
Berezin, Martin, 395
Bergman, A., 339, 342, 352
Bergmann, Martin S., *241–252*
Berkoff, Steven, 498
Berman, Emanuel, *491–499*
Bernard, Viola, 437
Bernardi, R., 320, 446
Bernfeld, Siegfried, 394, 397
Bernheim, Hippolyte, 377, 378, 387, 423
Bernstein, D., 45, 98
Bettelheim, Bruno, 454–455
Bibring, Edward, 235
Bibring, Grete, 251
Biddle, Sidney, 396
Binder, J. L., 473
Binger, Carl, 394, 396
Binswanger, Ludwig, 381
Bion, Wilfred R., 62, 66, 135, 136, 168, 178, 179, 206, 208, 220, 279, 366, 397, 402, 409, 411, 413, 417, 432, 437, 439
Bird, B., 205
Bisiach, E., 541
Blagys, M. D., 323, 325, 329, 330
Blatt, Sidney, 165, 219
Blecher, Jose, 440

Blechner, M., 209, 210
Blehar, M. E., 469–470
Bleiberg, Efrain, *173–183*
Bleuler, Eugen, 381, 389, 459
Bliwise, N. G., 473
Blos, Peter, 43, 440
Bluestone, H., 255
Blum, Harold, 242, 364
Boas, Franz, 479, 481
Boesky, D., 230, 232
Bohleber, Werner, 364
Bollas, Christopher, 105, 208, 284, 416, 508–509
Bonaparte, Marie, 423, 482, 495
Bond, J. A., 468
Bonge, D., 323
Bookwala, J. F., 471
Bornstein, Berta, 392
Bornstein, R. F., 465, 473
Boston Change Process Study Group, 85, 86, 88, 89, 220, 221
Bourdieu, Pierre, 484
Bowlby, John, 9, 119, 122, 138–139, 150, 159, 160–162, 163, 167, 182, 191, 337, 338, 339, 402, 408, 413, 457, 458, 468–469, 469, 485
Boyer, Bryce, 437, 484
Brakel, L. A. W., 468
Brandchaft, B., 123
Brazelton, T. Berry, 341
Breen, D., 101
Brenner, Charles, 232, 250, 285, 292
Bretano, Franz, 376
Bretherton, I., 162
Breton, André, 423
Breuer, Josef, 108, 194, 377
Briehl, Marie, 392, 397
Brierley, Marjorie, 408
Briggs, Jean, 487
Brill, A. A., 381, 388, 390, 391, 392
Britton, R., 193, 206
Bromberg, P. M., 138, 210, 211
Bronfman, E., 165
Brown, Jason, 539
Brücke, Ernst, 376, 459

Bruschweiler-Stern, N., 85
Bucci, Wilma, 119, *317–330*
Burke, Mark, 442
Burlingham, Dorothy, 337
Burnham, J. C., 390
Burrow, Trigant, 389
Burton, R. V., 483
Busch, F., 234
Butler, J., 94, 102, 106
Butler, Thomas, 531
Buxbaum, Edith, 394

Cabaniss, Deborah L., *255–265*
Cabernite, Leão, 443
Cameron, Ewen, 398
Canestri, Jorge, 364, 418
Cárcamo, Celes, 435, 436
Carranza, L. V., 471
Carroll, Lewis, 493
Carter, Jimmy, 526, 529
Casement, P., 221, 416
Cassidy, J., 470
Cath, S. H., 46
Cesio, Fidias, 439, 440
Chabert, Catherine, 431
Charcot, Jean-Martin, 376–377, 387,
    423
Chartrand, T., 542
Chasseguet-Smirgel, Janine, 96, 97, 440,
    444, 527
Chentrier, André, 398
Chodorow, Nancy, 18, 45, 94, 96, 99,
    101, 107, 485, 486
Chomsky, Noam, 485, 486
Chused, Judith, 274, 294
Cixous, H., 497
Claparede, Edouard, 466
Clarkin, J. F., 181
Coates, S., 101, 105
Cobb, Stanley, 398, 399
Cohen, Robert A., 399
Colarusso, C. A., 46
Cole, Thomas, 501–502
Colombo, Daria, *375–384*
Conway, Martin, 541, 542
Cooper, A. M., 11, 255, 379, 381, 384
Cooper, S. H., 322
Copernicus, 15
Corbett, K., 99, 100, 104–105
Coriat, Isador, 302, 389, 390, 391, 399
Craik, K., 161
Cranefield, Paul, 458
Crapanzano, Vincent, 487
Crews, Frederick, 457
Crisanto, Carlos, 447
Crits-Christoph, P., 325

Crittenden, P. M., 163, 166, 167
Cryanowski, J. M., 471
Cue, K. L., 472
Curtis, Homer, 400
Curtis, W. J., 134

Dahl, H., 310, 321, 322, 323, 326
Dahlheim, Luiz, 442
Dalheim, Luis Guimaraes, 437
Dalrymple, Leolia, 391
Damasio, Antonio, 139, 538, 544
Daniels, George, 396, 398
Darwin, Charles, 15, 105, 380, 480, 481,
    540
Davanzo, Hernán, 446
David, Christian, 426
Davidson, Donald, 519
Davies, J. M., 109, 211
Debbane, E. G., 324
Debbink, N. L., 251
de Beauvoir, Simone, 94
deCarufel, F. L., 324
de la Vega, Garcilaso, 447
de Leon de Bernardi, B., 207
Delgado, Honorio, 447
De Marneffe, D., 100
de Mijolla, A., 368
de M'uzan, Michel, 426
Denis, Paul, 364
Denktash, Rauf, 529
Dennis, Wayne, 337
de Oliveira, Walderedo, 437
Derrida, Jacques, 427, 497
Descartes, René, 361
Deutsch, Felix, 243, 393, 394,
    398
Deutsch, Helene, 383, 393
Devereux, George, 480, 484
Dewey, John, 505
Diatkine, René, 427
Dimen, Muriel, *93–110*
Dinnerstein, D., 94
Dollard, J., 464
Dolto, Françoise, 425
Dooley, Lucile, 389, 390
Doolittle, Hilda (H.D.), 203, 243–244
Dostoyevsky, Fyodor, 484, 492
Dozier, Mary, 165, 472
Drake, R., 322
Dreher, Anna Ursula, *361–371*
Drews, S., 364
Drummond de Andrade, Carlos, 447
Dunbar, Flanders, 394, 398
Dundes, Alan, 487
Dunn, J., 77
Durkeim, Emile, 479

Eagle, Morris, 166, 167, 457–458, 474, 508
Eames, V., 471–472
Eckhardt, Marianne, 395
Edelman, G. M., 85
Edes, Robert, 387
Eells, T., 321, 322
Ehrenberg, D. B., 209, 210, 211
Eifermann, R., 498
Einstein, Albert, 93, 527
Eissler, Kurt, 244, 393
Eissler, Ruth, 251
Eitingon, Max, 381, 383
Eizirik, Cláudio Laks, *435–448*
Eldred, S. H., 304
Elise, D., 99, 102
Ellenberger, Henri, 380, 383, 384, 455
Elliott, R., 324
Ellis, Havelock, 387
Emde, Robert N., *117–126*, 133, 321
Emerson, L. E., 389, 390
Engel, George, 394, 399
Erdelyi, M. H., 464
Erikson, Erik, 22–23, 46, 58, 59, 120,
    124, 126, 133, 150, 168, 282, 392,
    394, 398, 403, 457, 484, 494, 529
Erle, J. B., 305
Escalona, Sibylle, 339, 399
Esman, Aron, 456, 494
Etchegoyen, Horácio, 439, 440, 444
Ewers, Heinz, 492
Exner, Sigmund, 459
Ey, Henry, 430, 437
Eysenck, H. J., 465

Faimberg, H., 193
Fain, Michel, 426
Fairbairn, W. Ronald D., 32, 50, 58, 59,
    60, 62–63, 103, 104, 136, 179, 226,
    397, 408, 413
Fast, I., 101
Favez-Boutonier, Juliette, 425
Fechner, Gustav, 459
Feder, Luis, 445
Federn, Paul, 242, 381, 391
Feldman, F., 303
Feldman, M., 62, 206, 418
Felman, Shoshana, 493, 495–496
Fempner, Salomé, 441
Fenichel, Otto, 204, 245, 247, 302, 397,
    441, 528
Ferenczi, Sandor, 77, 108, 135, 202–203,
    207, 208, 209, 210, 219, 222, 225,
    246, 249, 381, 383, 388, 391, 392,
    408, 409, 481, 494, 497
Ferro, Antonio, 279
Feske, U., 471

Feuerbach, Ludwig, 376
Fine, B. D., 368
Fischer, N., 48
Fiske, John, 394
Fleigel, Z. O., 96
Fleming, J., 123, 397
Fliess, Wilhelm, 378, 379, 424, 491, 492
Fonagy, Peter, 58, 119, *131–140*, 166, 167–168, 208, 224–225, 246, 269, 277, 301, 321, 364, 370, 419, 444, 465, 469, 470, 471, 472
Forrester, John, 459
Forsyth, Dan, 486
Fosshage, J., 210
Foucault, Michel, 109, 283
Foutopoulou, Katerina, 542
Fraiberg, Selma, 126, 166
Frank, Jerome, 537
Frazer, James G., 480, 481
Freedman, N., 326
Freidman, Stanford, 243
Freidman, Susan, 243
Freud, Anna, 10, 24, 28, 29, 120, 134, 135, 150, 162, 167, 174, 176, 196, 234, 236, 274, 276, 277, 335, 337, 339, 379, 382, 383, 392, 393, 394, 399, 412, 413, 416, 494, 502
Freud, Sigmund, 3–18, 21–35, 40, 43, 47, 48, 49, 59, 84, 93, 95–100, 102–105, 109–110, 119–120, 126, 131–133, 135, 149, 159, 168, 173–174, 175, 189–191, 193, 194–195, 201–204, 205, 217–219, 222, 223, 225, 226, 232, 233–234, 241–251, 281–288, 290, 291, 317, 318, 328, 329, 352, 362, 364, 366, 367, 368, 375–384, 387, 389, 390, 391, 393, 402, 403, 408, 409, 410, 412, 413, 423, 424, 431, 435, 444, 447, 453–454, 458–459, 463–464, 465, 479, 480, 481, 482, 484, 486, 491–493, 494, 497, 502, 503–505, 506, 508, 509, 520, 522, 525, 526–527, 531, 535–537, 540, 541, 542, 543–544
Friedman, L., 133, 234
Fries, Margaret, 394
Frink, H. W., 391
Fromm, Erich, 209, 282, 395, 396
Fromm-Reichmann, Frieda, 60, 65, 393–394, 399
Frosch, J., 48
Furman, E., 42

Gabbard, Glen O., 178, 206, 211–212, 220, 223, 224, 231, 232, 267, 292, 293, 294, 319

Gagnon, J., 100
Galatzer-Levy, R., 307, 308
Gallagher, D., 325
Ganzarain, Ramón, 446
Garcia, Antonio, 445
Gardiner, Muriel, 391
Gardner, M. Robert, 397
Garfield, R., 45
Garma, Angel, 436, 442, 444, 446, 448
Garma, Elizabeth, 437
Gaskill, Herbert, 400
Gaston, L., 325
Gay, Peter, 376, 455
Gazzaniga, M. S., 541
Geahchan, Dominique, 427
Gedo, J. E., 317
Geertz, Clifford, 102
Gehring, George, 387, 394
Gergely, G., 269
Gerö, Georg, 442
Gesell, Arnold, 394
Ghent, E., 211
Gifford, Sanford, *387–403*
Gill, Merton, 150, 210, 234, 321, 496
Gillespie, W., 408
Gilman, Sander, 95
Gilmore, David, 487
Gitelson, Frances, 437
Gitelson, M., 121
Glas de Langer, Marie, 436
Glover, Edward, 217–219, 225, 246, 247, 250, 303, 413
Goethe, Johann Wolfgang von, 491
Goldberg, D. A., 305
Goldner, Virginia, *93–110*
González, Avelino, 437
Goodman, S., 119
Gorbachev, Mikhail, 529
Gorer, Geoffrey, 484
Göring, Erna, 443
Gosliner, B. J., 43
Goya, Francisco, 506, 507
Graf, Max, 381
Graff-Radford, Neill, 543
Granoff, Wladimir, 426
Gray, Paul, 205, 234
Green, André, 78, 79, 102, 242, 249, 366, 407, 432, 440, 444
Greenacre, Phyllis, 175, 456, 507, 508
Greenberg, H. R., 59, 60, 65, 66
Greenberg, J. R., 236
Greenberg, Jay, 212, *217–226*
Greenson, Ralph, 204, 212, 397
Greenspan, Stanley I., *335–355*
Greenwald, A. G., 464
Gregor, Thomas, 487

Gribinski, Michel, 431
Grinberg, León, 437
Grinker, Roy, 395, 399
Grinstein, A., 491
Groddeck, Georg, 394
Grossmann, K., 469
Grotjahn, Martin, 393, 394, 399, 493
Grotstein, James, 291
Guntrip, H., 60, 63, 135, 179, 226

Hadley, Ernest, 392
Haith, Marshall, 121
Hale, N. G., Jr., 390
Hall, Clark, 457
Hall, G. Stanley, 387, 388, 389, 394
Halton, A., 15
Hamilton, C., 469, 470
Hamilton, Victoria, 458
Hardy, G. E., 471
Hargreaves, Ronald, 457
Harlow, Harry, 457–458
Harris, Adrienne, 95, 101, *201–213*
Hartmann, Heinz, 6, 10, 12, 18, 50, 66, 118, 120, 133, 224, 282, 283, 383, 393, 394, 403, 424, 494, 502
Haynal, A., 79
Haynal-Reymond, V., 79
Hazen, N., 165
H.D. (Hilda Doolittle), 203, 243–244
Healy, William, 391
Heimann, Paula, 195, 207, 208, 221, 416, 418, 437, 496
Heinicke, Christoph, 160
Heller, Hugo, 381
Heller, M., 79
Hendrick, Ives, 10, 282, 391, 393, 396, 458
Henry, W. P., 310
Hernández, Max, 447
Herrmann, Fábio, 444
Herzog, J., 44
Hesse, E., 166
Hill, C., 324
Hilsenroth, M. J., 325, 329, 330
Hinde, Robert, 457, 458
Hinkle, Beatrice, 390
Hinz, H., 418
Hirsch, I., 209, 210
Hitler, Adolf, 393
Hoch, Paul, 437
Hoffman, Irwin, 138, 211, 212, 221, 282, 321
Hoffmann, E. T. A., 492
Holland, N. N., 494, 498
Holt, R., 455
Horney, Karen, 96, 98, 204, 209, 383, 395–396, 398

Horowitz, Donald, 531
Horowitz, Mardi J., 119, 321, 322, 325
Hughlings Jackson, John, 191
Hurvich, M., 326
Hurwitz, Rosetta, 392
Hussein, Saddam, 530
Husserl, Edmund, 82
Huxley, Julian, 457
Hyman, H., 302

Inderbitzen, L. B., 236
Ingham, John, 486
Ingres, Jean, 506
Inhelder, Barbel, 457
Irigaray, L., 99
Isaacs, Susan, 408
Isham, Mary, 390
Iverson, Margaret, 502

Jacobovitz, D., 165
Jacobs, T., 205–206
Jacobson, D., 492–493
Jacobson, Edith, 6, 50, 58, 59, 60, 66,
    120, 133, 135, 443
James, Henry, 495
James, William, 387, 388, 463–464
Janet, Pierre, 377, 387
Jelliffe, Smith Ely, 387, 389, 394, 537
Jessner, Lucie, 393
Joffe, W. G., 416
Johnson, Allen, 486
Johnson, M., 268
Johnson, Samuel, 400
Jones, E. E., 323, 329, 330
Jones, Enrico, 312
Jones, Ernest, 96, 98, 244, 282, 285, 302,
    381–382, 388, 389, 392, 393, 398,
    408, 412, 413, 436, 441, 442, 443,
    459, 481, 492
Joseph, Betty, 194, 206, 207, 411, 412,
    416, 417, 444
Jung, Carl, 149, 219, 366, 381, 384, 388,
    389, 390, 395, 454, 459, 487
Jurist, E. L., 269

Kächele, H., 301, 310, 321
Kafka, Franz, 498
Kaftal, E., 99
Kamm, Bernard, 394
Kandel, Eric, 473–474, 539, 540
Kant, Immanuel, 506, 519
Kantrowitz, Judith, 307, 317, 318, 319,
    320, 363
Kaplan, N., 470
Kaplan-Solms, Karen, 539, 540
Karazić, Radovan, 530

Kardiner, Abram, 396, 398, 482–483
Karpman, Ben, 392
Katz, A. L., 307
Kaufman, M. Ralph, 391, 394, 395, 398
Kemper, Katrin, 442, 443
Kemper, Werner, 442–443
Kempf, Edward J., 389, 399
Kenworthy, Marion, 390
Kernberg, Otto F., 8, 15, 50, 57–74, 110,
    137–138, 174, 181–182, 312, 339,
    349, 402, 440, 444, 446, 527
Kernberg, Paulina, 181, 446
Kerr, John, *453–460*
Kessel, L., 302
Kessler, S., 96
Kestenberg, J., 98
Kilmann, P. R., 471
King, Pearl, 412
Kirsner, Douglas, 397
Kizer, Manuel, 445
Klein, G. S., 10, 16, 29–30, 150
Klein, Melanie, 50, 58, 59, 60, 61–62,
    64, 96, 106, 135, 136, 178–179, 190,
    192, 195, 196, 206, 246–247, 274,
    366, 382, 397, 399, 402, 408–413,
    414, 415, 417, 418, 437, 439, 444,
    468, 495, 503
Kluckhohn, Clyde, 398, 484
Kluckhohn, Florence, 398
Kluckhohn, R., 483
Knapp, P. H., 304
Knight, Robert P., 303, 394, 399, 403
Koch, Adelheid Lucy, 440, 441
Kohut, Heinz, 6, 12, 17, 32, 60, 65, 123,
    124, 137, 180, 241, 282, 283, 293,
    339, 349, 366, 368, 394, 402, 440, 495
Koolhaas, Gilberto, 446
Korsgaard, Christine, 519
Koslowski, B., 341
Kracke, Waud, 487
Kramer, Selma, 119
Krause, R., 301, 321
Kravitz, Henry, 398
Kris, Ernst, 8, 239, 244, 368, 393, 394,
    399, 494, 502, 505–507
Kris, Marianne, 399
Kristeva, Julia, 109, 485, 502
Kroeber, Alfred, 398
Krutch, Joseph Wood, 493
Kuhn, Thomas, 363, 403

LaBarre, Weston, 484, 486
Lacan, Jacques, 60, 95, 97, 107–108,
    110, 196, 209, 249, 366, 402, 424–
    426, 427–429, 430, 431, 432, 440,
    444, 445, 446, 495

Laforgue, René, 423
Lagache, Daniel, 424, 425, 426, 430,
    431, 442
Laing, R. D., 498
Lakoff, G., 268
Langer, Susanne, 505
Langer, Walter, 392
Laplanche, Jean, 103, 109, 110, 368,
    426, 430–431, 444
Lasky, R. H., 326
Laswell, Harold, 526
Laughlin, J. E., 471
Lax, R., 45
Layton, L. B., 106
Lear, Jonathan, *513–522*
Leavy, Barbara Fass, 455
Lebovici, Serge, 427, 437
Leclaire, Serge, 430, 440
LeDoux, Joseph, 538, 541–542
Leigh, T., 470, 471
Lemmertz, José, 444
Lester, E. P., 294
Levenson, Edgar, 209, 210, 224
Levin, Fred, 538
Levin, Kenneth, 455
Levin, S., 304, 394
Lévi-Strauss, Claude, 485
Levy, A. T., 236
Levy, Kenneth N., *463–474*
Lewes, K., 98
Lewicki, P., 466–467
Lewin, Bertram, 396, 403
Lewis, J. M., 138
Liberman, David, 440, 444, 448
Libet, B., 542
Lichtenberg, J. D., 10, 17
Lieberman, Alicia, 166
Limentani, Adam, 437
Lin, Maya, 502
Lins de Almeida, José, 444
Linton, Ralph, 396, 398, 483
Lipton, Samuel, 203, 244
Little, Margaret, 207, 208, 496
Lizarazo, Arturo, 447
Lloyd, A., 486
Lobo, Amilcar, 443
Loewald, Hans, 4, 5, 17, 43, 59, 121,
    124, 125, 133, 205, 220, 232, 236,
    247
Loewenberg, Peter, 397
Loewenstein, Rudolph, 235, 393, 424
Lopez-Ballesteros, Luis, 447
Lorenz, Konrad, 9, 457, 460
Luborsky, L., 119, 321, 322, 325, 329,
    365
Lyons-Ruth, Karlen, 85, 165, 166, 167

Macalpine, Ida, 204, 437
MacIntyre, Alasdair, 289–290, 368
Mack Brunswick, Ruth, 242, 243, 251
MacLeod, Alastair, 398
Macnaughton, Dorothy, 398
Madow, Leo, 396
Maeder, LeRoy, 396
Maenchen, Anna, 394
Magritte, René, 506
Mahler, Margaret, 6, 43, 58, 59, 60, 66, 67, 80, 120, 134, 135, 150, 175, 176–178, 249, 335, 339, 342, 352, 363, 393, 440, 495, 503, 509
Mahony, P., 497
Mailloux, Noel, 398
Main, Mary, 166, 341, 469, 470
Major, René, 427
Malinowski, Bronislaw, 481, 485
Mannoni, Octave, 201, 502
Marcondes, Durval, 441
Marcovitz, Eli, 437
Marcus, Eric R., 229–239
Marcus, Steven, 95, 497
Margolin, Sydney, 394, 398
Marmor, Judd, 396
Maroda, K., 210, 211
Marti, Pierre, 426, 440
Martins, Cyro, 444
Martins, Mario Alvarez, 440, 442, 444
Martins, Zaira, 442, 444
Marucco, Norberto, 444
Masling, J. M., 465, 473
Masson, J. M., 379
Masten, A. S., 134
Masterson, J. F., 135, 177
Matte Blanco, Ignácio, 446, 448
Mayer, E. L., 98
Mayes, Linda C., 147–155
McCarter, R. H., 304
McDevitt, J. B., 15
McDougall, J., 106, 109, 407
McLaughlin, F., 251
McLaughlin, J., 138
Mead, Margaret, 398, 457, 483
Mechnikov, Elie, 459
Meissner, W. W., 21–36
Meltzer, Donald, 62, 106, 437
Meltzoff, A. N., 81
Menninger, Karl, 248
Menninger, William, 395
Mergenthaler, E., 323, 324
Merleau-Ponty, Maurice, 108, 431
Merrick, S., 470
Meyer, Adolf, 387, 388, 389, 390
Meyer, B., 471
Meyer, J. K., 251

Mezan, Renato, 444
Michaels, J. J., 394
Mill, J. S., 287
Miller, Jacques-Alain, 427, 428
Miller, N., 321, 464
Millet, John A. P., 396, 399
Milner, Marion, 413, 503
Milosević, Slobodan, 530
Mirsky, Arthur, 437
Mitchell, Juliet, 485
Mitchell, S., 22, 59, 60, 65, 66, 138, 209, 210
Mitscherlich, Alexander, 528
Modell, A., 10, 65, 135
Mom, Jorge, 438, 440
Mondrian, Piet, 455–456, 507
Money, John, 94, 100
Money Kyrle, Roger, 408, 415
Moore, B. E., 368
Moore, M. K, 81
Moran, G. S., 135
Moran, Richard, 519
Morgan, A., 85
Morrison, Amy, 294
Mosheim, R., 471
Müller-Braunschweig, Carl, 442
Münsterberg, Hugo, 387
Murphy, Gardner, 399
Murphy, Lois, 150
Murphy, Robert, 487
Murphy, Ruth, 399
Murray, John, 391, 395
Mushatt, Cecil, 398

Nacht, Sacha, 424
Nadel, J., 83
Nagel, Thomas, 519
Nahum, J., 85
Nathansohn, Amalia, 376
Navarro, Allende, 446
Nemiah, J. C., 426
Nesse, Randolph, 486
Nietzsche, Friedrich, 459, 522
Noble, Douglas, 398
Normand, W., 255

Oberndorf, Clarence, 390, 391, 394, 396
Obeyesekere, Gananath, 486, 487
Ogden, T., 123, 138, 206, 208
Oliveira, Walderedo, 442
O'Malley, Mary, 389
Orlan, 505
Ornstein, A., 232
Ornstein, P. H., 232
Orr, D. W., 204, 209
O'Shaughnessy, E., 193, 206

Ostow, Mortimer, 537
Ovesey, L., 100

Pacella, B., 48
Panksepp, Jaak, 538, 543, 544
Paolitto, F., 307
Parens, H., 15
Parkin, Alan, 398
Parsons, E., 165
Parsons, Talcott, 398
Paul, Robert A., 479–488
Payne, Sylvia, 408
Peck, Martin, 391, 393
Peirce, C. S., 361
Peña, Saul, 447
Perestrello, Danilo, 442
Perestrello, Marialzira, 442
Pérez Pastorini, Valentín, 446
Perrier, François, 428
Perron, R., 318, 319
Perry, J. C., 322
Person, Ethel, 16, 18, 85, 100, 102
Peterfreund, E., 175
Pfeffer, Arnold, 305–306, 538–539
Piaget, Jean, 122, 149, 340, 457
Picasso, Pablo, 506
Pichon Rivière, Enrique, 436
Pilkonis, P. A., 471
Pine, Fred, 3–18, 223, 339, 342, 352
Piper, W. E., 324
Pizer, S., 210
Plata Mujica, Carlos, 447
Plato, 514, 516, 517, 518, 520
Poe, Edgar Allan, 492, 495
Poetzl, O., 466
Pollack, S. S., 99
Pollen, William, 399
Pollock, George, 400
Pontalis, Jean-Bertrand, 103, 110, 368, 426, 430, 431
Prados, Miguel, 398
Pratt, Joseph, 399
Price-Williams, Douglass, 486
Prince, Morton, 387, 388, 389
Prince Lazar of Serbia, 530–531
Proietti, J. M., 471
Pruett, K., 44
Prunes, Celestino, 444
Puget, Janine, 440
Pulos, S. M., 323, 329, 330
Pulver, S. E., 368
Putnam, Irmarita, 391
Putnam, James Jackson, 387, 388, 389, 390, 391
Putnam, Marian, 394

Quijada, Hernán, 445
Quinn, S., 395
Quinodoz, Jean Michel, 407, 418

Racamier, P.-C., 427
Racker, Enrique, 440, 444
Racker, Heinrich, 73, 195, 205, 206,
    207, 291, 412, 448, 496
Rado, Sandor, 383, 391, 396
Ramachandran, V., 541
Rangell, Leo, 306, 397, 437
Rank, Otto, 381, 384, 390, 391, 395,
    453, 481, 492, 507
Rapaport, David, 14, 16, 394, 403, 464
Rascovsky, Arnaldo, 436, 442
Reber, A. S., 466
Redl, Fritz, 399
Reed, G. S., 79
Reese, Michael, 399
Reich, Wilhelm, 234
Reik, Theodor, 481
Rembrandt, 507
Remus, Estela, 445
Renik, Owen, 40, 138, 206, 210, 212,
    293
Resnick, Salomón, 437
Rickman, John, 408, 484
Ricouer, Paul, 319
Rie, H. E., 175
Riesemberg, Ruth, 446
Riggs, Austen, 387, 394
Riggs, S., 165
Riklin, Franz, 453, 455
Rinsley, D., 135, 177
Riviere, Joan, 408, 414
Robbins, Arnold, 396
Robbins, Bernard, 395
Robertson, James, 160
Rocha Barros, Elias, 444
Rochlin, G., 175
Róheim, Géza, 481–482, 483, 487
Rolland, Jean-Claude, 431
Rolland, Romain, 287
Romano, John, 394, 399
Roose, Steven P., 255–265
Rosenblatt, A. D., 46
Rosenfeld, Herbert, 62, 66, 167, 193,
    206, 409, 411, 417, 418, 437
Rosolato, Guy, 440
Ross, David, 285
Ross, J. M., 44, 45, 99
Roth, A., 471–472
Roth, T., 472
Rothenberg, A., 124
Royce, Josiah, 387, 389
Rubin, Gayle, 96, 97, 106

Rubino, G., 472
Rubovits-Seitz, P., 454
Ruddick, Bruce, 398
Rudnytsky, Peter, 459
Rusconi, M., 541
Rüütel, Arnold, 526

Sachs, Hanns, 391, 394
Samberg, Eslee, 229–239
Sampson, H., 317, 321
Sandell, Rolf, 310
Sander, L., 85, 89
Sandler, A.-M., 119, 416–417
Sandler, Joseph, 4, 5, 40, 59, 60, 119,
    120, 123, 135, 168, 195, 207, 208,
    221, 363, 364, 367, 413, 416–417,
    418, 419, 444
Sapir, Edward, 395
Sartre, Jean-Paul, 431, 519
Sashin, J. I., 304
Scarfone, Dominique, 423–432
Schacht, T. E., 310
Schachter, J., 457
Schaefer, M., 498
Schafer, Roy, 16, 28, 105, 205, 221, 233, 497
Scharf, L., 471
Schilder, Paul, 391, 399, 493, 494, 537
Schneider, W., 466
Schore, Allan, 538
Schuengel, C., 165
Schuker, E., 106
Schwaber, Evelyn, 213
Schwartz, James, 538–539
Scott, W. Clifford M., 398
Searles, Harold, 65–66, 67, 211
Segal, Hanna, 62, 178, 206, 219, 409,
    411, 418, 437, 444, 446, 503
Semrad, Elvin, 399
Sequin, Carlos Alberto, 447
Settlage, Calvin F., 119
Severn, Elizabeth, 203
Shakow, D., 464
Shane, Morton, 119
Shanker, Stuart G., 335–355
Shapiro, David, 292
Shapiro, T., 245, 321
Sharpe, Ella, 247, 248, 408
Sharpe, S. A., 46
Sherwood, M., 244
Shevrin, Howard, 466, 467, 468, 542
Shiffrin, R. M., 466
Shmueli-Goetz, Yael, 166
Sidis, Boris, 387, 389
Siedmann de Armesto, Mónica, 435–448
Siegel, P., 322
Sifneos, Peter, 426

Silverberg, William, 395, 396
Silverman, Lloyd, 467–468
Simmel, Ernst, 393, 394, 397
Simon, B., 499
Singer, Isaac Bashevis, 509
Singer, J., 321, 322
Skinner, B. F., 464
Skolnikoff, A. Z., 307, 308
Slade, Arietta, 164, 166–167
Slavson, S. R., 399
Smith, Henry, 206, 230, 273
Smith, J., 26
Socarrás, José Francisco, 447
Socrates, 513–518, 521
Sokolnicka, Eugénie, 423
Solms, Mark, 402, 535–545
Sophocles, 459, 492
Spain, David, 486
Spangler, G., 469
Spence, D. P., 323, 465, 497
Spezzanno, C., 211
Spiegel, John, 395
Spielrein, Sabina, 454
Spillius, Elizabeth B., 62, 136, 206, 279,
    417, 418
Spiro, Melford E., 485, 486, 487,
    488
Spitz, Ellen Handler, 493, 501–509
Spitz, René, 5, 47, 120, 124, 133, 150, 176,
    337, 339, 393, 394, 399, 424, 441
Sroufe, Alan, 161, 163, 469
Stechler, G., 15
Steele, H., 470, 472
Steele, M., 470, 471, 472
Stein, R., 109
Steinberg, Leo, 502
Steiner, John, 193, 206, 411, 444
Steiner, Ricardo, 535
Stekel, Wilhelm, 381, 392
Stengel, B., 322
Stengel, Erwin, 537
Stephen, Adrian, 408
Stephen, Karin, 408
Sterba, R., 230, 248
Stern, Adolf, 391
Stern, Daniel, 9, 77–90, 119, 139, 180–
    181, 209, 220, 221, 224, 225
Stiles, W., 324, 471
Stimmel, B., 102
Stoller, Robert, 94, 99, 100
Stolorow, R., 123, 182, 210
Stone, L., 204
Strachey, Alix, 408
Strachey, James, 5, 219–220, 236, 248,
    284, 408, 414, 442
Strupp, H., 310, 324

Sullivan, Harry Stack, 50, 59, 60, 65–66, 138, 209, 392, 395–396, 398, 399
Sulloway, Frank, 384, 455
Sultan Murat I, 530
Suomi, Steven, 458
Sutherland, J. D., 63
Swales, Peter, 459
Szpilka, Jaime, 440

Tacchi, P., 542
Taneyhill, G. Lane, 389
Target, Mary, 119, 135, *159–169*, 277, 370, 469
Tausk, Victor, 381
Taylor, E. W., 387
Teague, G. B., 472
Teller, V., 321, 322, 326
Teruel, Guillermo, 445
Tessman, L. H., 45
Thom, Douglas, 394
Thomä, H., 310, 321
Thompson, Clara, 138, 392, 395, 396
Thompson, L., 325
Ticho, Ernst, 293
Titchener, Edward Bradford, 463
Titian, 506
Travis, L. A., 473
Treboux, D., 470
Tuckett, David, 320, *407–419*
Tulving, E., 367
Turkle, Sherry, 423
Tustin, Francis, 82
Tuzin, Donald, 487, 488
Tyrrell, C. L., 472
Tyson, P., 119, 137, 174, 250
Tyson, R., 119, 137

Vaillant, G. E., 322
Valabrega, Jean-Paul, 428
Valenstein, A., 219
Vallar G., 541
van Amerongen, S. T., 304
van der Leeuw, J. J., 244
van der Leeuw, Peter, 437
Van Gogh, Vincent, 507
van IJzendoorn, M., 165
Velasquez, Diego, 506
Viderman, S., 319
Viederman, Milton, 456
Vischer, F. T., 282
Volkan, Vamık D., 525–532
von Bertalanffy, Ludwig, 121, 457
von Rochau, Ludwig, 526
Vygotsky, L. S., 123

Waelder, Robert, 11, 25, 248, 393, 394, 494, 527
Waelder-Hall, Jenny, 251, 393
Wall, S., 469–470
Wallace, Anthony F. C., 484
Wallerstein, Robert, 119, *301–313*, 317, 321, 325, 327, 330, 400, 401, 444
Wallon, Henri, 425
Wallwork, Ernest, *281–295*
Waters, Everett, 161, 469, 470
Watson, John, 335, 464, 466
Weber, Max, 282
Weinberger, Joel, *463–474*
Weinstein, Ed, 537
Weiss, Edoardo, 249, 380–381
Weiss, J., 321, 322
Werman, D. S., 24

Westen, D., 131–133, 220, 223, 224, 232, 267, 322
White, Robert, 458
White, William Allanson, 388, 389–390, 392, 399
Whiting, John, 483, 485
Widlöcher, Daniel, 426
Wilde, Oscar, 492
Will, Otto, 65
Williams, Bernard, 522
Williams, Paul, *189–197*
Wilson, Edmund, 495, 496
Winnicott, Donald, 5, 16, 17, 41, 48, 59, 60, 63–65, 103, 123, 132, 135, 136–137, 154, 168, 179–180, 183, 207–208, 211, 220, 247, 290, 291, 366, 402, 408, 413–416, 432, 437, 444, 495, 496, 503, 504, 508
Wolf, E. S., 137
Wolheim, Richard, 522
Wolitzky, D. L., 465
Wolstein, B., 209–210
Worcester, Elwood, 388
Wynne, Lyman, 399

Yankelovich, D., 285
Yanof, Judith A., *267–279*
Yehoshua, A. B., 498
Yeomans, F., 181

Zachhuber, U., 471
Zavitzianos, George, 398
Zetzsel, Elizabeth, 244, 437
Ziehen, Theodore, 459

Subject Index

Page numbers printed in *italic* type refer to chapters in this volume.

AAI. *See* Adult Attachment Interview
Abadi, Mauricio, 440
Abend, Sander M., 222–223, 235, *375–384*
Aberastury, Arminda, 436, 437
Ablon, J. S., 323, 329
ABP (Brazilian Psychoanalytic Association), 440
Abraham, Karl, 46, 247, 381, 383, 453
Abrams, S., 119, 230
Academy of Psychoanalysis, 396
Accordion phenomenon in politics and diplomacy, 531
Ackerman, Nathan, 437
Ackerman, S. J., 323, 325, 329, 330
Adaptation
    exercise of capacities and, 10–11
    forward-looking aspects of, in developmental orientation for psychoanalysis, 118–119
Adler, Alfred, 135, 149, 282, 381, 384, 390, 395
Administrative red tape, 402
Adolescence
    child's relationship with parental couple during, 45
    use of inanimate objects during, 48
Adult Attachment Interview (AAI), 119, 163, 164–166, 469, 470
    coding of, 164
    effect of attachment status on psychotherapy process and outcome, 472–473
    elements of, 164
    prediction of child's early attachment security by, 164
Affect(s). *See also* Emotions
    child's progress to internal representations from, 353–354
    as communicators, 120
    contributions to mental functioning, 21, 22
    in dreams, 34
    Freud's trauma-affect model, 190

Functional Emotional Developmental Approach, 339–340
    history of psychoanalytic thinking about, 120
    integration of, 58–59
    Jacobson's focus on, 66
    Kernberg's concept of, 68
    mother's contingent mirroring of infant's affect, 58, 123
    negative, 11
    regulatory role of, 120, 122
    signal functions of, 11, 120, 354
    therapeutic availability and regulation of, 123–124
    as tool of ego function, 11
Affect flooding, 11
Affective mirroring, 58, 123
Affective monitoring, 122
Affective scaffolding, 123
Affirmative empathy, 124
Agency, 10, 16, 22
    psychic determinism and, 24–25
Aggression
    in countertransference, 208
    destructive, 15
    Freud's theory of, 4, 5, 14–15, 17, 382
        "love commandment" as antidote, 288
        object relations theory and, 59
    intrapsychic conflict and, 28
    motivation and, 14–15, 17, 22, 23
    nonhostile, 15
    object constancy and, 15
    proactive vs. reactive status of, 14–15
    sexuality and, 15
    sources of, 15
Agorio, Rodolfo, 446
Aguayo, J., 408
Ainsworth, Mary, 150, 161, 163, 469–470
    categorization of babies' behavior in Strange Situation, 163–164, 469
        anxious/avoidant babies, 163, 469
        anxious/resistant babies, 163, 469

        disorganized/disoriented babies, 163, 165, 469
        maternal warmth and, 469–470
        parents' reflective function and, 470
        secure babies, 163, 469
Akhtar, Salman, 9, 17, *39–51*
Albee, Edward, 8–9
Albers, Josef, 507
Alexander, Franz, 222, 302, 383, 391, 394, 395, 396, 397, 399, 426
Alexithymia, 426
Alice in Wonderland (Lewis Carroll), 493, 494
Allan Memorial Hospital (Montreal), 398
Allison, George, 400
Alpha function, 136, 206
Althusser, Louis, 428
Alvarez, A., 207
Amacher, Peter, 458–459
American Institute of Psychoanalysis, 395
American Psychiatric Association
    Israeli–Egyptian dialogues sponsored by, 532
    Principles of Medical Ethics With Annotations Especially Applicable to Psychiatry, 319
    proposal for specialty board in psychoanalysis, 396
American Psychoanalytic Association
    admission of women to, 390
    analytic organizations established outside of, 396
    Central Fact-Gathering Committee of, 303
    Collaborative Analytic Multi-Site Program of, 325
    early years of, 388–390, 391–393
    ethical principles of, 282, 288–289
        confidentiality guidelines, 289
        Principles of Ethics for Psychoanalysts, 319
    institutional splitting and, 395–397

American Psychoanalytic Association
  (*continued*)
    from 1968 to present, 399, 403
      antitrust suit and end of lay-
        analysis controversy, 400–401
    study groups on politics and
      diplomacy, 532
American Psychopathological
  Association, 388
American Therapeutic Society, 388
Amnesia, infantile, 133
Analytic attitude, 220
Analytic dyad, 232–233. *See also* Patient–
  analyst relationship
Analytic hour, 408
Analytic neutrality, 236
  ethical aspects of, 282, 284–285
  preclusion of social contracts
    between patient and analyst for,
    396
  psychotropic medications and, 260,
    262
Analytic Process Scales (APS), 312, 323
Analytic tact, 235, 290
Animals
  child's relationship with, 47
  imprinting in, 160
Anna Freud Centre, 304
Anna O. case (Breuer), 377
Anthony, A., 483
Anthropology and psychoanalysis, 398,
  479–488
  challenge of cultural anthropology,
    481–484
    Culture and Personality school,
      483–484
    Kardiner, 482–483
    Malinowski, 481
    Róheim, 481–482
    Whiting, 483
  contemporary developments, 484–
    488
    evolutionary psychology, 485–486
    gender, 487–488
    human universals and cultural
      variation, 485
    life history determinants and
      complex emotional factors,
      486–487
  differences between, 479–480
  Freud's early interdisciplinary foray,
    480–481
  parallels between, 479
Antidepressants, 259, 261, 262–263
Antisocial personality disorder,
  Kernberg's view of, 181

Antitrust suit against American
  Psychoanalytic Association,
  400–401
Anxiety
  castration, 96, 98
    among Normanby Islanders, 482
  in dreams, 34
  due to psychic conflicts, 192
  Freud's concept of kinds of anxiety-
    provoking situations, 28–29
    anticipation of danger, 29
    phase-specific danger situations,
      29
    threats to basic needs of organism,
      28–29
  intrapsychic conflict and, 28
  in Kleinian object relations theory,
    61
  persecutory, 193
  separation, 63
  signal, 11, 120
  "skin-color," 41
  stranger, 42, 47
  traumatic, 11
Anxiety disorders, 258, 259
  informing patient of possible
    treatments for, 260
  sequence of treatments for, 259
Anzieu, Didier, 108, 426, 430, 527
APF (Association Psychanalytique de
  France), 426
APM (Mexican Psychoanalytic
  Association), 445
Applied analysis
  development of, 454–455
    Freud and beginnings of, 453–454
    Freudian approach to literature, 491–
      493
Applied psychoanalytic research, 148
Après-coup, 194
APS (Analytic Process Scales), 312, 323
APU (Uruguayan Psychoanalytic
  Association), 446
Aquinas, Thomas, 287
Arafat, Yasser, 529
Araújo, Jaime, 445
Argentina, 435–440
  development of psychoanalysis in,
    435–439
    contemporary perspectives, 439
    growth and institutionalization,
      436–437
    new challenges, 437–439
  psychoanalytic thought in, 439–440
Argentine Association of Group
  Psychology and Psychotherapy, 437

Argentine Center for Research in
  Psychosomatic Medicine, 437
Argentine Child and Adolescent
  Psychiatry and Psychology
  Association, 437
Argentine Psychoanalytic Association,
  435, 436–439, 445
Argentine School of Psychotherapy for
  Graduates, 437
Argentine Society of Psychoanalysis, 439
Aristotle, 287, 514
Arlow, Jacob, 24, 124, 232, 236, 285, 527
Arnold Pfeffer Center for Neuro-
  Psychoanalysis, 539
Aron, Lewis, 101, 109, 206, 210, 211, 494
Arousal, infant's regulation of, 340–343
ARPAC (Monterrey Psychoanalytic
  Society), 445
Art Beyond the Pleasure Principle
  (Margaret Iverson). 502
Arts and psychoanalysis, 501–509
  ego psychology and, 502, 505–507
  Freud and, 502, 503–505
  object relations theory and, 503,
    508–509
  three-part paradigm for approach to,
    502–503
ASOVEP (Venezuelan Psychoanalytic
  Association), 445
Association for the Advancement of
  Psychoanalysis, 395, 396
Association Psychanalytique de France
  (APF), 426
Attachment
  Adult Attachment Interview, 119,
    163, 164–166, 469, 470, 472
  Child Attachment Interview, 166
  continuity in patterns of, 163
  definition of, 139
  to father, 43–45
  to grandparents, 46–47
  imprinting and, 160
  information processing–cognitive
    model of, 163
  intersubjectivity and, 82–83
  low concordance between siblings,
    164
  mentalizing and, 139–140, 182–183
  to mother, 41–43
  motivation and, 4, 9–10
  psychopathology and, 164–165, 470–
    471
  to siblings, 45–46
  to transitional object, 47, 48, 64, 415,
    508
  trauma and, 164, 165

Attachment-individuation theories of gender, 100–101
Attachment theory, 159–169
  Ainsworth's Strange Situation and, 163–164, 337, 469
    anxious/avoidant babies, 163, 469
    anxious/resistant babies, 163, 469
    disorganized/disoriented babies, 163, 165, 469
    maternal warmth and, 469–470
    parents' reflective function and, 470
    secure babies, 163, 469
  of Bowlby, 9, 138–139, 160–162, 338
    criticisms of, 161, 162
    developmental model, 139, 161
    evolutionary origin of, 338, 485–486
    homeostasis between attachment behavior and exploratory behavior, 161
    interdisciplinary influences and, 160, 457–458
    internal working models in, 161–162
    "proximity-seeking signals" in, 160
    psychology and, 468–469
    relation to depth psychology, 338
    relational approaches and, 182
    sequence of children's reactions to separation, 160
    set goal of attachment system, 161
    studies of effects of institutionalization on children, 160
    studies of prolonged separation of children from caregivers, 337
  bridging psychoanalysis and, 168–169
  criticisms of, 161, 162
  depth psychology and, 337–338
  disorganization of attachment, 163, 165
  of Dozier, 165
  early attachment as predictive of social development, 164–165
  empirical base for, 159
  infant's capacity for engagement, 343–345
  internal working models in, 161–162
  measurement of attachment between preschool years and early adulthood, 165–166
  protective effects of secure attachment, 344

  psychoanalytic views of, 166–168
    Eagle, 167
    Fonagy, 167–168
    Fraiberg, 166
    Lieberman, 166
    Lyons-Ruth, 167
    Slade, 166–167
  psychology and, 468–470
  psychopathology and, 470–471
  psychotherapy and, 471–473
    attachment status and psychotherapy outcome, 471, 472–473
    attachment status and psychotherapy process, 471–472
  reception within psychoanalysis, 162
  research findings of, 162–163
  of Stern, 139
  unifying, life-span perspective of, 159–160
Atwood, G., 123, 182
Auden, W. H., 458
Audio recording for process research, 317
  intrusion of device for, 318
Augustine, 287
Aulagnier, Piera, 428, 432, 440
Autism
  child's inability to play due to, 272
  intersubjectivity and, 82
Autistic phase of development (Mahler), 58, 67, 134, 177, 342
Automaticity, 467
Axis I disorders, 256, 257–259
Axis II disorders, 256, 257

Babysitters, child's relationship with, 49
Bachrach, H. M., 307, 308
Bahia, Alcyon, 442
Bakermans-Kranenburg, M., 165
Balint, Michael, 135, 136, 195, 204, 207, 208, 413
Bandura, A., 464
Baranger, Madeleine, 437, 438, 440, 444, 446, 448
Baranger, Willy, 437, 438, 440, 444, 446, 448
Barber, J., 321, 325
Bargh, J., 542
Barke, C., 472
Barkham, M., 471
Barnett, L., 472
Barron, J. W., 465
Bassin, D., 101, 102, 107
Bateson, Gregory, 483

Beebe, B., 339
Behavioral organization of child, 348–349
Behrends, R., 219
Being and Nothingness (Jean-Paul Sartre), 519
Benedek, Tereza, 123, 441
Benedict, Ruth, 396, 398, 483, 484
Benign and tolerant curiosity, 291
Benjamin, Jessica, 18, 99, 109, 138, 399, 485
  gender theory of, 94, 101
  view of father–daughter relationship, 45
  view of transference and countertransference, 211
Berenstein, Isidoro, 440, 444
Beres, D., 124
Berezin, Martin, 395
Bergman, A., 339, 342, 352
Bergmann, Martin S., *241–252*
Berkoff, Steven, 498
Berlin Psychoanalytic Institute, 391, 393, 395
  outcome studies at, 302
Berman, Emanuel, *491–499*
Bernard, Viola, 437
Bernardi, R., 320, 446
Bernfeld, Siegfried, 394, 397
Bernheim, Hippolyte, 377, 378, 387, 423
Bernstein, D., 45, 98
Beta elements, 136
Bettelheim, Bruno, 454–455
Beyond the Pleasure Principle (Sigmund Freud), 382
"Bibliothèque de Psychanalyse," 426
Bibring, Edward, 235
Bibring, Grete, 251
Biddle, Sidney, 396
Binder, J. L., 473
Binger, Carl, 394, 396
Binghamton State Hospital (New York), 389
Binswanger, Ludwig, 381
Bion, Wilfred R., 62, 66, 135, 168, 178, 208, 220, 279, 366, 397, 402, 409, 413, 417, 432, 437, 439
  concept of alpha function, 136, 206
  concept of beta elements, 136
  concept of defensive organizations, 179
  concept of K and minus K, 136
  concept of thought, 411
  view of countertransference, 206
Bird, B., 205

Bisiach, E., 541
Blagys, M. D., 323, 325, 329, 330
Blatt, Sidney, 165, 219
Blecher, Jose, 440
Blechner, M., 209, 210
Blehar, M. E., 469–470
Bleiberg, Efrain, *173–183*
Bleuler, Eugen, 381, 389, 459
Bliwise, N. G., 473
Blos, Peter, 43, 440
Blue Cross/Blue Shield Federal
    Employees Program, 310
Bluestone, H., 255
Blum, Harold, 242, 364
Boas, Franz, 479, 481
Boesky, D., 230, 232
Bohleber, Werner, 364
Bollas, Christopher, 105, 208, 284, 416,
    508–509
Bonaparte, Marie, 423, 482, 495
Bond, J. A., 468
Bonge, D., 323
Bookwala, J. F., 471
Borderline personality disorder, 140, 197
    attachment status and, 470, 472
    defensive identification of victim
        with abuser in, 140
    developmental viewpoint of, 131
    Dialectical Behavior Therapy for, 465
    Kernberg's theory of, 68, 181
    Mahler's theory of, 67, 131, 177
    Masterson and Rinsley's theory of,
        177
    transference-focused psychotherapy
        for, 182
Bornstein, Berta, 392
Bornstein, R. F., 465, 473
Boston Change Process Study Group,
    85, 86, 88, 89, 220, 221
Boston Psychoanalytic Institute, 391
    outcome studies at, 304, 307
Boston Psychoanalytic Society, 389, 391,
    397
Boston Psychopathic Hospital, 388, 402
Bourdieu, Pierre, 484
Bowlby, John, 119, 122, 150, 159, 163,
    167, 182, 191, 337, 339, 402, 408,
    413, 468–469, 469, 485
    attachment theory of, 9, 138–139,
        160–162, 338
        criticisms of, 161, 162
        evolutionary origin of, 338, 485–
            486
        homeostasis between attachment
            behavior and exploratory
            behavior, 161

internal working models, 161–162
    "proximity-seeking signals," 160
    psychology and, 468–469
    relation to depth psychology, 338
    relational approaches and, 182
    sequence of children's reactions to
        separation, 160
    set goal of attachment system, 161
    studies of effects of
        institutionalization on
        children, 160
developmental model of, 139, 161
interdisciplinary collaboration and,
    160, 457–458
studies of prolonged separation of
    children from caregivers, 337
Boyer, Bryce, 437, 484
Brakel, L. A. W., 468
Brandchaft, B., 123
Brazelton, T. Berry, 341
Brazil, 440–445
    contemporary psychoanalysis in,
        444–445
    immigrant analysts and
        psychoanalysis in Rio de Janeiro,
        442–443
        Burke, 442
        Kemper, 442–443
    immigration and diversity of, 440
    periods of development of
        psychoanalysis in, 440
    psychoanalysis in Porto Alegre, 443–
        444
    psychoanalysis in São Paulo, 441–442
Brazilian Institute of Psychoanalysis,
    443
Brazilian Psychoanalytic Association
    (ABP), 440
Brazilian Society of Psychoanalysis of
    Rio de Janeiro, 440
Breen, D., 101
Brenner, Charles, 232, 250, 285, 292
Bretano, Franz, 376
Bretherton, I., 162
Breton, André, 423
Breuer, Josef, 108, 194, 377
Briehl, Marie, 392, 397
Brierley, Marjorie, 408
Briggs, Jean, 487
Brill, A. A., 381, 388, 390, 391, 392
British Psychoanalytic Society, 382, 401,
    408, 413
Britton, R., 193, 206
Bromberg, P. M., 138, 210, 211
Bronfman, E., 165
Brown, Jason, 539

Brücke, Ernst, 376, 459
Bruschweiler-Stern, N., 85
Bucci, Wilma, 119, *317–330*
Buenos Aires Psychoanalytic
    Association, 438, 439
Burke, Mark, 442
Burlingham, Dorothy, 337
Burnham, J. C., 390
Burrow, Trigant, 389
Burton, R. V., 483
Busch, F., 234
Butler, J., 94, 102, 106
Butler, Thomas, 531
Buxbaum, Edith, 394

Cabaniss, Deborah L., *255–265*
Cabernite, Leão, 443
Cameron, Ewen, 398
CAMP (Collaborative Analytic Multi-
    Site Program), 325
Canadian psychoanalysis, 398, 429–430
Canadian Psychoanalytic Society and
    Institute, 398
Canestri, Jorge, 364, 418
Caracas School of the Freudian Field,
    445
Cárcamo, Celes, 435, 436
Carranza, L. V., 471
Carroll, Lewis, 493
Carter, Jimmy, 526, 529
Case report, 317
Casement, P., 221, 416
Cassidy, J., 470
Castration anxiety
    among Normanby Islanders, 482
    Freud's concept of, 96, 98
Cath, S. H., 46
Causality, psychic, 23–25
    multicausality, 25
CCRT (Core Conflictual Relationship
    Theme), 321, 322, 325–326, 365
Center for the Study of Mind and
    Human Interaction, 532
Cesio, Fidias, 439, 440
CGI (Clinical Global Impression)
    Improvement Scale, 263
Chabert, Catherine, 431
Change
    analysis of resistance as catalyst for,
        233
    capacity for, 231
    equilibria and, 250
    interpretation vs. relationship in
        bringing about, 236
    philosophy and psychic change, 518–
        519, 521

resistance to, 233
homeostatic motivation power of,
11–12
Charcot, Jean-Martin, 376–377, 387,
423
Chartrand, T., 542
Chasseguet-Smirgel, Janine, 96, 97, 440,
444, 527
Chentrier, André, 398
Chestnut Lodge (Rockville, MD), 399,
401
Chicago Plan, 400
Chicago Psychoanalytic Clinic, outcome
studies at, 302
Chicago Psychoanalytic Institute, 391,
394, 399
Child Attachment Interview, 166
Child psychiatry, in America, 394, 399
Child psychoanalysis, 267–279. *See also*
Play
children who cannot play, 272–273
compared with adult analysis, 267–
268
development and, 267, 276–277
Freud's view of, 175
interpretation and insight in, 270,
273–274
multiple functions of analyst to child
in, 276
other theoretical models of, 278–279
Ferro, 279
modern Kleinians, 279
relational theorists, 279
patient–analyst relationship for, 267
play process in, 270–272
purpose of, 267
role of play in, 267–269
transference in, 274–276
work with parents in, 268, 277–278
working within the play, 270
Child Study Center at Yale University,
394
Children
development of ability to mentalize,
269
developmental levels of emotional
functioning, 340–353
1: self-regulation and interest in
the world: 0–3 months, 340–
343
2: forming relationships,
attachment, and engagement:
2–7 months, 343–345
3: two-way, purposeful
communication: 3–10
months, 345–347

4: behavioral organization,
problem solving, and
internalization: 9–18 months,
347–349
5: representational capacity: 18–
30 months, 349–351
6: representational differentiation:
30–48 months, 351–353
early relationships of, 39–51 (*See also*
Early relationships)
hermaphroditic, 94
imaginary companions of, 84
observations of, 175–178, 335
Anna Freud, 176
under extreme clinical challenges,
337
Mahler, 176–178
in normative situations, 336–337
Spitz, 176
"psychic equivalence" mode of
thinking, 269
use of "pretend mode" by, 269
Chile, 446–447
Chilean Psychoanalytic Association, 446
Chodorow, Nancy, 18, 45, 107, 485, 486
concept of masculinity, 99
gender theory of, 94, 101
Chomsky, Noam, 485, 486
Chrysanthemum and the Sword, The (Ruth
Benedict), 484
Chused, Judith, 274, 294
Cixous, H., 497
Claparede, Edouard, 466
Clark University lectures by Freud, 381,
387, 388, 463
Clarkin, J. F., 181
Clergy, child's relationship with, 49
Clinical Global Impression (CGI)
Improvement Scale, 263
Coates, S., 101, 105
Cobb, Stanley, 398, 399
Cognition during sleep, 32
Cognitive assimilation, 122
Cognitive psychology, 537
Cohen, Robert A., 399
Colarusso, C. A., 46
Cole, Thomas, 501–502
Collaborative Analytic Multi-Site
Program (CAMP), 325
Colombia, 447
Colombian Psychoanalytic Society, 447
Colombo, Daria, *375–384*
Columbia Psychoanalytic Center,
outcome studies at, 304–305
Columbia University Psychoanalytic
Clinic, 396

Commitment to analytic process, 231
Commonwealth Fund, 399
Comparative Psychotherapy Process
Scale (CPPS), 323
Competence, 10
Complementary identification in
countertransference, 73
Computer-assisted process research
measures, 323
caveat for use of, 323
Text Analysis System, 323
Therapeutic Cycles Model, 323
Conceptual research, 361–371
aim of, 362
application of hermeneutic methods
to, 370
change and clarification of concepts,
363–364, 370
vs. conceptual reflection, 368–369,
371
definition of, 361–362
elastic meaning-space of concepts, 364
transference, 364–365
essentials of process for, 369
Freud's thoughts on development of
concepts, 362
further sources of variety in concept
use, 366
history and practice in
psychoanalysis, 366–368
concept study groups, 368
panel discussions, 368
integration of "new" knowledge in,
362–363
interdependent cooperation with
empirical research, 370
methodological problems with, 369–
371
operationalization of concepts, 370
as a research program, 362, 368, 371
specific features of psychoanalytic
concepts, 365–366
Concordant identification in
countertransference, 73
Condensation in dreams, 33
Confidentiality guidelines, 289
Configurational analysis, 321, 322
Conflict, intrapsychic, 28–29, 192
defenses against, 192–193
object relations theories of, 69
Confrontations (discussion forum), 427
Conscience, 7, 49. See also Superego
Conscious(ness), 189, 190, 379. See also
Unconscious
core, 139
extended, 139

Consciousness raising, 18
Constancy principle, 25
Constitutional factors, 40
Contemporary Psychoanalysis (journal), 319
Control-Mastery theory, 322
Conway, Martin, 541, 542
Cooper, A. M., 11, 255, 379, 381, 384
Cooper, S. H., 322
COPAL (Cousejo de las Organizaciones Psicoanaliticos de America Latina), 436, 437
Copernicus, 15
Corbett, K., 99, 100, 104–105
Córdoba Study Group, 438
Core Conflictual Relationship Theme (CCRT), 321, 322, 325–326, 365
Coriat, Isador, 302, 389, 390, 391, 399
Corrective empathy, 123–124
Cost of psychoanalysis, 402
Countertransference, 40, 194–195, 201–213. *See also* Patient–analyst relationship; Transference
  in analytic process, 231–232
  complementary identification in, 73
  concordant identification in, 73
  evolution of concept of, 204–212
    American ego psychology, 204–206
    Freud, 194–195, 201, 222
    interpersonal tradition, 209–210
    Kleinian tradition, 206–207
    Lacanian models, 209
    object relations theory, 59, 60, 61, 73, 195, 207–209
    relational models, 210–212
    self psychology, 210
  hostility and hatred in, 202
  Latin American tradition on, 207
  one-way intersubjectivity and, 80
  projective identification and, 193
  real relationship and, 203–204, 212
  reevaluation of, 496, 497
  related to prescription of psychotropic medications, 260, 261
  sexuality and, 108–109
  status of influence in, 203
Cousejo de las Organizaciones Psicoanaliticos de America Latina (COPAL), 436, 437
CPPS (Comparative Psychotherapy Process Scale), 323
CRA, 324
Craik, K., 161

Cranefield, Paul, 458
Crapanzano, Vincent, 487
Crews, Frederick, 457
Crisanto, Carlos, 447
Crits-Christoph, P., 325
Crittenden, P. M., 163, 166, 167
Cryanowski, J. M., 471
Cuadernos de Psicoanálisis (journal), 445
Cue, K. L., 472
Cultural factors. *See also* Anthropology and psychoanalysis
  patient's reports of early experiences and, 41
Culture and Personality school of anthropology, 483–484
Curiosity of analyst, benign and tolerant, 291
Curtis, Homer, 400
Curtis, W. J., 134

DAAP (Discourse Attributes Analysis System), 324
Dahl, H., 310, 321, 322, 323, 326
Dahlheim, Luiz, 442
Dalheim, Luis Guimaraes, 437
Dalrymple, Leolia, 391
Damasio, Antonio, 139, 538, 544
Daniels, George, 396, 398
Darwin, Charles, 15, 105, 380, 480, 481, 540
Davanzo, Hernán, 446
David, Christian, 426
Davidson, Donald, 519
Davies, J. M., 109, 211
DBT (Dialectical Behavior Therapy), for borderline personality disorder, 465
de Beauvoir, Simone, 94
de la Vega, Garcilaso, 447
de Leon de Bernardi, B., 207
De Marneffe, D., 100
de Mijolla, A., 368
de M'uzan, Michel, 426
de Oliveira, Walderedo, 437
Death instinct, 5, 27, 246, 382
  in Kleinian object relations theory, 61
Debbane, E. G., 324
Debbink, N. L., 251
deCarufel, F. L., 324
Decision making, moral, 289, 294–295
Declarative (explicit) memory, 132, 223, 466
Defense Mechanism Rating Scales (DMRS), 322

Defense mechanisms, 190, 192–193
  affective expression in dreams and, 34
  in Kleinian object relations theory, 61–62
  maladaptive, 192–193
  plasticity of, as requirement for analytic process, 231
  psychopathology and, 174
  symptom formation and, 34–35
Delgado, Honorio, 447
Denial, 193
Denis, Paul, 364
Denktash, Rauf, 529
Dennis, Wayne, 337
Depression
  antidepressants for, 259, 261, 262–263
    split treatment, 260
  childhood, 175
  informing patient of possible treatments for, 259
  psychological mindedness and, 259
  rating scales for, 263
  remission status and optimal treatment for, 263
  self-esteem and, 137
  sequence of treatments for, 259
  signal, 120
Depressive position, in Kleinian object relations theory, 61, 62, 135–136, 178, 192, 410
Depth psychology, 335–336
  attachment research and, 337–338
    emotional signaling, 338
    Strange Situation, 337
  developmental framework for, 339–355 (*See also* Developmental research)
  developmental psychology and, 336
  observations of children under extreme clinical challenges, 337
  stages of mental (ego) development, 339–340
  vs. surface approaches, 336–338
Derrida, Jacques, 427, 497
Descartes, René, 361
Desire, sexual, 107–108
  multiplicities of, 106–107
Determinism
  Freud's view of, 23–24, 377
    ethics and, 285–286
  multiple, 25
  psychic, 23–25
Deutsch, Felix, 243, 393, 394, 398

Deutsch, Helene, 383, 393
Development, 191–192
  A. Freud's model of, 134, 176
  adult, 118
  basic motives of, 121–122
  Bowlby's model of, 139, 161
  of capacity for reflective functioning,
    118, 119
  child analysis and, 267, 276–277
  early relationships and their
    internalization, 39
  epigenetic theories of, 150
  Erikson's model of, 22–23, 133
  Hartmann's model of, 10, 120, 133
  increasingly organized complexity in,
    120
  Jacobson's model of, 133
  Kernberg's model of, 137–138
  Klein's model of, 61–62, 135–136,
    178
  across life span, 118
  Loweald's model of, 133–134
  motivation and developmental needs,
    16–17
  phase-specific danger situations
    during, 29
  S. Freud's model of, 132–133, 191–192
    phases of psychosexual
      development, 6, 13, 120, 191
  Sandler's model of, 135
  Sigmund Freud's model of, 132–133
  Spitz's model of, 120, 133
  Stern's model of, 139
Developmental, Individual-Difference,
  Relationship-Based Model
  (DIRtm), 339
Developmental orientation for
  psychoanalysis, 117–126, 173
  adaptation, forward-looking
    processes, and early
    relationships in, 118–119
  background of, 119–121
    child development, 120–121
    concepts of ego organization, 120
    entropy and negentropy, 120
    Freud's pleasure principle, 120
    Leowald's concept of therapeutic
      action, 121
    role of affects, 120
  contributions of other disciplines to,
    126
  early development and developmen-
    tal motives, 121–122
    activity, 121
    affective monitoring, 122
    cognitive assimilation, 122

  self-regulation, 121–122
  social fittedness, 122
  moving beyond, 126
  therapeutic availability and, 123–125
    affect regulation and empathy,
      123–124
    interpretation and shared aspects of
      therapeutic action, 124–125
    termination process, 125
  use of past in developmental present,
    117–118
Developmental psychoanalytic
  epistemology, 151–153
Developmental psychology, 336
  depth psychology and, 336
  methodology of, 336
  observations of children in normative
    situations, 336–337
  psychoanalysis and, 148–151
Developmental research, 335–355
  depth psychology, 335–336
    attachment research and, 337–338
    emotional signaling, 338
    Strange Situation, 337
  developmental framework for, 339
  developmental psychology and, 336
  observations of children under
    extreme clinical challenges,
    337
  vs. surface approaches, 336–338
  developmental levels of emotional
    functioning, 340–353
    1: self-regulation and interest in
      the world: 0–3 months, 340–
      343
      clinical observations, 341–342
      implications for mental (ego)
        functioning, 342–343
    2: forming relationships,
      attachment, and engagement:
      2–7 months, 343–345
      clinical observations, 344
      implications for mental (ego)
        functioning, 344–345
    3: two-way, purposeful
      communication:
      3–10 months, 345–347
      clinical observations, 345–346
      implications for mental (ego)
        functioning, 347
    4: behavioral organization, problem
      solving, and internalization:
      9–18 months, 347–349
      clinical observations, 347–348
      implications for mental (ego)
        functioning, 348–349

    5: representational capacity:
      18–30 months, 349–351
      clinical observations, 350
      implications for mental (ego)
        functioning, 350–351
    6: representational differentiation:
      30–48 months, 351–353
      clinical observations, 351–352
      implications for mental (ego)
        functioning, 352–353
    developmental pathway to formation
      of internal representations, 353–
      354
    evolution of, 335
    higher levels of mental functioning,
      353
    stages of mental (ego) development,
      339–340
Developmental Structuralist Theory, 339
Developmental theory, psychoanalytic,
  131–140
  beyond object relations, 138–140
    attachment theory, 138–139
    Sullivan, 65–66, 138
  British School of object relations and,
    135–137
    Fairbairn, 62–63, 136
    Klein, 61–62, 135–136
    Winnicott, 63–65, 136–137
  Freud and the classical tradition,
    132–133
  interface with other disciplines, 147–
    155
    developmental psychoanalytic
      epistemology, 151–153
    epistemologies of psychoanalysis
      and developmental
      psychology, 148–151
    models for collaboration, 153–155
  North American object relations and,
    137–138
    Kernberg, 67–68, 137–138
    Kohut, 137
  object relations theory and, 41, 132
  observation-based, 132, 149–150
  overview of psychoanalytic theories,
    132
  pushing classical developmental
    envelope, 133–135
    Anna Freud, 134
    Erikson, 22–23, 133
    Jacobson, 133
    Loewald, 133–134
    Mahler, 134–135
    Sandler, 135
    Spitz, 133

Devereux, George, 480, 484

Dewey, John, 505

Diagnosis of psychiatric disorders, 257–258

  decision to prescribe psychotropic medications based on, 258

  DSM-IV system for, 257–258

  relevance to recommendation for psychoanalysis, 257

Diagnostic and Statistical Manual of Mental Disorders (DSM-IV), 256–259

Diagnostic interview, 259

Dialectical Behavior Therapy (DBT), for borderline personality disorder, 465

Diatkine, René, 427

Dictionaries of analytic terms, 368

Dimen, Muriel, *93–110*

Dinnerstein, D., 94

DIRtm (Developmental, Individual-Difference, Relationship-Based Model), 339

Disavowal, 193

Discourse Attributes Analysis System (DAAP), 324

Discovery of the Unconscious (Henri Ellenberger), 455

Displacement in dreams, 33

Dissociation in the ego as requirement for analytic process, 230

Dissociative states, 197

DMRS (Defense Mechanism Rating Scales), 322

Dollard, J., 464

Dolto, Françoise, 425

Dooley, Lucile, 389, 390

Doolittle, Hilda (H.D.), 203, 243–244

Dostoyevsky, Fyodor, 484, 492

Dozier, Mary, 165, 472

Dr. Adams's Nervine Asylum (Boston), 387

Drake, R., 322

Dream analysis

  in analyzed persons, 248

  The Interpretation of Dreams (S. Freud), 32, 34, 35, 218, 375, 379, 402, 455, 502

  literary analysis and, 494

  neuroscientific research and, 544

  overdetermination in, 25

  Socrates' view that dreams are expressions of unconscious and illicit desires, 517

  working-through and, 195

Dream formation, 31–34

  affects in dreams, 34

  Fairbairn's concept of "state of affairs" dreams, 32

  Freud's concept of, 31–32

  Kohut's concept of "self-state dreams," 32

  latent content of dreams, 32

  mechanisms of representation in dream work, 32–33

    condensation, 33

    displacement, 33

    projection, 33

    secondary revision, 33

    symbolism, 33

  neurobiology of, 31

  posttraumatic dreams, 4, 27

  primary and secondary process in, 27–28

  punishment dream, 34

  stimuli associated with initiation of, 32

  symptom formation and, 34

Dreams and Myth (Karl Abraham), 453

Dreher, Anna Ursula, *361–371*

Drews, S., 364

Drives, 3, 4, 39

  Freud's concept of, 3, 4–6, 13–14, 17, 132, 382, 543

    psychopathology related to fixation and/or regression to, 174

  intersubjectivity and, 82–83

  Kernberg's concept of, 67–68

  motivations and, 13–15, 17

  neuroscientific research on instinctual mechanisms, 543–544

  object relations theory and, 58–59

  wishes and, 14

Drummond de Andrade, Carlos, 447

DSM-IV (*Diagnostic and Statistical Manual of Mental Disorders*), 256–259

Dunbar, Flanders, 394, 398

Dundes, Alan, 487

Dunn, J., 77

Duration of analysis, 195, 241

Durkeim, Emile, 479

Dynamics of Literary Response, The (N. N. Holland), 494

Eagle, Morris, 166, 167, 457–458, 474, 508

Eames, V., 471–472

Early experiences

  overemphasis on, 131

  psychopathology as maladaptive residues of, 131 (*See also* Developmental theory)

  Strange Situation and attachment in babies, 163–164, 337, 469

Early relationships, 39–51, 344–345. *See also* Attachment theory

  with animals, 47

  caveats related to, 39–41

    constitutional factors, 40

    cultural factors, 41

    element of subjectivity, 40

    multiplicity of roles and developmental overlays, 40–41

    unreliability of recall, 40

  with extended family, 48–49

  with father, 43–45

  forward-looking processes and, in developmental orientation for psychoanalysis, 118–119

  generalizations about lifelong psychic impact of, 39–40

  with God, 49

  with grandparents, 46–47

  with inanimate surround, 47–48

  internalization of, 49–51

    formal aspects of, 49–50

    metabolism of, 50–51

    processes of, 50

  with mother, 41–43

    mother's body, 41–42

    mother's mental contents, 42–43

    mother's presence, 42

    mother's relationships, 43

  with other significant persons, 49

  with parental couple, 45

  reasons for increasing interest in, 39

  with siblings, 45–46

  with stepfamilies, 48

Eckhardt, Marianne, 395

École Freudienne de Paris (EFP), 425–428

École Normale Supérieure, 428

Economic factors affecting psychoanalysis, 402–403

Edelman, G. M., 85

Edes, Robert, 387

EEA ("environment of evolutionary adaptedness"), 485–486

Eells, T., 321, 322

EFP (École Freudienne de Paris), 425–428

Ego
  anxiety arising in, 29
  capacities required for analytic
      process, 230–231
  as defense against expression of
      instinctual drives, 5
  definition of, 10
  developmental levels and functioning
      of, 339–340
    1: self-regulation and interest in
        the world: 0–3 months, 342–
        343
    2: forming relationships,
        attachment, and engagement:
        2–7 months, 344–345
    3: two-way, purposeful
        communication:
        3–10 months, 347
    4: behavioral organization,
        problem solving, and
        internalization: 9–18 months,
        348–349
    5: representational capacity:
        18–30 months, 350–351
    6: representational differentiation:
        30–48 months, 352–353
  dissociation in, as requirement for
      analytic process, 230
  vs. experiential self, 12
  Fairbairn's concept of, 62–63
  Freud's concept of, 7, 28, 190
  Hartmann's concept of, 10, 120, 133,
      174
  higher levels of functioning of, 353
  Klein's concept of, 62, 178
  motivations in functioning of, 4, 5,
      10–12
    anxiety signal, 11
    exercise of capacities, 10–11
    resistance to change, 11–12
  Spitz's concept of, 120
Ego analysis, 383
Ego and the Mechanisms of Defense, The
    (A. Freud), 383
Ego ideal
  Fairbairn's concept of, 63
  father's role in development of, 43,
      44
  Freud's concept of, 190
Ego identity, 50, 58
Ego psychology, 7, 196, 383
  arts and, 502, 505–507
  demise in United States, 138
  developmental concepts and, 133
  Kernberg's theory of, 60, 67–68,
      137–138

literary analysis and, 494
  New York school of, 394
  object relations theory and, 58, 59,
      60
  view of interpretation, 236, 237
  view of resistance, 234
  view of transference and
      countertransference, 204–206
Ego weakness, 138
Egoistic hedonism, 286
Egyptian–Israeli dialogues, 532
Ehrenberg, D. B., 209, 210, 211
Eifermann, R., 498
Einstein, Albert, 93, 527
Eissler, Kurt, 244, 393
Eissler, Ruth, 251
Eitingon, Max, 381, 383
Eizirik, Cláudio Laks, *435–448*
Eldred, S. H., 304
Elisabeth Von R. case (Freud), 377–378
Elise, D., 99, 102
Ellenberger, Henri, 380, 383, 384, 455
Elliott, R., 324
Ellis, Havelock, 387
Emde, Robert N., *117–126*, 133, 321
Emerson, L. E., 389, 390
Emmanuel Movement, 389
Emotional honesty of analyst, 291
Emotions. *See also* Affect(s)
  catastrophic, 354
  child's progress to internal
      representations from, 353–354
  development of multicause and
      triangular reasoning about, 353
  developmental levels of emotional
      functioning, 340–353
    1: self-regulation and interest in the
        world: 0–3 months, 340–343
    2: forming relationships,
        attachment, and engagement:
        2–7 months, 343–345
    3: two-way, purposeful
        communication:
        3–10 months, 345–347
    4: behavioral organization,
        problem solving, and
        internalization: 9–18 months,
        347–349
    5: representational capacity:
        18–30 months, 349–351
    6: representational differentiation:
        30–48 months, 351–353
  in dreams, 34
Functional Emotional
    Developmental Approach, 339–
    340

Empathy
  affirmative, 124
  corrective, 123–124
  empathic respect for patient, 290–
      291
  vs. intersubjectivity, 79
  Kohut's concept of, 124
  therapeutic availability and, 123–124
Engagement, infant's capacity for, 343–
    345
Engel, George, 394, 399
Entropy, 120
Environment, child's relationship with,
    47–48
"Environment of evolutionary
    adaptedness" (EEA), 485–486
"Equafinality," 121
Erdelyi, M. H., 464
Erikson, Erik, 46, 59, 120, 124, 126,
    150, 168, 282, 392, 394, 398, 403,
    457, 484, 529
  concept of ego identity, 58
  developmental model of, 22–23, 133
  literary dream analysis, 494
Erle, J. B., 305
Erotic transference, 194
Erotogenic zones, 6, 104, 174, 191
ERPs (event-related potentials),
    activation by stimuli, 468
Escalona, Sibylle, 339, 399
Esman, Aron, 456, 494
Estonia, 525–526
Etchegoyen, Horácio, 439, 440, 444
Ethical reflection, 281, 282
Ethics, 281–295
  deep ethical theory informing psy-
      choanalytic practice, 287–288
  definition of, 281
  of Freud, 281–283, 285–287
    determinism, 23–24, 285–286
    egoistic hedonism, 286
    ethical relativism, 281, 286–287
  in moral decision making, 289, 294–
      295
  vs. morality, 281
  as principles, rules, and guidelines,
      288–289
  related to publication of case material
      in journals, 319
  skepticism of psychoanalysts about,
      281, 282
  therapeutic goals and, 282–283, 292–
      293
  virtues and, 289–292
    benign and tolerant curiosity, 291
    definition of, 290

Ethics (continued)
  virtues and (continued)
    emotional honesty, 291
    empathic respect, 290–291
    openness and humility, 291
    problems with language of, 292
    restraint or self-control, 291–292
European outcome studies, 304
European psychoanalysis, 407–419
  British object relations and its
      reception in Continental
      Europe, 417–418
  contributions of Jones, 408
  diversity of, 407
  Freud and the early years, 375–384
  in Germany, 407
  interaction with Kleinian
      development, 413–417
    Sandler, 416–417
    Winnicott, 413–416
  Kleinian development, 408–413
    clinical evidence, 412–413
    clinical task, 412
    psychic reality and psychic
        conflict, 409–411
  public health and development of
      research, 418–419
Evaluation of patient for psychoanalysis,
    257–258
  vs. clinical psychiatric evaluation, 258
  goals of, 257, 258
  psychiatric diagnosis and, 257–258
Event-related potentials (ERPs),
    activation by stimuli, 468
Evolutionary origin of Bowlby's
    attachment theory, 338, 485–486
Evolutionary psychology, 485–486
Ewers, Heinz, 492
Exercise of capacities, 10–11
Exner, Sigmund, 459
Expectations, 119
Explicit (declarative) memory, 132, 223,
    466
Ey, Henry, 430, 437
Eysenck, H. J., 465

Faimberg, H., 193
Fain, Michel, 426
Fairbairn, W. Ronald D., 32, 50, 58, 59,
    60, 62–63, 103, 104, 136, 226, 397,
    408, 413
  concept of "masochistic defense," 63
  concept of schizoid phenomena, 50, 63
  concept of separation anxiety, 63
  concept of "state of affairs" dreams,
    32

followers of, 63
object relations theory of, 62–63, 136
psychoanalytic technique of, 63
view of psychopathology, 179
Family
  child's relationships with, 41–49
    extended family, 48–49
    father, 43–45
    grandparents, 46–47
    mother, 41–43
    parental couple, 45
    siblings, 45–46
    steprelatives, 48
  working with, in child analysis, 268,
    277–278
"Family Romances" (S. Freud), 509
Fantasy
  activity and passivity in the mind,
    521
  of child about mother's body, 42
  narcissistic, 30
  in relational models, 138
  role in internalization of self-object
      relations, 51
  self-reflective, 30
  of sexual gratification, 30
  unconscious, 29–30, 31, 51, 190, 409
    object relations theory and, 59–
      60, 409
Fast, I., 101
Father
  child's relationship with, 43–45
    boys, 43–44
    girls, 44–45
  developmental tasks of, 44
  establishment of incest barrier by, 43,
    44
  mother's relationship with, 43
Favez-Boutonier, Juliette, 425
Fechner, Gustav, 459
Feder, Luis, 445
Federn, Paul, 242, 381, 391
Feldman, F., 303
Feldman, M., 62, 206, 418
Felman, Shoshana, 493, 495–496
Femininity. See also Gender
  boyhood, 100, 101
  core gender and, 100
  Freud's view of, 95, 96, 97, 98
  Horney's view of, 98
  Jones's view of, 98
  primary, 98–99
  proto-femininity phase, 100
Feminism, psychoanalytic, 93, 94
Feminist critique, 104–105
Fempner, Salomé, 441

Fenichel, Otto, 204, 245, 247, 302, 397,
    441, 528
FEPAL (Brazil), 436, 444
Ferenczi, Sandor, 77, 108, 135, 202–203,
    207, 208, 209, 210, 222, 225, 246,
    249, 381, 383, 388, 391, 392, 408,
    409, 481, 494, 497
  concept of therapeutic action, 219
  view of transference, 202
Ferro, Antonio, 279
Feske, U., 471
"Fetishism," 509
Feuerbach, Ludwig, 376
Financial dealings with patients, 289
Financial support for process research,
    327
Fine, B. D., 368
First Idea, The (Stanley Greenspan), 338
Fischer, N., 48
Fiske, John, 394
Fleigel, Z. O., 96
Fleming, J., 123, 397
Flexner Report, 391
Fliess, Wilhelm, 378, 379, 424, 491, 492
Fluoxetine, 261
Follow-up studies, 310
Fonagy, Peter, 58, 131–140, 166, 246,
    277, 301, 321, 364, 370, 419, 444,
    465, 469
  concept of mentalization, 168, 269
  concept of reflective function, 118,
    119, 470
  psychoanalytic view of attachment
      theory, 167–168
  studies of attachment status and
      psychotherapy, 471, 472
  view of therapeutic action, 224–225
  view of transference and
      countertransference, 208
"Formulations on the Two Principles of
    Mental Functioning" (S. Freud),
    509
Forrester, John, 459
Forsyth, Dan, 486
Fosshage, J., 210
Foucault, Michel, 109, 283
Foutopoulou, Katerina, 542
Fraiberg, Selma, 126, 166
FRAMES (Fundamental Repetitive and
    Maladaptive Emotion Structures),
    321, 322, 324, 325–326
Frank, Jerome, 537
Frazer, James G., 480, 481
Free association, 35, 197
  Freud's method of, 35, 197, 378
  function of, 35

relation to children's play, 268–269
as requirement for analytic process, 230–231
unconscious motivation and, 15
Freedman, N., 326
Freidman, Stanford, 243
Freidman, Susan, 243
French psychoanalysis, 423–432
Association Psychanalytique de France, 426
Confrontations, 427
Freud and, 423
interaction with English approaches, 407
Lacan and, 424–425
École Freudienne de Paris, 425–428
Loewenstein and, 424
Marie Bonaparte and, 424
non-Lacanian, in early 1960s, 425–427
Organisation Psychanalytique de Langue Française (Fourth Group), 428, 429
post–World War II, 424
psychoanalytic thought, 430–432
Anzieu, 430
Aulagnier, 432
Green, 432
Laplanche, 430–431
Pontalis, 431
resistance to, 423
Société Psychoanalytique de Paris, 424, 425, 426–427, 428
stereotyped view of, 430
succession of schisms in, 427–428
training of analysts, 428–430
in World War II years, 424
Freud, Anna, 10, 24, 28, 29, 120, 135, 150, 162, 167, 174, 196, 234, 236, 274, 276, 277, 339, 379, 382, 392, 393, 394, 399, 412, 413, 416, 494, 502
developmental model of, 134, 176
The Ego and the Mechanisms of Defense, 383
observations of children, 176, 335
in war situations, 337
Freud, Biologist of the Mind (Frank Sulloway), 455
Freud, Sigmund, 3–18, 21–35, 40, 43, 47, 48, 49, 84, 93, 102–105, 109–110, 119–120, 126, 135, 149, 159, 168, 193, 194–195, 201–204, 205, 222, 223, 225, 226, 232, 233–234, 241–251, 281–288, 290, 291, 317,

318, 328, 329, 352, 362, 364, 366, 367, 368, 375–384, 387, 389, 390, 391, 403, 408, 409, 410, 412, 423, 424, 431, 435, 444, 447, 463–464, 465, 479, 480, 481, 482, 484, 486, 494, 497, 502, 506, 508, 509, 520, 522, 525, 531, 535–537, 540, 541, 542, 543–544
birth and family of, 376
classical developmental model of psychopathology, 132, 173–175
classical psychoanalytic tradition and, 132–133
concept of babies' protection from overstimulation, 175
concept of death instinct, 5, 27, 382
concept of dynamic unconscious, 21–35, 189–190, 375, 379–380
dream formation, 31–34
intrapsychic conflict, 28–29
multiple determinism, 25
multiple function, 25
pleasure principle, 4–5, 25–26, 120
primary and secondary process, 27–28, 189, 190
psychic determinism, 23–25, 285–286, 377
reality principle, 26, 411
repetition compulsion, 4–5, 27
unconscious motivation, 15–16, 22–23
concept of instinctual drives, 3, 4–6, 13–14, 17, 132, 382, 543
object relations theory and, 58–59
concept of narcissism, 4, 5, 175, 191–192
concept of overdetermination, 25, 494
concept of psychoanalytic process, 317–318
concept of repetition compulsion, 4–5, 195
concept of self, 5–6, 12
concept of symptom formation, 34–35
concept of therapeutic action, 217–219
death of, 413
development of psychoanalysis by, 375–384
later years and major foci of dissent, 383–384
theoretical revisions and the beginning of a movement, 380–383

developmental model of, 132–133, 191–192
dislike of America, 388, 402
education of, 376
emigration to London, 393
ethics of, 281–283, 285–288
determinism, 285–286
egoistic hedonism, 286
ethical relativism, 281, 286–287
influence on French psychoanalysis, 423
lectures at Clark University, 381, 387, 388, 463
neuroscience research of, 535–537
patients of
early cases, 377–378
Elisabeth Von R., 377–378
Hilda Doolittle (H.D.), 203, 243–244
Little Hans, 47, 175, 284
Rat Man, 47, 226, 244
van der Leeuw, 244
Wolf Man, 47, 242–243, 250, 251
publications of
"Analysis Terminable and Interminable," 217, 245–246, 248
On Aphasia: A Critical Study, 377
Beyond the Pleasure Principle, 382
Civilization and Its Discontents, 287
"Constructions in Analysis," 217
"Family Romances," 509
"Fetishism," 509
"Formulations on the Two Principles of Mental Functioning," 509
Future of an Illusion, 286
On the History of the Psychoanalytic Movement, 381
Inhibitions, Symptoms and Anxiety, 383
The Interpretation of Dreams, 32, 34, 35, 218, 375, 379, 402, 455, 502
"Leonardo da Vinci and a Memory of His Childhood," 509
"Moral Responsibility for the Content of Dreams," 286
"Mourning and Melancholia," 509
"New Introductory Lectures," 244
Papers in Applied Psychology, 377, 453, 455
Papers on Metapsychology, 382

Freud *(continued)*
publications of *(continued)*
"Papers on Technique," 234
"Project for a Scientific Psychology," 378, 384, 535–536
The Psychopathology of Everyday Life, 379
"Remembering, Repeating and Working-Through," 195
Studies on Hysteria, 217, 218, 377, 502
"The Note Upon 'The Mystic Writing Pad,'" 509
"The Splitting of the Ego in the Process of Defense," 509
"The Uncanny," 509
Three Essays on the Theory of Sexuality, 95, 103, 105, 219, 380, 454
Totem and Taboo, 480, 481, 482
"'Wild' Psycho-Analysis," 509
studies of hysteria, 376–379
technique of, 202, 234
free association, 35, 197, 378
hypnosis, 377, 378
observational method, 149, 377
"pressure technique," 378
termination, 242–246
transference and countertransference, 194–195, 201–204, 222, 232
transference resistance, 234, 378
theory of large-group psychology, 526–527
theory of motivation, 3, 4–6
aggression, 4, 5, 14–15, 17
dualism in, 4, 5
instinctual drives, 3, 6, 13–14
object relations theory and, 5
pleasure principle, 4–5, 25–26, 120
self-preserving instincts, 4, 5
sexuality, 4, 5, 6, 13–14, 17
species-preserving instincts, 4, 5
tension reduction, 5, 10
unconscious motivation, 15–16, 22–23
theory of primal crime, 481
theory of sexuality, 4, 5, 6, 13–14, 17, 93, 95–99, 191, 380
castration anxiety, 96, 98
childhood sexual trauma as origin of hysteria, 375, 377, 378, 379
erotogenic zones, 6, 104, 174, 191
fetishization of genitals, 96
heterosexuality and homosexuality, 105
idealization of phallic masculinity, 95, 99
infantile sexuality, 6, 14, 105, 132, 375, 380
as instinctual drive, 3, 6, 13–15
normality and illness, 105
Oedipus complex, 97–98, 174, 191, 378, 459
penis envy, 96, 98, 191
perversion and normality, 110
phases of psychosexual development, 6, 13, 120, 174, 191
view of femininity, 95, 96, 97, 98, 383
theory of the mind
structural, 7, 28, 190–191
topographical, 190, 244–245, 379–380
thoughts on development of concepts, 362
trauma-affect model of, 190
uses of interdisciplinary resources by, 453–460
anthropology, 480–481
arts, 502, 503–505, 509
beginnings of applied analysis, 453–454
development of applied analysis, 454–456
limitations of psychoanalytic data for interdisciplinary inquiry, 456–457
literature, 491–493
potential of psychoanalysis for interdisciplinary studies, 457–458
sources for psychoanalytic theory, 458–459
view of analytic process, 232
view of child psychoanalysis, 175
view of child's early relationships
with animals, 47
with father, 43
with mother, 41–42
view of happiness, 287
view of morality, 281
view of psychic reality, 193
view of psychoanalysis as value-free science, 281–282
Freud and Man's Soul (Bruno Bettelheim), 454
Friedman, L., 133, 234
Fries, Margaret, 394
Frink, H. W., 391
Fromm, Erich, 209, 282, 395, 396
Fromm-Reichmann, Frieda, 60, 65, 393–394, 399
Frosch, J., 48
Functional Emotional Developmental Approach, 339–340
Fundamental Repetitive and Maladaptive Emotion Structures (FRAMES), 321, 322, 324, 325–326
Furman, E., 42
Future-oriented mental processes, 126

Gabbard, Glen O., 178, 206, 220, 223, 224, 231, 267, 292, 293, 294, 319
view of analytic process, 232
view of transference and countertransference, 211–212, 234
Gagnon, J., 100
Galatzer-Levy, R., 307, 308
Gallagher, D., 325
Ganzarain, Ramón, 446
Garcia, Antonio, 445
Gardiner, Muriel, 391
Gardner, M. Robert, 397
Garfield, R., 45
Garma, Angel, 436, 442, 444, 446, 448
Garma, Elizabeth, 437
Gaskill, Herbert, 400
Gaskill Report, 400
Gaston, L., 325
Gay, Peter, 376, 455
Gay liberation, 18
Gazzaniga, M. S., 541
Geahchan, Dominique, 427
Gedo, J. E., 317
Geertz, Clifford, 102
Gehring, George, 387, 394
Gender, 93–102. *See also* Sexuality
attachment-individuation theories of, 100–101
child's awareness of, 100
core, 100
Freud's theory of, 95–97
the anatomical difference, 96
fetishization of genitals, 96
penis and phallocentrism, 96
view of femininity, 95, 96, 97
ideological, 97
nominal, 97
object relations theories of, 99
"over-inclusiveness," 101, 109
as personal idiom, 102
phallic masculinity/personal maleness, 99

polarity of, 94
postmodern studies of, 94–95
primary femininity, 98–99
psychoanalytic anthropology studies
    of, 487–488
    men's cults, 487–488
psychoanalytic feminism, 93, 94
psychological, 94, 95
relation to sexuality, 94, 102
self-designation of, 100
subjective, 97
as symbolic resource and relational
    strategy, 100–101
theoretical, 94
Gender dysphoria, 95
Gender identity, 50, 100
    from dualism to multiplicity, 102
    feminist critique and, 104–105
Gender Ideology and Psychological Reality
    (M. E. Spiro), 487
Gender nonconformity, 95
Genetic factors and psychopathology,
    180
"Genetic fallacy," 133
Genital anxiety, 99
Gergely, G., 269
German Psychoanalytical Association, 304
Gerö, Georg, 442
Gesell, Arnold, 394
Ghent, E., 211
Gifford, Sanford, *387–403*
Gill, Merton, 150, 210, 234, 321, 496
Gillespie, W., 408
Gilman, Sander, 95
Gilmore, David, 487
Gitelson, Frances, 437
Gitelson, M., 121
Glas de Langer, Marie, 436
Global Assessment of Functioning, 473
Glover, Edward, 217–219, 225, 246,
    247, 250, 303, 413
Goals of psychoanalysis, 235–236, 247,
    535
    ethics and, 282–283, 292–293
    life goals and, 293
God, child's belief in, 49
Goethe, Johann Wolfgang con, 491
Goldberg, D. A., 305
Goldner, Virginia, *93–110*
González, Avelino, 437
"Good enough" mother, 41, 64, 179,
    415
Goodman, S., 119
Gorbachev, Mikhail, 529
Gorer, Geoffrey, 484
Göring, Erna, 443

Göring Institute (Berlin), 443
Gosliner, B. J., 43
Goya, Francisco, 506, 507
Graf, Max, 381
Graff-Radford, Neill, 543
Grandparents
    child's relationship with, 46–47
    mother's relationship with, 43
Granoff, Wladimir, 426
Gray, Paul, 205, 234
Green, André, 78, 79, 102, 242, 249,
    366, 407, 432, 440, 444
    Le Discours Vivant, 432
    "The Dead Mother," 432
Greenacre, Phyllis, 175, 456, 507, 508
Greenberg, H. R., 59, 60, 65, 66
Greenberg, J. R., 236
Greenberg, Jay, 212, *217–226*
Greenson, Ralph, 204, 212, 397
Greenspan, Stanley I., *335–355*
    concept of stages of mental
        development, 339–340
    The First Idea, 338
    Functional Emotional Developmen-
        tal Approach, 339–340
Greenwald, A. G., 464
Gregor, Thomas, 487
Gribinski, Michel, 431
Grinberg, León, 437
Grinker, Roy, 395, 399
Grinstein, A., 491
Groddeck, Georg, 394
Grossmann, K., 469
Grotjahn, Martin, 393, 394, 399, 493
Grotstein, 291
Group therapy, 399
Guilt, 192
Guntrip, H., 60, 63, 135, 179, 226

Habit Clinic (Boston), 394
Hadley, Ernest, 392
Haith, Marshall, 121
Hale, N. G., Jr., 390
Hall, Clark, 457
Hall, G. Stanley, 387, 388, 389, 394
Halton, A., 15
Hamilton, C., 469, 470
Hamilton, Victoria, 458
Hamilton Depression Rating Scale, 263
Hamlet and Oedipus (Ernest Jones), 492
Hampstead Index Project, 363, 367
Happiness, 513, 522
    Freud's view of, 287
Hardy, G. E., 471
Hargreaves, Ronald, 457
Harlow, Harry, 457–458

Harris, Adrienne, 95, 101, *201–213*
Hartmann, Heinz, 6, 18, 50, 66, 118,
    224, 282, 283, 383, 393, 403, 424,
    494, 502
    concept of "average expectable
        environment," 18, 47, 48, 383
    concept of ego, 10, 120
    concept of "fitting together," 51
    concept of self, 12
    developmental model of, 10, 120, 133
    distinction of self and ego, 50
    "Ego Psychology and the Problems
        of Adaptation," 394
Hatred, in transference and
    countertransference, 202, 208
Haynal, A., 79
Haynal-Reymond, V., 79
Hazen, N., 165
H.D. (Hilda Doolittle), 203, 243–244
Health insurance coverage for
    psychoanalysis, 402–403
Healy, William, 391
Hedonism, egoistic, 286
Heimann, Paula, 195, 207, 221, 416,
    437, 496
    view of transference and
        countertransference, 208, 418
Heinicke, Christoph, 160
Heller, Hugo, 381
Heller, M., 79
Helplessness
    signal anxiety and, 120
    signal depression and, 120
Hendrick, Ives, 10, 282, 391, 393, 396,
    458
Henry, W. P., 310
Hermaphroditic children, 94
Hernández, Max, 447
Herrmann, Fábio, 444
Herzog, J., 44
Hesse, E., 166
Heterosexuality, 105. *See also* Sexuality
Hill, C., 324
Hilsenroth, M. J., 325, 329, 330
Hinde, Robert, 457, 458
Hinkle, Beatrice, 390
Hinz, H., 418
Hirsch, I., 209, 210
History of psychoanalysis
    in the French community, 423–432
    Freud and the early years, 375–384
        later years and major foci of
            dissent, 383–384
        theoretical revisions and the
            beginning of a movement,
            380–383

History of psychoanalysis (continued)
    in Great Britain and Continental
        Europe, 407–419
    in Latin America, 435–448
    in North America from 1895 to
        present, 387–403
Histrionic personality disorder,
    Kernberg's view of, 181
Hitler, Adolf, 393
Hoch, Paul, 437
Hoffman, Irwin, 138, 211, 212, 221,
    282, 321
Hoffmann, E. T. A., 492
"Holding environment," 64–65, 123,
    132, 415, 509
Holland, N. N., 494, 498
Holt, R., 455
Home for Little Wanderers (Boston),
    394
Homeostatic motivation power of
    resistance to change, 11–12
Homosexuality, 70, 105. See also
    Sexuality
    Freud's view of, 95, 105
    new narratives of, 106–107
    normality and illness, 105
Horney, Karen, 96, 204, 209, 383, 398
    in America, 395–396
    critique of Freud's oedipal thesis, 98
    view of femininity, 98
Horowitz, Donald, 531
Horowitz, Mardi J., 119, 321, 322, 325
Hostility
    in dreams, 34
    in transference and
        countertransference, 202, 208
Housekeepers, child's relationship with,
    49
HRAF (Human Relations Area Files),
    483
Hughlings Jackson, John, 191
Human Animal, The (Weston Labarre),
    486
Human Relations Area Files (HRAF),
    483
Humility of analyst, 291
Hurvich, M., 326
Hurwitz, Rosetta, 392
Hussein, Saddam, 530
Husserl, Edmund, 82
Huxley, Julian, 457
Hyman, H., 302
Hypnosis, Freud's use of, 377, 378
Hypochondriasis, Freudian view of, 175
Hysteria, Freud's studies of, 217, 218,
    376–379, 502

Id
    Freud's concept of, 7, 28, 190
    neuroscientific research on, 543–544
IDE, 442
Identity diffusion, 58
Idiosyncrasy of meaning, 521–522
IJP (Internal Journal of Psychoanalysis),
    319
Implicit learning, 466–467
    automated, 467
Implicit (procedural) memory, 132, 223–
    224, 367, 466
Implicit prejudice, 467
Imprinting, 160
Inanimate surround, child's relationship
    with, 47–48
Incest barrier, 45
    father's establishment of, 43, 44
Inderbitzen, L. B., 236
Individual psychology, 381
Infant. See also Children
    ability to infer intentions of others,
        81
    crying of, 11
    early relationships of, 39–51 (See also
        Early relationships)
    mother's contingent mirroring of
        affect of, 58, 123
    psychoanalytic observation of, 136
Infantile amnesia, 133
Infantile neurosis, 174
Infantile sexuality, 6, 14, 104, 105, 132,
    375, 380
Information processing, 21
    unconscious, 21–35
Informed consent, 289
    for publication of case material in
        journals, 319
    for use of patient information in
        presentations, 289
    for use of psychotropic medications,
        259
Ingham, John, 486
Ingres, Jean, 506
Inhelder, Barbel, 457
Inhibitions, Symptoms and Anxiety
    (S. Freud), 383
Initial consultation, 257
Institut Psychanalytique de Montréal,
    430
Institute for Juvenile Research
    (Chicago), 394, 399
Institute for Psychoanalytic Training
    and Research (IPTAR), 326, 402
Institute of Psychosomatics (IPSO),
    426

Institutes for analytic training. See also
    specific institutes
    establishment of, 391–393
    Europeanization of, 393–394
    splitting of, 395–397
Interdisciplinary studies in
    psychoanalysis
    anthropology, 479–488
    arts, 501–509
    Freud's uses of, 453–460
        beginnings of applied analysis,
            453–454
        interdisciplinary sources of
            psychoanalytic theory, 458–
            459
        limitations of psychoanalytic data
            for interdisciplinary inquiry,
            456–457
        pitfall and potential of applied
            analysis, 454–456
        potential of psychoanalysis for
            interdisciplinary studies,
            457–458
    literature, 491–499
    neuroscience, 535–545
    philosophy, 513–522
    politics and international relations,
        525–532
    psychology, 463–474
Internal Journal of Psychoanalysis (IJP),
    319
Internal (psychic) reality, 193–194
    après-coup and, 194
    definition of, 193
    Freud's view of, 193
Internal working models (IWMs), 161–
    162
    attachment security and, 164
    babies' behavior in Strange Situation
        and, 163
    definition of, 161
Internalization of psychoanalyst, 248–
    250
International Congress of Psychoanaly-
    sis, 381
International Journal of Psychoanalysis,
    408, 411, 441
International Psychoanalytical
    Association (IPA)
    Argentina and, 436, 437, 438, 439
    Brazil and, 440, 441, 442, 443,
        444
    Chile and, 446–447
    Colombia and, 447
    France and, 424, 425
    Mexico and, 445

North America and, 381, 388–389, 391–392, 400–401
Peru and, 447
Uruguay and, 446
Venezuela and, 445
Working Group on Terror and Terrorism, 532
International relations. *See* Politics, international relations, and psychoanalysis
International Training Commission, 391, 392, 401
Interpersonal object relations theory, 60
Interpersonal relationships
  attachment theory, 159–169 (*See also* Attachment; Attachment theory)
  psychology and, 468–473
  early relationships of child, 39–51 (*See also* Early relationships)
Interpersonal tradition, 138
  Sullivan's theory and, 65, 138
  view of interpretation, 237
  view of resistance, 234
  view of transference and countertransference, 209–210
Interpersonal World of the Infant, The (Daniel Stern), 139
Interpretation(s), 197, 235–238
  case example of, 237–238
  in child analysis, 270, 273–274
  claims of cure by, 217–218
  definition of, 235
  in developmental orientation, 124–125
  ego psychologists' view of, 236, 237
  ethics and, 288
  inexact, 219
  interpersonalists' view of, 237
  intersubjective analysts' view of, 237
  Loewald's view of, 236
  mutative, 220, 236
  neutrality of analyst in, 236
  object relations theorists' view of, 237
  vs. other technical interventions, 235
  of preconscious experience, 235
  process of, 236, 238
  vs. relationship in effecting change, 236
  relationship to therapeutic goals, 235–236
  reliability of, 237
  of resistance, 233, 235
  self psychologists' view of, 237
  sequence of preparation for, 235
  Strachey's view of, 236

validity of, 237
view of primacy in therapeutic action, 219
Interpretation of Dreams, The (S. Freud), 32, 34, 35, 218, 375, 379, 402, 455, 502
Intersex children, 96
Intersubjectivity, 77–90
  autism and, 81
  as basic and independent tendency of mind, 82–85
  children's imaginary companions and, 84
  clinical implications of, 85–90
    dialogue of relational moves, 86–87
    now moments and moments of meeting, 89–90
    sloppiness and co-creativity of analytic process, 88–89
  compared with classical approach to psychoanalysis, 77–78
  consciousness and, 79
  core, 80
  definitions of, 77, 78–80
  vs. empathy, 79
  falling in love and, 84–85
  imaginary, 80
  interpretation and, 237
  morality and, 83–84
  motivational system and, 83–85
  nature and development of, 80–82
  neurobiological mechanisms of, 80–81
  one-way, 79–80
  phenomenological philosophy and, 82
  in preverbal infant, 80–81
  psychological belongingness and, 83
  reflective consciousness and, 84
  role in species survival, 83–84
  schools of psychoanalysis based on, 77, 138, 182
  self-other differentiation and, 80
  of sexuality, 103
  transference, countertransference and, 80, 210
  two-way, 79
  verbal and nonverbal sources of, 80
Intrapsychic conflict, 28–29
  object relations theories of, 69
Inuit Morality Play (Jean Briggs), 487
IPA (International Psychoanalytical Association), 381, 388–389, 391–392, 400–401, 424, 425
IPSO (Institute of Psychosomatics), 426

IPTAR (Institute for Psychoanalytic Training and Research), 326, 402
Irigaray, L., 99
Isaacs, Susan, 408
Isham, Mary, 390
Israeli–Egyptian dialogues, 532
Iverson, Margaret, 502
IWMs. *See* Internal working models

J. J. Putnam Children's Center (Boston), 394
Jacobovitz, D., 165
Jacobs, T., 205–206
Jacobson, D., 492–493
Jacobson, Edith, 6, 50, 58, 59, 60, 66, 120, 133, 135, 443
  concept of superego, 66
  developmental model of, 133
  focus on affective processes, 66
  object relations theory of, 66
James, Henry, 495
James, William, 387, 388, 463–464
Janet, Pierre, 377, 387
Jelliffe, Smith Ely, 387, 389, 394, 537
Jessner, Lucie, 393
Joffe, W. G., 416
Johns Hopkins Medical School, 389
Johnson, Allen, 486
Johnson, M., 268
Johnson, Samuel, 400
Jones, E. E., 323, 329, 330
Jones, Enrico, 312
Jones, Ernest, 96, 244, 282, 285, 302, 388, 389, 459, 481
  formation of British Psychoanalytical Society by, 382
  Freud and, 381–382
  Hamlet and Oedipus, 492
  interaction with Klein, 408
  International Psychoanalytical Association and, 392, 393, 398, 412, 413, 436, 441, 442, 443
  view of femininity, 98
Jornal de Psicanálise, 442
Joseph, Betty, 194, 412, 416, 417, 444
  "close process" technique of, 412
  view of perversion, 207
  view of projective identification in consulting room, 411
  view of transference and countertransference, 206
Josiah Macy Foundation, 399
Journal of Nervous and Mental Disease, 389
Journal of the American Psychoanalytic Association, 368

Journals. *See also specific journals*
    ethics of publishing clinical material
        in, 319
Judge Baker Guidance Center (Boston),
        394, 399
Jung, Carl, 149, 219, 366, 381, 384, 388,
        389, 390, 395, 454, 459, 487
Jungian School of Psychoanalysis
        (Venezuela), 445
Jurist, E. L., 269

Kächele, H., 301, 310, 321
Kafka, Franz, 498
Kaftal, E., 99
Kamm, Bernard, 394
Kandel, Eric, 473–474, 539, 540
Kant, Immanuel, 506, 519
Kantrowitz, Judith, 307, 317, 318, 319,
        320, 363
Kaplan, N., 470
Kaplan-Solms, Karen, 539, 540
KAPP (Karolinska Psychodynamic
        Profile), 311
Karazić, Radovan, 530
Kardiner, Abram, 396, 398
    model of Basic Personality Structure,
        482–483
    studies of Marquesas Islanders, 483
Karolinska Psychodynamic Profile
        (KAPP), 311
Karpman, Ben, 392
Katz, A. L., 307
Kaufman, M. Ralph, 391, 394, 395, 398
Kemper, Katrin, 442, 443
Kemper, Werner, 442–443
Kempf, Edward J., 389, 399
Kenworthy, Marion, 390
Kernberg, Otto F., 8, 15, 50, *57–74*, 110,
        174, 312, 339, 349, 402, 440, 444,
        446, 527
    concept of affects, 68
    concept of borderline personality
        organization, 68
    concept of drives, 67–68
    concept of neurotic personality
        organization, 68
    concept of pathological grandiose
        self, 68
    concept of personality disorders, 68,
        181
    developmental model of, 137–138
    ego psychology–object relations
        theory of, 60, 67–68, 137–138
    view of psychopathology, 181–182
Kernberg, Paulina, 181, 446
Kerr, John, *453–460*

Kessel, L., 302
Kessler, S., 96
Kestenberg, J., 98
Kilmann, P. R., 471
King, Pearl, 412
Kirsner, Douglas, 397
Kizer, Manuel, 445
Klein, G. S., 10, 16, 29–30, 150
Klein, Melanie, 50, 58, 59, 60, 64, 96,
        106, 178, 190, 192, 195, 196, 206,
        246–247, 274, 366, 382, 397, 399,
        402, 408–413, 414, 415, 417, 418,
        437, 439, 444, 468, 495, 503
    concept of depressive position, 61,
        62, 135–136, 178, 192, 410
        manic defenses, 62
        pathological mourning, 62
        psychosis, 62
    concept of ego development, 62, 178
    concept of oedipal complex, 62
    concept of paranoid-schizoid
        position, 61–62, 135–136, 178,
        192, 409–410
    concept of projective identification,
        61, 136, 417–418
    concept of reparative impulses, 192
    concept of "total situation," 412
    concept of transference and
        countertransference, 62, 195,
        206–207, 412
    concept of unconscious fantasy, 190
    followers of, 62
    impact on psychoanalytic theory and
        practice in Europe, 409
    importance of clinical evidence to
        views of, 412–413
    Jones's interactions with, 408
    object relations theory of, 61–62,
        135–136
    view of mental function, 410–411
    view of psychic reality, 409–410
    view of psychopathology, 178–179
    Winnicott's modification of theories
        of, 414–415
Kluckhohn, Clyde, 398, 484
Kluckhohn, Florence, 398
Kluckhohn, R., 483
Knapp, P. H., 304
Knight, Robert P., 303, 394, 399, 403
Koch, Adelheid Lucy, 440, 441
Kohut, Heinz, 6, 17, 60, 65, 123, 180,
        241, 282, 283, 293, 339, 349, 366,
        368, 394, 402, 440, 495
    concept of empathy as "vicarious
        introspection," 124
    concept of "self-state dreams," 32

theory of self psychology, 12, 137
    interpersonal object relations
        theory and, 60
    Winnicott's object relations
        theory and, 65
Koolhaas, Gilberto, 446
Korsgaard, Christine, 519
Koslowski, B., 341
Kracke, Waud, 487
Kramer, Selma, 119
Krause, R., 301, 321
Kravitz, Henry, 398
Kris, Ernst, 8, 239, 244, 368, 393, 394,
        399, 494, 502
    theories in relation to arts and
        psychoanalysis, 505–507
Kris, Marianne, 399
Kristeva, Julia, 109, 485, 502
Kroeber, Alfred, 398
Krutch, Joseph Wood, 493
Kuhn, Thomas, 363, 403

LaBarre, Weston, 484, 486
Lacan, Jacques, 60, 95, 97, 107–108,
        110, 196, 209, 249, 366, 402, 424–
        426, 427–429, 430, 431, 432, 440,
        444, 445, 446, 495
    concept of mirror stage, 425
    death of, 428
    École Freudienne de Paris of, 425–
        428
    literary analysis and, 495–496
    proposal for training School Analyst,
        427–428
    Séminaire of, 424, 428
    "Speech and Language in
        Psychoanalysis," 430
    view of transference and
        countertransference, 209
Laforgue, René, 423
Lagache, Daniel, 424, 425, 426, 430,
        431, 442
Laing, R. D., 498
Laius complex, 44
Lakoff, G., 268
Langer, Susanne, 505
Langer, Walter, 392
Language of Psychoanalysis, The
        (Laplanche and Pontalis), 94
Laplanche, Jean, 103, 109, 110, 368,
        426, 430–431, 444
    concept of *étayage*, 431
    Psychanalyse à l'Université, 430
    theory of seduction, 430
    translation of Freud's works by, 430
    Vocabulaire de la Psychanalyse, 430, 431

Large-group psychology, 526–528
accordion phenomenon and, 531
minor differences and, 531
regression and rituals, 531
tent metaphor for, 529–531
chosen glories and chosen traumas, 529–530
time collapse, 530–531
Lasky, R. H., 326
Laswell, Harold, 526
Latency phase of development, child's relationship with parental couple during, 45
Latin American psychoanalysis, 196, 207, 435–448
in Argentina, 435–440
in Brazil, 440–445
in Chile, 446–447
in Colombia, 447
in Mexico, 445
in Peru, 447
in Uruguay, 446
in Venezuela, 445–446
Laughlin, J. E., 471
Lax, R., 45
Layton, L. B., 106
Lear, Jonathan, *513–522*
Learning, implicit, 466–467
Leavy, Barbara Fass, 455
Lebovici, Serge, 427, 437
Leclaire, Serge, 430, 440
LeDoux, Joseph, 538, 541–542
Leigh, T., 470, 471
Lemmertz, José, 444
"Leonardo da Vinci and a Memory of His Childhood," 509
Les Temps Modernes (journal), 431
Lester, E. P., 294
Levenson, Edgar, 209, 210, 224
Lévi-Strauss, Claude, 485
Levin, Fred, 538
Levin, Kenneth, 455
Levin, S., 304, 394
Levy, A. T., 236
Levy, Kenneth N., *463–474*
Lewes, K., 98
Lewicki, P., 466–467
Lewin, Bertram, 396, 403
Lewis, J. M., 138
Liberman, David, 440, 444, 448
Libet, B., 542
Libidinal development, 22–23
Libido theory. *See also* Sexuality
of Freud, 4, 5, 6, 13–14, 17, 380, 382

in one-person and two-person psychologies, 103
of Person, 103
Libres Cahiers Pour la Psychanalyse (journal), 431
Lichtenberg, J. D., 10, 17
Lieberman, Alicia, 166
Life instinct, in Kleinian object relations theory, 61
Limentani, Adam, 437
Lin, Maya, 502
Lins de Almeida, José, 444
Linton, Ralph, 396, 398, 483
Lipton, Samuel, 203, 244
Literature and psychoanalysis, 491–499
changing relationship between, 493–494
developments in psychoanalysis, 494–496
contemporary perspectives, 496
decline of reductionism, 494
ego psychology, 494
Lacan, 495–496
object relations, 495
reevaluation of countertransference, 496
new ways of reading literature, 496–497
Freud's applied analysis and, 491–493
elaboration and critique of, 492–493
Freud as sensitive listener and conquistador, 491–492
reaction to psychoanalytic literary analysis, 493
as mutual endeavor, 497–498
Little, Margaret, 207, 208, 496
view of countertransference, 208
Little Albert case (Watson), 466
Little Hans case (S. Freud), 47, 175, 284
Lizarazo, Arturo, 447
Lloyd, A., 486
Lobo, Amilcar, 443
Loewald, Hans, 4, 5, 17, 43, 59, 124, 125, 232, 247
concept of therapeutic action, 121
developmental model of, 133–134
view of analytic process, 232
view of analytic relationship and therapeutic action, 220
view of interpretation, 236
view of transference and countertransference, 205
Loewenberg, Peter, 397
Loewenstein, Rudolph, 235, 393, 424

London Hampstead Index Project, 363, 367
London Psycho-Analytical Society, 382
London Psychoanalytic Clinic, outcome studies at, 302
Lopez-Ballesteros, Luis, 447
Lorenz, Konrad, 9, 457, 460
Los Angeles Psychoanalytic Society, 397
Love
Freud's view of, 287–288
"love commandment" as antidote to aggression, 288
intersubjectivity and falling in love, 84–85
Luborsky, L., 119, 321, 322, 325, 329, 365
Lyons-Ruth, Karlen, 85, 165, 166
psychoanalytic view of attachment theory, 167
relational diathesis model of, 167

Macalpine, Ida, 204, 437
MacIntyre, Alasdair, 289–290, 368
Mack Brunswick, Ruth, 242, 243, 251
MacLeod, Alastair, 398
Macnaughton, Dorothy, 398
Madow, Leo, 396
Maeder, LeRoy, 396
Maenchen, Anna, 394
Magritte, René, 506
Mahler, Margaret, 6, 43, 58, 59, 60, 66, 67, 80, 120, 150, 175, 249, 335, 339, 342, 352, 363, 393, 440, 495, 503, 509
observations of children, 176–178
separation-individuation theory of, 58, 67, 134–135, 176–177
in analysis of borderline conditions, 67, 135, 177
criticisms of, 178
differentiation (hatching) subphase, 67, 134
Jacobson's theory and, 66
normal autism, 58, 67, 134, 177, 342
practicing subphase, 67
rapprochement subphase, 67, 134
role of father in child's development, 43
Searle's psychoanalytic approach and, 66
symbiosis, 58, 67, 134, 177
Mahony, P., 497
Mailloux, Noel, 398
Main, Mary, 166, 341, 469, 470
Major, René, 427

Malinowski, Bronislaw, 481, 485

Managed care, 402

Manhattan State Hospital (New York), 388, 389, 390

Manhood in the Making (David Gilmore), 487

Manic defenses, in Kleinian object relations theory, 62

Mannoni, Octave, 201, 502

MAOIs (monoamine oxidase inhibitors), 262

Mapping the Mind (Fred Levin), 538

Marcondes, Durval, 441

Marcovitz, Eli, 437

Marcus, Eric R., *229–239*

Marcus, Steven, 95, 497

Margolin, Sydney, 394, 398

Marmor, Judd, 396

Maroda, K., 210, 211

Marquesas Islanders, 483

Marti, Pierre, 426, 440

Martins, Cyro, 444

Martins, Mario Alvarez, 440, 442, 444

Martins, Zaira, 442, 444

Marucco, Norberto, 444

Masculinity, 99. *See also* Gender
core gender and, 100
Freud's view of, 95, 99

Masling, J. M., 465, 473

Massachusetts General Hospital, 389, 398, 399

Massachusetts Institute for Psychoanalysis (MIP), 402

Massachusetts Mental Health Center, 402

Masson, J. M., 379

Masten, A. S., 134

Masterson, J. F., 135, 177

Matriliny, among Normanby Islanders, 482

Matte Blanco, Ignácio, 446, 448

Mayer, E. L., 98

Mayes, Linda C., *147–155*

McCarter, R. H., 304

McDevitt, J. B., 15

McDougall, J., 106, 109, 407

McGlashan Semistructured Interview (MSI), 312

McLaughlin, F., 251

McLaughlin, J., 138

McLean Hospital (Massachusetts), 388, 401

Mead, Margaret, 398, 457, 483

Meaning-space, 364, 370
of transference, 364–365

Mechnikov, Elie, 459

Medications. *See* Psychotropic medications

Medusa's Hair (Gananath Obeyesekere), 487

Meissner, W. W., *21–36*

Melancholia, Freudian view of, 175

Meltzer, Donald, 62, 106, 437

Meltzoff, A. N., 81

Memory
declarative (explicit), 132, 223, 466
procedural (implicit), 132, 223–224, 367, 466
unreliability of recall of early experiences, 40

Mendoza Psychoanalytic Society, 438

Menninger, Karl, 248

Menninger, William, 395

Menninger Child and Family Program, The, 182–183

Menninger Clinic, The, 182–183, 394, 395
child research center at, 399
outcome studies at, 303
Psychotherapy Research Project, 307–309, 321
conclusions of, 308–309
goals of, 308
methodology of, 308

Menninger Foundation, The, 401

Men's cults, 487–488

Mental functioning
activity and passivity in the mind, 521
affect and, 21, 22
formative influence of early relationships on, 39–51
free association and, 35, 197
future-oriented, 126
motivation and, 3–18
primary and secondary process in, 27–28, 189, 190, 231
reflection function and psychic functioning, 519–520
unconscious, 21–35

Mental Mechanisms (William White), 389

Mentalization, 119
attachment theory and, 139–140, 182–183
by caregivers, 182
caregivers' responses and, 182
children's play and, 269
definition of, 182
Fonagy's concept of, 168, 269
Klein's depressive position and, 136, 415
Winnicott's theory of, 415

Mergenthaler, E., 323, 324

Merleau-Ponty, Maurice, 108, 431

Merrick, S., 470

Metapsychology, 24

Mexican Psychoanalytic Association (APM), 445

Mexican Study Group of Psychoanalytic Studies, 445

Mexico, 445

Meyer, Adolf, 387, 388, 389, 390

Meyer, B., 471

Meyer, J. K., 251

Mezan, Renato, 444

Michaels, J. J., 394

Military psychiatry in American after World War II, 395

Mill, J. S., 287

Miller, Jacques-Alain, 427, 428

Miller, N., 321, 464

Millet, John A. P., 396, 399

Milner, Marion, 413, 503

Milosević, Slobodan, 530

Mind
theory of, 7
unconscious functioning of, 21–35

Mind-cure movement, 387

MIO (MOMMY AND I ARE ONE) stimulus, 468

MIP (Massachusetts Institute for Psychoanalysis), 402

Mirror stage, 425

Mirsky, Arthur, 437

Mitchell, Juliet, 485

Mitchell, S., 22, 59, 60, 65, 66, 138, 209, 210

Mitscherlich, Alexander, 528

Modell, A., 10, 65, 135

Mom, Jorge, 438, 440

MOMMY AND I ARE ONE (MIO) stimulus, 468

Mondrian, Piet, 455–456, 507

Money, John, 94, 100

Money Kyrle, Roger, 408, 415

Monoamine oxidase inhibitors (MAOIs), 262

Monterrey Psychoanalytic Society (ARPAC), 445

Moore, B. E., 368

Moore, M. K., 81

Moral decision making, 289, 294–295
case discussions of, 295

Morality. *See also* Ethics
analytic neutrality and, 282, 284–285
vs. ethics, 281
Freud's view of, 281
intersubjectivity and, 83–84
naturalistic moral psychology, 522

of psychoanalytic practice, 281–282
standards of, 283, 286
superego and, 286
Moran, G. S., 135
Moran, Richard, 519
Morgan, A., 85
Morrison, Amy, 294
Mosheim, R., 471
Mother (caregiver)
child's relationship with, 41–43
mother's body, 41–42
mother's mental contents, 42–43
mother's presence, 42
mother's relationships, 43
contingent mirroring of infant's
affect by, 58, 123
"good enough," 41, 64, 179, 415
"phallic," 70
psychological transition to
parenthood, 154–155
role in child's developmental levels of
emotional functioning, 340–353
1: self-regulation and interest in
the world: 0–3 months, 340–
343
2: forming relationships,
attachment, and engagement:
2–7 months, 343–345
3: two-way, purposeful
communication:
3–10 months, 345–347
4: behavioral organization,
problem solving, and
internalization: 9–18 months,
347–349
5: representational capacity:
18–30 months, 349–351
6: representational differentiation:
30–48 months, 351–353
selective maternal attunement, 177
Motivation for change, 231
Motivation theory, 3–18
cultural forces and, 18
drives and, 13–15
aggression, 14–15
sexuality, 14, 22–23
ego functioning and, 10–12
anxiety signal, 11
exercise of capacities, 10–11
resistance to change, 11–12
of Freud, 3, 4–6
pleasure principle, 4–5, 25–26, 120
principle of entropy, 120
of Hartmann, 6
intersubjectivity and, 83–85
of Loewald, 4

modification of, 3
object relations and, 4, 5, 7–10
attachment, 9–10
internalized, 7–9
of Sandler, 4
superordinate concept, 15–17
agency, 16, 22
developmental needs, 16–17
unconscious motivation, 15–16,
22–23
Mourning
pathological, in Kleinian object
relations theory, 62
politics, diplomacy and, 531–532
"Mourning and Melancholia"
(S. Freud), 509
MSI (McGlashan Semistructured
Interview), 312
Müller-Braunschweig, Carl, 442
Multiple determinism, 25
Multiple function, 25, 494
Münsterberg, Hugo, 387
Murphy, Gardner, 399
Murphy, Lois, 150
Murphy, Robert, 487
Murphy, Ruth, 399
Murray, John, 391, 395
Mushatt, Cecil, 398
Mutuality, 125
Myth of the Birth of the Hero (Otto Rank),
453

Nacht, Sacha, 424
Nadel, J., 83
Nagel, Thomas, 519
Nahum, J., 85
Nannies, child's relationship with, 49
Narcissism, 196, 368
fantasies motivated by, 30
Freud's view of, 4, 5, 175, 191–192
Kohut's description of, 137
motivation and, 4, 5, 15, 22, 23
Narcissistic personality disorder, 140
Kernberg's view of, 181
Nathansohn, Amalia, 376
National Institute of Mental Health
(NIMH), 395, 399, 401
Naturalistic moral psychology, 522
Nature-nurture interaction, 40
Navarro, Allende, 446
Negentropy, 120
Nemiah, J. C., 426
Nesse, Randolph, 486
Neurasthenia, 377
Neuro-Psychoanalysis (journal), 538, 539–
540, 543

Neuro-Psychoanalysis Society, 539
Neuropsychoanalysis, 538–540
clinico-anatomical correlation in,
539, 540
direct observation of neurological
patients in psychoanalytic
setting, 539
Pfeffer's development of, 538–539
research approaches in, 540
Neuroscience and psychoanalysis, 196–
197, 535–545
advent of neuropsychoanalysis, 538–
540
future of, 544–545
historical background of, 535–537
cognitive psychology, 537
Freud, 535–537
major developments since Freud,
537–538
contributions from analyst-
neurologists, 537–538
contributions from nonanalytic
neuroscientists, 538
speculative syntheses, 538
research findings, 540–544
id, 543–544
meaning of dreams, 544
pleasure principle, 542–543
repression, 541–542
the unconscious, 540–541
Neurosis, 140
Freudian view of, 174
infantile, 174
transference, 194
Neurotic symptom formation, 34–35
Neutrality of analyst, 236
ethical aspects of, 282, 284–285
preclusion of social contacts between
patient and analyst for, 396
psychotropic medications and, 260,
262
New Criticism, 496
New Look, 464
New York Psychoanalytic Institute
Arnold Pfeffer Center for Neuro-
Psychoanalysis, 539
Ernst Kris Study Group, 368
Horney's defection from, 395
opposition to nonmedical analysts,
391–392, 400
outcome studies at, 305–306
New York Psychoanalytic Society, 390,
391, 392, 393
Nietzsche, Friedrich, 459, 522
Night terrors, 34
Nightmares, 34

NIMH (National Institute of Mental Health), 395, 399, 401
Noble, Douglas, 398
Normanby Islanders, 482
Normand, W., 255
North American psychoanalysis, 387–403
    analytic training abroad and first institutes (1925–1938), 391–393
    analytic treatment of psychosis, 399
    beginnings of analysis in America (1895–1909), 387–388
        first American Freudians, 388
        Freud's lectures at Clark University, 381, 387, 388, 463
    child psychiatry and, 394, 399
    early decades (1909–1925), 388–391
        American Psychoanalytic Association, 388–390
        antipathy to lay analysis, 390
        Baltimore and Washington, D.C., 389
        Boston, 389
        New York City, 390
    group therapy and, 399
    hospital psychiatry and, 388, 389, 390, 398–399
    immigration and Europeanization of American analysis (1933–1946), 393–394
    lean years (1968–present), 399–402
        economic factors, 402–403
        end of lay-analysis controversy, 400–401
        recent changes in American analysis, 401–402
        waning influence of psychoanalysis, 403
    postwar expansion and institutional splits (1946–1968), 395–399
        analysis in Canada, 398–399
        controversies and institutional splitting, 395–397
        link with anthropology, 398
        military psychiatry and spread of analysis, 395
        in retrospect, 398–399
        psychosomatic medicine and, 394, 398, 399
"Note Upon 'The Mystic Writing Pad,' The" (S. Freud), 509
Nouvelle Revue de Psychanalyse (journal), 431

Oberndorf, Clarence, 390, 391, 394, 396
Obeyesekere, Gananath, 486, 487

Object constancy, 351
    aggression and, 15
    infant–mother dyad and, 43
    in Mahler's separation-individuation theory, 58, 67
Object permanence, 48
Object Relations Inventory (ORI), 312
Object relations theories, 57–74, 135–138, 196
    arts and, 503, 508–509
    attachment theory and, 138–139
    basic concepts of, 57–59
        conditions of low affect activation, 57
        conditions of peak affect activation, 57–58
    British School of, 59, 61–65, 135–137, 196, 417–418
    comparison of, 59–61
    of countertransference, 195
    definition of, 7, 59
    on development of psychopathology, 178–180
        Fairbairn, 179
        Klein, 178–179
        Kohut, 180
        Winnicott, 179
    developmental overlays and, 41, 132, 135–138 (See also Developmental theory)
    ego psychology and, 58, 59, 60
    of Fairbairn, 62–63
    Freud's drive theory and, 58–59
    of gender, 99
    internalization of self-object relations, 49–51
    interpersonal, 60
    intersubjectivity and, 82
    intrapsychic conflict and, 28
    of Jacobson, 66
    of Kernberg, 67–68, 137–138
    of Klein, 61–62, 135–136, 192, 408–413
    of Kohut, 137
    Lacanian psychoanalysis and, 60
    literary analysis and, 495
    of Mahler, 58, 67, 342
    mainstream psychoanalysis and, 60
    motivations and, 4, 5, 7–10, 17
        attachment, 9–10
        internalized object relations, 7–9
    in North America, 137–138
    psychoanalytic technique and, 69–73
        countertransference, 73
        intrapsychic conflict, 69

    oedipal and preoedipal conflicts and their condensation, 70–71
    principles of, 69–70
    transference regression and reconstruction of past, 71–73
    role of aggression in, 59
    role of unconscious fantasy in, 59–60
    of Sandler, 416–417
    Socrates' theory of transmission of pathology, 516
    of Sullivan, 65–66, 138
    terminology in, 7
    transference, countertransference and, 59, 60, 61
    view of interpretation, 237
    of Winnicott, 63–65, 136–137, 413–416
Observation-based methods, 132, 149–150, 377
Oedipus complex, 13, 97–98
    in anthropological studies
        human universals and cultural variation, 485, 486, 487
        Malinowski's studies of Trobriand Islanders, 481, 485
        Whiting's Human Relations Area Files, 483
    child's relationship with parental couple, 45
    child's use of inanimate objects in mastery of, 48
    father–son relationship and, 43
    feminist critiques of, 98
    Freud's concept of, 97–98, 174, 191, 378, 459
    ideological gender and, 97–98
    infantile amnesia and, 133
    Jones's analysis of, 492
    neurosis and, 174
    object relations theory and, 70–71
        Klein, 62
Oedipus in the Trobriands (M. E. Spiro), 485, 486
Oedipus Ubiquitous (Johnson and Price-Williams), 486
"Offset" research, 310
Ogden, T., 123, 138, 206, 208
Oliveira, Walderedo, 442
O'Malley, Mary, 389
On the History of the Psychoanalytic Movement (S. Freud), 381
One-person and two-person psychologies
    in developmental process of psychoanalysis, 121
    libido theory and, 103

OPD (Operationalisierte Psychodynamische Diagnostik), 312
Openness of analyst, 291
Operationalisierte Psychodynamische Diagnostik (OPD), 312
Organisation Psychanalytique de Langue Française (OPLF), 428, 429
ORI (Object Relations Inventory), 312
Orlan, 505
Ornstein, A., 232
    view of analytic process, 232
Ornstein, P. H., 232
Orr, D. W., 204, 209
O'Shaughnessy, E., 193, 206
Ostow, Mortimer, 537
Outcome research, 301–313
    central questions in, 301–302
    criteria for, 301
    first-generation research: early statistical studies, 302–303, 321
        Berlin Institute, 302
        Central Fact-Gathering Committee of the American Psychoanalytic Association, 303
        Chicago Psychoanalytic Clinic, 302
        London Psychoanalytic Clinic, 302
        The Menninger Clinic, 303
        methodological flaws in, 303
        Southern California Psychoanalytic Institute, 303
    fourth-generation research: divergence of directions, 310–312, 321
        focus on postanalytic phase, 310
        integration of process and outcome studies, 310
        "offset" research, 310
        Problem-Treatment-Outcome Congruence, 310, 311
        structural change measures, 310–312
            Analytic Process Scales, 312, 323
            Karolinska Psychodynamic Profile, 311
            McGlashan Semistructured Interview, 312
            Object Relations Inventory, 312
            Operationalisierte Psychodynamische Diagnostik, 312

Psychotherapy Process Q-Set, 312, 322–323
            Scales of Psychological Capacities, 311
            Shedler-Westen Assessment Procedure, 312
            Structured Interview of Personality Organization, 312
    second-generation research: formal and systematic studies, 303–306, 321
        American group-aggregated studies, 304–305
            Boston Psychoanalytic Institute, 304
            Columbia Psychoanalytic Center, 304–305
            New York Psychoanalytic Institute, 305
        American individually focused studies, 305–306
        European studies, 304
    third-generation research: combined process and outcome studies, 306–309, 321
        newer Boston Psychoanalytic Institute studies, 307
        Psychotherapy Research Project of The Menninger Clinic, 307–309, 321
Outlines of Psychiatry (William White), 389
Overdetermination, 25, 494
Ovesey, L., 100

Pacella, B., 48
Panic disorder, 258
Panksepp, Jaak, 538, 543, 544
Paolitto, F., 307
Papers in Applied Psychology (monograph series), 377, 453, 455
Papers on Metapsychology (S. Freud), 382
Paranoid personality disorder, Kernberg's view of, 181
Paranoid-schizoid position, in Kleinian object relations theory, 61–62, 135–136, 178, 192, 409–410
Parens, H., 15
Parents/parenting. *See also* Father; Mother
    childhood psychopathology and, 180
    child's relationship with parental couple, 45
    distortions in mentalizing related to, 182–183

psychological transition to parenthood, 154–155
    work with parents in child analysis, 268, 277–278
Parkin, Alan, 398
Parsons, E., 165
Parsons, Talcott, 398
Pathological mourning, in Kleinian object relations theory, 62
Patient capacities required for analytic process, 230–231
    ability to self-observe, 230
    dissociation in the ego, 230
    evolution of, 231
    free association, 230–231
    motivation and commitment, 231
    plasticity of defenses, 231
    psychotherapy for stabilization or expansion of, 231
    reality testing, 230
Patient privacy, 289
    process research as threat to, 320
Patient–analyst relationship. *See also* Psychoanalyst
    for child analysis, 267
    co-construction of meaning in, 196, 210
    ethics of, 281–282, 288
    Freud's view of, 219
    Loewald's view of, 220
    preclusion of social contacts, 249, 251–252, 396
    requirements for analytic process, 232–233
    resistance and, 234
    Strachey's view of, 220
    therapeutic action and, 219–220
    therapeutic alliance, 197
    therapeutic availability in developmental orientation, 123–125
        affect regulation and empathy, 123–124
        interpretation and shared aspects of therapeutic action, 124–125
    transference, countertransference, and the real relationship, 194–195, 201–213 (*See also* Countertransference; Transference)
Patient's Experience of the Relationship with the Therapist (PERT), 321
Paul, Robert A., *479–488*
Payne, Sylvia, 408
PDDs (pervasive developmental disorders), 272

Peck, Martin, 391, 393
Peirce, C. S., 361
Peña, Saul, 447
Penis and phallocentrism, 96, 98–99
Penis envy, 96, 98, 191
Penser/Rêver (journal), 431
PEP (Psychoanalytic Electronic
    Publishing) CD-ROM, 197
Perceptual defense, in New Look
    studies, 464
Perceptual vigilance, in New Look
    studies, 464
Perestrello, Danilo, 442
Perestrello, Marialzira, 442
Pérez Pastorini, Valentín, 446
Perrier, François, 428
Perron, R., 318, 319
Perry, J. C., 322
Person, Ethel, 16, 18, 85, 100, 102
    concept of gender role identity, 100
    concept of libido, 103
Personality
    Culture and Personality school of
        anthropology, 483–484
    development of, 39
    Kardiner's Basic Personality
        Structure model, 482–483
    Socrates' dynamic theory of
        personality organization, 516
    Structured Interview of Personality
        Organization, 312
Personality disorders, 197. *See also*
    specific personality disorders
    in DSM-IV, 256, 257
    Kernberg's view of, 181
    The Menninger Clinic and
        Menninger Child and Family
        Program studies of, 182–183
    Socrates' dynamic theory of typical
        pathologies of personality
        organization, 516
PERT (Patient's Experience of the
    Relationship with the Therapist),
    321
Peru, 447
Peruvian Psychoanalytic Society, 447
Pervasive developmental disorders
    (PDDs), 272
Perversion, 197
    Green's view of, 249
    Joseph's view of, 207
Peterfreund, E., 175
Pfeffer, Arnold
    development of neuropsychoanalysis
        by, 538–539
    outcome research of, 305–306

"Pfeffer phenomenon," 306
"Phallic monism," 97
Phallocentrism, 96, 98–99
Pharmacology. *See* Psychotropic
    medications
Philadelphia Association for
    Psychoanalysis, 396
Philadelphia Psychoanalytic Society, 396
Philosophy and psychoanalysis, 513–522
    abandonment of the therapeutic
        ideal, 518
    future investigations, 520–522
        activity and passivity in the mind,
            521
        idiosyncrasy of meaning, 521–522
        naturalistic moral psychology, 522
        nature of human happiness and
            freedom, 522
        psychic change through
            conversation, 521
        transference, 521
    Plato, 514, 516, 517, 518, 520
    psychic change, 518–519
    reflection function and psychic
        functioning, 519–520
    Socrates, 513–518, 521
        contributions to dynamic
            psychological thinking, 516–
            517
        Republic, 513, 515–518
        Socratic method, 514–515
Phipps Clinic at Johns Hopkins
    University Hospital, 388, 389
Phobias, 34
Piaget, Jean, 122, 149, 340, 457
Picasso, Pablo, 506
Pichon Rivière, Enrique, 436
Pilkonis, P. A., 471
Pine, Fred, *3–18*, 223, 339, 342, 352
PINE (Psychoanalytic Institute of New
    England), 397, 402
Piper, W. E., 324
Pizer, S., 210
Plan Formulation method, 321, 322
Plata Mujica, Carlos, 447
Plato, 514, 516, 517, 518, 520
Play, 267–279
    accessing and communicating affect
        through, 268
    children who cannot play, 272–273
    child's capacity for engagement in,
        270–271, 273
    child's comprehension of complex
        relationships in, 269
    child's movement into and out of play
        frame, 271

    definition of, 268
    interpretation and insight in process
        of, 270, 273–274
    mentalization and, 269
    process of, 270–272
    promotion of development by, 268
    relation to free association in adults,
        268–269
    role in child analysis, 267–269
    stereotyped, 273
    transference revealed in, 275
    use of conceptual metaphors in, 268
    working within, 270
Pleasure principle, 4–5, 25–26, 120
    vs. egoistic hedonism, 286
    neuroscientific research on, 542–543
    principle of entropy and, 120
    repetition compulsion and, 27
Poe, Edgar Allan, 492, 495
Poetzl, O., 466
Politics, international relations, and
    psychoanalysis, 525–532
    accordion phenomenon, 531
    background for concepts of
        collaboration in politics and
        diplomacy, 528–529
    difficulties in collaboration, 525–526
    factors limiting contributions of
        psychoanalysis to politics, 526–
        528
        analysts not working in
            interdisciplinary settings, 528
        not exploring analysts' own large-
            group sentiments during
            their training, 527–528
        not having a psychology of large
            groups in its own right, 526–
            527
    large-group identity: tent metaphor,
        529–531
        chosen glories and chosen
            traumas, 529–530
        time collapse, 530–531
    large-group regression and rituals,
        531
    minor differences, 531
    mourning, 531–532
Pollack, S. S., 99
Pollen, William, 399
Pollock, George, 400
Pontalis, Jean-Bertrand, 103, 110, 368,
    426, 430, 431
    Nouvelle Revue de Psychanalyse, 431
    Vocabulaire de la Psychanalyse, 430, 431
Porto Alegre Psychoanalytic Society
    (SPPA), 444

Posttraumatic dreams, 4, 27
Power of Feelings, The (Nancy Chodorow), 486
PQS (Psychotherapy Process Q-Set), 312, 322–323
Prados, Miguel, 398
Pratt, Joseph, 399
PRC (Psychoanalytic Research Consortium), 325
Preconscious, 189, 190, 379
Prejudice, implicit, 467
"Pretend mode," 269
Price-Williams, Douglass, 486
Primal crime theory, 481
Primary and secondary process, 27–28, 189, 190
  in dream formation, 32–33
  shifting of attention between, 231
Prince, Morton, 387, 388, 389
Prince Lazar of Serbia, 530–531
Principles of Ethics for Psychoanalysts (American Psychoanalytic Association), 319
Principles of Medical Ethics With Annotations Especially Applicable to Psychiatry (American Psychiatric Association), 319
Privacy of patient, 289
  process research as threat to, 320
Problem-solving capacity of child, 348–349
Problem-Treatment-Outcome (PTO) Congruence, 310, 311
Procedural (implicit) memory, 132, 223–224, 367, 466
Process of psychoanalysis, 229–233, 317
  definitions related to, 229–230
  Freud's concept of, 317–318
  requirements for, 230–233
    analyst capacities, 231–232
    analytic dyad, 232–233
    patient capacities, 230–231
  resistance to, 233–234
Process research, 301–302, 310, 317–330
  defining knowledge base for, 317–318
    audio recording, 317
    case report, 317
  evolution of empirical research, 320–321
  first-generation research:
    development of objective measures, 321–325
    characterization of problematic themes, 321–322

configurational analysis and Role Relationship Model, 321, 322
    Core Conflictual Relationship Theme, 321, 322, 325–326, 365
    Defense Mechanism Rating Scales, 322
    Fundamental Repetitive and Maladaptive Emotion Structures, 321, 322, 324, 325–326
    measure of social cognition and object relations, 322
    Patient's Experience of the Relationship with the Therapist, 321
    Plan Formulation method, 321, 322
  measures of therapeutic interaction, 322–325
    classification of therapeutic interventions, 324
    computer-assisted measures, 323
    effects of interventions, 324–325
    measures of referential process, 324
    process scales, 322–323
  future directions for, 329–330
  implications for clinical work, 329
  integration with outcome research, 310, 321
  objections to, 318–320
    impact on treatment, 318–319
      intrusion of recording device, 318
      intrusion of research perspective, 318
      threats to patient privacy, 319
    need for multiple perspectives, 320
    status of psychoanalytic "facts," 319–320
  problems and goals in, 327–328
    clinical issues, 327
    conceptual issues, 328
    institutional issues, 327–328
      need for financial support, 327
      organization and management of database, 327
      training and support of psychoanalytic researchers, 327–328
    methodological issues, 327

second-generation research:
    collaborative studies, 325–326
    coordination of results from, 325
    major studies, 325
    narrative as unifying feature of, 325–326
  third-generation research:
    broadening the scope of observation, 326–327
    direct clinical applications in supervision process, 326–327
    IPTAR single case study, 326
Program on Conscious and Unconscious Mental Processes, 325
Proietti, J. M., 471
"Project for a Scientific Psychology" (S. Freud), 378, 384, 535–536
Projection, 193
  in dreams, 33
Projective identification
  by analyst, 207
  as attunement between mother and infant, 193
  in Bion's object relations theory, 136
  definition of, 193
  European reception of concept of, 418
  vs. intersubjectivity, 80
  in Kleinian object relations theory, 61, 136, 417–418
Promise keeping, 281, 288
Protoself, 139
PRP. *See* Psychotherapy Research Project of The Menninger Clinic
PRP-II, 311
Pruett, K., 44
Prunes, Celestino, 444
Psychanalyse à l'Université (journal), 431
Psychiatry (journal), 396
Psychic determinism, 23–25
  agency and, 24–25
  vs. chance events, 24
  current concept of, 24
  Freud's concept of, 23–24, 377
  ethics and, 285–286
"Psychic equivalence," 269
"Psychic presence," 249
Psychic reality, 193–194
  après-coup and, 194
  definition of, 193
  Freud's view of, 193, 409
  Klein's view of, 409–410
  Winnicott's view of, 415
Psychic Retreat, 411

Psychoanalysis, 189–195
  administrative red tape affecting, 402
  attachment theory in, 159–169
  challenges to, 197
  of children, 267–279
  classical, 375
  conflicts and defenses in, 192–193
  cost of, 402
  developmental orientation for, 117–
    126, 173
  developmental theory of, 131–140,
    191–192
    interface with other disciplines,
      147–155
    object relations theories, 41, 132,
      135–138
  distinguishing features of, 190
  duration of, 195, 241
  dynamic unconscious in, 21–35, 189–
    190
  early relationships and their
    internalization in, 39–51
  economic factors affecting, 402–403
  epistemology of, 148–151
  ethics in, 281–295
  evolution of theory of, 3, 132
  free association in, 35, 197
  Freud and classical tradition of, 132–
    133, 189–191
  Freud's development of, 189
  goals of, 235–236, 247, 282–283,
    292–293, 535
  health insurance coverage for, 402–
    403
  history of
    in the French community, 423–432
    Freud and the early years, 375–
      384
    in Great Britain and Continental
      Europe, 407–419
    in Latin America, 435–448
    in North America from 1895 to
      present, 387–403
  initial evaluation of patient for, 257–
    258
  instinctual mental life and, 190–191
  interdisciplinary studies in
    anthropology, 479–488
    arts, 501–509
    Freud's uses of, 453–460
    literature, 491–499
    neuroscience, 535–545
    philosophy, 513–522
    politics and international
      relations, 525–532
    psychology, 463–474

  internal (psychic) reality and, 193–
    194
  interpretation in, 197, 235–238
  intersubjectivity in, 77–90
  motivational theory in, 3–18
  neuroscience and, 196–197, 535–545
  object relations theories in, 57–74
  outcome studies of, 301–313
  patient's assumption of moral
    responsibility in, 281
  problems treated by, 197
  process of, 229–233, 317
  psychotropic medications and, 255–
    265
  reanalysis, 251–252
  relevance of psychiatric diagnosis to
    recommendation for, 257
  resistance in, 233–234
  settings for, 197
  stalemate in, 246, 247
  as talking cure, 212–213, 377
  technique of, 229
  termination of, 241–251
  therapeutic action of, 217–226
  transference, countertransference,
    and the real relationship in,
    194–195, 201–213
  as value-free science, 281–284
  working-through in, 195
"Psychoanalysis as a Developmental
  Psychology," 394
Psychoanalyst(s), 196–197. See also
  Patient–analyst relationship
  analytic tact of, 235, 290
  authenticity of, 206, 212
  capacities required for analytic
    process, 231–232
  countertransference reactions of,
    194–195, 201–213, 231–232
  credentials of, 196
  ethical principles, rules, and
    guidelines for, 288–289
  in France, 196
  Freudian, 196
  internalization of, 248–250
  interpretation by, 197
  interpretations of, 235–238
  in Latin America, 196
  neutrality of, 236, 260
    ethical aspects of, 282, 284–285
    moral values and, 282
    preclusion of social contracts
      between patient and analyst
      for, 396
    psychotropic medications and,
      260, 262

  object relations school, 196
  personal analysis of, 391
  preclusion of social contacts between
    patients and, 249, 251–252, 396
  problems treated by, 197
  prohibition against financial dealings
    with patients, 289
  prohibition against sexual relations
    with patients, 289, 294
  "psychic presence" of, 249
  as psychopharmacologist, 262–263
  reanalysis and relationship of new
    therapist to previous therapist,
    251
  resource for publications by, 197
  theoretical orientation of, 196–197
  therapeutic availability in
    developmental orientation, 123–
      125
    affect regulation and empathy,
      123–124
    interpretation and shared aspects
      of therapeutic action, 124–
        125
  training of, 196, 231, 241 (See also
    Training of psychoanalysts)
  in United States, 196
  virtues of, 289–292
    benign and tolerant curiosity, 291
    definition of, 290
    emotional honesty, 291
    empathic respect, 290–291
    openness and humility, 291
    restraint or self-control, 291–292
  work with children, 267–279 (See also
    Child psychoanalysis)
Psychoanalytic Association of Argentina,
  326–327
Psychoanalytic Electronic Publishing
  (PEP) CD-ROM, 197
Psychoanalytic Institute of New
  England (PINE), 397, 402
Psychoanalytic process, 229–233, 317
  definitions related to, 229–230
  Freud's concept of, 317–318
  requirements for, 230–233
    analyst capacities, 231–232
    analytic dyad, 232–233
    patient capacities, 230–231
  resistance to, 233–234
Psychoanalytic psychology, 473
Psychoanalytic Research Consortium
  (PRC), 325
Psychoanalytic Review (journal), 389
Psychoanalytic schools, 196
Psychoanalytic Society of Caracas, 445

Psychoanalytic Society of Porto Alegre, 440
Psychoanalytic Society of Rio de Janeiro, 440
Psychoanalytic Society of São Paulo, 441–442
Psychoanalytic understanding of psychopathology, 173–183
    classical Freudian developmental model, 173–175
    classical model and observation of children, 175–178
        Anna Freud, 176
        Mahler, 176–178
        Spitz, 176
Psychodynamic psychology, 190
Psychological anthropology, 484
Psychological Anthropology Reconsidered (John Ingham), 486
Psychology and psychoanalysis, 463–474
    academic psychology, 463–464
        New Look studies, 464
        psychoanalytic psychology, 473
    evolutionary psychology, 485–486
    interpersonal relationships, 468–473
        attachment and psychopathology, 470–471
        attachment and psychotherapy, 471–473
            attachment status and psychotherapy outcome, 471
            attachment status and psychotherapy process, 471–472
            attachment status as psychotherapy outcome measure, 472–473
        attachment theory, 468–470
    psychotherapy, 464–465
    unconscious processes, 465–468
        automaticity, 467
        implicit learning, 466–467
        implicit memory, 466
        more directly psychoanalytic research into, 467–468
            activation of event-related potential by stimuli, 468
            subliminal psychodynamic activation, 467–468
Psychopathology
    attachment and, 164–165, 470–471
    childhood disturbances and, 131
    classical Freudian developmental model of, 132, 173–175

classical model and observations of children, 175–178
    Anna Freud, 176
    Mahler, 176–178
    Spitz, 176
genetic factors and, 180
Hartmann's view of, 133
integrating models of, 180
    Kernberg, 181–182
    The Menninger Clinic and Menninger Child and Family Program, 182–183
    relational school, 182
    Stern, 180–181
neurotic, 140
object relations view of, 178–180
parental rejection and, 180
psychoanalytic understanding of, 173–183
    classical model and observation of children, 175–178
Socrates' theories of, 516
Psychopharmacologist, 260–263. *See also* Psychotropic medications
    analyst as, 262–263
    in split treatment, 260–262
Psychosexual development, 104
    anal eroticism, 104
    Erikson's stages of, 22–23
    Freud's phases of, 6, 13
    genital eroticism, 104
    infantile sexuality, 6, 14, 104, 132, 375, 380
    oral eroticism, 104
Psychosis, 197
    autistic, 67
    depressive, in Kleinian object relations theory, 62
    symbiotic, 67
    transference, 194
Psychosomatic medicine, 394, 398, 399
Psychosomatic Medicine (journal), 394
Psychotherapy
    attachment status and outcome of, 471–473
    attachment status and process of, 471–472
    psychoanalysis and, 464–465
Psychotherapy Process Q-Set (PQS), 312, 322–323
Psychotherapy Research Project (PRP) of The Menninger Clinic, 307–309, 321
    conclusions of, 308–309
    goals of, 308
    methodology of, 308

"Psychotic core," 249
Psychotropic medications, 255–265
    for combined Axis I and Axis II disorders, 256
    combined treatment with psychoanalysis, 256
        rates of, 256–257
    determining effect of, 263
    documentation of use of, 264
    factors affecting decision to prescribe, 257–259
        among graduate analysts, 259
        among psychoanalytic candidates, 258–259
        psychiatric diagnosis, 257–258
    initial resistance of psychoanalytic community to, 255
    management in ongoing analysis, 263–265
    psychoanalyst as psychopharmacologist, 262–263
    split treatment, 260–262
    symbolic meanings to analysand, 261, 263
    training in use of, 264
    treatment recommendation and informed consent for use of, 259–260
PTO (Problem-Treatment-Outcome) Congruence, 310, 311
Publication of case material in journals, ethics of, 319
Puget, Janine, 440
Pulos, S. M., 323, 329, 330
Pulver, S. E., 368
Punishment dream, 34
Putnam, Irmarita, 391
Putnam, James Jackson, 387, 388, 389, 390, 391
Putnam, Marian, 394

Queer theory, 94, 96
Quijada, Hernán, 445
Quinn, S., 395
Quinodoz, Jean Michel, 407, 418

Racamier, P.-C., 427
Racker, Enrique, 440, 444
Racker, Heinrich, 73, 195, 205, 206, 207, 291, 412, 448, 496
Racker Center for Research and Psychoanalytic Assistance, 437
Rado, Sandor, 383, 391, 396
Ramachandran, V., 541
Rangell, Leo, 306, 397, 437

Rank, Otto, 381, 384, 390, 391, 395, 481, 492
   Myth of the Birth of the Hero, 453
   theories in relation to arts and psychoanalysis, 507
Rapaport, David, 14, 16, 394, 403, 464
Rascovsky, Arnaldo, 436, 442
Rat Man case (Freud), 47, 226, 244
Rating scales for depression, 263
Reader Response Criticism, 496
Reality, psychic, 193–194
   après-coup and, 194
   definition of, 193
   Freud's view of, 193
Reality attunement, 10
"Reality constancy," 48
Reality principle, 26, 411
   opposition to unrestrained libidinal pleasure seeking, 286
Reality testing
   exercise of capacities and, 10–11
   as requirement for analytic process, 230
Reanalysis, 251–252
   relationship of new therapist to previous therapist, 251
   of Wolf Man, 242–243, 251
Reber, A. S., 466
Redl, Fritz, 399
Reductionism, 494
Reed, G. S., 79
Reese, Michael, 399
Referential process, 324
   definition of, 324
   measures of Referential Activity, 324
      CRA, 324
      Discourse Attributes Analysis System, 324
      high vs. low Referential Activity language, 324
      Weighted Referential Activity Dictionary, 324
   phases of, 324
Reflective consciousness, intersubjectivity and, 84
Reflective function (RF), 118, 119, 470
Reflective Function Scale, 470
Reich, Wilhelm, 234
Reik, Theodor, 481
Reinterpreting Freud From a Modern Psychoanalytic Anthropological Perspective (Dan Forsyth), 486
Relational diathesis model, 167
Relational schools, 138
   intersubjectivity and, 77, 138, 182
   libido theory of, 103

view of psychopathology, 182
view of transference and countertransference, 210–212
Religion
   Freud's critique of, 286–287
   spiritual life of child, 49
   symbolism in, 31
Rembrandt, 507
Remus, Estela, 445
Renik, Owen, 40, 138, 206, 210, 212, 293
Reparative impulses, 192
Repetition compulsion, 4–5, 27
   shock trauma and, 8
   strain trauma and, 8
   working-through and, 195
Representational capacity of child, 350–351
Representational differentiation by child, 352–353
Repression, 21, 190, 193
   Freud's view of, 193
   neuroscientific research on, 541–542
Republic, 513, 515–518
Research, 147–148
   central questions in, 301–302
   conceptual, 361–371
   development in Europe, 418–419
   developmental, 335–355
   developmental psychoanalytic epistemology, 151–153
   epistemologies of psychoanalysis and developmental psychology, 148–151
   follow-up, 310
   integration of process and outcome studies, 310
   interdependent cooperation between traditions of, 370
   models for collaboration, 153–155
   neuroscientific, 540–544
   "offset," 310
   outcome, 301–313
   Problem-Treatment-Outcome Congruence in, 310
   process, 301–302, 310, 317–330
Resistance, 5, 233–234
   analysis of, 233–234
   to change, 233
      homeostatic motivation power of, 11–12
   countertransference view of, 233
   definition of, 233
   ego psychologists' view of, 234
   Freud's concept of, 234, 378
   interpersonal and behavioral manifestations of, 233

interpersonalists' view of, 234
relationship to analytic dyad, 234
sources of, 233
transference, 233, 234
unconscious nature of, 233
Resnick, Salomón, 437
Respect for patient, empathic, 290–291
Restraint of analyst, 291–292
Revista Brasileira de Psicanálise (journal), 442
Revista de Psicanálise da SPPA (journal), 444
Revista de Psicoanálisis (journal), 436
Revista Uruguaya de Psicoanálisis (journal), 446
Revue Française de Psychosomatique (journal), 426
Revue Neurologique (journal), 423
RF (reflective function), 118, 119, 470
Rickman, John, 408, 484
Ricouer, Paul, 319
Rie, H. E., 175
Riesemberg, Ruth, 446
Riggs, Austen, 387, 394
Riggs, S., 165
Righting response, 4, 13, 122
Riklin, Franz, 453, 455
Rinsley, D., 135, 177
Riviere, Joan, 408, 414
Robbins, Arnold, 396
Robbins, Bernard, 395
Robertson, James, 160
Rocha Barros, Elias, 444
Rochlin, G., 175
Róheim, Géza, 481–482, 483, 487
Role Relationship Model (RRM), 321, 322
Rolland, Jean-Claude, 431
Rolland, Romain, 287
Romano, John, 394, 399
Roose, Steven P., *255–265*
Rosenblatt, A. D., 46
Rosenfeld, Herbert, 62, 66, 167, 193, 206, 409, 411, 417, 418, 437
Rosolato, Guy, 440
Ross, David, 285
Ross, J. M., 44, 45, 99
Roth, A., 471–472
Roth, T., 472
Rothenberg, A., 124
Royce, Josiah, 387, 389
RRM (Role Relationship Model), 321, 322
Rubin, Gayle, 96, 97, 106
Rubino, G., 472
Rubovits-Seitz, P., 454

Ruddick, Bruce, 398
Rudnytsky, Peter, 459
Rusconi, M., 541
Rüütel, Arnold, 526

Sachs, Hanns, 391, 394
St. Elizabeths Hospital (Washington, D.C.), 388, 389, 399
Samberg, Eslee, *229–239*
Sampson, H., 317, 321
San Francisco Psychoanalytic Institute, 397
Sandell, Rolf, 310
Sander, L., 85, 89
Sandler, A.-M., 119, 416–417
Sandler, Joseph, 4, 5, 59, 60, 119, 120, 123, 168, 195, 207, 208, 221, 363, 364, 367, 413, 418, 419, 444
   concept of role responsiveness, 40
   development of clinical theory of, 416–417
   developmental model of, 135
São Paulo Society, 440
Sapir, Edward, 395
Sartre, Jean-Paul, 431, 519
Sashin, J. I., 304
"Scaffolding," 123, 124
Scales of Psychological Capacities (SPC), 311
Scarfone, Dominique, *423–432*
Schacht, T. E., 310
Schachter, J., 457
Schaefer, M., 498
Schafer, Roy, 16, 28, 105, 205, 221, 233, 234, 497
Scharf, L., 471
Schilder, Paul, 391, 399, 493, 494, 537
Schizoid personality disorder, 140
   Kernberg's view of, 181
Schizophrenia, analytic treatment of, 399
Schneider, W., 466
Schore, Allan, 538
Schuengel, C., 165
Schuker, E., 106
Schwaber, Evelyn, 213
Schwartz, James, 538–539
SCORS, 322
Scott, W. Clifford M., 398
Searles, Harold, 65–66, 67, 211
Second Sex, The (Simone de Beauvoir), 94
Secondary process, 27–28, 189
   in dream formation, 33
Secondary revision in dreams, 33
"Seduction theory," 109
Segal, Hanna, 62, 178, 206, 219, 409, 411, 418, 437, 444, 446, 503

Selective serotonin reuptake inhibitors (SSRIs), 261, 262
Self
   agency and, 25
   boundaries between other and, 12
   comfortable state of, 13
   core, 139
   ecological dimension of, 47
   emerging, 139
   experiential, 12–13
   false, 64, 179
   Freud's concept of, 5–6, 12
   genuineness of, 12
   Hartmann's concept of, 12
   internalization of self-object relations, 50
   Kohut's concept of, 12
   motivation and, 4, 12–13
     righting response, 4, 13, 122
   narrative, 139
   subjective, 139
   true, 64, 179
   unconscious fantasies of, 30
   wholeness and continuity of, 12
Self-actualization, 292
Self-control of analyst, 291–292
Self-esteem, 12
   childhood depression and, 175
   exercise of capacities and, 10–11
   psychological disturbance and, 137
Self-harm, 183
Self-objects, 60
Self-observation, as requirement for analytic process, 230
Self psychology, 132, 196
   interpersonal object relations theory and, 60
   intersubjectivity and, 77
   Kohut's theory of, 12, 137
   literary analysis and, 495
   view of interpretation, 237
   view of resistance, 234
   view of transference and countertransference, 210
Self-realization, 292
Self-regulation, 121–122
   Bowlby's theory of, 160
   of infant from 0–3 months, 340–343
Self representation, 6
Self-righting response, 4, 13, 122
Self-understanding, 292
Seminário Interdisciplinario de Estudios Andinos (SIDEA), 447
Semrad, Elvin, 399
Sensorimotor activity, 121

Sensory experiences of infants (0–3 months), 340–343
Separation anxiety, 63
Separation-individuation
   inanimate objects and, 48
   Jacobson's theory of, 66
   Mahler's theory of, 58, 67, 134–135, 176–177
     in analysis of borderline conditions, 67, 135, 177
     criticisms of, 178
     differentiation (hatching) subphase, 67, 134
     normal autism, 58, 67, 134, 177, 342
     practicing subphase, 67
     rapprochement subphase, 67, 134
     role of father in child's development, 43
     Searle's psychoanalytic approach and, 66
     symbiosis, 58, 67, 134, 177
   role of extended family in, 49
   termination of treatment and, 249
Sequin, Carlos Alberto, 447
Settings for psychoanalysis, 197
Settlage, Calvin F., 119
Severn, Elizabeth, 203
Sex and Repression, 485
Sex assignment, 96, 97
Sex reassignment, 100
Sexual relations with patients, prohibition of, 289, 294
Sexuality, 93, 102–110. *See also* Gender
   aggression and, 15
   component instincts of, 104
   as drive, aim, and object, 103–104
   enigmas of, 109
   Erikson's developmental stages of, 22–23
   evolution and, 14
   Fairbairn's theory of, 62–63
   fantasies of sexual gratification, 30
   feminist critique and, 104–105
   Freud's theory of, 4, 5, 6, 13–14, 17, 93, 95–96, 380
     castration anxiety, 96, 98
     childhood sexual trauma as origin of hysteria, 375, 377, 378, 379
     erotogenic zones, 6, 104, 174, 191
     fetishization of genitals, 96
     heterosexuality and homosexuality, 105
     idealization of phallic masculinity, 95, 99

Sexuality *(continued)*
  Freud's theory of *(continued)*
    infantile sexuality, 6, 14, 105, 132, 375, 380
    as instinctual drive, 3, 6, 13–15
    Oedipus complex, 97–98
    penis envy, 96, 98, 191
    phases of psychosexual development, 6, 13, 120, 174, 191
    Three Essays on the Theory of Sexuality, 95, 103, 105, 219, 380, 454
    view of femininity, 95, 96, 97, 98, 383
  heterosexuality, 105
  homosexuality, 70, 105
    Freud's view of, 95, 105
    new narratives of, 106–107
    normality and illness, 105
  infantile, 6, 14, 105, 132, 375
  intrapsychic conflict and, 28–29
  libido in one-person and two-person psychologies, 103
  motivation and, 13–14, 17, 22–23
  multiple paths to, 105
  new narratives of, 105–107
    multiplicities of desire, 106–107
    revising classical narrative, 106
    sexual idiom, 105–106
  normality and illness, 105
  perversion and normality, 109–110
  proactive status of, 14
  in psychoanalysis, 102–103
  relation to gender, 94, 102
  subjectivity of, 107–109
    body and bodymind, 108
    desire, 107–108
    sexual self states, 107
    transference and countertransference, 108–109
Sexuality of Christ in Renaissance Art and in Modern Oblivion (Leo Steinberg), 502
SFP (Société Française de Psychanalyse), 424, 425
Shakow, D., 464
Shame and Necessity (Bernard Williams), 522
Shane, Morton, 119
Shanker, Stuart G., *335–355*
Shapiro, David, 292
Shapiro, T., 245, 321
Sharpe, Ella, 247, 248, 408
Sharpe, S. A., 46

Shedler-Westen Assessment Procedure (SWAP), 312
"Shell shock" in World War I, 4, 8
Sheppard Pratt Hospital (Baltimore), 399
Sherwood, M., 244
Shevrin, Howard, 466, 467, 468, 542
Shiffrin, R. M., 466
Shmueli-Goetz, Yael, 166
Shock trauma, 8
Siblings, 45–46
  developmental distance between, 46
  factors affecting relationships among, 45–46
  rivalry among, 46
  stepsiblings, 48
SIDEA (Seminário Interdisciplinario de Estudios Andinos), 447
Sidis, Boris, 387, 389
Siedmann de Armesto, Mónica, *435–448*
Siegel, P., 322
Sifneos, Peter, 426
Sigmund Freud Institute (Frankfurt), 367
Signal affects, 11, 120, 254
  anxiety, 11, 120
  depression, 120
Silverberg, William, 395, 396
Silverman, Lloyd, 467–468
Simmel, Ernst, 393, 394, 397
Simon, B., 499
Singer, Isaac Bashevis, 509
Singer, J., 321, 322
"Skin-color anxiety," 41
Skinner, B. F., 464
Skolnikoff, A. Z., 307, 308
Slade, Arietta, 164, 166–167
Slavson, S. R., 399
Sleep
  cognitive activity during, 32
  dream formation during, 31–34
Sleep cycle, 31
Smith, Henry, 206, 230, 273
Smith, J., 26
Socarrás, José Francisco, 447
Social contacts between patient and analyst, prohibition of, 249, 251–252, 396
Social development, early attachment as predictor of, 164–165
Social fittedness, 122
Sociedade Brasileira de Psicanálise de Porto Alegre, 444
Société Française de Psychanalyse (SFP), 424
Sociéte Psychoanalytique de Montréal, 398, 429–430

Sociéte Psychoanalytique de Montréal (SPM), 398, 429–430
Société Psychoanalytique de Paris (SPP), 424, 425, 426–427, 428
Society of Medical Psychoanalysts, 396
Sociobiology, 485
Socrates, 513–518, 521
  contributions to dynamic psychological thinking, 516–517
    account of limits of psychological integration, 517
    dynamic theory of personality organization, 516
    dynamic theory of psychic structure, 516
    dynamic theory of typical pathologies of personality organization, 516
    object relations theory of transmission of pathology, 516
    theory of illusion and rudimentary theory of transference, 517
    theory of neurotic conflict, 516
    theory of psychic formation, 516
    view that dreams are expressions of unconscious and illicit desires, 517
  in the *Republic*, 513, 515–518
  Socratic method, 514–515
Sokolnicka, Eugénie, 423
Solms, Mark, 402, *535–545*
Sophocles, 459, 492
Sources of Normativity, The (Christine Korsgaard), 519
Southern California Psychoanalytic Institute, outcome studies at, 303
Southern California Psychoanalytic Society, 397
Southern California Society for Psychoanalytic Medicine, 397
Spain, David, 486
Spangler, G., 469
SPC (Scales of Psychological Capacities), 311
"Speech and Language in Psychoanalysis" (Jacques Lacan), 430
Spence, D. P., 323, 465, 497
Spezzanno, C., 211
Spiegel, John, 395
Spielrein, Sabina, 454
Spillius, Elizabeth B., 62, 136, 206, 279, 417, 418

Spiritual life of child, 49
Spiro, Melford E., 486, 488
   Gender Ideology and Psychological Reality, 487
   studies of human universals and cultural variation, 485
Spitz, Ellen Handler, 493, *501–509*
Spitz, René, 5, 47, 120, 124, 150, 339, 393, 394, 399, 424, 441
   concept of ego organization, 120
   developmental model of, 133
   observations of children, 176
   studies of institutionalized infants, 337
"Split brain," 540–541
Split treatment, 260–262
Splitting, 193
   in Kleinian object relations theory, 61–62
"Splitting of the Ego in the Process of Defense, The" (S. Freud), 509
SPM (Sociéte Psychoanalytique de Montréal), 398, 429–430
SPP (Société Psychoanalytique de Paris), 424, 425, 426–427, 428
SPPA (Porto Alegre Psychoanalytic Society), 444
Sroufe, Alan, 161, 163, 469
SSRIs (selective serotonin reuptake inhibitors), 261, 262
Stalemate of analysis, 246, 247
Standard Edition (S. Freud), 94
"State of affairs" dreams, 32
Stechler, G., 15
Steele, H., 470, 472
Steele, M., 470, 471, 472
Stein, R., 109
Steinberg, Leo, 502
Steiner, John, 193, 206, 411, 444
Steiner, Ricardo, 535
Stekel, Wilhelm, 381, 392
Stengel, B., 322
Stengel, Erwin, 537
Stepfamilies, 48
Stephen, Adrian, 408
Stephen, Karin, 408
Sterba, R., 230, 248
Stern, Adolf, 391
Stern, Daniel, 9, *77–90*, 85, 89, 119, 209, 225
   The Interpersonal World of the Infant, 139
   view of development of sense of self, 139, 180
   view of psychopathology, 180–181

view of therapeutic action, 220, 221, 224
"way-of-being-with" concept of, 139, 180
Stiles, W., 324, 471
Stimmel, B., 102
Stimulus-seeking, 10
STIPO (Structured Interview of Personality Organization), 312
Stockholm Outcome of Psychoanalysis and Psychotherapy Project (STOPPP), 310
Stoller, Robert, 94, 99, 100
Stolorow, R., 123, 182, 210
Stone, L., 204
STOPPP (Stockholm Outcome of Psychoanalysis and Psychotherapy Project), 310
Strachey, Alix, 408
Strachey, James, 5, 219–220, 284, 408, 414, 442
   concept of internalization of psychoanalyst, 248
   view of interpretation, 236
Strain trauma, 8
Strange Situation, 163–164, 337, 469
   Ainsworth's categorization of attachment behavior in, 163, 469
      anxious/avoidant babies, 163, 469
      anxious/resistant babies, 163, 469
      disorganized/disoriented babies, 163, 165, 469
      maternal warmth and, 469–470
      parents' reflective function and, 470
      secure babies, 163, 469
   depth psychology and, 337
   Sroufe's interpretation of baby's behavior in, 163–164
Stranger anxiety, 42, 47
Structural change measures, 310–312
   Analytic Process Scales, 312, 323
   Karolinska Psychodynamic Profile, 311
   McGlashan Semistructured Interview, 312
   Object Relations Inventory, 312
   Operationalisierte Psycho-dynamische Diagnostik, 312
   Psychotherapy Process Q-Set, 312, 322–323
   Scales of Psychological Capacities, 311
   Shedler-Westen Assessment Procedure, 312

Structured Interview of Personality Organization, 312
Structural theory of the mind
   A. Freud's contributions to, 134
   intrapsychic conflict and, 28–29
   S. Freud's development of, 7, 28, 190–191, 217
Structured Interview of Personality Organization (STIPO), 312
Structured interviews, 258
Strupp, H., 310, 324
Studies on Hysteria (Breuer and Freud), 217, 218, 377, 502
Subception, in New Look studies, 464
Subliminal priming, 466
Subliminal psychodynamic activation, 467–468
Substance use disorders, 259
Suicidality, attachment status and, 470
Sullivan, Harry Stack, 50, 59, 60, 209, 392, 395–396, 398, 399
   concept of "good me," "bad me," and "not me," 65
   concept of needs for satisfaction and security, 65
   followers of, 65–66
   object relations theory of, 65–66, 138
Sulloway, Frank, 384, 455
Sultan Murat I, 530
Suomi, Steven, 458
Superego
   belief in God and, 49
   Freud's concept of, 7, 28, 174, 190–191
   harsh, 50
   Jacobson's concept of, 66
   Kernberg's concept of, 137
   Klein's concept of, 62
   morality and, 286
   punishment dream and, 34
Sutherland, J. D., 63
Swales, Peter, 459
SWAP (Shedler-Westen Assessment Procedure), 312
Symbiotic phase of development (Mahler), 58, 67, 134, 177
Symbols, 30–31
   child's progress from affects to, 353–354
   definition of, 30
   in dreams, 33
   as expression of unconscious content, 31
   formation of, 31
   religious, 31
   signs and, 30–31

Sympathy, 290
Symptom formation, 34–35
Szpilka, Jaime, 440

Tacchi, P., 542
Tact, analytic, 235, 290
"Talking cure," 212–213, 377
Taneyhill, G. Lane, 389
Target, Mary, 119, 135, *159–169*, 277, 370, 469
TAS (Text Analysis System), 323
Tausk, Victor, 381
Taylor, E. W., 387
TCAs (tricyclic antidepressants), 262
TCM (Therapeutic Cycles Model), 323
Teague, G. B., 472
Teller, V., 321, 322, 326
Temperament, 342
    difficult, 342
    infant's self-regulation and, 342
    maternal mental content and, 43
Tension reduction, Freud's concept of, 5, 10
Termination of analysis, 241–251
    analysand's readiness for, 249
    as break in equilibrium, 250
    in developmental orientation, 125
    forced, 242, 249
    Freud and problem of, 242–246
        death instinct, 246
        Hilda Doolittle, 243–244
        Rat Man, 244
        Wolf Man, 242–243, 250, 251
    internalization of psychoanalyst, 248–250
    possible conclusions to, 250–251
    post-Freudian concepts of, 246–248
        Fenichel, 247
        Ferenczi, 246
        Glover, 246, 247
        Kleinian model, 246–247
        Sharpe, 248
        Waelder, 248
    preclusion of social contacts after, 249, 251–252, 396
    reanalysis and, 251–252
    separation-individuation and, 249
    sociological pressures affecting, 241
    terminal phase, 250–251
    working-through and timing of, 195
Teruel, Guillermo, 445
Tessman, L. H., 45
Text Analysis System (TAS), 323
Theory of the mind
    intersubjectivity and, 81
    structural, 7, 28, 190–191

A. Freud's contributions to, 134
    intrapsychic conflict and, 28–29
    S. Freud's development of, 7, 28, 190–191, 217
    topographical, 190, 217, 244–245, 379–380
Therapeutic action, 217–226
    Abend's concept of, 222, 223
    analytic relationship and, 219–220
    developmental analogies to explain relational contributions to, 219–220
    in developmental orientation, 124–125
        interpretation, 124–125
        mutuality, 125
        termination process, 125
    Fonagy's concept of, 224–225
    Freud's concept of, 217–219
    Glover's concept of, 217–219
    Heimann's concept of, 221
    interpretation-vs.-relationship debate on, 217–220, 267
        persistence of, 220–223
        significance of, 225–226
    Leowald's concept of, 121
    multiple models of, 223, 267
    multiple unconscious registers in, 223–225
    1961 Edinburgh conference on, 219, 221
    persistence of interpretation-vs.-relationship debate on, 220–223
    Segal's concept of, 219
    Stern's concept of, 220, 221
    Strachey's concept of, 219–220
    technical steadiness vs. flexibility and, 221–223
    therapeutic cure vs. analytic cure, 218
    transference, countertransference and, 212–213
    view of role of interpretation in, 219
    viewing change as evidence of progress, 222
Therapeutic alliance, 197. *See also* Patient–analyst relationship
Therapeutic ambition, 282–283
Therapeutic availability, 123–125
    affect regulation and empathy, 123–124
    interpretation and shared aspects of therapeutic action, 124–125
Therapeutic Cycles Model (TCM), 323
Therapeutic efficacy
    reasons for lack of progress in empirical evidence for, 147–148
    research on, 147

Therapeutic goals, 235–236, 247, 535
    ethics and, 282–283, 292–293
    life goals and, 293
Therapeutic ideal, abandonment of, 518
Therapist Intervention Rating System (TIRS), 324
Thom, Douglas, 394
Thomä, H., 310, 321
Thompson, Clara, 138, 392, 395, 396
Thompson, L., 325
Three Essays on the Theory of Sexuality (S. Freud), 95, 103, 105, 219, 380, 454
Ticho, Ernst, 293
TIRS (Therapist Intervention Rating System), 324
Titchener, Edward Bradford, 463
Titian, 506
Tolerance of analyst, 291
Topographical theory of the mind, 190, 217, 244–245, 379–380
Totem and Taboo (S. Freud), 480, 481, 482
Totemism and Exogamy (James Frazer), 480
Training of psychoanalysts, 196, 231, 241
    in America
        early years, 391–392
        establishment of first institutes, 391–393
        institutional splitting, 395–397
        opposition to lay analysts, 390, 400–401
    in Canada, 398, 429–430
    in France, 428–429
    International Training Commission, 391, 392, 401
    not exploring analysts' large-group sentiments during, 527–528
    researchers, 327–328
    in use of psychotropic medications, 264
Transference, 5, 194–195, 201–213.
    See also Countertransference;
        Patient–analyst relationship
    analysis of, 201
    in analytic process, 232
    in child psychoanalysis, 274–276
    as communication, 194
    definition of, 194
    distortions in, 124
    erotic, 194
    evolution of concept of, 204–212, 382–383

American ego psychology, 204–206
Ferenczi, 202, 383
Freud, 194–195, 201–204, 232, 382–383
interpersonal tradition, 209–210
Kleinian tradition, 62, 206–207, 412
Lacanian models, 209
object relations theory, 59, 60, 61, 207–209
relational models, 210–212
self psychology, 210
hostility and hatred in, 202
how it works, 212–213
meaning-space of, 364–365
nature and impact of, 194
one-way intersubjectivity and, 80
patient's reports of early experiences and, 40
positive affirmative aspects of, 124
psychoanalytic-philosophical investigation of, 521
psychoanalytic technique and, 71–73
real relationship and, 203–204, 212
related to prescription of psychotropic medications, 260, 261, 263
sexuality and, 108–109
Socrates' rudimentary theory of, 517
status of influence in, 203
"unobjectionable positive," 9
as vehicle for cure, 234
Transference-focused psychotherapy, 181–182
Transference neurosis, 194, 204, 274
Transference psychosis, 194
Transference resistance, 233, 234
interpretation of, 235
Transgender identity, 95
Transitional object, 47, 48, 64, 179, 415, 508
Transsexualism, 95
Trauma
attachment and, 164, 165
defensive identification of victim with abuser, 140
Freud's trauma-affect model, 190
posttraumatic dreams, 4, 27
shock, 8
strain, 8
Traumatic anxiety, 11
Travis, L. A., 473
Treboux, D., 470
Tricyclic antidepressants (TCAs), 262
Trobriand Islanders, 481, 485
Truthfulness, 281, 288
Tuckett, David, 320, *407–419*
Tuhami (Vincent Crapanzano), 487

Tulving, E., 367
Turkle, Sherry, 423
Turn of the Screw, The (Henry James), 495
Tustin, Francis, 82
Tuzin, Donald, 487, 488
Tyrrell, C. L., 472
Tyson, P., 119, 137, 174, 250
Tyson, R., 119, 137

"Uncanny, The" (S. Freud), 509
Unconscious, 21–35, 189–190
academic psychology's studies of, 465–468
activation of event-related potential by stimuli, 468
automaticity, 467
implicit learning, 466–467
implicit memory, 466
subliminal psychodynamic activation, 467–468
clarification of concept of, 367, 368
consciousness raising and, 18
declarative, 132, 223
definition of, 189
dream formation, 31–34
free association as medium for expression of, 15, 35
Freud's concept of, 21–35, 189, 375, 379–380
intrapsychic conflict, 28–29
multiple unconscious registers in therapeutic action, 223–225
neuroscientific research on, 540–541
procedural, 132, 223–224
regulatory principles of, 23–28
multiple determinism, 25
multiple function, 25
pleasure principle, 4–5, 25–26
primary and secondary process, 27–28, 189, 190, 231
psychic determinism, 23–25, 377
reality principle, 26
repetition compulsion, 4–5, 27
symbol formation, 30–31
symptom formation, 34–35
Unconscious fantasy, 29–30, 31, 51, 190
object relations theory and, 59–60
Unconscious motivation, 15–16, 22–23
University of Vienna, 391
Uruguay, 446
Uruguayan Psychoanalytic Association (APU), 446

VA (Veterans Administration) facilities, 395
Vaillant, G. E., 322

Valabrega, Jean-Paul, 428
Valenstein, A., 219
Vallar G., 541
Value-free methodology, 281–284
van Amerongen, S. T., 304
van der Leeuw, J. J., 244
van der Leeuw, Peter, 437
Van Gogh, Vincent, 507
van IJzendoorn, M., 165
Velasquez, Diego, 506
Venezuela, 445–446
Venezuelan Psychoanalytic Association (ASOVEP), 445
Veterans Administration (VA) facilities, 395
Viderman, S., 319
Viederman, Milton, 456
Vienna Psychoanalytic Society, 381, 459
Violence of Interpretation, The (Piera Aulagnier), 432
Virtues, 289–292
benign and tolerant curiosity, 291
definition of, 290
emotional honesty, 291
empathic respect, 290–291
openness and humility, 291
problems with language of, 292
restraint or self-control, 291–292
Vischer, F. T., 282
Vocabulaire de la Psychanalyse (Laplanche and Pontalis), 430, 431
Volkan, Vamık D., *525–532*
von Bertalanffy, Ludwig, 121, 457
von Rochau, Ludwig, 526
Vygotsky, L. S., 123

Waelder, Robert, 11, 248, 393, 394, 527
concept of multiple function, 25, 494
concept of termination, 247
Waelder-Hall, Jenny, 251, 393
"Waking screen," 48
Wall, S., 469–470
Wallace, Anthony F. C., 484
Wallerstein, Robert, 119, *301–313*, 317, 321, 325, 327, 330, 400, 401, 444
Wallon, Henri, 425
Wallwork, Ernest, *281–295*
Washington Psychoanalytic Association, 392
Washington Psychoanalytic Society, 389, 392
Washington School of Psychiatry, 392, 395–396
Washington–Baltimore Psychoanalytic Society, 392
Waters, Everett, 161, 469, 470

Watson, John, 335, 464
  case of Little Albert, 466
Weber, Max, 282
Wednesday Psychological Society, 381
Weighted Referential Activity Dictionary (WRAD), 324
Weinberger, Joel, *463–474*
Weinstein, Ed, 537
Weiss, Edoardo, 249, 380–381
Weiss, J., 321, 322
Werman, D. S., 24
Westen, D., 131–133, 220, 223, 224, 232, 267, 322
White, Robert, 458
White, William Allanson, 388, 389–390, 392, 399
Whiting, John, 483, 485
Widlöcher, Daniel, 426
"'Wild' Psycho-Analysis," 509
Wilde, Oscar, 492
Will, Otto, 65
William Allanson White Psychiatric Foundation, 392, 396
Williams, Bernard, 522
Williams, Paul, *189–197*
Wilson, Edmund, 495, 496
Winnicott, Donald, 5, 16, 17, 48, 59, 60, 103, 123, 132, 135, 168, 179–180, 183, 207–208, 211, 220, 247, 366, 402, 408, 413–416, 432, 437, 444, 495, 496, 503, 504
  concept of capacity for concern, 64
  concept of "good enough mother," 41, 64, 179, 415

concept of "holding environment," 64–65, 123, 132, 415, 509
concept of psychological transition to parenthood, 154–155
concept of transitional object, 47, 48, 64, 179, 415, 508
concept of true self and false self, 64, 179
Kohut's self psychology and, 65
modifications of Kleinian theory, 414–415
object relations theory of, 63–65, 136–137
role of illusion in theory of, 415
"The Use of an Object," 290, 291
theories in relation to arts and psychoanalysis, 508–509
view of countertransference, 208
view of psychopathology, 179
Wish(es), 14, 16–17
  as forward-looking concept, 119
  unconscious, 192
  ungratified, 247
Wish Fulfillment and Symbolism in Fairy Tales (Franz Riklin), 453, 455
Wolf, E. S., 137
Wolf Man case (Freud), 47, 242–243, 250, 251
Wolheim, Richard, 522
Wolitzky, D. L., 465
Wolstein, B., 209–210
Women's liberation, 18
Worcester, Elwood, 388
Worcester State Hospital (Massachusetts), 388, 389

Work of Culture, The (Gananath Obeyesekere), 486–487
Working-through, 195
World object, 343
World Psychoanalytic Association, 428
World War II years
  analysis in France during, 424
  analysis in North American after, 395–399
    Canada, 398
    controversies and institutional splitting, 395–397
    military psychiatry and spread of analysis, 395
    postwar expansion in retrospect, 398–399
  immigration and Europeanization of American analysis during, 393–394
WRAD (Weighted Referential Activity Dictionary), 324
Wynne, Lyman, 399

Yale Child Study Center, 399
Yankelovich, D., 285
Yanof, Judith A., *267–279*
Yehoshua, A. B., 498
Yeomans, F., 181

Zachhuber, U., 471
Zavitzianos, George, 398
Zetzsel, Elizabeth, 244, 437
Ziehen, Theodore, 459
Zoo Story, The (Edward Albee), 9